Adult Health Nursing

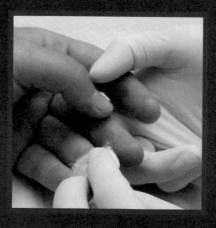

Barbara Lauritsen Christensen, RN, MS
Formerly, Nurse Educator
Mid-Plains Community College
North Platte, Nebraska

Elaine Oden Kockrow, RN, MS
Formerly, Nurse Educator
Mid-Plains Community College
North Platte, Nebraska

6th Edition

MOSBY

ELSEVIER

MOSBY
ELSEVIER

3251 Riverport Lane
St. Louis, Missouri 63043

ADULT HEALTH NURSING   ISBN: 978-0-323-05736-3
Copyright © 2011, 2006, 2003, 1999, 1995, 1991 by Mosby, Inc., an affiliate of Elsevier Inc.

Notices

Knowledge and best practice in this field are constantly changing. As new research and experience broaden our understanding, changes in research methods, professional practices, or medical treatment may become necessary.

Practitioners and researchers must always rely on their own experience and knowledge in evaluating and using any information, methods, compounds, or experiments described herein. In using such information or methods they should be mindful of their own safety and the safety of others, including parties for whom they have a professional responsiblity.

With respect to any drug or pharmaceutical products identified, readers are advised to check the most current information provided (i) on procedures featured or (ii) by the manufacturer of each product to be administered, to verify the recommended dose or formula, the method and duration of administration, and contraindications. It is the responsibility of practitioners, relying on their own experience and knowledge of their patients, to make diagnoses, to determine dosages and the best treatment for each individual patient, and to take all appropriate safety precautions.

To the fullest extent of the law, neither the Publisher nor the authors, contributors, or editors, assume any liability for any injury and/or damage to persons or property as a matter of products liability, negligence or otherwise, or from any use or operation of any methods, products, instructions, or ideas contained in the material herein.

The Publisher

Previous editions copyrighted 2006, 2003, 1999, 1995, 1991

Library of Congress Cataloging-in-Publication Control Number 2010921438

Vice President and Publisher: Tom Wilhelm
Managing Editor: Jill Ferguson
Associate Developmental Editor: Jennifer Hermes
Publishing Services Manager: Jeffrey Patterson
Senior Project Manager: Mary G. Stueck
Book Designer: Margaret Reid
Manuscript Copyeditor: Susan Hume

Printed in the United States of America

Last digit is the print number: 9 8 7 6 5 4 3 2 1

New Version Noted 03/07/15

e-Learning Resources

COMPANION CD

Body Spectrum Electronic Anatomy Coloring Book

Fluids and Electrolytes Tutorial

English/Spanish Audio Glossary

Animations

Abdominal Examination
Adrenal Function
Anatomy of Eye
Ankle Fracture
Asthma
Appendicitis, Symptoms
Brain Abscess
Brain Anatomy
Brain Lobes
Breast Cancer Spread; Metastasis
Cardiac Arrest, Ventricular Fibrillation, External Heart Monitor
Chemotherapy
Chest Pain Radiating to Arm
Congestive Heart Failure
Cranial Nerves
Eye: Aqueous Humor, Vitreous Humor
Function of the Heart
Generalized Seizure
Hemothorax
Hip Fracture, Femur Fracture, Femoral Fracture
Lymphocyte Function
Meningitis
Normal Cardiopulmonary Physiology
Normal Cardiopulmonary System
Organ Systems
Passage of Food through Digestive Tract
Pelvic Inflammatory Disease
Radiation Therapy
Renal Anatomy and Function
Retinal Detachment
Sickle Cell Anemia
Simple Pneumothorax and Tension Pneumothorax
Spine Structures
Structure of the Heart
Subarachnoid Hemorrhage
TIA, Transient Ischemic Attack; CVA, Cerebrovascular Accident; Stroke; Brain Blood Clot
Vascular Tree: Heart, Aorta, Major Branches
Visual Pathway

Video Clips

Auscultation: Abdomen, Bowel Sounds
Auscultation: Cardiac, with Diaphragm and Bell
Auscultation: Carotid Artery
Inspection: External Genitalia
Inspection: Fine Motor Coordination, Lower Extremities
Inspection: Fine Motor Coordination, Upper Extremities
Inspection: Gait
Inspection: General Muscular Strength
Inspection: Speculum Examination
Inspection and Palpation: Cardiac, Anterior Chest
Inspection and Palpation: Cardiac Auscultatory Landmarks
Inspection and Palpation: Breathing and Respiratory Excursion, Anterior Chest
Inspection and Palpation: Muscular Development
Inspection and Palpation: Pulses, Lower Extremities
Inspection and Palpation: Standing Position
Palpation: Tactile Fremitus, Posterior Chest
Percussion: Abdomen
Percussion: Anterior Thorax
Percussion: Liver
Percussion: Spleen

Audio Clips

Breath Sounds: Bronchial
Breath Sounds: Bronchovesicular
Breath Sounds: Vesicular
Crackles: High-Pitched
Crackles: Low-Pitched
Murmurs: Blowing, Harsh or Rough, and Rumble
Murmur: Diastolic
Murmurs: High, Medium, Low
Murmur: Systolic
Pericardial Friction Rub
Pericardial Friction Sounds
Pleural Friction Rub
S_1: Aortic Ejection
S_1 at Various Locations
S_1: Midsystolic Click
S_1: Pulmonic Ejection
S_2: Paradoxical Split
S_2 at Various Locations
S_2: Wide Split
The Fourth Heart Sound (S_4)
The Fourth Heart Sound (S_4) with Bell Held Lightly then Applied Firmly
The Third Heart Sound (S_3)
Stridor
Wheeze: High-Pitched
Wheeze: Low-Pitched

EVOLVE

In addition to the resources available on the Companion CD, the following resources are also available on the evolve website at **http://evolve.elsevier.com/Christensen/adult.**

Review Questions for the NCLEX® Examination (for each chapter)

Concept Map Creator

Calculators

Body Mass Index (BMI)
Body Surface Area Calculator
Fluid Deficit
Glasgow Coma Scale
IV Dosage Calculator: Infusion of a Dose
Units Conversion

Additional Animations

Acute Coronary Syndrome (ACS), Acute Myocardial Infarction (AMI), Coronary Ischemia, Coronary
Alzheimer's Disease
Artery Disease (Includes Use of Aspirin and Triglycerides)
Blood Clot Leading to Stroke
Brain Anatomy; Temporal Lobe, Brainstem, Cerebral Peduncle, Thalamus
Cerebral Infarct; Stroke
Parkinson's Disease
Pulmonary Embolus
Quadriplegia; Spinal Cord Injury
Ventricular Fibrillation

Additional Video Clips

Evaluation: Central Vision and Visual Acuity
Evaluation: Light Touch; Face, Upper and Lower Extremities, Cranial Nerve V—Trigeminal Nerve
Evaluation: Pupil Responses, Direct and Accommodation, Cranial Nerves III, IV, VI—Oculomotor, Trochlear, and Abducens Nerves
Evaluation: Pupil Responses, Direct and Consensual
Inspection: Ear Canal
Inspection: Female Breasts (Sitting Position)
Inspection: Female Breasts (Supine Position)
Inspection and Palpation: External Ear
Inspection and Palpation: External Eye
Inspection and Percussion: Diaphragmatic Excursion
Palpation: Abdomen Superficial and Deep
Palpation: Inguinal Hernia Evaluation
Percussion: Anterior Thorax

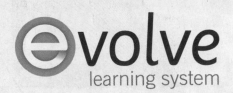
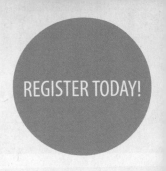
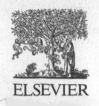

To my children and grandchildren: Jason Heath, Jennifer Holly, David Joseph,
Alexander Edison, Emma Elizabeth, Ava Louise, Jessica Heather, Eigo, Gus, and Mirabella.
Your love and support make my life a most pleasurable journey.

To my siblings: Shirlee, Ann, Lowell Chris, and Garnet.
A great joy in my life is the unconditional friendship of each of my siblings.

Barbara Lauritsen Christensen, RN, MS

To the brilliant health care providers who were responsible for the miraculous recovery
from my illness in 2008 and my continued good health:

North Platte, Nebraska
Janet Bernard, MD

Fort Walton Beach, Florida
Gregory Candell, MD
Patrick Anastasio, MD
Samuel Capra, MD
Christopher Dali, MD
Justin Philpott, MD
Larry Schatz, MD

Elaine Oden Kockrow, RN, MS

Acknowledgments

This edition has been completed through diligent research and response to reviewers, nurse educators, and student nurses. We are indebted to the nurse educators and student nurses who have used our text to assist in the achievement of excellence in the practice of nursing. Many thanks to current contributors, as well as those from past editions, including M. Christine Neff. We are grateful for the success of the past five editions and look forward to continuing to contribute to the education of student nurses.

For the completion of a textbook, one must have the cooperation of gifted and creative individuals. We wish to recognize those persons who have assisted with this text.

This text would not be possible without the superior effort of the talented editorial and production staff at Elsevier: Robin Levin Richman, Managing Editor, Philadelphia, for her cheerfulness and keen observations; Jacqueline Twomey, Developmental Editor, Philadelphia, for her attention to detail; Jill Ferguson, Managing Editor, St. Louis, for her gracious assistance in skillfully coordinating development; Jennifer Hermes, Associate Developmental Editor, St. Louis, for her thoroughness and punctuality; and Mary Stueck, Senior Project Manager, St. Louis, for her kind forbearance, organizational skills, and conscientious effort.

We are particularly grateful for the positive feedback and constructive reviews provided by our contributors and reviewers throughout the completion of this edition.

We wish to acknowledge Debbie Beebout, our typist, for her diligence and heedfulness to detail.

We would like to thank the administrators at Great Plains Regional Medical Center for their generous use of various GPRMC forms.

We wish to thank our siblings, children, and grandchildren for their love, kindness, and encouragement that provided us with vigor and inspiration to complete this labor of love.

Last, we wish to express to each other our gratitude for the gift of 35 years of friendship that is unique and has provided us with fortitude, stability, ardor, and purpose. We both share a love of family, community, teaching and the wonderful world of nursing.

Barbara Lauritsen Christensen
Elaine Oden Kockrow

Contributors and Reviewers

CONTRIBUTORS

Craig E. Nielsen, MS, NP, BC, ACRN
Assistant Professor of Medicine
Division of Infectious Disease
University of Colorado at Denver
Aurora, Colorado

Linda Y. North, PhD, RN
Dean of Health Sciences
Southern Union State Community College
Opelika, Alabama

Alita K. Sellers, MSN, PhD, RN
Chairperson, Health Sciences Division
West Virginia University at Parkersburg
Parkersburg, West Virginia

Martha E. Spray, MS, BSN, RN
Formerly, Practical Nursing Instructor
Mid-East Ohio Vocational School District
Zanesville, Ohio

REVIEWERS

Mary Ann Cosgarea RN, BSN, BA
Practical Nursing/Health Coordinator
Portage Lakes Career Center
W. Howard Nicol School of Practical Nursing
Green, Ohio

Brenda G. Holmes MSN/ED, RN
Assistant Professor
South Arkansas Community College
El Dorado, Arkansas

Laura Bevlock Kanavy, RN, BSN, MSN
Career Technology Center of Lackawanna County
    Practical Nursing Program
Scranton, Pennsylvania

Tammy Camille Killough, RN, BSN
Pearl River Community College–Forrest Co. Campus
Hattiesburg, Mississippi

Sue Parker, MSN, APN, FNP-BC, CNOR
Assistant Professor
University of Arkansas–Fort Smith
Fort Smith, Arkansas

Mary Russo, MSN, RN
Lincoln Land Community College
Springfield, Illinois

Rebecca S. Utz, RN, BSN
University of Arkansas Community College
    at Batesville
Batesville, Arkansas

LPN Advisory Board and Consultant

LPN ADVISORY BOARD

Shirley Anderson, MSN
Kirkwood Community College
Cedar Rapids, Iowa

M Gie Archer, MS, RN, C, WHCNP
Dean of Health Sciences
LVN Program Coordinator
North Central Texas College
Gainesville, Texas

Mary Brothers, MEd, RN
Coordinator, Garnet Career Center School of Practical
  Nursing
Charleston, West Virginia

Patricia A. Castaldi, RN, BSN, MSN
Union County College
Plainfield, New Jersey

Mary Ann Cosgarea, RN, BSN
PN Coordinator/Health Coordinator
Portage Lakes Career Center
Green, Ohio

Dolores Ann Cotton, RN, BSN, MS
Meridian Technology Center
Stillwater, Oklahoma

Lora Lee Crawford, RN, BSN
Emanuel Turlock Vocational Nursing Program
Turlock, California

Ruth Ann Eckenstein, RN, BS, MEd
Oklahoma Department of Career and Technology
  Education
Stillwater, Oklahoma

Gail Ann Hamilton Finney, RN, MSN
Nursing Education Specialist
Concorde Career Colleges, INC
Mission, Kansas

Pam Hinckley, RN, MSN
Redlands Adult School
Redlands, California

Deborah W. Keller, RN, BSN, MSN
Erie Huron Ottawa Vocational Education
School of Practical Nursing
Milan, Ohio

Patty Knecht, MSN, RN
Nursing Program Director
Center for Arts & Technology
Brandywine Campus
Coatesville, Pennsylvania

**Lieutenant Colonel (RET) Teresa Y. McPherson, RN,
  BSN, MSN**
LVN Program Director
Nursing Education
St. Philip's College
San Antonio, Texas

Frances Neu, MS, BSN, RN
Supervisor, Adult Ed Health
Butler Technology and Career Development Schools
Fairfield Township, Ohio

Dianna Danced Scherlin, MS, RN
National Director of Nursing
Lincoln Educational Services
West Orange, New Jersey

Beverley Turner, MA, RN
Director, Vocational Nursing Department
Maric College, San Diego Campus
San Diego, California

C. Sue Weidman, RN BSN
Brown Mackie College Nurse Specialist
Forest , Ohio

Sister Ann Wiesen, RN, MRA
Erwin Technical Center
Tampa, Florida

CONSULTANT

Emily Cannon, RN, MSN
Associate Professor of Nursing
Ivy Tech Community College
Terre Haute, Indiana

To the Instructor

The sixth edition of *Adult Health Nursing* was developed to educate the practical/vocational nursing student in medical-surgical nursing with an overview of anatomy and physiology. This full-color companion text to *Foundations of Nursing* continues to fill the needs of educators and students. It is accessible, accurate, up-to-date, clearly written, user-friendly, and portable. This new edition was revised to incorporate the most current and clinically-relevant information available. *Adult Health Nursing* and *Foundations of Nursing*, whether used together or separately, are the perfect texts to meet the educational needs of LPNs/LVNs in all health care settings.

Keeping the strengths of the first five editions, we have added new features to stay current with the many changes in the practice of nursing. The role of the LPN/LVN as health care provider continues to expand along with the needs of society and the technological advances in the health care system. With this revision, *Adult Health Nursing* will continue to be an excellent educational tool for providing the knowledge base necessary for the expanded role of LPNs/LVNs.

Finally, it is our belief that nursing will always be both an art and a science. This philosophy is reflected throughout the text.

ORGANIZATION AND STANDARD FEATURES

The organization of the sixth edition continues to follow the strengths of the previous edition, based on positive comments from educators and students.

TABLE OF CONTENTS

The text begins with an introductory chapter on anatomy and physiology to give students the basis for comprehension of the disorders content to follow. A chapter devoted to care of the surgical patient comes next, followed by chapters covering major disorders by body system. Systems disorders chapters are arranged in an orderly flow but can be studied in any order. New and additional content has been added to ensure that students have access to the most current information. The following are just a few of the many recent advancements in treatment and nursing interventions described in this new edition: recognizing blood loss in vital sign changes, new technologies including capsule endoscopy for diagnosis of gastrointestinal disorders and for clot-retrieval in patients with acute stroke, C-reactive protein testing for coronary artery disease and biventricular pacing to improve outcomes for heart failure, as well as new insulin and insulin-enhancing drugs.

CHAPTER ORGANIZATION

In disorders chapters, an overview of anatomy and physiology precedes the medical-surgical content, allowing the reader to easily correlate normal anatomy and physiology with disease conditions. Common disorders are then presented, typically organized with the following sections for more effective learning:
- Etiology and Pathophysiology
- Clinical Manifestations
- Assessment (with subjective and objective data)
- Diagnostic Tests
- Medical Management
- Nursing Interventions (including relevant medications)
- Nursing Diagnoses
- Patient Teaching
- Prognosis

NURSING PROCESS

The nursing process as applied to specific disorders is integrated throughout. A special nursing process summary section appears at the end of each chapter, enabling the reader to see more clearly its application to the chapter content as a whole. We have emphasized the role of the LPN/LVN in the nursing process as follows:
- The LPN/LVN will participate in planning care for the patient based on the patient's needs
- The LPN/LVN will review the patient's plan of care and recommend revisions as needed
- The LPN/LVN will follow defined prioritization for patient care
- The LPN/LVN will use clinical pathways, care maps, or care plans to guide and review patient care

REFERENCES AND SUGGESTED READINGS

These are grouped by chapter and listed at the end of the book for easy access. **Additional Resources** such as websites and agencies are included where applicable.

In the appendixes, **The Joint Commission's Lists of Dangerous Abbreviations, Acronyms, and Symbols** promotes safety in clinical practice in such areas as avoiding dosage errors, and **Common Abbreviations** and **Laboratory Reference Values** provide quick access to important information. **Answers to the Review Questions for the NCLEX® Examination** are provided in Appendix D.

LPN THREADS

The sixth edition of *Adult Health Nursing* shares some features and design elements with other Elsevier LPN/LVN textbooks. The purpose of these *LPN Threads* is to make it easier for students and instructors to use the variety of books required by the relatively brief and demanding LPN/LVN curriculum. *LPN Threads* include the following:

- A **reading level evaluation** is performed on every manuscript chapter during the book's development to increase the consistency among chapters and ensure the text is easy to understand.
- **Full-color design, cover, photos, and illustrations** are visually appealing and pedagogically useful.
- **Objectives** (numbered) begin each chapter and are divided into *Anatomy and Physiology* and *Medical-Surgical* categories. Chapter objectives provide a framework for content and are especially important in providing the structure for the TEACH Lesson Plans for the textbook.
- **Key Terms** with phonetic pronunciations and page number references are listed at the beginning of each chapter. Key terms appear in color in the chapter and are defined briefly, with full definitions in the **Glossary**. Simple phonetic pronunciations accompany difficult medical, nursing, or scientific terms or other words that may be difficult for students to pronounce. The goal is to help the student reader with limited proficiency in English to develop a greater command of the pronunciation of scientific and nonscientific English terminology. It is hoped that a more general competency in the understanding and use of medical and scientific language will result.
- A wide variety of **special features** related to critical thinking, clinical practice, care of the older adult, health promotion, safety, patient teaching, complementary and alternative therapies, communication, home health care, delegation and assignment, and more. Refer to the To the Student section of this introduction on pages xii and xiii for descriptions and examples of features from the pages of this textbook.
- **Critical Thinking Questions** with each Nursing Care Plan give students opportunities to practice critical thinking and clinical decision-making skills with realistic patient scenarios. Answers are provided in the Instructor Resources section on the Evolve website.
- **Key Points,** located at the end of chapters, follow the chapter objectives and serve as a useful chapter review.
- A full suite of **Instructor Resources** including TEACH Lesson Plans and Lecture Outlines, PowerPoint Lecture Slides, Test Bank, Image Collec-

tion, and Open Book Quizzes. Each of these teaching resources is described in detail below.
- In addition to consistent content, design, and support resources, these textbooks benefit from the advice and input of the **Elsevier LPN/LVN Advisory Board.**

TEACHING AND LEARNING PACKAGE

FOR STUDENTS

- A media-rich **Companion CD** is included with every book. Helpful features include animations and audio clips depicting physiologic processes, physical assessment video clips, an English/Spanish glossary with definitions and audio pronunciations, an anatomy coloring book, and a fluids and electrolytes tutorial.
- An **Evolve website** provides free student resources, including additional review questions for the NCLEX Examination for every chapter, calculators (Body Mass Index, IV Dosage, Unit Conversion, to name a few), and animations and video clips in addition to those provided on the book's Companion CD. All assets from the Companion CD are also available on the Evolve website.
- The *Study Guide for Adult Health Nursing* is designed to promote learning, understanding, and application of the content in the textbook. Each chapter ties specific activities to specific objectives rather than simply listing objectives and activities separately. Activities include hundreds of labeling, matching, and fill-in-the-blank questions, each with textbook page references; critical thinking questions with clinical scenarios; and multiple-choice and alternate-format questions for NCLEX review. Performance Checklists for every skill in the textbook are also available in the Study Guide. The complete answer key is provided in the Instructor Resources section of the Evolve website. *Sold separately.*
- *Virtual Clinical Excursions* is an interactive workbook/CD-ROM package that guides the student through a multifloor virtual hospital in a hands-on clinical learning experience. Students can assess and analyze information, diagnose, set priorities, and implement and evaluate care. NCLEX-style review questions provide immediate testing of clinical knowledge. *Sold separately.*

FOR INSTRUCTORS

The comprehensive **Evolve Resources with TEACH Instructor Resource** provides a rich array of teaching tools that includes the following:

- **TEACH Lesson Plans with Lecture Outlines,** based on the textbook learning objectives, provide ready-to-use lesson plans that tie together all of the text and ancillary components provided for *Adult Health Nursing*.

- A collection of more than 1000 text and graphic **PowerPoint Lecture Slides** are specific to the text.
- A **Test Bank,** delivered in ExamView and Partest, provides approximately 700 multiple-choice and alternate-format NCLEX-style questions. Each question includes the correct answer, rationale, topic, objective, cognitive level, step of the nursing process, NCLEX category of client needs, and textbook page references.

- An **Image Collection** contains nearly 300 images from the textbook, suitable for incorporation into classroom lectures, PowerPoint presentations, or distance-learning applications.
- An **Open-Book Quiz** for every chapter includes textbook page references for each question.
- **Answer Keys** are provided for the Critical Thinking Questions in Nursing Care Plans and for the activities in the Study Guide.

To the Student

Designed with you in mind, *Adult Health Nursing* presents medical-surgical nursing concepts in a visually-appealing and easy-to-use format. Here are some of the numerous special features that will help you understand and apply the material.

READING AND REVIEW TOOLS

Objectives introduce the chapter topics and are divided into *Anatomy and Physiology* and *Medical-Surgical* categories as appropriate.

Key Terms are listed with page number references, and difficult medical, nursing, or scientific terms are accompanied by simple phonetic pronunciations. Key terms are in color the first time they appear in the narrative and are briefly defined in the text, with complete definitions in the Glossary.

Each chapter ends with a *Get Ready for the NCLEX® Examination!* section. **Key Points** follow the chapter objectives and serve as a useful chapter review. An extensive set of **Review Questions for the NCLEX® Examination** provide immediate opportunity for testing your understanding of the chapter content. **Answers** are located in Appendix D in the back of the book.

ADDITIONAL LEARNING RESOURCES

The **Companion CD** included with your textbook contains animations, video clips, audio clips, an English/Spanish audio glossary, a Body Spectrum Electronic Anatomy Coloring Book, and a Fluids and Electrolytes tutorial. Your free online **Evolve Resources** at **http://evolve.elsevier.com/Christensen/adult** gives you access to all this *and* even more Review Questions for the NCLEX Examination, a Concept Map Creator, and much more.

CHAPTER FEATURES

Skills are presented in a logical step-by-step format with accompanying full-color illustrations. Clearly defined **nursing actions** followed by **rationales** in italicized type show you how and why skills are performed. These Skills also emphasize the importance of accurate, effective documentation of data.

1 **Nursing Care Plans,** developed around specific case studies, include nursing diagnoses with an emphasis on patient goals and outcomes and questions to promote **critical thinking**. These sample care plans are

valuable tools that can be used as a guideline in the clinical setting. The critical thinking aspect empowers you to develop sound clinical decision-making skills.

2 **Nursing diagnoses and interventions** are screened and set apart in the text in a clear, easy-to-understand format to help you learn to participate in the development of a nursing care plan. The most current NANDA International-approved nursing diagnoses are used.

3 **Evidence-Based Practice boxes,** *new to this edition,* summarize the latest research findings and highlight how they apply to LPN/LVN practice.

4 **Medication tables** developed for specific disorders provide quick access to action, dosage, side effects, and nursing considerations for commonly used medications.

5 **Safety Alert! boxes** emphasize the importance of maintaining safety in patient and resident care to protect patients, residents, family, health care providers, and the public from accidents and the spread of disease.

Health Promotion boxes emphasize a healthy lifestyle, preventive behaviors, and screening tests to assist in the prevention of accidents and disease.

Coordinated Care boxes throughout the text promote comprehensive patient care with other members of the health care team, focusing on prioritization, assignment, supervision, collaboration, and leadership topics.

Complementary and Alternative Therapies boxes in nearly every chapter give a breakdown of specific nontraditional therapies, along with precautions and possible side effects. A complete discussion of complementary and alternative therapies is given in Chapter 17 of *Foundations of Nursing.*

Cultural Considerations boxes explore select specific cultural preferences and how to address the needs of a culturally diverse patient and resident population when planning nursing care.

Communication boxes focus on communication strategies with real-life examples of nurse-patient dialogue.

Patient Teaching boxes appear frequently in the text to help develop awareness of the vital role of patient/family teaching in health care today.

6 **Life Span Considerations for the Older Adult boxes** bring a gerontologic perspective to nursing care, focusing on the nursing interventions unique to the older adult patient or resident.

Home Care Considerations discuss the issues facing patients and caregivers in the home setting.

1

Nursing Care Plan 7-1 The Patient with Leukemia

Ms. May is a 26-year-old patient diagnosed with acute lymphocytic leukemia. She is married and the mother of a 3-year-old daughter. Ms. May has been receiving chemotherapy and is immunocompromised, with a differential white blood cell (WBC) count revealing a neutrophil count of 22%. Her hemoglobin is 8.8 g/dL, and her platelets are $55,000/mm^3$. Her mouth appears edematous, and she complains of oral tenderness.

NURSING DIAGNOSIS *Risk for infection, related to leukopenia*

Patient Goals and Expected Outcomes	Nursing Intervention	Evaluation/Rationale
Patient or caregiver will identify measures to prevent or control infection	Inspect all body sites for infection at least daily; note and report fever, sore throat, purulent exudate, chills, cough, burning with urination, erythema, edema, tenderness, and pain.	Patient will remain free of infection.
Patient or caregiver will verbalize and report signs and symptoms of infection	Monitor vital signs. Obtain cultures as ordered. Monitor WBC counts and culture reports. Administer antibiotics on time as ordered. Promote and maintain hygiene integrity of skin and mucous membranes. Use aseptic technique in treatments. Teach the patient and family: • Necessity of avoiding crowds or people with infections while WBC count is ⊠ $1000/mm^3$ • Personal hygiene measures • Signs and symptoms of infection	Patient demonstrates no signs or symptoms of infection; temperature and WBC count are within normal range.

NURSING DIAGNOSIS *Ineffective coping, related to diagnosis and disease process*

Patient Goals and Expected Outcomes	Nursing Intervention	Evaluation
Patient and family will demonstrate measures to effectively cope by verbalizing role of family, significant others, and support groups in therapeutic coping	Assess coping capabilities of patient and significant others. Discuss disease process and expectations. Alleviate knowledge deficit. Encourage questions and self-expression: listen actively, demonstrate compassion, reassure with touch and personal contact. Assess fear of threat of death: allow time for personal expression and provide one-on-one discussion opportunity.	Patient and family express factors that are causing anxiety and powerlessness.

Critical Thinking Questions

1. What should the nurse do if a visitor with an obvious upper respiratory tract infection is seen approaching Ms. May's room?
2. What nursing interventions would be most appropriate in providing therapeutic oral hygiene for Ms. May?
3. What kind of a bath and activities of daily living would be most beneficial for Ms. May?

Clinical Manifestations

Skin and mucous membrane manifestations include petechiae and ecchymoses. Epistaxis and gingival bleeding are common. Circulatory hypovolemia is noted through hypotension; pallor; cool, clammy skin; and tachycardia. GI tract bleeding is common, with abdominal flank pain caused by internal bleeding. CNS involvement ranges from altered response and malaise to loss of consciousness or affected speech.

Assessment

Subjective data include a history of bleeding after surgical or dental procedures. Exposure to toxic or hazardous agents or to radiation may be revealed. Complaint of headache, extremity pain, and numbness is noted. Medications taken (e.g., aspirin) may lead to suspicion of toxicity.

Collection of **objective data** involves observation of pain on pressure to the abdomen, revealing liver and spleen tenderness and perhaps enlargement. Skin and mucous membranes may have petechiae, ecchymoses, and occasionally hematoma. Emesis and stool may show signs of bleeding. Joint examination reveals motion pain.

Diagnostic Tests

The platelet count is low. The RBC count is low with a decreased hemoglobin level. Coagulation time is altered. Bone marrow studies show abnormal cells.

orrhoids or marked protrusion. Surgical removal may be done by cautery, clamp, or excision. After removal of the hemorrhoid, wounds can be left open or closed, although closed wounds are reported to heal faster. Hemorrhoidectomy is not considered a major procedure, but pain may be acute, requiring opioids and analgesic ointments. Complications include hemorrhage, local infection, pain, urinary retention, and abscess.

Nursing Interventions and Patient Teaching

Rectal conditions can be embarrassing to the patient, and the nurse's direct but concerned attitude can decrease this embarrassment. Assess the knowledge level by asking patients about their condition, what they have been told about treatment, and what treatments have been done before surgery and why.

Observe the patient with a prolapsed hemorrhoid for edema, thrombosis, and ischemia. Ischemic tissue will be dark red to necrotic (black). Explain that a low-bulk diet can produce chronic constipation (see Evidence-Based Practice box).

For the surgical patient, take vital signs frequently for the first 24 hours to rule out internal bleeding. Sitz baths are given several times daily. Early ambulation and a soft diet facilitate bowel elimination. The patient may have a great deal of anxiety concerning the first defecation; open a discussion on this and provide an analgesic before the bowel movement to reduce discomfort. A stool softener such as docusate (Colace) is usually ordered for the first few postoperative days.

Nursing diagnoses and interventions for the patient with hemorrhoids include but are not limited to the following:

2

Nursing Diagnoses	Nursing Interventions
Pain, related to edema, prolapse, and surgical interventions	Instruct patient to wash anal area after defecation and pat dry. Sitz baths or local heat applied to site may be soothing. Use of local anesthetics (dibucaine ointment or Tucks pads) may give relief. Reinforce need for high-residue diet. Instruct patient on manual reduction of external hemorrhoids. Apply ice packs to hemorrhoids if thrombosed to prevent edema and pain. Use cushion for sitting postoperatively.
Anxiety, related to: • previous experiences • fear of first bowel movement postoperatively • lack of knowledge regarding diet	Establish a supportive relationship with patient. Explain need for high-residue diet. Administer laxatives and oil-retention enema as ordered. Give analgesics before first bowel movement and a sitz bath for pain relief.

3

Evidence-Based Practice Treatment of Chronic Constipation in Older Adults

Evidence Summary

The combined effect of decreased activity, change in diet, multiple diseases, and multiple drugs all put older adults at increased risk for constipation. Constipation is diagnosed when a person has two of the following criteria for 12 weeks during the past year: straining, pelletlike stools, sensation of incomplete evacuation, sensation of anal blockage, or using manual maneuvers, all for more than 25% of bowel movements; or having fewer than three bowel movements per week. Data are too limited in the older adult population to recommend one treatment over another. Because constipation in older adults is more likely to be a result of multiple physical and pathologic conditions, there is no consensus that fits all older adults. From a pharmacologic perspective, the ideal drug is selected in terms of effectiveness, tolerance, adverse effects, drug interactions, and cost-effectiveness.

Application to Nursing Practice

- When possible, replace a medication causing constipation with a substitute.
- Encourage older adults to increase physical activity when feasible.
- Give attention to the potential risk of fluid overload in older adult clients with congestive heart failure or renal failure.
- Encourage fiber intake of 20 g/day of wheat bran to start. Observe for bloating and flatulence in older adults.
- Stool softeners are no longer recommended for constipation.
- Fiber and bulk-forming laxatives are the first step in treating constipation in older adults.
- Osmotic laxatives are effective in the treatment of constipation in older adults because they are well tolerated and have no known interactions with other drugs.
- Stimulant laxatives are more effective than placebo, but concern remains regarding their adverse effects on older adults.
- Older adults who have mobility problems often need enemas to avoid an impaction. The tap water enema is the safest for regular use. Glycerol suppositories trigger the defecatory reflex and are sometimes useful in treating older adults.

From Potter, P.A., & Perry, A.G. (2009). *Fundamentals of nursing: concepts, process, and practice.* (7th ed.) St. Louis: Mosby. Adapted from Bosshard, W., Dreher, R., Schnegg, J.F., (2004). The treatment of chronic constipation in elderly people: an update, *Drugs Aging, 21*(14), 911-930.

4

Table 15-2 Medications for Immune Disorders

Generic (Trade)	Action	Side Effects	Nursing Implications
Diphenhydramine (Benadryl)	Antihistamine	Drowsiness, confusion, nasal stuffiness, dry mouth, photosensitivity, urine retention	Use cautiously with central nervous system depressants, including alcohol; give with food; it is a safe hypnotic for older adults; tell patient to avoid driving or hazardous activity due to drowsiness.
Loratadine (Claritin)	Nonsedating antihistamine	Slight sedation (more common with increased doses)	Store in tight container at room temperature. Teach patient and family to avoid driving or other hazardous activities if drowsiness occurs.
Fexofenadine (Allegra)	Nonsedating antihistamine	Headache, drowsiness, blurred vision, hypotension, bradycardia, tachycardia, dysrhythmias (rare), urinary retention, pancytopenia	
Dexamethasone (Decadron)	Corticosteroid		Do not use for extended period; use cautiously with patients with diabetes or peptic ulcers.
Flunisolide (AeroBid)	Corticosteroid (inhaled)	Headache, transient nasal burning, epistaxis, nausea, vomiting	Not effective for acute episodes; use regularly; teach care and cleaning of inhaler; if symptoms do not improve in 3 weeks, consult physician.
Epinephrine (Adrenalin Chloride, Sus-Phrine, EpiPen)	Bronchodilator	Nervousness, tremor, headache, hypertension, tachycardia, ventricular fibrillation, stroke	Do not use with monoamine oxidase inhibitor; use cautiously in patients with hyperthyroidism, hypertension, diabetes, and heart disease.

as leukotriene-receptor blockers, and zileuton (Zyflo) inhibits the production of leukotrienes.

Nursing Diagnoses

Nursing diagnoses for patients with hypersensitivity include (1) *risk for injury,* related to exposure to allergen; (2) *activity intolerance,* related to malaise; and (3) *risk for infection,* related to inflammation of protective mucous membranes.

Patient Teaching

Patient teaching should revolve around the specific diagnosis. Advise the patient with seasonal allergies to avoid offending allergens, and ensure he or she understands the therapeutic medication plan. Focus on health promotion and health teaching for self-care management (see Safety Alert box).

5

Safety Alert!

Treating the Patient with a Hypersensitivity Reaction

- List all of a patient's allergies on the chart, the nursing care plan, and the medication record.
- After an allergic disorder is diagnosed, therapeutic treatment is aimed at reducing exposure to the offending allergen; treating the symptoms; and, if necessary, desensitizing the person through immunotherapy.
- All health care workers must be prepared for the rare but life-threatening anaphylactic reaction, which requires immediate medical and nursing interventions.
- Instruct the patient to wear a medical-alert bracelet listing the particular drug allergy.
- For a patient allergic to insect stings, commercial bee sting kits contain epinephrine and a tourniquet. Teach the patient to apply the tourniquet and self-inject the subcutaneous epinephrine. The patient should wear a medical-alert bracelet and carry a bee sting kit whenever going outdoors.

toms. The major difficulty in symptomatic patients is gastroesophageal reflux, manifested as pyrosis (heartburn) after overeating. Complications of strangulation, infarction, or ulceration of the herniated stomach are serious and require surgical intervention. Factors contributing to the development of these hernias include obesity, trauma, and a general weakening of the supporting structures as a result of aging (see Life Span Considerations box).

Medical Management

The physician may perform (1) a posterior gastropexy, in which the stomach is returned to the abdomen and sutured in place; or (2) a laparoscopically performed Nissen fundoplication, in which the fundus is wrapped around the lower part of the esophagus and sutured in place (Figure 5-16). The use of laparoscopic techniques has reduced the overall morbidity, complications, and the cost of hospitalization associated with a thoracic or open abdominal approach. However, a thoracic or open abdominal approach may be used in selected cases.

Nursing Interventions

Nursing care of the patient after surgery is similar to that after gastric surgery or thoracic surgery, depending on the procedure performed.

6

Life Span Considerations

Older Adults

Gastrointestinal Disorders

- Loss of teeth and resultant use of dentures can interfere with chewing and lead to digestive complaints.
- Dysphagia is commonly seen in the older adult population and may be caused by changes in the esophageal musculature or by neurologic conditions.
- Hiatal hernias and esophageal diverticuli are significantly increased with aging because of changes in musculature of the diaphragm and esophagus.
- Older adults have decreased secretion of hydrochloric acid (hypochlorhydria and achlorhydria) from the parietal cells of the stomach. This results in an increased incidence of pernicious anemia and gastritis in the older adult population.
- Peptic ulcers are common, but often the symptoms are vague and go unrecognized until there is a bleeding episode. Medications such as aspirin, nonsteroidal antiinflammatory drugs, and steroids that are taken for the chronic degenerative joint conditions common with aging should be used with caution because they can contribute to ulcer formation.
- Frequency of diverticulosis and diverticulitis increases dramatically with aging and can contribute to malabsorption of nutrients.
- Constipation is a problem for many older adults. Inactivity, changes in diet and fluid intake, and medications can contribute to this problem. Monitor bowel elimination and establish a bowel regimen to prevent impaction.

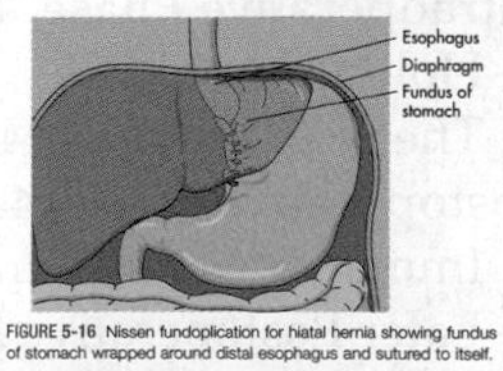

FIGURE 5-16 Nissen fundoplication for hiatal hernia showing fundus of stomach wrapped around distal esophagus and sutured to itself.

Prognosis

The prognosis for hernias is good because surgical intervention is usually successful. The result can be altered if the patient is a poor surgical risk or has other complications.

INTESTINAL OBSTRUCTION

Etiology and Pathophysiology

Intestinal obstruction occurs when intestinal contents cannot pass through the GI tract; it requires prompt treatment. The obstruction may be partial or complete. The causes of intestinal obstruction are classified as mechanical or nonmechanical.

Mechanical Obstruction

Mechanical obstruction may be caused by an occlusion of the lumen of the intestinal tract. Most obstructions occur in the ileum, which is the narrowest segment of the small intestine. Mechanical obstructions account for 90% of all intestinal obstructions. Mechanical obstructions include adhesions (Figure 5-17, *A*) or incarcerated hernias. Adhesions can develop after abdominal surgery. Other causes include impacted feces, diverticular disease, tumor of the bowel, intussusceptions, volvulus (Figure 5-17, *B*) (a twisting of bowel onto itself), or the strictures of inflammatory bowel disease. Residues from foods high in fiber, such as raw coconut or fruit pulp, can also obstruct the small bowel.

Nonmechanical Obstruction

Nonmechanical obstruction may result from a neuromuscular or vascular disorder. The cause is something that decreases the muscle action of the bowel and affects the ability of fecal matter and fluid to move through the intestines (Kent, 2007). Paralytic (adynamic) ileus (lack of intestinal peristalsis and bowel sounds) is the most common form of nonmechanical obstruction. It occurs to some degree after any abdominal surgery. Other causes include inflammatory responses (e.g., acute pancreatitis, acute appendicitis), electrolyte abnormalities (especially hypokalemia), and thoracic or lumbar spinal

Contents

1 Introduction to Anatomy and Physiology, 1

Barbara Lauritsen Christensen and M. Christine Neff

Anatomical Terminology, 1
  Body Planes, 2
  Body Cavities, 2
Abdominal Regions, 3
Abdominopelvic Quadrants, 3
Structural Levels of Organization, 3
  Cells, 5
  Tissues, 9
  Membranes, 12
  Organs and Systems, 12

2 Care of the Surgical Patient, 17

Elaine Oden Kockrow and Barbara Lauritsen Christensen

Perioperative Nursing, 18
  Influencing Factors, 19
  Psychosocial Needs, 20
  Socioeconomic and Cultural Needs, 20
  Medications, 21
  Education and Experience, 23
Preoperative Phase, 23
  Preoperative Teaching, 24
  Preoperative Preparation, 24
Intraoperative Phase, 43
  Holding Area, 43
  The Nurse's Role, 44
Postoperative Phase, 44
  Immediate Postoperative Phase, 44
  Later Postoperative Phase, 46
  Gastrointestinal Status, 52
  Fluids and Electrolytes, 52
Nursing Process for the Surgical Patient, 53
Discharge: Providing General Information, 55
  Ambulatory Surgery Discharge, 55

3 Care of the Patient with an Integumentary Disorder, 59

Linda Y. North

Anatomy and Physiology of the Skin, 59
  Functions of the Skin, 59
  Structure of the Skin, 60
  Appendages of the Skin, 61
Assessment of the Skin, 61
  Inspection and Palpation, 61
  Chief Complaint, 67
Psychosocial Assessment, 68

Viral Disorders of the Skin, 68
  Herpes Simplex, 68
  Herpes Zoster (Shingles), 72
  Pityriasis Rosea, 74
Bacterial Disorders of the Skin, 74
  Cellulitis, 74
  Impetigo Contagiosa, 75
  Folliculitis, Furuncles, Carbuncles, and Felons, 77
Fungal Infections of the Skin, 78
Inflammatory Disorders of the Skin, 79
  Contact Dermatitis, 79
  Dermatitis Venenata, Exfoliative Dermatitis, and Dermatitis Medicamentosa, 80
  Urticaria, 81
  Angioedema, 81
  Eczema (Atopic Dermatitis), 82
  Acne Vulgaris, 83
  Psoriasis, 84
  Systemic Lupus Erythematosus, 85
Parasitic Diseases of the Skin, 87
  Pediculosis, 87
  Scabies, 89
Tumors of the Skin, 90
  Keloids, 90
  Angiomas, 91
  Verruca (Wart), 91
  Nevi (Moles), 91
  Basal Cell Carcinoma, 91
  Squamous Cell Carcinoma, 91
  Malignant Melanoma, 92
Disorders of the Appendages, 94
  Alopecia, 94
  Hypertrichosis (Hirsutism), 94
  Hypotrichosis, 94
  Paronychia, 94
Burns, 94
Nursing Process for the Patient with an Integumentary Disorder, 103

4 Care of the Patient with a Musculoskeletal Disorder, 109

Martha E. Spray

Anatomy and Physiology of the Musculoskeletal System, 109
  Functions of the Skeletal System, 109
  Structure of Bones, 110
  Articulations (Joints), 110
  Divisions of the Skeleton, 110
  Functions of the Muscular System, 110

Laboratory and Diagnostic Examinations, 113
  Radiographic Studies, 113
  Aspiration, 116
  Endoscopic Examination, 116
  Electrographic Procedure, 117
  Laboratory Tests, 117
  Effects of Bed Rest on Mineral Content
    in Bone, 117
DISORDERS OF THE MUSCULOSKELETAL
  SYSTEM, 117
Inflammatory Disorders, 117
  Arthritis, 117
  Rheumatoid Arthritis, 118
  Ankylosing Spondylitis, 123
  Osteoarthritis (Degenerative Joint Disease), 125
  Gout (Gouty Arthritis), 127
Other Musculoskeletal Disorders, 128
  Osteoporosis, 128
  Osteomyelitis, 131
  Fibromyalgia Syndrome, 131
Surgical Interventions for Total Knee or Total Hip
  Replacement, 133
  Knee Arthroplasty (Total Knee Replacement), 133
  Unicompartmental Knee Arthroplasty, 133
  Hip Arthroplasty (Total Hip Replacement), 135
Fractures, 137
  Fracture of the Hip, 137
  Other Fractures, 142
  Fracture of the Vertebrae, 145
  Fracture of the Pelvis, 147
Complications of Fractures, 148
  Compartment Syndrome, 148
  Shock, 149
  Fat Embolism, 150
  Gas Gangrene, 150
  Thromboembolus, 151
  Delayed Fracture Healing, 152
Skeletal Fixation Devices, 152
  External Fixation Devices, 152
Nonsurgical Interventions for Musculoskeletal
  Disorders, 153
  Casts, 153
  Cast Removal, 156
  Traction, 156
  Orthopedic Devices, 157
Traumatic Injuries, 160
  Contusions, 160
  Sprains, 160
  Whiplash, 160
  Ankle Sprains, 161
  Strains, 161
  Dislocations, 162
  Airbag Injuries, 163
  Carpal Tunnel Syndrome, 163
  Herniation of Intervertebral Disk (Herniated
    Nucleus Pulposus), 164
  Tumors of the Bone, 166

  Amputation, 167
Nursing Process for the Patient with a
  Musculoskeletal Disorder, 169

5 Care of the Patient with a Gastrointestinal
   Disorder, 175
   Barbara Lauritsen Christensen

Anatomy and Physiology of the Gastrointestinal
  System, 175
  Digestive System, 175
  Accessory Organs of Digestion, 179
  Regulation of Food Intake, 180
Laboratory and Diagnostic Examinations, 180
  Upper Gastrointestinal Study (Upper GI Series,
    UGI), 180
  Tube Gastric Analysis, 180
  Esophagogastroduodenoscopy (EGD, UGI
    Endoscopy, Gastroscopy), 180
  Capsule Endoscopy, 181
  Barium Swallow and Gastrografin Studies, 181
  Esophageal Function Studies (Bernstein Test), 181
  Examination of Stool for Occult Blood, 182
  Sigmoidoscopy (Lower GI Endoscopy), 182
  Barium Enema Study (Lower GI Series), 182
  Colonoscopy, 182
  Stool Culture, 183
  Obstruction Series (Flat Plate
    of the Abdomen), 183
Disorders of the Mouth, 183
  Dental Plaque and Caries, 183
  Candidiasis, 184
  Carcinoma of the Oral Cavity, 184
Disorders of the Esophagus, 186
  Gastroesophageal Reflux Disease, 186
  Carcinoma of the Esophagus, 188
  Achalasia, 189
Disorders of the Stomach, 190
  Gastritis (Acute), 190
  Peptic Ulcers, 191
  Gastric Ulcers, 191
  Physiologic Stress Ulcers, 192
  Duodenal Ulcers, 192
  Cancer of the Stomach, 200
Disorders of the Intestines, 201
  Infections, 201
  Irritable Bowel Syndrome, 203
  Inflammatory Bowel Disease, 205
  Ulcerative Colitis, 205
  Crohn's Disease, 209
  Acute Abdominal Inflammations, 212
  Appendicitis, 212
  Diverticulosis and Diverticulitis, 213
  Peritonitis, 215
  Hernias, 216
  External Hernias, 216
  Hiatal Hernia, 217

Intestinal Obstruction, 218
Colorectal Cancer, 220
Hemorrhoids, 224
Anal Fissure and Fistula, 226
Fecal Incontinence, 226
**Nursing Process for the Patient with a
Gastrointestinal Disorder, 227**

**6 Care of the Patient with a Gallbladder,
Liver, Biliary Tract, or Exocrine Pancreatic
Disorder, 231**

Barbara Lauritsen Christensen

Laboratory and Diagnostic Examinations in
the Assessment of the Hepatobiliary and
Pancreatic Systems, 231
Serum Bilirubin Test, 231
Liver Enzyme Tests, 231
Serum Protein Test, 232
Oral Cholecystography, 232
Intravenous Cholangiography, 232
Operative Cholangiography, 232
T-Tube Cholangiography, 233
Ultrasonography of the Liver, the Gallbladder,
and the Biliary System, 233
Gallbladder Scanning, 233
Needle Liver Biopsy, 233
Radioisotope Liver Scanning, 234
Serum Ammonia Test, 234
Hepatitis Virus Studies, 234
Serum Amylase Test, 234
Urine Amylase Test, 234
Serum Lipase Test, 235
Ultrasonography of the Pancreas, 235
Computed Tomography of the Abdomen, 235
Endoscopic Retrograde
Cholangiopancreatography of the Pancreatic
Duct, 235
Disorders of the Liver, Biliary Tract, Gallbladder,
and Exocrine Pancreas, 236
Cirrhosis, 236
Liver Cancer, 241
Hepatitis, 243
Liver Abscesses, 247
Cholecystitis and Cholelithiasis, 248
Pancreatitis, 253
Cancer of the Pancreas, 255
**Nursing Process for the Patient with a
Gallbladder, Liver, Biliary Tract, or Exocrine
Pancreatic Disorder, 257**

**7 Care of the Patient with a Blood or Lymphatic
Disorder, 262**

Barbara Lauritsen Christensen

Anatomy and Physiology of the Hematologic
and Lymphatic Systems, 262
Characteristics of Blood, 262

Lymphatic System, 267
Laboratory and Diagnostic Tests, 269
Disorders of the Hematologic and Lymphatic
Systems, 269
Disorders Associated with Erythrocytes, 269
Anemia, 269
Disorders Associated with Leukocytes, 281
Agranulocytosis, 281
Leukemia, 282
Disorders of Coagulation, 284
Disorders Associated with Platelets, 286
Thrombocytopenia, 286
Clotting Factor Defects, 287
Hemophilia, 287
Von Willebrand's Disease, 289
Disseminated Intravascular Coagulation, 289
Disorder of Plasma Cells, 291
Multiple Myeloma, 291
Disorders of the Lymphatic System, 292
Lymphangitis, 292
Lymphedema, 293
Hodgkin's Disease, 293
Non-Hodgkin's Lymphoma, 297
**Nursing Process for the Patient with a Blood or
Lymphatic Disorder, 298**

**8 Care of the Patient with a Cardiovascular or a
Peripheral Vascular Disorder, 303**

Barbara Lauritsen Christensen

Anatomy and Physiology of the Cardiovascular
System, 304
Heart, 304
Blood Vessels, 306
Circulation, 307
Coronary Blood Supply, 307
Systemic Circulation, 307
Pulmonary Circulation, 308
Laboratory and Diagnostic Examinations, 308
Diagnostic Imaging, 308
Cardiac Catheterization and Angiography, 308
Electrocardiography, 308
Cardiac Monitors, 309
Thallium Scanning, 310
Echocardiography, 310
Positron Emission Tomography, 310
Laboratory Tests, 310
Disorders of the Cardiovascular System, 311
Normal Aging Patterns, 312
Risk Factors, 312
Cardiac Dysrhythmias, 314
Cardiac Arrest, 319
Disorders of the Heart, 320
Coronary Atherosclerotic Heart Disease, 320
Angina Pectoris, 321
Myocardial Infarction, 326
Heart Failure, 332
Pulmonary Edema, 340

Valvular Heart Disease, 340
Inflammatory Disorders of the Heart, 342
Rheumatic Heart Disease, 342
Pericarditis, 343
Endocarditis, 345
Myocarditis, 346
Cardiomyopathy, 346
Disorders of the Peripheral Vascular System, 348
Normal Aging Patterns, 348
Risk Factors, 348
Assessment, 349
Hypertension, 351
Disorders of the Arteries, 355
Arteriosclerosis and Atherosclerosis, 355
Peripheral Arterial Disease of the Lower
Extremities, 355
Arterial Embolism, 357
Arterial Aneurysm, 359
Thromboangiitis Obliterans (Buerger's
Disease), 360
Raynaud's Disease, 361
Disorders of the Veins, 362
Thrombophlebitis, 362
Varicose Veins, 365
Venous Stasis Ulcers, 366
**Nursing Process for the Patient with a
Cardiovascular Disorder,** 367

**9 Care of the Patient with a Respiratory
Disorder,** 373

Barbara Lauritsen Christensen

Anatomy and Physiology of the Respiratory
System, 374
Upper Respiratory Tract, 374
Lower Respiratory Tract, 377
Mechanics of Breathing, 377
Regulation of Respiration, 378
Assessment of the Respiratory System, 378
Laboratory and Diagnostic Examinations, 379
Chest Roentgenogram, 379
Computed Tomography, 380
Pulmonary Function Testing, 380
Mediastinoscopy, 380
Laryngoscopy, 381
Bronchoscopy, 381
Sputum Specimen, 381
Cytologic Studies, 382
Lung Biopsy, 382
Thoracentesis, 382
Arterial Blood Gases, 382
Pulse Oximetry, 383
Disorders of the Upper Airway, 384
Epistaxis, 384
Deviated Septum and Nasal Polyps, 385
Antigen-Antibody Allergic Rhinitis and
Allergic Conjunctivitis (Hay Fever), 386
Obstructive Sleep Apnea, 387

Upper Airway Obstruction, 388
Cancer of the Larynx, 389
Respiratory Infections, 391
Acute Rhinitis, 391
Acute Follicular Tonsillitis, 392
Laryngitis, 393
Pharyngitis, 394
Sinusitis, 394
Disorders of the Lower Airway, 395
Acute Bronchitis, 395
Legionnaires' Disease, 396
Severe Acute Respiratory Syndrome, 397
Anthrax, 398
Tuberculosis, 398
Pneumonia, 403
Pleurisy, 407
Pleural Effusion/Empyema, 408
Atelectasis, 410
Pneumothorax, 411
Lung Cancer, 413
Pulmonary Edema, 415
Pulmonary Embolism, 416
Acute Respiratory Distress Syndrome, 418
Chronic Obstructive Pulmonary Disease, 420
Emphysema, 421
Chronic Bronchitis, 424
Asthma, 426
Bronchiectasis, 428
**Nursing Process for the Patient with a
Respiratory Disorder,** 429

**10 Care of the Patient with a Urinary
Disorder,** 434

Alita K. Sellers

Anatomy and Physiology of the Urinary
System, 434
Kidneys, 434
Urine Composition and Characteristics, 438
Urine Abnormalities, 438
Ureters, 438
Urinary Bladder, 438
Urethra, 439
Normal Aging of the Urinary System, 439
Laboratory and Diagnostic Examinations, 439
Urinalysis, 439
Specific Gravity, 440
Blood (Serum) Urea Nitrogen, 440
Blood (Serum) Creatinine, 440
Creatinine Clearance, 440
Prostate-Specific Antigen, 440
Osmolality, 441
Kidney-Ureter-Bladder Radiography, 441
Intravenous Pyelogram or Intravenous
Urography, 441
Retrograde Pyelography, 441
Voiding Cystourethrography, 441
Endoscopic Procedures, 441

Renal Angiography, 442
Renal Venogram, 442
Computed Tomography, 442
Magnetic Resonance Imaging, 442
Renal Scan, 442
Ultrasonography, 442
Transrectal Ultrasound, 442
Renal Biopsy, 442
Urodynamic Studies, 442
Medication Considerations, 443
Diuretics to Enhance Urinary Output, 443
Medications for Urinary Tract Infections, 444
Nutritional Considerations, 445
Maintaining Adequate Urinary Drainage, 445
Types of Catheters, 445
Nursing Interventions and Patient Teaching, 446
Prognosis, 448
Disorders of the Urinary System, 448
Alterations in Voiding Patterns, 448
Urinary Retention, 448
Urinary Incontinence, 448
Neurogenic Bladder, 450
*Inflammatory and Infectious Disorders of the
Urinary System*, 451
Urinary Tract Infections, 451
Urethritis, 452
Cystitis, 453
Interstitial Cystitis, 453
Prostatitis, 454
Pyelonephritis, 455
Obstructive Disorders of the Urinary Tract, 456
Urinary Obstruction, 456
Hydronephrosis, 457
Urolithiasis, 457
Tumors of the Urinary System, 459
Renal Tumors, 459
Renal Cysts, 460
Tumors of the Urinary Bladder, 461
Conditions Affecting the Prostate Gland, 462
Benign Prostatic Hypertrophy, 462
Cancer of the Prostate, 464
Urethral Strictures, 466
Urinary Tract Trauma, 467
Immunologic Disorders of the Kidney, 467
Nephrotic Syndrome, 467
Nephritis, 468
Renal Failure, 470
Acute Renal Failure, 470
Chronic Renal Failure (End-Stage Renal
Disease), 471
Care of the Patient Requiring Dialysis, 474
Hemodialysis, 474
Peritoneal Dialysis, 475
Surgical Procedures for Urinary Dysfunction, 477
Nephrectomy, 477
Nephrostomy, 477
Kidney Transplantation, 478

Urinary Diversion, 478
**Nursing Process for the Patient with a Urinary
Disorder, 480**

**11 Care of the Patient with an Endocrine
Disorder, 484**

Barbara Lauritsen Christensen

Anatomy and Physiology of the Endocrine
System, 485
Endocrine Glands and Hormones, 485
Disorders of the Pituitary Gland
(Hypophysis), 489
Acromegaly, 489
Gigantism, 491
Dwarfism, 492
Diabetes Insipidus, 492
Syndrome of Inappropriate Antidiuretic
Hormone, 493
Disorders of the Thyroid and Parathyroid
Glands, 495
Hyperthyroidism, 495
Hypothyroidism, 498
Simple (Colloid) Goiter, 500
Cancer of the Thyroid, 501
Hyperparathyroidism, 502
Hypoparathyroidism, 503
Disorders of the Adrenal Glands, 504
Adrenal Hyperfunction (Cushing
Syndrome), 504
Adrenal Hypofunction (Addison's Disease), 506
Pheochromocytoma, 508
Disorders of the Pancreas, 509
Diabetes Mellitus, 509
**Nursing Process for the Patient with an
Endocrine Disorder, 528**

**12 Care of the Patient with a Reproductive
Disorder, 533**

Barbara Lauritsen Christensen

Anatomy and Physiology of the Reproductive
System, 534
Male Reproductive System, 534
Female Reproductive System, 535
Effects of Normal Aging on the Reproductive
System, 538
Human Sexuality, 538
Sexual Identity, 539
Taking a Sexual History, 540
Illness and Sexuality, 541
Laboratory and Diagnostic Examinations, 541
Diagnostic Tests for Women, 541
Diagnostic Tests for Men, 545
The Reproductive Cycle, 546
Menarche, 546
Disturbances of Menstruation, 546

Amenorrhea, 547
Dysmenorrhea, 547
Abnormal Uterine Bleeding (Menorrhagia and Metrorrhagia), 548
Premenstrual Syndrome, 550
Menopause, 551
Male Climacteric, 553
Erectile Dysfunction, 554
Infertility, 555
Inflammatory and Infectious Disorders of the Female Reproductive Tract, 556
Simple Vaginitis, 557
Senile Vaginitis or Atrophic Vaginitis, 557
Cervicitis, 558
Pelvic Inflammatory Disease, 558
Toxic Shock Syndrome, 559
Disorders of the Female Reproductive System, 560
Endometriosis, 560
Vaginal Fistula, 561
Relaxed Pelvic Muscles, 562
Leiomyomas of the Uterus, 563
Ovarian Cysts, 564
Cancer of the Female Reproductive Tract, 564
Cancer of the Cervix, 565
Cancer of the Endometrium, 567
Cancer of the Ovary, 567
Hysterectomy, 569
Vaginal Hysterectomy, 569
Abdominal Hysterectomy, 569
Disorders of the Female Breast, 570
Fibrocystic Breast Condition, 570
Acute Mastitis, 571
Chronic Mastitis, 571
Breast Cancer, 571
Inflammatory and Infectious Disorders of the Male Reproductive System, 583
Prostatitis, 583
Epididymitis, 584
Disorders of Male Genital Organs, 584
Phimosis and Paraphimosis, 584
Hydrocele, 585
Varicocele, 585
Cancer of the Male Reproductive Tract, 585
Cancer of the Testis (Testicular Cancer), 585
Cancer of the Penis, 586
Sexually Transmitted Infections, 586
Genital Herpes, 587
Syphilis, 588
Gonorrhea, 589
Trichomoniasis, 590
Candidiasis, 591
Chlamydia, 591
Acquired Immunodeficiency Syndrome, 592
Family Planning, 592
Nursing Process for the Patient with a Reproductive Disorder, 596

13 Care of the Patient with a Visual or Auditory Disorder, 601
Barbara Lauritsen Christensen
Anatomy and Physiology of the Sensory System, 602
Anatomy of the Eye, 602
Accessory Structures of the Eye, 602
Structure of the Eyeball, 602
Chambers of the Eye, 603
Physiology of Vision, 604
Anatomy and Physiology of the Ear, 604
External Ear, 604
Middle Ear, 604
Inner Ear, 605
Other Special Senses, 606
Taste and Smell, 606
Touch, 606
Position and Movement, 606
Normal Aging of the Sensory System, 606
Nursing Considerations for Care of the Patient with an Eye Disorder, 606
Laboratory and Diagnostic Examinations, 606
Disorders of the Eye, 607
Blindness and Near Blindness, 607
Refractory Errors, 610
Inflammatory and Infectious Disorders of the Eye, 613
Inflammation of the Cornea, 615
Noninfectious Disorders of the Eye, 615
Dry Eye Disorders, 615
Ectropion and Entropion, 616
Disorders of the Lens, 617
Disorders of the Retina, 618
Glaucoma, 623
Corneal Injuries, 627
Surgeries of the Eye, 629
Enucleation, 629
Keratoplasty (Corneal Transplant), 629
Photocoagulation, 630
Vitrectomy, 630
Nursing Considerations for Care of the Patient with an Ear Disorder, 631
Laboratory and Diagnostic Examinations, 631
Otoscopy, 631
Whispered Voice Test, 631
Tuning Fork Tests, 631
Disorders of the Ear, 633
Loss of Hearing (Deafness), 633
Inflammatory and Infectious Disorders of the Ear, 635
Noninfectious Disorders of the Ear, 640
Surgeries of the Ear, 644
Stapedectomy, 644
Tympanoplasty, 644
Myringotomy, 645
Cochlear Implant, 645
Nursing Process for the Patient with a Visual or Auditory Disorder, 645

14 Care of the Patient with a Neurologic Disorder, 650

Barbara Lauritsen Christensen

Anatomy and Physiology of the Neurologic System, 651
   Structural Divisions, 651
   Cells of the Nervous System, 651
   Central Nervous System, 652
   Peripheral Nervous System, 655
   Effects of Normal Aging on the Nervous System, 655
   Prevention of Neurologic Problems, 656
Assessment of the Neurologic System, 657
   History, 657
   Mental Status, 658
   Language and Speech, 659
   Cranial Nerves, 659
   Motor Function, 660
   Sensory and Perceptual Status, 661
Laboratory and Diagnostic Examinations, 661
   Blood and Urine Tests, 661
   Cerebrospinal Fluid, 661
   Other Tests, 662
Common Disorders of the Neurologic System, 665
   Headaches, 665
   Neuropathic Pain, 667
   Increased Intracranial Pressure, 668
   Disturbances in Muscle Tone and Motor Function, 672
   Disturbed Sensory and Perceptual Function, 675
Other Disorders of the Neurologic System, 676
   Conduction Abnormalities, 676
   Epilepsy or Seizures, 676
   Degenerative Diseases, 680
   Multiple Sclerosis, 680
   Parkinson's Disease, 683
   Alzheimer's Disease, 688
   Myasthenia Gravis, 690
   Amyotrophic Lateral Sclerosis, 693
   Huntington's Disease, 693
   Vascular Problems, 694
   Stroke, 694
   Cranial and Peripheral Nerve Disorders, 700
   Trigeminal Neuralgia, 700
   Bell's Palsy (Peripheral Facial Paralysis), 701
   Infection and Inflammation, 702
   Guillain-Barré Syndrome (Polyneuritis), 703
   Meningitis, 704
   Encephalitis, 705
   West Nile Virus, 705
   Brain Abscess, 706
   Acquired Immunodeficiency Syndrome, 706
   Brain Tumors, 707
   Trauma, 708
   Head Injury, 708

Spinal Cord Trauma, 710
Nursing Process for the Patient with a Neurologic Disorder, 713

15 Care of the Patient with an Immune Disorder, 719

Barbara Lauritsen Christensen

Nature of Immunity, 719
   Innate, or Natural, Immunity, 720
   Adaptive, or Acquired, Immunity, 720
   Humoral Immunity, 721
   Cellular Immunity, 722
Complement System, 722
Genetic Control of Immunity, 722
Effects of Normal Aging on the Immune System, 722
Immune Response, 723
Disorders of the Immune System, 724
   Hypersensitivity Disorders, 724
   Anaphylaxis, 726
   Latex Allergies, 728
   Transfusion Reactions, 729
   Delayed Hypersensitivity, 729
   Immunodeficiency Disorders, 730
   Primary Immunodeficiency Disorders, 730
   Secondary Immunodeficiency Disorders, 730
   Autoimmune Disorders, 730
   Plasmapheresis, 731

16 Care of the Patient with HIV/AIDS, 734

Craig E. Nielsen

Nursing and the History of HIV Disease, 734
   Significance of the Problem, 737
   Trends and Most Affected Populations, 737
Transmission of HIV, 738
   Sexual Transmission, 739
   Parenteral Exposure, 740
   Perinatal (Vertical) Transmission, 741
Pathophysiology, 742
   Influences on Viral Load and Disease Progression, 742
Spectrum of HIV Infection, 744
   Acute Retroviral Syndrome, 745
   Early Infection, 745
   Early Symptomatic Disease, 745
   AIDS, 746
Laboratory and Diagnostic Examinations, 747
   HIV Antibody Testing, 747
   CD_4^+ Cell Monitoring, 747
   Viral Load Monitoring, 747
   Resistance Testing, 749
   Other Laboratory Parameters, 749
Therapeutic Management, 749
   Pharmacologic Management, 749
Nursing Interventions, 757
   Adherence, 760

Palliative Care, 761
Psychosocial Issues, 762
Confidentiality, 763
Duty to Treat, 763
Ethical and Legal Principles, 763
Acute Intervention, 763
Prevention of HIV Infection, 769
HIV Testing and Counseling, 769
Risk Assessment and Risk Reduction, 771
Barriers to Prevention, 771
Reducing Risks Related to Sexual
Transmission, 771
Reducing Risks Related to Drug Abuse, 773
Reducing Risks Related to Occupational
Exposure, 773
Other Methods to Reduce Risk, 774
Outlook for the Future, 774

17 Care of the Patient with Cancer, 778

Barbara Lauritsen Christensen

Oncology, 778
Development, Prevention, and Detection of
Cancer, 780
Hereditary Cancers, 781
Genetic Susceptibility, 781
Cancer Risk Assessment and Genetic
Counseling, 781
Cancer Prevention and Early Detection, 781
Pathophysiology of Cancer, 785
Cell Mechanisms and Growth, 785
Description, Grading, and Staging
of Tumors, 785
Diagnosis of Cancer, 786
Biopsy, 786
Endoscopy, 787
Diagnostic Imaging, 787
Laboratory and Diagnostic Examinations, 788

Cancer Therapies, 789
Surgery, 789
Radiation Therapy, 790
Chemotherapy, 791
Biotherapy, 800
Bone Marrow Transplantation, 800
Peripheral Stem Cell Transplantation, 801
Nursing Interventions, 801
Advanced Cancer, 801
Pain Management, 801
Nutritional Therapy, 802
Communication and Psychological
Support, 802
Terminal Prognosis, 803

Appendixes

A **Common Abbreviations,** 808

B **The Joint Commission's Lists of Dangerous
Abbreviations, Acronyms, and Symbols,** 810

C **Laboratory Reference Values,** 811

D **Answers to Review Questions for the NCLEX®
Examination,** 820

References and Suggested Readings, R-1

Illustration Credits, IC-1

Glossary, G-1

Index, I-1

NANDA International-Approved Nursing
Diagnoses 2009–2011

Introduction to Anatomy and Physiology

Barbara Lauritsen Christensen and M. Christine Neff

http://evolve.elsevier.com/Christensen/adult/

Objectives

1. Define the difference between anatomy and physiology.
2. Define the term *anatomical position.*
3. List and define the principal directional terms and sections (planes) used in describing the body and the relationship of body parts to one another.
4. Use each word in a given list of anatomical terms in a sentence.
5. List the nine abdominopelvic regions and the abdominopelvic quadrants.
6. List and discuss in order of increasing complexity the levels of organization of the body.
7. Differentiate among tissues, organs, and systems.
8. Identify and define three major components of the cell.
9. Discuss the stages of mitosis and explain the importance of cellular reproduction.
10. Differentiate between active and passive transport processes that move substances through cell membranes, and give two examples of each.
11. Describe the four types of body tissues.
12. Discuss the two types of epithelial membranes.
13. List the 11 major organ systems of the body and briefly describe the major functions of each.

Key Terms

active transport (p. 8)
anatomy (p. 1)
cell (p. 4)
cytoplasm (CĪ-tō-plăzm, p. 6)
diffusion (dĬ-FŪ-zhŭn, p. 9)
dorsal (p. 1)
filtration (p. 9)
homeostasis (hō-mē-ō-STĀ-sĭs, p. 5)
membrane (p. 12)
mitosis (mĭ-TŌ-sĭs, p. 7)

nucleus (p. 6)
organ (pp. 5, 12)
osmosis (ŏz-MŌ-sĭs, p. 9)
passive transport (p. 9)
phagocytosis (făg-ŏ-sī-TŌ-sĭs, p. 8)
physiology (fĭz-ē-ŎL-ō-jē, p. 1)
pinocytosis (pī-nō-sī-TŌ-sĭs, p. 8)
system (p. 5)
tissue (p. 5)
ventral (p. 1)

Caring for a person with a disease process requires an understanding of the normal functioning of the human body, so the nurse must know basic human anatomy and physiology. **Anatomy** is the study, classification, and description of structures and organs of the body. **Physiology** explains the processes and functions of the various structures and how they interrelate. The normal, healthy human body is like a finely tuned machine, with each part performing a special function to accomplish a goal. As with the machine, when the body malfunctions, the repairer must understand how it works. Without the necessary repairs to return the body to homeostasis, illness, disease, or death may result.

ANATOMICAL TERMINOLOGY

Study of the human body first requires one to master certain terms that aid in locating specific structures. To understand the following terms, consider the body in a normal anatomical position, that is, standing erect with the face and palms facing forward (Figure 1-1):

Anterior (or **ventral**): To face forward; the front of the body. The chest is located anterior to the spine (Figure 1-2).

Posterior (or **dorsal**): Toward the back. The kidneys are posterior to the peritoneum.

Cranial: Toward the head. The brain is located in the cranial portion of the body.

Caudal: Toward the "tail"; the distal portion of the spine. A caudal anesthetic may be given.

Superior: Toward the head or above. The neck is superior to the shoulders.

Inferior: Lower, toward the feet, or below another. The foot is inferior to the ankle.

Medial: Toward the midline. The sternum (breastbone) is located in the medial portion of the chest.

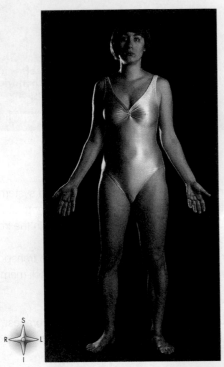

FIGURE 1-1 Anatomical position. The body is in an erect or standing posture with the arms at the sides and palms forward. The head and feet also point forward. The right and left sides of the body are mirror images of each other.

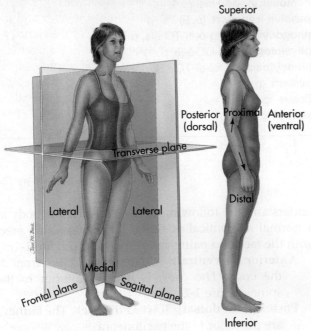

FIGURE 1-2 Directions and planes of the body.

Lateral: Toward the side. The outer area of the leg, the area located on the side, is called lateral.

Proximal: Nearest the origin of the structure; nearest the trunk. The elbow is proximal to the forearm.

Distal: Farthest from the origin of the structure; farthest from the trunk. The fingers are distal to the hand.

Superficial: Nearer the surface. The skin of the arm is superficial to the muscles below it.

Deep: Farther away from the body surface. The bone of the upper arm is deep to the muscles that surround and cover it.

BODY PLANES

To make it easier to study individual organs or the body as a whole, divide the body into three imaginary planes: the sagittal, the coronal (frontal), and the transverse (see Figure 1-2):

1. The **sagittal** plane runs lengthwise from the front to the back. A sagittal cut gives a right and a left portion of the body. A midsagittal cut gives two equal halves.
2. The **coronal** (frontal) plane divides the body into a ventral (front) section and a dorsal (back) section.
3. The **transverse** plane cuts the body horizontal to the sagittal and frontal planes, dividing the body into caudal and cranial portions.

BODY CAVITIES

From the outside, the body appears to be a solid structure, but it is not. It is made up of open spaces, or cavities, that contain compact, well-ordered arrangements of internal organs. The body has two major cavities that are, in turn, subdivided and contain compact, well-ordered arrangements of internal organs. The two major cavities are the ventral and the dorsal body cavities (Figure 1-3 and Table 1-1).

Ventral Cavity

The ventral cavity consists of the **thoracic** (or chest) cavity and the **abdominopelvic cavity** (see Figure 1-3), which are separated by the diaphragm (a muscle directly beneath the lungs).

The thoracic cavity contains the heart and the lungs. Its midportion is a subdivision of the thoracic cavity, the mediastinum, which contains the trachea, the heart, and the blood vessels. Its other subdivisions are the right and left pleural cavities, which contain the lungs.

The abdominal cavity contains the stomach, the liver, the gallbladder, the spleen, the pancreas, the small intestine, and parts of the large intestine. A subdivision called the **pelvic cavity** contains the lower portion of the large intestine (lower sigmoid colon, rectum), the urinary bladder, and the internal structures of the reproductive system. The abdominal and pelvic cavities are not separated by any structure and therefore are referred to as the abdominopelvic cavity (see Table 1-1).

Dorsal Cavity

The dorsal cavity is composed of the cranial and spinal body cavities. The cranial body cavity houses the brain, whereas the spinal cavity contains the spinal cord. The dorsal body cavity is smaller than the ventral cavity (see Table 1-1).

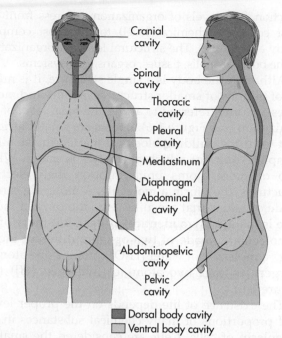

FIGURE 1-3 Location and subdivisions of the dorsal and ventral body cavities as viewed from the front (anterior) and the side (lateral).

Dorsal body cavity
Ventral body cavity

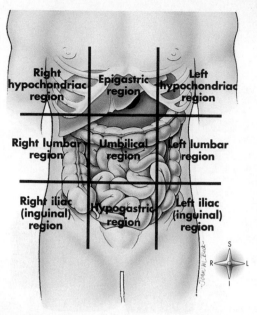

FIGURE 1-4 The nine regions of the abdominopelvic cavity. The most superficial organs are shown. Can you identify the deeper structures in each region?

Table 1-1	Body Cavities
BODY CAVITY	**ORGAN(S)**
VENTRAL BODY CAVITY	
Thoracic Cavity	
Mediastinum	Trachea, heart, blood vessels
Pleural cavities	Lungs
Abdominopelvic Cavity	
Abdominal cavity	Liver, gallbladder, stomach, spleen, pancreas, small intestine, parts of large intestine
Pelvic cavity	Lower (sigmoid) colon, rectum, urinary bladder, reproductive organs
DORSAL BODY CAVITY	
Cranial cavity	Brain
Spinal cavity	Spinal cord

ABDOMINAL REGIONS

For convenience in locating abdominal organs, anatomists divide the abdomen into nine imaginary regions. The nine regions (Figure 1-4), identified from right to left and from top to bottom, are the following:

1. Right hypochondriac region
2. Epigastric region
3. Left hypochondriac region
4. Right lumbar region
5. Umbilical region
6. Left lumbar region
7. Right iliac (inguinal) region
8. Hypogastric region
9. Left iliac (inguinal) region

The most superficial organs located in each of the nine abdominal regions are shown in Figure 1-4. The visible organs in each region are as follows: (1) right hypochondriac region, the right lobe of the liver and the gallbladder; (2) epigastric region, parts of the right and left lobes of the liver and a large portion of the stomach; (3) left hypochondriac region, a small portion of the stomach and large intestine; (4) right lumbar region, parts of the large and small intestine; (5) umbilical region, a portion of the transverse colon and loops of the small intestine; (6) left lumbar region, additional loops of the small intestine and a part of the colon; (7) right iliac region, the cecum and parts of the small intestine; (8) hypogastric region, loops of the small intestine, the urinary bladder, and the appendix; and (9) left iliac region, portions of the colon and the small intestine.

ABDOMINOPELVIC QUADRANTS

Health professionals frequently divide the abdomen into four quadrants to describe the site of abdominopelvic pain or locate an internal pathologic condition such as a tumor or abscess (Figure 1-5). Horizontal and vertical lines passing through the umbilicus (navel) divide the abdomen into **right** and **left upper quadrants** and **right** and **left lower quadrants**.

STRUCTURAL LEVELS OF ORGANIZATION

Before studying the structure and function of the human body and its many parts, think about how those parts are organized and how they might fit together into a functioning whole. Figure 1-6 illustrates the different levels of organization that influence body structure and

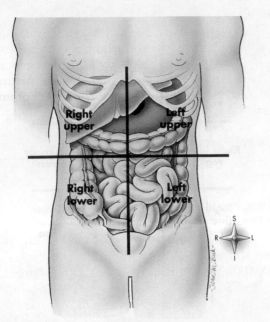

FIGURE 1-5 Horizontal and vertical line passing through the umbilicus (navel) divides the abdomen into right and left upper quadrants and right and left lower quadrants.

function. The levels of organization progress from the least complex (chemical level) to the most complex (body as a whole). The structural levels of organization in the body are cells, tissues, organs, and systems.

Although the body is a single structure, it is made up of billions of smaller structures. Atoms and molecules are often referred to as the chemical level of organization (see Figure 1-6). **Atoms** are small particles that form the building blocks of matter, the smallest complete units of which all matter is made. When two or more atoms unite through their electron structures, they form a **molecule.** A molecule can be made of atoms that are alike (e.g., the oxygen molecule is made of two identical atoms), but more often a molecule is made of two or more different atoms (e.g., a molecule of water [H_2O] contains one atom of oxygen [O] and two atoms of hydrogen [H]) (see Figure 1-6).

The existence of life depends on the proper levels and proportions of many chemical substances in the cytoplasm of cells. **Cells** are considered the smallest living units of structure and function in our body. Al-

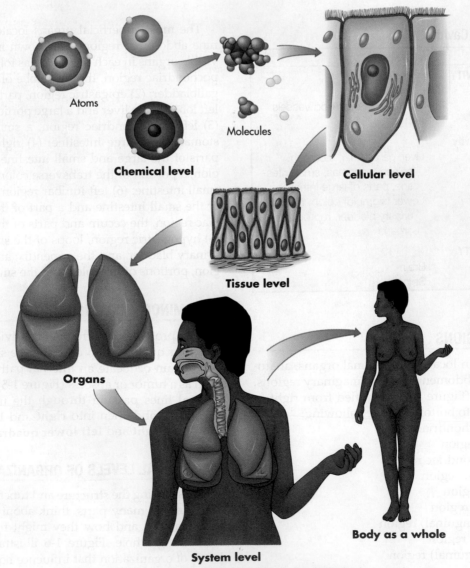

FIGURE 1-6 Structural levels of organization in the body.

Atoms

Chemical level

Molecules

Cellular level

Tissue level

Organs

System level

Body as a whole

though considered the simplest units of living matter, cells are far from simple; they are extremely complex.

Tissues are even more complex than cells. By definition a **tissue** is an organization of many similar cells that act together to perform a common function. Cells are held together and surrounded by varying amounts and types of gluelike, nonliving intercellular substances.

Organs are more complex than tissues. An **organ** is a group of several different kinds of tissues arranged to perform a special function. The lungs shown in Figure 1-6 are an example of organization at the organ level.

Systems are the most complex units that make up the body. A **system** is an organization of varying numbers and kinds of organs arranged to perform complex functions for the body. The organs of the respiratory system shown in Figure 1-6 permit air to enter the body and travel to the lungs, where oxygen and carbon dioxide are exchanged. Organs of the respiratory system include the nose, the windpipe (or trachea), and the complex series of bronchial tubes that permit passage of air into the lungs.

CELLS

Almost 350 years ago Robert Hooke discovered the first cell while examining plant fragments under the microscope. The structures reminded him of tiny, individual miniature prison cells, so he coined the term *cell* (the fundamental unit of all living tissue) (Figure 1-7). Many living things are so simple that they consist of just one cell. The human body, however, is so complex that it has trillions of these tiny powerhouses of life.

All cells are microscopic but differ widely in size and shape. Despite their differences, all cells exhibit five unique characteristics of life: growth, metabolism, responsiveness, reproduction, and homeostasis. **Homeostasis** is when the body's internal environment is relatively constant; this state is naturally maintained by adaptive responses that promote healthy survival.

Structural Parts of Cells

The three main parts of a cell are the plasma membrane, the cytoplasm, and the nucleus (see Figure 1-7).

Plasma Membrane

The plasma membrane encloses the cytoplasm and forms the outer boundary of the cell. It is an incredibly delicate structure—only about 7 nm (nanometers), or 3/10,000,000 inch, thick! Yet it has a precise, orderly structure.

Even though it seems fragile, the plasma membrane is strong enough to keep the cell whole and intact. It also performs other life-preserving functions for the cell, serving as a gateway between the fluid inside the cell and the fluid around it. The plasma membrane is **selectively permeable.** This means the membrane permits certain substances to enter and leave while not allowing other substances to cross. This membrane separates the cell contents from the dilute saltwater solution called interstitial fluid, or simply tissue fluid, which bathes every cell in the body. The plasma membrane also has distinct surface proteins that identify a cell as coming from one particular individual. This fact is the basis of **tissue typing,** a procedure performed before an organ from one person is transplanted into another. Carbohydrate chains attached to the surface of cells often help identify cell types.

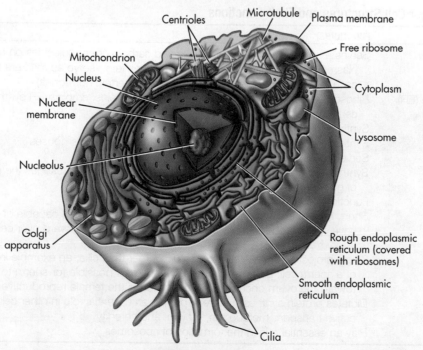

FIGURE 1-7 A typical cell.

Cytoplasm

Cytoplasm is the internal living material of cells. Cytoplasm (protoplasm) is a sticky, fluidlike substance that lies between the plasma membrane and the nucleus of the cell. Numerous organelles (tiny functioning structures) are located within the cytoplasm. Cells contain cytoplasm, or "living matter," a substance that exists only in cells. Cytoplasm is composed largely of a gel-like substance that contains water, food, minerals, enzymes, and other specialized materials. The term *cyto-* is a combining form from the Greek and denotes a relationship to a cell. These organelles were not discovered until the development of the powerful electron microscope.

Cytoplasm is composed of 70% water with traces of proteins, lipids, carbohydrates, minerals, and salts. (Table 1-2 lists major cell structures and their functions.)

Nucleus

The **nucleus** is the largest organelle within the cell. It is responsible for cell reproduction and control of the other organelles. The nucleus is surrounded by the nuclear membrane. It contains nucleoplasm, a refined form of cytoplasm. The nucleus contains two specialized structures: the nucleolus and the chromatin granules. The nucleolus is critical in the formation of protein. The chromatin granules are composed of protein and deoxyribonucleic acid (DNA). DNA contains the genetic code, or blueprint, of the body.

Endoplasmic Reticulum

Throughout the cytoplasm lies a system of membranes, or canals, called the endoplasmic reticulum (ER). ER functions as a miniature circulating system for the cell by carrying substances from one part of the cell to another.

There are two types of ER: (1) smooth, which is found in cells that deal with fatty substances; and (2) rough, which is found in cells that manufacture proteins.

Ribosomes

Ribosomes are tiny structures floating free in the cytoplasm or attached to the rough ER. They are called **protein factories** because they produce enzymes and other proteins.

Mitochondria

The mitochondria are the powerhouses of the cells. They are bean shaped with a folded interior membrane. They take food and convert it to a complex energy form, adenosine triphosphate (ATP), for use by the cell. ATP is described as the "energy currency" of the cells because it supplies the energy for all activities.

Lysosomes

Lysosomes are small saclike structures containing enzymes that digest food compounds and microbes that have invaded the cell.

Golgi Apparatus

The Golgi apparatus is usually located near the nucleus. It is the "packaging plant" of the cell. It packages certain carbohydrate and protein compounds into globules. Then it moves outward through the cell membrane, where it breaks open and releases its contents.

Centrioles

The centrioles are paired, rod-shaped organelles. During cell division (mitosis) they aid in the formation of the spindle, a structure necessary for cell reproduction.

Table 1-2	Some Major Cell Structures and Their Functions

CELL STRUCTURE	FUNCTION(S)
Plasma membrane	Serves as the cell's boundary; protein and carbohydrate molecules on outer surface of plasma membrane perform various functions (e.g., serve as markers that identify cells of each individual or as receptor molecules for certain hormones)
Endoplasmic reticulum (ER)	Ribosomes attach to rough ER to synthesize proteins; smooth ER synthesizes lipids and certain carbohydrates
Ribosomes	Synthesize proteins; the cell's "protein factories"
Mitochondria	Synthesize adenosine triphosphate (ATP); the cell's "powerhouses"
Lysosomes	Serve as cell's "digestive system"
Golgi apparatus	Synthesizes carbohydrate, combines it with protein, and packages the product as globules of glycoprotein
Centrioles	Function in cell reproduction
Cilia	Short, hairlike extensions on the free surfaces of some cells capable of movement; often have specialized functions such as propelling mucus upward over cells that line the respiratory tract
Flagella	Single projections of cell surfaces, much larger than cilia; an example in humans is the "tail" of a sperm cell; propulsive movement makes it possible for sperm to "swim" or move toward the ovum once they are deposited in the female reproductive tract
Nucleus	Dictates protein synthesis, thereby playing an essential role in other cell activities, namely, active transport, metabolism, growth, and heredity
Nucleoli	Play an essential role in the formation of ribosomes

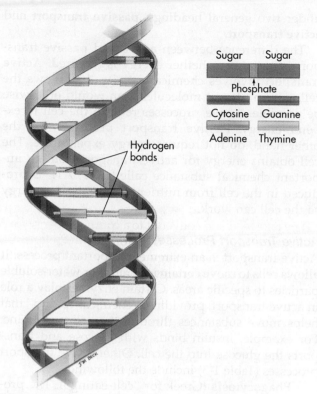

FIGURE 1-8 Deoxyribonucleic acid (DNA) molecule. Note that each side of the DNA molecule consists of alternating sugar and phosphate groups. Each sugar group is united to the sugar group opposite it by a pair of nitrogenous bases (adenine-thymine or cytosine-guanine). The sequence of these pairs constitutes a genetic code that determines the structure and function of a cell.

Protein Synthesis

Protein is a vital component of every cell in the body. Protein production relies on nucleic acids in the cell's cytoplasm and nucleus. Two important nucleic acids are (1) DNA (Figure 1-8), which is located in the nucleus; and (2) ribonucleic acid (RNA), which is located in the cytoplasm. The DNA encodes the message for protein synthesis and sends it to the RNA, which transports it to the ribosomes, where the protein is produced. Hence DNA is called the **chemical blueprint**, and RNA is called the **chemical messenger.**

Cell Division

All cells in the body, except sex cells, reproduce by mitosis. This is a type of somatic (pertaining to nonreproductive cells) cell division in which the original cell divides to form two daughters. Each daughter cell has the same characteristics (including both the nucleus and cytoplasm) as the original cell. Each daughter cell contains the same number of chromosomes as the parent cell. Each chromosome in the daughter cells contains the complete genetic information of the original chromosome because of duplication of the DNA molecule during interphase (Figure 1-9).

The chromosomes (spindle-shaped rods) in the cell's nucleus carry the genes that are responsible for the organism's traits, including such hereditary factors as hair and eye color. These chromosomes are composed of DNA. Each body cell in humans contains

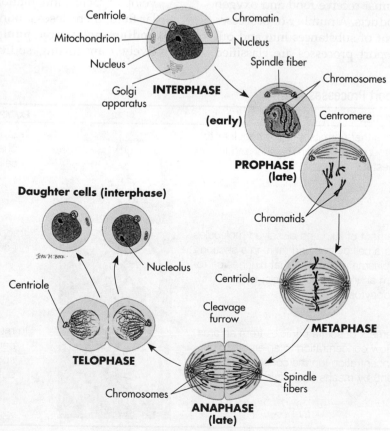

FIGURE 1-9 Mitosis.

46 chromosomes, which exist in pairs. At the time of fertilization, one member of each pair is received from the father and one is received from the mother. These paired chromosomes, except for the pair that determines sex, are alike in size and appearance and carry genes for the same traits.

During mitosis the cell goes through four phases: prophase, metaphase, anaphase, and telophase.

Prophase
In the nucleus the chromosomes form two strands called **chromatids.** In the cytoplasm the centrioles form a network of spindle fibers.

Metaphase
The nuclear membrane and nucleolus disappear, and the chromosomes are aligned across the center of the cell. The centrioles are at the opposite ends of the cell, and spindle fibers are attached to each chromatid.

Anaphase
The chromosomes are pulled to the opposite ends of the cell, and cell division begins.

Telophase
During this final phase of cell division, the two nuclei appear and the chromosomes disperse. At the end of the phase, two new daughter cells appear.

Movement of Materials Across Cell Membranes
For a cell to survive, it must receive food and oxygen and secrete its waste products. A number of processes allow for mass movement of substances into and out of the cells. These transport processes are classified under two general headings: **passive transport** and **active transport.**

The difference between active and passive transport is based on whether energy is required. **Active transport** involves chemical activity that allows the cell to admit larger molecules than would otherwise be possible. Active processes require the cell to expend energy. Passive transport processes, on the other hand, do not require energy expenditure. The cell obtains energy for active transport from an important chemical substance called ATP. ATP is produced in the cell from nutrients and releases energy so the cell can work.

Active Transport Processes
Active transport is an extremely important process. It allows cells to move certain ions or other water-soluble particles to specific areas. Certain enzymes play a role in active transport, providing a chemical "pump" that helps move substances through the cell membrane. For example, insulin binds with glucose and transports the glucose into the cell. Other active transport processes (Table 1-3) include the following:

- **Phagocytosis** (Greek for "cell-eating"): The process that permits a cell to engulf (or surround) any foreign material and to digest it. The white blood cells in the human body often perform this function.
- **Pinocytosis:** The process by which extracellular fluid is taken into the cell. The cell membrane develops a saclike indentation filled with extracellular fluid, then closes around it and digests it.
- **Sodium-potassium pump:** The process of actively transporting sodium ions (Na^+) out of

Table 1-3 Active Transport Processes

PROCESS	DESCRIPTION		EXAMPLES
Phagocytosis	Process that permits a cell to engulf or to surround any foreign material and to digest it		Trapping of bacterial cells by phagocytic white blood cells
Pinocytosis	Movement of fluid and dissolved molecules into a cell by trapping them in a section of plasma membrane that pinches off to form an intracellular vesicle; type of endocytosis		Trapping of large protein molecules by some body cell
Calcium pump	Movement of solute particles from an area of low concentration to an area of high concentration (up the concentration gradient) by means of a carrier molecule		In muscle cells, pumping of nearly all calcium ions to special compartments or out of the cell

Modified from Thibodeau, G.A., & Patton, K.T. (2007). *Anatomy and physiology* (6th ed.). St. Louis: Mosby.
ATP, Adenosine triphosphate. The energy required for active transport processes is obtained from ATP. ATP is in all active transport processes.

cells and potassium ions (K⁺) into cells. The sodium-potassium pump maintains a lower sodium concentration in intracellular fluid than in the surrounding extracellular fluid. At the same time, this pump maintains a higher potassium concentration in the intracellular fluid than in the surrounding extracellular fluid. This active transport pump operates in the plasma membrane of all human cells and is essential for healthy cell survival.

- **Calcium pump:** Active calcium carriers in the membranes of muscle cells (for example) that allow the cell to force nearly all of the intracellular calcium ions (Ca⁺⁺) into special compartments or out of the cell entirely. This is important because a muscle cell cannot operate properly unless the intracellular Ca⁺⁺ concentration is kept low during rest.

Active transport processes require cellular energy to move substances from a low concentration to a high concentration. In contrast, **passive transport** processes—the movement of small molecules across the membrane of a cell by diffusion—do not require cellular energy and move substances from a high concentration to a lower concentration.

Passive Transport Processes

The primary passive transport processes (Table 1-4) include the following:

- **Diffusion:** A process in which solid particles in a fluid move from an area of higher concentration to an area of lower concentration, resulting in an even distribution of the particles in the fluid (Figure 1-10).

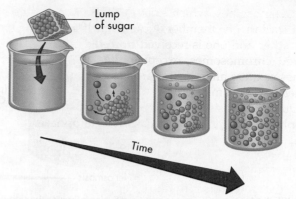

FIGURE 1-10 Diffusion. The molecules of a lump of sugar are very densely packed when they enter the water. As sugar molecules collide frequently in the area of high concentration, they gradually spread away from each other toward the area of lower concentration. Eventually the sugar molecules are evenly distributed.

- **Osmosis:** The passage of water across a selectively permeable membrane, with the water molecules going from the less concentrated solution to the more concentrated solution (Figure 1-11).
- **Filtration:** The movement of water and particles through a membrane by force from either pressure or gravity. This membrane contains spaces that allow liquid to pass but are too small to be permeated by solid particles. Movement is from areas of greater pressure to areas of lesser pressure.

TISSUES

Tissues are groups of similar cells that work together to perform a specific function. The body and its organs are composed of the following four main types of tissues (Table 1-5).

Table 1-4 Passive Transport Processes

PROCESS	DESCRIPTION		EXAMPLES
Simple diffusion	Movement of particles through phospholipid bilayer or through channels from an area of high concentration to an area of low concentration—that is, down the concentration gradient		Movement of carbon dioxide out of all cells; movement of sodium ions into nerve cells as they conduct an impulse
Filtration	Movement of water and particles through a membrane by force from either pressure or gravity; membrane contains spaces that allow liquid to pass but are too small to be permeated by solid material; movement from areas of greater pressure to areas of lesser pressure		During procedure called peritoneal dialysis, small solutes diffuse from blood vessels but blood proteins do not (thus removing only small solutes from the blood)
Osmosis	Passage of water across a selectively permeable membrane; water molecules move from a less concentrated solution to a more concentrated solution		Diffusion of water molecules into and out of cells to correct imbalances in water concentration

Modified from Thibodeau, G.A., & Patton, K.T. (2007). *Anatomy and physiology* (6th ed.). St. Louis: Mosby.

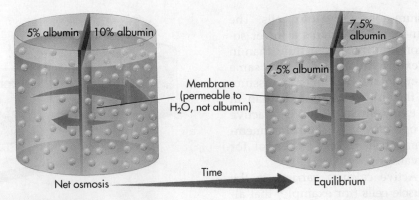

FIGURE 1-11 Osmosis. Osmosis is the diffusion of water through a selectively permeable membrane. The membrane shown in this diagram is permeable to water but not to albumin. Because there are relatively more water molecules in 5% albumin than in 10% albumin, more water molecules osmose from the more dilute into the more concentrated solution (as indicated by the *large arrow* in the diagram on the left) than osmose in the opposite direction. The overall direction of osmosis, in other words, is toward the more concentrated solution. Movement across the membrane continues until the concentrations of the solutions equalize.

Table 1-5   Tissues

TISSUE	LOCATION	FUNCTION
EPITHELIAL		
Simple squamous	Alveoli of lungs	Absorption by diffusion of respiratory gases between alveolar air and blood
	Lining of blood and lymphatic vessels	Absorption by diffusion, filtration, and osmosis
Stratified squamous	Surface of lining of mouth and esophagus	Protection
	Surface of skin (epidermis)	Protection
Simple columnar	Surface layer of lining of stomach, intestines, and parts of respiratory tract	Protection; secretion; absorption
Stratified transitional	Urinary bladder	Protection
CONNECTIVE*		
Areolar	Between other tissues and organs	Connection
Adipose (fat)	Under skin	Protection
	Padding at various points	Insulation; support; reserve food
Dense fibrous	Tendons; ligaments	Flexible but strong connection
Bone	Skeleton	Support; protection
Cartilage	Part of nasal septum; covering articular surfaces of bones; larynx; rings in trachea and bronchi	Firm but flexible support
	Disks between vertebrae	
	External ear	
Blood	Blood vessels	Transportation
Hematopoietic	Liquid matrix with dense arrangement of blood cell–producing cells located in red bone marrow	Blood cell formation
MUSCLE		
Skeletal (striated voluntary); see Figure 1-12, *A*	Muscles that attach to bones	Maintenance of posture, movement of bones
	Eyeball muscles	Eye movements
	Upper third of esophagus	First part of swallowing
Cardiac (striated involuntary); see Figure 1-12, *B*	Wall of heart	Contraction of heart
Smooth (nonstriated involuntary or visceral); see Figure 1-12, *C*	In walls of tubular viscera of digestive, respiratory, and genitourinary tracts	Movement of substances along respective tracts
	In walls of blood vessels and large lymphatic vessels	Changing diameter of blood vessels
	In ducts of glands	Movement of substances along ducts
	Intrinsic eye muscles (iris and ciliary body)	Changing diameter of pupils and shape of lens
	Arrector of muscles of hairs	Erection of hairs (gooseflesh)
NERVOUS	Brain; spinal cord; nerves	Irritability; conduction

*Connective tissues are the most widely distributed of all tissues.

1. Epithelial tissue
2. Connective tissue
3. Muscle tissue
4. Nervous tissue

Epithelial Tissue

Epithelial cells are packed closely together and contain no blood vessels. Epithelial tissue covers the outside of the body and some of the internal structures. The four types of epithelial tissue are (1) simple squamous, (2) stratified squamous, (3) simple columnar, and (4) stratified transitional (see Table 1-5).

Epithelial tissue serves several important functions in the body, including the following:

- **Protection:** Covering the body and many of its organs, it serves as a protective barrier against invasion.
- **Absorption:** Certain specialized epithelial cells can absorb material in the body (e.g., the lining of the small intestine can absorb digested nutrients).
- **Secretion:** Mucus is secreted in areas such as the respiratory and digestive tracts.

Connective Tissue

As the name suggests, connective tissue "connects," or joins, tissues or structures of the body, and it also supports and protects them. Connective tissue is the most abundant and widely distributed tissue in the body. It exists in varying forms: thin and delicate, tough and cordlike, or liquid (blood). Mast cells, plasma cells, and white blood cells are found in connective tissue; red blood cells are not unless blood vessels have been injured. Unlike the closely packed epithelial tissue, the connective tissue cells are spaced out and surrounded by intercellular fluid, which is composed of protein complexes and tissue fluid.

Some of the most important forms of connective tissue are **areolar** connective tissue, **adipose** (fat) tissue,

fibrous connective tissue, **bone, cartilage, blood,** and **hematopoietic** tissue (see Table 1-5).

Muscle Tissue

Muscle tissue is composed of cells that contract in response to a message from the brain or the spinal cord. The three types of muscle cells are (1) **skeletal** (striated, voluntary), (2) **cardiac** (striated, involuntary), and (3) **visceral** (smooth, involuntary) (Figure 1-12).

Skeletal muscle cells are striated (have a striped appearance) and attach to bones to produce voluntary movement. Skeletal muscle is also known as **voluntary muscle** because a person has voluntary control over skeletal muscle contractions (see Figure 1-12, *A*).

Cardiac muscle cells are striated with fibers that branch to form many networks, or webs. These networks are found only in the walls of the heart, and the regular contractions of cardiac muscle produce the heartbeat. Generally, cardiac muscle cells are involuntary, that is, a person cannot contract them at will (see Figure 1-2, *B*).

Smooth (visceral) muscle cells are nonstriated and appear in the viscera, or internal organs, such as the walls of blood vessels, the stomach, the intestines, and the uterus. Contractions of smooth muscle propel food and fluid through the digestive tract and help regulate the diameter of blood vessels. Contraction of smooth muscle in the tubes of the respiratory system, such as the bronchioles in the lungs, can impair breathing and result in asthma attacks and labored respiration. Generally, smooth muscles are involuntary, but some control can be exerted through the use of biofeedback techniques (see Figure 1-12, *C*).

Nervous Tissue

Nervous tissue allows rapid communication between the brain or spinal cord body structures and control of body functions. Nervous tissue is composed of two

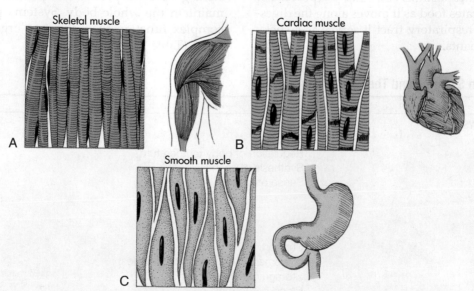

FIGURE 1-12 Types of muscles. **A,** Skeletal muscle. **B,** Cardiac muscle. **C,** Smooth muscle.

types of cells: neurons and glial cells. The neurons are the nerve cells and transmit impulses or messages. They are the system's functional or conducting units. The glial cells are connecting and supporting cells; they support and nourish the neurons.

Neurons have three parts: (1) dendrites, which carry impulses toward the cell body; (2) cell body; and (3) axons, which carry impulses away from the cell body (see Chapter 14, Figure 14-1).

MEMBRANES

Membranes are thin sheets of tissue that serve many functions in the body. They cover body surfaces, line and lubricate hollow organs, and protect and anchor organs and bones. The two major types of membranes are epithelial and connective tissue membranes.

Epithelial Membranes

Epithelial membranes are usually composed of a thin layer of epithelial cells with an underlying layer of connective tissue for strength. Epithelial membranes are divided into two subgroups: mucous membranes and serous membranes.

Mucous Membranes

Mucous membranes secrete **mucus** (a thick, slippery material), which keeps the membranes moist and soft and protects against bacterial invasion. Mucous membranes line the body surfaces that open to the outside environment. Examples include the nose; the mouth; and urinary, respiratory, gastrointestinal, and reproductive tracts. The type of epithelium in the mucous membrane varies, depending on its location and function. The esophagus, for example, contains a tough, abrasion-resistant, stratified squamous epithelium. A thin layer of simple columnar epithelium covers the walls of the lower segments of the digestive tract.

In addition to protection, the mucus produced by mucous membranes also serves other purposes. For example, it lubricates food as it moves along the digestive tract. In the respiratory tract it serves as a sticky trap for contaminants.

Serous Membranes

Serous membranes secrete a thin, watery fluid that prevents friction when organs rub against one another. These membranes line the body surfaces that do not open to the outside environment. Examples include the lungs (pleura), the intestines (peritoneum), and the heart (pericardium). Like epithelial membranes, serous membranes are composed of two distinct layers of tissue: (1) the epithelial sheet, a thin layer of simple squamous epithelium; and (2) the connective tissue layer, a very thin sheet that holds and supports the epithelial cells.

The serous membrane that lines body cavities and covers the surfaces of organs in those cavities is really a single, continuous sheet covering two different surfaces. The **parietal** membrane lines the wall of the cavity like wallpaper; the **visceral** membrane covers the surface of the viscera (organs within the cavity).

Connective Tissue Membranes (Synovial Membranes)

Connective tissue (or synovial) membranes are smooth and slick and secrete **synovial fluid** (a thick, colorless lubricating fluid). Synovial membranes line the joint spaces and prevent friction between the ends of the bones, thus allowing free movement of the joints. Synovial membranes also line small, cushionlike sacs called **bursae,** which are found between some moving body parts. Unlike serous and mucous membranes, connective tissue membranes do not contain epithelial components.

ORGANS AND SYSTEMS

When several kinds of tissues are united to perform a more complex function than any tissue alone, they are called **organs.** Examples are the heart, stomach, and kidneys. These organs working together for the same general purpose make up organ systems, which maintain the whole body. Systems perform a more complex function than any one organ can perform alone (Table 1-6).

Table 1-6   Organ Systems and Their Functions

STRUCTURE	FUNCTION
INTEGUMENTARY SYSTEM	
Skin	Protection
Hair	Regulation of body temperature
Nails	Synthesis of chemicals
Sense receptors	Sense organ
Sweat glands	
Oil glands	
SKELETAL SYSTEM	
Bones	Support
Joints	Movement (with joints and muscles)
	Storage of minerals
	Blood cell formation

Table 1-6	Organ Systems and Their Functions—cont'd
STRUCTURE	**FUNCTION**
MUSCULAR SYSTEM	
Voluntary or striated muscles	Movement
Involuntary or smooth muscles	Maintenance of body posture
	Production of heat
NERVOUS SYSTEM	
Brain	Contains body's control center
Spinal cord	Responsible for all the coordination of body's activities
Nerves	Communication
Sense organs	Integration
	Control
	Recognition of sensory stimuli
	System functions by production of nerve impulses caused by stimuli of various types
	Control is fast acting and of short duration
ENDOCRINE SYSTEM	
Pituitary gland	Secretion of special substances (hormones) directly into the blood
Pineal gland	Same as nervous system—communication, integration, control
Hypothalamus	Control is slow and of long duration
Thyroid gland	Examples of hormone regulation: growth, metabolism, reproduction, and
Parathyroid glands	fluid and electrolyte balance
Thymus gland	
Adrenal glands	
Pancreas	
Ovaries (female)	
Testes (male)	
CARDIOVASCULAR (CIRCULATORY) SYSTEM	
Heart	Transportation for nutrition, water, oxygen, and wastes
Blood vessels	Regulation of body temperature
	Immunity (body defense)
LYMPHATIC SYSTEM	
Lymph nodes	Protection
Lymphatic vessels	Maintains body's internal fluid environment by producing, filtering and conveying lymph
Thymus	
Spleen	Production of various blood cellsTransportation
Tonsils	
RESPIRATORY SYSTEM	
Nose	Exchange of waste gas (carbon dioxide) for oxygen in the lungs
Pharynx	Area of gas exchange in the lungs called alveoli
Larynx	Filtration of irritants from inspired air
Trachea	Regulation of acid-base balance
Bronchi	
Lungs	
DIGESTIVE SYSTEM	
Primary Organs	
Mouth	Mechanical and chemical breakdown (digestion) of food
Pharynx	Absorption of nutrients
Esophagus	Undigested waste product that is eliminated is called **feces**
Stomach	
Small intestine (duodenum, jejunum, ileum)	
Large intestine (ascending, transverse, descending, sigmoid)	
Rectum	
Anal canal	

Continued

Table 1-6	Organ Systems and Their Functions—cont'd	
STRUCTURE	**FUNCTION**
DIGESTIVE SYSTEM—cont'd	
Accessory Organs	
Teeth	
Salivary glands	
Tongue	
Liver	
Gallbladder	
Pancreas	
Appendix	Appendix is a structural but not a functional part of digestive system
URINARY SYSTEM	
Kidneys	Clearing or cleaning blood of waste products; waste product excreted from body is called **urine**
Ureters	
Urinary bladder	Electrolyte balance
Urethra	Water balance
	Acid-base balance
	Urethra has urinary and reproductive functions (in male)
REPRODUCTIVE SYSTEM	
Male	
Gonads (testes)	Survival of species
Genital ducts (epididymis, vas deferens, ejaculatory duct, urethra)	Production of sex cells (male are sperm; female are ova)
	Transfer and fertilization of sex cells
Accessory glands (prostate, seminal vesicles, Cowper's glands)	Development and birth of offspring
	Nourishment of offspring
Supporting structures (penis, scrotum)	Production of sex hormones
Female	
Gonads (ovaries)	
Accessory organs (uterus, fallopian tubes [oviducts], vagina)	
External genitalia (vulva)	
Mons pubis	
Labia majora	
Labia minora	
Clitoris	
Accessory glands	
Skene's glands	
Bartholin's glands	
Mammary glands (breasts)	

Get Ready for the NCLEX® Examination!

Key Points

- Anatomy is the study, classification, and description of structures and organs of the body. Physiology explains the function of the various structures and how they interrelate.
- The normal anatomical position of the body is standing erect with the face and the palms of the hands forward.
- For the purposes of study, the body is divided into three imaginary planes: sagittal, coronal (frontal), and transverse.
- The body is divided into two large groups of cavities: the dorsal and the ventral. The dorsal cavity contains the cranial and spinal cavities. The ventral cavity contains the thoracic, abdominal, and pelvic cavities.
- For the purposes of study, the abdominal region is divided into nine regions: right hypochondriac region, epigastric region, left hypochondriac region, right lumbar region, umbilical region, left lumbar region, right inguinal region, hypogastric region, and left inguinal region.
- The cell's major structures are the cytoplasm, nucleus, ER, ribosomes, mitochondria, lysosomes, Golgi apparatus, and centrioles.
- Organization is a fundamental characteristic of body structure.
- Cells are considered to be the smallest living units of structure and function in the body. Although long recognized as the simplest units of living matter, cells are extremely complex.
- Tissues are groups of similar cells that work together to perform a specific function.
- Organs are structures made up of two or more kinds of tissues organized so they can perform a more complex function than they could alone.

- Systems are groups of organs arranged so they can perform a more complex function than they could alone.
- To receive nutrition and oxygen and to rid itself of wastes, the cell performs passive transport (diffusion, osmosis, filtration) and active transport (phagocytosis and pinocytosis).
- The body is composed of four main types of tissues: epithelial, connective, muscle, and nervous tissues.
- The major systems of the body are integumentary, skeletal, muscular, nervous, endocrine, cardiovascular (circulatory), lymphatic, respiratory, digestive, urinary, and reproductive.

Additional Learning Resources

 Go to your Companion CD for an audio glossary, animations, video clips, and more.

evolve Be sure to visit the Evolve site at http://evolve.elsevier.com/Christensen/adult/ for additional online resources.

Review Questions for the NCLEX-PN® Examination

1. The anatomical term that refers to the distal portion of the spine is:
   1. medial.
   2. caudal.
   3. proximal.
   4. dorsal.

2. The trachea, the heart, the blood vessels, and the lungs are located in which body cavity? ·
   1. Dorsal
   2. Abdominopelvic
   3. Ventral
   4. Pelvic

3. A relative constant state in the body's internal environment naturally maintained by adaptive responses that promote healthy survival is called:
   1. homeostasis.
   2. mitosis.
   3. lysosomes.
   4. protein synthesis.

4. A process in which solid particles in a fluid move from an area of greater concentration to an area of lesser concentration, resulting in an even distribution of the particles in the fluid, is called:
   1. phagocytosis.
   2. pinocytosis.
   3. osmosis.
   4. diffusion.

5. The movement of materials across the membrane of a cell by means of chemical activity requiring the expenditure of energy by the cell is called:
   1. passive passport.
   2. active transport.
   3. telophase.
   4. transcription.

6. What type of tissue is composed of cells that contract in response to a message from the brain or spinal cord?
   1. Epithelial
   2. Connective
   3. Membrane
   4. Muscle

7. The thin sheets of tissue that secrete mucus and line the body surfaces that open to the outside environment are:
   1. mucous membranes.
   2. serous membranes.
   3. striated, involuntary.
   4. visceral, involuntary.

8. An active transport process that permits a cell to engulf or surround foreign material and digest it is called:
   1. mitosis.
   2. pinocytosis.
   3. phagocytosis.
   4. filtration.

9. A type of cell division of somatic cells in which each daughter cell contains the same number of chromosomes as the parent cell is called:
   1. flagella.
   2. mitosis.
   3. ER synthesis.
   4. mitochondria.

10. A group of several different kinds of tissues arranged so they can perform a special function together is called:
    1. cells.
    2. organ.
    3. tissue.
    4. system.

11. Groups of similar cells that work together to perform a specific function are called:
    1. cells.
    2. organ.
    3. tissue.
    4. system.

12. The hypogastric region of the abdominopelvic cavity is:
    1. inferior to the umbilical region.
    2. lateral to the left iliac region.
    3. medial to the right iliac region.
    4. both 1 and 3.

13. The two major cavities of the body are the:
    1. thoracic and abdominal.
    2. abdominal and pelvic.
    3. dorsal and ventral.
    4. anterior and posterior.

14. The structure that divides the thoracic cavity from the abdominal cavity is the:
    1. mediastinum.
    2. diaphragm.
    3. lungs.
    4. stomach.

Matching

Match the directional terms in Column B with its *opposite* term in Column A.

Column A

15. _____ Superior
16. _____ Distal
17. _____ Anterior
18. _____ Lateral
19. _____ Deep

Column B

a. posterior
b. superficial
c. medial
d. proximal
e. inferior

Match the function in Column B with the correct system in Column A.

Column A

20. _____ Integumentary
21. _____ Skeletal
22. _____ Muscular
23. _____ Nervous
24. _____ Endocrine
25. _____ Cardiovascular
26. _____ Lymphatic
27. _____ Respiratory
28. _____ Digestive
29. _____ Urinary
30. _____ Reproductive

Column B

a. Provides movement, body posture, and heat
b. Uses hormones to regulate body functions
c. Transports fatty nutrients from the digestive system to the blood
d. Makes physical and chemical change in nutrients and absorbs nutrients
e. Cleans the blood of metabolic wastes and regulates electrolyte balance
f. Protects underlying structures, provides for sensory reception, and regulates body temperature
g. Transports substances from one part of the body to another
h. Ensures the survival of the species rather than the individual
i. Uses electrochemical signals to integrate and control body functions
j. Exchanges oxygen and carbon dioxide and regulates acid-base balance
k. Provides a rigid framework for the body and stores minerals

Care of the Surgical Patient

Elaine Oden Kockrow and Barbara Lauritsen Christensen

http://evolve.elsevier.com/Christensen/adult/

Objectives

1. Identify the purposes of surgery.
2. Distinguish among elective, urgent, and emergency surgery.
3. Explain the concept of perioperative nursing.
4. Discuss the factors that influence an individual's ability to tolerate surgery.
5. Discuss considerations for the older adult surgical patient.
6. Describe the preoperative checklist.
7. Explain the importance of informed consent for surgery.
8. Explain the procedure for turning, deep breathing, coughing, and leg exercises for postoperative patients.
9. Differentiate among general, regional, and local anesthesia.
10. Explain conscious sedation.
11. Describe the role of the circulating nurse and the scrub nurse during surgery.
12. Discuss the initial nursing assessment and management immediately after transfer from the postanesthesia care unit.
13. Identify the rationale for nursing interventions designed to prevent postoperative complications.
14. List the assessment data for the surgical patient.
15. Identify the information needed for the postoperative patient in preparation for discharge.
16. Discuss the nursing process as it pertains to the surgical patient.

Key Terms

ablation (ăb-LĀ-shŭn, p. 18)
anesthesia (ăn-ĕs-THĒ-zē-ă, p. 37)
atelectasis (ă-tĕ-LĔK-tā-sĭs, p. 49)
cachexia (kă-KĔK-sē-ă, p. 48)
catabolism (kă-TĂB-ō-lĭsm, p. 52)
conscious sedation (sĕ-DĀ-shŭn, p. 40)
dehiscence (dē-HĬS-ĕns, p. 48)
drainage (p. 45)
embolus (ĔM-bō-lŭs, p. 33)
evisceration (ĕ-vĭs-ĕr-Ā-shŭn, p. 48)
extubate (ĕks-TŪ-bāt, p. 45)
exudate (ĔKS-ū-dāt, p. 45)
incentive spirometry (ĭn-SĔN-tĭv spĭ-RŎM-ĕ-trē, p. 28)
incisions (ĭn-SĬZH-ŭn, p. 35)

infarct (ĬN-fährkt, p. 33)
informed consent (p. 24)
intraoperative (ĭn-tră-ŎP-ĕr-ă-tĭv, p. 18)
palliative (PĂL-ē-ă-tĭv, p. 18)
paralytic ileus (păr-ă-LĬT-ĭk ĬL-ē-ŭs, p. 52)
perioperative (pĕr-ē-ŎP-ĕr-ă-tĭv, p. 18)
postoperative (pōst-ŎP-ĕr-ă-tĭv, p. 18)
preoperative (prē-ŎP-ĕr-ă-tĭv, p. 18)
prosthesis (prŏs-THĒ-sĭs, p. 41)
singultus (SĬNG-gŭl-tŭs, p. 52)
surgery (p. 17)
surgical asepsis (ā-SĔP-sĭs, p. 44)
thrombus (THRŎM-bŭs, p. 32)

Surgery is defined as that branch of medicine concerned with diseases and trauma requiring operative procedures. Surgery became a medical specialty in the mid-nineteenth century. It enabled physicians to treat conditions that were difficult or impossible to manage only with medicine. However, early surgeons had little knowledge of the principles of asepsis, and anesthetic techniques were primitive and unsafe. Indeed, a surgeon's success was based on speed. In the 1840s the discovery of anesthesia allowed surgeons to operate on a patient who was pain free.

Nurses working in the first operating rooms (ORs) cleaned the rooms and equipment, performed technical tasks such as obtaining supplies, and occasionally accompanied the patient to the surgical ward to deliver nursing care.

With the advent of antiseptic and later aseptic practices, surgery became a treatment of choice for many conditions. Safer anesthetic gases allowed surgeons to conduct longer operative procedures. All surgery was conducted in hospital settings. Although modern-day suites have moved surgery from the Dark Ages, patients still often view the surgical process as mysterious and frightening.

Surgery is classified as elective, urgent, or emergency. Elective surgery is not necessary to preserve life and may be performed at a time the patient chooses. Urgent surgery is required to keep additional health problems from occurring. Emergency surgery is performed immediately to save the individual's life or preserve the function of a body part. Surgical procedures may also be labeled as either major or minor, although all surgeries have an element of risk.

Surgery is performed for various purposes, including diagnostic, **ablation** (amputation or excision of any body part or removal of a growth or harmful substance), **palliative** (therapy to relieve or reduce uncomfortable symptoms without cure), reconstructive, transplant, constructive, and cosmetic (Table 2-1). See Table 2-2 for frequently used surgical terminology.

Traditionally, surgical procedures were performed in hospitals. With the discovery of new technologies and today's emphasis on decreasing health care costs, the surgical suite may now be in a variety of settings.

Although facilities use different terms for surgical settings and processes, some common variations exist (Box 2-1).

PERIOPERATIVE NURSING

Perioperative nursing refers to the nurse's role during the **preoperative** (before surgery), **intraoperative** (during surgery), and **postoperative** (after surgery) phases of a surgical experience. Perioperative nursing stresses the importance of providing continuity of care for the surgical patient using the nursing process. In many hospitals, perioperative nurses assess a patient's health status preoperatively, identify specific patient needs, teach and counsel, attend to the patient's needs in the OR, and then follow the patient's recovery. However, in other institutions, different nurses care for the patient during each phase. Nurses also may delegate certain aspects of perioperative nursing to appropriate personnel (Box 2-2). The nurse's major responsibility is safe, consistent, and effective nursing interventions during each phase of surgery.

Table 2-1   Classification for Surgical Procedures

TYPE	DESCRIPTION AND EXAMPLES
ADMISSION STATUS	
Ambulatory (outpatient)	Patient who enters setting, has surgical procedure, and is discharged on the same day (e.g., breast biopsy, cataract extraction, hemorrhoidectomy, scar revision)
Same-day admit	Patient who enters hospital and undergoes surgery on the same day and remains for convalescence (e.g., carotid endarterectomy, cholecystectomy, mastectomy, vaginal hysterectomy)
Inpatient	Patient who is admitted to hospital, undergoes surgery, and remains in hospital for convalescence (e.g., amputation, heart transplant, laryngectomy, resection of aortic aneurysm)
SERIOUSNESS	
Major	Involves extensive reconstruction or alteration in body parts; poses great risks to well-being (e.g., coronary artery bypass, colon resection, gastric resection)
Minor	Involves minimal alteration in body parts; often designed to correct deformities; involves minimal risks compared with those of major procedures (e.g., cataract extraction, skin graft, tooth extraction)
URGENCY	
Elective	Performed on basis of patient's choice (e.g., bunionectomy, plastic surgery)
Urgent	Necessary for patient's health (e.g., excision of cancerous tumor, removal of gallbladder for stones, vascular repair for obstructed artery [e.g., coronary artery bypass])
Emergency	Must be done immediately to save life or preserve function of body part (e.g., removal of perforated appendix, repair of traumatic amputation, control of internal hemorrhaging)
PURPOSE	
Diagnostic	Surgical exploration that allows physician to confirm diagnosis; may involve removal of tissue for further diagnostic testing (e.g., exploratory laparotomy [incision into peritoneal cavity to inspect abdominal organs], breast mass biopsy)
Ablation	Excision or removal of diseased body part (e.g., amputation, removal of appendix, cholecystectomy)
Palliative	Surgery for relief or reduction of intensity of disease symptoms; will not produce cure (e.g., colostomy, debridement of necrotic tissue)
Reconstructive	Restoration of function or appearance to traumatized or malfunctioning tissue (e.g., internal fixation of fractures, scar revision, breast reconstruction)
Transplant	Replacement of malfunctioning organs (e.g., cornea, heart, joints, kidney)
Constructive	Restoration of function lost or reduced as result of congenital anomalies (e.g., repair of cleft palate, closure of atrial-septal defect in heart)
Cosmetic	Alteration of personal appearance (e.g., rhinoplasty to reshape nose)

Table 2-2	Surgical Terminology	
TERM	**INTERPRETATION WITH EXAMPLE**
Anastomosis	Surgical joining of two ducts or blood vessels to allow flow from one to another; to bypass an area (e.g., *Billroth I*, joins stomach and duodenum)
-ectomy	Surgical removal of (e.g., *cholecystectomy*, removal of the gallbladder)
Lysis	Destruction or dissolution of (e.g., *lysis of adhesions*, removal of adhesions)
-orrhaphy	Surgical repair of (e.g., *herniorrhaphy*, repair of a hernia)
-oscopy	Direct visualization by a scope (e.g., *cystoscopy*, direct visualization of the urinary tract by means of a cystoscope)
-ostomy	Opening made to allow the passage of drainage (e.g., *ileostomy*, formation of an opening of the ileum onto the surface of the abdomen for passage of feces)
-otomy	Opening into (e.g., *thoracotomy*, surgical opening into the thoracic cavity)
-pexy	Fixation of (e.g., *cecopexy*, fixation or suspension of the cecum to correct its excessive mobility)
-plasty	Plastic surgery (e.g., *mammoplasty*, reshaping of the breasts to reduce, lift, reconstruct)

Box 2-1	Common Surgical Settings

- **Inpatient:** Patient hospitalized for surgery
- **One-day (same-day surgery):** Patient admitted the day surgery is scheduled and dismissed the same day
- **Outpatient:** Patient, not hospitalized, admitted either to a short-stay unit or directly to the surgical suite (sometimes referred to ambulatory surgery)
- **Short-stay surgical center ("surgicenter"):** Independently owned agency; surgery performed when overnight hospitalization is not required (also called ambulatory surgical center or one-day surgery center)
- **Short-stay unit:** Department or floor where a patient's stay does not exceed 24 hours (sometimes referred to as outpatient/observation unit)
- **Mobile surgery units:** Units that move from place to place; go to the patient instead of the patient traveling to the unit

Box 2-2	Delegation Considerations in Perioperative Nursing

- The skills of assessment that are part of preparing the patient for surgery require the critical thinking and knowledge application unique to a nurse. For these skills, delegation is inappropriate. Assistive personnel (AP) may obtain vital signs and weight and height measurements. Instruct AP on proper precautions for these delegated procedures as needed.
- The skills of preoperative teaching require the critical thinking and knowledge application unique to a nurse. For this skill, delegation is inappropriate. AP can reinforce and assist patients in performing postoperative exercises.
  —Review with AP any precautions for a particular patient (e.g., turning method).
  —Be certain staff knows when to inform the nurse if the patient is unable to perform the exercises correctly.
- Coordinating the patient's preparation for surgery requires the critical thinking and knowledge application unique to a nurse. However, AP may administer an enema or douche; obtain vital signs; apply antiembolic stockings; and assist patient in removing clothing, jewelry, and prostheses.
  —Instruct AP in proper precautions when preparing a patient for surgery.
  —Instruct AP in proper observations and precautions if the patient has an IV catheter in place.
- The skills of sterile gowning and gloving can be delegated to a surgical technologist or the nurse who has acquired the proper skills.
- The skill of initiating and managing postoperative care of the patient requires the critical thinking and knowledge application unique to a nurse. AP may obtain vital signs, apply nasal cannula or oxygen mask, and provide basic comfort and hygiene measures.

INFLUENCING FACTORS

Regardless of the surgical procedure, the process is stressful for the patient. Observing a patient's mannerisms and listening to questions help identify the patient's feelings and concerns. By helping patients express their concerns, the nurse can offer support, reassurance, and information—the best way to address fear of the unknown.

Numerous factors affect the individual's ability to tolerate surgery.

Age

The young and the old do not tolerate major surgical treatment as well as those in other age-groups. Their altered metabolic needs may not respond to physiologic changes quickly. Specific concerns center on the body's response to temperature changes, cardiovascular shifts, respiratory needs, and renal function. To assist patients in returning to their optimal level of health, nursing assessments and appropriate interventions should be ongoing (see Life Span Considerations box).

Physical Condition

Healthy patients have smoother and faster recovery periods than patients who have coexisting health problems. Assess each body system to identify actual and potential problems, then select measures to prevent postsurgical complications (Box 2-3).

Life Span Considerations

Older Adults

Undergoing Surgery

- Older adults undergoing surgery have higher morbidity and mortality rates than younger people.
- Surgery places a greater stress on older people than on younger people. Carefully evaluate the older patient's physiologic status and coexisting conditions before surgery. Medical management is often preferred unless a condition is life threatening. However, age is no longer a factor for determining the benefit an individual can achieve from a surgical procedure. Consequently, nurses are caring for many more surgical patients of advanced age and are required to know the age-related factors that affect a surgical procedure.
- Older patients tend to recover more slowly from surgery compared with younger patients. Recovery is affected by the level of mental functioning, individual coping ability, and the availability of support systems.

- Risks of aspiration, atelectasis, pneumonia, thrombus formation, infection, and altered tissue perfusion are increased in the older adult.
- Disorientation or toxic reactions can occur in the older adult after the administration of anesthetics, sedatives, or analgesics. These reactions are often present for days after administration of the medication.
- Preoperative and postoperative teaching may require extra time. Provide teaching at the older adult's level of understanding. Repeat and reinforce directions.
- When communicating with older adult patients, be aware of any auditory, visual, or cognitive impairment that may be present.

Box 2-3	**ABCDE Mnemonic Device to Ascertain Serious Illness or Trauma in the Preoperative Patient**

A Allergy to medications, chemicals, and other environmental products such as latex. All allergies are reported to anesthesia and surgical personnel before the beginning of surgery. Place an allergy band on the patient's arm immediately.

B Bleeding tendencies or the use of medications that deter clotting, such as aspirin or products containing aspirin, heparin, or warfarin sodium. Herbal medications may also increase bleeding times or mask potential blood-related problems.

C Cortisone or steroid use.

D Diabetes mellitus, a condition that not only requires strict control of blood glucose levels but is also known to delay wound healing.

E Emboli. Previous embolic events (such as lower leg blood clots) may recur because of prolonged immobility.

Patients whose immune systems are suppressed are at a much higher risk for development of postoperative infection and are less capable of fighting that infection.

Nutritional Factors

The body uses carbohydrates, proteins, and fats to supply energy-producing glucose to its cells. Carbohydrates and fats are the primary energy producers, and protein is essential to build and repair body tissue. During stressful conditions, the body's need for energy and repair increases. Nutritional needs are affected by a patient's age and physical requirements; patients who maintain a sound, nutritional diet tend to recover more quickly.

A complete diet history identifies the patient's usual eating habits, nutritional patterns, and food preferences. Dietary practices are influenced by a patient's ethnic, cultural, religious, and socioeconomic background. With this information, offer the patient appropriate foods that are high in energy-producing nutrients. Surgery may decrease a patient's appetite and alter metabolic functions, so observe the patient for signs of malnutrition. If malnutrition is promptly identified, tube feedings, intravenous (IV) therapy, or parenteral hyperalimentation can be initiated (see Chapter 21 in *Foundations of Nursing*).

PSYCHOSOCIAL NEEDS

As patients and families plan for surgery, they frequently express concern and fears about possible outcomes (Box 2-4). Preoperative fear has been linked to postoperative behavior. The preoperative anxiety level influences the amount of anesthesia required, the amount of postoperative pain medication needed, and the speed of recovery from surgery. Determine each patient's perceptions, emotions, behavior, and support systems that may help or hinder their progress through the surgical period. Patiently and actively listening to the patient, the family, and significant others invites confidence and helps reduce anxiety levels (Figure 2-1).

While the patient attempts to understand the approaching surgery, family members and support people are also trying to cope. Families may have additional burdens, such as financial obligations, living changes, and added personal responsibilities. In addition to nursing and medical personnel, ministerial staff, social workers, or patient advocates can provide support for patients and families during this stressful time (see Patient Teaching box).

SOCIOECONOMIC AND CULTURAL NEEDS

The United States is a nation of diverse individuals from different social, economic, religious, ethnic, and cultural origins. Even geographic location affects the way a patient responds to surgery. Therefore it is im-

Box 2-4 Common Fears Associated with Surgery

- **Fear of loss of control** is associated primarily with anesthesia. The patient becomes almost totally dependent on the health care team during the surgical experience—even for basic needs such as breathing and life support—while under the influence of anesthesia.
- **Fear of the unknown** may result from uncertainty about the surgical outcome or a lack of knowledge regarding the surgical experience.
- **Fear of anesthesia** may include fears of unpleasant induction of or emergence from anesthesia. The patient may fear waking up during the operation and feeling pain while under anesthesia. This fear is often related to loss of control and fear of the unknown.
- **Fear of pain or inadequate postoperative analgesia** is common. Reassure the patient and significant others that the pain will be controlled.
- **Fear of death** is a legitimate fear. Even with the great strides in surgery and anesthesia, no anesthetic or operation is perfectly safe for all patients.
- **Fear of separation from the usual support group** may arise because the patient is separated from spouse, family, or significant others, as well as other support groups, and is cared for by strangers during this highly stressful period.
- **Fear of disruption of life patterns** relates to surgery and recovery interfering in varying degrees with activities of daily living, social activities, work, and professional activities.
- **Fear of change in body image and mutilation** is not unusual. Surgery disrupts body integrity and threatens body image.
- **Fear of detection of cancer** produces a high anxiety level.

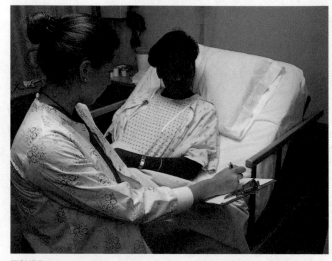

FIGURE 2-1 Often knowledge deficits occur when the patient is undergoing her first surgical experience.

portant to allow patients and families to express themselves openly.

Patients from different cultures (see Chapter 8 in *Foundations of Nursing*) may react to the preoperative experience in different ways. A multicultural perspective helps nurses approach patients with respect and

Patient Teaching

Preoperative Care

Examples of helpful information for preoperative patients and families are the following:
- Preoperative tests, reason, preparation
- Preoperative routines, sequence of events
- Special equipment needed
- Transfer to operating room (time, checking procedures)
- Medications
- Recovery room or postanesthesia care unit
  —Place where the patient will awaken
  —Frequent monitoring of vital signs
  —Return to room when vital signs are stable
- Probable postoperative therapies
  —Need for increased mobility as soon as possible
  —Need to keep respiratory passages clear
- Anticipated treatments (e.g., intravenous line, dressing changes, incentive spirometry)
- Pain medication routines (timing sequence, "as needed" [prn] status), other modalities of management such as patient-controlled analgesia and patient-controlled epidural

individually tailor care that promotes recovery (see Cultural Considerations box).

MEDICATIONS

Review of the patient's current medication regimen is essential. Polypharmacy (concurrent use of multiple medications) occurs in all age-groups but is more common with older adults. Studies have shown that patients age 65 and older use an average of two to six prescribed medications and one to three over-the-counter medications. The use of multiple medications can lead to adverse drug reactions and interactions with other medications in the perioperative setting.

During the surgical experience, health care providers use medications in a number of pharmacologic categories, including anesthesia agents, antimicrobials, anticoagulants, hemostatic agents, oxytocics, steroids, diagnostic imaging dyes, diuretics, central nervous system agents, and emergency protocol medications. A seriously ill patient may receive as many as 20 medications in a perioperative setting at one time. Large numbers of medications increase the chance of interactions.

Patients also frequently use herbal remedies as alternative or complementary medicines. Ask patients about their use of herbal remedies, either as dietary supplements or as medicines. Unless specifically asked, some patients may not consider their natural remedies as medicines. Even though herbs are natural products, they act like medications and may interact with or potentiate other medications or interfere with surgical procedures (Table 2-3).

Some medications may be stopped when a patient goes to surgery. However, it is important to know the purposes and actions of drugs, since they may be critical for patients with diseases such as diabetes. The anesthesiologist, in collaboration with the patient's

⊕ **Cultural Considerations**

The Surgical Patient

- Use of the patient's language helps put an anxious patient at ease. Use an interpreter when possible; learn some key phrases in foreign languages; and use references such as medical dictionaries, which usually have key phrases listed in an appendix.
- Because some Southeast Asians and Native Americans may avoid eye contact and consider it disrespectful, consider limiting eye contact when dealing with such patients.
- Chinese-Americans may not ask for pain medication and may need teaching to help explain how comfort and relief from pain promote healing and a quicker recovery.
- Native Americans are often stoic when ill. Complaints of pain to the nurse may be in general terms such as, "I am uncomfortable." Undertreatment of pain is common. The patient may lack basic trust.
- Among Arab-Americans, verbal consent often has more meaning than written consent because it is based on trust. Fully explain the need for written consent. The patient is expressive regarding pain; pain may cause intense fear. Prepare the patient for painful procedures, and develop a care plan to prevent pain.
- Blacks may be open to expression of pain but may avoid medication because of fear of addiction. For a terminal diagnosis, news is best expressed in a family care conference or by speaking with the patient's religious representative.
- For Vietnamese-American patients, having an interpreter (often a hired one) is important, depending on the sensitivity of the subject under discussion, because of modesty. A female family member is expected to be at the bedside to provide care and comfort. Men are the decision makers and support the family; therefore speaking with the male head of the family may be necessary.
- Russian-American patients often prefer an amiable nurse who has a friendly smile. Use open, inviting, nonverbal postures. A Russian-American patient is more willing to follow instruction if the nurse providing it is sincere, competent, and trustworthy. Russian-American families usually have a principal patriarch.

Table 2-3 **Preoperative Considerations for Commonly Ingested Herbs**

HERB	COMMON USES	PREOPERATIVE CONSIDERATIONS
Echinacea	Treat cold symptoms	Possible negative impact on the liver Subsequent interference with hepatic metabolism of certain anesthesia medications
Ephedra sinica	Decongestant Weight loss	Increased risk of cardiac dysrhythmias May reduce effectiveness of medications used to treat hypotension
Feverfew	Migraine prevention	Has anticoagulation factors; potential for increased bleeding Preoperative assessment should include clotting studies Discontinue before surgery
Garlic	Improved immunity High blood pressure and cholesterol	Potential for increased bleeding
Ginger	Motion sickness Cough Menstrual cramps Intestinal gas	Risk of prolonged clotting times Preoperative assessment should include clotting studies Discontinue before surgery
Ginkgo biloba	Brain function and alertness Tension Erectile dysfunction	Potential for increased bleeding
Ginseng	Overall well-being Diabetes	May increase anesthetic agent requirements Potential for hypoglycemia in patients taking insulin or oral diabetes agents
Guarana	Mental alertness Fatigue	May reduce the efficacy of warfarin May potentiate sympathetic nervous system stimulants, leading to cardiac complications May decrease cerebral blood flow
Kava	Sleep aid Anxiety, tension	May potentiate muscle relaxants May increase effects of certain antiemetics Potential for serious liver damage and subsequent decreased hepatic metabolism of certain anesthetic agents
Licorice	Asthma, eczema, rheumatoid arthritis Expectorant Gastritis	May cause hypertension Potential for hypokalemia and associated cardiac dysrhythmias
St. John's wort	Antidepressant Antiviral properties Antiinflammatory action	Should not be used with other psychoactive drugs, monoamine oxidase inhibitors, or serotonin reuptake inhibitors Discontinue before surgery because of possible drug interactions
Valerian root	Sedative or tranquilizer effect Sleep aid	Should not be used with sedatives or anxiolytics May increase effects of central nervous system depressants

physician and surgeon, determines whether these medications should be taken the day of surgery and postoperatively.

Remember to assess for allergies to drugs that may be given during any phase of the surgery. If patients say they are allergic to a drug, ask them exactly what happened when they took it. Also ask about nondrug allergies, including allergies to foods, chemicals, pollen, antiseptics used to prepare the skin for surgery, and latex rubber products. Patients with a history of allergic responsiveness are more likely to have hypersensitivity reactions to anesthesia agents. Many facilities require such patients to wear an allergy identification band during surgery. Flag the front of the patient's chart to alert all health care providers to the allergy status.

EDUCATION AND EXPERIENCE

As individuals age, life experiences influence problem-solving abilities and coping methods. Tailoring information to a patient's educational level enables understanding to replace fear. Encourage patients to repeat or summarize what has been presented. This process double checks what patients heard and how they interpreted it.

PREOPERATIVE PHASE

Before surgery, patients require a thorough health assessment. Acute or chronic diseases hinder the body's ability to repair itself or adjust to surgical treatment. Disorders of the systems identified in Table 2-4 present

Table 2-4	Surgical Effects on Body Systems
DISEASE OR DISORDER	**SURGICAL EFFECTS**
CARDIOVASCULAR (Chapter 8)	
Recent myocardial infarction, dysrhythmias, and heart failure Hypertension	Hypotension and cardiac dysrhythmias are the most common cardiovascular complications of the surgical patient. Early recognition and management before these complications become serious enough to diminish cardiac output depend on frequent assessment of the patient's vital signs.
ENDOCRINE (Chapter 11)	
Liver disease	Liver disease alters metabolism and elimination of drugs administered during surgery and impairs wound healing because of alterations in protein metabolism.
Diabetes mellitus	Diabetes increases susceptibility to infection and may impair wound healing from altered glucose metabolism and associated circulatory impairment. Fluctuating blood levels may cause central nervous system malfunction during anesthesia.
GASTROINTESTINAL (Chapter 5)	
Hiatal hernia Ulcers	Preoperative and postoperative medication may be necessary to control gastric acidity.
Esophageal varices	Risk of hemorrhage may increase due to intubation.
IMMUNE (Chapter 15)	
Acquired immunodeficiency syndromeAllergiesImmunodeficiency	Disease slows the body's ability to fight infection. Immunologic disorders increase risk of infection and delay wound healing after surgery. Hypothermia during surgery decreases immune function.
MUSCULOSKELETAL (Chapter 4)	Osteoporosis and increased risk for fractures in the older adult places patient at increased risk for injury.
NEUROLOGIC (Chapter 14)	
Seizures	Check the therapeutic levels of patient's medications.
Myasthenia gravis	Muscle relaxants may need to be excluded due to decreased ability to reverse their effects.
Cerebrovascular accident	Impaired verbal communication, defective perception of the body, paralysis, and visual disturbances place patient at high risk for injury.
Peripheral vascular disease	Patient has a decreased threshold for peripheral pain.
RESPIRATORY (Chapter 9)	
Tumors	Lung motility is decreased and gas exchange slowed.
Chronic obstructive pulmonary disease Emphysema Asthma	Anesthetic agents reduce respiratory function, increasing risk for severe hypoventilation.
URINARY (Chapter 10)	
Renal failure	Impaired kidney function decreases excretion of anesthesia and alters acid-base balance.
Tumors	Prostate enlargement may increase risk of urinary tract infection.

high-risk conditions for surgery. Each system is further affected by the patient's age, health, nutritional status, and mental state. Assessment questions regarding the patient's use of chemicals, alcohol, and recreational substances help the health team select medications. Postoperative care is also adjusted, when possible, to prevent potential complications. For example, a patient who smokes cigarettes may have impaired alveoli and reduced lung capacity. Mucus and anesthesia by-products may be trapped in the lung, causing atelectasis and pneumonia. After surgery, breathing exercises and treatments for the smoker aid in lung expansion and decrease the risk of respiratory complications.

Additional preoperative questions identify allergies, past surgeries, and infection and disease history. Ask the patient to name prescription drugs currently taken, over-the-counter drugs, and home remedies. Also record the patient's vital signs, height, and weight before surgery to have a baseline for postoperative comparison.

PREOPERATIVE TEACHING

Patient teaching before surgery helps decrease the patient's stress associated with fear of the unknown. Preoperative information helps reduce (1) anxiety, (2) the amount of anesthesia needed, (3) postsurgical pain, and (4) corticosteroid production. Decreasing postsurgical complications through preoperative teaching speeds wound healing.

In providing preoperative teaching, include the patient and family and remember that basic terminology and information are easier to understand than complex explanations. Stop frequently to verify the patient's understanding of information, ask questions, and encourage responses. Avoid questions that can be answered "yes" or "no." For example, "Do you have any questions?" is not as good as "What questions do you have?" If printed materials or videotapes are routinely used in preoperative teaching sessions, document what the patient read, heard, or saw. Older adults may have difficulty reading small print or hearing taped messages. If the patient does not understand English, an interpreter can explain information presented. Also emphasize that a nurse will be with the patient throughout the entire surgical experience.

For surgical procedures that have potential long-term effects, support groups can offer support preoperatively. Cancer organizations, amputation support groups, and enterostomal therapist associations are examples of large national organizations that offer peer support for surgical and nonsurgical patients.

Ideally, preoperative teaching is provided 1 or 2 days before surgery, when anxiety is not as high. In some instances, the patient may not be admitted to the hospital until early on the day of surgery. Most institutions have an established teaching program, often with a systematic preoperative teaching plan and checklist.

Begin by clarifying the sequence of preoperative and postoperative events. Generally, instruct the patient about the surgical procedure, informed consent, the method of skin preparation, and the gastrointestinal (GI) cleanser to be used. Clarify what the physician has explained. Review the time of the surgery and information about the recovery area (e.g., previously assigned units, intensive care, specialty units, or outpatient area). If a transfer is planned, it is helpful to take the patient and family on a tour of the new unit. Reinforce that vital signs, dressings, and tubes are assessed every 15 to 30 minutes until the patient is awake and stable.

PREOPERATIVE PREPARATION

Preparation for surgery depends on the patient's age and physical and nutritional status, the type of surgery, and the surgeon's preference. For surgery in a short-stay or ambulatory setting, the workup normally occurs a few days in advance. If the patient is admitted to the hospital, testing may be conducted to assess for potential problems. Preparation frequently includes both in-hospital testing and evaluation of test results that were completed in the physician's office.

Laboratory Tests and Diagnostic Imaging

Testing before surgery depends on the institution's policies, the physician's directives, and the patient's condition. Follow standing orders in completing this overall process. Laboratory tests commonly reviewed before surgery include a urinalysis; a complete blood count; and a blood chemistry profile to assess endocrine, hepatic, renal, and cardiovascular functions. Serum electrolytes are evaluated if extensive surgery is planned or the patient has associated problems. One essential electrolyte examined is potassium; if not enough potassium is available, dysrhythmias can occur during anesthesia and the patient's recovery may be delayed by general muscle weakness. A chest x-ray evaluation and electrocardiogram are used to identify disease processes or existing respiratory or cardiac damage. Additional tests are conducted to assess the organ involved in surgery. Blood chemistry profile (lactate dehydrogenase, γ-glutamyltransferase, alkaline phosphatase, total bilirubin) and urine bilirubin levels are used to assess hepatic function.

Informed Consent

The Patient's Bill of Rights affirms that patients must give **informed consent** (permission to perform a specific test or procedure) before the beginning of any procedure. In signing the consent form, the patient must be competent and agrees to have the procedure that is stated on the form. Information must be clear, the risks explained, expected benefits identified, and consequences or alternatives for the presenting problem stated. Witnesses are required to meet the state's legal requirements. A witness only verifies that this is the person who signed the consent and that it was a voluntary consent. The witness (often a nurse) does not verify that the patient understands the procedure. Ideally, the surgeon discusses the surgical procedure with the patient in advance. In some institutions, the surgical consent is completed in the physician's office or in the admissions department before the patient is admitted to the unit. Informed consent should not be obtained if the patient is disoriented, unconscious, mentally incompetent, or, in some agencies, under the influence of sedatives. Know agency policy (see Chapter 2, Figure 2-1 in *Foundations of Nursing*).

If the patient does not see or hear well, allow additional time to explain the surgery. For patients who do not understand English or are deaf, an interpreter may be necessary. Never coerce a patient into signing a consent that he or she does not understand or that contains information different from that originally given. If necessary, contact the physician and indicate that the patient does not understand the procedure.

In an emergency, the patient may not be able to give consent for surgery. Every effort is made to locate family members to assume this responsibility. Occasionally telephone permission may be obtained. Hospitals have standard guidelines for obtaining verbal consent. If the patient's life is in danger and family members cannot be located, the surgeon may legally perform surgery. If family members object to surgery that the physician believes is essential, a court order may be obtained for the procedure. This practice is used only in extreme circumstances, however (e.g., when a child's life is in danger). Know agency policy.

Gastrointestinal Preparation

At midnight before surgery, the patient is usually placed on nothing by mouth (NPO) status; this ensures the GI tract is empty when the patient is anesthetized, thereby decreasing the chance of vomiting or aspirating emesis after surgery. An NPO sign is posted over the patient's bed, and all fluids are removed from the room. Reinforce with both the patient and the family the importance of not ingesting foods or fluids. If the patient fails to comply with the NPO order, notify the physician. An order for NPO after midnight should apply to solid foods for patients scheduled for surgery in the morning. An early light breakfast is allowed for afternoon procedures. Clear liquid may be taken up to 3 hours before surgery.

Patients can have oral care while NPO, but caution them not to swallow fluids used. A wet cloth on the lips helps relieve dryness. If patients need to be hydrated or require special IV medications, the physician may order parenteral fluids or medication. Depending on the surgery, many patients resume foods and fluids the same day after surgery.

Because anesthesia relaxes the bowel, a bowel cleanser may be ordered to evacuate fecal material and lessen postoperative GI problems (nausea and vomit-

ing). A cleansing enema or a general laxative is frequently used. A GI lavage solution, GoLYTELY (an isosmotic solution), rapidly evacuates the bowel. Go-LYTELY is contraindicated, however, in patients with GI obstruction, gastric retention, bowel perforation, toxic colitis, or megacolon. If a bowel preparation is used, chart the type of preparation used, the patient's tolerance to the procedure, and results. Before bowel surgery, medication (neomycin, sulfonamides, erythromycin) may be given over a period of days to detoxify and sterilize the GI tract. This lessens the chance of fecal contamination during surgery.

Skin Preparation

Before surgery the patient may have hair removed at the surgical site. The operative site must be shaved carefully to remove the hair without injuring the skin (Skill 2-1). However, surgeons generally order hair removal only if it might interfere with exposure, closure, or dressing of the surgical site. Shaving the hair before surgery creates microscopic cuts that increase the risk of surgical site infection. The Centers for Disease Control and Prevention strongly recommends not removing hair at all unless it would interfere with the surgery (Nichols, 2001).

There is debate about the best method to remove hair. A lower rate of infection occurs with either no shave or use of electric clippers than with any other method. Use of a depilatory agent (a substance or procedure that removes hair) also has a low wound infection rate. In some cases, the patient showers after hair removal, unless contraindicated, using an antiseptic soap such as Hibiclens. If the surgical procedure involves the head, neck, or upper chest area, the patient also shampoos the hair.

If shaving is used, it should be performed close to the actual time of the surgical procedure to decrease the time for growth of bacteria and lower the potential for infection. Some surgical departments prepare the patient either in a surgical holding room or in the OR itself. Each agency or facility should have policies and protocols regarding the timing, the method, and the people responsible for the preoperative skin preparation of surgical patients.

Hospital policies differ regarding the description of skin areas to be prepped, or the surgeon may give specific orders. Review agency policy and the patient chart to determine the area to be shaved (Figure 2-2). Before the skin preparation, carefully assess the surgical site for skin impairment (e.g., infection, irritation, bruises, or lesions). Assess the patient for allergies. Record anything unusual and report it to the surgeon.

Once the patient is in the OR, scrub the skin thoroughly with a detergent solution and then apply an antiseptic solution to kill more adherent and deeper-residing bacteria. The surgeon may place a transparent sterile drape directly over the skin before making an incision.

Skill 2-1   Performing a Surgical Skin Preparation

Nursing Action (Rationale)

1. Refer to medical record, care plan, or Kardex for special interventions. (*Provides basis for care.*)
2. Obtain equipment. (*Organizes procedure.*)
   a. Appropriate light
   b. Operating room prep kit
      - Basin
      - Razor
      - Sponge with soap
      - Waterproof pad
      - Cotton-tipped applicators
   c. Clean gloves
3. Introduce self. (*Decreases patient's anxiety.*)
4. Identify patient. (*Identifies correct patient for procedure.*)
5. Explain procedure to patient. (*Seeks cooperation and decreases anxiety.*)
6. Wash hands and, if appropriate, don clean gloves. Know agency policy and guidelines from the Centers for Disease Control and Prevention (CDC) and the Occupational Safety and Health Administration (OSHA). (*Reduces spread of microorganisms.*)
7. Prepare patient for intervention:
   a. Close door to room or pull curtain. (*Provides privacy.*)
   b. Drape for procedure if necessary and position patient. (*Promotes proper body mechanics.*)
8. Raise bed to comfortable working level. (*Promotes proper body mechanics.*)
9. Place towel or waterproof pad under area to be shaved. (*Protects bed and linen from soiling.*)
10. Fill basin with warm water. (*Allows nurse to lather soap and rinse skin.*)
11. Place bath blanket over patient. (*Exposes only area to be shaved.*)
12. Adjust lighting. (*Allows thorough assessment of skin and helps decrease chance of skin impairment.*)
13. Lather skin with antiseptic soap and warm water. (*Cleanses skin, softens hair, and reduces friction from razor.*)

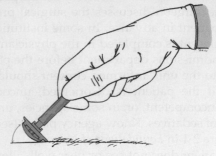

Step **14**

14. Hold razor at a 30- to 45-degree angle to skin. (*Minimizes chances of cutting or nicking skin.*)
    a. Shave small areas while holding skin taut.
    b. Use short, smooth strokes. (*Prevents pulling skin.*)
    c. Shave hair in same direction it grows (see illustration). (*Removes hair close to skin surface.*)
15. Rinse razor frequently. (*Removes accumulation of hair from razor and prevents contamination from dirty water.*)
16. If entire area is shaved, cleanse it with a washcloth and clean, warm water. Dry skin. (*Removes excess shaved hair, body oils, and soil on skin. Reduces number of microorganisms. Promotes patient comfort.*)
17. Reassess skin for cuts, nicks, or hair. (*Prevents growth of microorganisms and possible infections from skin impairment.*)
18. Return patient to appropriate position. (*Provides patient comfort and safety.*)
19. Clean and dispose of equipment. (*Reduces spread of microorganisms.*)
20. Remove and dispose of soiled gloves and wash hands. (*Reduces spread of microorganisms.*)
21. Document. (*Verifies procedure.*)

Special concerns for patients undergoing a surgical skin preparation are as follows:

- Small children may be easily frightened by this procedure, and it may need to be done in the OR.
- Older adults need a detailed explanation to relieve their anxiety.
- Older adults have less subcutaneous tissue, less skin elasticity, and more delicate skin tissue. Take extreme care when shaving the older adult.
- Older adults are usually more susceptible to infections.

Latex Allergy Considerations

Focused assessment of risk factors helps identify patients with the nursing diagnosis of risk for latex allergy response. Assessing the patient's experience helps identify those at risk for a systemic reaction; for example, patients may relate stories of complicated anesthesia events, hives from blowing up a balloon, or severe swelling of the labia with a urinary catheterization.

With the advent of Universal Precautions (now called *Standard Precautions*) in the late 1980s, the use of latex gloves dramatically increased, and latex allergies became much more common. Basically, every health care

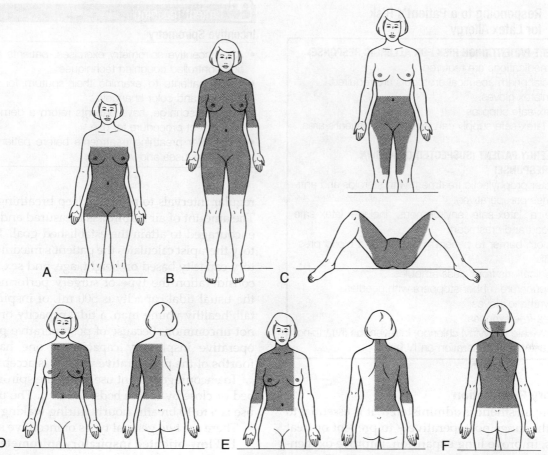

FIGURE 2-2 Skin preparation for surgery on various body areas. The shading indicates the area that could be shaved. **A,** Abdominal surgery. **B,** Open heart surgery. **C,** Perineal surgery. **D,** Chest or thoracic surgery. **E,** Breast surgery. **F,** Cervical spine surgery.

worker wears gloves. Most gloves are powdered to make them easier to put on. The powder absorbs protein allergens from the latex and deposits them on skin and into surgical wounds; it also aerosolizes the protein allergens. Aerosolized latex allergens are carried in ventilation systems, requiring further preventive measures.

Latex allergy is classified in three categories: irritant reaction and types IV and I allergic reactions. The irritant reaction, which is most commonly seen, is actually a nonallergic reaction. The type IV allergic reaction to latex is a cell-mediated response to the chemical irritants found in latex products. The true latex allergy is the type I allergic reaction, and it occurs shortly after exposure to the proteins in latex rubber. The type I reaction is an immunoglobulin E–mediated systemic reaction that occurs when latex proteins are touched, inhaled, or ingested.

Factors influencing the risk for latex allergy response are the person's susceptibility and the route, duration, and frequency of latex exposure. Risk factors include the following:

- History of anaphylactic reaction of unknown etiology during a medical or surgical procedure
- Multiple surgical procedures (especially from infancy)
- Food allergies (specifically kiwi, bananas, avocados, chestnuts)
- A job with daily exposure to latex (health care, food handlers, tire manufacturers)
- History of reactions to latex (balloons, condoms, gloves)
- Allergy to poinsettia plants
- History of allergies and asthma

To provide a latex-safe environment for susceptible patients, all surgical patients should be screened for the risk for latex allergy response before admission. Identification of patients at risk is the first step in preventing a reaction.

When a patient with a suspected or known latex allergy is scheduled for surgery, all latex use is avoided and the patient is admitted directly to the OR as the first case of the day, if possible. Many facilities have converted isolation rooms into latex-safe environments for patients with latex allergy. Ensure that everyone on the health care team is aware that a patient is, or may be, latex allergic. Place a medical alert or allergy band around the patient's wrist, and clearly flag the patient's status on the chart. Remove all natural rubber latex products from the area. Use latex-free measures to prepare the patient's medication. Have a crash cart standing by stocked with latex-free equipment, supplies, and drugs for treating anaphylaxis. As ordered, give preoperative prophylactic treatment with glucocorticoid steroids and antihistamines. Box 2-5 lists interventions for the perioperative care of patients with risk for latex allergy response.

Box 2-5 Responding to a Patient's Risk for Latex Allergy

LATEX-ALERT PATIENT (HIGH RISK FOR ALLERGIC RESPONSE)
- No premedications are required.
- No special pharmaceutical protocols are required.
- Use nonlatex gloves.
- Use latex-safe supplies.
- Keep a latex-safe supply cart available in patient's area.

LATEX-ALLERGY PATIENT (SUSPECTED OR KNOWN ALLERGIC RESPONSE)
- Administer prophylactic treatment with steroids and antihistamines preoperatively.
- Prepare a latex-safe environment, include latex-safe supply cart and crash cart.
- Apply cloth barrier to patient's arm under a blood pressure cuff.
- Use medications from glass ampules.
- Do not puncture rubber stoppers with needles.
- Wear synthetic gloves.
- Use latex-free syringes.
- Use latex-safe (polyvinyl chloride) intravenous (IV) tubing.
- Do not use latex preparation on IV bags.

Patient Teaching

Incentive Spirometry
- After incentive spirometry exercises, patients should practice controlled coughing techniques.
- Teach patients to examine their sputum for consistency, amount, and color changes.
- Before discharge, have patients return a demonstration of the correct procedure for use.
- Administer breathing treatments before patients' meals to prevent nausea and vomiting.

Respiratory Preparation

If a general anesthetic is administered, it is essential to ventilate the lungs postoperatively to prevent or treat atelectasis, improve lung expansion, improve oxygenation, and prevent postoperative pneumonia. Because the lungs do not expand fully during surgery, mucus and gases remain in the lungs until expelled. Pulmonary exercises can assist in expanding the lungs and removing these by-products. Preoperative introduction to the use of the incentive spirometer is of great value to the patient.

In spirometry, referred to as **incentive spirometry,** the patient uses a device (spirometer) at the bedside at regular intervals to promote deep breathing (Skill 2-2). The amount of air inspired is measured and the patient encouraged to attain the established goal. The respiratory therapist calculates the patient's maximum inspiratory capacity based on height, age, and sex, taking into consideration the type of surgery performed. At rest, the usual tidal capacity is 500 mL of inspired air. In a tall, healthy young man, a tidal capacity of 4300 mL is not uncommon. Because of postoperative pain, a postoperative inspiratory capacity of one half to three fourths of the preoperative volume is acceptable.

To encourage patient use, place the spirometer in the bed or close by on the bedside stand. The usual rate of use is 8 to 10 breaths hourly during waking hours.

There are two general types of incentive spirometers:
1. **Flow-oriented inspiratory spirometer:** This type of incentive spirometer is inexpensive and measures inspiration. It contains one or more clear plastic cylinder chambers that contain freely movable, colored, lightweight plastic balls. Instruct the patient to place the mouthpiece in the mouth and inhale slowly and deeply; this raises the balls in the cylinders. Encourage the patient to keep the colored balls floating as long as possible. The degree of elevation is marked on the

Skill 2-2 Incentive Spirometry or Positive Expiratory Pressure Therapy and "Huff" Coughing

Nursing Action (Rationale)

1. Refer to physician's orders, care plan, or Kardex. (*Health care facilities frequently require a medical order for incentive spirometry.*)
2. Assess patient's respiratory status and lung sounds. Indications for spirometry are (a) asymmetric chest wall movement, (b) increased respiratory rate, (c) increased production of sputum, and (d) diminished lung expansion postoperatively. (*Alerts health care personnel to those patients at risk for respiratory complications during illness or after surgery.*)
3. Explain procedure, and instruct patient in the correct use of the spirometer. Frequently the respiratory therapist will do this. However, it may be the nurse's responsibility to follow up and promote proper technique. (*Understanding improves compliance with use.*)
4. Obtain supplies and equipment. (*Organizes procedure.*)
   a. Incentive spirometer or positive expiratory pressure (PEP) therapy device
   b. Emesis basin
   c. Tissues
   d. Bedside trash bag
   e. Clean gloves (if soiling is likely)
5. Wash hands and don gloves (if soiling is likely). Know agency policy and guidelines from the Centers for Disease Control and Prevention and the Occupational Safety and Health Administration. (*Reduces spread of microorganisms.*)

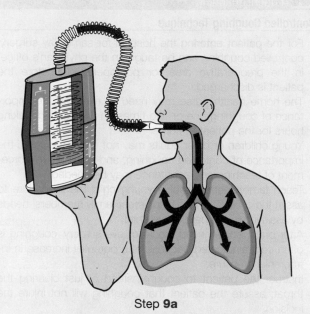

Step **9a**

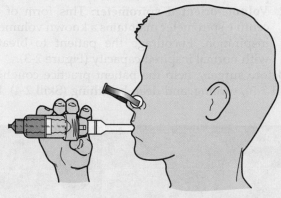

Step **10c**

6. Place prescribed incentive spirometer at the bedside. (*Prepares equipment for procedure.*)
7. Place patient in semi-Fowler's or full Fowler's position. (*Promotes optimal lung expansion.*)
8. Place tissues, emesis basin, and bedside trash bag within easy reach. (*Enables sanitary disposal of respiratory secretions expectorated during procedure.*)
9. Incentive spirometry
   a. Instruct patient to completely cover mouthpiece with lips (use a noseclip if patient is unable to breathe through the mouthpiece) and to (a) inhale slowly until maximum inspiration is reached, (b) hold breath 2 or 3 seconds, and (c) slowly exhale (see illustration). (*Promotes maximum inspiration.*)
   b. Instruct patient to relax and breathe normally for a short time. (*Prevents patient from hyperventilating and prevents fatigue.*)
   c. Instruct and encourage patient to gradually increase depth of inspiration. (*Promotes maximum lung expansion.*)
   d. Offer oral hygiene after spirometry is completed. (*Patients often find this refreshing.*)
   e. Store spirometer in an appropriate place, such as the bedside table, until next scheduled time. (*Provides a convenient place for repeated use.*)
10. PEP therapy and "huff" coughing
   a. Wash hands. (*Reduces transmission of microorganisms.*)
   b. Set PEP device for setting ordered. (*The higher the setting, the more effort required.*)
   c. Instruct patient to assume semi-Fowler's or high Fowler's position, and place noseclip on

patient's nose (see illustration). (*Promotes optimum lung expansion and expectoration of mucus.*)
   d. Instruct patient to place lips around mouthpiece and (1) take a full breath and exhale two or three times longer than inhalation and (b) repeat this pattern for 10 to 20 breaths. (*Ensures that all breathing is done through the mouth and that the device is used properly.*)
   e. Remove device from mouth, and have patient take a slow, deep breath and hold for 3 seconds. (*Promotes lung expansion before coughing.*)
   f. Instruct patient to exhale in quick, short, forced "huffs." (*"Huff" coughing, or forced expiratory technique, promotes bronchial hygiene by increasing expectoration of secretions.*)
11. Position patient as desired or as ordered. (*Helps maintain patient comfort and promotes maximum chest expansion.*)
12. Place call light within easy reach. (*Maintains patient safety.*)
13. Remove and dispose of soiled gloves and wash hands. (*Reduces spread of microorganisms.*)
14. Assess respiratory status and evaluate patient's response to spirometry. (*Provides a basis for repeated use.*)
15. Document in nurse's notes patient's respiratory status before and after incentive spirometry, type of spirometry, and any adverse effects from the procedure. (*Verifies patient care. Some agencies require such documentation for third-party reimbursements.*)
16. Carry out patient teaching (see Patient Teaching box, Incentive Spirometry).

cylinders so that this, plus the length of time the patient maintains elevation, can be recorded.

2. **Volume-oriented spirometer:** This form of incentive spirometer maintains a known volume of inspiration. Encourage the patient to breathe with normal inspired capacity (Figure 2-3).

Before surgery, help the patient practice coughing (Skill 2-3), turning, and deep breathing (Skill 2-4). Be-

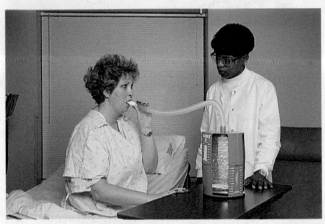

FIGURE 2-3 Volume-oriented spirometer.

 Patient Teaching

Controlled Coughing Technique

- For the patient entering the hospital for same-day surgery, controlled coughing can be taught in the physician's office, in the preoperative area, or postoperatively before the patient is discharged.
- The home health nurse may need to reinforce the importance of coughing one or two times an hour during waking hours for the patient at home.
- Young children or older adults may not fully understand the importance of controlled coughing, and continual reinforcement of teaching and assistance may be needed.
- Teach family members of a young child the procedure to assist the child. This also helps meet family members' needs by assisting in the care of the child.
- After brain, spinal, head, neck, or eye surgery, coughing is often contraindicated because of a potential increase in intracranial pressure.
- Instruct the patient to cough instead of just clearing the throat; assure the patient that coughing will not injure the incision.
- Teach the patient to examine the sputum for odor, consistency, amount, and color changes.

Skill 2-3 Teaching Controlled Coughing

Nursing Action (Rationale)

1. Refer to medical record, care plan, or Kardex for special interventions. (*Provides basis for care.*)
2. Obtain equipment. (*Organizes procedure.*)
   a. Pillow or bath blanket
   b. Gloves
   c. Emesis basin
   d. Facial tissues
   e. Chair or bed
3. Introduce self. (*Decreases patient's anxiety.*)
4. Identify patient. (*Ensures correct patient for procedure.*)
5. Explain procedure. (*Seeks cooperation.*)
6. Wash hands and don clean gloves according to agency policy and guidelines from the Centers for Disease Control and Prevention and the Occupational Safety and Health Administration. (*Reduces spread of microorganisms.*)
7. Assist patient to upright position. Place pillow between bed or chair and patient. (*Facilitates deep breathing and optimum chest expansion.*)
8. Demonstrate coughing exercise for patient (see illustration). (*Allows patient to observe nurse and to ask questions.*)
   a. Take several deep breaths. (*Deep breaths expand lungs fully so that air moves behind mucus and facilitates effect of coughing.*)

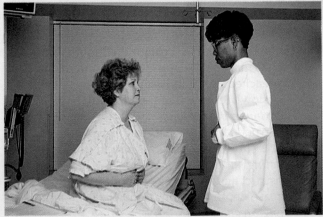

Step **8**

   b. Inhale through nose.
   c. Exhale through mouth with pursed lips.
   d. Inhale deeply again and hold breath for count of three.
   e. Cough two or three consecutive times without inhaling between coughs. (*Consecutive coughs remove mucus more effectively and completely than one forceful cough.*)
9. Caution patient against just clearing the throat instead of coughing. (*Clearing the throat does not remove mucus from deep in airways.*)

10. Abdominal or thoracic incision can be splinted before coughing with hands, pillow, towel, or rolled bath blanket (see illustration). (*Surgical incision cuts through muscles, tissues, and nerve endings. Deep breathing and coughing place additional stress on suture line and cause discomfort. Splinting incision provides firm support and reduces incisional pulling.*)

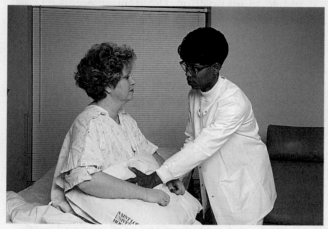

Step **10**

11. Encourage patient to practice coughing while splinting incisional area once or twice an hour during waking hours. Assist patient as indicated. (*Helps effectively expectorate mucus with minimal discomfort.*)
12. Remind patient to use tissues and emesis basin for any mucus expectorated. (*Reduces spread of microorganisms.*)
13. Teach patient to examine sputum for consistency, amount, and color change. (*Changes could indicate respiratory complications such as pneumonia.*)
14. Provide wash cloth and warm water for washing hands and face, provide for oral hygiene, and return patient to comfortable position. (*Provides for patient comfort.*)
15. Remove and dispose of soiled gloves and wash hands. (*Reduces spread of microorganisms.*)
16. Document exercises performed and patient's ability to perform them independently. (*Verifies care given and patient teaching.*)
17. Carry out patient teaching (see Patient Teaching box, Controlled Coughing Technique).

Skill 2-4 Teaching Postoperative Breathing Techniques, Leg Exercises, and Turning

Nursing Action (Rationale)

1. Refer to medical record, care plan, or Kardex for special interventions. (*Provides basis for care.*)
2. Obtain equipment. (*Helps organize procedure.*)
   a. Support pillow, towel, or folded bath blanket
   b. Gloves
   c. Emesis basin
   d. Facial tissues
3. Introduce self. (*Decreases patient's anxiety.*)
4. Identify patient. (*Verifies correct patient for procedure.*)
5. Explain procedure to patient. (*Improves cooperation and decreases anxiety.*)
6. Wash hands and don clean gloves. Know agency policy and guidelines from the Centers for Disease Control and Prevention and the Occupational Safety and Health Administration. (*Reduces spread of microorganisms.*)
7. Prepare patient for intervention.
   a. Close door to room or pull curtain. (*Provides privacy.*)
   b. Drape for procedure if necessary.

8. Raise bed to comfortable working level. (*Promotes proper body mechanics.*)
9. Premedicate with pain medication, if indicated. (*Elicits patient compliance.*)

Postoperative Breathing Techniques

10. Place pillow between patient and bed or chair. (*Allows for fuller chest expansion. [Bed or chair itself is too firm to provide expansion.]*)
11. Sit or stand facing patient. (*Allows patient to observe nurse.*)
12. Demonstrate taking slow, deep breaths. Avoid moving shoulders and chest while inhaling. Inhale through nose. (*Prevents panting and hyperventilation. Moistens, filters, and warms inhaled air.*)
13. Hold breath for a count of three, and slowly exhale through pursed lips. (*Allows for gradual expulsion of air.*)
14. Repeat exercise three to five times. Have patient practice exercise. (*Allows patient to observe appropriate technique. Allows nurse to assess patient's technique and correct errors.*)

Continued

15. Instruct patient to take 10 slow, deep breaths every 2 hours until ambulatory. (*Helps prevent postoperative complications.*)
16. If there is an abdominal or chest incision, instruct patient to splint incisional area using pillow or bath blanket, if desired, during breathing exercises. (*Provides support and additional security for patient.*)

Leg Exercises

17. Lifting one leg at a time and supporting joints, gently flex and extend leg 5 to 10 times (see illustration). (*Stimulates circulation and helps prevent thrombi formation.*)
18. Repeat exercise with opposite extremity. Lifting leg while supporting joints, gently flex leg 5 to 10 times. (*Stimulates circulation and helps prevent thrombi formation.*)
19. Alternately point toes toward the chin and toward the foot of the bed four or five times. (*Uses additional muscle flexion and contraction to stimulate circulation.*)
20. Make circle with ankles of both feet four or five times to the left and four or five times to the right (see illustration). (*Further stimulates circulation through muscle contraction and flexion.*)

21. Assess pulse, respiration, and blood pressure. (*Aids in determining complications from exercise.*)

Turning Exercises

22. Instruct patient to assume supine position to right side of bed. Have side rails on both sides of bed in up position. (*Positioning begins on right side of bed so that turning to left side will not cause patient to roll toward bed's edge. Side rails in the raised position promote patient safety.*)
23. Instruct patient to place left hand over incisional area to splint it. (*Supports and minimizes pulling on suture line during turning.*)
24. Instruct patient to keep left leg straight and flex right knee up and over left leg. (*Straight leg stabilizes patient's position. Flexed right leg shifts weight for easier turning.*)
25. Instruct patient to turn every 2 hours while awake. (*Reduces risk of vascular and pulmonary complications.*)
26. Remove and dispose of soiled gloves and wash hands. (*Reduces spread of microorganisms.*)
27. Document. (*Records patient education and verifies procedure.*)

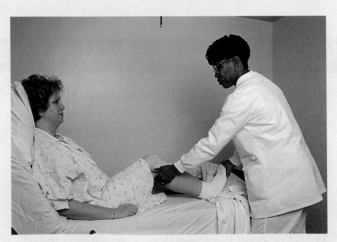

Step **17**

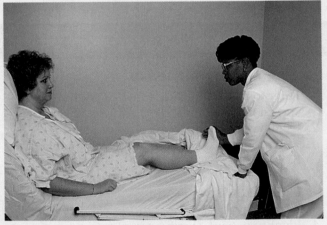

Step **20**

cause coughing increases intracranial pressure, it is usually contraindicated in cranial and spinal-related surgeries. Coughing is also contraindicated for patients having cataract surgery (Box 2-6). Some physicians believe coughing may actually cause alveolar collapse and order only incentive spirometry. Patients frequently ambulate within a few hours of surgery to return cardiovascular and respiratory functions to normal more quickly.

Cardiovascular Considerations

Accompanying the need to turn, cough, and deep breathe is the need to practice leg exercises (see Skill 2-4). Because blood stasis occurs when the patient lies flat, encourage him or her to do leg exercises to assist venous blood flow. With the venous blood slowing, a **thrombus** (an accumulation of platelets, fibrin, clotting factors, and cellular elements of the blood attached to the anterior wall of a vessel, sometimes oc-

| Box 2-6 | Surgeries for Which Coughing Is Contraindicated or Modified |

- **Intracranial:** Coughing increases intracranial pressure (ICP), leading to cerebrospinal fluid leak.
- **Eye:** Coughing increases ICP, which then increases intraocular pressure, causing pressure on suture line.
- **Ear:** Mouth must be kept open if coughing occurs to prevent pressure backup through eustachian tube to middle ear, causing pressure on suture line.
- **Nose:** Mouth must be kept open if coughing occurs to prevent dislodgment of a clot with subsequent bleeding.
- **Throat:** Vigorous coughing may dislodge a clot with subsequent bleeding.
- **Spinal:** Coughing increases spinal canal pressure.

 Patient Teaching

Use of Thromboembolic Deterrent Stockings and Sequential Compression Devices

- Teach patient to correctly apply antiembolism stockings.
- Teach patient appropriate care of the stockings. (Wash in warm water and mild soap, do not wring dry, and lay over flat surface to dry.)
- Instruct patient not to massage legs because of the risk of dislodging a thrombus.
- Teach patient the signs of possible complications. (If stockings or devices are too restrictive, edema and pain could result.)

- Postoperative patients with abdominal or thoracic incisions will not be able to bend and pull on their own stockings.
- Stockings may be difficult to fit and maintain in obese or very thin patients.
- Stockings may be difficult to apply for elderly patients; the nurse or family members will need to assist.

Vital Signs

Vital signs mirror the body's response to anesthesia and surgery. Instruct the patient before surgery that it is normal for blood pressure, temperature, pulse, and respiration to be monitored until stable. The schedule

cluding the lumen) may form. If a thrombus is dislodged, it can travel as an **embolus** to the lungs, the heart, or the brain, where the vessel can be occluded. Without an adequate blood supply, an **infarct** (localized area of necrosis) can occur. Antiembolism stockings (thromboembolic deterrent stockings), a Jobst pump, or sequential compression devices (SCDs) with intermittent external pneumonic compression system may be ordered to provide support and to prevent venous thrombus in the lower extremities (Skill 2-5).

Consider the following points when applying antiembolism stockings.

Skill 2-5 Applying Thromboembolic Deterrent Stockings and Sequential Compression Devices

Nursing Action (Rationale)

1. Refer to medical record, care plan, or Kardex for special interventions. (*Provides basis for care.*)
2. Obtain equipment. (*Organizes procedure.*)
   a. Thromboembolic deterrent stockings (TEDs) or sequential compression devices (SCDs)
   b. Clean gloves (when appropriate)
   c. Tape measure
3. Introduce self. (*Decreases patient's anxiety.*)
4. Identify patient. (*Identifies correct patient for procedure.*)
5. Explain procedure. (*Seeks cooperation and decreases anxiety.*)
6. Wash hands and, if appropriate, don clean gloves. Know agency policy and guidelines from the Centers for Disease Control and Prevention and the Occupational Safety and Health Administration. (*Reduces spread of microorganisms.*)
7. Prepare patient.
   a. Close door to room, pull curtain, and drape for procedure, if necessary. (*Provides privacy.*)
8. Raise bed to comfortable working level. (*Promotes proper body mechanics.*)

9. Examine legs and assess risk for conditions. (*Helps nurse determine presence of pigmentation around ankles, pitting edema, or peripheral cyanosis, which may indicate inadequate circulation.*)
10. Assess patient for calf pain or positive Homans' sign. (*May indicate presence of thrombophlebitis.*)
11. Measure legs for stockings according to agency policy, and order stockings. (*Promotes the correct size to accomplish purpose of stockings.*)

Thromboembolic Deterrent Stockings

12. Assist patient to supine position to apply stockings before patient rises. Patient should be recumbent for at least 30 minutes before application. (*Prevents veins from becoming distended or edema from occurring.*)
13. Turn stockings inside out as far as heel. Place thumbs inside foot part, and slip stocking on until heel is correctly aligned (Figure 2-4, *A* and *B*). (*Positions stocking for appropriate application.*)

Continued

Skill 2-5 Applying Thromboembolic Deterrent Stockings and Sequential Compression Devices—cont'd

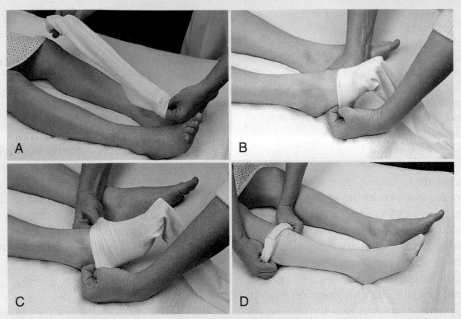

FIGURE 2-4 Applying antiembolism stockings. **A,** Turn the elastic stocking inside out by placing one hand into the sock, holding the toes of the sock with the other hand, and pulling. **B,** Place the patient's toes into the foot of the elastic stocking, making sure that the sock is smooth. **C,** Slide remaining portion of the sock over the patient's foot, making sure that the toes are covered. Sock will now be right-side out. **D,** Slide the sock up over the patient's calf until the sock is completely extended. Be sure that the sock is smooth with no ridges.

14. Gather fabric and ease it over ankle and up the leg (Figure 2-4, C). *(Prevents bunching of stocking, which can cause local pooling of blood.)*
15. Pull leg portion of stocking over foot and up as far as it will go, making certain that gusset lies over femoral artery. Adjust stocking to fit evenly and smoothly with no wrinkles (Figure 2-4, D). *(Allows appropriate fit and application, which are vital for maintaining even pressure. Prevents irritation and impediments to circulation.)*
16. Repeat steps 12 to 15 for opposite extremity. *(Ensures appropriate application.)*

Sequential Compression Devices (Figure 2-5)

17. Place sleeve under patient's leg, with fuller portion at top of thigh. *(Ensures correct fit.)*
18. Apply sleeve with opening at front of knee and closed portion behind knee. *(Ensures appropriate placement and desired effect.)*
19. When the SCD is in place, make sure there are no wrinkles or creases in stockings. Fold Velcro strips over to secure stockings. *(Allows proper functioning of stockings and prevents irritation.)*
20. Attach tubing to SCD after both sleeves are applied. Align arrows for correct connection and appropriate effect. Plug in unit. *(Allows air to inflate stockings in sequential order.)*

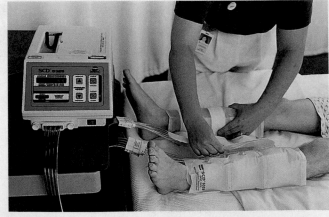

FIGURE 2-5 Application of sequential compression devices.

21. Assess patient periodically. *(Determines presence of edema or cyanosis.)*
22. Assess stocking at regular intervals. *(Ensures that top has not rolled down or loosened and that no wrinkles are present.)*
23. Remove and dispose of soiled gloves and wash hands. *(Reduces spread of microorganisms.)*
24. Document. *(Verifies patient care.)*
25. Carry out patient teaching (see Patient Teaching box, Use of Thromboembolic Deterrent Stockings and Sequential Compression Devices, p. 33).

for monitoring vital signs depends on the hospital's protocol and the patient's stability. Preoperative vital signs serve as the baseline for deciding when stability has returned or problems arise. Postoperative vital signs are discussed later in this chapter.

Genitourinary Considerations

After general anesthesia, the urinary bladder's tone is decreased. Therefore you should know the patient's normal bladder habits and identify when the bladder is full and distended. Inform the patient preoperatively that the lower part of the abdomen will be palpated at intervals to check for bladder fullness (Figure 2-6). Once patients are awake and tolerating fluids, encourage an adequate intake. Occasionally a urinary catheter is inserted to monitor urinary output. This procedure is normally reserved for patients undergoing urinary surgery or those who may have difficulty voiding. The catheter is usually removed 1 or 2 days postoperatively to reduce the chance of bladder infection. Once it is removed, encourage the patient to drink 8 ounces of fluids per hour while awake unless contraindicated. Also, monitor intake and output (I&O) values until the patient's normal voiding pattern returns. Urinary retention and urinary tract infections are common postoperative complications.

Surgical Wounds

With today's technologies, incisions (cuts produced surgically by a sharp instrument to create an opening into an organ or body space) are closed in a variety of ways: sutures, staples, Steri-Strips, or transparent strips. Knowing the type of closure enables you to explain its appearance to the patient. Some surgeries require the removal of exudate, often with a drain. Explain the purpose of the drain and the need for close monitoring. Although not all incisions require dressings, assess the wound's appearance. Wound care, dressing changes, and drainage systems are described in more detail in Chapters 12, 13, and 20 in *Foundations of Nursing*.

Pain

Patients fear pain more than any other postsurgical complication. Emphasize to the patient that pain relief is an important part of care. Various methods are used to reduce discomfort. If the patient is considering non-pharmacologic analgesia (e.g., imagery, biofeedback, relaxation techniques), review these techniques and allow practice time. The majority of patients choose traditional analgesia. Postoperative pain is what the patient says it is, so it is important to reassure patients that addiction to analgesics rarely occurs in the time frame needed for comfort. For the patient who is apprehensive about intermittent injections, patient-controlled analgesia (PCA) and opioids injected into the epidural space (patient-controlled epidural) are safe and effective for postoperative pain management. When the patient is allowed oral intake, oral analgesics coupled with nontraditional methods are often effective (see Chapter 16 in *Foundations of Nursing*).

Tubes

Depending on the surgery, patient teaching includes information about nasogastric (NG) tubes, wound evacuation units, and IV and oxygen therapy. Allowing patients to view these items and understand their purposes lessens the fear associated with each. (See Chapters 13 and 20 in *Foundations of Nursing* for more detailed discussion of the tubes and drains used in the postoperative patient.)

Preoperative Medication

Preoperative medication reduces the patient's anxiety, decreases the amount of anesthetic needed, and reduces respiratory tract secretions. Provide the patient with information on what to expect from preoperative medications. Barbiturates and tranquilizers (phenobarbital and diazepam [Valium]) are sometimes given for sedation to reduce the amount of the anesthetic required. Opioid analgesics (meperidine and morphine) may be administered by intermittent injection or PCA if the patient has pain before surgery; this also reduces the amount of anesthetic required. An introduction to PCA preoperatively helps patients understand the concept and how the equipment works. Anticholinergics such as atropine reduce spasms of smooth muscles and decrease gastric, bronchial, and salivary secretions (Table 2-5).

The patient frequently becomes drowsy, notices a dry mouth, and experiences vertigo after receiving the

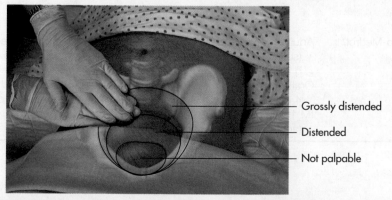

Grossly distended

Distended

Not palpable

FIGURE 2-6 Assess the bladder by palpating the lower abdomen for distention.

Table 2-5 Medications for the Perioperative Period

Generic (Trade)	Dose and Route	Action	Nursing Implications
BENZODIAZEPINES			
Midazolam (Versed, Valium, Ativan)	Dose depends on the amount of adequate sedation necessary for surgery	Decreases anxiety and produces sedation Induces amnesia	Monitor for respiratory depression, hypotension, drowsiness, and lack of coordination.
Diazepam	5-20 mg po		
Lorazepam	44 mcg/kg to 2 mg IV		
OPIOID ANALGESICS			
Morphine (Morphine)	5-15 mg IM, IV	Decreases anxiety	Monitor for respiratory depression,
Fentanyl citrate (Sublimaze)	50 mcg/mL IM or slow IV	Allows decreased anesthetics	nausea, vomiting, orthostatic hypotension, and pruritus.
H₂ RECEPTOR ANTAGONISTS			
Famotidine (Pepcid)	20 mg IV	Reduces gastric acid volume and concentration	Monitor for confusion and dizziness in older adults.
Ranitidine (Zantac)	50 mg IV		
ANTIEMETICS			
Metoclopramide (Reglan)	10 mg IV or IM	Enhances gastric emptying	Monitor for sedation and extrapyramidal reaction (involuntary movement,
Droperidol (Inapsine)	2.5-10 mg	Tranquilizer	muscle tone changes, and abnormal
Ondansetron HCl (5-HT₃ receptor antagonist) (Zofran)	4 mg IV	Prevents postoperative nausea and vomiting	posture). Instruct patient to report any difficulty breathing.
ANTICHOLINERGICS			
Atropine sulfate (Atropine sulfate)	0.4-0.6 mg IM or IV	Reduces oral and respiratory secretions to decrease risk of aspiration Decreases vomiting and laryngospasm	Monitor for confusion, restlessness, and tachycardia. Prepare patient to expect dry mouth.
Glycopyrrolate (Robinul)	0.1-0.3 mg IM or IV		
ANTIBIOTICS			
Cefazolin sodium (Ancef)	1-2 g q6h Maximum 12 g/day	Bactericidal Wound infection Minimizes risk of wound infection	If large doses are given, therapy is prolonged or patient is at high risk, monitor for signs and symptoms of superinfection, including abdominal
Cefotaxime sodium (Claforan)	1 g IM or IV 30-90 min preoperative	Bactericidal	pain, moderate to severe diarrhea, severe anal or genital pruritus, and
Ceftriaxone (Rocephin)	1 g IM or IV 0.5-2 hr preoperative	Bactericidal as perioperative prophylaxis	severe mouth soreness. Determine patient's history of allergies. If dosing continues, space drug evenly around the clock. Advise patient to complete therapy.
ADRENOCORTICAL STEROID			
Methylprednisolone (Depo-Medrol, Solu-Medrol)	Adults: 10-250 mg (succinate) IV q 4-6 hr Oral 2-60 mg in 4 divided doses IM 10-80 mg (acetate)	Decreases inflammation	Determine whether patient has hypersensitivity to drug. Determine whether patient has diabetes mellitus, and anticipate an increase in antidiabetic drug regimen because of raised blood glucose level.

Table 2-5   Medications for the Perioperative Period—cont'd

Generic (Trade)	Dose and Route	Action	Nursing Implications
NONSTEROIDAL ANTIINFLAMMATORY DRUG (NSAID)			
Ketorolac (Toradol)	50 mg/mL IM; 30 mg/mL IV push over at least 15 sec	Reduces intensity of pain Reduces inflammation	Assess the duration, location, onset, and type of pain the patient is having. Evaluate patient for therapeutic response.
ANTICOAGULANTS			
Enoxaparin sodium (Lovenox)	30 mg/0.3 mL to 150 mg/mL subQ in prefilled syringes	Produces anticoagulation Prevents new clot formation or secondary embolic complications	Do not give IM, but give subQ. Tell the patient not to take aspirin or similar over-the-counter drugs.
Heparin sodium (Heparin)	10 units/mL to 15,000 units/ 500 mL subQ Heparin sodium flush syringes: 10 units/ mL, 100 units/mL; vials (most use saline for the flush) 10 units/mL ≤100 units/mL; vials 10- 100 units/mL		Cross-check heparin dose with another nurse before administering. Use constant rate IV infusion pump. Monitor the patient's partial thromboplastin time diligently. Assess patient's gums for erythema and gingival bleeding; skin for bruises or petechiae; and urine for hematuria.
Warfarin sodium (Coumadin)	5 mg vials IM; 1-10 mg po tablets or IV		Observe patient for evidence of hemorrhage such as abdominal or back pain, decreased blood pressure, increased pulse rate, and severe headache. Urge patient to not ingest alcohol or make drastic dietary changes. If administration continues, urge patient to notify the physician if he or she experiences black stools; bleeding; brown, dark, or red urine; coffee-ground vomitus; or red-speckled mucus from a cough.

preoperative medication. Ask the patient to void beforehand. If preoperative medication is given on the nursing unit, the patient must remain in bed. Institute safety measures, such as putting the bed in low position and raising side rails, and monitor the patient every 15 to 30 minutes until the patient leaves for surgery. Reassure the patient and provide a quiet environment on the nursing unit while waiting for transport to the surgical suite. In many institutions, the preoperative medication is given by the anesthesiologist or anesthesia provider in the preoperative holding area.

Surgery cancels all medications ordered before surgery, except for medications for long-term conditions, such as phenytoin (Dilantin) for seizure control (Table 2-6). The surgeon reorders medication necessary after surgery.

Anesthesia

Anesthesia means the absence of feelings (pain) (*an*, meaning "without," plus *esthesia*, meaning "awareness of feeling"). Anesthesia is divided into three categories: general, regional, and local.

General Anesthesia

Modern anesthetics are much easier to reverse and allow the patient to recover with fewer unwanted effects than in the past. **General anesthesia** results in an immobile, quiet patient who does not recall the surgical procedure. The patient's amnesia acts as protection from the unpleasant events. General anesthesia is used for major surgery requiring extensive tissue manipulation.

An anesthesiologist gives general anesthetics by IV and inhalation routes through the four stages of anesthesia. In **Stage I** the patient is awake and the administra-

Table 2-6	Medications with Special Implications for the Surgical Patient
DRUG CLASS	**EFFECTS DURING SURGERY**
Antibiotics	Antibiotics potentiate action of anesthetic agents. If taken within 2 weeks before surgery, aminoglycosides (gentamicin, tobramycin, neomycin) may cause mild respiratory depression from depressed neuromuscular transmission.
Antidysrhythmics	Antidysrhythmics can reduce cardiac contractility and impair cardiac conduction during anesthesia.
Anticoagulants	Anticoagulants alter normal clotting factors and thus increase risk of hemorrhaging. They should be discontinued at least 48 hours before surgery. Aspirin is a commonly used medication that can alter clotting mechanisms.
Anticonvulsants	Long-term use of certain anticonvulsants (e.g., phenytoin [Dilantin], phenobarbital) can alter metabolism of anesthetic agents.
Antihypertensives	Antihypertensives interact with anesthetic agents to cause bradycardia, hypotension, and impaired circulation. They inhibit synthesis and storage of norepinephrine in sympathetic nerve endings.
Corticosteroids	With prolonged use, corticosteroids cause adrenal atrophy, which reduces the body's ability to withstand stress. Before and during surgery, dosage may be temporarily increased.
Insulin	Diabetic patient's need for insulin after surgery is reduced because nutritional intake is decreased. Stress response and intravenous administration of glucose solutions can increase dosage requirements after surgery.
Diuretics	Diuretics potentiate electrolyte imbalances (particularly potassium) after surgery.
Nonsteroidal antiinflammatory drugs (NSAIDs)	NSAIDs inhibit platelet aggregation and may prolong bleeding, increasing susceptibility to postoperative bleeding.
Herbal therapies (ginger, ginkgo, ginseng)	These herbal therapies can affect platelet activity and increase susceptibility to postoperative bleeding. Ginseng may increase hypoglycemia with insulin therapy. (See Chapter 17 in *Foundations of Nursing*, Complementary and Alternative Therapies.)

Adapted from Potter, P.A., & Perry, A.G. (2007). *Basic nursing: essentials for practice* (6th ed.). St. Louis: Mosby.

tion of anesthetic agents begins. The stage is completed when the patient loses consciousness. **Stage II** begins with the loss of consciousness and ends with the onset of regular breathing and loss of eyelid reflexes. This is referred to as the excitement or delirium phase because it is often accompanied by involuntary motor activity. The patient must not receive any auditory or physical stimulation during this period because it can stimulate a release of catecholamines, which can raise heart rate and blood pressure. **Stage III** begins with the onset of regular breathing and ends if respirations cease This stage is known as the operative or surgical phase. **Stage IV** begins with the cessation of respirations and must be avoided, or it will necessitate the initiation of cardiopulmonary resuscitation and may lead to death. These stages were defined in the past when ether was used and may be less clear with newer anesthetic agents.

A more useful designation of stages includes the three phases of induction, maintenance, and emergence. The **induction phase** includes the administration of agents and endotracheal intubation. The **maintenance phase** includes positioning the patient, preparing the skin for incision, and performing the surgery. Appropriate levels of anesthesia are maintained during this phase. During the **emergence phase,** anesthetics are decreased and the patient begins to awaken. Because of the short half-life of today's medications, emergence often occurs in the OR.

Anesthesia is often induced intravenously, although an inhalation agent may be used. The patient is unconscious 10 to 20 seconds after the dose. Barbiturates provide sedation, amnesia, and hypnosis but must be used with other agents to relieve pain and relax muscles. To prevent aspiration and other respiratory complications, the anesthesiologist puts an endotracheal tube into the patient's airway. Endotracheal intubation is usually performed after administration of short-acting or, occasionally, long-acting muscle relaxants (Figure 2-7).

An anesthesia provider or OR nurse may assist with cricoid pressure during induction of general anesthesia and endotracheal cuff inflation during intubation. Cricoid pressure reduces the risk of aspirating stomach contents by compressing the esophagus to prevent passive regurgitation. (This technique cannot, however, stop active vomiting.) The maneuver is begun while the patient is awake. Patient reassurance is important during this period of mild discomfort. Once initiated, pressure must be held constant until the cuff has been inflated or aspiration can happen rapidly.

When induction is completed, anesthesia may be maintained through a combination of inhalation and IV medications. The patient also receives a continuous supply of oxygen and adjunct medications such as opioid analgesics and muscle relaxants. A combination of smaller amounts of several medications can mean a significant reduction in the dose compared with using a single medication.

The duration of anesthesia depends on the length of surgery. Surgical risks influence the duration of surgery. The greatest risks from general anesthesia are the side effects of anesthetic agents, including cardiovascular depression or irritability, respiratory depression, and liver and kidney damage.

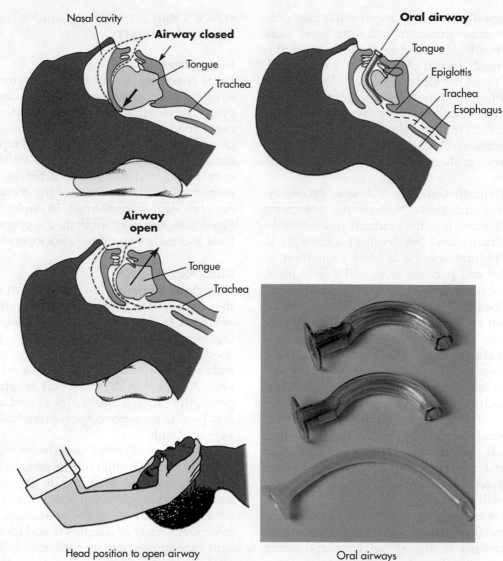

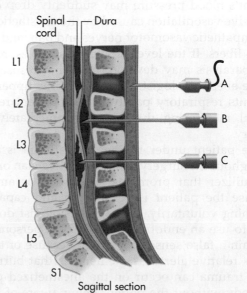

FIGURE 2-7 Possible airways used during surgery.

Emergence from anesthesia occurs when the procedure is completed and reversal agents are given. The oropharynx is suctioned to decrease the risk of aspiration and laryngeal spasm after extubation. Extubation is often accomplished before transfer to the postanesthesia care unit (PACU).

Regional Anesthesia

Induction of **regional anesthesia** results in loss of sensation in an area of the body. The portion of sensory pathways that is anesthetized depends on the method of induction. The patient does not lose consciousness with regional anesthesia, but is usually sedated. The anesthesiologist gives regional anesthetics by infiltration and local application. Figure 2-8 demonstrates common locations for the induction of medication to achieve the regional block.

Infiltration of anesthetic agents may involve one of the following induction methods:

- **Nerve block:** Local anesthetic is injected into a nerve (e.g., brachial plexus in the arms), blocking the nerve supply to the operative site.

FIGURE 2-8 Spinal column—side view with spinal and epidural anesthesia needle placement. *A,* Epidural catheter. *B,* Single injection epidural. *C,* Spinal anesthesia. (Interspaces most commonly used are L4-L5, L3-L4, and L2-L3.)

- **Spinal anesthesia:** The anesthesiologist performs a lumbar puncture and introduces local anesthetic into the cerebrospinal fluid in the subarachnoid space. Anesthesia can extend from the tip of the xiphoid process down to the feet. Positioning of the patient influences movement of the anesthetic agent up or down the spinal cord. Spinal anesthesia is often used for lower abdominal, pelvic, and lower extremity procedures; urologic procedures; or surgical obstetrics.
- **Epidural anesthesia:** This is a safer procedure than spinal anesthesia because the anesthetic agent is injected into the epidural space outside the dura mater and the depth of anesthesia is lighter. Epidural anesthesia blocks sensation in the vaginal and perineal areas and thus is often used for obstetric procedures. The epidural catheter may be left in so that the patient can receive medication via continuous epidural infusion after surgery.
- **IV regional anesthesia (Bier block):** Local anesthetic is injected via an IV line into an extremity below the level of a tourniquet after blood has been withdrawn. The drug is allowed to infiltrate only tissues in the intended surgical area. The extremity is pain free while the tourniquet is in place. Advantages include a short onset and short recovery time. However, the tourniquet may be inflated for only 2 hours or tissue damage will occur.

Infiltrative anesthesia involves risks, particularly with spinal anesthesia, because the anesthetic agent may move upward in the spinal cord and affect breathing. This migration of anesthetic depends on the drug type and amount and patient position. The patient's blood pressure may suddenly drop due to extensive vasodilation caused by the anesthetic block to sympathetic vasomotor nerves and pain and motor nerve fibers. If the level of anesthesia rises, respiratory paralysis may develop, requiring resuscitation by the anesthesiologist. Elevation of the upper body prevents respiratory paralysis. The patient requires careful monitoring during and immediately after surgery.

The patient under regional anesthesia is awake throughout the surgery unless the physician orders a tranquilizer that promotes sleep and/or amnesia. Because the patient is responsive and capable of breathing voluntarily, the anesthesiologist does not need to use an endotracheal tube. OR personnel often gain a false sense of security because of the patient's relative alertness. Remember that burns and other trauma can occur on the anesthetized part of the body without the patient being aware of the injury. It is therefore necessary to frequently observe the position of extremities and the condition of the

skin. OR staff also must use caution regarding topics discussed in surgery.

Local Anesthesia

Local anesthesia involves loss of sensation at the desired site (e.g., growth on the skin or the cornea of the eye). The anesthetic agent (e.g., lidocaine) inhibits nerve conduction until the drug diffuses into the circulation. It may be injected or applied topically. The patient loses sensation of pain and touch, and control over motor and autonomic activities (e.g., bladder emptying). Local anesthesia is commonly used for minor procedures performed in ambulatory surgery. Physicians also may infiltrate the operative area with local anesthetics to promote postoperative pain relief.

Conscious Sedation

Conscious sedation is the administration of drugs that depress the central nervous system or provide analgesia to relieve anxiety or provide amnesia during surgical diagnostic procedures. It is routinely used for procedures that do not require complete anesthesia but rather a depressed level of consciousness. A patient under conscious sedation must independently retain a patent airway and airway reflexes and be able to respond appropriately to physical and verbal stimuli.

Advantages of conscious sedation include adequate sedation and reduction of fear and anxiety with minimal risk, amnesia, relief of pain and noxious stimuli, mood alteration, elevation of pain threshold, enhanced patient cooperation, stable vital signs, and rapid recovery. A variety of diagnostic and therapeutic procedures are appropriate for conscious sedation; these include burn dressing changes, cosmetic surgery, and pulmonary biopsy and bronchoscopy.

Nurses assisting with the administration of conscious sedation must be knowledgeable about anatomy, physiology, cardiac dysrhythmias, procedural complications, and pharmacologic principles related to the administration of individual conscious sedation agents. Nurses must also be able to assess, diagnose, and intervene in the event of untoward reactions and demonstrate skill in airway management and oxygen delivery. Resuscitation equipment must be readily available.

Positioning the Patient for Surgery

During general anesthesia the nursing personnel and surgeon often wait to position the patient until he or she is completely relaxed. The choice of position is usually determined by the surgical approach (Figure 2-9). Ideally the patient's position provides good access to the operative site and sustains adequate circulatory and respiratory function. It should not impair neuromuscular structures. The patient's comfort and safety must be considered. The team must take

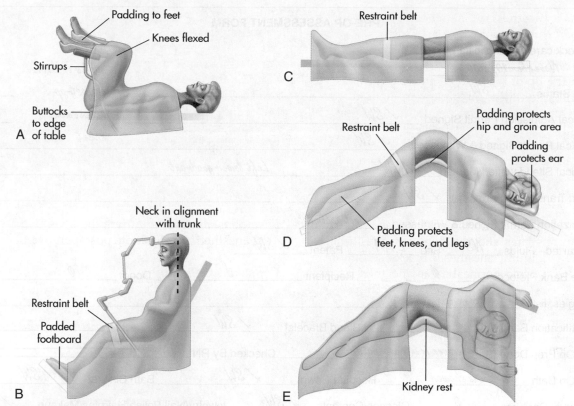

FIGURE 2-9 Common perioperative positions and the padding provided to relieve pressure in each position. **A,** Lithotomy position, used for vaginal and perineal procedures. **B,** Sitting position, used for neurologic procedures. **C,** Supine position (the most common position). Potential pressure points are the occiput, scapula, olecranon, thoracic vertebrae, sacrum, coccyx, and calcaneus. **D,** Jackknife position, used for gluteal and anorectal surgeries. **E,** Lateral kidney position, used for procedures requiring a retroperitoneal approach.

into account age, weight, height, nutritional status, physical limitations, and preexisting conditions and document them for staff who care for the patient postoperatively. Sometimes nurses in postoperative divisions fail to appreciate the discomfort a patient may feel after surgery (e.g., discomfort of the left arm or side of a patient whose right kidney was removed).

An alert person maintains normal range of joint motion by pain and pressure receptors. If a joint is extended too far, pain reminds the person that muscle joint strain is too great. In a patient who is anesthetized, however, normal defense mechanisms cannot guard against joint damage, muscle stretch, and strain. The muscles are so relaxed that it is relatively easy to place the patient in a position he or she could not assume while awake. The patient often remains in a given position for several hours. Although it may be necessary to place a patient in an unusual position, attempt to maintain correct alignment and protect the patient from pressure, abrasion, and other injuries (e.g., corneal abrasion). Attachments to the OR table allow protection and padding of extremities and bony prominences. Positioning should not interfere with normal movement of the diaphragm or circulation to body parts. If restraints are necessary, pad the area to be restrained to prevent skin trauma (see Chapter 14 in *Foundations of Nursing*).

Preoperative Checklist

Complete the preoperative checklist before the patient leaves the nursing unit (Figure 2-10). Signing the preoperative checklist means that you assume responsibility for all areas of care included on the list. If the preoperative medication is to be given on the nursing unit, complete the preoperative checklist before administering the medication. Any **prosthesis** (an artificial replacement for a missing part of the body), contact lenses, dentures, jewelry, and other valuables are removed and either given to family members or placed in a secure area. Some hospitals allow dentures to be worn while in surgery and removed later. If the patient wears rings, they should be secured with tape and noted in the chart. The patient should void before the preoperative medication is administered, or 1 hour before surgery is scheduled. Although most patients become drowsy after administration of a preoperative medication, a few either become hyperactive or demonstrate no side effects. Remind the patient to remain in bed, and raise the side rails. Place the call light within reach and point it out to the patient.

PRE-OP ASSESSMENT FORM

(Please check carefully and initial)

Extra copies on back of post-op assessment sheet

Date *November 10, 2010*

1. DNR Status ✓ *SW*

2. Medical Admission Permit Signed ✓ *SW*

3. Surgical Permit Signed & Witnessed ✓ *SW*

4. Surgical Site Identified/Marked ✓ *SW*   *Left lower quadrant*

5. Blood Transfusion Permit ✓ *SW*

6. Sterilization Permit Signed & Witnessed *not applicable*

7. IV Started - Fluids *NS* Site *L.7.A* Patent ✓ *SW*

8. Bone Bank Protocol *∅*   Recipient *∅*   Donor *∅*

9. Allergies, list: *penicillin*

10. Identification Band ✓ *SW*   Blood Bracelet ✓ *SW*

11. Pre-Op Prep Done *to be done in intraoperative*   Checked By RN _____

12. Pre-Op Bath *Hibiclens shower*   Hospital Gown ✓ *SW*   Bath Blanket ✓ *SW*

13. Remove: Dentures *∅*   Glasses/Contacts ✓ *SW*   Jewelry/Nail Polish/Hairpins/Makeup ✓ *SW*

14. TED stockings when ordered ✓ *SW*   Side Rails Up ✓ *SW*   Patient Labels ✓ *SW*

15. Pre-Op Vital Signs Time: *1000* T *98⁶* P *80* R *20* BP *120/80* Pain Intensity 0-10 *∅ SW*

16. Pre-Op Medications *to be administered in intraoperative*

17. Insert Foley Catheter ✓ *SW*

18. Physical Disability, such as Amputations, Glass Eye, etc. *∅*

19. Systemic Diseases *type 2 diabetes mellitus*   *SW*

20. History and Physical ✓ *SW*

    See Guidelines for pre-op testing policy number 600 - P 118. Testing completed per policy.

21. Lab Reports: *CBC, Basic metabolic profile*

ECG *on chart* *SW*   Chest X-Ray *on chart* *SW*

NURSING STAFF IDENTIFICATION
SW Susan Welker RN

22. Infectious Process Present _____ Yes ✗ No

    Type of Infection _____

23. Additional Comments *pre- & post-op nursing interventions explained*

24. Chart Signed Off ✓ *SW* *RN*

Great Plains Regional
Medical Center
601 West Leota Street - P.O. Box 1167
North Platte, Nebraska 69103-1167

LABEL

FIGURE 2-10 Preoperative assessment form.

Eliminating Wrong Site and Wrong Procedure Surgery

In 2006, The Joint Commission (TJC) established Universal Protocol guidelines to prevent surgeons from performing surgery on the wrong site or performing the wrong procedure (TJC, 2009a). If an invasive surgical procedure is planned, this protocol must be implemented regardless of location (ambulatory surgery centers, hospital, or health care provider's office). The protocol consists of three main principles:

1. Obtain a preoperative verification that guarantees all relevant documents and studies are available and that they meet the patient's expectations.
2. Mark the operative site with indelible ink, including marking left or right, multiple structures (e.g., toes), and levels of the spine.
3. Just before the start of the procedure, all members of the surgical and procedure team have a time-out to verify they have the correct patient, procedure, site, and any implants.

A legally designated representative or an active patient must be included in all the protocol steps. If the representative or patient refuses to allow marking of the operative site, this must be noted on the procedure checklist (Ridge, 2008).

Transport to the Operating Room

Personnel in the OR notify the nursing unit when it is time for surgery. The transporter checks the patient's identification bracelet against the patient's medical record to be sure the correct person is going to surgery. For transportation on a gurney, the nurses and transporter help the patient safely transfer from bed to gurney. The ambulatory surgery patient may walk to the OR, allowing more control over the event. The trip to surgery should be as smooth as possible so that the sedated patient does not experience nausea or dizziness.

Allow the family to visit before the patient is transported to the OR, then direct the family to the appropriate waiting area. If family members plan on leaving the facility during the procedure, ensure there is a way to contact them and give them phone numbers of the nurse's station and patient's room.

Preparing for the Postoperative Patient

If the patient was hospitalized before surgery and will return to the same nursing unit, prepare the bed and room for the patient's return. Arrange furniture so that the gurney can easily be brought to the bedside. Place the bed in the high position with the bed rails down on the receiving side and up on the other side. A postoperative bedside unit should include the following:

- Sphygmomanometer, stethoscope, and thermometer
- Emesis basin
- Clean gown
- Wash cloth, towel, and facial tissues
- IV pole and pump

- Suction equipment
- Oxygen equipment
- Extra pillows for positioning
- Bed pads to protect bed linen from drainage
- PCA pump

INTRAOPERATIVE PHASE

Intraoperative (within the surgical suite) care centers on care and protection of the patient. When the patient enters the OR (Figure 2-11), identify the patient both verbally and by the identification band and medical records. Nursing interventions include warm, personal contact with the patient to humanize the OR's often cold, aseptic, and highly technical environment. During surgery and particularly anesthesia, patients cannot protect themselves from many sources of possible harm. Essential elements for monitoring and promoting patient safety are being aware of the potential for harm, recognizing body areas most susceptible to injury, strictly adhering to principles of positioning and asepsis, and monitoring sites for impairment or early signs of injury. Do not leave small or potentially dangerous objects such as needles and syringes near the patient. Use side rails and safety straps, even for the fully conscious patient; safety reminder devices may be necessary to protect the delirious, semicomatose, or disoriented patient from injury.

HOLDING AREA

In many hospitals the patient enters a surgical care unit called a **preanesthesia care unit** (or holding area) outside the OR, where the nurse completes the preoperative preparations. Nurses in this unit are usually part of the OR staff and wear surgical scrub suits.

The nurse or anesthesiologist inserts an IV catheter into the patient's vein to establish a route for fluid re-

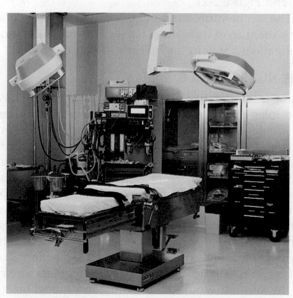

FIGURE 2-11 Traditional operating room.

Box 2-7	Responsibilities of the Circulating Nurse and the Scrub Nurse

RESPONSIBILITIES OF THE CIRCULATING NURSE

- Prepares operating room with necessary equipment and supplies and ensures that equipment is functional
- Arranges sterile and unsterile supplies; opens sterile supplies for scrub nurse
- Sends for patient at proper time
- Visits with patient preoperatively; explains role, identifies patient, verifies operative permit, and answers any questions
- Performs patient assessment
- Confirms patient assessment
- Checks medical record for completeness
- Assists in safe transfer of patient to operating room table
- Positions patient on operating room table in accordance with type of procedure and surgeon's preference
- Places conductive pad on patient if electrocautery is to be used
- Counts sponges, needles, and instruments with scrub nurse before surgery
- Assists scrub nurse and surgeons by tying gowns
- May prepare patient's skin
- Assists scrub nurse in arranging tables to create sterile field
- Maintains continuous astute observations during surgery to anticipate needs of patient, scrub nurse, surgeons, and anesthesiologist
- Provides supplies to scrub nurse as needed
- Observes sterile field closely for any breaks in aseptic technique, and reports accordingly

- Cares for surgical specimens according to institutional policy
- Documents operative record and nurse's notes
- Counts sponges, needles, and instruments when closure of wound begins
- Transfers patient to gurney for transport to recovery area
- Accompanies patient to the recovery room and provides a report

RESPONSIBILITIES OF THE SCRUB NURSE

- Performs surgical hand scrub
- Dons sterile gown and gloves aseptically
- Arranges sterile supplies and instruments in manner prescribed for procedure
- Checks instruments for proper functioning
- Counts sponges, needles, and instruments with circulating nurse
- Gowns and gloves surgeons as they enter operating room
- Assists with surgical draping of patient
- Maintains neat and orderly sterile field
- Corrects breaks in aseptic technique
- Observes progress of surgical procedure
- Hands surgeon instruments, sponges, and necessary supplies during procedure
- Identifies and handles surgical specimens correctly
- Maintains count of sponges, needles, and instruments so none will be misplaced or lost in wound

placement and IV medications. Use a large-bore IV catheter for optimal infusion of all fluids and possible blood products. Administer preoperative medications.

If hair around the surgical site needs to be removed, this is done in a private area near the OR immediately before surgery. Consult the physician's order sheet and the agency policy and procedure manual (see Skill 2-1 and Figure 2-2).

The temperature in the OR is usually cool, so offer the patient an extra blanket for warmth and relaxation. The patient's stay in the holding area is brief.

THE NURSE'S ROLE

In the intraoperative phase, the nurse assumes one of two roles during the surgical procedure: scrub nurse or circulating nurse (Box 2-7). Everyone (nurses, physicians, anesthesia providers) in the OR must prevent contamination of sterile items and aid in maintaining aseptic conditions. Personnel practice **surgical asepsis** (using sterile technique to protect against infection before, during, or after surgery) to prevent microbial contamination of the operative site. The goal of surgical asepsis is to prevent or minimize postoperative wound infections. The patient is at risk for introduction of infecting organisms through catheters, drains, or the surgical wound. Standards and guidelines for surgical scrubs and skin preparation should be strictly followed. The operation's success and ease greatly de-

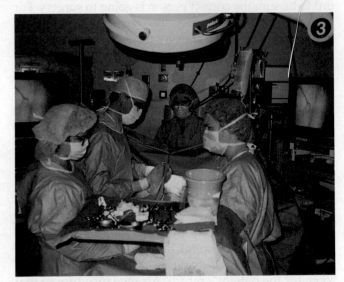

FIGURE 2-12 Safe, effective intraoperative care requires a team effort.

pend on group dynamics as professionals work to achieve common goals (Figure 2-12).

POSTOPERATIVE PHASE

IMMEDIATE POSTOPERATIVE PHASE

During the postoperative phase the OR nurse assists in transferring the patient to the PACU (Figure 2-13), the recovery room, or the intensive care area. Review with

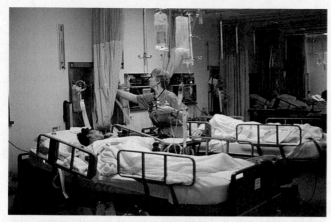

FIGURE 2-13 Nurse in a postanesthesia care unit.

the staff information about the patient's status, including IV fluids, medications, and blood products administered; the surgical dressing; any complication in the OR; and unusual risks for hemorrhage or cardiac irregularities. The OR nurse is an important resource in planning the patient's postoperative care.

Immediate postoperative observation and interventions follow the ABCS of airway, breathing, consciousness, circulation, and systems (Table 2-7). Assess vital signs every 15 minutes during the recovery period, and monitor respiratory and GI functions. Evaluate the

wound for any **drainage** (the removal of fluids from a body cavity, wound, or other source of discharge by one or more methods) or **exudate** (substances [e.g., perspiration, pus, serum] that slowly seep from cells or blood vessels through small pores or breaks in cell membranes). Once the patient has a patent airway and stable vital signs, is conscious, and responds to stimuli, the anesthesia provider or surgeon approves transfer to the nursing unit. As the patient regains consciousness, relief of pain is often the first need expressed. Frequently, medication is given in the recovery area. Staff on the nursing unit review documentation from the surgical suite and recovery room to assess how well the patient tolerated the surgical process.

Carefully monitor body temperature. Hypothermia, a core temperature of less than 98.6° F (37° C), occurs in 60% to 80% of all postoperative patients. Contributing factors include body exposure in a cold OR, the effects of cold solutions, and a consequence of some anesthetics. The heat loss that occurs in the OR can continue in the PACU if the patient is not warmed sufficiently. Warm blankets are used, especially around the feet; adding warmth around the head is helpful. A newer method is convective warming therapy, in which a disposable cover inflated with warm air from a heating unit is placed over the patient; warm air passes out through the underside, so the warm air is constantly

Table 2-7	Interventions Associated with the ABCS of Immediate Recovery
ASSESSMENT MODE	**INTERVENTION**
A: Airway	Maintain patency: keep head tilted up and back; may position on side with the face down and the neck slightly extended.
	Note presence or absence of gag or swallowing reflex; stay at bedside until gag reflex returns.
	Suction until awake and alert.
	Provide oxygen if necessary.
B: Breathing	Evaluate depth, rate, sounds, rhythm, and chest movement.
	Assess color of mucous membranes.
	Place hand above patient's nose to detect respirations if shallow.
	Initiate coughing and deep breathing exercises as soon as patient is able to respond.
	Chart time oxygen is discontinued.
	Monitor oxygen saturation levels (SaO_2) by pulse oximetry checks.
C: Consciousness	**Extubate** patient (remove endotracheal tube from airway).
	Patient responds to commands.
	Patient verbalizes responses.
	Patient reacts to stimuli.
C: Circulation	Monitor temperature, pulse, respirations, and blood pressure every 10 to 15 minutes; take axillary, tympanic, or rectal temperature if warranted.
	Assess rate, rhythm, and quality of pulse.
	Evaluate color and warmth of skin and color of nailbeds.
	Check peripheral pulses as indicated.
	Assess incision and dressing (monitor wound drainage output).
	Monitor intravenous lines: solution, rate, site.
	Cardiac monitors are usually in place for patients who had general anesthesia.
S: System review	Assess neurologic functions, muscle strength, and response.
	Monitor drains, tubes, and color and amount of output.
	Check for pressure, type, and condition of dressings.
	Evaluate pain response; may need to give analgesic and monitor patient response.
	Observe for allergic reactions.
	Assess urinary output if Foley catheter is in place.

moving. In the PACU, monitor the patient's temperature and vital signs every 15 minutes until vital signs are stable, or more frequently if they are unstable. The frequency and duration of monitoring are dictated by facility PACU policy. Patients are monitored until they are discharged from the PACU, usually at least 1 hour. Before discharge, their minimum temperature must be greater than 96.8° F (36° C). Warming requires the maintenance of temperature without overwarming and excessive vasodilation, which can cause fluid shifts and a decrease in blood pressure.

The PACU nurse must be aware that malignant hyperthermia can occur in the PACU and repeatedly assess the patient for signs of this condition. Malignant hyperthermia is a genetic disorder characterized by uncontrolled skeletal muscle contractions leading to potentially fatal hyperthermia. It occurs in patients predisposed to the disorder when they receive a combination of certain anesthetic agents. Unless the triggering event is stopped and the body is cooled, death results.

LATER POSTOPERATIVE PHASE

Immediate Assessments

When the patient returns to the nursing unit, a thorough postsurgical assessment follows. Review vital signs, the IV and incisional sites, any tubes, and postoperative orders. A review of each body system identifies when body functions return and provides a guideline

for further assessments. Unless otherwise indicated, monitor vital signs and make general assessments using the "times-four" factor—every 15 minutes times 4 (for 4 hours); every 30 minutes times 4; every hour times 4; then every 4 hours, or until assessments are within expected ranges. The times-four gauge is the maximal time that should elapse between assessments. Table 2-8 details body temperature responses to surgery. A postoperative flow sheet (Figure 2-14) is frequently used to document the patient's progress. Significant observations are critical for the patient after surgery.

Although the patient may respond, the level of functioning is impaired. Keep the side rails up and the call light within reach. Until the patient is fully conscious, do not place a pillow under the head. Either position the patient on the side, depending on the type of surgery, or raise the head of the bed to a 45-degree angle. Positioning the head higher than the chest reduces the chance of the patient aspirating vomitus. Because nausea and vomiting are normal in the first 12 to 24 hours, keep an emesis basin at the bedside. If the patient vomits, measure the amount and carefully describe it in the documentation. Report any red or coffee-ground emesis immediately. Frequently the patient remains on NPO status for the first few hours after surgery. Introduce fluids gradually. The physician usually orders ice chips followed by clear or full liquids.

Postoperative complications can occur suddenly; therefore note any change. Because the patient is often

---

Table 2-8	Temperature Assessment and Intervention
CAUSE	**ASSESSMENT AND INTERVENTION**
HYPOTHERMIA **Within First 12 Hours**	
Response to surgery, anesthesia, and body exposure	Monitor temperature readings. Assess for warmth. Provide warm blankets. Do not expose for long periods. Assess orientation.
HYPERTHERMIA **24-48 Hours**	
Dehydration Decreased lung activity Inflammatory response to surgery	Monitor temperature readings. Monitor intravenous rate. Encourage fluids. Assess intake and output (I&O). Have patient turn, cough, and breathe deeply. Provide incentive spirometer. Assess lung sounds. Observe incision.
After Day 2	
Infection: respiratory, wound, urinary, or circulatory	Monitor temperature readings. Assess lung sounds and expectoration of sputum. Evaluate incision and drainage. Monitor I&O. Encourage fluids of 6-8 oz/hr unless contraindicated. Note urine color, odor, amount, and consistency, and patient's complaints of burning on micturition. Perform leg exercises every 2 hours, and ambulate every 4 hours.

POST-OP ASSESSMENT FORM

SURGEON: *Dr. J. Bernard*	REPORT FROM: *S Welker RN*	ALLERGIES: *NKA*

Date: *1-27-10*	Anesthesia Note: *General*	PROCEDURE: *Reverse colostomy-sigmoid colostomy*
ARRIVAL ON FLOOR *1440*	BLOCK LEVEL: _____	
		CBI CREDIT ———— *resection (seg mem)*

PRE-OP MEDS	INTRA OP MEDS	POST OP MEDS	CBI INTAKE ————	IV FLUIDS & CREDITS
Versed 2 mg	*Fentanyl 250 mcg*	*Versed 1 mg*	OUTPUT *Foley 650 mL*	*NS – 125 mL*
pepcid 20 mg	*Flagyl 750 mg*	*Morphine 1 mg*		*700 mL*
	Zofran 4 g	*q 10 min/6 mg/*	DRAINS *Jackson Pratt* ∅ EBL	
			PACKS *NA* IV INTAKE *3300 mL*	

Time	BP-P-R		TEMP	PAIN INTENSITY 0-10	SAO₂	NURSING OBSERVATIONS
1440	144/83	84-12	96⁶	∅	95%	*1440 Returned from pacunit to Room 356 B per gurney—awake—alert—*
1500	166/82	86-16	96⁸	5	94%	*oriented x 4. Color pink—skin warm and dry. Normal saline infusing in left—*
1515	152/82	86-16			96%	*wrist @ 125 mL/hr with MS. PCA present. Site without edema or erythema.—*
1530	145/78	84-18	96⁹	4	96%	*Pedal pulses 4 bilaterally. Capillary refill < 2 seconds.———*
1545	140/79	86-16	96³	4	96%	*Lung sounds clear. O2 4L per nasal Cannula. Incentive spirometer to 1500 mL.—*
1600	139/73	86-18	96⁴	4	97%	*Abd. dressings dry & intact ō SM am't of serosanguineous exudate. Area*
1630	144/80	87-18	96⁸	4	95%	*marked. Bowel sounds absent. 44 Jackson Pratt draining serosanguineous—*
1730	149/78	87-18	97²	4	90%	*exudate. Foley catheter draining light, yellow urine. TED hose on bilaterally—*
1830	129/71	86	97⁵	4	99%	*flowtrons in place.———*
						1600 active ROM to lower extremities.
						1730 Walked 100 feet ō assistance. C/o dizziness & nausea —
						returned to bed.
						1800 IV NS changed to D5 ½ NS @ 125 mL/hr. Site s̄
						erythema or edema. Luann Richardson SPN————
						1900 Above assessment remains unchanged. ———
						Luann Richardson SPN.

NURSING STAFF SIGNATURE AND INITIALS
LR Luann Richardson SPN

Great Plains Regional Medical Center
601 West Leota Street - P.O. Box 1167
North Platte, Nebraska 69103-1167

N-12 (Rev. 7/03)

topel

LABEL

FIGURE 2-14 Postoperative assessment form.

Box 2-8	Possible Causes of Postoperative Shock

- Movement of patient from operating table to gurney
- Patient (gurney) being jarred during transport
- Reactions to drugs and anesthesia
- Loss of blood and other body fluids
- Cardiac dysrhythmias
- Cardiac failure
- Inadequate ventilation
- Pain

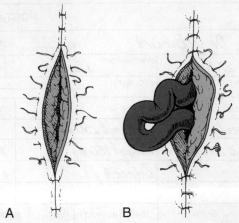

A   B

FIGURE 2-15 A, Wound dehiscence. **B,** Evisceration.

cold, provide additional blankets for comfort, without leading to sweating. Vital signs, coupled with the patient's behavior, are first-line observations. A pulse that increases and becomes thready—coupled with a declining blood pressure, cool and clammy skin, reduced urinary output, and restlessness—may signal hypovolemic shock. Hypovolemic shock in the postoperative period is frequently caused by internal hemorrhage, a life-threatening emergency (Box 2-8). A drop in blood pressure slightly below a patient's preoperative baseline reading is common after surgery. However, a significant drop in blood pressure, accompanied by an increased heart rate, may indicate hemorrhage, circulatory failure, or fluid shifts. Do not diagnose impending hypovolemic shock on the basis of one low blood pressure reading. If you are concerned about a dropping blood pressure, measure pressure every 5 minutes for 15 minutes to determine the variability. Decreased blood pressure can also mean that the anesthetic is wearing off or that the patient is experiencing severe pain.

In addition to hypotension, manifestations of shock include tachycardia; restlessness and apprehension; and cold, moist, pale, or cyanotic skin. When a patient appears to be going into shock, take the following steps: (1) administer oxygen or increase its rate of delivery, (2) raise the patient's legs above the level of the heart, (3) increase the rate of IV fluids (unless contraindicated because of fluid excretion problems), (4) notify the anesthesia provider and the surgeon, (5) provide medications as ordered, and (6) continue to assess the patient and response to interventions.

Incision

Monitor the incisional dressing, since bleeding or excessive drainage may also signal postoperative hemorrhage. Normally dressings are not changed but are reinforced during the first 24 hours. To accurately measure the amount of drainage, circle the drainage markings on the dressing and write the time and date. **Dehiscence** (the separation of a surgical incision or rupture of a wound closure) may occur 3 days to more than 2 weeks postoperatively. Wound separation in the first 3 days is usually related to technical factors, such as the sutures. Separation from 3 to 14 days postoperatively is usually associated with postoperative complications such as distention, vomiting, excessive coughing, dehydration, or infection. Wound separation after

2 weeks is usually associated with metabolic factors, such as **cachexia** (ill health, malnutrition, and wasting as a result of chronic disease), hypoproteinemia, increased age, malignancy, radiation therapy, and obesity. Wound **evisceration** (protrusion of an internal organ through a wound or surgical incision, especially in the abdominal wall) may also occur. Both wound dehiscence and evisceration require prompt attention (Figure 2-15). If the patient feels a sudden "give," sutures may have broken. Contact the physician immediately. Cover the wound with a sterile towel moistened with sterile physiological saline (warm). Tension on the abdomen may be decreased by placing the patient in Fowler's position with the knees slightly flexed. Reassure the patient regarding the situation, and tell him or her that surgery will be required. Prepare the patient for surgery. Sterile technique procedures—including dressing change and care of the surgical incision with phases of wound healing—are discussed in Chapters 12 and 13 in *Foundations of Nursing*.

Ventilation

Immediate postoperative hypoventilation can result from drugs (anesthetics, narcotics, tranquilizers, sedatives), incisional pain, obesity, chronic lung disease, or pressure on the diaphragm. Inadequate ventilation leads to hypoxemia. Monitor arterial oxygenation saturation (SaO_2), either by arterial blood gas measurements or by pulse oximetry.

Because lung ventilation is vital, help the patient turn, cough, and breathe deeply every 1 to 2 hours until the chest is clear. Having practiced this combination preoperatively, the patient is usually able to adequately remove trapped mucus and surgical gases. To ease the pressure on the incision, help the patient support the surgical site with a pillow, rolled bath blanket, or the heel of the hand. Administer analgesics, as prescribed, to control pain before coughing and deep breathing exercises. Early mobility and frequent position changes facilitate secretion clearance and improve the ventilation and perfusion in the lungs. Respiratory infections are frequently caused by shallow breathing and poor coughing. Listen for wheezing or crowing sounds from patients who have undergone head or neck surgery; this response occurs when edema places pressure over the trachea, resulting in respiratory insufficiency.

If the patient feels chest pain or has a fever, productive cough, or dyspnea, **atelectasis** (an abnormal condition characterized by the collapse of lung tissue) or pneumonia may be developing. Sudden chest pain along with dyspnea, tachycardia, cyanosis, diaphoresis, and hypotension is a sign of a pulmonary embolism. Raise the head of the bed to decrease dyspnea, and immediately report signs and symptoms. Frequently oxygen therapy is instituted to assist with breathing.

Whenever air exchange is reduced, postoperative recovery slows. Medication, suctioning, and oxygen therapy may be needed to assist the patient in respiratory distress. Mechanical devices, such as incentive spirometers, are used to stimulate deep breathing (see Skill 2-2). Frequently the incentive spirometer is used when the patient can deep breathe independently; the instrument visually measures the amount of air inhaled. Volume-oriented spirometers assist patients in deep breathing. Patients are encouraged to take 10 deep breaths every hour while awake.

If respiratory complications develop, the physician may order respiratory therapy to provide intermittent positive pressure breathing (IPPB) treatments to deliver a mixture of air and oxygen; medication can be added to enhance respirations. Chest percussion and postural drainage—a form of chest physiotherapy that combines positioning and percussion movements to lung areas to help dislodge and move secretions—are also used. Do not leave patients unattended during postural drainage, since they may experience respiratory distress.

Pain
Internal organs do not have many nerve endings, but a skin incision produces painful responses. Because pain is normal postoperatively, offer patients prescribed analgesics. Ask patients every 3 to 4 hours if they need something for pain because some patients will not ask for an analgesic. Acute pain begins to subside within 24 to 48 hours, and pain medication is adjusted as necessary. In the early stages of recovery, comfort interventions help ease pain. Anxiety may affect pain perception. After the acute phase, comfort measures may be the only interventions required (Box 2-9).

A patient's level of pain can be difficult to evaluate. Ask the patient to rate the pain on a scale of 0 to 10. There are standard pain indexes (restlessness, moaning, grimacing, diaphoresis), but some patients may not outwardly exhibit signs. Objective pain factors are signs that the body is responding to "pain"; these include vital sign changes (blood pressure lowers in the immediate postoperative period and elevates in response to

---

Box 2-9 **Postoperative Comfort Measures for Pain**

DECREASE EXTERNAL STIMULI
- Darken room; close drapes.
- Keep TV and radio off or low.
- Monitor hall traffic and noise.
- Assess staff interruptions.
- Check room for noise—dripping water, buzzing lights, constant intercom messages.

REDUCE INTERRUPTIONS
- Plan care to allow rest.
- Post "Do Not Disturb" sign.
- Unplug telephone.
- Restrict visitors.
- Pull curtains around bed.

ELIMINATE ODORS
- Discuss offending odors and assess elimination.
- Remove from room all dressings that are soiled with exudate.
- Post "No Smoking" sign.
- Alert housekeeping to omit room-cleaning products.
- Install air-circulating unit.
- Alert dietary department to reduce foods with odors.

NURSING INTERVENTIONS
- Ask patient about normal relaxation patterns and practices.
- Have patient practice deep-breathing and relaxation techniques.
- Plan rest periods.
- Provide back rub.
- Engage patient in conversation; ask about concerns and fears.
- Encourage diversional activities.
- Reposition and support with pillows, bed rolls.
- Check tube placement.
- Offer warm fluids if indicated.
- Reduce room clutter.
- Provide restful environment.

---

pain after about 12 hours, and pulse increases), restlessness, diaphoresis, and pallor. The patient's description of discomfort represents subjective pain factors. The way the pain affects the patient emotionally is termed **suffering.** Pain behaviors are influenced by the patient's culture and past experiences. Behaviors include moaning, grimacing, and favoring a body area.

The effectiveness of analgesic measures differs with each person; if relief is not obtained, changing the medication or administration schedule may provide effective pain control. Each patient interprets pain differently and has a personal pain tolerance level. Remember that only the patient bearing the pain is an expert about that pain. McCaffery and Pasero (1999) states, "Pain is whatever the experiencing person says it is, existing whenever he says it does."

The success of pain management depends on the surgery, the patient's emotional state, and postopera-

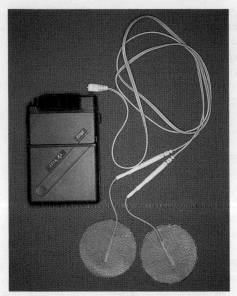

FIGURE 2-16 Transcutaneous electric nerve stimulation (TENS) unit.

tive complications. Patients experiencing chronic pain may have more difficulty obtaining relief than individuals with acute episodes. Commonly used analgesic measures are nurse-administered narcotics, patient-controlled IV medications (see Chapter 16 in *Foundations of Nursing*), and pain control via a transcutaneous electric nerve stimulation (TENS) unit (Figure 2-16). Attached to the skin, the TENS unit applies electric impulses to the nerve endings and blocks transmission of pain signals to the brain. The PCA system is a pump that is programmed to dispense only a given amount of medication. The patient can self-administer an analgesic by pressing a control button. Monitor the PCA system every 3 to 4 hours.

Urinary Function
Anesthesia retards urinary function. Assess the bladder area every 2 hours for distention and changes in renal function. It routinely takes 6 to 8 hours for voiding to occur after surgery. If patients do not void within 8 hours, catheterization may be necessary, but it should be used as a last measure. Have the patient listen to running water, place the hands in warm water, or walk to the bathroom, if able, to facilitate voiding. Helping male patients stand often encourages voiding. Serum blood urea nitrogen may be measured daily until patient has recovered. Usually I&O are measured while a Foley catheter is in place, while the patient is receiving IV therapy, and immediately after a Foley catheter has been removed. Continue urine measurement until the patient is voiding without difficulty.

Fluid deficit may result from inadequate replacement of body fluids lost during surgery or from continued fluid losses. Fluid excess may occur from large amounts of IV fluids when kidney function is inadequate (evidenced by oliguria). A urinary output of 30 mL per hour is considered acceptable postoperatively. Unless the patient has had urinary tract surgery, urine should be clear and yellow and have an ammonia odor.

Venous Stasis
Venous stasis (a disorder in which the normal flow of fluid through a vessel of the body is slowed or halted) is the underlying cause of thrombus formation. Performing leg exercises every 2 hours and using intermittent pneumatic compression devices and compression stockings aid the circulatory system and help prevent deep-vein thrombosis. Assessment of the feet and legs includes palpating for pedal pulse and noting the skin's color and temperature. If edema, aching or cramping, sensitivity, or pain occurs in the calf (Homans' sign) or leg, the patient will complain of calf pain on dorsiflexion of the foot, and a thrombus should be suspected. Have the patient remain in bed until the physician can perform an evaluation. Teach the patient not to cross legs when in bed, and encourage sitting up as another means of preventing venous stasis. Do not use a knee gatch.

Surgical patients are at the greatest risk of developing life-threatening deep-vein thrombosis and pulmonary embolism. Not only does surgery injure blood vessels, but anesthesia and inactivity also cause venous stasis. Surgery, however, is not the only risk factor. Others include pregnancy, myocardial infarction, heart failure, stroke (brain attack), cancer, sepsis, and immobility. The most effective method of preventing deep-vein thrombosis is with low-dose subcutaneous heparin therapy. Heparin is an anticoagulant but is contraindicated in trauma and general surgery patients. Antiembolism stockings and ambulation are also useful preventive measures.

The external intermittent pneumatic compression system (SCD) (see Skill 2-5) is used on patients who are at risk of developing deep-vein thrombosis and pulmonary embolism. This device includes an air pressure pump and cuffs, one for each calf or foot. Continuous inflation and deflation of the cuffs decreases pooling of venous blood in the legs and improves venous return to the heart. The pressure cuffs automatically inflate to 40 mm Hg or the prescribed setting and deflate in cycles, with inflation lasting about 12 seconds and deflation lasting about 48 seconds. This system is contraindicated for any patient with acute thrombophlebitis or deep-vein thrombosis.

When ambulating the patient, disconnect the pump tubing, although sometimes the cuffs are kept in place on the calves. Do not disconnect the device for more than 30 minutes. If the patient has diagnostic examinations that require leaving the nursing unit for longer than 30 minutes, the compression pump, the cuffs or sleeves, and the instructions on operation should travel with the patient.

The treatment continues for 72 hours postoperatively or until the patient is ambulating well. Remove the cuffs once a day to assess skin integrity and provide skin care. Document the use of the intermittent external pneumatic compression system and any reaction such as numbness or tingling (see Figure 2-5).

Activity

Early ambulation is a significant factor in hastening postoperative recovery and preventing postoperative complications. The exercise of getting in and out of bed and walking during the early postoperative period has numerous benefits (Box 2-10). Ambulation is usually contraindicated for patients with severe infection or thrombophlebitis.

Assessment

Before helping the patient ambulate for the first few times after major surgery, assess the following:

1. Level of alertness: Ask the patient simple questions or to follow simple commands.
2. Cardiovascular status (orthostatic hypotension)
   a. Assess pulse and respiratory rate and depth while patient is supine, then after sitting.
   b. Observe skin color for pallor while patient is sitting.
   c. Note complaints of vertigo while patient is sitting.
3. Motor status
   a. Assess muscle strength of patient's legs.
   b. Assess sitting ability.
      (1) Help patient to sitting position on side of bed.
      (2) Ask patient to maintain an erect position while being gently pushed sideways.

It is also important to know of any preoperative limitations to ambulation. The patient with arthritis or arteriosclerosis may take longer to move and to adjust to standing and walking. The patient who used a walker preoperatively needs assistance for a longer time before using the walker again. Family members are important in assisting patients with any physical limitation and in providing emotional support during postoperative recovery.

Nursing Interventions

Nursing interventions are as follows:

1. Encourage muscle-strengthening exercises before ambulation:
   a. Have patient bend knees, lower knees, press back of knees hard against bed.
   b. Have patient alternately contract and relax calf and thigh muscles 10 times using the following cycle: contract, relax, rest.
2. Have patient sit on side of bed (legs dangling) to become accustomed to upright position before ambulating the first time. Be certain that pulse has stabilized (returned to baseline) before patient attempts ambulation.
3. Clamp NG tube while patient ambulates, and then reconnect.
4. Keep urinary tube connected to drainage bag; carry bag or pin bag to inside of robe. Keep drainage receptacle below level of bladder to prevent reflux of urine.
5. Attach IV bag to a movable pole.
6. Use two people to assist in ambulating an unsteady patient receiving IV fluids (Figure 2-17).
7. Encourage patient to walk farther at each ambulation.

Box 2-10	Effects of Early Postoperative Ambulation

- Increased rate and depth of breathing
  —Prevention of atelectasis and hypostatic pneumonia
  —Increased mental alertness from increased oxygenation to brain
- Increased circulation
  —Nutrients required for healing are more available to wound
  —Prevention of thrombophlebitis
- Increased micturition (urinary elimination)
  —Increased kidney function
  —Prevention of urinary retention
- Increased metabolism
  —Prevention of loss of muscle tone
  —Restoration of nitrogen balance
- Increased peristalsis
  —Promotion of expulsion of flatus
  —Prevention of abdominal distention and gas pain
  —Prevention of constipation
  —Prevention of paralytic ileus

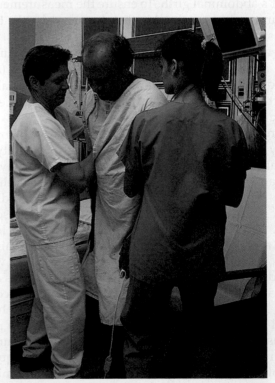

FIGURE 2-17 Progression in levels of postoperative activity promotes tissue perfusion.

The word *ambulate* means to move from place to place—to walk. Sitting in a chair is not ambulation. After ambulating, the patient may sit in a chair, but should be advised to stand and walk at intervals and to elevate the legs while sitting to prevent venous pooling in the extremities. The patient should avoid sitting in a chair for long periods. Also see Chapter 15 in *Foundations of Nursing*.

GASTROINTESTINAL STATUS

Abdominal distention frequently occurs after surgery. Because anesthesia and surgical manipulation slow peristalsis, it may take 3 or 4 days for bowel activity to return. Ask the patient if he or she is nauseated or hungry (a more accurate assessment of gastrointestinal activity than the presence of bowel sounds). Listening for bowel sounds in the lower abdomen can help gauge the return of function. Normal peristalsis is indicated by hearing 5 to 30 gurgles per minute. Listen for bowel sounds in all four quadrants for 1 minute. A **paralytic ileus** (a decrease in or absence of intestinal peristalsis that may occur after abdominal surgery, peritoneal trauma, severe metabolic disease, and other conditions) may also develop. If inactivity continues, the physician usually orders an NG or nasointestinal tube to be placed to help remove the gas formed in the stomach and small intestine. When listening for bowel sounds in patients who have an NG or nasointestinal tube, turn off the suction machine but *never* leave the room without turning the machine back on.

Verify abdominal distention by measuring the patient's abdominal girth. To ensure the measurement is accurate, mark on the skin the placement for the tape measure, which is at the level of the umbilicus. Assess and chart the expelling of flatus, bowel sounds, and abdominal girth. Occasionally analgesics (meperidine) and other medications may slow peristalsis; charting the patient's GI habits helps identify etiologic factors.

Encouraging movement (turning every 2 hours, early ambulation) assists in restoring GI activity. A rectal tube may be inserted, or the physician may order an "up and down" flush (Harris flush) to relieve pain from intestinal gas. A Harris flush is a mild colonic irrigation using 100 to 200 mL of enema solution. After instillation, the enema container is lowered and the solution siphoned back into the container. This process may be repeated. For the patient who has difficulty with flatus, limiting iced beverages and offering warm liquids may help resolve the discomfort. The patient may have fluids and food withheld until flatus is expelled. As the patient returns to previous eating habits, bowel function slowly resumes its preoperative state. Constipation is also a frequent problem after surgery. The same aids for abdominal distention assist in alleviating constipation. If the patient does not pass feces within 2 or 3 days after resuming solid foods, a suppository or tap water enema may be ordered. Again, encourage ambulation to promote peristalsis.

Singultus (hiccup) is an involuntary contraction of the diaphragm followed by rapid closure of the glottis. Singultus results from irritation of the phrenic nerve. The condition is seen most often in men. Sedatives may be necessary in extreme cases. Because abdominal distention may be the cause, assess the patient's abdomen for proper GI function. Abdominal distention usually is caused by gas in the intestinal tract, but may be related to internal bleeding. Evaluate the patient for signs of shock, vital signs, skin condition, and level of consciousness.

FLUIDS AND ELECTROLYTES

Fluid is lost during surgery through blood loss and increased insensible fluid loss through the lungs and skin. For at least the first 24 to 48 hours after surgery, the body retains fluids as part of the stress response to trauma and the effect of anesthesia.

Sodium and potassium depletion can occur after surgery as a result of the loss of blood or body fluids during surgery or the loss of GI secretion because of vomiting and NG tubes. Potassium is also lost during **catabolism** (tissue breakdown), especially after severe trauma or crush injuries. Loss of gastric secretions can result in chloride loss, producing metabolic alkalosis. Electrolytes are often added to the IV solution in the form of potassium chloride (KCl). However, potassium may irritate the vein when administered by an IV route. Advise the patient that a stinging sensation may occur.

Closely monitor fluid tolerance and electrolyte values during the postoperative period. When the patient returns from the recovery room, therapy will be in progress. Until the patient is past the nausea and vomiting period and can tolerate oral fluids, maintain parenteral therapy. Observe the IV line for patency and ordered fluid rate, and monitor the IV site for erythema, edema, heat, and pain. The IV solution may become infiltrated because of movement or inadvertent dislodgment of the needle when the patient ambulates; therefore it is necessary to assess the site every 1 to 2 hours or when the patient complains of discomfort. The assessment for rate of infusion is extremely important for older patients, who may quickly experience fluid overload and pulmonary edema.

Muscles and nerves require ongoing nourishment to function adequately, and parenteral fluids contain the necessary glucose and electrolytes. Depending on the type of surgery and the patient's nutritional needs, IV therapy lasts from a few hours to a few days. As long as the patient is receiving parenteral fluids, record the patient's I&O. If the patient's overall nutritional state is in question, weigh the patient daily. Also see Chapter 22 in *Foundations of Nursing*.

As oral fluids are introduced, encourage patients to drink small amounts frequently (6 to 8 ounces per hour). Review the diet history to note fluids normally enjoyed. Unless otherwise ordered, patients usually begin by ingesting clear liquids (7-Up, water, tea, broth, gelatin) and progress as the GI system returns to normal functioning. If the patient has difficulty drinking the amount of fluid recommended, offer fluids more frequently and without a straw. (A straw, although convenient, reduces the amount of fluids ingested.) Unless the patient has other problems (e.g., decreased renal excretion because of renal failure or advanced age), encourage the patient to drink 2000 to 2400 mL in 24 hours. Because iced and carbonated beverages cause GI disturbances in some individuals, patients should avoid these fluids until active peristalsis is noted. If nausea and vomiting persist, an antiemetic such as promethazine (Phenergan), benzquinamide (Emete-Con), or prochlorperazine (Compazine) is usually ordered to be administered intravenously or rectally.

❖ NURSING PROCESS *for the Surgical Patient*

The role of the licensed practical nurse/licensed vocational nurse (LPN/LVN) in the nursing process is that the LPN/LVN will:

- Participate in planning care for patients based on patient needs
- Review patients' care plans and recommend revisions as needed
- Review and follow defined prioritization for patient care
- Use clinical pathways, care maps, or care plans to guide and review patient care

▪ Assessment

General assessment of the preoperative patient includes obtaining a nursing history. This consists of any prior surgery, allergies, current medications, use of other drugs or alcohol, and smoking status. Also assess the patient's physical condition, at-risk data, emotional status of the patient and family members, and preoperative diagnostic data. It is important for the patient and family to understand the surgical procedure and the expected outcomes. In the intraoperative stage, complete any procedures such as skin preparation or catheterization. During surgery and recovery, continually assess the patient's condition. Also provide postoperative care to prevent and detect complications and return the patient to wellness.

▪ Nursing Diagnosis

Nursing diagnoses establish direction for the care that is provided during one or all surgical phases (Boxes 2-11 and 2-12). Nursing diagnoses may focus on preoperative, intraoperative, and postoperative risks. Preventive care is essential for effective management of the surgical patient.

| Box 2-11 | Preoperative Nursing Diagnoses |

- **Airway clearance, ineffective,** related to:
  —Diminished cough
  —Increased pulmonary congestion
- **Anxiety (specify level),** related to:
  —Knowledge deficit of impending surgery
  —Threat of loss of body part
- **Coping, compromised family,** related to:
  —Temporary role change of patient
  —Impending severity of surgery
- **Fear,** related to:
  —Impending surgery
  —Anticipation of postoperative pain
- **Knowledge, deficient regarding implications of surgery,** related to:
  —Lack of experience with surgery
  —Information misinterpretation
- **Nutrition, imbalanced: less than body requirements,** related to:
  —Preoperative malnourishment
- **Nutrition, imbalanced: more than body requirements,** related to:
  —Excess intake of food
- **Powerlessness,** related to:
  —Emergency nature of surgery
- **Skin integrity, risk for impaired,** related to:
  —Preoperative radiation
  —Immobilization during surgery
- **Sleep deprivation,** related to:
  —Fear of surgery
  —Preoperative hospital routines

▪ Expected Outcomes and Planning

The care plan begins before surgery and follows through the postoperative period to provide the best nursing interventions possible. It is important to include the patient in health care planning. A patient informed about the surgical experience is less likely to be fearful and is better able to prepare for expected outcomes.

Goals and expected outcomes for the surgical patient may include the following:

Goal: Patient achieves physical comfort.
Outcome: Patient verbalizes relief of pain.

▪ Implementation

Nursing interventions before surgery physically and psychologically prepare the patient for the surgical procedure. Act as an advocate for the patient during and after surgery to ensure that the patient's dignity and rights are protected at all times (Nursing Care Plan 2-1).

▪ Evaluation

Evaluate the effectiveness of the care plan and revise the plan as needed. An example of a goal and an evaluative measure is the following:

Goal: Patient achieves physical comfort.
Evaluative measure: Observe patient for nonverbal signs of discomfort, such as guarding the painful area and grimacing.

Box 2-12 **Postoperative Nursing Diagnoses**

- **Airway clearance, ineffective,** related to:
  —Diminished cough
  —Retained secretions
  —Prolonged sedation
- **Body temperature, hypothermia,** related to:
  —Lowered metabolism
- **Breathing pattern, ineffective,** related to:
  —Incisional pain
  —Analgesia effects on ventilation
- **Communication, impaired verbal,** related to:
  —Endotracheal tube placement
  —Airway tube placement
- **Coping, ineffective,** related to:
  —Constraints imposed by surgery
  —Postoperative therapies
- **Fluid volume, risk for deficient,** related to:
  —Wound drainage
  —Inadequate fluid intake
- **Grieving, anticipatory,** related to:
  —Patient's critical condition
- **Infection, risk for,** related to:
  —Surgical wound incision
  —Presence of Foley catheter and wound drainage tubes
- **Mobility, impaired bed,** related to:
  —Pain
  —Postoperative activity restrictions
  —Casts or dressings
  —Surgical incision
  —Nasogastric (NG) tube placement
- **Oral mucous membrane, impaired,** related to:
  —Irritation of NG or endotracheal tube
  —NPO status
- **Self-care deficit, bathing/hygiene, dressing/grooming, feeding, toileting,** related to:
  —Postoperative activity restrictions
  —Pain
- **Skin integrity, risk for impaired,** related to:
  —Wound exudate
  —Impaired mobility
  —Decrease in nutritional intake

⭐ Nursing Care Plan 2-1 **The Postoperative Patient**

Mr. Sanders is a 40-year-old obese patient weighing 280 lb, who was admitted with bowel obstruction and a scheduled right hemicolectomy. Mr. Sanders has hypertension and a history of poor wound healing.

NURSING DIAGNOSIS *Ineffective airway clearance, related to incisional pain*

Patient Goals and Expected Outcomes	Nursing Interventions	Evaluation and Rationale
Patient will cough deeply in 24 hours	Medicate with analgesia to control pain.	Providing pain relief enables patient to cough and breathe deeply without discomfort.
Patient's lung sounds will clear after coughing	Raise head of bed to full Fowler's position during exercises.	In Fowler's position the diaphragm falls, which permits lung expansion.
	Splint incision with rolled bath blanket.	Splinting incision provides abdominal support during coughing.
	Have patient turn, cough, and deep breathe every hour while awake.	Turning, coughing, and deep breathing aid in mobilizing secretions.
	Use incentive spirometer hourly.	Adequate lung expansion can prevent atelectasis.
	Take vital signs q4h and note evidence of dyspnea or restlessness.	
	Monitor intravenous fluids.	
	Offer sips of fluid every hour if permissible.	Increased fluid intake helps prevent thickening of mucus.

NURSING DIAGNOSIS *Ineffective breathing pattern, related to poor body mechanics*

Patient Goals and Expected Outcomes	Nursing Interventions	Evaluation and Rationale
Patient will effectively use incentive spirometer	Encourage deep breathing q1-2h while awake.	Adequate lung expansion helps prevent atelectasis.
Patient's respirations will be even and unlabored	Reposition q2h; support joints and incision.	Turning promotes lung expansion.
	Continue oxygen at 2 L per cannula; cleanse nares q4h; post "No Smoking" sign.	Additional oxygen ensures adequate tissue oxygenation. "No Smoking" sign promotes safety.
	Encourage use of incentive spirometer.	Adequate lung expansion helps prevent atelectasis.

Nursing Care Plan 2-1   The Postoperative Patient—cont'd

Patient Goals and Expected Outcomes	Nursing Interventions	Evaluation and Rationale
	Record respirations q4h, noting depth, rate, and quality.	Regular assessments helps detect early signs and symptoms of respiratory complications. A change in color of skin and nailbeds signals poor oxygenation.
	Assess skin and nailbed q4h; report slow blanching color and condition.	
	Darken room; decrease stimuli, monitor pain, and offer analgesic prn.	Comfort measures promote rest and relaxation and decrease pain level.

NURSING DIAGNOSIS *Risk for infection, related to open surgical incision and draining wound*

Patient Goals and Expected Outcomes	Nursing Interventions	Evaluation and Rationale
Patient's wound will not be erythematous or produce purulent exudate	Use good handwashing technique.	Handwashing helps prevent transmission of microorganisms.
Patient's vital signs will remain within normal range	Monitor wound q4h, noting amount and color of drainage; assess skin for warmth, color, and sensation.	Regular assessments reveals early signs and symptoms of wound infection.
	Mark drainage on dressing q4h; reinforce prn.	Containing wound drainage within dressing provides comfort to the patient and enables the nurse to correctly determine the type of drainage.
	Use surgical asepsis when changing dressing.	Surgical asepsis prevents the transmission of microorganisms.
	Monitor vital signs q4h.	Regular assessments of vital signs reveal early signs and symptoms of wound infection.
	Monitor white blood cell (WBC) level as ordered.	Elevation of WBCs indicates an infectious process and its severity.

Critical Thinking Questions

1. On the second postoperative day, Mr. Sanders is taking shallow breaths and having difficulty complying with coughing and deep breathing. His temperature is 101.8° F (38.8° C), and he has adventitious breath sounds bilaterally in the bases. List several nursing interventions to assist Mr. Sanders.
2. In his third postoperative day Mr. Sanders has an erythematous incision with moderate amounts of purulent exudate from the Penrose drain site. List the correct nursing interventions.
3. What signs and symptoms would the nurse note when assessing Mr. Sanders for dehydration secondary to elevated temperature and decreased fluid intake?

DISCHARGE: PROVIDING GENERAL INFORMATION

Preparation for the patient's discharge is an ongoing process throughout the surgical experience, beginning during the preoperative period. The informed patient is therefore prepared as events unfold and gradually assumes greater responsibility for self-care during the postoperative period. As discharge approaches, be certain the patient has vital information (Box 2-13). If the physician has not provided information about diet or activity prescriptions or restrictions, either obtain this information or encourage the patient to do so. Attention to complete discharge instruction may prevent needless distress for the patient. Written instructions

are important for reinforcing verbal information. Specifically document in the record the discharge instructions provided to the patient and family (Figure 2-18). Document information related to patient's mental status (ability to understand importance of teaching for patient and family members). For the patient, the postoperative phase of care continues into the recuperative period. Assessment and evaluation of the patient after discharge may involve a follow-up call or a visit from a home health nurse.

AMBULATORY SURGERY DISCHARGE

The patient leaving an ambulatory surgery setting must be able to provide a degree of self-care and must be mobile and alert. Postoperative pain and nausea and

Box 2-13   **Vital Information for the Discharged Patient**

- Care of wound site and any dressings
- Action and possible side effects of any medications; when and how to take them
- Activities allowed and prohibited; when various physical activities can be resumed safely (e.g., driving a car, return to work, sexual intercourse, leisure activities)
- Dietary restrictions or modifications
- Symptoms to be reported (e.g., development of incisional tenderness or increased drainage, discomfort in other parts of the body)
- Where and when to return for follow-up care
- Answers to any individual questions or concerns (allow time for questions)

vomiting must be controlled. Overall, the patient must be stable and near the same level of functioning as before surgery. On discharge, give the patient and family both specific and general instructions—verbally and reinforced with written directions. The patient may not drive and must be accompanied by a responsible adult at the time of discharge. Telephone the patient for a follow-up evaluation and to address any specific questions and concerns.

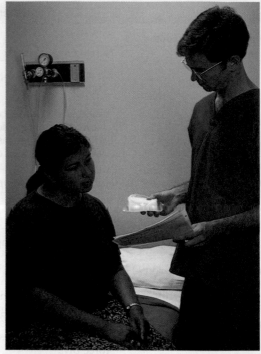

FIGURE 2-18 Reviewing discharge planning instructions.

Get Ready for the NCLEX® Examination!

Key Points

- The time before, during, and after surgery is the perioperative period. It is divided into preoperative, intraoperative, and postoperative phases.
- Perioperative nursing interventions take place before, during, and after surgery.
- The ability to tolerate surgery is influenced by nursing interventions, previous illness, and past surgeries.
- Older adult patients are at surgical risk from their declining physiologic status.
- All medications taken before surgery are automatically discontinued after surgery unless a physician reorders the medications, except for medications for long-term conditions such as phenytoin for seizure control.
- Family members are important in assisting patients with physical limitations and in providing emotional support during the postoperative recovery.
- Preoperative assessment of vital signs and physical findings provides an important baseline for comparing perioperative and postoperative assessment data.
- A patient's feelings about surgery can have a significant effect on relationships with nursing staff and the patient's ability to participate in care.
- Nursing diagnoses of the surgical patient may require interventions during one or all phases of surgery.
- Informed consent should not be obtained if a patient is confused, unconscious, mentally incompetent, or under the influence of sedatives. Know agency policy.
- Structured preoperative teaching positively influences postoperative recovery.

- A routine preoperative checklist is a guide for final preparation of the patient before surgery.
- Nurses in the OR focus on protecting the patient from potential harm.
- Assessment of the postoperative patient centers on the body systems most likely to be affected by anesthesia, immobilization, and surgical trauma.
- Because a surgical patient's condition may change rapidly during immediate postoperative recovery, monitor the patient's status at least every 15 minutes.
- The PACU nurse reports to the nurse on the postoperative unit information pertaining to the patient's current physical status and risk for postoperative complications.
- From the time of admission, plan for the surgical patient's discharge.
- Discharge planning identifies home care measures to promote recovery that involve both patient and family.
- Evaluation of all perioperative care is at times difficult, since the patient may be discharged from the nurse's care before the outcome is certain.

Additional Learning Resources

Go to your Companion CD for an audio glossary, animations, video clips, and more.

evolve Be sure to visit the Evolve site at http://evolve.elsevier.com/ Christensen/adult/ for additional online resources.

Review Questions for the NCLEX® Examination

1. The patient has cancer of the larynx and is scheduled for a laryngectomy. This is an example of which type of surgery?
   1. Minor
   2. Elective
   3. Emergency
   4. Major

2. The patient is being discharged, and the nurse is teaching her how to do daily dressing changes at home. The most important point to include in the teaching plan is:
   1. discussion of surgical asepsis.
   2. discussion of hand hygiene.
   3. instruction in sterilization.
   4. demonstration of gloving.

3. To assist the patient in the prevention of postoperative pulmonary complications, preoperatively the nurse should:
   1. ask his physician to prescribe IPPB treatment.
   2. teach him to do leg exercises.
   3. teach him to use an incentive spirometer.
   4. tell him that if he does not cough, he may need to be suctioned.

4. The patient underwent surgery for lysis of adhesions. He is transferred from the PACU to his own room on the surgical floor. During the immediate postoperative period on the surgical floor, measure blood pressure, pulse, and respirations every:
   1. 15 minutes.
   2. 5 minutes.
   3. 20 minutes.
   4. 30 minutes.

5. The nurse is assessing the bowel sounds of her patient who had a suprapubic prostatectomy 2 days ago. To determine that he does not have bowel sounds present, the nurse would need to auscultate each quadrant for:
   1. 1 minute.
   2. 3 minutes.
   3. 10 minutes.
   4. 15 minutes.

6. The patient is recovering from a right lobectomy. The nurse is going to assist in splinting the patient's incision so she can cough and breathe deeply. The most therapeutic administration of an analgesic would be:
   1. after the procedure so she can rest.
   2. 15 minutes before the procedure.
   3. 1 hour before the procedure.
   4. 30 minutes before the procedure.

7. A patient reports being allergic to penicillin. Which question would elicit the most useful information?
   1. When did the reaction occur?
   2. What infection did you have that required penicillin?
   3. What type of allergic reaction did you have?
   4. Did you notify your physician of the allergy?

8. Which patient is at greatest risk for surgical and anesthetic complications?
   1. A 3-year-old patient scheduled for hernia repair
   2. An 80-year-old patient scheduled for exploratory laparotomy
   3. An 18-year-old patient scheduled for emergency appendectomy
   4. A 42-year-old patient scheduled for breast biopsy

9. An alert 75-year-old patient is to undergo elective surgery. The operative permit must be signed in the presence of a witness by:
   1. the patient.
   2. the patient and the patient's spouse.
   3. either the patient or the patient's spouse.
   4. the patient and the surgeon.

10. A nursing intervention to help a patient cope with fear of pain would be to:
    1. describe the degree of pain expected.
    2. explain the availability of pain medication.
    3. inform the patient of the frequency of pain medication.
    4. divert the patient when talking about pain.

11. A patient tells the nurse that "blowing into this tube thing [incentive spirometer] is a waste of time." The nurse explains that the specific purpose of the therapy is to:
    1. directly remove excess secretions from the lungs.
    2. increase pulmonary circulation.
    3. promote lung expansion.
    4. stimulate the cough reflex.

12. When preparing a patient for surgery, the nurse should:
    1. provide sips of water for a dry mouth.
    2. remove the patient's makeup and nail polish.
    3. remove the patient's gown before transport to the OR.
    4. leave all of the patient's jewelry on.

13. A patient who is being prepped for surgery asks the nurse to explain the purpose of the preoperative medications he has been given. The nurse should inform the patient that these particular medications:
    1. reduce preoperative fear.
    2. promote gastric emptying.
    3. reduce body secretions.
    4. facilitate the induction of anesthesia.

14. A patient who receives general or regional anesthesia in an ambulatory surgery center:

    1. will remain in the unit longer than a hospitalized patient.
    2. is allowed to ambulate as soon as being admitted to the recovery area.
    3. must be near the level of preoperative functioning before dismissal.
    4. is immediately given liberal amounts of fluid to promote excretion of the anesthesia.

15. After abdominal surgery, a patient is suspected of having internal bleeding. Which finding is most indicative of this complication?

    1. Increased blood pressure
    2. Incisional pain
    3. Abdominal distention
    4. Increased urinary output

16. An obese patient is at risk for poor wound healing postoperatively because:

    1. ventilatory capacity is reduced.
    2. fatty tissue has a poor blood supply.
    3. the risk for dehiscence is increased.
    4. resuming normal physical activity is delayed.

17. The nurse should ask each patient preoperatively for the name and dosage of all prescription and over-the-counter medications (including herbal remedies) taken before surgery because they:

    1. may cause allergies to develop.
    2. are automatically ordered postoperatively.
    3. may create a greater risk for complications or interact with anesthetic agents.
    4. should be taken the morning of surgery with sips of water.

18. A patient who smokes two packs of cigarettes per day is most at risk postoperatively for:

    1. infection.
    2. pneumonia.
    3. hypotension.
    4. cardiac dysrhythmias.

19. Family members should be included when the nurse teaches the patient preoperative exercises so that they can:

    1. supervise the patient at home.
    2. coach the patient postoperatively.
    3. practice with the patient while waiting for transport to the OR.
    4. relieve the nurse by getting the patient to exercise every 2 hours.

20. When deep breathing and coughing, the patient should be sitting because this position:

    1. facilitates expansion of the thorax.
    2. is more comfortable.
    3. increases the patient's view of the room and is more relaxing.
    4. helps the patient to splint with a pillow.

21. The nurse is checking a patient 2 hours after he returns from surgery. Which assessment finding requires immediate attention?

    1. The nasogastric tube drained 50 mL of tea-colored urine.
    2. The patient's skin is pale, cool, and dry.
    3. The Foley catheter drained 30 mL of urine during the past 2 hours.
    4. The patient is drowsy, but responds promptly to voices.

22. A postoperative abdominal surgery patient complains that he "felt something give way" in his incision. On assessing the wound, the nurse notes a large amount of serosanguineous drainage and that wound edges are not approximated. Intestines are protruding from the wound. The nurse immediately:

    1. encourages the patient to turn, cough, and deep breathe while splinting the opening.
    2. covers the protruding internal organs with sterile gauze moistened with normal saline.
    3. paints the open wound with an antimicrobial solution to prevent infection.
    4. reinserts the organs and applies a pressure dressing to prevent further organ protrusion.

23. On admission of a patient to the PACU from surgery, the nurse places the highest priority on assessing the:

    1. patient's level of consciousness.
    2. condition of the surgical site.
    3. adequacy of airway and breathing.
    4. fluid and electrolyte balance.

24. The patient arrives on the unit after undergoing extensive abdominal surgery. He is awake and alert. He refuses to be repositioned in bed. What should the nurse assess first to determine the reason for the patient's refusal?

    1. Consciousness
    2. Maturation
    3. Knowledge related to complications of immobility
    4. Pain

25. The nurse is admitting a patient into the room on the surgical unit after abdominal surgery. There is a 1.5-cm–diameter spot of serosanguineous drainage on the dressing. What should the nurse do at this time?

    1. Notify the physician of bleeding from the wound.
    2. Note the amount of drainage and continue to monitor.
    3. Remove the dressing to check for bleeding from the suture line.
    4. Apply gentle pressure to the site for 5 minutes.

Care of the Patient with an Integumentary Disorder

Linda Y. North

Objectives

Anatomy and Physiology

1. Discuss the primary functions of the integumentary system.
2. Describe the differences between the epidermis and dermis.
3. Discuss the functions of the three major glands located in the skin.

Medical-Surgical

4. Discuss the general assessment of the skin.
5. Discuss the viral disorders of the skin.
6. Discuss the bacterial, fungal, and inflammatory disorders of the skin.
7. Identify the parasitic disorders of the skin.

8. Describe the common tumors of the skin.
9. Identify the disorders associated with the appendages of the skin.
10. State the pathophysiology involved in a burn injury.
11. Identify the methods used to classify the extent of a burn injury.
12. Discuss the stages of burn care with appropriate nursing interventions.
13. Discuss how to use the nursing process in caring for patients with skin disorders.
14. Identify general nursing interventions for the patient with a skin disorder.

Key Terms

alopecia (ăl-ō-PĒ-shē-ă, p. 94)
autograft (ĂW-tō-grăft, p. 100)
contracture (kŏn-TRĂK-chŭr, p. 98)
Curling's ulcer (KŬR-lĭngz ŬL-sĕr, p. 98)
debridement (dă-BRĒD-mōń, p. 99)
eschar (ĔS-kăr, p. 99)
excoriation (ĕks-kŏr-ē-Ā-shŭn, p. 72)
exudate (ĔKS-ū-dāt, p. 69)
heterograft (xenograft) (HĔT-ĕr-ō-grăft; ZĒ-nō-grăft, p. 100)
homograft (allograft) (HŌ-mō-grăft; ĂL-ō-grăft, p. 100)
keloids (KĒ-loydz, p. 90)
macules (MĂK-ūlz, p. 76)

nevi (NĒ-vī, p. 91)
papules (PĂP-ūlz, p. 79)
pediculosis (pĕ-dĭk-ū-LŌ-sĭs, p. 87)
pruritus (proo-RĪ-tŭs, p. 61)
pustulant vesicles (PŬS-tū-lănt VĔS-ĭ-kŭlz, p. 76)
rule of nines (p. 96)
suppuration (sūp-ū-RĀ-shŭn, p. 77)
urticaria (ŭr-tĭ-KĂ-rē-ă, p. 81)
verruca (vĕ-RŪ-kă, p. 91)
vesicle (VĔS-ĭ-kl, p. 68)
wheals (wēlz, p. 81)

The skin, or **integument** is a major organ and the outer covering of the body. Together with its appendages—hair, nails, and special glands—it makes up the integumentary system. Skin is essential to life. Society has long held healthy skin in high esteem, probably because it is so visible to others. People spend many hours grooming their hair, cleansing their skin, and manicuring their nails. But beyond its social aspect, the integument is the body's protector, its first line of defense against infection and injury.

ANATOMY AND PHYSIOLOGY OF THE SKIN

FUNCTIONS OF THE SKIN

Although the skin covers the outside of the body, its main function is homeostasis and protection of the internal organs. Each day it is subjected to temperature

and humidity changes, trauma, ecchymosis, abrasions, contact with pathogens, and wear and tear. The skin carries out the numerous functions to protect and maintain the body (Box 3-1).

Box 3-1 Functions of the Skin

- Protects from pathogenic organisms and foreign substances; provides a natural barrier against infection
- Regulates temperature
- Prevents excessive water loss (dehydration)
- Aids in excretion of waste products
- Synthesizes vitamin D
- Insulates body and protects from trauma through subcutaneous layer of fat
- Has nerve endings that provide sensory perception to the brain related to pain, heat and cold, touch, pressure, and vibration

Protection

Sensory receptors within the skin receive information about the environment. Messages about heat, cold, pressure, and touch are received and relayed to the central nervous system for interpretation. Healthy skin protects the body from absorbing many chemicals and foreign substances. Additionally, as long as it remains intact, skin provides a barrier to many microorganisms in the environment. Internal organs are cushioned and protected by a subcutaneous layer of adipose (fat) tissue. The skin aids in elimination of waste products, prevents dehydration, and serves as a reservoir for food and water.

Temperature Regulation

Skin assists the body in maintaining a constant temperature under varying internal and external conditions. It allows blood vessels near the surface to constrict when the environment is cold to preserve heat and allows them to dilate when it is hot to release excess body heat. Sweat glands release moisture, which cools the body as it evaporates. A layer of adipose tissue works as an insulator by retaining heat.

Vitamin D Synthesis

Cholesterol compounds in the skin are converted to vitamin D when exposed to the sun's ultraviolet rays. Vitamin D is necessary for healthy bone development. Prolonged exposure to the sun's rays, which is ultraviolet radiation, should be avoided because of the increased risk of developing skin cancer.

STRUCTURE OF THE SKIN

Skin consists of two layers: the outer epidermis and inner dermis, or corium. Beneath these layers of skin lies the subcutaneous layer, or superficial fascia (Figure 3-1).

Epidermis

The **epidermis,** the superficial fascia (avascular layers of the skin), is composed of stratified squamous (from the Latin *squama,* meaning "scale") epithelium. The cells of the epidermis are tightly packed and have no distinct blood supply. The epidermis is divided into layers, or strata: an outer, dead, cornified portion and a deep, living, cellular portion. The inner layer is called the **stratum germinativum;** it is the only layer of the epidermis able to undergo cell division and reproduce itself. It receives its blood supply and nutrition from the underlying dermis through a process called **diffusion.** This provides a constant new supply of cells for the upper layers and enables the skin to repair itself after injury. As these cells push their way to the surface, their internal structures are destroyed and the cells die. When they reach the outermost layer, called the **stratum corneum,** they are flat and the cell structure is filled with a protein called **keratin** (horn). The stratum corneum is sometimes called the horny layer. The keratin makes the cells dry, tough, and somewhat waterproof.

Another layer in the epidermis contains highly specialized cells called **melanocytes.** These cells give rise to the pigment **melanin,** a black or dark brown pig-

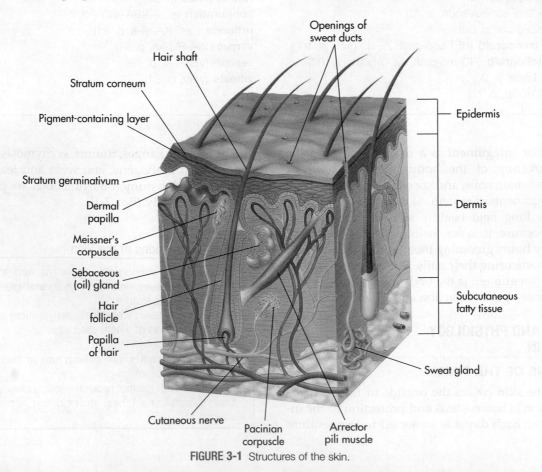

FIGURE 3-1 Structures of the skin.

ment occurring naturally in the hair, the skin, and the iris and choroid of the eye. Melanin is responsible for the skin's color. The greater the concentration of melanin, the darker the skin. Sometimes irregular patches with greater concentrations of melanin occur, producing freckles. The amount of melanin a person has is inherited from the parents. Although skin color is inherited, exposure to the sun and other factors can influence skin color.

Dermis

The **dermis,** or **corium,** is often called the true skin. It is well supplied with blood vessels and nerves and also contains glands and hair follicles. It varies in thickness throughout the body but tends to be thickest in the palms and soles. The dermis is composed of connective tissue with cells scattered among collagen and elastic fibers. The dermis receives strength from the collagen and flexibility from the elastic connective fibers. The cells throughout this layer are bathed in tissue fluid called interstitial fluid. The skin wrinkles with the normal aging process, as the dermis loses some of its elastic connective fibers and the subcutaneous tissue directly beneath it loses some of its adipose tissue. Located in the upper portion of the dermis are small fingerlike projections called **papillae** that project into the lower epidermal layer. Without the dermal papillae, the epidermal layer would be unable to survive.

Subcutaneous Layer

The subcutaneous layer, sometimes called the **superficial fascia,** is the layer of tissue directly beneath the dermis that connects the skin to the muscle surface. This layer is composed of adipose tissue and loose connective tissue. It serves several important functions: (1) stores water and fat, (2) insulates the body, (3) protects the organs lying beneath it, and (4) provides a pathway for nerves and blood vessels. The distribution of subcutaneous tissue throughout the body provides shape and contour. A woman's body usually contains more subcutaneous tissue than a man's; thus her body is softer and more rounded.

APPENDAGES OF THE SKIN

Sudoriferous Glands

The **sudoriferous** (sweat) **glands** are coiled, tubelike structures located in the dermis and subcutaneous layers. The tubes open into pores on the skin surface. Approximately 3 million sweat glands are located throughout the integumentary system. These glands excrete sweat, which cools the body's surface. Sweat is composed of water, salts, urea, uric acid, ammonia, sugar, lactic acid, and ascorbic acid.

Ceruminous Glands

Ceruminous glands are modified sudoriferous glands. They secrete a waxlike substance called **cerumen** and are located in the external ear canal. Cerumen is thought to protect the canal from foreign body invasion.

Sebaceous Glands

The **sebaceous** (oil) **glands** secrete **sebum** (an oily secretion) through the hair follicles distributed on the body. Their function is to lubricate the skin and hair that covers the body. Sebum also inhibits bacterial growth.

Hair and Nails

Hair is composed of modified dead epidermal tissue, mainly keratin. It is distributed all over the body in varying amounts. The root of the hair is enclosed in a follicle deep in the dermis. The shaft of the hair protrudes from the skin. Surrounding the hair follicle is a band of muscle tissue called **arrector pili** (see Figure 3-1). A sensation of cold or fear causes these muscles to contract, making the hair stand upright and dimpling the skin surrounding it. The effect is called piloerection, or "gooseflesh."

Nails are also composed mainly of keratin, but the keratin is more compressed. The base of the nail, the root, is made up of living cells and is mostly covered by the cuticle. Part of the root, the lunula, is exposed and looks like a white crescent. The remainder of the nail is called the **nail body.** It appears pink because of the blood vessels lying immediately beneath it.

ASSESSMENT OF THE SKIN

INSPECTION AND PALPATION

A thorough assessment of the skin helps identify many diseases that result from an outside organism penetrating the skin. However, remember that recognizing skin conditions by inspection takes time and experience.

Begin the assessment by obtaining a careful health history from the patient. Ask the patient about (1) recent skin lesions or rashes, (2) where the lesions first appeared, and (3) how long the lesions have been present. Also ask about a personal or family history of asthma, seasonal rhinitis, or drug allergies. Explore all complaints of pain, **pruritus** (the symptom of itching), tingling, or burning. Ask the patient about personal skin care and about (1) any recent skin color changes; (2) exposure to the sun, with or without sunscreen; and (3) family history of skin cancer.

Assess the skin under natural lighting, and use the senses of sight, touch, and smell while inspecting and palpating the skin. Expose the area to be assessed while maintaining privacy. Remember to wear gloves when inspecting the skin, mucous membranes, and any involved area. In the hospital, the morning bath provides an excellent opportunity to assess the patient's skin without exposure or embarrassment.

Observe the color of the skin. The color depends on many physiologic factors, including the following:
- Amount of hemoglobin in the blood
- Oxygen saturation in the blood
- Amount of substances such as bilirubin, urea, or other chemicals in the blood

- Quality and quantity of blood circulating in the superficial blood vessels
- Amount of melanin in the epidermis

Assessment of specific skin lesions, their appearance, and their location assists the dermatologist in diagnosing skin disorders and the nurse in providing care. Most disorders have only one or two types of lesions. Some of the typical clinical manifestations of skin disorders are shown in Table 3-1.

Assessment also includes the presence of rashes, scars, lesions, or ecchymoses and the distribution of hair. Assess temperature and texture by touch, using

Text continued on p. 67

Table 3-1   Primary Skin Lesions

DESCRIPTION	EXAMPLES		
MACULE Flat, circumscribed area that is a change in the skin color; <1 cm in diameter	Freckles, flat moles (nevi), petechiae, measles, scarlet fever		Measles[a]
PAPULE Elevated, firm, circumscribed area; <1 cm in diameter	Wart (verruca), elevated moles, lichen planus		Lichen planus[b]
PATCH Flat, nonpalpable, irregularly shaped macule; >1 cm in diameter	Vitiligo, port-wine stains, mongolian spots, café-au-lait spots		Vitiligo[b]
PLAQUE Elevated, firm, and rough lesion with flat top surface; >1 cm in diameter	Psoriasis, seborrheic and actinic keratoses		Plaque[a]

Modified from Thompson, J., & Wilson, S. (1995). *Health assessment for nursing practice.* St. Louis: Mosby.
Sources: [a]Habif, T.P. (1996). *Clinical dermatology* (3rd ed.). St. Louis: Mosby; [b]Weston, W.L., et al. (1996). *Color textbook of pediatric dermatology.* St. Louis: Mosby.

Table 3-1 **Primary Skin Lesions—cont'd**

DESCRIPTION	EXAMPLES
WHEAL Elevated irregularly shaped area of cutaneous edema; solid, transient; variable diameter	Insect bites, urticaria, allergic reaction

Wheal[c]

DESCRIPTION	EXAMPLES
NODULE Elevated, firm, circumscribed lesion; deeper in dermis than a papule; 1-2 cm in diameter	Erythema nodosum, lipomas

Hypertrophic nodule[d]

DESCRIPTION	EXAMPLES
TUMOR Elevated and solid lesion; may or may not be clearly demarcated; deeper in dermis; >2 cm in diameter	Neoplasms, benign tumor, lipoma, hemangioma

Hemangioma[b]

DESCRIPTION	EXAMPLES
VESICLE Elevated, circumscribed, superficial, not into dermis; filled with serous fluid; <1 cm in diameter	Varicella (chickenpox), herpes zoster (shingles)

Vesicles caused by varicella[c]

Sources: [b]Weston, W.L., et al. (1996). *Color textbook of pediatric dermatology.* St. Louis: Mosby; [c]Farrar, W.E., et al. (1994) *Infectious diseases* (2nd ed.). London: Gower; [d]Goldman, M.P., & Fitzpatrick, R.E. (1994). *Cutaneous laser surgery: The art and science of selective photo thermolysis.* St. Louis: Mosby.

Continued

Table 3-1 Primary Skin Lesions—cont'd

DESCRIPTION	EXAMPLES		
BULLA Vesicle >1 cm in diameter	Blister, pemphigus vulgaris		_Blister[e]_
PUSTULE Elevated, superficial lesion; similar to a vesicle but filled with purulent fluid	Impetigo, acne		_Acne[b]_
CYST Elevated, circumscribed, encapsulated lesion; in dermis or subcutaneous layer; filled with liquid or semisolid material	Sebaceous cyst, cystic acne		_Sebaceous cyst[b]_
TELANGIECTASIA Fine, irregular red lines produced by capillary dilation	Telangiectasia in rosacea		_Telangiectasia[d]_

Sources: [b]Weston, W.L., et al. (1996). _Color textbook of pediatric dermatology._ St. Louis: Mosby; [d]Goldman, M.P., & Fitzpatrick, R.E. (1994). _Cutaneous laser surgery: The art and science of selective photo thermolysis._ St. Louis: Mosby; [e]White, G.M. (1994). _Color atlas of regional dermatology._ St. Louis: Mosby.

Table 3-1 **Primary Skin Lesions—cont'd**

DESCRIPTION	EXAMPLES		
SCALE Heaped-up keratinized cells; flaky skin; irregular; thick or thin; dry or oily; variation in size	Flaking of skin with seborrheic dermatitis after scarlet fever, or flaking of skin following a drug reaction; dry skin		 Fine scaling[f]
LICHENIFICATION Rough, thickened epidermis secondary to persistent rubbing, itching, or skin irritation; often involves flexor surface of extremity	Chronic dermatitis		 Stasis dermatitis in an early stage[g]
KELOID Irregularly shaped, elevated, progressively enlarging scar; grows beyond the boundaries of the wound; caused by excessive collagen formation during healing	Keloid formation after surgery		 Keloid[b]
SCAR Thin to thick fibrous tissue that replaces normal skin after injury or laceration to the dermis	Healed wound or surgical incision		 Hypertrophic scar[d]

Sources: [b]Weston, W.L., et al. (1996). *Color textbook of pediatric dermatology.* St. Louis: Mosby; [d]Goldman, M.P., & Fitzpatrick, R.E. (1994). *Cutaneous laser surgery: The art and science of selective photo thermolysis.* St. Louis: Mosby; [f]Baran, R., et al. (1991). *Color atlas of the hair, scalp, and nails.* St. Louis: Mosby; [g]Marks, J.G., Jr., & DeLeo, V.A. (1991). *Contact and occupational dermatitis.* St. Louis: Mosby.

Continued

Table 3-1 **Primary Skin Lesions—cont'd**

DESCRIPTION	EXAMPLES		
EXCORIATION Loss of the epidermis; linear hollowed-out crusted area	Abrasion or scratch, scabies		Scabies[b]
FISSURE Linear crack or break from the epidermis to the dermis; may be moist or dry	Athlete's foot, cracks at the corner of the mouth		Fissures[d]
EROSION Loss of part of the epidermis; depressed, moist, glistening; follows rupture of a vesicle or bulla	Varicella, variola after rupture		Erosion[h]
ULCER Loss of epidermis and dermis; concave; varies in size	Pressure sores, stasis ulcers		Stasis ulcer[a]

Sources: [a]Habif, T.P. (1996). *Clinical dermatology* (3rd ed.). St. Louis: Mosby; [b]Weston, W.L., et al. (1996). *Color textbook of pediatric dermatology.* St. Louis: Mosby; [d]Goldman, M.P., & Fitzpatrick, R.E. (1994). *Cutaneous laser surgery: The art and science of selective photo thermolysis.* St. Louis: Mosby; [h]Cohen, B.A. (1993). *Pediatric dermatology.* London: Wolfe;

Table 3-1	Primary Skin Lesions—cont'd

DESCRIPTION	EXAMPLES
CRUST	
Dried serum, blood, or purulent exudate; slightly elevated; size varies; brown, red, black or tan	Scab on abrasion, eczema

Scab[g]

ATROPHY	
Thinning of skin surface and loss of skin markings; skin translucent and paperlike	Striae; aged skin

Aged skin[g]

Source: [g]Marks, J.G., Jr., & DeLeo, V.A. (1991). *Contact and occupational dermatitis.* St. Louis: Mosby.

the palms of the hands to compare opposite body areas. For example, feel both legs before concluding that the left leg is cold. Use a cotton-tipped applicator to touch the sole of the foot and assess sensation. Inspect the nails for normal development, color, shape, and thickness. Clubbing (broadening) of the fingertips indicates decreased oxygen (hypoxemia) and should be reported. Inspect the hair for thickness, dryness, or dullness. Assessment also includes inspecting the mucous membranes for pallor or cyanosis. Document profuse sweating or any sign of impaired skin integrity. Examine the ceruminous and sebaceous glands for overactivity or underactivity using appropriate questions, such as, "Tell me how often the physician has had to remove the wax from your ears."

Assessment of Dark Skin

The color of a person's skin, and how dark or light it is, is genetically determined. Dark skin color results from the reflection of light as it strikes the underlying skin pigment. Melanocytes have increased activity and produce large amounts of melanin, which accounts for the darker skin color. This increased melanin forms a natural sun shield, accounting for the lower incidence of skin cancer in people with dark skin.

The structures of dark skin are no different from those of lighter skin, but they are more difficult to as-

sess. Practice and comparison are necessary. Assessment is easier in areas where the epidermis is thin, such as the lips and mucous membranes. Rashes are often difficult to observe and may need to be palpated.

Dark skin is predisposed to certain skin conditions, including pseudofolliculitis, keloids, and mongolian spots. For some persons with dark skin, color cannot be used as an indicator of systemic conditions (e.g., flushed skin with fever) (see Cultural Considerations box).

CHIEF COMPLAINT

When skin lesions are found accompanying a skin disorder, document the exact location, length, width, general appearance, and name. A helpful mnemonic for assessing the chief complaint is to remember the following letters:

P: **P**rovocative and **P**alliative factors (factors that cause the condition)

Q: **Q**uality and **Q**uantity (characteristics and size) of the skin problem

R: **R**egion of the body

S: **S**everity of the signs and symptoms

T: **T**ime (length of time the patient has had the disorder)

An important objective in skin assessment is to identify possible malignancies. The three most common are melanoma, basal cell carcinoma, and squamous cell carcinoma. When assessing growths or

Skin Care

- The darker a person's skin, the more difficult it is to assess for changes in color. Establish a baseline in natural lighting if possible or with at least a 60-watt light bulb.
- Assess baseline skin color in areas with the least pigmentation, such as palms of the hands, soles of the feet, underside of forearms, abdomen, and buttocks.
- All skin colors have an underlying red tone. Pallor in black-skinned individuals is seen as ashen or gray. Pallor in brown-skinned individuals appears as yellowish. Assess pallor in mucous membranes, lips, nailbeds, and conjunctivae of the lower eyelids.
- To assess rashes and skin inflammation in dark-skinned individuals, rely on *palpation* for warmth and *induration* rather than observation.
- Some folk remedies may be misdiagnosed as injuries. Three folk practices of Southeast Asia can leave marks on the body that can be mistaken for signs of abuse or violence. *Cao gio* is the rubbing of the skin with a coin to produce dark blood or ecchymotic strips; it is done to treat a thrombus or the symptoms of the flu. *Bat gio* is skin pinching on the temples to treat headaches or on the neck for a sore throat. The treatment is considered a success if petechiae or ecchymosis appears. *Paua* is the burning of the skin with the tip of a dried weedlike grass. It is believed the burning will cause the noxious element that causes the pain to leave the body.

changes in a mole, ask the following questions, using the mnemonic device **ABCDE**:

    A: Is the mole **A**symmetrical?
    B: Are the **B**orders irregular?
    C: Is the **C**olor uneven or irregular?
    D: Has the **D**iameter of the growth changed recently?
    E: Has the surface area become **E**levated?

Promptly report a positive finding of any of these characteristics to a physician. After completing the assessment, document the findings. Proper assessment and identification serve as a baseline for evaluating nursing care and determining whether changes are needed.

PSYCHOSOCIAL ASSESSMENT

The person with an integumentary disorder may have a chronic or acute condition. Regardless of the severity, recovery may be lengthy with little visible outward improvement. A person's body image and self-esteem may be affected. Society's reaction to a skin condition has a significant effect on the patient. Personal appearance is a primary concern to many individuals, and others may think the condition is infectious and may socially isolate the patient. An integumentary disorder can have a negative effect on a patient's self-concept because of the value society places on a person's physical characteristics.

Assess the patient's coping abilities by using open-ended questions to encourage him or her to talk and ventilate feelings. Also assess the patient's interaction with family and others. Nonverbal behavior such as covering the involved area and avoiding eye contact may indicate a self-image problem. Validate or correct a patient's knowledge base. Rarely are skin diseases fatal, and few are contagious. Nurses need to work through their own feelings about a patient's skin appearance before they can be a source of encouragement. The nurse's attitude and interventions should be nonjudgmental, warm, and accepting. The nurse must be skilled and knowledgeable about skin care.

A patient with a skin disorder may have a problem with anxiety. Decrease the patient's anxiety by implementing the following interventions:

- Provide patients with consistent information related to their care plan.
- Include the family in the treatment plan. The family may be able to support instructions given, which helps to decrease anxiety.
- Provide positive feedback concerning the patient's efforts and progress, no matter how large or small.
- Refer the patient to a support group as soon as possible (if appropriate).

VIRAL DISORDERS OF THE SKIN

HERPES SIMPLEX

Etiology and Pathophysiology

The herpetovirus *Herpesvirus hominis* is the cause of herpes simplex. Two types of the virus are known:

- Type 1, the most common, causes the common cold sore and is usually associated with febrile conditions. The virus is self-limiting with no cure.
- Type 2 causes lesions in the genital area known as genital herpes. Type 2 is the same virus as type 1 and is discussed with sexually transmitted infections in Chapter 12.

Both types of virus may be transmitted by direct contact with any open lesion. However, in type 2, the primary mode is through sexual contact. The lesions are usually present for 2 to 3 weeks and are most painful during the first week. Complications may be severe if the disease spreads to other body areas.

Clinical Manifestations

Type 1 herpes simplex is characterized by a **vesicle** (circumscribed elevation of skin filled with serous fluid; smaller than 0.5 cm) at the corner of the mouth, on the lips, or on the nose. It is commonly known as a **cold sore** (Figure 3-2). At first the involved area is usually erythematous and edematous. The vesicle then appears, ulcerates, and encrusts. When the vesicle ruptures, it produces a burning pain. The patient experiences general malaise and fatigue. Usual occurrence is during an acute illness or infection.

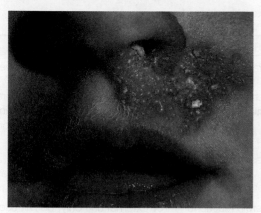

FIGURE 3-2 Herpes simplex.

Type 2, genital herpes, produces various types of vesicles that rupture and encrust, causing ulcerations. The cervix is the most common site in women, and the penis is the most common area in men. Flulike symptoms occur 3 or 4 days after the vesicles erupt. Headache, fatigue, myalgia, fever, and anorexia are common.

Assessment

Assessment primarily involves inspection of the skin. Obtain a complete health history to support assessment data. **Subjective data** include complaints of fatigue along with pruritus and burning pain in the mouth for herpes simplex type 1 and in the genital area for herpes simplex type 2.

Objective data for herpes simplex type 1 include an edematous, erythematous area at the corner of the lip. In herpes simplex type 2, the labia, vulva, or penis will appear edematous and erythematous. The vesicular lesions may rupture and develop a dried **exudate** (fluid, cells, or other substances that have been slowly exuded, or discharged, from cells or blood vessels through small pores or breaks in cell membranes).

Diagnostic Tests

Diagnosis of herpesvirus is made by laboratory assessment of cultures from the lesion. Inspection and health history support the diagnosis. Patients should also be assessed for human immunodeficiency virus (HIV).

Medical Management

Herpesvirus has no cure, but treatment is aimed at relieving symptoms. Acyclovir (Zovirax) is an antiviral agent that can alter the course of the disease. Acyclovir can be administered orally, topically, or intravenously (Table 3-2). These drugs inhibit viral reproduction but are not a cure (Lewis et al., 2007).

Nursing Interventions and Patient Teaching

Nursing interventions primarily focus on treating symptoms and preventing spread of the disease. The patient can use warm compresses to relieve pain and severe pruritus. He or she should keep the lesions dry and avoid direct contact. Analgesics such as acetamin-

ophen (Tylenol) are effective in pain control. The specific nursing diagnoses for herpes are based on assessment data gathered. Type 2 herpesvirus, genital herpes, remains transferable during remission. Teach patients to take precautions such as using condoms during sexual activity (Lewis et al., 2007).

Nursing diagnoses and interventions for the patient with herpes include but are not limited to the following:

Nursing Diagnoses	Nursing Interventions
Pain, related to pruritus	Assess factors that precipitate pruritus. Apply local anesthetic, such as Orabase, for pain. Apply drying agent to lesions. Apply warm compresses. Have patient wear loose-fitting, cotton clothing that does not constrict movement or occlude circulation.
Impaired skin integrity, related to open lesions	Inspect lesions for drainage, color, and location. Wash hands before and after contact. Keep area dry. Administer antiviral agents as ordered. In genital herpes, use of a hair dryer can dry the lesions and promote patient comfort.
Risk for infection, related to skin excoriation	Use body substance precautions. Teach patient proper skin care. Wash hands before and after care. Keep area dry. Administer antiviral drugs as ordered.

Preventing infection remains the top priority when caring for a patient with an open skin lesion. Patient teaching focuses on the principles of medical asepsis and includes specific measures to prevent spread of the disease. Using good hygiene in all areas of care is critical in preventing secondary infections. Include the complications and precipitating factors in patient teaching and discharge planning.

Prognosis

Herpes simplex has no cure. The prognosis for type 1 is healing within 10 to 14 days, and possible recurrence with depression of the immune system. For type 2, lesions are usually present for 7 to 14 days. Unfortunately, 75% of all patients have at least one recurrence, and two thirds have one to five recurrences annually.

Table 3-2 Medications for the Integumentary System

Generic (Trade)	Action	Side Effects	Nursing Implications
Acyclovir (Zovirax)	Antiviral	Topical: Burning, rash, pruritus, stinging Systemic: Headache, seizures, renal toxicity, phlebitis at IV site	Topical: Use glove to apply; cover lesion completely. Systemic: Ensure adequate hydration to prevent crystallization in kidneys; administer IV dose for at least 1 hour
Alpha Keri	Emollient	Local irritation, allergic reactions	For external use only; exercise caution when using in tub to avoid slipping
Aluminum acetate solution (Burow's solution)	Astringent	Local irritation, allergic reactions	For external use only; do not use with occlusive dressings
Antihistamines, including: Diphenhydramine (Benadryl) Hydroxyzine (Vistaril, Atarax)	Blocks histamine at H_1 receptor site, inhibiting many allergic reactions	Drowsiness, dizziness, confusion, dry mouth, urinary retention	If drowsiness occurs, avoid activities that require concentration; avoid using with alcohol or other CNS depressants
Benzoyl peroxide	Antiacne agent	Excessive drying of skin, allergic reactions	Discontinue use if excessive drying or peeling occurs; avoid contact with hair or fabric
Chlorhexidine gluconate (Hibiclens)	Antimicrobial skin cleanser	Irritation, dermatitis, allergic reactions	For external use only; do not use on broken skin unless directed by a physician
Calamine lotion	Astringent	Local irritation	For external use only
Coal tar (Estar-Gel, Psori-Gel, others)	Treatment of pruritic dermatoses, including eczema and psoriasis	Photosensitivity, dermatitis, allergic reactions	Avoid exposure to sunlight for 72 hours after use; may stain clothes and bathtub; for external use only
Corticosteroids (topical), including: Fluocinonide (Lidex) Triamcinolone (Kenalog) Betamethasone (Valisone)	Antiinflammatory agent	Local irritation, maceration, superinfection, atrophy, itching, and drying of skin (more severe local reactions and systemic effects possible with higher doses and potency or when used with occlusive dressings)	Do not use occlusive dressings unless directed by a physician; washing or soaking area before application increases drug penetration
Crotamiton (Eurax)	Scabicidal and antipruritic	Local irritation, allergic reactions	For external use only; do not apply to severely irritated skin
Curel, Eucerin, Lubriderm	Emollient	Local irritation, allergic reactions	For external use only
Fluconazole (Diflucan)	Antifungal	Headache, nausea, vomiting, diarrhea	May elevate liver function test; monitor BUN, creatinine
Griseofulvin (Fulvicin, Grisactin, Grifulvin, others)	Antifungal agent	Hypersensitivity reactions, photosensitivity, nausea, fatigue, mental confusion	Avoid exposure to sunlight; drug absorption increased when given with meals; clinical response may appear only after full course of therapy

BUN, Blood urea nitrogen; *CNS,* central nervous system; *IV,* intravenous; *PT,* prothrombin time; *UVA,* ultraviolet A.

Table 3-2 Medications for the Integumentary System—cont'd

Generic (Trade)	Action	Side Effects	Nursing Implications
Isotretinoin (Accutane)	Antiacne agent	Severe dryness of skin, mouth, eyes, mucous membranes, nose, and nails; skin fragility; epistaxis; joint and muscle pain; nausea; abdominal pain	Absolutely contraindicated in pregnant women or women contemplating pregnancy; women of childbearing age must practice contraception during therapy and 1 month before and after therapy; give drug with meals; do not give vitamin supplements containing vitamin A; avoid exposure to sunlight
Itraconazole (Sporanox)	Antifungal agent	Hypertension, headache, nausea, anorexia	Give with food; check hepatic function; can increase PT level
Lindane (Kwell)	Scabicide, ovicide	Local irritation, dizziness, seizures (rare)	For external use only; avoid applying to open skin lesions
Lubriderm	Emollient	Local irritation, allergic reactions	For external use only; exercise caution when using in tub to avoid slipping
Methoxsalen (Oxsoralen, Oxsoralen-Ultra, 8-MOP)	Skin pigmenting agent	Severe photosensitivity, nausea, nervousness, insomnia, headache, hypopigmentation	Avoid all exposure to sunlight for 8 hours after oral ingestion and for several days after topical application; wear UVA-absorbing sunglasses for 24 hours after oral ingestion; use sunscreens to prevent exposure to sunlight; give agent with food or milk or in divided doses; clinical response may not appear for several months
Povidone-iodine (Betadine)	Topical antimicrobial agent	Local irritation	For external use only; may stain skin and clothing
Pyrethrin (RID, others)	Pediculicide	Local irritation	For external use only; do not use for infestations of eyebrows or eyelashes
Salicylic acid	Keratolytic agent	Local irritation, erythema, scaling	For external use only; may damage clothing, plastic, wood, and other materials on contact
Terbinafine (Lamisil)	Antifungal	Pruritus, local burning, erythema	For external use only; do not use occlusive dressings unless directed by a physician
Tetracycline	Antibacterial agent	Topical: Stinging, burning, slight yellowing of skin may occur. Systemic: Nausea, diarrhea, photosensitivity	Topical: Avoid contact with sunlight. Systemic: Give on empty stomach; avoid concomitant administration of dairy products, laxatives, antacids, and products containing iron; avoid contact with sunlight; may cause permanent tooth discoloration when used in children
Tolnaftate (Tinactin, Aftate, others)	Antifungal agent	Local irritation	For external use only

BUN, Blood urea nitrogen; *CNS,* central nervous system; *IV,* intravenous; *PT,* prothrombin time; *UVA,* ultraviolet A.

The recurrences, however, are milder and of shorter duration than the primary infection.

HERPES ZOSTER (SHINGLES)

Etiology and Pathophysiology

Herpes zoster, commonly known as **shingles,** is caused by the same virus that causes chickenpox (herpes varicella or herpesvirus type 3). The lesions are located along the nerve fibers of spinal ganglia. The virus causes an inflammation of the spinal ganglia. It is believed that the virus responsible for shingles lies dormant in patients until their resistance to infections has been lowered. The virus then advances to the skin by way of the peripheral nerves. At the skin surface the virus multiplies and forms an erythematous rash of small vesicles along a spinal nerve pathway (Figure 3-3). Sometimes the virus may affect a single nerve such as the trigeminal nerve.

Clinical Manifestations

The eruption of the vesicles is preceded by pain. The rash generally occurs in the thoracic region; the vesicles erupt in a line along the involved nerve. The vesicles rupture and form a crust, and the serous fluid in the vesicle may become purulent. The virus can also affect the lumbar, cervical, or cranial areas. The course of this painful condition runs from 7 to 28 days.

The pain associated with herpes zoster is severe; most patients describe it as burning and knifelike. Extreme tenderness and pruritus occur in the affected area. Patients with herpes zoster request analgesic medications at frequent intervals during the acute episode.

Herpes zoster is usually not permanently disabling to healthy adults. The greatest risk is for patients who have a lowered resistance to infection, such as those receiving chemotherapy or large doses of prednisone. In these patients, with compromised immune systems, the disease could be fatal

Assessment

Assessment of the patient should include both subjective and objective data. A good health history and thorough inspection skills are necessary to gather relevant data.

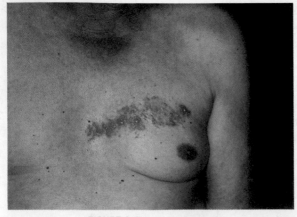

FIGURE 3-3 Herpes zoster.

Subjective data include (1) sharp, burning pain, usually on one side; (2) severe pruritus of the lesions; (3) general malaise; and (4) a history of chickenpox (varicella).

Objective data include (1) evidence of skin **excoriation** (injury to the surface layer of skin caused by scratching or abrasion) related to scratching, (2) patches of vesicles on erythematous skin following a peripheral nerve pathway, and (3) demonstration of tenderness to touch in the involved area. Other objective signs may include frequent requests for analgesics.

Diagnostic Tests

The diagnostic test for herpes zoster is a culture that isolates the virus. Other diagnostic measures are physical examinations and a thorough health history obtained on admission to the health care facility.

Medical Management

Medical interventions are directed at controlling the pain and preventing secondary complications. Analgesics, often opioids, are given for the pain. Steroids may be given to decrease inflammation and edema. Lotions (Kenalog, Lidex) may be used to relieve pruritus, and corticosteroids may be used to relieve pruritus and inflammation. Oral and intravenous acyclovir, when administered early, reduces the pain and duration of the virus. Recovery generally occurs in 2 to 3 weeks. Approximately 20% of patients experience some form of neuralgia following the episode. A vaccine available to prevent herpes zoster called Zostavax is now available. It is recommended for adults over 60 years who have had varicella (chickenpox) (Lewis et al., 2007).

Nursing Interventions and Patient Teaching

Nursing interventions are directed at relieving pain and pruritus and at preventing secondary complications. Tranquilizers such as lorazepam (Ativan) and hydroxyzine HCl (Atarax) are prescribed to decrease the anxiety associated with severe pain. Analgesics are given to control pain. The nurse needs to understand and be able to apply the principles of pain management to provide nursing interventions. Medicated baths and warm compresses may be ordered to soothe the skin. Use aseptic technique when caring for open lesions (Nursing Care Plan 3-1).

Nursing diagnoses and interventions for the patient with herpes zoster include but are not limited to the following:

Nursing Diagnoses	Nursing Interventions
Acute pain, related to inflammation of the involved nerve pathways	Assess pain and pruritus for necessary relief measures. Administer medications for pain and pruritus. Teach stress relaxation techniques, and offer diversional activities.

Continued on page 74

⭐ Nursing Care Plan 3-1 The Patient with Herpes Zoster

Ms. Lares, a 28-year-old teacher, is admitted with herpes zoster located around her left orbital area. She has several vesicles that have crusted and several vesicles that are still intact. She is complaining of pruritus and pain. She keeps asking the nurse if the lesions will leave a scar.

NURSING DIAGNOSIS *Impaired tissue integrity related to the open lesions around the left eye*

Patient Goals and Expected Outcomes	Nursing Interventions	Evaluation and Rationale
Patient's tissue integrity will improve as shown by:		
No signs of infection such as erythema, purulent drainage, and elevated white blood cell count during hospitalization	Assess skin, especially eye area, for changes in color, texture, or turgor or increase in lesion size.Assess lesions for signs of infection.Monitor albumin and white blood cell levels as ordered.	The patient showed no signs of erythema or purulent drainage. The patient showed improvement of vesicles.
Remaining skin showing no signs of impairment during hospitalization	Use principles of aseptic technique.	No skin impairment noted in remaining skin
Decrease in the number of lesions within 72 hours	Monitor status of lesions for 12 hours.	The number of lesions increased during the first day of hospitalization but decreased during the next 48 hours.
Patient stating pain level has decreased from a "9" to a "4" within 24 hours	Administer or apply medications as ordered to decrease pain or pruritus. Teach patient importance of using medical asepsis in care of lesions.	Patient stated that pain was a "3" within 24 hours of medication administration.

NURSING DIAGNOSIS *Disturbed body image, related to location of lesions as manifested by continual remarks to the nurse, "Will these sores leave a scar?"*

Patient Goals and Expected Outcomes	Nursing Interventions	Evaluation and Rationale
The patient will verbalize and demonstrate acceptance of appearance as manifested by: • Verbalizing positive feelings about body image • Participating in normal activities	Assess patient's feelings about personal appearance by encouraging patient to express her feelings. Encourage patient to ask questions about her health problem. Provide reliable information, and reinforce the information already given. Clarify any misconceptions about the care the patient is receiving. Provide privacy, and avoid criticism. Teach patient about the disease and the course of the disease.	The goal was met. The patient stated she believed that lesions would not be permanent. The patient returned to work after dismissal from the hospital before the lesions had completely healed. The goal was met.

Critical Thinking Questions

1. Ms. Lares turns on her call light. She is crying and states she is in severe pain. She describes the pain as a burning, stabbing pain over her left forehead and eye. She rates her pain as a 7 on the pain scale of 0 to 10. She also complains of pruritus. What would be the most appropriate nursing interventions to provide comfort and pain control for Ms. Lares?
2. Ms. Lares tells the nurse that a friend told her she could not visit because she has not had chickenpox. Her friend is afraid she might "catch chickenpox" from Ms. Lares's shingles. Give the accurate patient teaching in response to Ms. Lares' statements.

Nursing Diagnoses	Nursing Interventions
Risk for infection, related to tissue destruction	Assess factors that contribute to infection, such as an immunocompromised patient (one who has decreased white blood cell count). Monitor for signs of infection, such as pyrexia and leukocytosis. Stress aseptic hand hygiene technique. Maintain aseptic technique when providing care. Limit visitors. Don gloves when caring for lesions.

Begin patient teaching by assessing the patient's knowledge and readiness. Areas to cover include (1) methods for controlling pain, (2) application of medication and wet dressings, (3) methods for inhibiting the spread of disease, (4) techniques to prevent secondary infections, and (5) proper diet with vitamin C to promote healing.

Prognosis

The prognosis is generally good; however, older adults are more susceptible to complications such as post-therapy neuralgia, which may persist for several months after the skin lesions have cleared. Evidence indicates that the herpes zoster virus remains latent in the body of a person once infected. A person lacking varicella (chickenpox) immunity can acquire chickenpox from someone who has shingles.

PITYRIASIS ROSEA

Pityriasis rosea is a skin rash that usually affects people between 6 and 30 years of age. The rash begins as a single pink, scaly patch that resembles a large ringworm. It ranges from 1 to 3 inches in diameter.

Etiology and Pathophysiology

Most sources note that pityriasis rosea is caused by a virus. The rash generally disappears without treatment (*Mosby's dictionary of medical, nursing, and health professions*, 8th ed., 2009).

Clinical Manifestations

Pityriasis rosea begins as a single lesion, known as a herald patch, that is scaly, has a raised border, and has a pink center. Seven to 14 days after the initial eruption, smaller matching spots become widespread on both sides of the body. The rash consists of pink oval-shaped spots that are ¼ to ½ inch across. The rash appears mainly on the chest, abdomen, back, groin, and axillae (Figure 3-4).

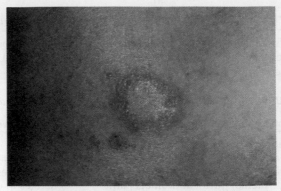

FIGURE 3-4 Pityriasis rosea herald patch.

Assessment

Assessment involves inspecting the skin and gathering a detailed health history. Ask questions related to the objective data.

Diagnostic Tests

Diagnosis of rosea stems from inspection and subjective data from the patient. No specific laboratory tests support a definitive diagnosis.

Medical Management

Generally, rosea requires no treatment, but preventive interventions can control secondary infections related to pruritus. If the skin becomes dry, moisturizing cream may help. For pruritus, the patient should use 1% hydrocortisone cream two or three times a day. Ultraviolet light, such as sunbathing for 30 minutes, shortens the course of pityriasis rosea.

Nursing Interventions

The nursing interventions for pityriasis rosea include symptomatic relief of the symptoms such as pruritus. Analgesics and Aveeno baths may be ordered to help decrease the pain and pruritus. Antihistamines and topical steroids may be used to control the pruritus. Sun exposure aids in the resolution of the lesions.

Prognosis

The disease is thought to be viral. Teach the patient that the disease is self-limiting and resolves in a few weeks.

BACTERIAL DISORDERS OF THE SKIN

CELLULITIS

Etiology and Pathophysiology

Cellulitis, a potentially serious infection, involves the underlying tissues of the skin. Although it is not contagious, the bacteria that cause cellulitis can be spread by direct contact with an open area on a person who has an infection. The most common causes in adults are group A streptococci and *Staphylococcus aureus*; *Haemophilus influenzae* type B is more common in children. The risk is increased by venous insufficiency or stasis; diabetes mellitus; lymphedema; surgery; malnutrition; substance abuse; presence of another infection; compromised immune function due to HIV; treatment with steroids or cancer chemotherapy; or autoimmune diseases, such as lupus erythematosus.

Cellulitis develops as an edematous, erythematous area of skin that feels hot and tender. It occurs when bacteria enter the body through a break in the skin, such as a cut, scratch, or insect bite that is not cleansed with soap and water. The infection usually affects skin on the lower extremities or face, although cellulitis can occur on any part of the skin. The infection is usually superficial, but cellulitis may spread and become life threatening as the infection invades the deeper tissues, lymph nodes, and bloodstream. Thus it is known by the lay term *blood poisoning*.

Clinical Manifestations

Cellulitis is an infection of the skin and underlying subcutaneous tissues. The affected areas become erythematous, edematous, tender, and warm to the touch. Often a fever accompanies the other symptoms. The first signs and symptoms generally are erythema, pain, and tenderness over an area of skin. These signs and symptoms are caused by bacteria themselves and by the body's attempts to halt the infection. The infected skin may look slightly pitted, like an orange peel. Over time, the area of erythema spreads and small red spots may appear. Vesicles may form and burst, or large bullae may appear on the infected skin. As the infection spreads, nearby lymph nodes may become enlarged and tender (lymphadenitis). Erysipelas is one form of streptococcal cellulitis in which the skin is bright red and noticeably edematous and the edges of the infected area are raised. Edema occurs because the infection occludes the lymphatic vessels in the skin. Most patients with cellulitis feel only mildly ill, but some have fever, chills, tachycardia, headache, hypotension, and confusion.

Assessment

Assessment primarily involves inspection of the skin. Collect a health history to support assessment data. **Subjective data** include complaints of fatigue, tenderness, pain, limited movement of the involved extremity, and general malaise. **Objective data** include edema, erythema, and areas that are warm to touch. Vesicles may be present. An elevated temperature accompanied by tachycardia and leukocytosis often occurs.

Diagnostic Tests

The physician diagnoses cellulitis based on its appearance and signs and symptoms. If a patient is seriously ill, cultures may be needed from blood, purulent exudate, or tissue specimens for laboratory identification of the bacteria. A complete blood count (CBC) reveals leukocy-

tosis. A Gram stain may be done to determine the appropriate antibiotic therapy. Occasionally the physician performs tests to differentiate cellulitis from deep-vein thrombosis of the lower extremity because the signs and symptoms of these disorders are similar. X-ray examination, ultrasound, computed tomography, or magnetic resonance imaging may be used to determine the extent of inflammation and to identify abscess formation.

Medical Management

Prompt treatment with antibiotics can prevent cellulitis from spreading rapidly and reaching the blood and organs. Most cases are treated with antibiotic therapy that is effective against both streptococci and staphylococci. Patients with mild cellulitis may take oral antibiotics. If the patient has rapidly spreading cellulitis, high fever, or other evidence of a serious infection, the physician will order intravenous antibiotics.

Nursing Interventions and Patient Teaching

Nursing interventions involve treating signs and symptoms and preventing spread of the disease. Administer the antibiotic, monitor the patient's progress, assess pain, administer an analgesic, change dressings, and monitor the patient's nutrition and hydration status. The affected body part, when possible, remains immobile and is elevated to help reduce edema. Warm, moist dressings applied to the infected area may relieve discomfort.

Signs and symptoms of cellulitis usually disappear after a few days of antibiotic therapy. However, signs and symptoms often worsen before they improve, probably because the death of the bacteria releases substances that cause tissue damage. When this occurs, the body continues to react even though the bacteria are dead. Antibiotics are continued for a minimum of 10 days. Teach patients that it is important to take the entire prescription of antibiotics and to monitor for signs and symptoms of secondary diseases such as yeast infections. The specific nursing diagnoses for cellulitis depend on the assessment data gathered and the extent of the infection. Analgesics such as acetaminophen or oxycodone-acetaminophen (Percocet) help control the pain and fever associated with cellulitis.

Prognosis

Cure is possible with 7 to 10 days of treatment. Cellulitis may be more severe in people with chronic diseases and those who are susceptible to infection such as those with immunosuppression. Complications from cellulitis include sepsis, meningitis, and lymphangitis.

IMPETIGO CONTAGIOSA

Etiology and Pathophysiology

Impetigo is caused by *S. aureus*, streptococci, or a mixed bacterial invasion of the skin. It is a highly contagious inflammatory disorder, seen at all ages but particularly common in children. The lesions start as **macules** (small, flat blemishes that are flush with the skin surface), develop into **pustulant vesicles** (small, circumscribed elevations of the skin that contain pus), and then rupture and form a dried exudate. The crust is honey colored and easily removed. Under the dried exudate is smooth, red skin (Figure 3-5).

Clinical Manifestations

The exposed areas of the body most often affected are the face, hands, arms, and legs. The pustulant lesions are distributed randomly over the involved area. The honey-colored dried exudate ranges from pinpoint to the size of a nickel or larger. Impetigo is highly contagious to a person who directly contacts the exudate of a lesion. The disease may be spread by touching personal articles, linens, and clothing of the infected person.

Assessment

Subjective data include symptoms of (1) pruritus, (2) pain, (3) malaise, (4) spreading of the disease to different body parts, and (5) other diseases present.

Objective data include all or some of the following: (1) focal erythema; (2) pruritic areas; (3) honey-colored crust over dried lesions; (4) smooth, red skin under the crust; (5) low-grade fever; (6) leukocytosis; (7) positive culture for streptococcus or *S. aureus*; and (8) purulent exudate.

Diagnostic Tests

The diagnosis is made by taking a culture of the exudate and identifying the specific bacterium. Inspection and symptoms are the standard means of identifying the condition.

Medical Management

The physician prescribes systemic antibiotics (such as erythromycin, dicloxacillin, or a cephalosporin) based on the culture and sensitivity test. Topical antibiotics such as mupirocin (Bactroban) have proven effective when started early in the treatment, but most physicians include a systemic antibiotic as well. Retapamu-

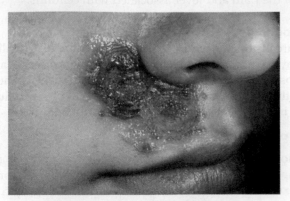

FIGURE 3-5 Impetigo and herpes simplex.

lin (Altabax) was approved by the U.S. Food and Drug Administration (FDA) for topical treatment of impetigo (GlaxoSmithKline, 2007). Medical treatment emphasizes the use of antiseptic soaps to remove crusted exudate and cleansing agents to thoroughly clean the involved area before applying an antibiotic cream, ointment, or lotion. A primary goal is preventing glomerulonephritis (inflammation of the glomerulus of the kidney), which may occur after streptococcal infections.

Nursing Interventions and Patient Teaching

Interventions are aimed at disrupting the course of the disease and preventing the spread of infection. Antibiotics are used to arrest the disease process. Systemic parenteral penicillin is one of the most commonly used antibiotics. Ceftriaxone sodium (Rocephin) is widely used as well. Other antibiotics such as cephalosporins may be used. Don gloves and wash the lesions with special cleansing agents, such as povidone-iodine (Betadine) and chlorhexidine gluconate (Hibiclens).

The lesions are usually soaked with an antiseptic solution, and the dried exudate is removed using special instruments. Topical antibiotics are applied several times a day using sterile technique.

Nursing diagnoses and interventions for the patient with impetigo include but are not limited to the following:

Nursing Diagnoses	Nursing Interventions
Impaired skin integrity, related to crusted, open lesions	Inspect lesions every day for drainage, size, and extent of body area covered. Keep area clean and dry. Don gloves when giving direct patient care.
Deficient knowledge, related to the cause and spread of the disease	Assess patient's knowledge level and readiness to learn. Demonstrate appropriate care and application of topical medications. Stress importance of individual personal items, such as linens and towels. Involve family in patient teaching.

Assess the patient's level of knowledge, and instruct the patient and family members in the principles of hygiene. When demonstrating home care techniques, reinforce correct information and stress the importance of preventing the spread of the disease by contact.

Prognosis

With proper treatment the prognosis is good. Emphasize that the patient should take all of the prescribed antibiotic.

FOLLICULITIS, FURUNCLES, CARBUNCLES, AND FELONS

Etiology and Pathophysiology

Folliculitis is an infection of a hair follicle, generally from *S. aureus* bacteria. The infection may involve one or several follicles. It often occurs after men or women shave. A stye is an example of folliculitis.

A **furuncle** (boil) is an inflammation that begins deep in the hair follicles and spreads to the surrounding skin. Irritation is a common predisposing factor to a furuncle. Common locations are the posterior area of the neck, the forearm, buttocks, and the axillae (Figure 3-6).

A **carbuncle** is a cluster of furuncles. It is an infection of several hair follicles that spreads to surrounding tissue. Obesity, poor nutrition, untreated diabetes mellitus, and poor hygiene contribute to the formation of carbuncles.

A **felon** is an infection of the soft tissue under and around an area such as the fingernail. The involved finger becomes erythematous, edematous, and tender to touch.

Clinical Manifestations

The involved area is usually edematous, erythematous, painful, and pruritic. After several days, the infected area becomes localized. The exact area may get shiny, point up; for a furuncle or carbuncle, the center turns yellow. Carbuncles can have four or five cores with spontaneous rupture of the core. The pain stops immediately on rupture. A surgical incision and drainage can be performed if the core does not rupture.

Assessment

Collection of **subjective data** includes asking questions about the patient's general symptoms, such as tenderness and pain with movement. Ask about a family history of diabetes mellitus or the wearing of improperly fitting clothing. Collection of **objective data** includes noting erythema and edema in the involved area. The patient is often overweight and may have poor body hygiene.

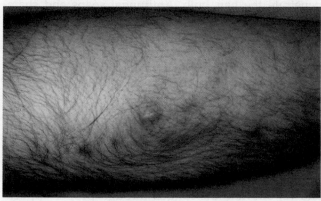

FIGURE 3-6 Furuncle of the forearm.

Diagnostic Tests

Diagnosis is based primarily on a thorough physical examination, health history, and inspection of the area. A culture of the drainage may be done.

Medical Management

Medical treatment is aimed at preventing the spread of infection. Patients in the hospital are isolated, using wound and secretion precautions. Surgical treatment may include draining the lesion and applying topical antibiotics.

Nursing Interventions and Patient Teaching

Warm soaks, two or three times a day, can be used to speed the process of **suppuration** (production of purulent material). When the lesion ruptures, discontinue the soaks to prevent damage of the surrounding skin and spread of the infection. Use good medical asepsis while caring for these patients. In the hospital, follow isolation procedures for drainage and secretion. If the lesion is incised and drained, use sterile technique to apply topical antibiotics. The affected part needs to be immobilized to prevent pain and elevated to decrease the edema.

Nursing diagnoses and interventions for the patient with bacterial disorders include but are not limited to the following:

Nursing Diagnoses	Nursing Interventions
Impaired skin integrity, related to exudates from wound	Assess wound daily for exudates and excoriation.
	Don gloves when providing care; use correct isolation technique.
	Apply skin protectant to opening.
Pain, related to edema	Assess area for edema and tenderness.
	Elevate involved body part above the level of the heart.
	Apply hot soaks, and immobilize affected part.

Teach patients not to touch the exudate. Meticulous hand hygiene is a must before and after contact with the lesions. Demonstrate good hygiene practices and ask for return demonstrations by the patient and the family. The entire family needs individual toilet items and bath linens and should be encouraged to use bacteriostatic soap and shampoo. Demonstrate proper disposal and cleaning of contaminated articles.

Prognosis

Patients make a full recovery when they follow the treatment plan. A follow-up examination with a physician may be needed to identify any underlying disease process, such as diabetes mellitus.

FUNGAL INFECTIONS OF THE SKIN

Fungal infections, which are known as **dermatophytoses,** are superficial infections of the skin. The most common types are tinea capitis, tinea corporis, tinea cruris, and tinea pedis.

Etiology and Pathophysiology

Tinea capitis is commonly known as ringworm of the scalp. *Microsporum audouinii* is the major fungal pathogen. The fungus is spread by contact with infected articles. Trauma or irritation breaks the skin and facilitates spread of the infection (Figure 3-7).

Tinea corporis is known as ringworm of the body. It occurs on parts of the body with little or no hair.

Tinea cruris is known as jock itch. It is found in the groin area.

Tinea pedis is the most common of all fungal infections. Commonly known as athlete's foot, it occurs between the toes of people whose feet perspire heavily. The fungus can also be spread from contaminated public bathroom facilities and swimming pools.

Clinical Manifestations

Tinea capitis is usually an erythematous, round lesion with pustules around the edges (see Figure 3-7). Temporary alopecia occurs at the site, and infected hairs turn blue-green under a Wood's light (an ultraviolet light).

Tinea corporis produces flat lesions that are clear in the center with erythematous borders. Scaliness also occurs, and pruritus is severe (Figure 3-8).

Tinea cruris has brownish red lesions that migrate out from the groin area. Pruritus and skin excoriation from scratching are found.

Tinea pedis produces more skin maceration than the others. Commonly seen are fissures and vesicles around and below the toes, with occasional discoloration of the infected area.

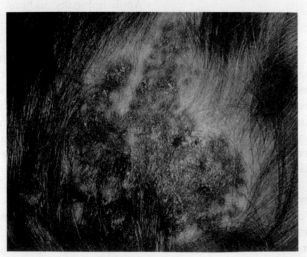
FIGURE 3-7 Tinea capitis.

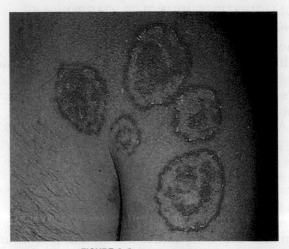
FIGURE 3-8 Tinea corporis.

Assessment

Subjective data include any symptoms of extreme pruritus and tenderness from excoriation of the area. Collection of **objective data** for tinea capitis includes an inspection and location of a round, scaled lesion that has pustules around the edges of the scalp. The involved area is erythematous and has no hair. In tinea corporis, the lesions are flat with clear centers and erythematous borders on nonhairy body parts. In tinea cruris, the groin area reveals brown to red lesions that radiate outward, with skin excoriation from intense scratching. In tinea pedis, fissures between the toes and soft skin are accompanied by vesicular lesions and thick toenails.

Diagnostic Tests

The diagnosis is primarily by visual inspection and, for tinea capitis, use of a Wood's light. The light causes hairs infected by the fungus to become brilliantly fluorescent. No other tests are performed, but a thorough health history supports the diagnosis of all fungal infections of the skin.

Medical Management

Medical treatment involves the use of topical or oral antifungal drugs. Griseofulvin (Fulvicin, Grifulvin) is the most common oral drug given; topical drugs do not penetrate the hair bulb. Antifungal soaps and shampoos are recommended. Antifungal agents such as tolnaftate 1% (Tinactin), miconazole (Lotrimin AF), (Monistat Derm, Desenex), and butenafine (Mentax) can be applied directly. Treatment may last from 2 to 6 weeks. See Table 3-2 for a list of drugs commonly used for fungal and other integumentary infections.

Nursing Interventions and Patient Teaching

Nursing interventions for fungal infections involve two primary principles: (1) protect the involved area from trauma and irritation by keeping it clean and dry, and (2) alleviate the fungus through proper application of medications and warm compresses.

Tinea pedis should be treated with warm soaks using Burow's solution and topical antifungal agents. Excellent foot care is stressed. The feet should be cleaned and dried thoroughly, paying special attention to the toes. Wearing sandals or going barefoot helps decrease foot moisture. Footwear, such as stockings, needs to be of an absorbent material.

A nursing diagnosis and interventions for the patient with fungal infections include but are not limited to the following:

Nursing Diagnosis	Nursing Interventions
Impaired skin integrity, related to: • increased moisture • pruritus	Keep involved area clean and dry. Have patient wear loose-fitting clothing and shoes. Apply medications as directed.

Patient education involves teaching proper skin care and comfort measures to relieve pruritus. Review the medications to be taken and the procedures for the patient to do at home, emphasizing that fungal skin disorders may take months to cure. Stress general information about athlete's foot and clarify the many misconceptions.

Prognosis
Prognosis for recovery is good. Few complications result when treatment is followed.

INFLAMMATORY DISORDERS OF THE SKIN
Superficial infection of the skin is known as **dermatitis.** It can be caused by numerous agents, such as drugs, plants, chemicals, metals, and food. Regardless of the precipitating factor, the lesions associated with dermatitis develop along the same pattern. The nurse first observes erythema and edema, followed by the eruption of vesicles that rupture and encrust. Pruritus is always present, which promotes further skin excoriation.

CONTACT DERMATITIS
Etiology and Pathophysiology
Contact dermatitis is caused by direct contact with agents in the environment to which a person is hypersensitive. The epidermis becomes inflamed and damaged by the repeated contact with the physical and chemical irritants. Common causes of dermatitis are detergents, soaps, industrial chemicals, and plants such as poison ivy.

Clinical Manifestations
Lesions appear first at the point of contact with the irritant. Usually the patient feels burning, pain, pruritus, and edema. The involved area is soon erythematous, with **papules** (small, raised, solid skin lesions less than 1 cm in diameter) and vesicles appearing most often on the dorsal surfaces.

Assessment
Thoroughly research the patient's activities. If necessary, ask the patient to write a log of activities for the 48 hours before development of symptoms.

Collection of **subjective data** usually reveals that the patient has (1) tried a new soap, (2) been traveling and using different personal items, or (3) been working with plants or flowers. The patient may have severe pruritus and difficulty moving the involved area.

Collection of **objective data** should reveal (1) erythema, (2) papules and vesicles that generally ooze and weep a clear fluid, (3) scratch marks resulting from intense pruritus, and (4) edema of the area.

Diagnostic Tests
The primary diagnostic test is an accurate health history to identify the agent. Intradermal skin testing may identify plants and environmental agents, and elimination diets are used to identify food allergies. Elevated serum immunoglobulin E (IgE) levels and eosinophilia support the diagnosis. Both tests are thought to be related to abnormalities of T-cell function.

Medical Management
Medical intervention involves identifying the cause of the hypersensitive reaction. Symptomatic treatment for the inflammation, edema, and pruritus may include application of corticosteroids and the oral administration of antihistamines such as diphenhydramine (Benadryl). If the patient has a history of asthma (reactive airway disease), he or she may have an acute asthmatic episode. Hydroxyzine (Atarax) and inhalation treatments provide prophylactic treatment for asthma.

Nursing Interventions and Patient Teaching
The primary goal is to identify the offensive agent to protect the skin from further damage. Identify the cause by first describing the pattern of the reaction.

Wet dressings, using Burow's solution, help promote the healing process. To prevent infection, use aseptic technique to apply the corticosteroids to the open lesions.

Pruritus is responsible for most of the discomfort. A cool environment with increased humidity decreases the pruritus. Cold compresses may be applied to reduce circulation to the area (vasoconstriction). The patient should take daily baths with an application of oil to cleanse the skin. Fingernails should be cut at the level of the fingertips to decrease excoriation from scratching. Clothing should be lightweight and loose to decrease trauma of the involved area.

Nursing diagnoses and interventions for the patient with inflammation of the skin include but are not limited to the following:

Nursing Diagnoses	Nursing Interventions
Impaired skin integrity, related to scratching	Assess for signs of scratching. Have patient keep fingernails short and wear mittens. Apply medications as directed.
Pain, related to pruritus	Assess degree of pruritus and discomfort every shift. Keep environment cool. Apply cold compresses.

Teach the patient to keep an accurate history of possible predisposing offensive agents. As soon as the primary irritant has been identified, the patient should avoid it, as well as soaps, excessive heat, and rubbing of the area. Any time the skin is exposed to the primary irritant, the affected area should be washed thoroughly. Topical creams may be applied only as directed by a physician.

Prognosis

Removal of the offensive agent results in full recovery. Desensitizing the individual may be necessary if recurrences are frequent.

DERMATITIS VENENATA, EXFOLIATIVE DERMATITIS, AND DERMATITIS MEDICAMENTOSA

Etiology and Pathophysiology

Dermatitis venenata results from contact with certain plants, commonly **poison ivy** and poison oak. The signs and symptoms include mild to severe erythema with pruritus. On first exposure the body undergoes a sensitizing antigen formation. This results in an immunologic change in certain lymphocytes. Subsequent exposure to the antigen causes the lymphocytes to release irritating chemicals, leading to inflammation, edema, and vesiculation. The lesions are mainly found on the body part exposed to the sensitizing agent.

Exfoliative dermatitis can be caused by the infestation of certain heavy metals, such as arsenic or mercury, or by antibiotics, aspirin, codeine, gold, or iodine. The skin sloughs off, and the area becomes edematous and erythematous. Severe pruritus with fever occurs, and most patients require hospitalization. Treatment is individualized. If the cause can be determined, it should be removed or treated appropriately. Careful monitoring is essential to prevent secondary infection, avoid further irritation, and maintain fluid balance.

Dermatitis medicamentosa occurs when people are given a medication to which they are hypersensitive. Any drug can cause a reaction, but the common agents are penicillin, codeine, and iron.

Clinical Manifestations

Clinical manifestations range from mild to severe erythema with vesicular eruptions. In severe reactions, respiratory distress may occur. Any type of lesion may be found.

Assessment

Collection of **subjective data** for dermatitis involves questions about pruritus and a burning pain in the involved area.

Collection of **objective data** reveals lesions that are white in the center and red on the periphery. Vesicles are common in dermatitis venenata. Patients with dermatitis medicamentosa may have severe dyspnea caused by respiratory distress.

Diagnostic Tests

A careful patient history is of prime importance in the diagnosis of dermatitis venenata, exfoliative dermatitis, and dermatitis medicamentosa. A laboratory examination for serum IgE and eosinophilia is ordered.

Medical Management

The medical treatment for dermatitis ranges from therapeutic baths to administration of corticosteroids. The medical treatment is directed at the cause.

Nursing Interventions and Patient Teaching

Pruritus is the primary symptom in all types of dermatitis. Calamine lotion is a common over-the-counter medication used. Therapeutic baths using colloid solution, lotions, and ointments also help relieve the pruritus. Emotional support is necessary. The patient's physical appearance is difficult for the patient and family members to accept.

In dermatitis venenata, instruct the patient to wash the affected part immediately after contact with the offending allergen. After the lesions appear, only cool, open, wet dressings should be used.

In dermatitis medicamentosa, identifying the drug and discontinuing its use are paramount. If the offending allergen cannot be pinpointed, no drugs should be given. Notify the physician. The lesions will disappear after the medication is discontinued. More specific nursing intervention is directed by individual patient symptoms.

Nursing diagnoses and interventions for the patient with dermatitis include but are not limited to the following:

Nursing Diagnoses	Nursing Interventions
Impaired skin integrity, related to crusted, open lesions	Inspect lesions every day for exudate, size, and specific body area involved. Keep area clean and dry. Don gloves when giving direct patient care.

Nursing Diagnoses	Nursing Interventions
Risk for infection, related to break in skin	Assess skin for signs of infection. Identify interventions to prevent or reduce the risk of infection. Monitor vital signs; assess for elevated temperature. Stress medical aseptic hand hygiene technique. Use aseptic technique, and keep involved areas dry when providing care.
Deficient knowledge, related to the cause and spread of the disease	Assess patient's knowledge level and readiness to learn. Demonstrate appropriate care and application of topical medications. Stress importance of individual personal items, such as linens and towels. Involve family in patient teaching.

Advise the patient to wear a medical-alert bracelet or necklace showing the name of the allergen and to notify all health care personnel of the medication allergy.

Prognosis
Full recovery occurs when the offending agent is removed.

URTICARIA
Etiology and Pathophysiology
Urticaria refers to the presence of wheals or hives in an allergic reaction commonly caused by drugs, food, insect bites, inhalants, emotional stress, or exposure to heat or cold. The wheals (round elevation of the skin; white in the center with a pale red periphery) (see Table 3-1) of urticaria appear suddenly. Urticaria or hives is caused by the release of histamine in an antigen-antibody reaction.

Clinical Manifestations
The increased histamine causes the capillaries to dilate, resulting in increased permeability. Respiratory involvement may occur.

Assessment
Subjective data include pruritus, edema, a burning pain, and sometimes dyspnea.

Collection of objective data identifies transient wheals of varying shapes and sizes with well-defined erythematous margins and pale centers. Intense scratching may be seen, and in some cases respiration may be compromised. Assessment of

respiratory status provides a baseline for future assessments.

Diagnostic Tests
A detailed health history is the primary tool to identify the cause of hives. An allergy skin test may be performed using minute quantities of the antigen to identify the allergic substances. A serum examination for IgE elevation may be ordered.

Medical Management
Relief from urticaria can be achieved by administering an antihistamine and sometimes epinephrine. Identification of the cause of the urticaria is important to prevent recurrence.

Nursing Interventions and Patient Teaching
Nursing interventions include helping the patient identify the cause and decreasing the discomfort from the pruritus. Teach the patient about possible causes and prevention methods. Explain medications thoroughly, and demonstrate therapeutic baths. Review the signs and symptoms of an anaphylactic reaction, including shortness of breath, wheezing, and cyanosis.

Prognosis
Patients recover fully when the offending agent is determined and avoided. Compliance with the therapeutic regimen influences the outcome.

ANGIOEDEMA
Etiology and Pathophysiology
Angioedema is a form of urticaria and is caused by the same offenders. It occurs in the subcutaneous tissue, whereas urticaria is a skin and mucous membrane lesion. Angioedema is characterized by local edema of an entire area, such as an eyelid, hands, feet, tongue, larynx, gastrointestinal (GI) tract, genitalia, or lips. Only a single edematous area usually appears at one time.

Assessment
Subjective data include symptoms of burning, pruritus, acute pain if in the GI tract, or respiratory distress if in the larynx.

The collection of objective data reveals lesions that have a normal appearance on the outer skin with edema.

Diagnostic Tests
A careful patient history is essential in the diagnosis of angioedema. Patients with a history of allergies are more likely to have angioedema.

Medical Management
Treatment to relieve angioedema may include antihistamine drugs such as diphenhydramine. Epinephrine and corticosteroids such as methylprednisolone (Solu-Medrol) may also be given.

Nursing Interventions

A cold pack or cold compress may be used. Continual respiratory assessment is essential to detect respiratory distress. Tell patients to wear a medical-alert bracelet. Education is the key to preventing recurrent episodes.

Prognosis

With treatment, the prognosis is excellent.

ECZEMA (ATOPIC DERMATITIS)

Etiology and Pathophysiology

Eczema is primarily a disease of infants and is associated with allergies, commonly to chocolate, eggs, wheat, and orange juice. The allergen causes histamine to be released, and an antigen-antibody reaction occurs.

Clinical Manifestations

Papular and vesicular lesions appear and are surrounded by erythema. The vesicles generally rupture, discharging a yellow, tenacious exudate that dries and encrusts. If the lesions become infected, the skin loses its pigment and become shiny with dry scales.

Assessment

Subjective data include pruritus and scratching. Children are generally fussy and irritable, and anorexia is common. The skin is sensitive to touch. A family history of allergies and asthma supports the findings in many cases.

Objective data include vesicles and papules found on the scalp, the forehead, the cheeks, the neck, and the surfaces of the extremities. The involved area is erythematous and dry. Tiny cracks in the epithelium allow fluid to escape and further promote dryness. The primary signs result from the scratching from pruritus. Scales accompanied by dryness in the involved area are a distinguishing characteristic of eczema.

Diagnostic Tests

The diagnosis is generally made during a thorough health history that reveals a family history of eczema, since heredity is a prominent factor. Diet elimination and skin testing may be used to identify the specific substance to which the patient is hypersensitive. IgE serum tests provide data related to allergic response.

Medical Management

Medical treatment involves reducing the amount of allergen exposure. The eruptions and pruritus can be relieved if the aggravating factor is identified and controlled. The primary goal is to break the inflammation cycle.

Hydration of the skin is the key to treatment. The skin is dry because of tiny cracks that allow body fluids to escape. The skin may be hydrated by soaking the affected area in warm water for 15 to 20 minutes and then applying an occlusive ointment to retain the water. Examples of occlusive preparations are petrolatum, corticosteroid ointments, and vegetable shortening. The skin should be patted dry after the bath and the occlusive preparation applied immediately to the damp skin.

Nursing Interventions and Patient Teaching

Nursing interventions are directed toward treatment of symptoms for the eczematous patient. Administer the therapeutic bath and occlusive preparations as directed. Use wet dressings to maximize hydration of the skin. Apply topical steroids to relieve discomfort.

When the lesions begin to heal, a lotion such as Eucerin, Alpha Keri, Lubriderm, or Curel should be applied three or four times a day to add moisture to the skin. Wet wraps and occlusive preparations only hold water already present.

The emotional impact of having eczema ranges from anger to depression. The nurse provides an emotional outlet for these patients. Encourage the patient to share emotions by using effective listening skills and open-ended questions. This provides a means to establishing a therapeutic rapport with the patient.

Before the development of steroids, coal tar products were used to reduce the skin inflammation. Coal tar products do not decrease inflammation as quickly as steroids, but they last longer and have fewer side effects. Therefore coal tar preparations are recommended for chronic eczema. Preparations such as Estar-Gel and Psori-Gel are applied once a day at bedtime with a moisturizer.

Nursing diagnoses and interventions for the patient with eczema include but are not limited to the following:

Nursing Diagnoses	Nursing Interventions
Impaired skin integrity, related to open lesions	Assess skin for signs of secondary infection. Monitor CBC for elevated white blood cell count. Apply ordered medications using medical aseptic technique.
Risk for situational low self-esteem, related to change in body image	Assess patient's mental status. Be an active listener. Encourage verbalization of concerns the patient may be experiencing. Observe interaction with family and staff members and assist in establishing a therapeutic rapport.
Risk for infection, related to open lesion	Report at once the signs of wound infection such as erythema, especially beyond the wound margins. Increasing edema, purulent exudates, change in the description of the pain or increased pain, and increased warmth in the involved area are signs and symptoms of infection.

ACNE VULGARIS

Etiology and Pathophysiology

Acne is an inflammatory papulopustular skin eruption that involves the sebaceous glands; it occurs primarily in adolescents. The exact cause is unknown. However, several factors that may contribute are diet, stress, heredity, and overactive hormones. Hygiene has not been found to be a significant factor in the development of acne.

Acne develops when the oil glands become occluded. At puberty, androgens secreted increase the size of the oil glands, causing the sebum to combine more readily with epithelial cells and bacteria. Sebum may then occlude a hair follicle, forming a comedo (plural, *comedones*). A comedo is a blackhead. It is dark because of the effect of oxygen on sebum, not because of the presence of dirt.

Clinical Manifestations

Acne is found most often on the face, neck, upper chest, shoulder, and back (Figure 3-9). The first symptom is usually tenderness and edema in the area, followed by the comedo. The skin is oily and shiny, and the lesions last up to 10 days. Scarring results from large lesions that are traumatized when the person tries to rupture the comedo.

Assessment

Collection of **subjective data** includes asking the adolescent how acne affects lifestyle: Does it affect your participation in activities or group communication? Most patients acknowledge that acne affects their self-image. Common locations for acne lesions are the face and chin, which are highly visible areas. Lesions increase with emotional upsets and stress.

Collection of **objective data** includes noting the presence of edema in the involved area. Comedones (blackheads) are found on the skin of the face, back, or chest.

Diagnostic Tests

The medical diagnosis is primarily made by inspection of the lesions and a health history that supports the diagnosis. Sometimes blood samples are drawn to measure hormone levels.

Medical Management

The medical management can involve topical, systemic, or intralesional medications. Topical therapy peels away the superficial skin layer to prevent sebum occlusions. A common topical medication is benzoyl peroxide gel (such as Clearasil). Effective topical therapy requires the use of special cleansing agents followed by applications of vitamin A acids, antibiotics, and sulfur-zinc lotions.

Systemic antibiotic therapy, combined with topical therapy, helps decrease the scarring associated with acne. Systemic antibiotics such as tetracycline are used. Isotretinoin (Accutane), a form of vitamin A, is also used frequently. Accutane reduces the sebum production and abnormal keratinization of gland ducts. Accutane must be prescribed with extreme caution in adolescent females because of its destructive effect on fetal development. Depression is a side effect of the drug. Changes in behavior should be noted and the patient referred for assistance. All patients taking the drug must have monthly liver function tests to determine if the drug is hepatotoxic.

Nursing Interventions and Patient Teaching

In planning nursing interventions, be aware that most adolescents do not comply with long-term treatment regimens. Assess and consider what acne means to them. The actual extent of the condition is not as important as the adolescent's feelings. When an adolescent's face constantly has ugly black and white lesions, it is hard to maintain a healthy self-esteem.

In addition to psychological concerns, focus on preventive nursing interventions. The important areas are skin care, compliance, and emotional support. Prevention stresses identification of factors that directly increase acne. Although poor hygiene may not be a cause, cleanliness decreases infection rate and promotes healing. The patient should keep the hands and hair away from the face, wear clothes that do not restrict affected areas, wash the hair daily, and wash the skin two or three times a day with medicated soap. Cosmetics need to be water based, and products that have wax esters should be avoided. Compliance is difficult because improvement is slow. Often 3 weeks of treatment are required before the patient, the family, or friends notice improvement (see Health Promotion box).

Nursing diagnoses and interventions for the patient with acne vulgaris include but are not limited to the following.

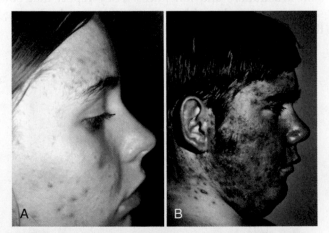

FIGURE 3-9 Acne vulgaris. **A,** Comedones with a few inflammatory pustules. **B,** Papulopustular acne.

Nursing Diagnoses	Nursing Interventions
Impaired skin integrity, related to occluded oil glands	Assess extent of occluded oil glands by inspecting lesions for size, color, and location. Monitor for signs of infection. Wash involved areas two or three times a day. Apply medications to decrease occlusion of oil glands.
Situational low self-esteem, related to physical appearance	Assess primary cause of low self-esteem and depth of feelings. Assess family support. Encourage verbalization of feelings about cosmetic appearance and ways to deal with the situation. Observe nonverbal communication to discover patient's perception of the illness. Stress the importance of not comparing oneself with others. Have patient list current successes and strengths. Give positive reinforcement.
Social isolation, related to decreased self-esteem	Assess extent and feelings of isolation. Assess factors that contribute to sense of helplessness. Listen to and spend time with patient. Involve patient in support group. Focus on patient's strengths.

Health Promotion

Healthy Skin

- Adequate nutrition (especially fluids; protein; vitamins A, B complex, and C; iron; adequate calories; and unsaturated fatty acids) promotes healthy skin.
- Refrain from smoking to improve skin color and prevent circulation difficulties.
- Drink eight glasses of water per day to help rid the skin of waste products.
- Exercise increases circulation and dilates blood vessels. In addition to the healthy glow produced by exercise, the psychological effects can improve one's appearance and mental outlook. However, caution must be used to protect against overexposure to heat, cold, and sun during outdoor exercise.
- In general, the skin and hair should be washed often enough to remove excess oil and excretions and to prevent odor.
- The use of neutral soaps and avoidance of hot water and vigorous rubbing can noticeably decrease local irritation and inflammation.
- Older adults should avoid using harsh soaps and shampoos because of the increased dryness of their skin.
- Moisturizers should be used after bath or shower, while the skin is still damp, to seal in this moisture.
- Obesity has an adverse effect on the skin. Increased subcutaneous fat can lead to stretching and overheating. Overheating causes an increase in perspiring, which can impair normal or inflamed skin.

Teaching should center on the patient's physical and emotional needs. Address diet, hygiene, stress reduction, makeup, and medications. Coping skills may need to be retaught and counseling referrals made. The extensive treatment time should be covered in minute detail because this disease is chronic and exacerbations will occur. Helping the adolescent communicate about feelings will decrease any long-term effects that acne may have on his or her personality. Patients taking isotretinoin will develop dry skin; teach patients measures to prevent it.

Prognosis

Prognosis for acne is good. However, lasting psychological effects can occur from the scarring that may result. In extreme cases eczema may develop from taking medications for acne, such as isotretinoin.

PSORIASIS

Etiology and Pathophysiology

Psoriasis is a noninfectious skin disorder; it is a hereditary, chronic, proliferative disease involving the epidermis and can occur at any age. No specific predisposing factors are known. The skin cells divide much more rapidly than normal. The normal time for the entire skin to be replaced, through sloughing and generation of new cells, is 28 days; in psoriasis the time may decrease to 7 days. Severe scaling results from the rapid cell division.

Clinical Manifestations

The lesions appear as raised, erythematous, circumscribed, silvery scaling plaques. The primary lesion is papular. The papules become plaques, which are located on the scalp, the elbows, the chin, and the trunk (Figure 3-10). The disease may be classified as mild, moderate, or severe.

Assessment

Collection of **subjective data** initially reveals only mild pruritus. Sometimes patients express feelings of depression, frustration, and loneliness. They report that observers stare and avoid contact with them, increasing their self-consciousness about their appearance.

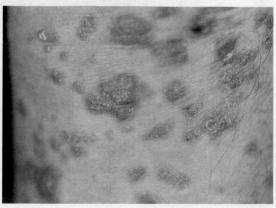

FIGURE 3-10 Psoriasis.

Collection of **objective data** includes observing dull, erythematous, sharply outlined plaques covered with silvery scales on the elbows, the knees, and the scalp. Fingernails can be affected and will show pitting with yellowish discoloration.

Diagnostic Tests

No specific diagnostic tests exist for psoriasis. Primary diagnosis is made by observing the patient and the symptoms displayed.

Medical Management

Medical management is aimed at slowing the proliferation of epithelial layers of the skin. Topical steroids and keratolytic agents are used in occlusive wet dressings to decrease inflammation. Keratolytic agents such as tar preparations and salicylic acid (Calicylic) decrease shedding of the outer layer of the skin. Topical steroids used are hydrocortisone and betamethasone valerate (Valisone).

Another treatment, photochemotherapy, involves the use of a drug enhanced by exposure to light. This therapy combines methoxsalen (Oxsoralen), which is given orally, and the concurrent use of ultraviolet light A (UVA).

Methotrexate and vitamin D reduce epidermal proliferation in some cases. The systemic medications approved by the FDA also include antimetabolite (methotrexate), immunosuppressant (cyclosporine), and retinoid (acitretin). Infliximab (Remicade) is used to control the severe plaque form of the disease (Lewis et al., 2007).

Nursing Interventions and Patient Teaching

Nursing interventions include proper administration of the treatment modality. Additional rest and measures to promote psychological well-being, such as counseling, are necessary. The patient's emotional needs are as important as the physical needs. Because this disease is chronic, encourage the patient to focus on positive attributes.

Nursing diagnoses and interventions for the patient with psoriasis include but are not limited to the following:

Nursing Diagnoses	Nursing Interventions
Impaired skin integrity, related to proliferation of epithelial cells	Assess extent of the scaliness. Administer treatment method correctly. Use medical aseptic technique.
Situational low self-esteem, related to appearance	Assess patient's concept of body. Help patient focus on positive aspects. Discuss with patient ways to conceal obvious lesions.

Nursing Diagnoses	Nursing Interventions
Social isolation, related to decreased self-esteem	Assess activity pattern and social outlets. Demonstrate ways to conceal lesions with clothes. Involve patient in support group.

The primary points in patient teaching include the nature of the disease, correct application of the treatment modality, and compliance with medical care. Stress that patients should not treat themselves. Inform patients that the disease is not curable.

Prognosis

Psoriasis is a chronic disease. The clinical course is variable, but less than half of the patients have a prolonged remission. Severity ranges from a minimal cosmetic problem to a life-threatening emergency.

SYSTEMIC LUPUS ERYTHEMATOSUS

Lupus is the Latin word for "wolf," used since AD 1230 to describe the cutaneous skin changes that resemble the zygomatic erythema of a red wolf (Figure 3-11). Lupus erythematosus affects the skin and may become systemic. Discoid lupus is an inflammatory condition with skin manifestation that can lead to the autoimmune disease, systemic lupus erythematosus (SLE).

Etiology and Pathophysiology

SLE is an autoimmune disorder characterized by inflammation of almost any body part. It is a chronic, multisystem inflammatory disorder that occurs when the body produces antibodies against its own cells. The resulting antigen and antibody complexes damage connective tissues. SLE is a disease of exacerbations and remissions. It is distinguished by an inflam-

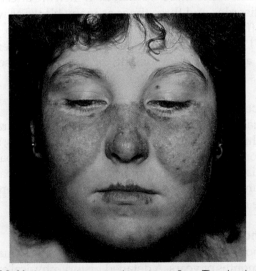

FIGURE 3-11 Systemic lupus erythematosus flare. The classic butterfly rash occurs over the nose and cheek area in 10% to 50% of patients with acute cutaneous lupus erythematosus.

Box 3-2   Pathogenic Conditions and Clinical Manifestations in Body Systems of Persons with Systemic Lupus Erythematosus

MUSCULOSKELETAL

Inflammation of vessels, tendons, and muscle tissue occurs because of deposits of fibrin. Polyarthralgia and polyarteritis occur in approximately 90% to 95% of patients.

GASTROINTESTINAL

Ulceration occurs on mucosal membranes because of degeneration of collagen tissue, with gastrointestinal manifestations of hemorrhage, abdominal pain, pancreatitis, cholecystitis, and bowel infarction.

RENAL

Glomerular sclerosis and glomerulonephritis occur with persistent proteinuria or cellular casts in urine.

HEMATOLOGIC

Cells are destroyed, and interference with coagulation occurs because of circulating antibodies. Anemia, leukopenia, lymphopenia, thrombocytopenia, and elevated erythrocyte sedimentation rate result.

CARDIOVASCULAR

Pericarditis is the most common cardiac manifestation. It often is the first clinical problem the patient manifests. Pericar-dial rub, commonly associated with pericarditis, can lead to dysrhythmias. Vasculitis in the small vessels may occur.

PULMONARY

Pleurisy and pleural effusions resulting from inflammation of the pleura are relatively common.

INTEGUMENTARY

Classic characteristics include the erythematous butterfly rash over the bridge of the nose and on the cheeks and linear erythema along the eyelids (see Figure 3-11). Other features may include bullae, patchy areas of purpura, urticaria, and subcutaneous nodules.

NEUROLOGIC

Mental and neurologic signs and symptoms occur in 35% to 40% of patients with systemic lupus erythematosus. Signs and symptoms relate to the central nervous system, not to the peripheral nerves. Mental and behavioral changes may occur, as well as seizures, headaches, and strokes.

---

matory lesion that affects several organ systems: the skin, the joints, the kidneys, and serous membranes.

SLE is a chronic, incurable, and multicausal disease. Although the syndrome's origin is a mystery, increasing evidence suggests that immunologic, hormonal, genetic, and possibly viral factors may contribute to its onset. Genetic predisposition seems to play a role in most cases, coupled with a precipitating agent or factor. The person with SLE has a decreased number of T-suppressor cells; those T-suppressor cells that remain function in a limited manner. Antibodies develop against other antigens.

SLE is most prevalent in women of childbearing age. Nine times more women than men are affected by this disorder, and three times as many blacks as whites are affected. Survival rates have increased to more than 15 years after diagnosis with this disorder. Despite advances in treatment, SLE remains a serious illness.

Clinical Manifestations

Clinical manifestations include oral ulcers, arthralgias or arthritis, vasculitis, rash, nephritis, pericarditis, synovitis, organic brain syndromes, peripheral neuropathies, anemia, leukopenia, thrombocytopenia, coagulopathies, immunosuppression, and dermatitis. Anemia tends to be the most common complication (Box 3-2).

Diagnostic Tests

Diagnosis of SLE may require extensive evaluations over months or years. A detailed history, physical examination, and results of laboratory findings are required to obtain a diagnosis (Lewis et al., 2007). Diagnostic tests for SLE (Box 3-3) often have positive results in the presence of inflammatory disease. No single test is considered conclusive for diagnostic purposes. However, positive results of one or more diagnostic tests along with at least three other criteria lead to the diagnosis of SLE. Criteria for diagnosis include the following:

- Erythematous butterfly rash (see Figure 3-11) over the nose and cheeks and along the eyelids
- Alopecia (hair loss), with frontal alopecia seen more frequently in women

Box 3-3   Diagnostic Tests for Systemic Lupus Erythematosus

- Antinuclear antibody (ANA)
- DNA antibody
- Anti-Sm antibody
- Complement
- Complete blood count (CBC)
- Erythrocyte sedimentation rate (ESR)
- Sedimentation rate (not diagnostic, but used to monitor disease activity and effectiveness of therapy)
- Coagulation profile
- Rheumatoid factor (RF)
- Rapid plasma reagin (RPR)
- Skin and renal biopsy
- C-reactive protein (CRP)
- Coombs' test
- Lupus erythematosus cell preparation (LE cell prep)
- Urinalysis
- Chest radiographic study

- Other skin features, including bullae, patchy areas of purpura, thickening of epidermis
- Photosensitivity
- Oral ulcers
- Polyarthralgias and polyarthritis
- Pleuritic pain, pleural effusion, pericarditis, and vasculitis
- Renal disorders as evidenced by protein or cellular casts in the urine
- Neurologic signs, such as seizures of unknown cause
- Hematologic disorders—such as hemolytic anemia, leukopenia, lymphopenia, or thrombocytopenia—in the absence of other diagnostic reasons
- Immunologic disorder identified with positive lupus erythematosus prep, antinuclear antibody (ANA), or double-stranded DNA
- Positive ANA in the absence of patient use of drugs known to cause drug-induced lupus erythematosus

Medical Management

SLE treatment goals include relief of the symptoms. The outcomes of the medical plan include remission of the disease, early alleviation of exacerbations, and prevention of untoward complications. Additional outcomes include therapeutic management of the signs and symptoms of the syndrome and suppression of inflammation.

Drug therapy includes nonsteroidal antiinflammatory agents, such as acetylsalicylic acid (ASA) and ibuprofen (Motrin); antimalarial drugs (hydroxychloroquine [Plaquenil] or chloroquine); and corticosteroids (such as prednisone) in low doses given several times a day. Methylprednisolone may be used intravenously in cases of exacerbation. Peak amounts of steroids help to achieve remission. The steroid doses are decreased slowly until a maintenance dose is reached. Topical corticosteroid creams are used for the rash of SLE. Antineoplastic drugs such as azathioprine (Imuran), cyclophosphamide (Cytoxan), or chlorambucil (Leukeran) may be used therapeutically to achieve remission or to control signs and symptoms.

Antimalarial drugs (hydroxychloroquine) are used to control discoid and other skin lesions and rheumatic manifestations. Because retinal toxicity may occur at high doses, patients should receive pretreatment and annual ophthalmic examinations.

Antiinfective agents are used both to treat and to prevent infections in the patient with SLE. The specific antibiotic depends on the infection site. Urinary tract infections respond well to ciprofloxacin (Cipro).

Peritoneal dialysis or hemodialysis may be indicated in patients who have moderate to severe renal involvement. Laboratory tests such as assessing blood urea nitrogen (BUN) and serum creatinine provide information regarding kidney function. Analgesics and diuretics may be used to treat symptoms often found in patients with SLE. Supportive therapy—such as a balanced diet, a balance between rest and activity, and reduced exposure to the sun—may also be indicated.

Nursing Interventions and Patient Teaching

Because SLE is a multisymptom disease, a thorough assessment is indicated. Tailor the care plan to include (1) skin care, including teaching avoidance of direct sunlight and use of protective clothing and sunscreen; (2) balance between rest and activity; (3) recognition of signs of exacerbation (i.e., fever, rash, cough, or increasing muscle and joint pain); (4) early recognition of signs and symptoms of infection; (5) stress reduction and management; and (6) balanced nutrition and reduction of sodium intake. Because the disease is one of exacerbation and remissions, each exacerbation will intensify the patient's stress and decrease his or her ability to cope. Provide psychosocial, emotional, and spiritual support for the patient.

Patients with impaired immune system function must endure the consequences of chronic or incurable disease. A caring, gentle, and understanding approach to patient care will help reduce the burden and stress of SLE (Nursing Care Plan 3-2). The nurse's responsibilities in patient education are related to the information needed for the patient to live a normal life. Focus on activity level, prevention of infection, and potential complications.

Prognosis

SLE has no known cure. Management of the disease depends on the nature and severity of the manifestations and the organs affected. Treating SLE earlier in its course has contributed to a better prognosis.

PARASITIC DISEASES OF THE SKIN

PEDICULOSIS

Etiology and Pathophysiology

Pediculosis (lice infestation) is a parasitic disorder of the skin that many associate with poor living conditions and poor personal hygiene. This is not always the case, however; pediculosis can occur anywhere. Lice obtain their nutrition from the blood of their victims. They leave their eggs (nits) on the skin surface attached to the shaft of the hair (Figures 3-12 and 3-13).

Humans have three types of lice: the head louse, the body louse, and the pubic louse. In pediculosis capitis, the head louse attaches itself to the hair shaft and lays 8 to 16 eggs per day. The eggs are visible at the back of the neck as gray, shiny, oval bodies.

In pediculosis corporis, the body louse is found around the neck, waist, and thighs. The louse is generally found in the seams of clothing and causes severe pruritus and pinpoint hemorrhages.

The pubic louse, the parasite involved in pediculosis pubis, does not resemble the head or body louse. It looks like a crab with sharp pincers that attach to the

Nursing Care Plan 3-2   **The Patient with Systemic Lupus Erythematosus**

Ms. Templeton, age 34, is experiencing an acute exacerbation of systemic lupus erythematosus. She is admitted to the medical unit with severe joint pain, butterfly rash, generalized edema, and Sjögren syndrome.

NURSING DIAGNOSIS *Impaired skin integrity, related to skin rash (butterfly across face), hair loss, skin atrophy, discoid lesions involving other parts of the body*

Patient Goals and Expected Outcomes	Nursing Interventions	Evaluation and Rationale
Patient will verbalize understanding of skin care regimen and positioning schedule	Develop positioning schedule. Use appropriate devices such as air mattress, eggcrate mattress, sheepskin, or foam padding, where indicated.	Patient verbalizes understanding of the purpose of changing positions every 2 hours to prevent skin impairment.
Patient will demonstrate behaviors to promote skin healing	Assess and monitor skin and mucous membranes and describe lesions' size, characteristics, and changes noted. Assess nutritional status and areas at risk for pressure. Measure intake and output. Provide optimum nutrition.	Patient states she understands skin care regimen to promote skin healing.
Patient will experience improved wound and lesion healing	Monitor for signs of infection. Encourage patient to minimize sun exposure by wearing long-sleeved blouses or shirts and wide-brimmed hats and by using sunscreens with a sun protection factor of 15. Teach skin care maintenance.	Patient's skin lesions are beginning to show signs of healing.

NURSING DIAGNOSIS *Disturbed body image, related to baldness and pathologic skin pattern conditions*

Patient Goals and Expected Outcomes	Nursing Interventions	Evaluation and Rationale
Patient will verbalize understanding of altered body image. Patient will have a positive, accepting, and realistic body image. Patient will perform self-care activities within level of own ability. Patient will identify personal community resources that can provide assistance	Assess patient's perception of body image; investigate what aspects are not pleasing and how she perceives changes as deviating from social norms. Teach patient ways to improve body image (e.g., improving personal hygiene, wearing makeup, changing type of clothes, protecting self from sun). Encourage family members and significant others to maintain open communication with patient. Record emotional changes. Set limits on maladaptive behavior.	Patient states she understands that skin changes and hair loss are part of the disease process of systemic lupus erythematosus. Patient talks about importance of open communication with her family and significant other concerning her feelings of body image disturbance.

Critical Thinking Questions

1. Ms. Templeton has painful, edematous joints that greatly decrease her mobility. She has 4+ pitting edema to the lower extremities secondary to the loss of protein through her kidney. What are the most appropriate nursing interventions to decrease Ms. Templeton's pain level and to increase her mobility?
2. On entering the room, the nurse notes Ms. Templeton crying. She says that her lifestyle is severely altered because she is unable to be in the sun to work in her beloved garden. What nursing interventions would be most beneficial?
3. Ms. Templeton confides that she fears that this severe increase in her symptoms will lead to an early death. What initial response to this statement would be of greatest assistance?

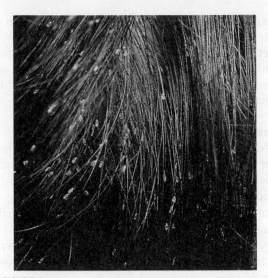

FIGURE 3-12 Eggs of pediculus attached to shafts of hair.

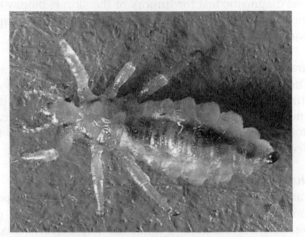

FIGURE 3-13 Lice have six legs and are wingless.

pubic hair. Transmission can be through sexual contact, bed linens, or bath towels.

Clinical Manifestations

Nits or lice can be seen on the body. Pinpoint, raised red macules, pinpoint hemorrhages, and severe pruritus confirm the diagnosis. Excoriation is common because of the intense pruritus.

Assessment

Subjective data include complaints of pruritus in the area involved. Tenderness and difficulty wearing clothes are also noted.

Objective data include erythema, petechiae, and skin excoriation in the area.

Diagnostic Tests

The diagnostic test is a physical examination of the involved area. A health history supports the diagnosis. Removal of the parasite confirms the diagnosis.

Medical Management

A topical pediculicide such as lindane (Kwell) or pyrethrins (RID) is applied in any contaminated area. The specific technique for applying these products varies and should be followed closely to control the lice.

Nursing Interventions and Patient Teaching

The primary nursing intervention involves applying the medication to rid the patient of lice. Identify involved people and appropriate health teaching. Stress the nature and transmission of the disease. Assess each family member for nits, and teach measures to reduce pruritus, such as cool compresses and corticosteroid ointments. Any furniture or nonwashable materials with which the patient has come in contact should be properly cleaned to prevent reinfection. Bed linens should all be washed in hot water and dried in a dryer. Assessment of the patient's emotional needs is also important. Society often associates a lice infestation with poor hygiene practices.

Prognosis

The prognosis is good; proper treatment results in full recovery.

SCABIES

Etiology and Pathophysiology

Scabies is caused by the female itch mite (*Sarcoptes scabiei*). The mite penetrates the skin and makes a burrow. Once under the skin, the mite lays eggs that mature and rise to the skin surface. Scabies is transmitted by prolonged contact with an infected area. Overcrowded living conditions, poverty, changing sexual behaviors, and world travel have increased the incidence of scabies. Scabies occurs in all age-groups and socioeconomic classes.

Clinical Manifestations

Scabies causes wavy, brown, threadlike lines on the body, especially the hands, arms, body folds, and genitalia (Figure 3-14). Pruritus is severe, and secondary infections are common from the excoriation caused by scratching.

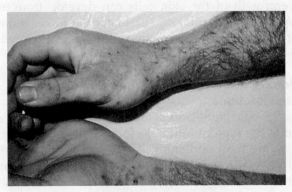

FIGURE 3-14 Scabies.

Assessment

Subjective data include the severe pruritus associated with scabies and the skin excoriation resulting from scratching.

Collection of **objective data** includes finding the wavy brown lines on the body and severe erythema from the scratching.

Diagnostic Tests

The condition can be confirmed by microscopic examination of infected skin. A health history and characteristic signs and symptoms support the diagnosis.

Medical Management

Medical treatment attempts to eliminate the mite and prevent complications. Drug therapy is basically the same as for pediculosis. Two additional drugs used are crotamiton (Eurax) and a 4% to 8% solution of sulfur in petrolatum.

Nursing Interventions and Patient Teaching

Nursing interventions for restoring skin integrity involve using medical aseptic techniques to improve hygiene and to apply medications. Proper application of medication is essential to destroy the parasite. The patient's emotional well-being is another focus of nursing care. Using open-ended questions and listening skills help provide support.

A primary concern is educating family members about the transmission of scabies. Each family member needs to treat the whole body with a scabicide. Clothing, bed linens, and bath articles should be washed in hot water and dried in a dryer. If clothes are line dried, they should be ironed. Stress the importance of compliance with the treatment. Also, teach the family that scabies infestations can happen to anyone. Conveying a nonjudgmental attitude is important.

Prognosis

The prognosis is good; with adequate treatment, full recovery results.

TUMORS OF THE SKIN

Overgrowth of the skin cells can develop from any layer or its appendages. The majority of skin tumors are benign. Many outgrowths or tumors can be predisposing factors for skin cancer.

Etiology, Pathophysiology, and Clinical Manifestations

The specific signs and symptoms of skin tumors relate to the type of tumor. Keloids, which originate in scars, are hard and shiny. Angiomas resemble birthmarks. Warts (verrucae) are located on the arms and hands. Nevi are thought to predispose a person to cancer, and patients become anxious when they notice a color change. Skin cancers may be life threatening and occur wherever exposure to the sun was greatest.

Report any changes in a skin lesion to a physician, including changes in size, color, border, surface, or elevation. Also report the development of pain, bleeding, or pruritus.

Assessment

Collection of **subjective data** includes a good health history. First assess the patient's risk factors, such as lifestyle, occupation, family history, and geographic location.

Collection of **objective data** includes describing the lesion in detail. The size, the location, and any pain are significant factors in determining the type of skin tumor. The lesion's appearance can take several forms.

Diagnostic Tests

The diagnostic test for tumors of the skin is biopsy of the lesion. A health history and visual inspection support the diagnosis.

Medical Management

The primary medical intervention for skin tumors is surgical removal. Other treatment modalities are radiation therapy to decrease the tumor size and application of topical medications such as corticosteroids to decrease the size and inflammation.

Nursing Interventions and Patient Teaching

Patients are understandably concerned about the potential threat of malignancy. Careful explanations of treatments, medications, and tests help decrease anxiety. Nursing interventions center on preparing the patient for the treatment needed. Skin tumors may be a threat to the patient's self-concept. Emotional care is important; encourage the patient to verbalize feelings of fear or anxiety.

Nursing diagnoses and interventions discussed with malignant melanoma are applicable to most skin cancers. Although the tumors previously mentioned are not all malignant, the problems posed are the same until a definitive diagnosis is made.

Discharge instructions include skin care, dressing changes, and follow-up care. Involve the family in teaching so they can support the patient. Discuss the signs and symptoms of infection for patients who have tumors surgically removed.

KELOIDS

Keloids (an overgrowth of collagenous scar tissue at the site of a wound of the skin) are seen more often in blacks than in whites. Collagen tissue becomes raised, hard, and shiny. Keloids usually originate from a scar and can be located anywhere on the body (Figure 3-15). The sternum, the ears, the neck, and the arms are common locations. Keloids are usually surgically excised

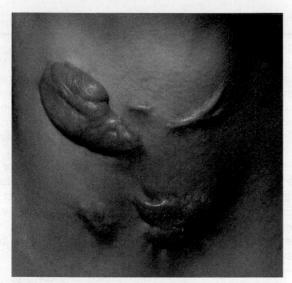

FIGURE 3-15 Keloids.

but may recur. Steroids and radiation therapy are two treatment measures.

ANGIOMAS

An angioma develops when a group of blood vessels dilate and form a tumorlike mass. A common angioma is a birthmark, such as the port-wine birthmark. This stain is not elevated and may be found on one side of the face or any part of the body. Treatment involves electrolysis or radiation.

A spider angioma or telangiectasis is associated with liver disease. A group of venous capillaries dilate and branch out like a spider. Spider angiomas usually resolve as the disease improves.

VERRUCA (WART)

A **verruca** is a benign, viral, warty skin lesion with a rough, papillomatous (nipplelike) growth occurring in many forms. Verrucae may occur singly or in groups and are thought to be contagious. Common locations are the hands, arms, and fingers, but warts can occur anywhere on the body. The plantar wart develops on the sole of the foot and is extremely painful. Treatment of warts depends on the type, location, and number. Cauterization, solid carbon dioxide, liquid nitrogen, and preparations of salicylic acid are used to remove warts.

NEVI (MOLES)

Nevi (singular, *nevus*; a pigmented, congenital skin blemish that is usually benign but may become cancerous), or moles, are nonvascular tumors, also called **birthmarks.** There are many types of nevi, and several may become malignant, especially if traumatized. The raised, black nevus is considered one of the most threatening, and removal is recommended to prevent it from becoming malignant. Any change in color, size, or texture or any bleeding or pruritus deserves investigation.

BASAL CELL CARCINOMA

Basal cell carcinoma is one type of skin cancer. Factors related to the development of skin cancer include frequent contact with certain chemicals, overexposure to the sun, and radiation treatment. Fair-skinned people are more likely to develop skin cancer, possibly because they have less melanin on the skin surface.

Basal cell carcinomas arise in the basal cell layer of the epidermis. They are often found on the face and upper trunk and are not noticed by the patient. Metastasis is rare, but underlying tissue destruction can progress to include vital structures. Basal cell carcinoma is usually scaly in appearance. It may be a pearly papule with a central crater and waxy, pearly border.

With early detection and complete removal, the outcome is favorable; however, this type of cancer recurs in 40% to 50% of patients treated (Figure 3-16).

SQUAMOUS CELL CARCINOMA

Squamous cell carcinoma arises in the epidermis. This cancerous neoplasm is a firm, nodular lesion topped with a crust or a central area of ulceration and indurated margins (Figure 3-17). Ten percent of patients have rapid invasion with metastasis by way of the lymphatic system; therefore early detection and treatment are important. Larger tumors are more prone to metastasis.

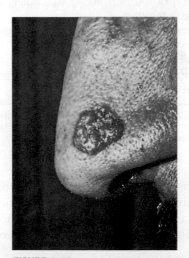

FIGURE 3-16 Basal cell carcinoma.

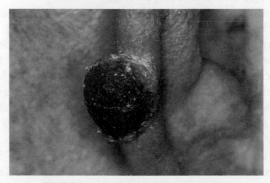

FIGURE 3-17 Squamous cell carcinoma.

🔍 **Evidence-Based Practice** | Skin Cancer Prevention

Research Summary

What is cancer? More specifically, what is skin cancer? Cancer by definition is an "uncontrolled growth and spread of abnormal cells" (ACS, 2006). Therefore skin cancer is characterized by abnormal skin cells, which can spread and invade other tissues. More importantly, what can we do about skin cancer? As nurses, it becomes our responsibility to assess for and educate our patients about all types of skin cancers, especially for the most serious form called melanoma. There are several risk factors for melanoma. Major factors are positive family history of melanoma, a prior melanoma, and multiple or unusual moles. Other factors include fair complexion/skin that is sensitive to the sun; excessive exposure to the sun (especially before age 18), and the use of tanning beds/booths.

Research has indicated that skin cancer, when detected early and treated properly, is highly curable. Overall survival rates for melanoma at the 5-year mark are 92%, with 98% for localized melanoma; when it is grouped in regional and distant stages, the survival rates dramatically decrease (ACS, 2006). Therefore early intervention is of utmost importance.

Application to Nursing Practice

The results from the research studies have made it a nursing responsibility to screen and intervene for our patients' best interest. It is a necessity that we promote self-screening for all patients and their family members. We must also educate the general public.

- Instruct patients to conduct a complete monthly self-examination of the skin and scalp, noting moles, blemishes, and birthmarks.
- Perform the examination after a bath or shower, including a head-to-toe check.
- Use a well-lit room and mirrors to examine all skin surfaces. If necessary, have the patient ask a family member/significant other to aid in the investigation.

- The ACS (2006) outlines the warning signs of skin cancer using the ABCD mnemonic: *A* is for Asymmetry—look for uneven shape; *B* is for Border irregularity—look for edges that are blurred, notched, or ragged; *C* is for Color—pigmentation is not uniform; blue, black, brown variegated and areas of pink, white, gray, blue, or red are abnormal (Hayes, 2003); and *D* is for Diameter, greater than the size of a typical pencil eraser.
- Teach your patients to contact their health care provider if a skin lesion or mole starts to bleed or ooze or feels different (swollen, hard, lumpy, itchy, or tender to the touch). Especially instruct older adults, who tend to have delayed wound healing.
- Inform your patients of ways to prevent skin cancer by avoiding overexposure to the sun:
  —Wear wide-brimmed hats and long sleeves.
  —Apply broad-spectrum sunscreens with SPF of 15 or greater to protect against ultraviolet B (UVB) and ultraviolet A (UVA) rays approximately 15 minutes before going into the sun and after swimming or perspiring.
  —Avoid tanning under the direct sun at midday (10 AM to 4 PM).
  —Do not use indoor sunlamps, tanning parlors, or tanning pills.
- Inform patients who are on medications that make the skin more sensitive to the sun (e.g., oral contraceptives, antibiotics, antiinflammatories, antihypertensives, immunosuppressives) to take extra precautions when spending time in the sun.
- Inform patients to protect their children from the sun. Severe sunburns in childhood greatly increase melanoma risk later in life (ACS, 2006).
- These interventions will provide the patient with self-screening measures to detect, prevent, and seek early treatment for skin cancer.

From Potter, P.A., & Perry, A.G. (2009). *Fundamentals of nursing: concepts, process, and practice* (7th ed.). St. Louis: Mosby. Data from American Cancer Society (2006). *Cancer facts and figures 2006*, Atlanta: Author; and Hayes, J.L. (2003). Are you assessing for melanoma? *RN*, 66(2), 36. *ACS*, American Cancer Society.

Sun-exposed areas, especially the head, neck, and lower lip, are common places of occurrence. The cancer also occurs on sites of chronic irritation or injury (scars, irradiated skin, burns, and leg ulcers).

MALIGNANT MELANOMA

Etiology and Pathophysiology

A malignant melanoma is a cancerous neoplasm in which pigment cells (melanocytes) invade the epidermis, dermis, and sometimes the subcutaneous tissue. Several types of melanoma occur, and they are categorized by location and description. Most melanomas arise from melanocytes in the epidermis, but some may appear in preexisting moles. Melanoma can metastasize to any organ, including the brain and heart.

This is the most deadly skin cancer, and its incidence has doubled in the past two decades, a faster rate of growth than any other cancer (Figure 3-18). The increased occurrence is associated with recreational exposure to the sun (see Evidence-Based Practice box). Heredity is also a factor, and any person who has a large number of moles with a variety of sizes and colors should be monitored. The person who has a history of skin cancer is at greater risk.

Clinical Manifestations

Basically, malignant melanomas are divided into four types: (1) superficial spreading melanomas, (2) malignant lentigo melanomas, (3) nodular melanomas, and (4) acral lentiginous melanomas.

Superficial spreading melanomas are the most common and occur anywhere on the body. These melanomas are slightly elevated, irregularly shaped lesions in a varying hues; common colors are tan, brown, black, blue, gray, and pink. **Lentigo melanomas** are usually found on the heads and necks of older adults. Characteristically these appear as tan, flat lesions that

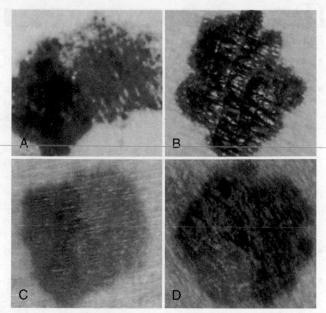

FIGURE 3-18 The ABCDs of melanoma. **A,** Asymmetry (one half unlike the other). **B,** Border (irregularly scalloped or poorly circumscribed border). **C,** Color varied from one area to another; shades of tan and brown, black, and sometimes white, red, or blue; change in shape, size, or color of mole. **D,** Diameter larger than 6 mm as a rule (diameter of a pencil eraser).

change shape and size. **Nodular melanomas** appear as a blueberry-type growth, varying from blue-black to pink. The patient often describes the lesion as a blood blister that fails to resolve. Nodular melanomas grow and metastasize faster than the other types. **Acral lentiginous melanomas** occur in areas not exposed to sunlight and where no hair follicles are present. Common locations are the hands, the soles, and the mucous membranes of dark-skinned people.

Assessment
The collection of **subjective data** should include a thorough health history related to skin cancer. Patients at greatest risk have fair complexions, blue eyes, red or blond hair, and freckles.

Objective data include the location, color, and appearance of the lesions.

Diagnostic Tests
Diagnosis primarily depends on tissue biopsy. The patient is also examined thoroughly for suspicious lesions. Monitor any lesion that is variegated in color, has an irregular border, or has an irregular surface. The tumor thickness at the time of diagnosis is a key factor in the prognosis of malignant melanoma. The two measurements to determine the thickness of the melanoma are Breslow measurement and Clark level. The thicker the tumor, the poorer the prognosis (Lewis et al., 2007).

Medical Management
Medical management depends on the site, level of invasion, thickness of the melanoma, and the patient's age and general health.

A wide, surgical excision of the primary lesion with a margin of normal skin is the treatment of choice. Skin grafts are sometimes needed. Subsequent treatment modalities such as chemotherapy, nonspecific immunotherapy, chemoimmunotherapy, and radiation may be planned, depending on the stage of the disease. Gene therapy is currently being examined as another treatment option (Lewis et al., 2007).

Nursing Interventions and Patient Teaching
The major goals of nursing care include pain relief, reduction of anxiety, and palliative treatment of the disease. Fear of the unknown is a major concern for the patient with a melanoma. Explaining procedures and diagnostic tests in terms that the patient can understand may help decrease anxiety.

Nursing diagnoses and interventions for the patient with melanomas include but are not limited to the following:

Nursing Diagnoses	Nursing Interventions
Pain, related to lesion	Assess pain using the five PQRST variables of the chief complaint.
	Provide nursing comfort measures, such as back rubs, to decrease pain.
	Administer pain medication as needed.
	Teach relaxation techniques.
Anxiety, related to cancer, its treatment, and prognosis	Listen to and accept expression of anger, sadness, and helplessness.

Discharge instructions include wound care, medication, cleansing, and follow-up care. Assess the family's knowledge about the seriousness and treatment of the disease. Explain to the patient the need for regular physical examinations and regular skin self-assessment. Encourage the patient to protect skin from the sun by using sunscreens and protective clothing and by limiting exposure. Stress the use of medical aseptic techniques to prevent a secondary infection.

Prognosis
The key prognostic factor in malignant melanoma is the thickness of the lesion. Individuals with lesions less than 0.76 mm thick have a survival rate of almost 100%, whereas those with lesions 3 mm thick or thicker have survival rates of less than 50%. If the cancer spreads to regional lymph nodes, the patient has a 50% 5-year survival rate. The tumor may metastasize by vascular or lymphatic spread, with rapid movement of melanoma cells to other parts of the body. If metastasis occurs, treatment is largely palliative.

DISORDERS OF THE APPENDAGES

ALOPECIA

Alopecia is the loss of hair. The cause can be aging, drugs such as antineoplastics, anxiety, or disease processes. Unless it is related to aging, alopecia is usually not permanent; the hair usually grows back but can take several months. Any time a patient loses hair, body image and self-esteem are threatened.

HYPERTRICHOSIS (HIRSUTISM)

Hypertrichosis is an excessive growth of hair in a masculine distribution. It can be hereditary or acquired as a result of hormone dysfunction and medications. The treatment is removal by dermabrasion, electrolysis, chemical depilation, shaving, tweezing, or rubbing with pumice. Treatment of the cause usually stops growth of additional hair.

HYPOTRICHOSIS

Hypotrichosis is the absence of hair or a decrease in hair growth. Skin disease, endocrine problems, and malnutrition are associated factors. Treatment involves identifying and treating the cause.

PARONYCHIA

Paronychia is a disorder of the nails. The nails get soft or brittle, and the shape can change as they grow into the soft tissue (ingrown nails). In paronychia, an infection of the nail develops and spreads around the nail, thus giving it the nickname "runaround." The nails are painful as they loosen and separate from the tissue. Wet dressings or topical antibiotics may be used. Sometimes a surgical incision and drainage of the infected area are performed.

BURNS

Etiology and Pathophysiology

Each year more than 1 million people in the United States seek medical attention for burns. About 70,000 of them need to be hospitalized, and one third require extensive care services. An estimated 4500 of these people die annually as a direct result of their burns (CDC, 2009). The incidence of burns has decreased slightly and the number of deaths resulting from burn injury has also decreased (CDC, 2009). This decrease stems from the creation of regional burn centers, a national focus on fire safety, the use of smoke detectors, and occupational safety mandates.

Burns may result from thermal or nonthermal causes. Thermal burns are caused by flames, scalds, and thermal energy (heat). Thermal burns are the most common type of burn injury. Nonthermal burns result from electricity, chemicals, and radiation. Skin destruction depends on the burning agent, the temperature of the burning agent, the condition of the skin before the injury, and the duration of the person's contact with the agent.

 Safety Alert

Prevention of Burns

- The major cause of fires in the home is carelessness with cigarettes. Preventive education is imperative.
- Other causes of burns include hot water from water heaters set higher than 140° F (60° C), cooking accidents, space heaters, combustibles such as gasoline and charcoal lighter fluid, steam from radiators, and chemicals.
- Most burns can be prevented. The nurse as a citizen and health care provider is in a good position to conduct home safety assessments and to educate people about burn injuries before accidents occur. Home safety measures include using smoke alarms and fire extinguishers. Families should have fire drills, and each family member should know where to go and what to do in case of a fire.
- Local fire departments can inform the public of regional fire codes and perform home safety checks.
- Knowledge of potential sources of burn injury allows problem solving for burn prevention.

Teaching people proper use of appliances (e.g., space heaters, electrical cords, wiring, outlets, outdoor grills, and water heaters) can prevent burn injury.

Burns cause dramatic changes in most physiologic functions of the body, beginning in the first few minutes to the first 12 to 24 hours after the burn injury. The burn's effect depends on two factors: the extent of the body surface burned and the depth of the burn injury. The extent of burn is measured in terms of the total body surface area (TBSA) injured. Burns exceeding 20% TBSA result in massive evaporative water losses and fluid loss into the interstitial spaces. Depth depends on the layers of the skin involved.

With any burn injury, a pathophysiologic process ensues. In the damaged area, the capillaries dilate, resulting in capillary hyperpermeability that lasts for about 24 hours. The increased cell permeability causes the fluid to shift from the capillaries into the surrounding tissues (interstitial spaces), resulting in edema and vesiculation (blistering). A larger burned area results in a more rapid shift of fluid from the intravascular area into the interstitial area (sometimes known as *third spacing*). This shift poses the greatest threat to life because the cells become dehydrated. As a result, the body experiences hypovolemic shock and hyperviscosity. Blood pressure and blood flow to the kidneys decrease, symptoms of hypovolemic shock develop, and acute renal failure may result.

The pathophysiology and care of burns may be divided into three stages. The emergent phase, stage 1, is from the onset of the injury until the patient stabilizes. Hypovolemic shock is the major concern for up to 48 hours after a major burn. Stage 2, the intermediate or acute (or diuretic) phase, begins 48 to 72 hours after the burn injury. In this stage the greatest concern is circulatory overload. Circulatory overload may result from the fluid shift back from the interstitial spaces into the capillaries. The acute phase begins when the kidneys excrete large volumes of urine (hence the name *diuretic stage*). Stage 3, the long-term rehabilitation phase, begins at the same time as burn wound treatment. In the third stage, the patient care outcome involves returning the patient to as normal a state as possible. A second outcome is freedom from wound infection.

In a burn injury, usually the greatest fluid loss occurs within the first 12 hours. The proteins, plasma, and electrolytes shift from the vascular compartment to the interstitial compartment. Red blood cells tend to remain in the vascular system, causing increased viscosity of the blood and a falsely elevated hematocrit level. Acute dehydration is present, and renal perfusion is seriously compromised. This fluid shift and the loss of intravascular fluids may lead to the development of burn shock. The rapid loss of fluid places a strain on the heart because the blood volume diminishes and the heart can no longer supply enough blood to perfuse the vital organs. The body responds by increasing the peripheral resistance. Burn shock is characterized by hypotension; decreased urinary output; increased pulse (tachycardia); rapid, shallow respirations (tachypnea); and restlessness. Most deaths from burns result directly from burn shock.

Fluids begin to shift back to the vascular compartment in approximately 48 to 72 hours. Fluid return denotes the end of the hypovolemic stage and the beginning of the diuretic stage. Reabsorption of the interstitial fluid back into the intravascular area causes an increased blood volume. As the blood volume increases, the cardiac output increases, resulting in increased renal perfusion. The result includes diuresis. However, the patient is at risk of fluid overload because of the rapid movement of fluid back into the intravascular space. Carefully monitor the patient's vital signs, urinary output, and consciousness. Patients with preexisting cardiac problems, as well as the very young and very old, run the greatest risk for circulatory overload.

A burn victim may experience smoke inhalation damage from breathing the chemicals produced by the burn. The fumes damage the cilia and the mucosa of the respiratory tract. Alveolar surfactant decreases, and atelectasis can occur. Breathing difficulties may take several hours to appear. While assessing a patient who has sustained any burn to the upper chest, the neck, and the face, consider the patient at high risk for respiratory distress. Signs of respiratory difficulty include a hoarse voice or a productive cough. Other physical findings suggesting an inhalation injury include the following:
- Singed nasal hairs
- Agitation, tachypnea, flaring nostrils, or intercostal retractions
- Brassy cough, grunting, or guttural respiratory sounds
- Erythema or edema of the oropharynx or nasopharynx
- Sooty sputum

Clinical Manifestations
Traditionally, burns were classified as first, second, or third degree (Table 3-3). However, using only the visual characteristics of the burn wound results in an inaccurate description. A more accurate classification is superficial thickness injuries, partial-thickness injuries, and full-thickness injuries; these terms graphically describe the burn and indicate the depth and severity of the tissue injury (Figures 3-19 to 3-21).

Assessment
The nursing assessment includes (1) depth of the burn, (2) causative agent, (3) temperature and duration of contact, and (4) skin thickness. The patient's age and

Table 3-3 | **Causes and Factors Determining Depth of Burn Injury**

DEPTH	CAUSE	APPEARANCE	COLOR	SENSATION
Superficial (first degree)	Flash flame, ultraviolet light (sunburn)	Dry, no vesicles Minimal or no edema Blanches with fingertip pressure, and refills when pressure removed	Increased erythema	Painful
Partial thickness (second degree)	Contact with hot liquids or solids Flash flame to clothing Direct flame Chemicals Ultraviolet light	Large, moist vesicles that increase in size Blanches with fingertip pressure, and refills when pressure removed	Mottled with dull, white, tan, pink, or cherry red areas	Very painful
Full thickness (third degree)	Contact with hot liquids or solids Flame Chemicals Electrical contact	Dry with leathery eschar Charred vessels visible under eschar Vesicles rare, but thin-walled vesicles that do not increase in size may be present No blanching with pressure	White, charred, dark tan Black Red	Little or no pain Hair easily pulls out

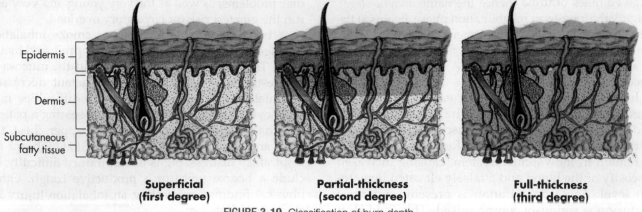

| Epidermis |
| Dermis |
| Subcutaneous fatty tissue |

Superficial (first degree) **Partial-thickness (second degree)** **Full-thickness (third degree)**

FIGURE 3-19 Classification of burn depth.

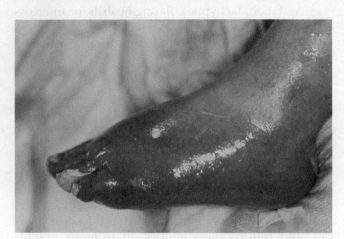

FIGURE 3-20 Superficial partial-thickness injury.

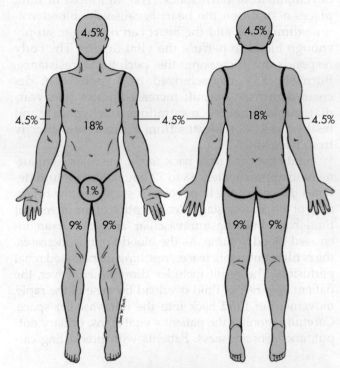

FIGURE 3-22 Rule of nines.

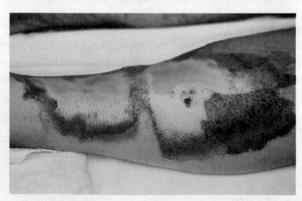

FIGURE 3-21 Full-thickness thermal injury.

other disease processes affect the outcome of the burn. The **rule of nines** determines the TBSA burned (Figure 3-22). The rule of nines divides the body into multiples of nine. The entire head is 9%; the anterior and posterior aspects of the arms are a total of 9% each; the legs are 9% anterior and 9% posterior; the chest and back are 18% each; and the perineum is 1%.

The rule of nines does not take into account the different levels of growth and is not accurate for children.

Collection of **subjective data** reveals the causative agent, other diseases present, the temperature and du-

ration of contact, and the patient's age. If the patient is able to communicate, ask him or her to rate the pain on a scale from 0 to 10.

Objective data include the depth of the burn, the skin thickness involved, the percentage of TBSA burned, the specific location, and any other injuries sustained. Any time a patient has a burn that involves the face, the neck, or the chest, observe for respiratory difficulty. Determine whether the victim has had a tetanus booster in the past 5 years.

The severity of the burn depends on several factors. Major burns require the most skilled nursing interventions. Moderate and minor burns require fewer nursing interventions. Factors determining a major, moderate, or minor burn are the (1) percentage of the TBSA burned, (2) victim's age, (3) specific location of the burn, (4) cause of the burn, (5) other diseases present, (6) depth of the burn, and (7) injuries sustained during the burn (Box 3-4).

Diagnostic Tests

The primary diagnostic test is a physical examination to determine the amount of burned area. Blood assessments—such as those for electrolytes, CBC, serum chemistries, and arterial blood gases—may be done to establish the severity of the dehydration. In inhalation burns, carboxyhemoglobin level is evaluated. Most fatalities occur among survivors with severe asphyxiation or carbon monoxide intoxication. Carbon monoxide (CO) binds to hemoglobin with greater affinity than does oxygen, resulting in tissue hypoxia.

Medical Management

The medical treatment of burns is divided into three phases with differing priorities. Remember that these phases are not always clearly defined and may overlap.

Emergent Phase

The primary concern in the emergent phase is to stop the burning process using the "stop, drop, and roll" technique. Also, removing clothing and shoes from the victim may eliminate the source of the burn to arrest skin damage. Do not apply ice to burns because it can cause rapid vasoconstriction, which may cause more trauma to the tissues by increasing the depth of the burn.

Box 3-4 **Classification of Severity of Burns**

MAJOR BURN INJURIES
- Greater than 25% total body surface area (TBSA) (greater than 20% in children less than 10 years and adults more than 40 years of age)
- Greater than 10% TBSA, full thickness
- Involvement of face, eyes, ears, hands, feet, perineum
- Electrical burns
- Burns complicated by inhalation injury or major trauma
- Burns in patients with preexisting disease (diabetes, heart failure, or chronic renal failure)

MODERATE BURN INJURIES
- 15% to 25% TBSA in adults, partial thickness (10% to 20% TBSA in children less than 10 years and adults more than 40 years of age)
- Less than 10% TBSA, full thickness
- Burns with no concurrent injury
- Burns in patients with no preexisting disease

MINOR BURN INJURIES
- Less than 15% TBSA in adults (less than 10% in children or older adults)
- Less than 2% TBSA, full thickness
- Burns in patients with no preexisting disease

The second step is to provide an open airway; third is to control bleeding. Fourth, remove all nonadherent clothing and jewelry (rings, watches). Fifth, cover the victim with a clean sheet or cloth. Sixth, transport the victim to the hospital. In the case of a chemical burn, it is important to rinse the skin generously with water to remove all chemicals. Electrical burns have an entry point and an exit point that need to be identified. Most electrical burns result in cardiac arrest, and the patient requires cardiopulmonary resuscitation or astute cardiac monitoring.

During the primary survey assessment, quickly assess the ABCs (airway, breathing, and circulation) and look for life-threatening injuries, such as blunt chest trauma. Assessment of the patient's airway becomes and remains the priority of nursing care. Suspect an inhalation injury, especially if the burn occurred in a closed or confined area. Signs and symptoms of inhalation injury include singed facial hair, black-tinged sputum, soot in the throat, hoarseness, and neck or face burns. Stridor is a life-threatening sign.

CO poisoning is likely if the patient was in an enclosed area. CO displaces oxygen from hemoglobin. Do not rely on pulse oximetry to rule out CO poisoning. Oximeters cannot distinguish between oxyhemoglobin and carboxyhemoglobin. The carboxyhemoglobin level should be measured, when feasible, per blood sample. Early signs of CO poisoning include headache, nausea, vomiting, and unsteady gait. Treatment includes administering 100% oxygen.

Once the patient is in the hospital, the severity of the burn dictates the care given. Perform a thorough assessment every 30 minutes to 1 hour in the emergent phase. Patients with major burns generally are transferred to burn care centers or units for treatment but must be stabilized first. Patients with moderate to severe burns are treated using the following steps:

1. Establish airway. Administer oxygen as ordered. Often the physician inserts an endotracheal tube to ensure a patent airway (Figure 3-23).
2. Initiate fluid therapy. Begin intravenous fluid therapy with Ringer's lactate solution immediately. The amount of fluid given is related to the percentage of TBSA burned. Weigh the patient so the physician can determine the amount of fluids needed.
3. Insert Foley catheter for hourly urinary output. An hourly output of 30 to 50 mL is recommended. Intravenous fluids are given to maintain renal perfusion (Box 3-5).
4. Insert a nasogastric tube to prevent aspiration. Patients with severe burns often develop a paralytic ileus as a result of trauma.
5. Administer analgesics intravenously in small, frequent doses for pain control. Morphine may be used. Any degree of hypovolemia can increase the effects of medications. Carefully assess

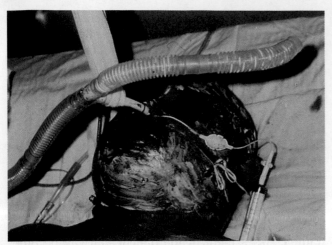

FIGURE 3-23 Endotracheal intubation for patient with severe edema 5 hours after a burn injury.

Box 3-5 Indications for Fluid Resuscitation

- Burns greater than 20% total body surface area (TBSA) in adults
- Burns greater than 10% TBSA in children
- Patient older than 55 or younger than 4 years of age
- Patient with preexisting disease that would reduce normal compensatory responses to minor hypovolemia (cardiac or pulmonary disease, diabetes)
- Electrical burns

---

the patient's respiratory status when administering morphine.

6. Maintain airway and fluid status, and monitor vital signs.
7. Give tetanus immunization prophylaxis as needed. (Patients who have been immunized against tetanus do not need a tetanus toxoid booster unless the last injection was more than 5 years ago. If the patient has never had a tetanus immunization, administer tetanus serum and active immunization in the emergency department.)

The first 72 hours require diligent medical care. The primary goals in the emergent phase are to maintain respiratory integrity and to prevent hypovolemic shock, which may result in death (Box 3-6).

Acute Phase

The acute phase begins when fluids shift back to the intravascular compartment, usually 72 hours after the burn. During the acute phase, the patient's metabolism increases. Urinary output also increases as the fluid shifts back into the blood circulation. As the urinary output increases, the edema in the tissues begins to decrease. The acute phase may last from 10 days to months. The two primary treatment goals are treatment of the burn wound and prevention and management of complications. Infection is the most common complication and cause of death after the first 72 hours. Other

---

Box 3-6 Nursing Diagnoses for the Emergent Phase of Burns

- Ineffective airway clearance, related to edema of the respiratory passages
- Deficient fluid volume (dehydration), related to shift of body fluids
- Deficient fluid volume, related to capillary hyperpermeability with fluid moving out of the cells into the interstitial area
- Acute anxiety, related to injury
- Acute pain, related to loss of skin
- Risk for infection, related to impairment of skin integrity
- Impaired skin integrity, related to damage by the burns
- Decreased cardiac output, related to hypovolemia
- Risk for aspiration, related to decreased peristalsis
- Impaired swallowing, related to mucosal edema
- Impaired verbal communication, related to breathing difficulties
- Disturbed sleep pattern, related to hospital environment

---

complications include heart failure, renal failure, **contractures** (shortening or tension of muscles that affects extension), paralytic ileus causing gastric dilation, and **Curling's ulcer** (a duodenal ulcer that develops 8 to 14 days after severe burns on the surface of the body; the first sign is usually vomiting of bright red blood).

Nursing interventions. Prioritizing nursing care using the ABCs remains the most important nursing intervention. After completing the ABCs, gather data in the head-to-toe assessment concerning (1) respiratory pattern, (2) vital signs, (3) circulation, (4) intake and output, (5) ambulation, (6) bowel sounds, (7) inspection of the wound itself, and (8) mental status.

Fluid-reshifting complications may also develop during the acute phase if renal damage has occurred. Monitor the patient for signs of acute renal failure such as elevated serum creatinine and BUN. Heart failure may develop as a result of the rapid increase in blood volume from the return of fluid from the interstitial spaces into the intravascular vessels. The primary goals in the acute phase include proper care of the burn wound to promote healing and prevent infection as well as preventing and treating complications. Assessment for an infection of the burn wound includes observing the wound for increasing erythema, odor, or a green or yellow exudate. Local and systemic infections complicate recovery and increase recovery time (Figure 3-24). Wound cultures and sensitivities help pinpoint the type of organism present and the most effective antibiotic for treatment. Any signs of an infection should be reported.

Once the patient's vital signs and urinary output stabilize and the acute phase begins, complete a nutritional assessment. Provision for adequate nutrition remains a cornerstone of burn care during the acute phase. Increased amounts of protein, calories, and vitamins help repair the damaged tissue; encourage oral

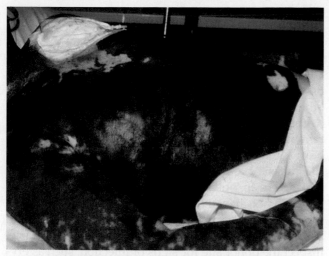

FIGURE 3-24 Postburn *Pseudomonas* infection.

intake of nutrients as soon as possible. The nutritional challenge includes providing enough nutrients to meet the body's increased metabolic requirement. Monitor nutritional status through daily measurement of weight, serum electrolytes, and serum albumin and through urinalysis. Adequate nutrition decreases healing time, whereas weight loss increases healing time. Skin grafts will not be successful unless nutrition is adequate.

Nursing interventions include measures to control pain and to support the patient's psychological well-being. Intravenous opioids in small, frequent doses provide relief from pain, but care must be taken to avoid jeopardizing respiratory integrity. Specific interventions include verbal support, unhurried care, truthful explanations, and effective listening. Excellent communication skills are essential.

Without an intact first line of defense—that is, the skin—the protective mechanisms function abnormally. Thus protective isolation is necessary. Wear gowns, masks, caps, and gloves during each contact with a patient with major burns. Follow strict surgical aseptic technique during dressing changes. Use of proper equipment and cleaning procedures is imperative. Hydrotherapy (e.g., whirlpool) can be a source of infection.

The standard treatment for partial-thickness burns includes debriding the wound, applying topical antibiotics, and changing dressings twice a day. A new treatment for burns includes temporary skin substitutes. Made from a variety of materials, skin substitutes promote faster healing for burn wounds and can eliminate painful dressing changes and minimize scarring. In 1997, TransCyte, a temporary bioengineered skin substitute, became the first such product to be approved by the FDA for burn treatment. TransCyte is designed as an alternative both to silver sulfadiazine (Silvadene) for patients with partial-thickness burns and to cadaver skin for full-thickness burns and deep partial-thickness burns requiring surgical debride-

ment. It is made from neonatal human fibroblast cells. The fibroblasts secrete human derma, collagen, matrix proteins, and growth factors. All of these factors promote wound healing. TransCyte is typically applied only once, thus avoiding the frequent, painful dressing changes. TransCyte provides a temporary covering that helps protect against fluid loss and reduces the risk of infection.

A new and highly successful skin replacement therapy called Integra Dermal Regeneration Template is being used in the treatment of life-threatening, full-thickness or deep partial-thickness burn wounds. Within the first few days of admission, the patient goes to surgery, the wound is debrided, and the Integra artificial skin is applied. The wound is then wrapped with dressings. The artificial skin stimulates regeneration of new dermis by the body. During a second surgical procedure, the artificial skin is removed and replaced by the patient's own autografts (Lewis et al., 2007).

Traditional wound care involves the removal of the eschar that forms. Eschar is a black leathery crust (i.e., a slough) that the body forms over burned tissue; eschar can harbor microorganisms and cause infection. It may also compromise circulatory status. An escharotomy is often done to relieve the circulatory constriction (Figure 3-25). Daily debridement (removal of damaged tissue and cellular debris from a wound or burn to prevent infection and to promote healing) and special cleansing support regeneration of the tissues. Hydrotherapy softens the eschar to make removal less painful. It also promotes range of motion to decrease contractures.

The specific wound care method depends on the severity of the burn. The open or exposure method may be used for burns of the face, neck, ears, and perineum. The area is cleaned and exposed to air. A hard crust forms, and regeneration of tissue follows.

Proper positioning and range-of-motion exercises (facilitated by the nurse and physical therapist) are vi-

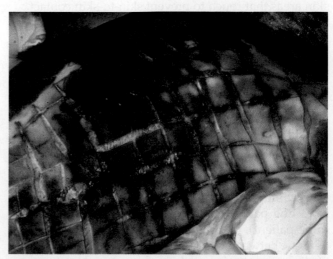

FIGURE 3-25 Grid escharotomy used to alleviate circulatory and pulmonary constriction.

tal for the burn patient's well-being. Special bed equipment is needed to prevent the burn from touching the linens. A bed cradle, a CircOlectric bed, or a Clinitron bed is recommended. Chilling may be controlled by keeping the room temperature at 85° F (29.4° C) and providing lights or heat lamps for additional warmth. Humidity should be between 40% and 50%.

Advantages to the open method are that (1) the wound can be observed more easily, (2) movement in bed is less restricted, (3) circulation of the body part is not restricted, and (4) exercises can be done more easily to prevent contractures. Disadvantages are (1) pain; (2) chilling; (3) contamination of wound by the health care provider; (4) unattractive appearance, which causes emotional distress; and (5) the need for protective isolation precautions for the immunocompromised patient.

Control the pain with intravenously administered opioids in the early days of the acute phase. However, considering the long-term nature of a burn, addiction is a potential problem. Diazepam (Valium) has been found to be effective, but morphine is commonly used.

The closed (or occlusive) method involves cleaning the burn, applying the prescribed medication, and dressing the wound as ordered. Advantages of the closed method are that (1) it protects the burn area from injury, and (2) it prevents contamination of the area by the health care provider. Circulation checks are important with pressure dressings to assess for adequate arterial perfusion to the involved areas.

The topical medications used to hasten healing and prevent infection vary. Topical administration is preferred because the capillaries are coagulated by the burn. Mafenide (Sulfamylon), silver sulfadiazine, and silver nitrate are common drugs used in burn care. Each drug has specific advantages and disadvantages (Table 3-4).

Burn care essentials include a lightweight dressing. A single layer of gauze covered with medication and a single wrap of Kerlix provide adequate coverage. When applying gauze to the burn area, place gauze between skin areas that touch to prevent skin-to-skin contact.

Changing burn dressings is painful; therefore 30 minutes before the procedure, administer an analgesic, either 5 to 10 mg of intravenous morphine sulfate or a sedative. Most dressings are changed after hydrotherapy. Remove all old medication and eschar before applying any new medication. Failure to debride promotes infection, delays healing, and increases scarring.

Skin grafts are used as soon as possible to cover full-thickness burns. Grafting promotes healing and prevents infection. Grafting generally occurs during the first 3 weeks of care. Four types of grafts may be used: (1) an **autograft** (surgical transplantation of any tissue from one part of the body to another location in the same patient), (2) a **homograft (allograft)** (the transfer of tissue between two genetically dissimilar individuals of the same species, such as skin transplant from another person who is not an identical twin [often a ca-

daver]), (3) a **heterograft (xenograft)** (tissue from another species, such as a pig or a cow, used as a temporary graft), or (4) a synthetic graft substitute. The autograft is permanent, whereas the other types are temporary.

Grafts are applied by either the **pedicle method** (the tissue is left partially attached to the donor site and the other portion of the tissue is attached to the burn site) or the freestanding method (the tissue is completely removed from the donor site and is attached to the burn site).

Graft sites are a nursing challenge. Any movement that results in pulling the graft area can dislodge the graft. Do not change dressings until ordered. The donor site resembles a partial-thickness burn after the graft. Donor site care is as important as care of the burn site. Inspect the donor site for signs of infection, such as erythema and malodor (see Patient Teaching box). Pain is a primary complaint after the graft and should be treated.

The nutritional aspect of burn care is another nursing challenge. Destroyed body proteins and fluid loss present problems as the body increases metabolism to meet the extra demands. Therefore the body requires enough energy to maintain homeostasis while meeting the increased need for repairing the injury.

Burn patients should eat by mouth as soon as their condition permits. Protein requirements are greater than normal. Normal protein intake encompasses 0.8 grams per kilogram of body weight, whereas the burned patient requires 1.5 to 3.2 grams per kilogram of body weight. Thus a normal 150-pound person needs 55 grams of protein per day; if burned, the same person needs 102 to 158 grams of protein, depending on the extent of the burn. Daily caloric requirements range from 2000 calories to more than 6000 calories, depending on the burn. Meeting these enormous requirements requires diligent nursing interventions. Concentrated, high-calorie foods need to be offered frequently. The body also requires additional amounts of vitamins A, B, and C to promote digestion, absorption, and repair of tissue. Increased amounts of calcium, zinc, magnesium, and iron are needed. Vitamin C and zinc aid in wound healing, and added B complex vitamins aid metabolism of the extra protein and

---

Patient Teaching

Skin Grafts

- Do not remove dressing unless ordered.
- Report changes in the graft (hematoma, fluid collection) to physician.
- Protect grafted skin from direct sunlight with a sunscreen lotion for at least 6 months.
- Keep surface of healed graft moistened daily with skin lotion for 6 to 12 months. (Grafted skin does not perspire; it dries and cracks easily.)
- Wear a strong elastic stocking for 4 to 6 months for grafts on lower extremities.

Table 3-4 Topical Medications for Burn Therapy Skin Grafts

Generic (Trade)	Advantages	Disadvantages
Mafenide (Sulfamylon)	Bacteriostatic against gram-negative and gram-positive organisms Penetrates thick eschar	Metabolic acidosis Pain on application Allergic rash
Silver sulfadiazine (Silvadene)	Broad antimicrobial activity against gram-negative, gram-positive, and *Candida* organisms No electrolyte imbalances Painless and somewhat soothing Not nephrotoxic	With repeated application, skin may develop slimy, grayish appearance, simulating an infection despite negative cultures Prolonged use may cause skin rash and depress granulocyte formation
Silver nitrate	Bacteriostatic effect Lessens pain and eliminates odor Reduces evaporative water loss from burns	Electrolyte imbalances Stains everything it comes into contact with Does not penetrate eschar Pain on application
Nitrofurazone (Furacin)	Inhibits enzymes necessary for bacterial metabolism Broad spectrum of activity Effective against *Staphylococcus aureus* Not absorbed systemically Low incidence of sensitivity	Contact dermatitis in unaffected skin Urine turns a reddish color
Gentamicin sulfate (Garamycin)	Broad antimicrobial activity Painless	Ototoxicity Nephrotoxicity Development of resistant bacterial strains
Neomycin	Broad antimicrobial activity Causes miscoding in the messenger RNA of bacterial cells	Serious toxic effects Ototoxicity Nephrotoxicity
Scarlet red	Nonantiseptic (applied to gauze soaked with oil-based red dye) Drying agent Applied to donor site Promotes epithelialization	No antimicrobial effects Stains and irritates skin Infection may develop beneath scarlet red gauze, which may have systemic effects
Xeroform	Nonantiseptic Debrides and protects donor site Protects graft	Removal may be painful, because it sometimes adheres to wound Neither antiseptic nor antimicrobial
Sodium hypochlorite (Dakin's solution)	Chlorine-based solution that is bactericidal Aids in debriding wounds Aids cleaning of copious drainage	Dissolves blood clots May inhibit clotting May irritate the skin
Sutilains ointment (Travase)	Topical enzymatic agent Dissolves necrotic tissue by proteolytic action Facilitates removal of eschar and purulent drainage	Mild, transient pain on application Paresthesia, bleeding, dermatitis Dressing must be kept moist at all times

RNA, Ribonucleic acid.

carbohydrate intake. Adding oral supplements such as Ensure, Sustacal, and Carnation Instant Breakfast can increase vitamin, mineral, and protein intake. Total parenteral nutrition provides an alternative to oral intake of proteins if the patient is unable to take in adequate nutrients by mouth.

The daily calorie requirement is estimated by the use of the formula (25 kilocalories × body weight in kilograms) + (40 kilocalories × %TBSA burned) = kilocalories per day required. Most burn victims have poor appetites; therefore getting the patient to eat is difficult. Small, frequent feedings of high-calorie, high-protein, low-volume foods are the best way to meet

the patient's nutritional needs. Some patients develop Curling's ulcer 8 to 14 days after the burn injury because of increased gastric acidity. The first sign is vomiting of bright red blood. The prophylactic treatment involves intravenous or oral administration of cimetidine (Tagamet), ranitidine (Zantac), omeprazole (Prilosec), or famotidine (Pepcid). See Box 3-7 for nursing diagnoses for the acute phase of burn care.

Rehabilitation Phase
Rehabilitation of the burn patient begins at admission. However, the third phase of burn care begins when 20% or less of the TBSA remains burned. The goal becomes

Box **3-7**	**Nursing Diagnoses for the Acute Phase of Burns**

- Acute anxiety, related to change in body image
- Fear, related to chronic illness
- Chronic pain, related to procedures performed
- Risk for infection, related to open skin wounds
- Imbalanced nutrition: less than body requirements, related to increased metabolic demands
- Social isolation, related to perceived change in body image
- Impaired physical mobility, related to burns
- Self-care deficit in activities of daily living (ADLs), related to area of burn involved
- Deficient knowledge in all areas, related to expected care
- Interrupted family processes, related to long-term hospitalization
- Disturbed body image, related to disfigurement from burns
- Deficient diversional activity, related to confinement during care
- Ineffective coping, related to:
  —Seriousness of injury
  —Perceived role changes
- Powerlessness, related to:
  —Prolonged recovery
  —Loss of income
  —Loss of physical attractiveness

Box **3-8**	**Nursing Diagnoses for the Rehabilitation Phase of Burns**

- Ineffective airway clearance, related to edema of the respiratory passages
- Impaired physical mobility, related to:
  —Splinting
  —Dressings
  —Pain
- Activity intolerance, related to prolonged bed rest
- Anxiety, acute to moderate, related to role change
- Disturbed body image, related to scarring
- Deficient knowledge, related to impaired home maintenance management
- Self-care deficit (in ADLs), related to:
  —Pain
  —Fatigue
- Fear, related to impending surgery
- Risk for disuse syndrome, related to noncompliance
- Post-trauma syndrome, related to the cause of the burn
- Impaired adjustment
- Ineffective coping, related to long-term rehabilitation
- Disturbed personal identity, related to inability to return to previous lifestyle for prolonged period
- Caregiver role strain, related to prolonged recovery period
- Ineffective management of therapeutic regimen, related to complexity and chronicity of rehabilitation
- Anticipatory grieving, related to loss of wellness

to promote independence so the patient may have a productive life. The rehabilitation process addresses both social and physical skills and may take years.

Mobility limitations constitute the major concerns. The patient requires a comprehensive physical therapy program for positioning, skin care, exercise, ambulation, and activities of daily living (ADLs). Contractures remain a concern in the care of a burn patient. Although physical therapists provide most of the rehabilitative care, the nurse assists in providing continuity of care. When planning the care, set realistic, short-term goals to motivate patients to try to achieve more.

Maintaining or restoring the patient's independence remains the primary rehabilitative goal. Given the possibility of a changed body image, encourage the patient to talk about fears and concerns. Working with others such as social workers and counselors, develop a holistic care plan to provide the comprehensive care needed. During visiting hours, assess family interactions. Helping the family cope with the changes in their loved one is a major nursing intervention.

Numerous nursing diagnoses apply to burn victims, encompassing family, patient, and social roles (Box 3-8).

Patient Teaching
Before discharge, the burn patient and family need education. Provide written instructions that are complete, comprehensive, easy to understand, and realistic. Return demonstrations are the best way to determine that learning has taken place. The major topics to cover are (1) wound care, (2) signs and symptoms

 Home Care Considerations

Burns

- Bathe twice a day with mild soap.
- Test the water temperature before getting into the shower because your skin is sensitive to extremes of hot and cold.
- Be certain to clean the tub well before each bath.
- If itching becomes severe, take a lukewarm bath with Alpha Keri lotion added to the bath water.
- Do not use lotions that contain lanolin or alcohol because they will cause blisters.
- Avoid direct sunlight. Wear light clothing to cover areas that have been burned because these areas burn easily.
- Discoloration and scarring are normal during healing. The color of the scar may remain red because of the healing process. Usually within 6 months to a year the scar loses its red color and becomes softer. Normal color to the area may take several months to return.
- Report to the physician:
  —Any signs of infection
  —Fever greater than 101° F (38.3° C)
  —Feeling of inability to cope

of complications, (3) dressings, (4) exercises, (5) clothing, (6) ADLs, and (7) social skills (see Home Care Considerations box).

Evaluation
Evaluation depends on meeting the stated goals. In evaluating the burn patient, ask the following questions:
- Can the patient take care of self?
- Can the patient ambulate without difficulty?

- Can the patient cope?
- Can the family cope?
- Does the patient have contractures?
- Does the patient understand the treatment process?

Burn care is extensive, and the exact nursing interventions for each patient are individualized. Many times the patient must change vocations, and family relationships change. The degree of scarring—emotionally and physically—cannot be predicted; nor can the patient's acceptance by society.

Prognosis

The outcome for the patient with burns depends on the size of the burn; depth of the burn; the victim's age; the body part involved; the burning agent; and history of cardiac, pulmonary, endocrine, renal, or hepatic disease and other injuries sustained at the time of the burn.

❖NURSING PROCESS *for the Patient with an Integumentary Disorder*

The role of the licensed practical nurse/licensed vocational nurse (LPN/LVN) in the nursing process as stated is that the LPN/LVN will:

- Participate in planning care for patients based on patient needs
- Review patient care plan and recommend revisions as needed
- Review and follow defined prioritization for patient care
- Use clinical pathways, care maps, or care plans to guide and review patient care

■ Assessment

Assessment of the skin is an important aspect of patient care. Skin changes can reflect specific skin disorders, but they may also alert the nurse to a systemic disorder. Skin assessment allows the identification of obvious and subtle changes in the patient's state of health. Effective skin assessment takes a critical eye and knowledge of the expected normal findings.

Because the skin is usually assessed at the same time as other body systems, nurses tend to underestimate the valuable information that can be obtained. Assessing the skin provides a baseline knowledge of the patient's hygiene measures, nutritional status, circulatory status, and sensory perception. The skin is the first line of defense against infection. Therefore ongoing assessment of the skin is important in the maintenance of health and the prevention of infection.

Assessment of the older adult can be challenging for the health care professional. The normal changes that occur related to aging are important for the nurse to know. The older patient population is growing, as are the opportunities for the student to assess the older patient (see Life Span Considerations box).

 Life Span Considerations

Older Adults

Effects of Aging on the Integumentary System

- Physiologic changes make the skin of the older adult more fragile and susceptible to impairment.
- Aging changes include decreases in tissue fluid, subcutaneous fat, and sebaceous secretions. This results in dryness, flaking, pruritus, loss of elasticity, altered turgor, and a wrinkled appearance.
- Hyperkeratotic changes are typically seen in the nails, which make them thick and difficult to care for. Podiatric care is recommended for older adults, particularly those with circulatory impairment.
- Circulatory changes and decreased mobility increase the risk of senile purpura and decubitus ulcers.
- Significant hair and scalp changes can occur with aging:
  —Loss of pigmentation leading to graying
  —Decreased hair thickness or balding
  —Increased incidence of seborrheic dermatitis of the scalp requiring special care
  —Growth of facial hair on women, which can damage self-image
- Localized clusters of melanocytes surrounded by areas of decreased pigmentation result in "age spots."
- The incidence of basal and squamous cell carcinoma increases with age, particularly in individuals who have had excessive sun exposure. Inspect aging skin closely for changes in the appearance of moles or warts.

■ Nursing Diagnosis

Assessment provides data to identify the patient's problems, strengths, potential complications, and learning needs. After defining the diagnoses, start formulating a care plan that meets the patient's needs prioritizing problems from most to least important. Being able to prioritize nursing interventions contributes to a more predictable recovery for the patient. Possible nursing diagnoses that should be considered for the patient with a skin disorder are as follows:

Nursing Diagnoses	Nursing Interventions
Anxiety, related to altered appearance	Assess anxiety level every shift.
	Observe verbal and nonverbal behavior.
	Encourage the patient to share feelings.
	Teach relaxation techniques.
	Assess patient for pain.
Pain, related to loss of superficial skin layers	Initiate nursing measures to minimize or relieve pain.
Deficient knowledge, related to cause of skin disorder	Assess patient for learning needs daily.
	Involve patient in setting goals.
	Use audiovisuals as teaching aids.
	Evaluate patient's success.

Continued

Nursing Diagnoses	Nursing Interventions
Risk for infection, related to impaired skin integrity	Assess patient daily for risk factors such as abrasions, elevated white blood cell count, and temperature.
	Implement nursing measures, such as using good hand hygiene and keeping patient's nails trimmed, to decrease risk factors.
Deficient knowledge, related to treatment of pruritus	Assess factors contributing to pruritus.
	Promote hydration of the skin by having patient avoid hot showers and apply emollients after bathing.
	Encourage adequate fluid intake.
	Implement nursing measures to decrease skin irritation, such as avoiding clothes made of rough weave.
	Encourage patient to stop scratching by rubbing or applying pressure to the area.
	Administer prescribed medications for pruritus such as corticosteroids and antihistamines.
Risk for trauma, related to excessive scratching	Assess onset and contributing factors of episodes of pruritus.
	Encourage patient to stop scratching by rubbing or by applying pressure to the involved area.
Social isolation, related to anticipated or actual response of others to disfiguring skin disorders	Encourage patient to discuss feelings of loneliness.
	Identify available support systems to patient.
Situational low self-esteem, related to disfigured skin	Assess patient's feelings of self-worth by having patient describe feelings about self.
	Implement nursing measures to assist patient in dealing with body image.
	Accept feelings of anger or hostility from patient.
	Suggest clothing to conceal changes in skin integrity.

■ Expected Outcomes and Planning

When planning patient care, look at the nursing diagnoses and establish the cause of the nursing problem. Determining the cause enables you to develop a care plan that includes nursing interventions to eliminate the cause if possible. Include the patient in this planning. Ascertain the patient's preferences and capabilities. Including the patient is one way to promote compliance. Most skin problems are chronic, and progress is often slow. Also, many patients are older and require more time for healing.

Planning includes the development of realistic goals and outcomes that stem from the identified nursing diagnoses. Establish short- and long-term goals. Examples of measurable goals include the following:

Goal 1: Patient shows no signs of infection in abdominal wound as evidenced by the wound remaining free of erythema, purulent drainage, odor, and localized tenderness.

Goal 2: Patient is able to change dressing correctly as evidenced by the patient following the written guidelines during demonstration.

Goals should have a date when they will be evaluated. Failure to attain a goal means the nurse should reevaluate the chosen interventions and determine why the goals have not been met.

■ Implementation

When providing nursing interventions related to the skin, (1) include ways to prevent skin problems, (2) provide education in home care management, and (3) provide safety tips for the patient. Patients with skin diseases are usually managed at home and need to be aware of the potential for infection because the skin is not intact (see Box 3-1 and Home Care Considerations box).

Nursing measures for the skin include a variety of simple or complex interventions, including applying medications, dressings, and heat or cold and teaching the patient how to perform these measures at home. The principles of surgical and medical asepsis are important when providing nursing interventions. Also incorporate nutritional guidelines for the patient to follow. Patients need extra nutrients, such as protein, for the building and repair of tissues.

Consider the patient's cultural beliefs, personal values, and economic resources when selecting the appropriate care. More people are using other forms of treat-

🏠 Home Care Considerations

Home Care Guidelines for Baths and Soaks

- The water temperature should be comfortable—usually 90° to 100° F (32° to 38° C).
- Dissolve medication completely while tub is filling.
- The soak should last 20 to 30 minutes.
- When oils are added, patients are assisted out of the water to prevent slipping.
- Pat the skin dry, rather than rubbing, to avoid skin irritation.
- Apply creams or ointments immediately after the bath to retain moisture.
- Drain water from the tub before the patient gets out.
- The door should not be locked, and a helper should be within hearing distance.
- Use a bath mat to prevent slipping.
- Hand rails may be needed in the shower or tub.
- A seat may be needed in the shower or tub.
- After a medicated bath, pour 1 cup of bleach into used tub water; let stand 5 minutes; wipe sides and bottom of tub; drain tub, and clean as usual.

ment for integumentary disorders besides traditional medical therapy (see Complementary and Alternative Therapies box). To promote compliance with planned treatment, consider the patient's independence, dignity, privacy, and physical strengths and limitations.

▪ Evaluation

During and after the planned nursing interventions, determine the outcomes. This is an ongoing process of continually trying to establish the most effective care plan.

Economic and home care implications are important. Today patients are being discharged from the health care facility more quickly, and insurance companies are more selective in how they pay for the care and supplies the patient needs. Creativity and critical thinking are important skills to meet the needs of today's patient.

Evaluation involves determining whether the established goals have been met. The nurse and patient evaluate the goals to see whether the criteria for measurement have been met. For example, the goal is that the patient's wound would not become infected, as demonstrated by a lack of erythema, purulent drainage, and odor. If at the end of the designated time frame the wound shows no signs of infection, the goal has been met.

Complementary and Alternative Therapies

Integumentary Disorders

- The management of integumentary disorders is often difficult. Nutritional and herbal approaches to the treatment of skin problems have been shown to be effective for some disorders, often with fewer side effects than with conventional methods.
- Chinese herbs have long been used in Asian countries for the treatment of skin diseases. A landmark study in England showed the effectiveness of Chinese herbs in treating atopic dermatitis. This study was undertaken after dermatologists were impressed by the results in their patients who were also under the care of a Chinese herbalist. Participants in the study who received the active herbal formula reported decreases in the number of lesions and itching, as well as improved sleep.
- A traditional Australian plant remedy, tea tree oil (from *Melaleuca alternifolia*), has been effective in the treatment of acne.
- A topical mixture of the essential plant oils of thyme, rosemary, lavender, and cedarwood, in a carrier of jojoba and grapeseed oils, has been found to have significant effect in the treatment of alopecia areata.
- A published report from Taiwan states that acupuncture has been effective in the treatment of urticaria (hives).

From Sheehan, M.P., Rustin, M.H., Atherton, D.J., et al. (1992): Efficacy of traditional Chinese herbal therapy in adult atopic dermatitis. *Lancet, 340*(8810), 13-17.

Get Ready for the NCLEX® Examination!

Key Points

- The skin, including nails, hair, and glands, makes up the integumentary system.
- The main functions of the integumentary system are protection, temperature regulation, and vitamin D synthesis.
- The two layers of true skin are the epidermis and dermis.
- The layer of tissue directly beneath the skin is the subcutaneous layer; it is composed of adipose tissue and loose connective tissue.
- The sudoriferous (sweat) glands release perspiration through the skin.
- The sebaceous (oil) glands secrete sebum, which lubricates the skin and prevents invasion of bacteria through the skin.
- Any injury to the skin poses a threat to a person's self-concept.
- It is important to establish a therapeutic relationship to meet the patient's psychological needs.
- Most skin disorders are not contagious and are rarely fatal. They are often chronic.
- Sterile technique and isolation techniques are required with any open, draining lesion.
- Wet dressings need to be checked frequently. Constant moisture softens the skin and contributes to skin maceration.
- Medicines must be applied to clean skin.
- The nursing interventions for a skin disorder depend on the cause; however, common problems are decreased skin integrity, risk for infection, lack of knowledge concerning the disease, and ineffective coping.
- A primary nursing intervention is teaching the patient about the mode of transmission of the particular disease.
- The assessment of patients with skin disorders includes collection of both subjective and objective data.
- Wet dressings and baths may be done to soothe, vasoconstrict, debride, or decrease pruritus.
- Before initiating heat and cold therapy, understand normal body responses to local temperature variations, assess the integrity of the body part, determine the patient's ability to sense temperature, and ensure proper operation of equipment.
- Prevent malignant skin diseases by educating the public about causes.
- Burns can be classified by depth and TBSA involved.
- The pathophysiology and care of burns involve three stages: the hypovolemic, or emergent, phase; the acute, or diuretic, phase; and the long-term, or rehabilitation, phase.
- The three phases of burn care overlap, with different goals and nursing interventions in each.
- A primary nursing intervention for the burn patient in the emergent phase is to establish and maintain an open airway.
- The treatment method for a burn patient depends on age, body surface area involved, location, depth, and other diseases present.

- The primary causes of death in burn victims are hypovolemic shock in the first 72 hours and infection during the acute phase.
- Suspect inhalation injury if the burn injury occurred in a closed or confined area.
- A treatment for burns is use of temporary skin substitutes derived from human fibroblast cells.

Additional Learning Resources

 Go to your Companion CD for an audio glossary, animations, video clips, and more.

evolve Be sure to visit the Evolve site at http://evolve.elsevier.com/Christensen/adult/ for additional online resources.

Review Questions for the NCLEX® Examination

1. The physician has ordered oral griseofulvin for tinea capitis. The mother asks the nurse why an oral medication is used rather than a cream. The best reply is that:
   1. topical creams do not reach the root of the hair to kill the fungus.
   2. oral medications are more economical.
   3. topical medications cause more pain when applied.
   4. it is more convenient to take the medication once a day rather than applying the cream once a day.

2. The most important nursing intervention for the patient with a skin disorder is:
   1. patient teaching.
   2. prevention of secondary infections.
   3. application of medications.
   4. referral for counseling.

3. The physician instructs a mother to take her child out in the sun for approximately an hour or until the skin turns red (not sunburned). This is a common medical treatment for:
   1. atopic dermatitis.
   2. acne vulgaris.
   3. pityriasis rosea.
   4. psoriasis.

4. Which of the following assessments should the nurse report to the physician immediately for an adult patient with partial-thickness burns over 25% of his body?
   1. Complaints of pain every 4 to 6 hours
   2. Decreasing appetite
   3. Hourly urinary output of 10 to 15 mL
   4. Edema at the IV site

5. The patient has a rash on her back that began about 10 days ago with a raised, scaly border and a pink center. Now she has similar eruptions on both sides of her back. From these signs, the nurse would determine the rash to be:
   1. impetigo contagiosa.
   2. pityriasis rosea.
   3. contact dermatitis.
   4. infantile eczema.

6. A patient complains of a burning pain on his lower thoracic area. On inspection, the area is found to be erythematous and edematous with a cluster of vesicles. The nurse suspects the patient has:
   1. herpes zoster.
   2. herpes simplex.
   3. varicella.
   4. impetigo.

7. A patient complains that he has basal cell carcinoma and is going to die. The nurse knows that:
   1. basal cell carcinoma is rarely terminal.
   2. without proper medication it can result in melanoma.
   3. it is a hereditary disorder caused by decreased melanin.
   4. treatment involves strong chemotherapeutic agents.

8. It is important to teach the patient the warning signs of skin cancer. Which is a warning sign of skin cancer?
   1. Border irregularity
   2. Smooth surface
   3. Decreasing diameter
   4. Mole symmetry

9. A patient has an inhalation burn injury. Which of the following is a medical emergency?
   1. Singed facial hair
   2. Neck or face burns
   3. Pallor
   4. Respiratory stridor

10. Which method of assessing burn size applies only to adults?
    1. Lund-Browder
    2. Rule of nines
    3. Parkland method
    4. Primary survey

11. The nurse just finished an assessment for a patient with SLE. Which clinical manifestation would the nurse expect to find?
    1. Oral ulcers and erythematous rash over the nose and cheeks
    2. Leukocytosis and urticaria
    3. Anemia and jaundice
    4. Diarrhea and hypokalemia

12. The physician has scheduled a debridement for a patient who has partial-thickness burns on his chest and right upper leg. Which nursing intervention is most important?
    1. Ambulate the patient to increase the blood flow to the area.
    2. Administer an opioid analgesic intravenously before the debridement.
    3. Teach the patient to remove the old dressings using clean technique.
    4. Explain to the patient that the procedure will be painful.

13. A patient is admitted with partial- and full-thickness burns on his right lower extremity. Plan for the patient to have a(n):
    1. closed dressing change every 3 hours.
    2. open dressing.
    3. temporary skin cover.
    4. incision and drainage of the wound.

14. A patient is admitted with partial-thickness burns on his upper chest and face. It would be most important for the nurse to initially monitor the patient for:
    1. respiratory problems.
    2. burn shock.
    3. infection of the wound.
    4. cellulitis of the affected area.

15. An electrical burn must be assessed for:
    1. infection.
    2. cardiac irregularities.
    3. burn depth.
    4. hypovolemic shock.

16. A patient is admitted with herpes zoster. The nurse should plan to administer which medication on a frequent basis?
    1. Acyclovir (Zovirax)
    2. Cefaclor (Ceclor)
    3. Acetaminophen (Tylenol)
    4. Cimetadine (Tagamet)

17. The most common symptom of scabies is:
    1. nausea.
    2. nocturnal pruritus.
    3. localized pain.
    4. skin paresthesia.

18. It is most important to assess the adolescent with acne for:
    1. suicidal tendencies.
    2. low self-esteem.
    3. increased intake of fatty foods.
    4. change in weight.

19. A patient with thermal burns over 30% of his body has maintained a urinary output of 250 mL for the past 8 hours. From this information, the nurse might suspect that the:
    1. patient is not improving as expected.
    2. stage of hypovolemic burn shock is resolving.
    3. pain is decreasing.
    4. nutritional status is improving.

20. The patient tells the nurse she has not gone out of the house for weeks because she could not cover the lesions on her face with makeup. The most appropriate nursing diagnosis would be:
    1. Disturbed body image, related to change in personal appearance
    2. Defensive coping, related to lack of social contact
    3. Anxiety, related to the fear of permanent disfigurement
    4. Activity intolerance, related to lack of exercise

21. When inspecting the skin, the nurse remembers that the skin provides a primary:
    1. source for vitamin D storage.
    2. protective device against microorganisms.
    3. means of preventing overhydration.
    4. defense against hyperthermia.

22. When teaching a patient to care for herpes zoster lesions at home, the most important instruction for the nurse to give is:
    1. clean the lesions with sterile saline daily.
    2. wash hands for at least 1 to 2 minutes before applying medication.
    3. report to the physician when the lesions are crusted.
    4. launder all clothes in vinegar.

23. A nurse is reviewing the history for a patient who has been admitted with cellulitis. Which condition would predispose the patient to cellulitis? (Select all that apply.)
    1. Malnutrition, substance abuse
    2. Treatment with steroids or chemotherapy
    3. Coronary artery disease
    4. Infectious tonsillitis

24. A parent tells the dermatologist that her daughter seems to be losing interest in school. Which medication could have caused the patient's change in behavior?
    1. Isotretinoin (Accutane)
    2. Minocycline (Minocin)
    3. Tazarotene (Tazorac)
    4. Penicillin

25. A black patient is seen with impending shock after an accident. How would the nurse expect the skin to appear during the assessment of the patient?
    1. Ruddy blue
    2. Generalized pallor
    3. Ashen, gray, or dull
    4. Whitish, blue, or bright

26. The nurse's assessment shows that the patient has a solid, elevated, circumscribed lesion that is less than 1 cm in diameter. In the documentation, the nurse would chart this as a _____.

27. A 28-year-old electrical lineman is brought to the emergency department after coming in contact with a live overhead wire. He has two quarter-size burns on his right hand. He is admitted to the hospital. What is the most important rationale for admission to the hospital?
    1. The skin provides the least resistance to the flow of electricity.
    2. The evident skin injury seldom represents the full extent of the damage.
    3. Ventricular fibrillation may follow within 48 hours after the burns.
    4. Lethal arc burns may develop after a burn.

28. A new student nurse, whose mother recently died from malignant melanoma, asks the faculty member, "What can I do to prevent malignant melanoma from developing?" The best response by the faculty member is:

    1. malignant melanoma is a relatively rare type of skin cancer.
    2. the patient is at high risk for melanoma because of family history.
    3. avoiding excessive sun exposure will decrease risk.
    4. individuals with fair skin and blue eyes are at increased risk.

29. The nurse planning the care for a patient who has impetigo expects to administer which topical drug to the patient?

    1. Acetaminophen
    2. Retapamulin
    3. Nystatin
    4. Corticosteroids

30. A patient who has developed a severe contact dermatitis of the lower extremities states, "The itching is terrible, I just cannot keep from scratching." Which statement should the nurse include in teaching the patient? (Select all that apply.)

    1. Take cool or tepid baths several times daily to decrease pruritus.
    2. Use cool, wet cloths or dressings to reduce itching.

    3. Add oil to the bath water to aid in moisturizing the affected skin.
    4. Use an OTC antihistamine with sedative effects to reduce scratching.

31. When teaching home care to a patient with recurrent herpes simplex genitalis infection, it is important to include that:

    1. the infection is contagious only when lesions are visible.
    2. antiviral agents are curative in the majority of cases.
    3. the patient will need to take antiviral agents daily for life.
    4. the patient will need to use protection even when no lesions are evident.

32. On admission, a patient is noted to have impaired skin integrity related to severe dermatitis. Which nursing intervention to enhance patient comfort should be included when planning the patient's care? (Select all that apply.)

    1. Keeping the environment cool
    2. Using cool compresses
    3. Applying heat for 20 minutes three times per day
    4. Using bath oils to decrease dryness

Care of the Patient with a Musculoskeletal Disorder

Martha E. Spray

Objectives

Anatomy and Physiology

1. List the five basic functions of the skeletal system.
2. List the two divisions of the skeleton.
3. Describe the location of major bones of the skeleton.
4. Describe the location of the major muscles of the body.
5. List the types of body movements.
6. Describe three vital functions muscles perform when they contract.

Medical-Surgical

7. List diagnostic examinations for musculoskeletal function.
8. Compare medical regimens for patients suffering from gouty arthritis, rheumatoid arthritis, and osteoarthritis.
9. Discuss nursing interventions for rheumatoid arthritis.
10. Describe nursing interventions for degenerative joint disease (osteoarthritis).
11. List at least four healthy lifestyle measures people can practice to reduce the risk of developing osteoporosis.
12. Describe the surgery for arthritis of the hip and knee.
13. Describe nursing interventions for the patient undergoing a total hip or knee replacement.
14. Discuss nursing interventions for a patient with a fractured hip after open reduction with internal fixation and bipolar hip prosthesis (hemiarthroplasty).
15. Discuss the physiology of fracture healing (hematoma, granulation tissue, and callus formation).
16. Describe the signs and symptoms of compartment syndrome.
17. List nursing interventions for a fat embolism.
18. List at least two types of skin and skeletal traction.
19. Compare methods for assessing circulation, nerve damage, and infection in a patient who has a traumatic insult to the musculoskeletal system.
20. List four nursing interventions for bone cancer.
21. Describe the phenomenon of phantom pain.
22. Define lordosis, scoliosis, and kyphosis.

Key Terms

ankylosis (ăng-kĭ-LŌ-sĭs, p. 124)

arthrocentesis (ăr-thrō-sĕn-TĒ-sĭs, p. 116)

arthrodesis (ăr-thrō-DĒ-sĭs, p. 133)

arthroplasty (ĂR-thrō-plăs-tē, p. 133)

bipolar hip replacement (hemiarthroplasty) (hĕ-mē-ĂR-thrō-plăs-tē, p. 139)

blanching test (p. 170)

callus (p. 144)

Colles' fracture (KŎL-ēz FRĂK-shŭr, p. 144)

compartment syndrome (p. 148)

crepitus (KRĔP-ĭ-tŭs, p.144)

fibromyalgia (fī-brō-mĭ-ĂL-jă, p. 131)

kyphosis (kĭ-FŌ-sĭs, p. 170)

lordosis (lŏr-DŌ-sĭs, p. 170)

open reduction with internal fixation (ORIF) (p. 145)

paresthesia (păr-ĕs-THĒ-zē-ă, pp. 132, 163)

scoliosis (skō-lē-Ō-sĭs, p. 170)

sequestrum (sĕ-KWĔS-trŭm, p. 131)

subluxation (sŭb-lŭk-SĀ-shŭn, p. 162)

tophi (TŌ-fī, p. 127)

Volkmann's contracture (VŎLK-mănz kŏn-TRĂK-shŭr, p. 149)

ANATOMY AND PHYSIOLOGY OF THE MUSCULOSKELETAL SYSTEM

Bones and joints form the framework of the body, and muscles contract and relax to allow movement. All movement of the body is orchestrated by the functioning of the bones, the joints, and the muscles attached to the bones. This chapter discusses the structure and the function of bones and muscles and how they serve the body.

FUNCTIONS OF THE SKELETAL SYSTEM

The human skeletal system is composed of 206 bones. The skeletal system has five basic functions: support, protection, movement, mineral storage, and hematopoiesis.

Support

The skeleton is the the body framework that supports internal tissues and organs.

Protection

The skeleton forms a firm, cagelike structure that protects many internal structures. The cranium (skull) protects the brain, the vertebrae protect the spinal cord, the ribs and the sternum (breastbone) protect the lungs and the heart, and the pelvis protects the digestive and reproductive organs.

Movement

Skeletal muscles are attached to the bones, which enables the bones to provide leverage for movement. As a muscle contracts, it pulls on the bone and movement occurs.

Mineral Storage

The bones serve as a storage area for various minerals, particularly calcium and phosphorus. When the body's intake of these minerals is inadequate, the bones release the minerals.

Hematopoiesis

Hematopoiesis (blood cell formation) takes place in the red bone marrow. The red bone marrow is spongy bone found in the ends of the long bones. A child's bones contain a proportionately larger amount of red bone marrow than an adult's. As a person ages, much of the red bone marrow converts to yellow bone marrow, which is composed of fat cells.

STRUCTURE OF BONES

Bones are classified into four groups, based on their form and shape: long, short, flat, and irregular. Long bones are found in the extremities, short bones are found in the hands and feet, flat bones are found in the skull and sternum, and irregular bones make up the vertebrae (backbone).

ARTICULATIONS (JOINTS)

Bones cannot bend without damage. To allow movement, individual bones articulate (join together) at joint sites (Figure 4-1). Bones are held together by flexible connective tissue. The joint is the point of contact between the individual bones. The structure of the individual bones depends on the function of the area. Every bone in the body (except the hyoid bone, which anchors the tongue) connects, or articulates, with at least one other bone.

Joints perform two important functions: they hold the bones together to form the skeleton, and they allow movement and flexibility of the skeleton.

The most common way to classify joints is according to the degree of movement they permit. There are three types of joints:

1. **Synarthrosis:** no movement
2. **Amphiarthrosis:** slight movement
3. **Diarthrosis:** free movement

A goniometer measures the angle of a joint. It is used to determine the degree of joint mobility (Lewis et al., 2007).

DIVISIONS OF THE SKELETON

The skeleton is divided into the axial and the appendicular skeletons (Box 4-1). The axial skeleton is composed of the skull, hyoid bone in the neck, vertebral column, and thorax (chest). The appendicular skeleton

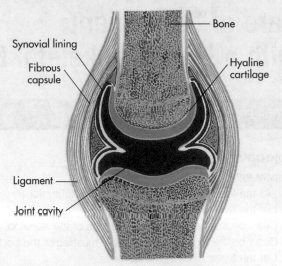

FIGURE 4-1 Structure of a freely movable (diarthrotic) joint. Note these typical features: joint capsule, joint cavity lined with synovial membrane, and articular (hyaline) cartilage covering the end surfaces of the bones within the joint capsule.

Box **4-1** **Main Parts of the Skeleton**	
AXIAL SKELETON	**APPENDICULAR SKELETON**
Skull	**Upper Extremities**
Cranium	Shoulder (pectoral) girdle
Ear bones	Arms
Face	Wrists
	Hands
SPINE	
Vertebrae	**Lower Extremities**
	Hip (pelvic) girdle
THORAX	Legs
Ribs	Ankles
Sternum	Feet

is composed of the upper extremities, lower extremities, shoulder girdle, and pelvic girdle (excluding the sacrum) (Figures 4-2 and 4-3).

FUNCTIONS OF THE MUSCULAR SYSTEM

The bones and joints provide the framework of the body, but the muscles are necessary for movement. This motion results from contraction and relaxation of the individual muscles. The body has more than 600 muscles, making up approximately 40% to 50% of the total body weight. They usually act in groups to execute a body movement (Table 4-1).

As muscles contract, they perform three vital functions: motion, maintenance of posture, and production of heat. Contraction also assists in return of venous blood and lymph to the right side of the heart.

All body movements rely on the integrated functioning of the bones, joints, and muscles. Muscle tissue is under voluntary or involuntary control. Voluntary muscle is under conscious control, whereas involuntary muscle tissue responds to internal commands without any conscious control of it. Involuntary motions include activities conducted by the internal organs, such as the heart beating, the gallbladder releasing bile, and the stomach churning food.

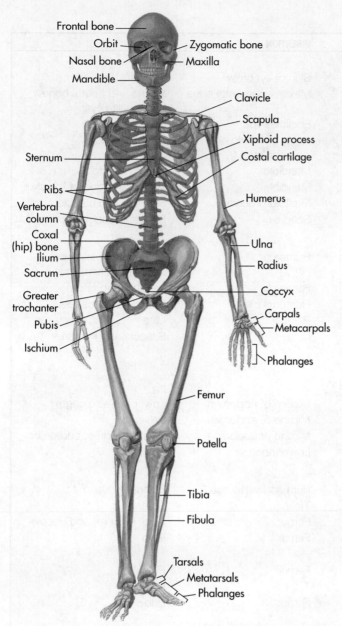

FIGURE 4-2 Skeleton, anterior view. Axial skeleton is shown in blue. Appendicular skeleton is bone colored.

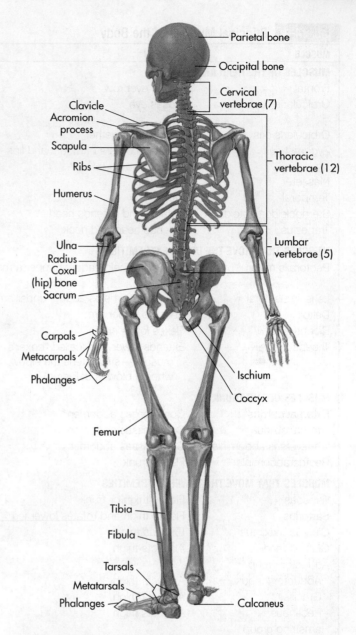

FIGURE 4-3 Skeleton, posterior view. Axial skeleton is shown in blue. Appendicular skeleton is bone colored.

The contraction of certain skeletal muscles gives the body proper posture. These muscles pull on various bones, allowing the body to sit or stand.

As skeletal muscles contract, they produce body heat. Approximately 85% of all body heat is generated by the contraction of the skeletal muscles.

Skeletal Muscle Structure

A skeletal muscle is composed of hundreds of muscle fibers (cells). Each skeletal muscle is surrounded by a covering of connective tissue called the **epimysium.** The epimysium joins with two other inner coverings, the perimysium and the endomysium, and extends beyond the muscle to form a tough cord of connective tissue known as a **tendon.** Tendons anchor muscles to bones. As a muscle contracts, it pulls the corresponding tendon and bone toward it. This is how movement occurs. Tendons in the ankle and wrist are enclosed in

tendon sheaths, which are sleeves or tubelike structures of connective tissue. Tendon sheaths contain synovial fluid and permit the tendons to slide easily; the sheaths also keep the tendons in place. All the tendons, ligaments, and aponeuroses of the body are composed of connective tissue in various sizes, shapes, and densities. These are collectively known as **fasciae.**

Nerve and Blood Supply

Because of the physical demands placed on the skeletal muscles, they need a constant supply of oxygen and nutrition. They are well supplied with blood vessels that carry oxygen and nutrition to the area and remove the waste products of metabolism.

The skeletal muscles are voluntary, so they need a constant source of information. Nerve cells or fibers continuously send impulses that stimulate the muscle cells. These impulses enter at the neuromuscular junc-

Table 4-1   Principal Muscles of the Body

MUSCLE	FUNCTION	INSERTION	ORIGIN
MUSCLES OF THE HEAD AND NECK			
Frontal	Raises eyebrow	Skin of eyebrow	Occipital bone
Orbicularis oculi	Closes eye	Maxilla and frontal bone	Maxilla and frontal bone (encircles eye)
Orbicularis oris	Draws lips together	Encircles lips	Encircles lips
Zygomaticus	Elevates corners of mouth and lips	Angle of mouth and upper lip	Zygomatic bone
Masseter	Closes jaw	Mandible	Zygomatic arch
Temporal	Closes jaw	Mandible	Temporal region of the skull
Sternocleidomastoid	Rotates and extends head	Mastoid process	Sternum and clavicle
Trapezius	Extends head and neck	Scapula	Skull and upper vertebrae
MUSCLES THAT MOVE THE UPPER EXTREMITIES			
Pectoralis major	Flexes and helps adduct upper arms	Humerus	Sternum, clavicle, and upper rib cartilages
Latissimus dorsi	Extends and helps adduct upper arm	Humerus	Vertebrae and ilium
Deltoid	Abducts upper arm	Humerus	Clavicle and scapula
Biceps brachii	Flexes lower arm	Radius	Ulna
Triceps brachii	Extends lower arm (called "boxer's muscle"—straightens the elbow when a blow is delivered)	Ulna	Scapula and humerus
MUSCLES OF THE TRUNK			
External oblique	Compresses abdomen	Midline of abdomen	Lower thoracic cage
Internal oblique	Compresses abdomen	Midline of abdomen	Pelvis
Transversus abdominis	Compresses abdomen	Midline of abdomen	Ribs, vertebrae, and pelvis
Rectus abdominis	Flexes trunk	Lower ribcage	Pubis
MUSCLES THAT MOVE THE LOWER EXTREMITIES			
Iliopsoas	Flexes thigh or trunk	Ilium and vertebrae	Femur
Sartorius	Flexes thigh and rotates lower leg	Tibia	Ilium
Gluteus maximus	Extends thigh	Femur	Ilium, sacrum, and coccyx
Gluteus medius	Abducts thigh	Femur	Ilium
Adductor group			
Adductor longus	Adducts thigh	Femur	Pubis
Gracilis	Adducts thigh	Tibia	Pubis
Pectineus	Adducts thigh	Femur	Pubis
Hamstring group			
Semimembranosus	Flexes lower leg	Tibia	Ischium
Semitendinosus	Flexes lower leg	Tibia	Ischium
Biceps femoris	Flexes lower leg	Fibula	Ischium and femur
Quadriceps group			
Rectus femoris	Extends lower leg	Tibia	Ischium
Vastus lateralis, intermedius, and medialis	Extends lower leg	Tibia	Femur
Tibialis anterior	Dorsiflexes foot	Metatarsals (foot)	Tibia
Gastrocnemius	Plantar flexes foot	Calcaneus (heel)	Femur
Soleus	Plantar flexes foot	Calcaneus (heel)	Tibia and fibula
Peroneus group			
Peroneus longus and brevis	Plantar flexes foot	Tarsals and metatarsals (ankle and foot)	Tibia and fibula

tion, the point of contact between the nerve ending and the muscle fiber. As a nerve impulse passes through this junction, chemicals are released that cause the muscle to contract.

Usually one artery, two veins, and one nerve penetrate a particular muscle. Each muscle cell comes in contact with several capillaries and a portion of a nerve cell. The muscle cells, in union with the nerve cell that controls them, are called a **motor unit.**

The impulse from the nerve cell must travel across a small gap because the nerve cell and the muscle cell do not directly touch each other. This small gap is called a **synaptic cleft** and is filled with tissue fluid. A special chemical **(neurotransmitter)** travels through the fluid to stimulate the muscle fiber. Acetylcholine is the neurotransmitter for skeletal muscle tissue. An enzyme called **cholinesterase** breaks down the acetylcholine once it has transferred the message. This allows the muscle cell to relax between impulses.

Muscle Contraction

Muscle Stimulus

Muscle cells are governed by the "all or none" law; that is, when a muscle cell is adequately stimulated or shocked, it will contract completely. Because each skeletal muscle is composed of thousands of muscle cells that react to many different nerve cells, the muscle as a whole contracts according to the principle of graded response. The strength of the muscle contraction, therefore, depends on the number of individual muscle cells responding. These muscle responses allow us to tenderly brush a baby's cheek or swat an irritating mosquito.

Muscle Tone

The skeletal muscles are in a constant state of readiness for action. At any given time, several muscle cells within a certain muscle are contracted; the remainder of the muscle cells are relaxed. Muscle tone is necessary for good posture but does not provide movement. To understand the importance of muscle tone, observe an extremity that has become paralyzed; the muscles are flaccid, limp, or atrophied (wasted) and incapable of producing movement because the cells no longer receive stimuli from the nerve fibers.

Types of Body Movements

Some muscles can move some body parts in only two directions, whereas others can move certain body

| Box **4-2** | Types of Body Movement |

- **Flexion:** A movement allowed by certain joints of the skeleton that decreases the angle between two adjoining bones. For example, bending the arm at the elbow decreases the angle between the humerus and the ulna.
- **Extension** (see Figure 4-4): A movement allowed by certain joints of the skeleton that increases the angle between two adjoining bones. For example, extending the leg increases the angle between the femur and the tibia. If the extension angles more than 180 degrees, the extremity is **hyperextended.**
- **Abduction:** A movement of an extremity away from the midline of the body.
- **Adduction:** A movement of an extremity toward the axis of the body.
- **Rotation:** A movement of a bone around its longitudinal axis (e.g., a pivot motion, such as shaking the head "no").
- **Supination:** A movement of the hand and forearm that causes the palm to face upward or forward.
- **Pronation:** A movement of the hand and forearm that causes the palm to face downward or backward.
- **Dorsiflexion:** A movement that causes the top of the foot to elevate or tilt upward.
- **Plantar flexion:** A movement that causes the bottom of the foot to be directed downward.

parts in several directions. The body's more common movements include flexion, extension, abduction, adduction, rotation, supination, pronation, dorsiflexion, and plantar flexion (Table 4-2; Box 4-2; Figure 4-4).

Skeletal Muscle Groups

Skeletal muscles are usually classified into two broad categories: axial and appendicular. The axial muscle groups are located on the head, face, neck, and trunk. The appendicular muscle groups are in the extremities. Figures 4-5 and 4-6 show the location of the muscles of the body.

LABORATORY AND DIAGNOSTIC EXAMINATIONS

RADIOGRAPHIC STUDIES

The diagnostic study most often used for determining musculoskeletal system integrity is the radiographic, roentgenographic, or (as it is more commonly known) x-ray examination or diagnostic imaging.

A radiographic examination of a joint reveals fluid, irregularity of the joint with spur formation, or changes

Table **4-2**	Muscles Grouped According to Function			
PART MOVED	**FLEXORS**	**EXTENSORS**	**ABDUCTORS**	**ADDUCTORS**
Upper arm	Pectoralis major	Latissimus dorsi	Deltoid and latissimus dorsi contracting together	Pectoralis major
Lower arm	Biceps brachii	Triceps brachii	None	None
Thigh	Iliopsoas and sartorius	Gluteus maximus	Gluteus medius	Adductor group
Lower leg	Hamstrings	Quadriceps group	None	None
Foot	Tibialis anterior	Gastrocnemius and soleus	Peroneus longus	Tibialis anterior

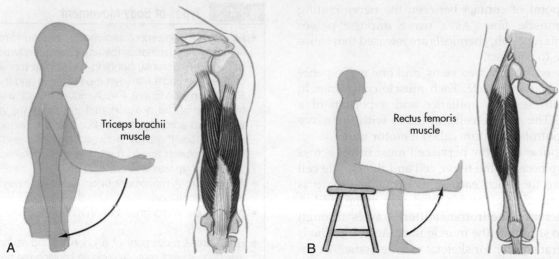

FIGURE 4-4 Extension of the lower arm and lower leg. **A,** When the triceps brachii muscle *(right)* contracts, it extends the lower arm at the elbow joint *(left).* **B,** When the rectus femoris muscle (part of the quadriceps femoris muscle group) *(right)* contracts, it extends the lower leg at the knee joint *(left).*

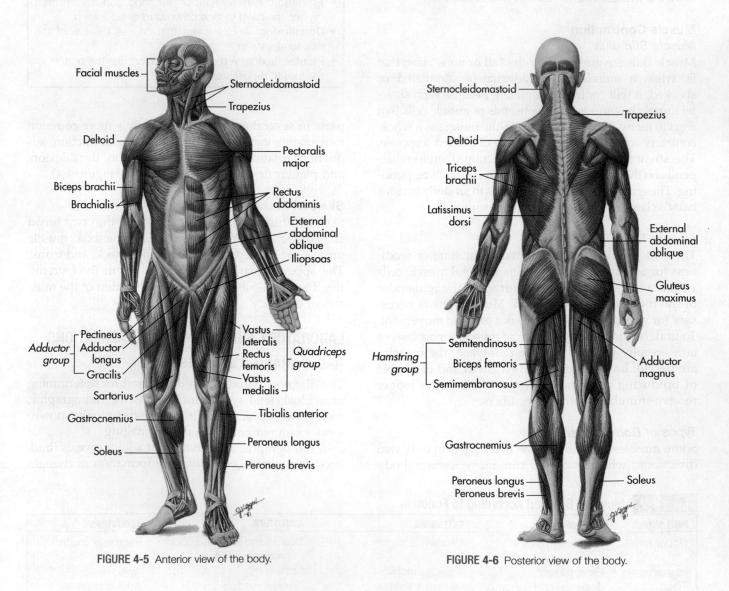

FIGURE 4-5 Anterior view of the body.

FIGURE 4-6 Posterior view of the body.

in the size of the joint contour. Radiographic examination is used to determine presence of a skeletal fracture. It is important to ask women of childbearing age if there is any possibility that they are pregnant before performing x-ray examinations because pregnant women should not be exposed to radiation except in emergencies because of potential damage to the fetus.

Laminography or **planography** (also called **body section roentgenography**) is useful in locating small cavities, foreign bodies, and lesions that are overshadowed by opaque structures.

Scanography, a method of producing a radiograph of internal body organs using a series of parallel beams that eliminate size distortion, allows accurate measurement of bone length.

Myelogram

Myelographic examination involves injection of a radiopaque dye into the subarachnoid space at the lumbar spine to x-ray the spinal cord and the vertebral column to detect herniated disk syndrome (herniated nucleus pulposus) or spinal tumors. The test involves the same procedure as a lumbar puncture (spinal tap), which is discussed in Chapter 14. Contrast medium causes allergic reactions in patients with allergies to iodine and seafood. Notify the physician about such allergies so that a nonionic contrast agent can be used or medications such as steroids or antihistamines can be given before the examination to minimize any reaction to the radiographic dye.

This examination may involve the entire spine or just the cervical or lumbar area. After the myelogram, oil-based dye is removed through the spinal needle to prevent meningeal irritation. Water-soluble dye is used most often and does not need to be removed; the body absorbs it and excretes it in urine. Inform the patient that the test is performed with the patient on a tilting table that is moved during the test to allow contrast medium to flow up to the cervical area.

The most common discomfort after a myelogram is headache. If water-soluble dye is used, the patient should lie quietly in a semi-Fowler's position for approximately 8 hours. Patient positioning is important to keep the dye in the lower spine. During this time, encouraging fluids helps the body absorb the dye from the spinal column. If oil-based dye is used, the patient rests in a flat position for up to 12 hours. Tell the patient to inform the nurse if he or she has a headache, stiff neck, leg weakness, or difficulty voiding. Rare complications include seizure, infection, drowsiness, severe headache, numbness, and paralysis.

Patients needing a myelogram fear the needle will be inserted into the spinal canal and damage the cord. Inform the patient that the tap is done in the lumbar region of the spine at approximately the fourth or fifth lumbar space (L4-L5). The spinal cord starts at the level of the foramen magnum and ends at the second lumbar space (L2) (lower border of ribcage).

Nuclear Scanning

Nuclear scanning tests are done in the nuclear medicine department, which has scanners or camera detectors that record images on radiographic film. Diagnostic tests use low dosages of radioactive isotopes; precautionary measures that are required for radium therapy are not necessary.

Nursing interventions required when patients are scheduled for nuclear scanning procedures involve (1) obtaining written consent from the patient, (2) informing the patient that the radioactive isotopes will not affect family or visitors, and (3) following the nuclear medicine department's instructions for special preparations for specific scans.

Magnetic Resonance Imaging

Musculoskeletal magnetic resonance imaging (MRI) assists in diagnosing abnormalities of bones and joints and surrounding soft tissue structures, including cartilage, synovium, ligaments, and tendons. The test uses magnetism and radio waves to make images of cross-sections of the body. MRI can give much more detailed pictures of fluid-filled soft tissue and blood vessels than any other test.

In preparation, have the patient remove any metal, such as jewelry, clothing with metal fasteners, glasses, and hair clips. Patients with metal prostheses such as heart valves, orthopedic screws, or cardiac pacemakers cannot undergo MRI.

The standard machine looks like a narrow tunnel which completely encloses the patient. Patients are required to lie still in this machine for 45 to 60 minutes. The patient enters the tunnel head first and may feel some anxiety or claustrophobia. The procedure is painless; however, if the patient is extremely anxious, a sedative is given. Encourage patients to use relaxation techniques, such as imagery, during the test. New MRI machines called open MRI are designed to be less confining and more comfortable than the traditional machine. Because the procedure requires the patient to be motionless, relaxation techniques that require flexing and relaxing the muscles are not appropriate.

After the test, take routine vital sign measurements and allow the patient to resume pretest activities. There are no adverse effects.

Computed Tomography

Body sections can be examined from many different angles using a computed tomography (CT) scanner, which uses a narrow x-ray beam and produces a three-dimensional picture of the structure being studied. The CT scanner is approximately 100 times more sensitive than the radiograph machine and should not be used unnecessarily because of radiation exposure. Iodine contrast dye is sometimes used. CT scan is used for the head and body. It is useful in locating injuries to the ligaments or tendons, tumors of the soft tissue, and fractures in areas difficult to define by other means.

Patient preparation includes (1) having the patient sign a consent form authorizing the examination if not included on the initial hospital consent form, (2) questioning the patient regarding allergies (e.g., iodine and seafood), (3) keeping the patient on NPO (nothing by mouth) status 3 to 4 hours before the test (in case contrast dye is used, since the dye can cause nausea and vomiting), (4) measuring vital signs to be used as a baseline, (5) having the patient void before the test, (6) removing metal articles such as jewelry and hairpins, and (7) telling the patient that he or she must lie still during the test and may feel warm and slightly nauseated for a few minutes when dye is injected.

After the test, observe the patient for delayed allergic reactions (if contrast dye was used). Encourage fluids unless contraindicated. Pretest diet and activity can usually be resumed.

Bone Scan

The bone scan test is especially valuable in detecting metastatic and inflammatory bone disease (osteomyelitis). This test involves the intravenous (IV) administration of nuclides (atomic material) approximately 2 to 3 hours before the test is scheduled. There are no food or fluid restrictions, and patients are encouraged to drink water over the next 1 to 3 hours to aid renal clearance of any radioisotope not picked up by the bone. After the patient has voided, a scanning camera reveals the degree of radionuclide uptake; areas of concentrated nucleotide uptake may represent a tumor or other abnormality. These areas of concentration can be detected days or weeks before an ordinary radiograph reveals a metastatic lesion. The test takes approximately 30 to 60 minutes and requires the patient to lie still.

ASPIRATION

An aspiration procedure is done to obtain a specimen of body fluid. The physician inserts a needle into a cavity with the patient under local anesthesia. This procedure is performed using sterile technique. Commonly the physician takes a biopsy of tissue while doing the aspiration procedure. Nursing interventions are similar for all aspiration tests, with special emphasis on (1) having the consent form signed; (2) reinforcing the physician's explanation of the procedure; (3) encouraging the patient to remain immobile during the procedure; (4) having the patient void before the procedure; (5) maintaining sterile technique; (6) supporting the patient emotionally; (7) applying a sterile pressure dressing to the puncture site and maintaining the dressing until bleeding has stopped; (8) assisting with collecting, labeling, and transporting a specimen to the laboratory immediately; and (9) observing for emotional and physical distress after the procedure.

Synovial Fluid Aspiration

Arthrocentesis is the puncture of a patient's joint with a needle and the withdrawal of synovial fluid for diagnos-

tic purposes. It is helpful in diagnosing trauma, systemic lupus erythematosus, gout, osteoarthritis, and rheumatoid arthritis (RA). It may also be used to instill medications for the patient with septic arthritis or to remove fluid from joints to relieve pain. Normally a patient's synovial fluid is straw colored, clear, or slightly cloudy. If trauma or a disease is present, the synovial fluid appears cloudy, milky, sanguineous, yellow, green, or gray.

After the procedure, provide proper support to the affected extremity. Placing it on a pillow and maintaining joint rest for approximately 12 hours may be indicated. Apply ice to the affected joint for 24 to 48 hours unless otherwise ordered. An antiinfective or corticosteroid may be prescribed. Assess the patient for signs of infection. After the pressure dressing is removed from the site, an adhesive bandage can be used.

ENDOSCOPIC EXAMINATION

For endoscopy, a lighted tube is used to visualize inside a body cavity. Although some procedures require general anesthesia, most require only local anesthesia. Emotional support and complete explanations help relieve the patient's anxiety. Preparation for an endoscopic examination is similar to that for surgical preparation: (1) have the patient sign a consent form; (2) complete a preoperative checklist with special attention to removing jewelry, dentures, and contact lenses; (3) initiate NPO status 6 to 12 hours before the examination; (4) give premedications, such as atropine and a sedative; (5) encourage the patient to void; (6) record vital signs; and (7) maintain bed rest with side rails up after giving the premedication.

Arthroscopy

Arthroscopy is an endoscopic examination that enables direct visualization of a joint. The procedure is used to (1) explore the joint to determine the presence of a disease process, (2) drain fluid from the joint cavity, and (3) remove damaged tissue or foreign bodies.

This examination is most commonly done on the knee joint, with the synovium, articular surfaces, and meniscus (a curved, fibrous cartilage in the knee) visualized through the scope. The procedure involves insertion of a large-bore needle into the suprapatellar pouch and saline instillation into the joint. Arthroscopy can also be done on the hip or shoulder. The patient may be given a general or local anesthetic agent. After the arthroscopic examination, advise the patient to limit activities for several days.

Endoscopic Spinal Microsurgery

Surgeons can perform spinal surgery with less damage to surrounding tissues by passing endoscopic equipment through small incisions. Special scopes enable surgeons to successfully treat spinal column disorders (e.g., herniated disk, spinal stenosis) and spinal deformities (e.g., scoliosis, kyphosis). Spinal microsurgery can be performed with the patient under local anesthesia; discharge occurs after a brief stay. Candidates for microsurgery procedures are evaluated on information obtained from x-ray examinations, MRI scans, CT scans, and bone scans.

ELECTROGRAPHIC PROCEDURE

Electrographic procedures use electrodes to measure electrical activity in specific areas of the body.

Electromyogram

An electromyogram involves insertion of needle electrodes into the skeletal muscles so that electrical activity can be heard, seen on an oscilloscope (an instrument that displays a graphic representation of electron beams), and recorded on paper at the same time. Muscles do not produce an electrical charge at rest, but with neuromuscular disorders unusual patterns can be observed. Nerves can be observed for neuropathy and muscles for myopathy. Electromyography can be used to detect chronic low back pain based on muscle fatigue patterns.

LABORATORY TESTS

Specific laboratory tests are ordered when musculoskeletal disorders are suspected (Table 4-3).

EFFECTS OF BED REST ON MINERAL CONTENT IN BONE

Studies done on people confined to bed rest reveal a loss of body calcium. Immobilization results in bone resorption—the bone tissue becomes less dense. Prolonged bed rest puts the patient at risk for pathologic fractures (Potter & Perry, 2009). This rate of loss over several weeks is a serious concern for an older adult in terms of regaining mobility; it also increases the risk of fracture.

DISORDERS OF THE MUSCULOSKELETAL SYSTEM

INFLAMMATORY DISORDERS

ARTHRITIS

Arthritis is a disease involving an inflammation of the joint. An estimated 50 million Americans are affected by arthritis, and 4 million of these are dependent and unable to work, attend school, or participate in social functions. There are many types of arthritis, but the most common are RA, rheumatoid spondylitis, osteoarthritis (degenerative joint disease [DJD]), and gout

Table 4-3	Laboratory Tests for Musculoskeletal Disorders
NORMAL VALUE	**POSSIBLE CAUSE FOR INCREASE OR DECREASE**
Calcium: 9.0-10.5 mg/dL	Increased in metastatic tumor to the bone, Addison's disease, Paget's disease of the bone, acromegaly, acute osteoporosis, hyperparathyroidism, vitamin D deficiency, renal failure, malabsorption, and rickets
Phosphorus: 2.5-4.5 mg/dL	Increased in acromegaly, bone metastases, excessive levels of vitamin D, hypocalcemia, renal failure Decreased in acute gout, hypercalcemia, vitamin D deficiency
Vitamin D 25-dihydroxy: 6-52 ng/mL	Increased in vitamin D intoxication Decreased in bowel resection, malabsorption, rickets
Vitamin D₁, 25-dihydroxy: 15-60 pg/mL	Increased in liver disease; bone disease; healing fractures; metastatic tumor in bone; osteogenic sarcoma; osteoporosis; cancer of breast, colon, lung, or pancreas Decreased in severe anemia, folic acid deficiency, pernicious anemia
Alkaline phosphatase: 30-120 units/L	Increased in skeletal muscle injury or myocardial infarction
Myoglobin: 5-70 mcg/dL	Decreased in rheumatoid arthritis
Erythrocyte sedimentation rate (ESR) Males: up to 15 mm/hr Females: up to 20 mm/hr	A nonspecific test used to detect inflammatory, neoplastic, infectious, and necrotic processes Indicates the presence of inflammation as seen in rheumatoid arthritis and rheumatic fever One of the most objective measurements of rheumatoid arthritis severity Increased as the disease worsens Increased in multiple myeloma, acute myocardial infarctions, toxemia, bacterial infections, and gout Decreased in congestive heart failure, sickle cell anemia, polycythemia vera, infectious mononucleosis, degenerative arthritis, and angina pectoris
Lupus erythematosus (LE) preparation: no LE cells seen	Lupus erythematosus, rheumatoid arthritis, scleroderma, and drug sensitivities
Rheumatoid factor (RF): <60 units/mL	An immunoglobulin found in approximately 80% of adults with rheumatoid arthritis; other diseases such as systemic lupus erythematosus may cause a positive RF
Uric acid (blood) Males: 2.1-8.5 mg/dL Females: 2.0-6.6 mg/dL	Increased in patients with gout, kidney failure, alcoholism, leukemia, metastatic cancer, multiple myeloma, or dehydration

(gouty arthritis). See Table 4-4 for a comparison of RA and osteoarthritis.

RHEUMATOID ARTHRITIS

Etiology and Pathophysiology

RA, the most serious form of the arthritis, leads to severe crippling. It is a chronic, systemic disease that affects 3% of the general population. RA can strike anyone; however, some people are more susceptible than others. Of the approximately 6 million Americans who have RA, 75% are women. Although RA can occur at any age, it most often occurs in women of childbearing age. RA is thought to be an autoimmune disorder, although there is evidence of genetic predisposition. Smoking significantly increases the risk of RA in both men and women who are genetically predisposed to the disease.

RA can affect many organ systems (lungs, heart, blood vessels, muscles, eyes, and skin). RA is characterized by a chronic inflammation of the synovial membrane (synovitis) of the diarthrodial joints (also called synovial joints: the freely movable joints in which continuous bony surfaces are covered by cartilage and connected by ligaments lined with synovial membrane).

Clinical Manifestations

RA is believed to involve an immune reaction that will not shut off because of an immune system failure; agents that should protect the body attack joint tissues instead and cause a chronic inflammatory reaction in the synovial membrane. This in turn damages the affected joint and surrounding tissue, possibly leading to gross deformity and loss of function (Figure 4-7).

RA is characterized by periods of remission and exacerbation. Some patients report a precipitating stressful event such as infection, work stress, physical exertion, childbirth, surgery, or emotional upset. During remission the inflammation, pain, stiffness, and edema subside, and progression of tissue damage is halted. (The patient may experience residual joint dysfunction even with remission.)

Table 4-4	Comparison of Rheumatoid Arthritis and Osteoarthritis	
	RHEUMATOID ARTHRITIS (RA)	**OSTEOARTHRITIS (OA)**
Pathophysiology	Inflammation of synovial membrane; destruction of bones, ligaments, tendons, cartilage, and joint capsule.	Degeneration of cartilage from wear and tear; bone spur formation.
Joints most commonly affected	Symmetrical joint involvement noted in wrists, knees, and knuckles.	Often only one side of body affected with changes noted in hands, spine, knees, and hips.
Clinical signs and symptoms	Edema, erythema, heat, pain, tenderness, nodule formation, fatigue, stiffness, muscle aches, and fever. Systemic manifestations occur. Vasculitis (inflammation of blood vessels) may be responsible for a variety of systemic complications, including peripheral neuropathy, myopathy, cardiopulmonary involvement, and ischemic ulcerations of the skin. Potential complications include infection, osteoporosis, and Sjögren syndrome. Dry mouth and decreased tearing occur in Sjögren syndrome.	Localized pain, stiffness, bony knobs of end joints of fingers (Heberden's nodes), edema (not as pronounced as in RA). No systemic involvement is present. Constitutional symptoms such as fatigue or fever are not present. Other organ involvement is absent as well, which is an important differentiation between OA and RA.
Age at onset	Children nearing adolescence. Adults between 20 and 50.	Ages 45-90. Most people have some features with increasing age.
Sex	Females affected more often than males, with a ratio of 3:1.	Males and females affected equally.
Heredity	Familial tendency.	The form with knobby fingers can be hereditary.
Diagnostic tests	Rheumatoid factor (RF) found in serum of about 85% of patients with RA. Erythrocyte sedimentation rate, C-reactive protein, complete blood count, x-rays, examination of joint fluid RF positive in 80% of patients.	X-rays; no specific laboratory abnormalities are useful in diagnosing OA. RF negative.
Treatment	Control inflammation and pain with medications. Balance exercise with rest. Provide joint protection; encourage weight control and stress reduction. Surgically replace joints.	Maintain activity level. Control pain with medication. Encourage exercise, joint protection, weight control, stress reduction. Surgical joint replacement may be necessary.

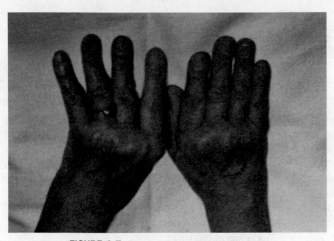

FIGURE 4-7 Rheumatoid arthritis of hands.

Assessment

Collection of **subjective data** includes noting the patient's complaints of malaise, muscle weakness (especially grip strength), loss of appetite, and generalized aching.

Collection of **objective data** includes observing the joints for edema, tenderness, subcutaneous nodules, limitation in range of motion (ROM) (morning stiffness especially), symmetrical joint involvement, and fever.

Diagnostic Tests

No single test is definitive for RA. Diagnosis is based on patient history and physical examination. The four classic symptoms most frequently reported are morning stiffness, joint pain, muscle weakness, and fatigue. Radiographic studies reveal loss of articular cartilage and change in subchondral bone. The following laboratory tests are often used in confirming a diagnosis and in ruling out other diseases:

- Erythrocyte sedimentation rate (ESR): An increase indicates the presence of inflammatory reaction somewhere in body.
- Rheumatoid factor (RF): An elevation indicates abnormal serum protein concentration. Positive RF occurs in approximately 80% of RA patients.
- Antinuclear antibody (ANA) titers and elevated C-reactive protein (CRP): These are seen in some RA patients.
- Latex agglutination test: This test detects presence of the immunoglobulin M version of RF, the anti–immunoglobulin G antibodies.
- Red blood cell count: This detects anemia, which is often present during chronic infection.
- Synovial fluid aspiration: Normal fluid is usually clear and highly viscous; however, when inflammation is present, fluid is cloudy, yellow, and less viscous and contains increased protein.
- Synovial fluid biopsy: The biopsy shows changes in tissue.

Table 4-5 Medications for Rheumatoid Arthritis

Generic (Trade)	Action	Side Effects/Toxic Effects	Nursing Implications
SALICYLATES			
Aspirin, salsalate (Disalicid, Asaphen) Choline salicylate (Arthropan) Choline magnesium trisalicylate (Trillisate)	Antiinflammatory, analgesic, antipyretic; act by inhibiting synthesis of prostaglandins	GI irritation (dyspepsia, nausea, ulcer, hemorrhage) Prolonged bleeding time Exacerbation of asthma (aspirin-sensitive asthma) Tinnitus, dizziness with repeated large doses	Administer drug with food, milk, antacids as prescribed, or full glass of water; may use enteric-coated aspirin. Report signs of bleeding (e.g., tarry stools, bruising, petechiae, nosebleeds).
NONSTEROIDAL ANTIINFLAMMATORY DRUGS (NSAIDs)			
Indomethacin (Indocin)	Analgesic, antiinflammatory	Headache, vertigo, insomnia; confusion, GI irritation, can decrease effect of ACE inhibitors	Give with food, milk, or antacid. Discontinue if CNS symptoms develop and notify physician. Monitor BP. Report signs of bleeding.
Ibuprofen (Motrin, Advil)	Analgesic, antiinflammatory	Same as indomethacin but believed less irritating to GI tract Fluid retention Can cause hypertension	Know that delayed absorption occurs if taken with food. Monitor BP.
Tolmetin sodium (Tolectin)	Analgesic, antiinflammatory	Same as ibuprofen	Give with food or milk.

From Lewis, S.L., et al. (2007). *Medical-surgical nursing: Assessment and management of clinical problems* (7th ed.). St. Louis: Mosby.
ACE, Angiotensin-converting enzyme; *BP,* blood pressure; *CNS,* central nervous system; *GI,* gastrointestinal.

Continued

Table 4-5   Medications for Rheumatoid Arthritis—cont'd

Generic (Trade)	Action	Side Effects/Toxic Effects	Nursing Implications
NONSTEROIDAL ANTIINFLAMMATORY DRUGS (NSAIDs)—cont'd			
Naproxen (Naprosyn)	Analgesic, antiinflammatory	Same as ibuprofen Causes drowsiness	Give with food, milk, or antacid. Tell patient to avoid driving until dosage effect is established.
Meloxicam (Mobic)	Antiinflammatory, analgesic, antipyretic	Dizziness, headache, insomnia, seizures, dysrhythmias, heart failure, hemorrhage, diarrhea, indigestion, nausea, pancreatitis, renal failure, leukopenia, thrombocytopenia, asthma, bronchospasm, angioedema. Drug is contraindicated in women who are pregnant or plan to become pregnant.	Monitor BP. Instruct patient to avoid using aspirin or products containing aspirin. Assess patient for history of allergic reactions to aspirin or other NSAIDs before starting drug. Tell patient the drug can be taken without regard to meals. Advise patient to report signs and symptoms of GI ulcers and bleeding. Advise patient to report any skin rash, weight gain, or edema. Alert patient with history of asthma that asthma may recur while taking the drug. Advise patient to avoid alcohol and tobacco products while taking the drug. NSAIDs can cause fluid retention; closely monitor patients with hypertension, edema, or heart failure. Inform patient that consistent pain relief may take several days of drug administration.
Nabumetone (Relafen)	Analgesic, antiinflammatory	Dizziness, anxiety, depression, gastric irritation, edema, prolonged bleeding, rash	Give with meals or antacids. Advise patient to avoid alcohol, aspirin, or aspirin products or acetaminophen without physician's consent. Arthritic relief noted in 1-2 weeks.
Meclofenamate (Meclofen)	Analgesic, antiinflammatory	Gastric irritation, headache, dizziness, edema	Advise patients to avoid aspirin and aspirin products. Give 30 minutes before or 2 hours after eating.
COX-2 INHIBITOR			
Celecoxib (Celebrex)	Analgesic, antiinflammatory	Mild to moderate indigestion, risk of GI bleeding, diarrhea, abdominal pain. Has been linked to an increased risk of cardiovascular events, such as MI or stroke (U.S. Food and Drug Administration, 2006)	Give medication orally. It can be taken with or without food. Celebrex is indicated for relief of the signs and symptoms of osteoarthritis and RA. Do not administer to patients who have asthma, urticaria, or allergic reactions to aspirin or other NSAIDs. Do not give to patients who are allergic to sulfonamide. Use cautiously with ACE inhibitors, warfarin, lithium, and furosemide. Monitor patients for signs of GI bleeding.
POTENT ANTIINFLAMMATORY AGENTS			
Adrenocorticosteroids (e.g., prednisone)	Interfere with body's normal inflammatory responses	Fluid retention, sodium retention, potassium depletion, hypertension, decreased healing potential, increased susceptibility to infection, GI irritation, hirsutism, osteoporosis, fat deposits, diabetes mellitus, myopathy. Adrenal insufficiency or adrenal crisis if abruptly withdrawn	Give with food, milk, or antacid. Do not increase or decrease dosage without physician supervision. Give in morning if given once a day.

ACE, Angiotensin-converting enzyme; *BP,* blood pressure; *GI,* gastrointestinal; *MI,* myocardial infarction; *NSAIDs,* nonsteroidal antiinflammatory drugs; *RA,* rheumatoid arthritis.

Table 4-5   Medications for Rheumatoid Arthritis—cont'd

Generic (Trade)	Action	Side Effects/Toxic Effects	Nursing Implications
POTENT ANTIINFLAMMATORY AGENTS—cont'd			
Corticosteroids intraarticular injections (methylprednisolone [Depo-Medrol])	Suppression of inflammation and modification of the normal immune response	Decreased wound healing and increased susceptibility to infection	Check injection site for signs of infection. Inform patient joint improvement can last weeks to months. Advise patient to avoid overuse of joint.
SLOW-ACTING ANTIINFLAMMATORY AGENTS			
Antimalarials			
Hydroxychloroquine (Plaquenil)	Antiinflammatory (mechanism unknown); effect not expected to be noted for 6-12 months after beginning therapy	GI disturbances Retinal edema that may result in blindness	Instruct patient to obtain eye examination before beginning therapy and every 6 months thereafter. Monitor CBC.
Gold Salts (IM)			
Gold sodium thiomalate (Myochrysine)	Antiinflammatory; effect not noted for 3-6 months after beginning therapy	Renal and hepatic damage, corneal deposits, dermatitis, ulcerations in mouth, hematologic changes	Monitor urinalysis and CBC before each injection. Report dermatitis, metallic taste in mouth, or lesions in mouth to physician.
Oral gold salts auranofin (Ridaura)	Antirheumatic	Stomatitis (lesions in mouth); thrombocytopenia and leukopenia	Minimize exposure to sunlight and provide meticulous oral hygiene.
Antineoplastic			
Methotrexate (Folex, Rheumatrex, Trexall)	Alters the way the body uses folic acid, which is necessary for cell growth; decreases inflammation	Upset stomach, nausea, vomiting, anorexia, diarrhea, or sore mouth; headache, blurred vision, dizziness	Drug is taken orally or by injection. Monitor vital signs, WBC, platelets, I&O, appetite. Advise patient to avoid pregnancy while on drug and to not get vaccinations without physician's consent. Keep patient well hydrated.
DISEASE-MODIFYING ANTIRHEUMATOID DRUGS (DMARDs)			
Etanercept (Enbrel)	Blocks the normal and inflammatory immune responses seen in RA; binds tumor necrosis factor (TNF), which is involved in immune and inflammatory reactions	Pain at injection site, upper respiratory tract infections and sinusitis; in severe cases, tuberculosis possible	Give twice weekly subcutaneously in the thigh, abdomen, or upper arm. Refrigerate, but never freeze medication. Use with caution in patients with chronic infections. May cause or aggravate systemic lupus erythematosus.
Leflunomide (Arava)	Reduces signs and symptoms of RA and retards structural bone damage	Diarrhea, elevated liver enzymes, alopecia, rash	Medication is taken orally. Monitor urinary output. Do not use with patients with hepatic impairment or positive for hepatitis B or C.
Infliximab (Remicade)	An antibody that binds specifically to proinflammatory enzymes that are produced by the synovial cells	Upper respiratory tract infections, headache, nausea, sinusitis, rash, cough	Administer intravenously at 2 and 6 weeks initially, then every 8 weeks thereafter. Do not give to patients with a clinically active infection.

CBC, Complete blood count; *I&O*, intake and output; *RA*, rheumatoid arthritis; *TNF*, tumor necrosis factor; *WBC*, white blood cell count.

Continued

Table 4-5 Medications for Rheumatoid Arthritis—cont'd

Generic (Trade)	Action	Side Effects/Toxic Effects	Nursing Implications
DISEASE-MODIFYING ANTIRHEUMATOID DRUGS (DMARDs)—cont'd			
Adalimumab (Humira)	Reduces infiltration of inflammatory cells	Increased risk of infection, headaches and rash; neutropenia; injection site reaction	Assess for signs of infection before injection. Do not give to patients with active infections. Monitor new infections closely.
Sulfasalazine (Azulfidine, Salazopyrin)	Sulfonamide; anti-inflammatory; blocks prostaglandin synthesis	GI effects (anorexia, nausea, vomiting); bleeding, bruising, jaundice; headache; rash, urticaria, pruritus	Advise patient that drug may cause orange-yellow discoloration of urine or skin. Space doses evenly around the clock, taking drug after food with 8 oz water. Treatment may be continued even after symptoms are relieved. Monitor CBC.
Penicillamine (Cuprimine, Depen)	Antiinflammatory; exact mechanism of action in RA unknown but may suppress cell-mediated immune response	GI irritation (nausea, vomiting, anorexia, diarrhea); reduced or altered taste; rash; proteinuria, hematuria; iron deficiency (especially in menstruating women)	Monitor WBC count, platelets, urinalysis. Advise patient to take medication 1 hour before or 2 hours after meals or at least 1 hour away from any other drug, food, or milk.
Anakinra (Kineret)	Blocks the action of interleukin-1, thus decreasing the inflammatory response	Injection site reaction, leukopenia, headache, abdominal pain, rash	Evaluate for relief of pain, swelling, stiffness; increase in joint mobility. Advise patient that injection site reaction generally occurs in first month of treatment and decreases with continued therapy. Evaluate renal function. Monitor for infection. Do not give drug with other TNF inhibitors.
Abatacept (Orencia)	Modulates T-cell activation; suppresses immune response	Headache, upper respiratory tract infection, nausea, sore throat, injection site reaction	Not recommended for concomitant use with TNF inhibitors. Evaluate for relief of pain, swelling, stiffness and increase in joint mobility.
Rituximab (Rituxan)	Monoclonal antibody that targets B cells	Dizziness, palpitations, fever, itching, difficulty breathing, sore throat	Give in combination with methotrexate. Monitor for infection and bleeding. Advise patient to not receive the virus vaccines with treatment. Monitor for low BP if also taking BP medication.
IMMUNOSUPPRESSANT			
Azathioprine (Imurant) Cyclophosphamide (Cytoxan)	Inhibits DNA, RNA, protein synthesis	GI irritation (nausea, vomiting, anorexia with large doses), rash	Evaluate for relief of pain, swelling, stiffness; increase in joint mobility. Advise patient to immediately report unusual bleeding or bruising. Advise patient that therapeutic response may take up to 12 weeks. Advise women of childbearing age to avoid pregnancy.
TOPICAL ANALGESICS			
Capsaicin cream (Zostrix, Capzasin) 5% lidocaine	Depletes substance P from nerve endings, interrupting pain signals to the brain (Substance P may participate directly or indirectly in the transmission process of certain neurons.)	Rash, urticaria, localized burning sensation, erythema	Must be used regularly over time for maximal effect. Aloe vera cream may moderate burning sensation. Advise patient not to use cream with external heat source (heating pad) because of risk of burns. Available in OTC and prescription strengths. Advise patient to wear gloves when applying cream to other joints and to wash hands; avoid touching damaged or irritated skin, eyes, nose and mouth.

BP, Blood Pressure; *CBC,* complete blood count; *DNA,* deoxyribonucleic acid; *GI,* gastrointestinal; *OTC,* over the counter; *RA,* rheumatoid arthritis; *RNA,* ribonucleic acid; *TNF,* tumor necrosis factor; *WBC,* white blood cell.

Medical Management

The RA patient benefits from aggressive treatment early in the course of the disease. The medical management of RA is directed toward (1) controlling the disease activity by administering disease-modifying and antiinflammatory drugs (Table 4-5); (2) providing pain relief (see Table 4-5); (3) reducing clinical symptoms in days to weeks with the rapid antiinflammatory effect of methotrexate (Rheumatrex); (4) prolonging joint function (often with physical therapy, traction, and splints); and (5) slowing the progression of joint damage by promoting activities of daily living (ADLs), an exercise program, and weight management.

Advances in cell and molecular biology have influenced the treatment of RA. Current medications actually target the pathophysiology of the disease. Disease-modifying antirheumatoid drugs (DMARDs) offer wider treatment options. These medications target an enzyme known as tumor necrosis factor (TNF). TNF is produced by the synovial cells and other cells of the body and is a proinflammatory substance—that is, it has the ability to produce signs and symptoms of inflammation (see Table 4-5). Complementary therapies to decrease inflammation include capsaicin (Capsin), a nonopioid topical analgesic, fish oil, and antioxidants (vitamins C and E and beta-carotene). Musculoskeletal surgery in the form of joint replacement is another option.

Nursing Interventions and Patient Teaching

Patient education is essential to help the patient and family understand what is happening and what to expect as the disease progresses. Fatigue is a major problem, so sleeping 8 to 10 hours a night and taking a 2-hour nap during the day are recommended. Exercise helps prevent the joints from "freezing" and the muscles from weakening. A typical exercise program calls for two or three 10- to 15-minute daily sessions of "quiet" exercise that gently puts joints through ROM. Heat is often used to relax and soothe muscles. Hot packs, heat lamps, and applications of hot paraffin wax are helpful. Rehabilitation is aimed at helping the patient adapt to physical limitations and promoting normal daily activities.

Nursing diagnoses and interventions for the patient with RA include but are not limited to the following:

Nursing Diagnoses	Nursing Interventions
Pain, related to joint inflammation	Administer prescribed salicylate or nonsteroidal antiinflammatory drugs (NSAIDs).
	Assist patient with an exercise program prescribed by a physical therapist, including proper body mechanics and use of a walker or cane.

Nursing Diagnoses	Nursing Interventions
	During acute stages of disease, encourage patient to rest inflamed joints.
	Maintain bed rest as ordered; maintain proper body alignment.
	Assist and teach patient to extend joints as possible and to avoid external rotation of extremities; use sandbags or trochanter rolls.
	Avoid use of pillow under knees.
	Immobilize and/or support joints.
Chronic low self-esteem, related to negative self-evaluation about self or capabilities	Encourage patient to express feelings about health problems, progress, and prognosis concerning diagnosis.
	Encourage patient to explore ways to remain active while experiencing limited mobility (e.g., doing tasks while sitting as opposed to standing or walking).

As with any chronic illness, patient teaching is perhaps the most important aspect of nursing interventions. Patient teaching includes information about joint protection and energy conservation techniques, proper balance of rest and activity, proper use of medications (i.e., names of drugs, dosages, precautions in administration, and side effects or toxic effects), plans for implementation of the exercise program prescribed by the physician or physical therapist, proper application of heat or cold packs, proper use of walking aids, safety measures to prevent injury, basics of good nutrition and importance of avoiding weight gain, and the danger of following programs that promise a "cure."

Prognosis

The course of RA is variable but is most frequently marked by remissions and exacerbations. The prognosis is based on a variety of clinical and laboratory findings. Stage I represents early effects. Stage IV, the terminal category, includes marked joint deformity, extensive muscle atrophy, soft tissue lesions, bone and cartilage destruction, and fibrous or bony ankylosis.

ANKYLOSING SPONDYLITIS

Etiology and Pathophysiology

Ankylosing spondylitis (AKS) is a chronic, progressive disorder of the sacroiliac and hip joints, the synovial joints of the spine, and the adjacent soft tissues. It can affect both sexes but is seen more often in young men. The presence of human leukocyte antigen A and B27 (HLA-B27) in the serum of 90% of whites and 50% of blacks with AKS suggests a hereditary factor. The most common age for onset of AKS is between 15 and 35 years of age. The highest incidence rate is among 25- to 34-year-olds (Lewis et al., 2007). Women develop a milder form of AKS than men, and fusion of the spine is rarely seen. It is sometimes referred to as **rheumatoid spondylitis.**

Clinical Manifestations

AKS involves inflammation of the spine that results in the bones of the spine growing together. This is termed **ankylosis,** the fixation of a joint, often in abnormal position. It usually results from destruction of articular cartilage and subchondral bone.

AKS involves inflammation in which the ligament or tendon attaches to the bone; it does not affect the synovial membrane, as seen in RA. AKS affects joints such as the neck, jaw, shoulders, knees, and hips. The disease process causes the ligaments to become ossified (hardened). The cardiovascular system can be involved, and heart enlargement and pericarditis can occur. If the costovertebral joints are affected, kyphosis can occur and alter respirations. The patient may have difficulty expanding the ribcage while breathing. Many patients with the disease also have inflammatory bowel disease. Vision loss occurs with chronic AKS, and blindness may result from glaucoma and pupil damage.

Assessment

Subjective data include patient complaints of low backache, stiffness, and alternating or bilateral "sciatica pain" that lasts for a few days and then subsides. Pain is more pronounced when the patient is in an erect position. Inactivity exacerbates the pain, and exercise gives relief. Complaints of weight loss, abdominal distention, visual problems, and fatigue are common. AKS is present in 3% to 10% of patients with inflammatory bowel disease.

Collection of **objective data** includes assessment for tenderness over the spine and sacroiliac region. Peripheral joint edema and decreased ROM may be seen. Assessment of vital signs may indicate elevated temperature, tachycardia, and hyperpnea. Respiratory difficulties arise if there is limited expansion of the chest, as is often seen in kyphosis.

Diagnostic Tests

Patients with AKS often have the following laboratory test results: (1) low hemoglobin and hematocrit, indicative of anemia; (2) elevated ESR and CRP, which are common in chronic inflammatory disease; (3) elevated serum alkaline phosphatase levels in patients who are immobilized or have bone resorption; and

(4) presence of the HLA-B27 antigen. Radiographic examination often reveals sacroiliac joint and intervertebral disk inflammation with bony erosion and joint space fusion.

Medical Management

The physician usually prescribes oral analgesics and NSAIDs. Etanercept (Enbrel) is a biologic agent that is useful in decreasing symptoms of AKS and improving patient role performance (Lewis et al., 2007). Additional biologic agents, such as infliximab (Remicade) and adalimumab (Humira), may be effective. Exercise programs (swimming and walking) help prevent demineralization of bone.

Surgery may be necessary to replace fused joints (commonly the hip or the knee). Cervical or lumbar osteotomy can be done for severe kyphosis.

Endoscopic microsurgery can be performed on select candidates. In microsurgery, the bone or tissue that is putting pressure on the spinal nerves is removed by using endoscopic equipment placed through small incisions. Most patients leave the hospital within 24 hours and start physical therapy within a few days.

Nursing Interventions and Patient Teaching

Nursing interventions are aimed at maintaining alignment of the spine. Providing a firm mattress, bed board, and back brace helps provide support. Postural and breathing exercises help compensate for the possibility of impaired gas exchange caused by the changes in posture and chest cavity size. Encouraging the patient to lie on the abdomen for at least 15 to 30 minutes four times daily helps extend the spine. Turning and positioning every 2 hours helps prevent pressure sores.

A nursing diagnosis and interventions for the patient with AKS include but are not limited to the following:

Nursing Diagnosis	Nursing Interventions
Chronic low self-esteem, related to body image	Encourage patient to share fears and anxiety about the disease process. Deal with behavior changes: denial, powerlessness, anxiety, and dependence. Be supportive and kind but firm in setting goals. Encourage independence. Be aware of limitations, and encourage discussion of feelings and concerns.

Teach the patient the appropriate use of prescribed medications, postural exercises, and methods of applying heat to back and hips. Promote correct posture and prevent complications by encouraging the patient to use a firm mattress, sleep without a pillow, and do respiratory exercises.

Prognosis

AKS is a chronic disease occurring in persons younger than age 30 that generally burns itself out after a course of 20 years, leaving permanent, irreversible systemic involvement.

OSTEOARTHRITIS (DEGENERATIVE JOINT DISEASE)

Etiology and Pathophysiology

Osteoarthritis is also known as DJD, hypertrophic arthritis, osteoarthrosis, or senescent arthritis. Osteoarthritis is a nonsystemic, noninflammatory disorder that progressively causes bones and joints to degenerate. Almost everyone past 40 years of age has hypertrophic changes in the joints (Box 4-3). The disease is an almost inevitable consequence of aging and is a major cause of severe chronic disability. Osteoarthritis takes two forms: primary (cause is unknown) and secondary (caused by trauma, infections, previous fractures, RA, stress on weight-bearing joints from obesity, or such occupations as coal mining or boxing). A comparison of RA and osteoarthritis is found in Table 4-4.

Clinical Manifestations

This disorder affects the joints of the hand, knee, hip, and cervical and lumbar vertebrae (Figure 4-8). Osteoarthritis appears to be related to aging, but researchers are unclear as to the cause. Nearly all people older

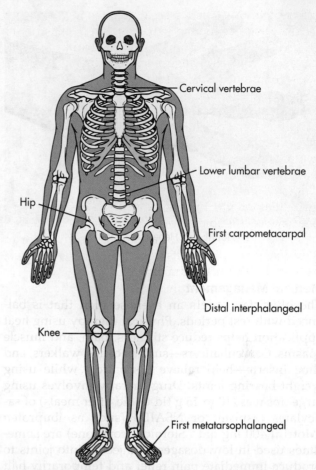

FIGURE 4-8 Joints most frequently involved in osteoarthritis.

than 60 years show osteoarthritic changes, with women being affected more often than men. The disease affects the hands in women more often, whereas in men the hips are affected.

Assessment

Collection of **subjective data** includes questioning the patient about pain and stiffness (rest usually relieves pain in the early stages). Past illnesses, surgical procedures, or trauma may be relevant, and information about excessive weight gain and occupation may be significant. Complaints of muscle spasms and reduced grip strength are common.

Collection of **objective data** includes assessment for joint edema, tenderness, instability, and deformity. **Heberden's nodes** appear on the sides of the distal joints of fingers (Figure 4-9), and **Bouchard's nodes** appear on the proximal joints of fingers; these nodes are hard, bony, and cartilaginous enlargements. The patient's gait reveals a limp, especially if the hips or legs are affected.

Diagnostic Tests

There is no specific test to diagnose osteoarthritis. However, radiographic studies, arthroscopy, synovial fluid examination, and bone scans are used to provide information.

Box 4-3	Osteoarthritis

- Osteoarthritis is the most common form of arthritis and the leading cause of disability in people older than age 65. Under age 55, men and women are affected equally. In older individuals, osteoarthritis of the hip is more common in men and osteoarthritis of the interphalangeal joints and the thumb is more common in women. Osteoarthritis occurs more frequently in people who are obese or who experience repetitive stress to the joints.
- More than 70% of total hip and knee replacements are for osteoarthritis.
- Overweight people have a higher risk of knee and hip osteoarthritis.
- Weight-loss programs for overweight older adults lessen symptoms in those with the disease.
- Acetaminophen is recommended by the American College of Rheumatology for osteoarthritis pain because of fewer gastrointestinal and renal side effects compared with other drugs.
- Bicycling and swimming are considered good exercises for people with osteoarthritis of the knee; walking should be done on level ground.
- People with osteoarthritis of the knee or hip should avoid climbing stairs, bending, stooping, or squatting.

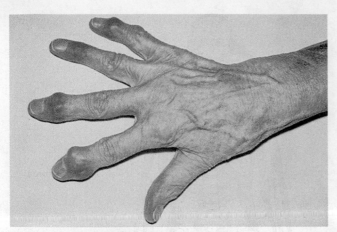

FIGURE 4-9 Heberden's nodes.

Medical Management

The physician orders an exercise plan that is balanced with rest periods. Physical therapy using heat application helps reduce stiffness, pain, and muscle spasms. Gait enhancers—such as canes, walkers, and shoe inserts—help relieve discomfort while using weight-bearing joints. Drug therapy involves using large dosages (10 to 15 g tid to qid after meals) of salicylates (aspirin) or NSAIDs (such as ibuprofen [Motrin] 400 mg qid). Steroids (cortisone) are sometimes used in low dosages or injected into joints to produce immediate pain relief and temporarily halt the destructive process. Patients with hypertension must be screened carefully while taking NSAIDs because certain NSAIDs elevate blood pressure. Patients need to inform their physician so that a safe and effective combination of drugs can be chosen. Indomethacin (Indocin) can decrease the effect of enalapril (Vasotec) (an angiotensin-converting enzyme inhibitor used for hypertension), and the combination of ibuprofen and lisinopril (Prinivil, Zestril) can trigger a hypertensive response. Acetaminophen is commonly used as an analgesic and does not affect the blood pressure. Tramadol hydrochloride (Ultram) is a synthetic analgesic used for moderate to severe pain and can be used for patients taking antihypertensives.

Alternatives to NSAIDs

The discomfort associated with acute or chronic RA, osteoarthritis, gouty arthritis, and AKS may also be decreased through the use of nonpharmacologic measures. Measures such as relaxation techniques, massage therapy, imagery, and therapeutic touch have been proven effective in reducing discomfort and decreasing the need for NSAIDs.

Glucosamine is found in the body as a lubricant and shock absorber necessary for repairing and maintaining healthy joint function. The aging process has been linked to the loss of glucosamine and other substances in the cartilage. Taking supplements to natu-

---

Complementary and Alternative Therapies

Musculoskeletal Disorders

- Alternative therapies being considered in the treatment of osteoarthritis include compounds such as glucosamine and chondroitin. These substances appear to provide pain relief, perhaps even slowing the disease process. Glucosamine apparently stimulates cartilage cells to manufacture proteoglycans, whereas chondroitin inhibits enzymes that break down cartilage. Few adverse effects have been seen with glucosamine used up to 3 years.
- Chiropractic adjustment has been effective in patients with some types of back pain. Many insurance companies allow for this form of therapy.
- Other manual healing methods—therapy that includes touch and manipulation of soft tissues or realignment of body parts to correct a dysfunction that affects other body parts—include the following:
  —Massage and other physical healing methods
  —Acupuncture
  —Reflexology (a system of treating certain disorders by massaging the soles of the feet or the palms of the hands)
  —Rolfing (a technique of deep massage intended to realign the body by altering the length and tone of myofascial tissues)

---

ral glucosamine enables the body to manufacture collagen and proteoglycans and resupply lubricant found in the synovial fluid necessary for restoring healthy cartilage (see Complementary and Alternative Therapies box). Glucosamine supplements have been linked with reductions in articular pain, joint tenderness, and restricted joint movement in people suffering from arthritis. People allergic to shellfish, those with chronic medical problems, or women who are pregnant or lactating should not take supplemental glucosamine without conferring with a health care provider (Lewis et al., 2007).

Surgical intervention, such as osteotomy, may help correct malalignment. Joint replacement may be necessary to replace all or part of the joint's articulating surface. Arthroplasty of the hip and knee is the most common surgical intervention.

Nursing Interventions and Patient Teaching

Nursing interventions include encouraging the patient to maintain ADLs and adapt to limitations of the disease. Alternating sitting, walking, and standing with periods of rest can help reduce joint discomfort and deterioration. Older patients may be physically capable of turning and moving in bed but may forget to do so because of alteration in their level of orientation. Assist the patient with a weight-reduction plan if obesity is a problem. If splints are used to support a painful joint, assess for neurovascular impairment above and below the site of application. Also check gait enhancers for safety considerations, such as rubber tips on ends, proper size, and patient knowledge about use. If the patient has been taking aspirin over a period of time, gastrointestinal (GI) bleeding may occur. It may be necessary to perform a guaiac test on stool and emesis to determine the presence of occult blood.

As with RA, teaching the person with osteoarthritis about the disease process and the steps to control that process is the most important aspect of nursing interventions. Patient teaching should include the same information as for RA.

Prognosis

Osteoarthritis is a chronic disease that ultimately causes permanent destruction of affected cartilage and underlying bone with variable pain and disability.

GOUT (GOUTY ARTHRITIS)

Etiology and Pathophysiology

Gout is a metabolic disease resulting from an accumulation of uric acid in the blood. It is an acute inflammatory condition associated with ineffective metabolism of purines. Gout can be primary (linked with hereditary factors), secondary (resulting from use of certain medications or complication of another disease), or idiopathic (of unknown origin). It affects men approximately eight times more frequently than women and usually occurs in middle life. It does not occur before puberty in the male or before menopause in the female. For primary disease, it takes approximately 20 years for sufficient urates to accumulate in the body before causing signs and symptoms. Of all people with gout, 85% have a genetic tendency to develop the disease. **Tophi** (calculi containing sodium urate deposits that develop in periarticular fibrous tissue, typically in patients with gout) result in inflammation of the joint; it is unclear why this occurs. Typically the big toes are involved, but other joints can also be affected.

Clinical Manifestations

Onset occurs at night, with excruciating pain, edema, and inflammation in the affected joint. The pain may last a short time but return at intervals, or it may be severe and continuous for 5 to 10 days. The patient may have repeated attacks or only one attack in a lifetime. Tophi are seen around the rim of the ear and can disfigure the ear. Surgical removal may be necessary.

Assessment

Collection of **subjective data** includes noting a complaint of pain occurring at night involving the great toe or other joints. Take a dietary history, with specific questions on consumption of alcohol and foods high in purines, such as organ meats (brain, kidney, liver, and heart), anchovies, yeast, herring, mackerel, and scallops.

Collection of **objective data** includes assessment of joints (especially the great toe) for signs of edema, heat, discoloration (may appear erythematous or purple), and limited movement. Vital sign data may reveal an elevated temperature and hypertension, tachycardia, and tachypnea. Carefully assess urinary output because tophi can form in the kidneys and alter kidney function. Assess the patient for tophi (typically seen on the earlobes, fingers, hands, and toes).

Diagnostic Tests

Laboratory tests used to diagnose gout include serum (see Table 4-3) and urinary uric acid levels (elevation is significant), complete blood count (CBC) (leukocytosis and anemia may be present), and elevated ESR. Radiographic studies reveal cysts and toe bone pockets. Synovial fluid contains urate crystals.

Medical Management

Several drugs are used to treat gout. For acute attacks, colchicine is administered orally or intravenously. The oral dosage is 0.5 mg hourly for 12 doses. The drug is discontinued if GI symptoms develop or pain is not relieved. Indomethacin (Indocin SR) is an affective antiinflammatory drug in treating gout. Corticosteroids can be administered orally, intravenously, or intraarticularly and will relieve signs and symptoms within 12 hours. The physician may order allopurinol (Zyloprim) to decrease the production of uric acid; probenecid (Probalan), inhibits renal tubular resorption of uric acid to increase secretion of uric acid by the kidneys; and sulfinpyrazone (Anturane) to prevent the development of tophi in various parts of the body, including the kidneys. Aspirin inactivates the effect of uricosurics (probenecid), resulting in urate retention, and should be avoided while patients are taking uricosuric drugs.

Nursing Interventions and Patient Teaching

Nursing intervention is aimed at giving medications prescribed by the physician for relief of pain and inflammation. When giving colchicine, it is important to observe for side effects, such as diarrhea, nausea, and vomiting. Increasing the patient's fluid intake to at least 2000 mL daily helps eliminate the excess urinary urates. Approximately 10% to 20% of patients with gouty arthritis have uric acid kidney stones. Carefully document intake and output (I&O). Advise the patient to avoid excessive use of alcohol and consumption of foods high in purine. Maintain bed rest and joint immobilization while the patient is symptomatic. Bed cradles prevent pressure from bed linens on the affected joints.

Nursing diagnoses and interventions for the patient with gout include but are not limited to the following:

Nursing Diagnoses	Nursing Interventions
Pain, related to disease process	Maintain patient in a position of comfort with foot supported and in alignment; place bed cradle over foot; no weight bearing.
	Apply cold packs as ordered, keeping pressure off joint.
	Administer analgesics and antigout and antiinflammatory agents as ordered; observe for side effects.
Deficient knowledge, related to lack of information concerning medications and home care management	Provide medication schedule, including name, dosage, purpose, and side effects.
	Discuss importance of diet, exercise, and rest program.
	Encourage follow-up visits with physician.

Patient teaching is aimed at giving information about the disease and stressing the importance of keeping the serum uric acid levels within normal range by taking the prescribed medications; following the prescribed diet; and avoiding infections, lack of sleep, and stress. The patient may need to take colchicine, probenecid, and allopurinol as a maintenance dose even when signs and symptoms are not present.

Prognosis
The signs and symptoms are recurrent; episodes become longer each year. The disorder is disabling and, if untreated, can progress to the development of tophi and destructive joint changes.

OTHER MUSCULOSKELETAL DISORDERS

OSTEOPOROSIS
Etiology and Pathophysiology
Osteoporosis is a disorder that results in reduction in the mass of bone per unit of volume. This reduction is sufficient to interfere with the mechanical support function of the bone. The cause of osteoporosis is not completely known. Women between the ages of 55 and 65 years are identified as a high-risk group for postmenopausal osteoporosis, and many researchers believe that this is related to the loss of the female hormone estrogen. An increase of postmenopausal osteoporosis suggests estrogen deficiency is connected with increased bone resorption and sensitivity to parathyroid hormone (substance that weakens bone by increasing calcium movement from bone into ex-

tracellular fluid). Senile osteoporosis is seen in people between ages 70 and 85 years and affects twice as many women as men. One in two women compared with one in eight men will have osteoporosis-related fractures in their lifetime (Lewis et al., 2007). Genetic and environmental factors, such as small bone structure and lack of exercise, can contribute to the rate of bone loss. Osteoporosis affects the vertebrae, neck of the femur, pelvis, hands, and wrists. Individuals most at risk for developing osteoporosis are small-framed, white (European descent) or Asian race, nonobese, menopausal women who smoke. Other contributing factors are steroids, anticonvulsants or heparin, diets low in calcium throughout life, excessive caffeine intake, alcoholism, and too much protein in the diet (see Cultural Considerations box).

Clinical Manifestations
The disorder develops slowly, beginning with a complaint of backache. As the disease progresses, the bones become porous and brittle due to a lack of calcium.

Assessment
Collection of **subjective data** includes questioning the patient about lifestyle practices and complaints of pain (low thoracic and lumbar) that worsens with sitting, standing, coughing, sneezing, and straining.

Collection of **objective data** includes assessing the patient for dowager's hump (spinal deformity and height loss that result from repeated spinal vertebral fractures) and increased lordosis, scoliosis, and kyphosis (Figure 4-10). Also assess gait impairment associated with inability to maintain erect posture.

Diagnostic Tests
The physician orders a CBC; serum calcium, phosphorus, and alkaline phosphatase; blood urea nitrogen (BUN); creatinine level; urinalysis; and liver and thy-

---

 Cultural Considerations

Osteoporosis

- White and Asian women have a higher incidence of osteoporosis than black women.
- Black women have 10% more bone mass than white women.
- Postmenopausal women are at the highest risk regardless of cultural background or ethnic group.
- Black men have dense bones and a low incidence of osteoporosis.
- Hispanic women have a lower incidence of osteoporosis than white women.

From Lewis, S.L., Heitkemper, M.M., Dirksen, S.R., et al. (2007). *Medical-surgical nursing: Assessment and management of clinical problems* (7th ed.). St. Louis: Mosby.

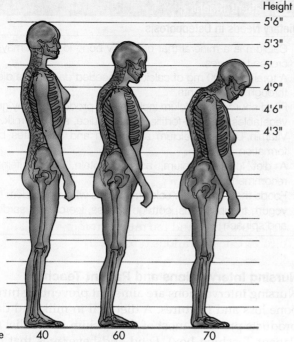

Height
5'6"
5'3"
5'
4'9"
4'6"
4'3"

Age   40   60   70

FIGURE 4-10 A normal spine at age 40 years and osteoporotic changes at ages 60 and 70 years. These changes can cause a loss of as much as 6 inches in height and can result in the so-called dowager's hump *(far right)* in the upper thoracic vertebrae.

roid function tests. A bone mineral density (BMD) measurement is recommended for women around the time of menopause. BMD is performed by a dual energy x-ray absorptiometry (DEXA). The BMD test assesses the mass of bone per unit volume, or how tightly the bone is packed. Usually the hip and the spine are measured. The test takes about 10 minutes and has low

amounts of radiation. The World Health Organization has defined criteria for adult women as follows:

- Normal bones have a BMD within 1 standard deviation of the young adult average.
- Low bone mass (osteopenia) is 1 standard deviation below the young adult average.
- Osteoporosis is 2.5 standard deviations below the young adult average (www.who.int).

Medical Management

The physician orders a treatment regimen aimed at increasing bone density and retarding bone loss. Calcium supplements that bring the total calcium intake per day to 1,000 mg for men and 1,500 mg for postmenopausal women are recommended (as well as vitamin D, 50,000 international units once or twice per week). Weight-bearing exercise programs to improve muscle tone, such as walking, have been effective in preventing further bone loss and stimulating new bone formation. Treatment may include adequate doses of estrogen. Estrogen will not correct the condition but will help to prevent fractures and may be approved for women at significant risk.

Alendronate (Fosamax), etidronate (Didronel), pamidronate (Aredia), tiludronate (Skelid), and ibandronate (Boniva) are bone resorption inhibitors (Table 4-6). These drugs absorb calcium phosphate crystal in bone and are given orally to treat symptoms of osteoporosis. Administer these drugs first thing in the morning with 6 to 8 ounces of water at least 30 minutes before other medications, beverages, or food. Caution patient to remain upright for 30 minutes after a dose to facilitate passage to stomach and minimize risk of esophageal irritation.

Table 4-6 | Medications for Osteoporosis

Generic (Trade)	Action	Side Effects/Toxic Effects	Nursing Implications
Biphosphates: alendronate (Fosamax), risedronate (Actonel), etidronate (Didronel), pamidronate (Aredia), tiludronate (Skelid), ibandronate (Boniva)	Slow bone loss and increase bone density	Difficulty in swallowing, chest pain, severe or recurring heartburn	Administer first thing in the morning with 6-8 oz plain water, 30 minutes before other medications, beverages, or food.
Calcitonin-salmon injection (Miacalcin) or calcitonin-salmon nasal spray (Fortical)	Increases bone mass, particularly in the spine	Injection site reaction, nasal irritation	Monitor for injection site reaction. Advise patient to take medication exactly as directed.
Estrogen receptor modulator: raloxifene (Evista)	Prevents bone loss and spinal fractures	May increase tendency for deep-vein thrombosis, myocardial infarcts, uterine bleeding, and breast abnormalities	Administer without regard to meals.
Parathyroid hormone: teriparatide (Forteo)	Prevents bone loss; promotes bone growth	Increased heart rate or dizziness	Administer subcutaneously into thigh or abdominal wall once daily.

Risedronate (Actonel) is another bone resorption inhibitor. The drug absorbs calcium phosphate crystal in bone and inhibits bone resorption without inhibiting bone formation or mineralization. It is given orally. The patient should sit upright for 30 minutes after a dose to prevent esophageal irritation. Another type of drug used in treating osteoporosis is selective estrogen receptor modulators, such as raloxifene (Evista). These drugs mimic the effect of estrogen on bone by reducing bone resorption.

Teriparatide (Forteo) is a form of parathyroid hormone that is approved for postmenopausal women who are at increased risk for osteoporosis fractures or who cannot use other treatments. The drug prevents sloughing of osteoblasts (bone cells that form new bone) in porous or spongy bones and increases bone mass in the spine and hip. Teriparatide treatment requires a daily subcutaneous injection of the drug and is limited to a 24-month period. The drug must be kept refrigerated. The most common side effects are nausea, dizziness, leg cramps, hypercalcemia, and orthostatic hypotension. The drug is not recommended for patients with an increased risk of osteosarcoma.

Surgical Interventions for Osteoporosis

Women with severe osteoporosis who are unresponsive to an analgesic may be candidates for a surgical procedure to relieve the pain. Vertebroplasty and kyphoplasty are 90% successful in relieving pain from compression fractures of the spine. Vertebroplasty (plastic surgery on a vertebra) involves high-pressure injection of polymethyl methacrylate cement into the spine, which pushes the vertebrae apart. The procedure is done with the patient under a general or local anesthetic. Major complications involve damage to the posterior vertebral walls from the high pressure used to inject the cement and movement of the cement out of vertebral spaces into the spinal canal.

Kyphoplasty (plastic surgery on dowager's hump) involves inserting a balloon into the center of the collapsed vertebrae, which restores the position of the vertebrae and creates a space for injection of polymethyl methacrylate cement. Porous bone is packed around the outside edge. This procedure is less risky than vertebroplasty because the balloon removes the need to use high pressure for the cement placement.

Nursing Considerations

Patients are admitted to the hospital and required to stay up to 23 hours after the procedure. Flat bed rest is ordered for the first 4 hours postoperatively; then patients are allowed to ambulate as able. A small dressing covers the operative site, and antibiotics and steroids are typically ordered for three doses following the procedure.

 Patient Teaching

Dietary Needs in Osteoporosis

- Calcium is a mineral that can slow bone loss and may decrease fractures.
- A total of 1,500 mg of calcium is needed daily in the diet or through supplements.
- Food sources of calcium include milk products, many green vegetables, calcium-fortified orange juice, and soy milk.
- Vitamin D helps calcium absorption and stimulates bone formation.
- A diet low in sodium, animal protein, and caffeine is recommended.
- Foods that are high in calcium include whole and skim milk, yogurt, turnip greens, cottage cheese, ice cream, sardines, and spinach.

Nursing Interventions and Patient Teaching

Nursing interventions are aimed at preventing further bone loss and fractures. A diet rich in milk and dairy products provides most of the calcium in the diet (see Patient Teaching box). Food and beverages that contain caffeine also contain phosphorus, which contributes to bone loss. Teach patients relaxation techniques and encourage them to stop smoking. Patients who take estrogen need information about the higher risk for thromboembolism, endometrial cancer, and possibly breast cancer. Hormone replacement must be prescribed at the lowest dose possible and for a short duration. Safety measures, such as side rails, hand rails, bedside commodes with seat elevators, and rubber mats in showers, can help prevent falls in older adults. Efforts are made to keep patients with osteoporosis ambulatory to prevent further loss of bone substance as a result of immobility. Encourage weight-bearing exercise to increase bone density.

A nursing diagnosis and interventions for the patient with osteoporosis include but are not limited to the following:

Nursing Diagnosis	Nursing Interventions
Deficient knowledge, related to issues of home care	Stress importance of activity and rest; provide aerobic management exercise schedule; caution patient to avoid jogging. Advise patient to take recommended medications. Instruct patient in how to maintain a healthy diet.

To prevent osteoporosis, advise women to have an adequate daily intake of calcium and vitamin D; to avoid smoking; to decrease caffeine intake; to decrease excess protein in the diet; and to engage in moderate activity such as walking, bike riding, or swimming at least 3 days a week.

After menopause, the usual recommended daily allowance is 1,000 mg of calcium in postmenopausal women taking estrogen and 1,500 mg in postmenopausal women who are not taking estrogen. Vitamin D, which increases calcium absorption, may be added to the daily regimen of postmenopausal women according to the physician's orders. Encourage the patient to make follow-up visits to the physician for guidance on medication, diet, and exercise regimen.

Prognosis

Osteoporosis is a chronic disorder, but vitamin D and calcium may help stop the rate of bone loss. In postmenopausal women, therapy with estrogen decreases the rate of bone resorption, but does not increase bone formation. Prevention of osteoporosis should begin before bone loss has occurred.

OSTEOMYELITIS

Etiology and Pathophysiology

Osteomyelitis (local or generalized infection of bone and bone marrow) can occur from bacteria introduced through trauma, such as a compound fracture or surgery. Also, bacteria may travel by the bloodstream from another site in the body to a bone, causing an infection. Staphylococci are the most common causative agents. Other invading organisms include *Streptococcus viridians, Escherichia coli, Mycobacterium tuberculosis, Neisseria gonorrhoeae, Pseudomonas* organisms, salmonellae, and fungi (Crowley, 2004).

Bacteria invade the bone, and bone tissue degenerates. If osteomyelitis becomes chronic, the bone tissue often is weak and predisposed to spontaneous fractures. Osteomyelitis can become chronic as a result of inadequate acute treatment. It is either a continuous persistent problem or a process of exacerbations and remissions. Over time, granulation tissue turns to scar tissue. This avascular scar tissue provides an ideal site for continued microorganism growth and is impenetrable to antibiotics.

Clinical Manifestations

The patient with osteomyelitis is subject to contractures in the affected extremity if positioned incorrectly. A new focus of infection can develop months and sometimes years after the initial infection is diagnosed.

Assessment

Collection of **subjective data** includes a complete history of injuries, surgical procedures, and diseases. Assess the patient's complaints of persistent, severe, and increasing bone pain and tenderness, as well as regional muscle spasm. Also inquire about any allergies, especially to medications, because antibiotics are given long term.

Collection of **objective data** includes careful inspection of any wounds. Assess the drainage for color, amount, and odor. Monitor vital signs for signs of infection (temperature elevation, tachycardia, and tachypnea). Note any edema, especially in joints with limited mobility.

Diagnostic Tests

Take a complete history, along with a physical examination. The physician orders radiographic studies and bone scan, CBC (leukocytosis may be present), ESR, and cultures of blood and drainage (if present).

Medical Management

Vigorous and prolonged intravenous antibiotic therapy will be used. Numerous antibiotics may be used depending on the pathogen. These antibiotics may include penicillin, nafcillin (Nafcil), neomycin, cephalexin (Keflex), cefoxitin (Mefoxin), and gentamicin (Garamycin) (Lewis et al., 2007). Parenteral antibiotics are usually necessary for several weeks but may be as long as 3 to 6 months. Bed rest is usually prescribed. For some patients, surgery may be performed to remove a fragment of necrotic bone that is partially or entirely detached from the surrounding or adjacent healthy bone (sequestrum).

Nursing Interventions and Patient Teaching

Nursing interventions include gentleness in moving and manipulating the diseased extremity, since pain is severe in the early phase of infection. The affected part may need absolute rest, with careful positioning using pillows and sandbags for good alignment. Often wounds are irrigated with hydrogen peroxide or other antiseptic or antibiotic solution and then covered with a sterile dressing, using strict surgical asepsis. Patients are placed on drainage and secretion precautions. Dietary planning includes a diet high in calories, protein, and vitamins.

Teaching includes information about the signs of infection, such as elevated temperature. Because chronic osteomyelitis may last a lifetime, warn the patient of the recurrence of signs and symptoms. Patients must avoid trauma to the affected bone because pathologic fractures are common.

Prognosis

Acute osteomyelitis may respond to treatment after several weeks. Chronic osteomyelitis may persist for years with exacerbations and remissions.

FIBROMYALGIA SYNDROME

Etiology and Pathophysiology

Fibromyalgia is a chronic syndrome of unknown etiology that causes pain in the muscles, bones, or joints. It is associated with soft tissue tenderness at multiple characteristic sites. It contributes to poor sleep, headaches, altered thought processes, and stiffness or muscle aches. Fibromyalgia affects more women than men, with up to 5% of the population affected. The disorder is more common in people between ages 20 and 50. Fibromyalgia has been referred to as **fibrositis, fibro-**

myositis, myofascial pain syndrome, and **psychogenic rheumatism.** Clinical symptoms of fibromyalgia syndrome (FMS) can overlap those of chronic fatigue syndrome (Hellmann, 2007). It is not considered life threatening and does not cause permanent damage. Stress response appears hyperactive in FMS patients (Lewis et al., 2007).

Clinical Manifestations
Patients with FMS frequently complain of a generalized achiness in axial locations, such as the neck and lower back, accompanied by stiffness that is worse in the morning. Factors that aggravate the condition include cold or humid weather, physical or mental fatigue, excess physical activity, and anxiety or stress.

Patients with FMS also experience irritable bowel syndrome, tension headaches beginning with neck discomfort, **paresthesia** (sensation of numbness or tingling) of the upper extremities with normal nerve conduction studies, and the sensation of edematous hands with no visible signs of edema. Complaints of fatigue are often associated with dysfunctional sleep. Patients complain of nonrestorative or nonrefreshing sleep.

Assessment
Collection of **subjective data** includes questioning the patient about muscle pain, often described as muscle ache; tension or migraine headaches; premenstrual tension; jaw pain; excessive fatigue; anxiety; and depression. Include questions about sensations of numbness, tingling, and perception of insects crawling on or under the skin. Complaints of being forgetful and unable to recall recent information—such as appointments, location of parked car, or how to get to familiar places—are significant.

Collection of **objective data** includes noting periodic limb movement, especially at night, or a persistent need to move the lower extremities day and night.

Ask about sleep deprivation and the patient's ability to complete self-care activities.

Diagnostic Tests
No specific laboratory and radiographic tests diagnose FMS. Blood chemistry screening, a CBC, and ESR are normal in patients with FMS. A sleep study may be ordered in patients with a history suggestive of particular types of sleep disturbances; however, sleep study findings are typically normal in FMS patients.

Medical Management
The primary treatment approach includes patient education and reassurance. Inform the FMS patient that this is not a psychiatric disturbance and that symptoms are not uncommon in the general population. Although FMS has no single treatment, combining pharmacologic agents has been helpful. Tricyclic antidepressants are used in the treatment of uncontrollable pain disorders. Benefits of these agents include (1) antidepressant results, (2) antiinflammatory features, (3) central skeletal muscle relaxation, and (4) pain inhibition through suppression of serotonergic and noradrenergic pathways (Table 4-7).

Nursing Interventions and Patient Teaching
Nursing interventions are individualized, holistic, and goal oriented. Management of FMS focuses on functional goals that enable the patient to live as normal a life as possible. Treatment programs include education, exercise, and relaxation techniques. Patients are taught the basic principles of good sleep hygiene (see Patient Teaching box). Exercise programs consist of gentle, progressive stretching, beginning with a muscle warm-up through either gentle exercise or warm baths. Stretching helps release tight muscles. Nonimpact exercise such as swimming, walking, or stationary cycling is helpful.

Table 4-7	Medications for Fibromyalgia Syndrome
Medication	**Action**
Amitriptyline (Elavil, Endep)	Diminishes local pain and stiffness; improves sleep pattern
Cyclobenzaprine (Flexeril)	Diminishes local pain, improves sleep pattern, and decreases number of tender points
Clonazepam (Klonopin)	Decreases symptoms of constant leg movement, especially at night
Acetaminophen and tramadol	Used together or given alone for management of moderate to severe pain. Binds opioid receptors, inhibits reuptake of norepinephrine and serotonin.
Pregabalin (Lyrica)	An anticonvulsant that decreases pain severity and improves fatigue, sleep, and physical functioning
Tizanidine (Zanaflex)	Eases pain by lowering the substance (P) that participates in the transmission process of certain neurons; improves sleep and physical functioning
Sodium oxybate (Xyrem)	Improves deep sleep and growth hormone levels and helps reduce pain and fatigue
Duloxetine hydrochloride (Cymbalta)	Reduces pain in patients with fibromyalgia with or without having symptoms of major depression

Prognosis

Prognosis is generally excellent.

SURGICAL INTERVENTIONS FOR TOTAL KNEE OR TOTAL HIP REPLACEMENT

Surgical procedures can prevent progressive deformities; relieve pain; improve function; and correct deformities resulting from RA, osteoarthritis, or other disorders. Tendon transplants can replace damaged muscles. Patients with RA may need a synovectomy (excision of synovial membrane) to maintain joint function. An osteotomy (cutting into bone to correct bone or joint deformities) can improve function and relieve pain. **Arthrodesis** (surgical fusion of a joint) can be performed when severe joint destruction has occurred. Total joint replacement **arthroplasty** (repair or refashioning of one or both sides, parts, or specific tissue within a joint) is often required on the elbow, hip, knee, or shoulder joint to restore or increase mobility.

KNEE ARTHROPLASTY (TOTAL KNEE REPLACEMENT)

The knee joint may be replaced to restore motion, relieve pain, or correct deformity. Figures 4-11 and 4-12 show the tibial and femoral components of a knee

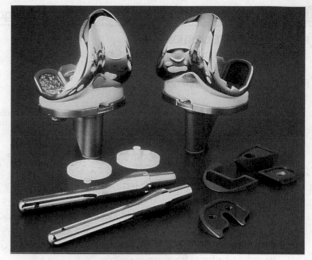

FIGURE 4-12 Total joint replacements: knee.

prosthesis. Nursing interventions for the patient undergoing total knee replacement are shown in Box 4-4 (Figure 4-13).

UNICOMPARTMENTAL KNEE ARTHROPLASTY

Unicompartmental knee replacement is also referred to as partial knee replacement. This modified surgical procedure is performed when only one of the compartments of the knee is affected by arthritic changes. If both sides of the bones in the knee, including the underside of the patella, are damaged, a total knee replacement is necessary (see Figure 4-12).

The knee has three compartments: (1) media, or inside, compartment; (2) lateral, or outside, compartment; and (3) patellofemoral compartment, which is where the kneecap rests. Minimally invasive knee surgery removes only the most damaged areas of cartilage; a small plastic disk replaces the worn cartilage, providing a new cushion between the bones.

The surgery is recommended for select patients ages 50 and older. Patients with RA or lupus erythematosus arthritis are not candidates for the surgery. The long-term benefits of the surgery will last from 5 to 15 years, compared with 20 to 30 years for a total knee procedure. Patients undergoing a unicompartmental knee replacement may eventually need a total knee replacement; at that point, the total knee replacement may be more difficult.

The partial knee surgery involves making a small incision over the knee and exposing the worn-out cartilage. The rough edges of the distal area of the femur and superior area of the tibia are cut flat and cleaned, and the unicompartmental device is put into place. Some of the devices are cemented in place.

Because the kneecap is not disrupted, the patient can resume walking 3 to 4 hours after the operation. There is minimal blood loss and reduced risk of deep-vein thrombosis. The surgery is performed in the hospital with the patient under a spinal block or

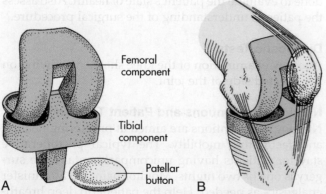

FIGURE 4-11 A, Tibial and femoral components of total knee prosthesis. Patellar button, made of polyethylene, protects the posterior surface of the patella from friction against the femoral component when the knee is moved through flexion and extension. **B,** Total knee prosthesis in place.

Box 4-4 | Nursing Interventions for the Patient Undergoing Total Knee Replacement

PREOPERATIVE INTERVENTIONS
Same as for any major surgery (see Chapter 2).

POSTOPERATIVE INTERVENTIONS
1. Positioning
   a. Elevate the operative leg on pillows to enhance venous return for the first 24 hours only. Place pillows with caution to avoid flexing the knee.
   b. The patient may be turned from side to back to side.
2. Wound care
   a. Care of drains (usually Hemovac) as for total hip replacement
   b. Assess patient for systemic evidence of loss of blood (hypotension, tachycardia) if bulky compression dressing is used because it may hold large quantities of drainage before drainage is visible.
   c. Remove bulky dressings before the patient begins continuous passive motion (CPM) flexion greater than 20 degrees.
3. Activity
   a. Passive flexion in a CPM machine within prescribed flexion-extension limits may be started in the postanesthesia care unit (see Figure 4-13). Patient's leg should remain in machine as much as tolerated (up to 22 hours per day) to facilitate even healing of tissue. The physical therapist increases extension on CPM as patient tolerates. (Once the large bulky dressing is replaced with a smaller dressing, flexion degree is in-

creased.) When CPM is not occurring, patient's leg is extended with no pillow under leg.
   b. Encourage patient to perform active dorsiflexion of the ankles; quadriceps setting; and, after the drain is removed, straight leg–raising exercises.
   c. Patient begins active flexion exercises three or four times a day about the fifth postoperative day.
   d. Light weight bearing with an assistive device may be started as early as the first postoperative day and increased as the patient tolerates.
   e. Sitting in a chair with the leg elevated may be started on the first postoperative day.
   f. Encourage patient to wear a resting knee extension splint (immobilizer) on the operated leg until able to demonstrate quadriceps control (independent straight leg raising).
4. Pain control
   a. For initial control of pain, use opioids (usually with a patient-controlled epidural or patient-controlled analgesia) and positioning; gradually decrease medication to nonopioid analgesics as patient tolerates.
   b. Encourage patient to use cool applications at 40° F continuously on knee.
5. Discharge instructions
   a. Patient must observe partial weight-bearing restriction and use ambulatory aid for approximately 2 months after discharge.
   b. Patient should continue active flexion and straight leg–raising exercises at home.

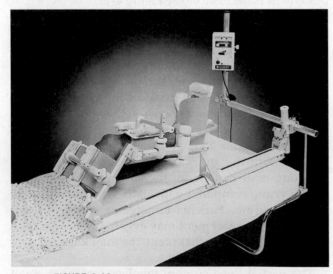

FIGURE 4-13 Continuous passive motion machine.

general anesthetic and takes approximately 60 to 90 minutes.

Assessment
Subjective data include a medical history of home medications, allergies, past surgeries, and significant medical problems such as RA or lupus erythematosus arthritis. Patients with these conditions are not candi-

dates for the surgery. Assess the patient for complaints of pain on one side of the knee with weight bearing. Also gather information on the effectiveness of conservative treatments such as medications, cortisone injections, strengthening exercises, weight loss, and use of gait enhancers.

Objective data include vital signs and weight. Patients who are obese or have significant inflammation are not candidates for the surgery. Blood tests, electrocardiogram (ECG), and chest x-ray examination are done to evaluate the patient's state of health. Also assess the patient's understanding of the surgical procedure.

Diagnostic Tests
An x-ray examination of the knee shows narrowing on the affected side of the joint.

Nursing Interventions and Patient Teaching
Nursing interventions are aimed at promoting healing and facilitating mobility. The typical postoperative stay for patients having unicompartmental knee surgery is one or two nights. Monitor pain and administer analgesics as needed. Help the patient do deep breathing and coughing every 2 hours. Also encourage use of an incentive spirometer. Begin clear liquids and advance to regular diet as tolerated. Monitor IV fluids and antibiotics. Change the dressing as needed.

Patients resume weight bearing 3 to 5 hours postoperatively. Assess their ability to use a gait enhancer such as crutches. The first day after surgery the physical therapist begins teaching basic postoperative exercises. Before discharge, the patient must practice going up and down stairs. Also instruct the patient that prophylactic antibiotics are recommended before routine dental cleaning or any dental procedure up to 2 years following the surgery.

HIP ARTHROPLASTY (TOTAL HIP REPLACEMENT)

Hip arthroplasty, or total hip replacement, is commonly performed when arthritis involves the head of the femur and acetabulum. A Vitallium cup is cemented into the arthritic acetabulum to receive the head of the femur. Total hip replacement was originally developed by John Charnley, a British orthopedic surgeon. Several variations are now practiced, but each uses similar equipment. The Bechtol total hip system involves a white plastic cup cemented in place to replace the damaged acetabulum. A stainless steel or Vitallium ball on a stem replaces the head of the femur, which is surgically removed. The stem is cemented into the femoral canal, and the new head fits precisely into the plastic acetabulum, providing friction-free movement in the joint. The cement used is a soft, surgical bone cement that hardens quickly and stabilizes the prosthesis to prevent erosion of surrounding bone (Figure 4-14).

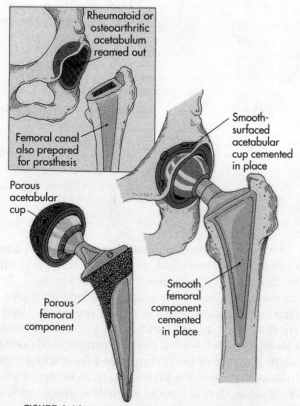

FIGURE 4-14 Hip arthroplasty (total hip replacement).

Assessment

Collection of **subjective data** includes assessing the patient's level of orientation because older adults can become disoriented from a change in the environment (home to hospital setting). Complaints of pain and numbness, tingling, or paresthesia indicate neurovascular impairment.

Collection of **objective data** includes assessment of the patient's compliance with nursing interventions to promote circulation; prevent impairment of skin integrity; and prevent hypostatic pneumonia by such means as coughing, turning (to the unaffected side; additional pillows are used to keep the affected leg abducted), deep breathing every 2 hours, and using an incentive spirometer. Assess vital signs for evidence of excessive bleeding, including hypotension, tachycardia, and tachypnea. Decreased urinary output is indicative of hypovolemia. Carefully assess drainage of the surgical wound at least every 4 hours. Hemovacs or other suction devices are placed in the wound during surgery to provide closed-wound suction. Assess approximation of the incision line and signs of inflammation (erythema, edema, fever, and pain). Also assess traction (if used) for the correct amount of weight, the proper alignment, and maintenance of the affected leg in an abducted position. Look for any reaction to the cement, signs of phlebitis (edema, erythema, and pain), and urinary retention (indwelling catheters may be used for the first 24 to 48 hours).

Nursing Interventions and Patient Teaching

Nursing interventions are aimed at promoting healing and facilitating mobility. Teach the patient to do isometric exercises on the quadriceps and gluteal muscles of the affected extremity by keeping the toes pointed up, flexing the ankles, and flexing and extending the knee of the unaffected extremity. Carefully document the patient's I&O. Apply thigh-high antiembolism stockings before or during surgery. The physician will order a plan of weight bearing and physical therapy; help explain this to the patient.

Additional nursing activities include emptying and recording Hemovac drainage every 4 hours (if ordered) or as needed. Give oxygen at 1 to 2 L per nasal cannula as needed. Instruct the patient in the use of the incentive spirometer every 2 to 4 hours, and help the patient do deep breathing and coughing every 2 hours.

Perform neurovascular checks every hour for 24 hours, then every 2 hours for the next 24 hours, and then every 4 hours. Check vital signs every 4 hours. Also carefully assess the patient for pain control. This includes monitoring patient-controlled epidural (PCE), patient-controlled analgesia (PCA), or oral medications, whichever is prescribed.

Change the dressing using surgical asepsis after 24 to 48 hours as ordered; reinforce the dressing if necessary. Maintain the position of the operative area with a splint, an abduction pillow (Figure 4-15), an immobilizer, or a brace; turn the patient to the unoperated side.

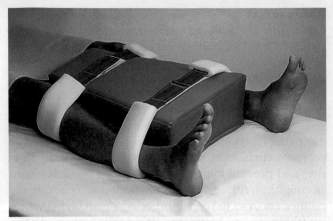

FIGURE 4-15 Maintaining postoperative abduction after total hip replacement.

Begin clear liquids, and advance to regular diet as tolerated. Encourage fluid intake and high-fiber foods (if tolerated) to prevent constipation; administer rectal suppository if needed to empty rectum.

Maintain bed rest for 24 to 48 hours (depending on the security of the replacement prostheses and physician's choice). The patient should be up but not bearing weight on the operative limb after the bed rest order expires. Some physicians may permit touch-down weight bearing. Physical therapy exercises begin on the second postoperative day. The exercises are either active or passive to all joints, excluding the operated joint, and include quadriceps setting, straight leg raising, flexion and extension, or other individually prescribed exercises. The patient should be up with walker or crutches four times daily; increase ambulation as the patient is able with up to 25 pounds of weight bearing on the operative limb, gradually increasing to full weight bearing with crutches or a walker.

Have the patient sit in a chair for only 10 to 15 minutes two or three times daily for the first week, then for 20 to 30 minutes four times daily. The patient should wear antiembolism hose or a pneumatic stocking pump system. Use of a toilet-seat riser prevents hyperflexion of the hip after total replacement.

Nursing diagnoses and interventions for the patient with a total hip replacement include but are not limited to the following:

Nursing Diagnoses	Nursing Interventions
Pain, related to: • preoperative arthritic pain necessitating surgery • postoperative hip incisional pain secondary to bone • soft tissue trauma of surgery	Explain analgesic therapy, including medication, dose, and schedule. If patient is a candidate for PCA or PCE, explain the concept and routine.
	Respond quickly to pain complaints. Obtain pain rating scale from patient. Instruct patient to request analgesic before pain is severe. Administer analgesics as ordered and per hospital policy or procedure.
	Encourage use of analgesics 30 to 45 minutes before therapy. Unrelieved pain hinders rehabilitation progress.
	Provide eggcrate mattress. Change position (within hip precautions) every 2 hours.
	Document all responses to analgesics.
Impaired physical mobility, related to surgical procedure and discomfort	Allow patient to dangle feet at bedside several minutes before getting out of bed.
	Reinforce physical therapist's instructions for exercises and ambulation techniques and devices. Maintain weight-bearing status on affected extremity as prescribed. Consistent instructions from interdisciplinary team members promote safe, secure rehabilitation environment.
	Keep abduction pillow between legs while turning in bed (see Figure 4-15).
	Do not have the patient lie on the operative side. Maintain the leg in abduction when the patient is lying supine or on the nonoperative side.
	Use trapeze in bed to assist in mobility.

Discharge instructions include teaching the patient to use an ambulatory aid, avoid adduction, and limit hip flexion to 90 degrees for approximately 2 to 3 months. A raised toilet seat is obtained and used at home until flexion restrictions are removed. The patient may need a long-handled shoehorn and reacher to facilitate ADLs within flexion restriction. Be certain patient is aware of the lifelong need for antibiotic prophylaxis to protect the prosthesis from bacterial infection during dental work, intrusive procedures, or surgery.

FRACTURES

FRACTURE OF THE HIP

Etiology and Pathophysiology

Hip fractures are the most common type of fracture treated in the hospital (see Life Span Considerations box and Health Promotion box). Women may be at a higher risk because of their increased risk for osteoporosis and longer life expectancy compared with men. Fractures of the hip include intracapsular fracture, when the femur is broken inside the joint, and fractures of the femoral head or neck that are contained within the hip capsule (Figure 4-16, *A* to *C*). Intracapsular fractures may disrupt the blood supply to the head of the femur, which subsequently develops avascular necrosis (Figures 4-17 and 4-18). Therefore fractures of the head or proximal femoral neck may be treated with insertion of a femoral prosthesis (Figure 4-19). The more common type of hip fracture is an extracapsular fracture, one that occurs outside the hip joint capsule. These are referred to as intertrochanteric or subtrochanteric fractures (Figure 4-16, *D*). These fractures heal well without vascular necrosis with the use of compression screws or nails because the blood supply to the fracture site comes from the surrounding vessels outside the capsule (see Figures 4-17 and 4-18).

Life Span Considerations

Older Adults

Musculoskeletal Disorder

- Physiologic changes of aging result in decreased joint flexibility and muscular strength.
- Changes in bone mass, particularly in older women, increase the risk of fractures. Hip fractures and compression fractures of the spine are most common.
- Degenerative joint disease related to "wear and tear" on joints is common. Joint replacement is increasingly common and has done much to improve mobility and the quality of life.
- Changes in the foot can occur from a lifetime of use, poorly fitted shoes, or heredity. Bunions and hammertoe are commonly seen in older adults. These may cause pain and lead to decreased mobility. Encourage older adults to wear properly fitted shoes to reduce discomfort. If discomfort is severe, surgical correction may be necessary.
- Check the homes of older adults for safety hazards such as rugs that could cause falls.
- Older adults should avoid climbing unsteady or uneven surfaces because coordination and balance change with age and falls may result.
- Instruct older adults in the correct use of assistive devices such as canes or walkers. Encourage them to use these regularly to prevent injury.

Health Promotion

Hip Fracture

- Factors that contribute to the incidence of hip fracture in older adults include a propensity to fall, inability to correct a postural imbalance, inadequacy of local tissue shock absorbers (e.g., fat, muscle bulk), and underlying skeletal weakness.
- Factors that increase the risk of older adults falling include gait and balance problems, decreased vision and hearing, diminished reflexes, orthostatic hypotension, and medication use.
- Leading hazards that increase the risk of falls are loose rugs and slippery or uneven surfaces.
- Many falls are associated with getting in or out of a chair or bed.
- Falls to the side, the most common type in the frail elderly, are more likely to result in a hip fracture than forward falls.

- Two important factors influencing the amount of force imposed on the hip are the presence of energy-absorbing soft tissue over the greater trochanter and the state of leg muscle contraction at the time of the fall.
- Many older adults have poor muscle tone, an important factor in the severity of a fall.
- Older women often have osteoporosis and accompanying low bone density, which increases the risk of hip fracture.
- Targeted interventions to reduce hip fractures in older adults include a variety of strategies. Calcium and vitamin D supplementation, estrogen replacement, and drug therapy have been shown to decrease bone loss or increase bone density and decrease the likelihood of fracture. Be vigilant in planning interventions for the older adult that are known to reduce the incidence of hip fracture.

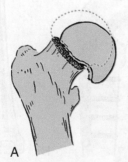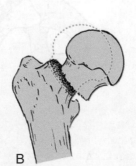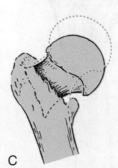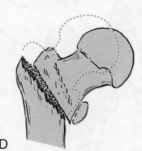

FIGURE 4-16 Fractures of the hip. **A,** Subcapital fracture. **B,** Transcervical fracture. **C,** Impacted fracture of the base of the neck. **D,** Intertrochanteric fracture.

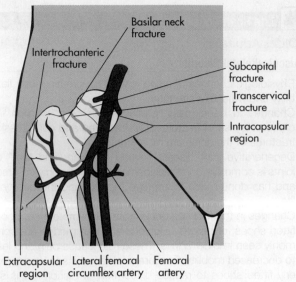

FIGURE 4-17 Femur with location of various types of fractures.

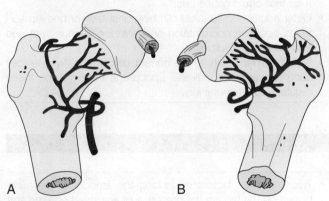

FIGURE 4-18 **A,** Anterior arterial blood supply to hip joint. **B,** Posterior arterial blood supply to hip joint.

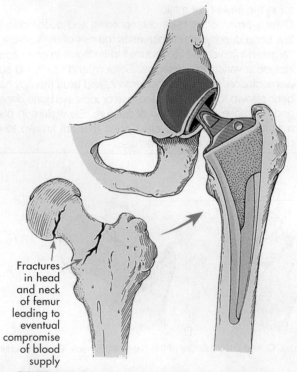

FIGURE 4-19 Bipolar hip replacement (hemiarthroplasty).

Side plates attached to the nails help maintain a stable reduction while healing progresses (Figure 4-20, *A*). An intertrochanteric fracture occurs below the lesser trochanter and is frequently seen in younger patients suffering from hip trauma (see Figure 4-16, *D*).

Clinical Manifestations

Signs and symptoms of hip fracture are severe pain and tenderness in the region of the fracture site or inability to move the leg voluntarily, and shortening or external rotation of the leg.

Assessment

Subjective data include an accurate history of the events before the injury. Assess the patient's level of orientation. Disorientation can occur, especially in older adults when they are in pain, are anxious, or are in an unfamiliar environment. The patient's medical and surgical history is significant, as is any family history of bone disease. Patients with gastroesophageal reflux disease who are taking antacids or using proton pump inhibitors are at increased risk of hip fractures, since these drugs cause a malabsorption of calcium.

Signs and symptoms of a fracture vary with the type and location of the break. Usually the patient has some degree of discomfort that may be more pronounced with slight movement of the affected part. Most patients complain of pain in the affected leg after sustaining a fractured hip, although patients suffering from an impacted intracapsular fracture have little pain, if any, immediately after the fracture. Assess for edema, tenderness, muscle spasms, deformity, and loss of function. Patients may say they heard a "snap" or "pop" at the time the bone was injured. Impaired sensation may indicate nerve damage from the bone fragments "pinching" or severing the nerve.

Collection of **objective data** includes assessment for soft tissue injury with erythema or ecchymosis noted.

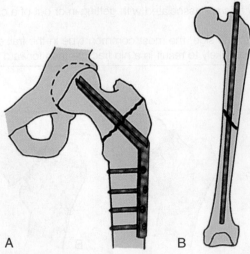

FIGURE 4-20 **A,** Neufeld nail and screws in repair of intertrochanteric fracture. **B,** Küntscher nail (intramedullary rod) used in repair of midshaft femoral fracture.

Look for differences between the injured limb and the uninjured limb. A change in the curvature or length of bone may indicate fracture. The affected leg is shorter, usually externally rotated approximately 90 degrees, and slightly flexed after an extracapsular hip fracture. With an intracapsular fracture, the upper thigh is more edematous than the area below it, and the affected leg is shortened with external rotation. Subtrochanteric fractures cause excessive bleeding into the soft tissue, and the affected leg is shortened and rotated anteriorly. Crepitus may be felt or heard as the broken bone ends rub together. Assess neurovascular status of the extremity (Box 4-5).

Keep the injured part still because movement of a fractured bone can cause additional damage and may turn a closed fracture into an open fracture. Also assess the patient's nutritional status. Both thin and obese patients are at risk for impaired skin integrity if bed rest is ordered. After the fracture is reduced, regularly inspect skin areas in contact with cast edges or traction apparatus for signs of neurovascular compromise. Also note that patients suffering from any trauma are at risk for shock. Treating the shock takes precedence over treating the fracture.

Box 4-5	Circulation Check (Neurovascular Assessment)

- Circulation check is also known as a neurovascular assessment. The mnemonic CMS indicates the need to check circulation, motion, and sensation. The assessment is made on patients following musculoskeletal trauma; postoperatively if damage to nerves and blood vessels is suspected; and after casting, splinting, or bandaging.
- Assess the patient every 15 to 30 minutes for several hours and every 3 to 4 hours thereafter, with proper documentation of the findings.
- **Subjective data** include complaints of numbness or tingling not relieved by flexing the fingers and toes and repositioning the extremity. **Objective data** include cool, pale, or cyanotic skin above or below the altered site; edema; greater than 2 seconds capillary refill time; and absent or diminished pulses.
- Remember the seven Ps when completing the assessment:
  1. Pulselessness
  2. Paresthesia (numbness or tingling sensation)
  3. Paralysis or paresis
  4. Polar temperature
  5. Pallor
  6. Puffiness (edema)
  7. Pain
- Complaints of numbness or tingling may result from general decreased mobility and may be relieved by flexing the fingers and toes and repositioning the extremity. However, if the numbness and tingling are not relieved by these measures and the extremity feels cool to the touch, is slow in capillary refill, has diminished or absent pulses, and appears pale or cyanotic, these are significant symptoms of neurovascular impairment and the findings must be reported immediately.

Diagnostic Tests

Diagnosis is confirmed by radiographic examination of the injured part. Blood tests, such as hemoglobin values, often show decreased laboratory values because of bleeding at the fracture site; the blood glucose level may be elevated because of the stress of the trauma.

Medical Management

Surgical repair is the preferred method of managing intracapsular and extracapsular hip fractures. Surgical treatment enables the patient to get out of bed sooner and decreases the major complications associated with immobility.

The affected extremity may be temporarily immobilized by either Buck's or Russell's traction until the patient's physical condition is stabilized and surgery can be scheduled. The choice of fixation device depends on the fracture location and the potential for avascular necrosis of the femoral head and neck. The use of these devices is called internal fixation. Prosthetic implants, such as the **bipolar hip replacement (hemiarthroplasty)** (see Figure 4-19), are used to replace the femoral head and neck in fractures when the vascular supply to the femoral head may be compromised. A Neufeld nail and screws are used in the repair of intertrochanteric fractures (see Figure 4-20, *A*). A Küntscher nail (intramedullary rod) is used to repair midshaft femoral fractures (see Figure 4-20, *B*). Sliding nails are used in repair of intertrochanteric fractures. Sliding nails usually permit the patient to bear weight to some degree because they "give" slightly without shifting their placement or penetrating the femur. Bone grafts, either autograft (patient's bone) or allograft (cadaver bone), may be used with internal fixation devices when excessive bone is lost at the fracture site. If a stable reduction cannot be achieved, the physician may do an arthroplasty (surgical reconstruction of a joint). Immobilization devices, such as casts or splints, may also be used with open reduction.

Nursing Interventions and Patient Teaching

Nursing interventions for a fractured hip are concerned with preventing shock and further complications. A primary concern is maintaining proper alignment through traction and abduction of the hip when turning a patient with a fractured hip from side to side. Some physicians do not want patients turned onto their sides for several days after surgery; others may order the patient to be turned only on the unoperated side. It is important to know the orders and to educate patients about activity restrictions. Patients who have had internal fixation for a fractured hip should avoid elevating the affected extremity when sitting. Elevate the head of the bed a maximum of 45 degrees to avoid acute flexion of the hip and strain on the fixation device. Instruct the patient *not* to cross the legs because this can adduct the affected extremity and dislocate the hip. Limit weight bearing on the hip by providing walking assists such as a walker or crutches.

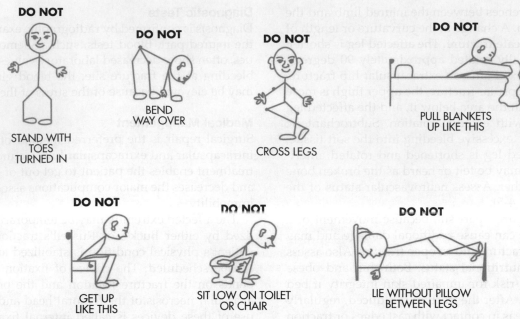

DO NOT

STAND WITH
TOES
TURNED IN

DO NOT

BEND
WAY OVER

DO NOT

CROSS LEGS

DO NOT

PULL BLANKETS
UP LIKE THIS

DO NOT

GET UP
LIKE THIS

DO NOT

SIT LOW ON TOILET
OR CHAIR

DO NOT

LIE WITHOUT PILLOW
BETWEEN LEGS

FIGURE 4-21 Instruction sheet for the patient with a bipolar hip replacement (hip prosthetic implant).

Postoperative interventions for a patient with hip fracture repair include wound assessment with special attention to color, amount, and odor of exudate. Assess vital signs, as well as the suture line for approximation of skin edges and intact sutures or staples, at least every 8 hours. Jackson-Pratt drainage tubes or Hemovacs are often used and must be assessed for amount and color of wound drainage at least every 4 hours. Document I&O to help the physician establish the need for IV fluid therapy. Encourage the use of incentive spirometers to aid in adequate respiratory ventilation and prevent pneumonia. Turning and moving the patient on schedule will maintain skin integrity and promote circulation.

Leg manipulation during surgery and immobility afterward place the patient at risk for deep-vein thrombosis and pulmonary embolism. Antiembolism stockings, Ace wraps, or pneumatic compression stockings and foot and leg exercises increase venous flow to the heart. Remove the stockings once each shift to assess for compression points and skin integrity. Anticoagulation therapy with enoxaparin (Lovenox), aspirin, or warfarin (Coumadin) is often prescribed.

Special postoperative instructions regarding proper positioning, sitting, and turning are required for patients who have had a prosthetic implant or bipolar hip replacement (Figure 4-21 and Patient Teaching box on postoperative care of the patient who had a fractured hip). Isometric exercises are done on the quadriceps and gluteal muscles to strengthen the muscles used for walking (see Patient Teaching box on quadriceps setting exercises).

Nursing interventions also involve use of an abduction splint (a wedge-shaped foam bolster or pillow) for 7 to 10 days to ensure postoperative maintenance of leg abduction and to prevent dislocation of the pros-

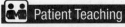

Patient Teaching

Quadriceps Setting Exercises

Quadriceps and gluteal muscles must be strong for ambulation. The quadriceps muscles stabilize the knee joint. Teach the patient to do the following exercises 10 to 15 times hourly:

- To strengthen quadriceps muscles, push the knee down against the mattress while raising the heel of the foot off the bed; maintain the contraction for a count of five and relax for a count of five.
- For gluteal setting exercises, contract, or "pinch," the buttocks together for a count of five, then relax for a count of five.
- Strengthen the unaffected leg by pushing down against the footboard, holding for a count of five, releasing for a count of five, and repeating.

thesis. Place the abduction splint between the patient's legs when in a supine position. Turn the patient with the extremities maintained in proper alignment by using the log-rolling procedure with the assistance of at least two nurses. Most physicians order the patient to be turned toward the unoperated side; check each order by the physician. Transfer the patient from bed to chair on the unoperated side by pivoting on the unaffected leg. The injured leg is kept extended forward to avoid extreme hip flexion and possible dislocation of the prosthesis. Provide a chair with a firm, nonreclining seat and arms; elevate the sitting surfaces as necessary with pillows or foam cushions to keep the angle of the hip within the prescribed limits when the patient is sitting. In general, patients who have had *any* kind of internal fixation for a fractured hip should avoid elevation of the operated leg when sitting in a chair, since this puts excessive strain on the fixation device (Nursing Care Plan 4-1).

Nursing Care Plan **4-1**   **The Patient with a Fractured Hip**

Ms. Drake, age 72, fell in her kitchen while removing cookies from the oven. She sustained a subcapital fracture of the right hip. Ms. D. is scheduled in the morning for a bipolar (hemiarthroplasty) prosthesis.

NURSING DIAGNOSIS *Ineffective tissue perfusion, related to vascular injury or interruption of arterial and venous flow secondary to edema*

Patient Goals and Expected Outcomes	Nursing Interventions	Evaluation and Rationale
Patient's circulation will be maintained to fulfill body requirements	Palpate site for warmth. Observe site for color. Apply moderate pressure to nailbed, and subsequently observe speed of capillary refill. Assess pedal pulse bilaterally every 4 hours. Question patient regarding pain and paresthesia in injured part. Apply antiembolism stockings as ordered.	Distal pulses palpable; toes symmetrical, warm, dry, and pink; sensation and mobility intact
	Help and teach patient to cough every 2 hours and deep breathe every hour. Monitor vital signs every 2 to 4 hours.	Able to cough and deep breathe with assistance; oxygen saturation 92%, lungs clear

NURSING DIAGNOSIS *Deficient knowledge, related to home care management*

Patient Goals and Expected Outcomes	Nursing Interventions	Evaluation and Rationale
Patient and/or significant other will demonstrate understanding of home care and follow-up instructions through interactive discussion and return demonstration	Stress importance of prescribed rehabilitation plan of activity, rest, and exercise.	Patient demonstrates ambulation with walker, exercises, transfers, and precautions, verbalizes understanding of discharge instructions and home care.
	Provide diet instructions on type and amount of food to eat, and advise patient to avoid weight gain if applicable.	Discusses correct foods to eat for therapeutic results.
	Discuss medications: name, purpose, schedule, dosage, and side effects.	Verbalizes knowledge of medications for purpose, dosage, side effects and correct schedule to prevent any drug errors.
	Discuss signs and symptoms to report to physician: severe pain; changes in temperature, color, or sensation in extremity; malodorous drainage from wound.	Verbalizes knowledge of need to report abnormalities to the physician including severe pain, abnormal temperature, color or tingling in affected extremity as well as abnormal wound drainage.
	Stress home safety factors such as elimination of throw rugs, use of safety bars on the bathtub, elevated toilet seats.	Discusses home preparations for safety to include: removal of throw rugs, placement of safety bars on bathtub and availability of toilet riser. Safety knowledge will prevent accidents
	Encourage follow-up visits with physician.	Notes the importance of postoperative follow-up visits with physician. Promotes postoperative recovery.

Critical Thinking Questions

1. The first postoperative evening, Ms. Drake is restless and disoriented. What nursing interventions are needed to prevent dislocation of her bipolar hip prosthesis?
2. Ms. Drake is in her third postoperative day, and the nurse notes an erythematous area on her coccyx. What therapeutic measures can prevent skin impairment?
3. On Ms. Drake's third postoperative day, she complains of pain in her right calf when the nurse performs dorsiflexion. What is the most appropriate immediate action by the nurse?

Prognosis

Complications of hip fractures are the most common cause of death after age 75. Hip fractures in older adults are often complicated by other medical conditions such as diabetes mellitus, cardiac problems (e.g., heart failure), and neurologic disorders (e.g., stroke). A large bone such as the hip heals slowly in older patients, and this predisposes them to various complications. They are at high risk for pneumonia, deep-vein thrombosis, fat embolus, pulmonary embolus, impaired skin integrity, urinary retention, constipation, mental disorientation, and depression.

OTHER FRACTURES

Etiology and Pathophysiology

A fracture is a traumatic injury to a bone in which the continuity of the tissue of the bone is broken. Most fractures result from an insult to the bone, such as a forceful blow (twisting or crushing), which places more stress on the bone than it can absorb. Fractures that occur without trauma are referred to as pathologic or spontaneous fractures and can be caused by a weakening of the bone by osteoporosis, metastatic cancer and tumors of the bone, Cushing's syndrome, malnutrition, and complications of long-term steroid therapy.

Fractures may result from (1) direct force, which causes a fracture at the site of the trauma; (2) torsion, as in a twisting injury in which the fracture occurs at a point remote from the trauma (e.g., forceful twisting of the wrist may fracture the arm); or (3) violent contractions involving highly developed muscles (e.g., severe muscle spasms may cause a fracture in a paraplegic patient).

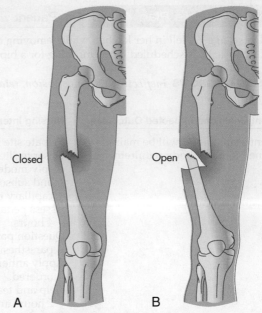

Closed   Open

A   B

FIGURE 4-22 A, Closed fracture. **B,** Open fracture with bone protruding through skin.

The more than 150 types of fractures can be classified in various ways. First, they are described as either closed (simple) or open (compound) (Figure 4-22). In a closed fracture, the bone has not protruded through the skin; in an open fracture, it has. Open fractures are more serious because they involve more soft tissue damage, require surgical treatment to repair, and are prone to infections. A bullet wound (where the injury is directed inward) that has fractured a bone is another example of an open fracture. A closed fracture does not involve a break in the

 Patient Teaching

Postoperative Care for the Patient Who Had a Fractured Hip

OPEN REDUCTION WITH INTERNAL FIXATION

Teaching for patients who had a fractured hip and received an internal fixation with nails or pins would include the following (see Figure 4-20, *A*):

- Assess patient's ability to understand instructions and limitations.
- Help patient dangle feet at bedside on first postoperative day, then to pivot to chair with no weight on operative leg, or touch-down weight if allowed.
- Stress that the operative foot should be placed on floor but weight should be borne on the unoperative leg (refer to limb as either left or right leg so the patient understands) to maintain safety in care.
- Turn patient every 2 hours; prop with pillows between legs or under the back to maintain position.
- Assist with range-of-motion exercises to maintain muscle strength.
- Help physical therapist walk patient with walker and with limited weight placed on operative limb (if assistance is needed) for comfort and safety.
- Encourage patient and family members to walk together for patient's safety. Instruct family about weight-bearing techniques for clarity and safety.

- If a stable plate and screw fixation is used to repair the fractured hip, the patient should not bear weight for 6 weeks to 3 months to protect the fracture site.
- A telescoping nail fixation allows minimal to partial weight bearing during the first 6 weeks to 3 months.

HIP PROSTHETIC IMPLANT

Teaching for patients who had a fractured hip and received a hip prosthetic implant (hemiarthroplasty) includes the following (see Figure 4-19):

- Avoid hip flexion beyond 60 degrees for approximately 10 days.
- Avoid hip flexion beyond 90 degrees for 2 to 3 months.
- Avoid adduction of the affected leg beyond midline for 2 to 3 months.
- Maintain partial weight-bearing status for approximately 2 to 3 months.
- Avoid positioning on the operative side in bed.
- Maintain abduction of the hip by using a wedge-shaped foam bolster or pillows arranged in a wedge; this will require nursing assistance.

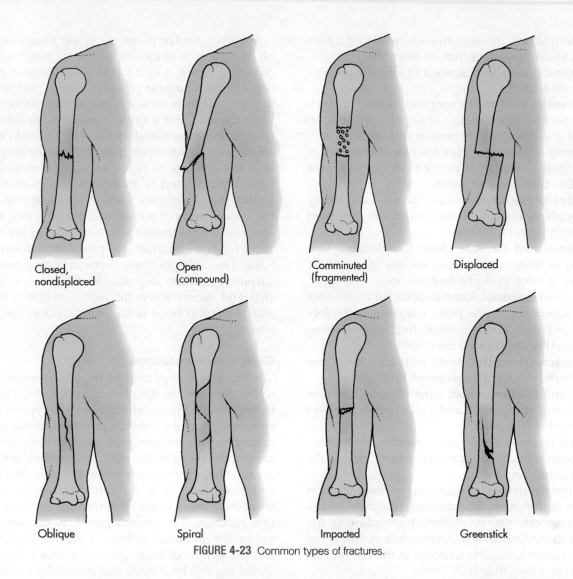

Closed, nondisplaced

Open (compound)

Comminuted (fragmented)

Displaced

Oblique

Spiral

Impacted

Greenstick

FIGURE 4-23 Common types of fractures.

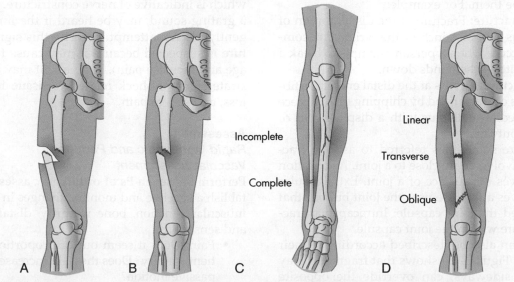

Incomplete

Complete

Linear

Transverse

Oblique

A   **B**   **C**   **D**

FIGURE 4-24 Bone fractures. **A,** Open. **B,** Closed. **C,** Incomplete and complete. **D,** Linear, transverse, and oblique.

skin. These fractures can sometimes be realigned by external manipulation, rather than invasive surgery.

Fractures can also be described in terms of appearance (Figure 4-23):

- **Greenstick fracture:** Incomplete fracture in which the fracture line extends only partially through the bone. The bone is broken and bent but still secured at one side. This fracture is common in children because their bones are softer and more flexible than those of adults.
- **Complete fracture:** Fracture line extends entirely through the bone, with the periosteum disrupted on both sides of the bone.
- **Comminuted fracture:** Bone is splintered into three or more fragments at the site of the break. There is more than one fracture line.
- **Impacted fracture:** Sometimes called a *telescoped* fracture because one bone fragment is forcibly wedged into another bone fragment. In long bones, this can shorten the extremity.
- **Transverse fracture:** Break runs directly across the bone, at a right angle to the bone's axis.
- **Oblique fracture:** Break runs diagonally across the bone, at approximately a 45-degree angle to the shaft of the bone.
- **Spiral fracture:** Break coils around the bone. This is sometimes called a torsion fracture and results from a twisting force.

Fractures are described according to their location on the bone—for example, proximal, midshaft, or distal. Fractures can also be classified according to the force that caused the break. An example of this is the marching fracture, which can occur in the metatarsals as a result of a long march.

Fractures sometimes are named after the first physician to describe them. For example:

- **Colles' fracture:** Fracture of the distal portion of the radius within 1 inch of the wrist joint; commonly occurs when a person attempts to break a fall by putting the hands down.
- **Pott's fracture:** Occurs at the distal end of the fibula and is characterized by chipping off of a piece of the medial malleolus with a displacement of the foot outward.

Fractures are sometimes referred to as joint fractures if they involve or are close to a joint. Articulation fracture involves the surface of a joint. Extracapsular fracture involves a fracture near the joint but one that has not entered the joint capsule. Intracapsular fracture is a fracture within the joint capsule.

Fractures can also be described according to their displacement. Figure 4-24 shows that fragments may be displaced sideways, can override the opposite fractured surface, may angulate or create a bend in the bone, and may rotate away from the fracture site. When a bone is displaced, the bone fragments can cause soft tissue damage. The patient experiences severe pain, edema, and muscle spasms in the early stages of healing.

Bone is vascular; therefore, when a fracture occurs, bleeding occurs at the site of the fracture and in surrounding tissue. A clot forms at the ends of the fractured bone. The next phase of healing occurs when the hematoma becomes organized as fibroblasts invade the area and a fibrin meshwork is formed. Inflammation is localized as the white blood cells wall off the area. Osteoblasts enter the fibrous area to help hold the union firm. Blood vessels develop, and collagen strands start to incorporate calcium deposits. **Callus** (bony deposits formed between and around the broken ends of a fractured bone during healing) forms when the osteoblasts continue to lay the network for bone buildup and osteoclasts destroy dead bone. The collagen strengthens and continues to incorporate calcium deposits. Remodeling is the final step and occurs when the excess callus is resorbed and trabecular bone is laid down along the lines of stress.

Clinical Manifestations

The signs and symptoms of fractures vary according to the location and function of the involved bone, the strength of its muscle attachment, the type of fracture sustained, and the amount of related damage. Signs and symptoms include pain; warmth over the injured area; ecchymosis of the skin surrounding the injured area, which may not be present for several days; and soft tissue edema in the injured area. In addition, there may be an obvious deformity and loss of normal function. The injured part may be incapable of voluntary movements; have a change in the curvature or length of bone (for a fractured hip, the affected leg will be shorter and externally rotated); and have a loss of sensation or paralysis distal to injury, which is indicative of nerve constricture. **Crepitus**, or a grating sound, may be heard if the limb is moved gently (do not attempt to verify this sign when fracture is suspected because it may cause further damage and increase pain). The patient may also demonstrate signs of shock related to tissue injury, blood loss, and severe pain.

Assessment
Rapid Orthopedic and Peripheral Vascular Assessment
Perform the **seven Ps of orthopedic assessment** to establish a baseline and monitor changes in the patient's muscular function, bone integrity, distal circulation, and sensation:

- Pain: Does it seem out of proportion to the patient's injury? Does the pain increase on active or passive motion?
- Pallor
- Paresthesia, or numbness
- Paralysis
- Polar temperature: Is the extremity cold compared with the opposite extremity?
- Puffiness from edema or a hematoma

- Pulselessness: A Doppler ultrasound device may be useful to determine the presence or absence of blood flow if unable to palpate distal pulses

Subjective data include pain at the site of the injury, loss of sensation or movement of the affected part, and cause of injury.

Objective data include warmth, edema, and ecchymosis; obvious deformity; loss of normal function in the injured part; signs of systemic shock; and signs of any circulatory, motor, or sensory impairment.

Diagnostic Tests

An accurate diagnosis of the fracture is made by radiographic examination or fluoroscopy.

Medical Management

Immediate management includes splinting and elevation to prevent edema of the affected part. Preservation of body alignment is also critical. Apply cold packs (during the first 24 hours) to reduce hemorrhage, edema, and pain. Administer analgesics as ordered. Observe the injured part for change in color, sensation, or temperature. Also observe the patient for signs of shock.

Secondary management for a closed fracture begins with optimal reduction: replacing bone fragments in their correct anatomical position. This can be accomplished through (1) closed reduction, which involves manual manipulations—moving bony fragments into position by applying traction and pressure to distal fragments; (2) traction; (3) **open reduction with internal fixation (ORIF),** a surgical procedure allowing fracture alignment under direct visualization while using various internal fixation devices applied to the bone; or (4) immobilization. Immobilization can be achieved through one or a combination of the following: (1) external fixation with a cast or splint; (2) traction; or (3) internal fixation devices such as pins, plates, screws, wires, and prostheses (see Figure 4-20).

For an open fracture, additional measures are taken. The wound undergoes surgical debridement to remove dirt, foreign materials, devitalized tissue, and necrotic bone. Administer tetanus toxoid. Take a culture of the wound and begin treatment with antibiotics. Observe the wound for signs of osteomyelitis, tetanus, or gangrene. Closure of the wound occurs when there is no sign of infection. Reduction and immobilization of the fracture then take place. Finally, observe for and treat any complications.

Nursing Interventions and Patient Teaching

The nursing interventions for patients with fractures are essentially the same as for any surgical patient. The care of the patient in traction and in a cast is discussed later in this chapter. The patient needs a well-balanced diet, but opinions differ on the value of vitamin and mineral supplements in hastening bone repair. Encourage fluids. Exercise of the unaffected joints, muscle-setting exercises, skin care, and elimination are important considerations in patient care. Internal fixation

has simplified nursing intervention for many patients with fractures and shortened the period of hospitalization, but many patients require longer periods of hospitalization. If activity is restricted, anticipate and prevent the complications that result from immobility.

Patient teaching includes (1) how to move comfortably in bed; (2) how to transfer safely in and out of bed; (3) weight-bearing restrictions and activity limitations, including how long these need to be observed; (4) proper use of ambulatory assistive devices; (5) how to avoid edema in the affected part by proper elevation; (6) how to control pain or discomfort in the affected part; (7) exercises to perform to maintain strength and enhance circulation; and (8) proper method of cleansing pins, using surgical asepsis per physician's protocol.

Prognosis

Bone production and fracture healing depend on the patient's age and general health. Presence of other systemic diseases complicates the healing process.

FRACTURE OF THE VERTEBRAE

Etiology and Pathophysiology

Injuries such as diving accidents or blows to the head or body can result in fractures of the vertebrae. Patients with osteoporosis and metastatic cancer are at risk for vertebral fractures. Motorcycle and car accidents (especially head-on collisions) occur more frequently with young men (ages 16 to 30 years).

Fractures of the vertebrae may involve the vertebral body, lamina, and articulating processes and may occur with or without displacement. If the fracture has displaced the vertebral structures, pressure may be placed on spinal nerves. The sharp bone fragments may also sever the spinal cord nerves, causing permanent paralysis from the point of injury downward.

Clinical Manifestations

Signs and symptoms of vertebral fracture include pain at the site of the injury; partial or complete loss of mobility or sensation below the level of the injury; and evidence of fracture or fracture dislocation on routine radiographic examination, myelography, or CT scans.

Assessment

Collection of **subjective data** includes assessment for pain (if the fracture has injured the spinal cord, pain may not be present), numbness, tingling, and inability to move extremities from below the level of the trauma site.

Collection of **objective data** includes careful assessment of neurologic function, such as pupillary reaction to light, hand grip, ability to move extremities, level of orientation, vital signs, and reaction to painful stimuli (see Chapter 14). Observe for fecal and urinary retention and for signs of hemorrhage such as hypotension, tachycardia, tachypnea, and decreased renal functioning.

Diagnostic Tests

Radiographic studies are done to determine whether the vertebral bodies are compresssed. A spinal cord injury may result from a fracture or dislocation of a vertebra; if this is suspected, the physician performs a spinal tap to evaluate the spinal fluid. Spinal fluid is normally clear, and the presence of blood indicates trauma (see Chapter 14).

Medical Management

Stable injuries to the vertebrae that are not a threat to spinal cord integrity are treated with pain medication and muscle relaxants. Anticoagulant therapy may be ordered as a prophylaxis for thromboembolic complications. Maintaining erect posture can be enhanced by the use of a back support, corset brace, or a cast. The patient may be allowed to ambulate with assistance (gait enhancers) once discomfort subsides.

Unstable fractures that involve displacement are more serious. Treatment is aimed at fracture reduction through postural positioning and traction. Cranial skeletal traction is used with cervical spine fractures (see Chapter 14). A halo brace (Figure 4-25), an external immobilization device in which a plaster or plastic brace that incorporates metal struts attached to pins is inserted into bone, is used to allow the patient to be mobile. Pelvic traction is used for lumbar spinal fractures. An open reduction may be necessary with internal fixation using a Harrington rod. After this surgical procedure, the patient is placed in a body cast.

Nursing Interventions and Patient Teaching

Nursing interventions are aimed at maintaining the stability of the fracture fixation by (1) log-rolling the patient for position changes; (2) following the correct procedure for turning a patient in a special bed, such as a Stryker frame or Foster bed; (3) elevating the head of the bed no more than 30 degrees; (4) using stabilization devices for the head and back; and assess the continuity of traction (e.g., weights hanging free and ropes not twisted) and skin integrity (e.g., erythema, tenderness, and edema), as well as surrounding traction equipment.

Nursing diagnoses and interventions for the patient with a vertebral fracture include but are not limited to the following:

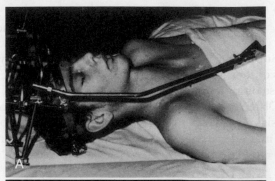

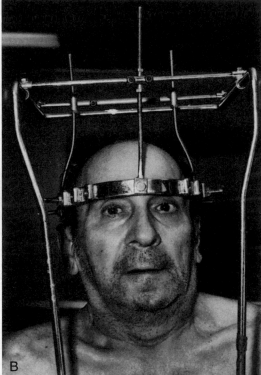

FIGURE 4-25 **A,** Halo attached to body cast. Metal strut will be anchored firmly into body cast with additional plaster. **B,** Metal ring, or halo, that attaches to skull.

Nursing Diagnoses	Nursing Interventions
Powerlessness, related to: • decreased mobility • pain	Use active listening, and permit verbalization of anger and helplessness. Assist patient in identifying coping mechanisms that will reduce feeling of powerlessness; use those that have been successful in the past.

Nursing Diagnoses	Nursing Interventions
	Offer positive recognition for increased activity level. Assist patient in identifying areas over which he or she has control. Involve patients in decision-making process for their own care.
Risk for infection, related to immobility and/or surgical intervention	Monitor patient for signs and symptoms of infection (elevated temperature, increased pulse rate, malodorous exudates, erythema, cloudy urine, diminished breath sounds, and crackles and wheezes).

Nursing Diagnoses	Nursing Interventions
Risk for infection, related to immobility and/or surgical intervention—cont'd	Monitor laboratory values (such as CBC) and blood and wound cultures.
	Protect patient from cross-contamination by practicing good handwashing techniques, maintaining surgical asepsis when changing dressings, and using strict surgical asepsis with catheter care.
	Encourage coughing, deep breathing, and leg exercises.
	Encourage use of incentive spirometer.
	Prevent people with infectious processes from coming in contact with patient.
Impaired physical mobility, related to: • neuromuscular skeletal impairment • pain • discomfort	Maintain bed rest in correct body alignment; avoid lifting or twisting body.
	Place patient in immobilization device as ordered, such as cervical head halter, skeletal traction, Stryker frame, or Circ-Olectric bed; maintain cervical spine in extension.
	Assess neurovascular status every 2 hours; monitor pulse, color, temperature, sensation, and mobility of all extremities.
	Perform passive ROM or assist with and teach active ROM exercises for all extremities every 2 hours.
	As fracture heals, traction is replaced with cast.
	Assist patient with ambulation when ordered; monitor for vertigo and weakness; progress slowly.

Patient teaching includes how to support the back by (1) using a firm mattress; (2) sitting in straight, firm chairs (for no longer than 20 to 30 minutes), when allowed; (3) using proper lifting techniques (using the leg muscles, not the back); and (4) doing back exercises to strengthen spinal extensor muscles.

Prognosis

Stable injuries to the vertebrae that are not a threat to spinal cord integrity have an excellent prognosis with full recovery. Unstable fractures are more serious, and prognosis is guarded when spinal cord injury is involved.

FRACTURE OF THE PELVIS

Etiology and Pathophysiology

Most pelvic fractures result from trauma involving great force, such as falls from extreme heights, automobile accidents, or crushing accidents. When trauma is severe enough to fracture the pelvis, vital abdominal organs may also be damaged, such as the bladder, vagina, uterus, liver, spleen, intestines, or kidneys. Because the pelvis has a rich blood supply, a fracture can result in extensive blood loss (as much as 1 to 4 L).

Clinical Manifestations

The patient with a fractured pelvis is unable to bear weight without discomfort. Local tenderness and edema are common at the trauma site. Hematuria (blood in the urine) may result from trauma to the bladder. Hemorrhage is by far the most life-threatening complication to a patient with a pelvic fracture.

Assessment

Subjective data include complaints of pelvic pain or tenderness and backache. Complaints of restlessness, anxiety, and progressive disorientation may be signs of shock.

Collection of **objective data** includes assessment of muscle spasms in the pelvic region; ecchymosis over the pelvis, perineum, groin, or suprapubic area; inability to raise the legs when supine; and external foot rotation on the affected side with noticeable shortening of one leg. Vital sign assessment may indicate shock (hypotension, tachycardia, tachypnea, oliguria, and diaphoresis). Careful observation for fat embolism syndrome is especially pertinent for patients with pelvic fractures. Assess bowel sounds in all four quadrants and document the findings; large bowel and rectal lacerations are possible in patients with pelvic fractures. Assess color and amount of urinary output because of the possibility of laceration of the bladder.

Diagnostic Tests

Abdominal radiographic studies are done with the patient in the supine and lateral positions. CT provides an evaluation of both the bony pelvis and intraabdominal contents. Intravenous pyelogram is performed to determine kidney damage. Interpretation of laboratory values for hemoglobin and hematocrit, urinalysis, and stool for occult blood helps determine whether the patient is bleeding and anemic.

Medical Management

The patient often remains on bed rest for 3 weeks and then walks with crutches for approximately 6 weeks. If the patient has a symphysis pubis fracture and an iliac fracture on the same side, the physician performs surgery. After surgery, skeletal traction is applied for approximately 6 weeks to maintain the leg position. When traction is released, the patient may ambulate without bearing weight for approximately 3 months. For a bilateral fracture of the pelvis, the physician may order a pelvic sling to support the fracture. To treat severe fractures that totally disrupt the pelvic ring and dislocate the sacroiliac joints, the physician may apply an external skeletal fixation device. He or she may also apply a spica or body cast to support the fracture.

Nursing Interventions and Patient Teaching

Nursing interventions involve monitoring the patient for signs of progressive shock (hypotension, tachycardia, tachypnea, and decreased urinary output). Measure the abdominal girth at least every 8 hours for signs of increased abdominal pressure that could result from internal hemorrhaging. Monitor I&O for signs of hypovolemia, laceration of the bladder, and potential kidney trauma. Insert a Foley catheter for monitoring urinary output and color. Implement nursing interventions appropriate for impaired mobility, impaired skin integrity, fluid volume deficit, and pain management.

A nursing diagnosis and interventions for the patient with a pelvic fracture include but are not limited to the following:

Nursing Diagnosis	Nursing Interventions
Risk for ineffective tissue perfusion, related to: • hemorrhage • hypovolemia • shock	Assess for ecchymosis over pelvis and perineum. Monitor vital signs every 15 minutes for evidence of shock until stable. Insert a Foley catheter per physician's order to monitor color and amount of urinary output. Monitor parenteral fluids per physician's order. Provide quiet, therapeutic environment. Administer oxygen per physician's order. Maintain bed rest per physician's order. Monitor bowel sounds and measure abdominal girth to ascertain possible lacerated bowel.

Reinforce the reasons for immobility and not bearing full weight; the patient may be too anxious to hear or understand initial explanations. Also explain measures for dealing with acute pain and changes in medications as pain decreases. In addition, explain turning and moving techniques to prevent skin impairment.

Prognosis

Hemorrhage is by far the most life-threatening complication. The long-term prognosis depends on the severity of the fracture, the patient's age, and the presence of other systemic disorders.

COMPLICATIONS OF FRACTURES

COMPARTMENT SYNDROME

Compartment syndrome is a pathologic condition caused by the progressive development of arterial vessel compression and reduced blood supply to an extremity. Fractures of the forearm or tibia usually precede the onset of muscle edema within the fasciae, which form compartments for the muscles of the forearm and lower leg. With severe trauma, such as fractures or compression of blood vessels as a result of a tight cast or dressing, muscle ischemia (decreased blood supply to the muscles) can occur. Irreversible muscle ischemia can occur within 6 hours as a result of compression of the arteries, nerves, and tendons entering the compartment. Paralysis and sensory loss follow, with contracture and permanent disability of the extremity seen within 24 to 48 hours.

Assessment

Collection of **subjective data** includes pain assessment. Usually the patient complains of sharp pain that increases with passive movement of the hand or foot. The patient experiences deep, unrelenting, progressive, and poorly localized pain unrelieved by analgesics or elevation of the extremity. Numbness or tingling in the affected extremity is common.

Collection of **objective data** includes assessment of the patient's inability to flex the fingers or toes, coolness of the extremity, and absence of pulsation in the affected extremity. Assess skin color for signs of pallor or cyanosis. Gentle palpation of the extremity will reveal slowing of the capillary refill time (blanching). Close monitoring and proper documentation of vital signs are essential (especially temperature to detect signs of tissue necrosis) (see Box 4-5).

Medical Management

Most cases require a fasciotomy (incision into the fascia) to relieve pressure and allow return of normal blood flow to the area. This is done immediately (within 30 minutes). The incision is often left open to heal by granulation (healing by second intention) (Figure 4-26).

Nursing Interventions

Nursing interventions include administration of analgesics with careful documentation of relief ob-

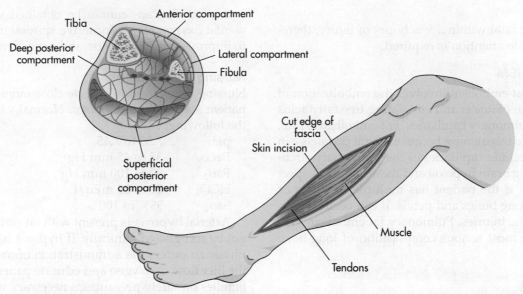

FIGURE 4-26 Compartment syndrome. Often more than one compartment is involved, and anterior compartment is especially vulnerable. Causes include trauma, severe burn, or excessive exercise. A single incision may open more than one compartment.

tained. To slow further circulatory compromise, elevate the affected limb, no higher than heart level, to maintain arterial pressure. Apply cold packs and remove any constricting material, such as an elastic bandage. The most common complication when decompression is delayed is infection as a result of tissue necrosis. Purulent drainage from the dressing is a sign of infection and must be reported immediately. If drainage and secretion isolation are required, provide careful instructions to the patient, who may feel isolated. Encourage patients to express their fears and emotional needs. **Volkmann's contracture** is a permanent contracture (with clawhand, flexion of wrist and fingers, and atrophy of the forearm) that can occur as a result of compartment syndrome. Proper positioning and alignment can reduce the risk of this complication.

Prognosis
Compartment syndrome can result in a permanent contracture deformity of the hand or foot.

SHOCK
Shock can occur as a result of blood loss from a fractured bone (bone is vascular) or from severed blood vessels, seen especially in open fractures. Pain and fear can also cause shock.

Assessment
Collection of **subjective data** includes monitoring the patient's level of consciousness. Restlessness or complaints of anxiety may suggest a decrease in cerebral perfusion, resulting in brain hypoxia. Complaints of weakness and lethargy are common.

Collection of **objective data** includes monitoring vital signs. Typical signs of shock include hypotension, tachycardia, and tachypnea. As shock progresses, hy-

pothermia occurs. The patient may have pale, cool, moist skin. Oliguria (diminished urinary output) is present with shock.

Medical Management
The physician's main concern is restoring blood volume to ensure a rapid return of oxygen to the tissues. Blood volume can be expanded with IV fluids (lactated Ringer's solution or 5% dextrose in normal saline). Whole blood, plasma, or plasma substitutes may also be given. Respiratory assistance may be given by administering oxygen. A central venous catheter may be inserted for accurate monitoring of vital signs to prevent pulmonary edema. Shock trousers may be applied. These are pneumatic trousers designed to counteract hypotension associated with internal or external bleeding and hypovolemia.

Nursing Interventions
Nursing interventions for IV fluid administration include checking (1) the contents and IV flow rate against the physician's orders, and (2) the infusion site for signs of infiltration (erythema, edema, pain, and induration [hardening of tissue]). Monitor the patient's vital signs every 15 minutes until stable. Monitor urinary output every hour. Less than 30 mL of urine per hour indicates decreased renal perfusion. The patient should remain flat in bed. If there are no head injuries, raise the lower extremities slightly to improve venous return. Avoid the Trendelenburg position because it tends to push the abdominal organs against the diaphragm, reducing the effectiveness of heart and lung functions. Keep the patient warm, but avoid external heat. Give nothing by mouth, and avoid sedatives, tranquilizers, and narcotics. Be aware that the patient's family will be anxious and provide them with brief explanations of the patient's condition.

Prognosis

Shock can be fatal within a few hours of injury; therefore immediate attention is required.

FAT EMBOLISM

Pulmonary fat embolism involves the embolization of tissue fat with platelets and circulating free fatty acids within the pulmonary capillaries. Fat embolism is rare, but can be life threatening because the fat droplets can effectively occlude capillaries of the pulmonary circulation, causing brain hypoxia and tissue death. Suspect fat embolism if the patient has multiple fractures or fractures of long bones and pelvis. It can occur within 48 hours of the injuries. Pulmonary fat embolism syndrome is the most serious complication of long bone fractures.

Assessment

Collection of **subjective data** includes assessment of mental disturbances, such as irritability, restlessness, disorientation, stupor, and coma. These symptoms can result from effects of severe hypoxemia. The patient may complain of chest pain, especially on inspiration, and of localized muscle weakness, spasticity, and rigidity.

Collection of **objective data** includes assessing for tachypnea, dyspnea, hypoxemia, and auditory crackles and wheezes in the lung field. As the lung filters and traps embolic material, ventilation is disturbed. Assess the apical pulse to detect dysrhythmias. Patients are placed on cardiac monitoring for observation of dysrhythmias and cardiovascular collapse. Assess the patient for petechiae (especially in the buccal membranes, conjunctival sacs, hard palate, chest, and anterior axillary folds) caused by occlusion of capillaries. The appearance of petechiae on the conjunctiva of the eye, the neck, chest, or axillary region is a typical sign of a fat embolism (Lewis et al., 2007).

Diagnostic Tests

The diagnosis is based on clinical signs and symptoms, which appear within 24 to 48 hours of injury. Blood gases indicate hypoxemia. Hemoglobin and hematocrit laboratory values are decreased. Fat is present in the blood and urine. The sedimentation rate is increased, and the platelet count is decreased.

Medical Management

Treatment for fat embolism is directed at prevention. Careful immobilization of a long bone fracture is probably the most important factor in the prevention of fat embolism. The physician orders the administration of IV fluids to prevent shock and dilute free fatty acids. Use of corticosteroids to prevent or treat fat embolism is controversial. Digoxin is often ordered to increase the patient's cardiac output. Oxygen is administered if the Po_2 is less than 70 mm Hg. Intubation or intermittent positive pressure ventilation may be considered if

a satisfactory Pao_2 cannot be obtained with supplemental oxygen alone. Incentive spirometry is ordered to improve lung expansion and oxygenation.

Nursing Interventions

Nursing interventions include close monitoring of the patient's arterial blood gases. Normal values include the following:

pH	7.35 to 7.45
$Paco_2$	35 to 45 mm Hg
Pao_2	80 to 100 mm Hg
HCO_3	21 to 28 mEq/L
Sao_2	95% to 100%

Arterial hypoxia is present with fat emboli and may not be recognized clinically. If hypoxia is present, the physician orders the administration of oxygen. Check the liter flow of oxygen and educate patients and their families on safety precautions necessary when oxygen is administered (e.g., no smoking or use of electrical equipment). Respiratory failure is the most common cause of death. Careful stabilization and immobilization of long bone fractures are important steps in preventing fat embolism syndrome. Careful support when turning and positioning the patient can prevent the manipulation of the fracture and reduce the risk of fat embolism syndrome. Reposition the patient as little as possible before fracture immobilization because of the danger of dislodging more fat droplets into the general circulation. An accurate record of I&O and daily weights is essential to monitor fluid balance.

Prognosis

Fat embolism can be life threatening.

GAS GANGRENE

Gas gangrene is a severe infection of the skeletal muscle caused by gram-positive *Clostridium* bacteria, particularly *Clostridium perfringens*, which may occur in the presence of open fractures and lacerated wounds. These injuries can produce exotoxins that destroy tissue. The onset is usually sudden, generally 1 to 14 days after injury. These organisms are anaerobic (grow and function without oxygen) and spore formers. They are normally found in soil and the intestinal tracts of humans. As the clostridia bacteria invade devitalized tissue (especially where blood supply is diminished), they multiply and produce toxins that cause (1) hemolysis (breakdown of red blood cells and release of hemoglobin); (2) vessel thrombosis; and (3) damage to the myocardium, the liver, the kidneys, and the brain.

Assessment

Collection of **subjective data** includes observation of pain, which is usually sudden and severe at the site of the injury. A characteristic finding is toxic delirium.

Collection of **objective data** includes careful inspection of the skin for gas bubbles at the site of the wound.

The various *Clostridium* species produce a characteristic cellulitis in which gas is present under the skin. This causes crepitation (a crackling sensation when the skin is touched). Observe for signs of infection, including elevated temperature, tachycardia, tachypnea, and edema around the wound. The skin around the wound becomes necrotic and ruptures, revealing necrotic muscle. The wound discharge is thin, watery, and foul smelling. Carefully document the patient's response to antibiotic therapy (e.g., decline in temperature and decrease in amount of wound drainage).

Medical Management

Treatment of gas gangrene involves establishing a larger wound opening to admit air and promote drainage. Antibiotics, such as penicillin G or cephalothin, are ordered intravenously and must be administered as scheduled. Observe the patient for adverse reactions.

Nursing Interventions

Nursing interventions include wound care using strict medical asepsis. Spore-forming bacteria are not destroyed by ordinary disinfecting methods. Therefore all contaminated equipment and linens must be autoclaved. Follow drainage and secretion isolation procedures to prevent the spread of the infection to other patients.

Prognosis

If left untreated, gas gangrene is rapidly fatal. Prompt treatment, including excision of gangrenous tissue and administration of penicillin G intravenously, saves 80% of patients. If massive gangrene develops, amputation is necessary.

THROMBOEMBOLUS

Etiology and Pathophysiology

Thromboembolus is a condition in which a blood vessel is occluded by an embolus carried in the bloodstream from the site of formation of the clot. It is associated with reduced skeletal muscle contractions and bed rest. The person suffering from pelvic and hip fractures is at high risk for this complication.

Clinical Manifestations

The area supplied by an obstructed artery may tingle and become cold, numb, and cyanotic. An embolus in the lungs causes a sudden, sharp thoracic or upper abdominal pain, dyspnea, cough, fever, and hemoptysis.

Assessment

Collection of **subjective data** includes careful investigation of complaints of pain in the lower extremities (especially the calf). A complaint of tenderness over the area is common. The patient may complain of a sharp pain in the thoracic area when an embolus is in the lung.

Collection of **objective data** includes assessing for a positive Homans' sign, which indicates thromboembolus. Homans' sign is pain in the calf of the affected leg on dorsiflexion of the foot. The affected area may be erythematous, warm to touch, and edematous. Assess for differences in leg size (circumference) bilaterally from thigh to ankle. Also observe the patient for dyspnea and blood in the sputum if pulmonary embolus is present. When anticoagulant therapy is ordered, assess for signs of bleeding, such as petechiae, epistaxis, hematuria, hematemesis, and occult or gross blood in the stool.

Diagnostic Tests

A complete history is taken and a physical examination is performed. In addition to checking Homans' sign, obtain a prothrombin time (PT), International Normalized Ratio (INR), D-dimer, and CBC. Diagnostic tests for deep-vein thrombosis may include Doppler ultrasonography or duplex scanning. A spiral CT scan of the lung, a ventilation/perfusion scan, or a pulmonary arteriogram may be ordered to rule out pulmonary embolism.

Medical Management

Treatment includes administration of anticoagulants, such as heparin, enoxaparin or warfarin. A surgical procedure known as thrombectomy (removal of a thrombus from a blood vessel) may be done.

Nursing Interventions

Nursing interventions involve caring for the patient on activity restriction. Many times this involves bed rest with the foot of the bed elevated to aid venous return. Teach the patient to do active exercise, such as dorsiflexion (pointing backward) and plantar flexion (pointing forward) of the toes, several times each hour. This exercise stimulates circulation to the legs. Continuous hot, moist compresses are usually ordered. Antiembolism stockings and intermittent pneumatic compression devices are ordered while the patient is on bed rest and are maintained even after the patient is ambulatory. Assess lung sounds every 4 hours and adhere to the activity ordered. If the patient is receiving anticoagulants, closely monitor PT, INR, and partial thromboplastin times.

Prognosis

Obstruction of the pulmonary artery or one of its branches may be fatal. A thrombus in an extremity usually resolves with treatment, and a favorable prognosis is noted.

 Safety Alert!

Thromboembolus

Never massage a patient's lower extremities. Thromboembolus can be present without clinical signs and symptoms.

DELAYED FRACTURE HEALING

A **delayed union** is a fracture that fails to heal within the usual time. The healing is impaired but has not completely stopped and will eventually repair itself. **Nonunion** is when the ends of the fractured bone fail to unite and produce a stable union after 6 to 9 months. The calcification of cartilage and bone formation do not occur. Bone grafting, prosthetic implant, internal fixation, external fixation, or a combination of these methods can be used to correct the problem of delayed union or nonunion of bone fractures. Physicians are using electrical stimulation as a new method of promoting healing of nonunion fractures. The use of electrical probes on bone stimulates bone production.

Prognosis

Bone production and fracture healing depend on the patient's age and general health. The presence of other systemic diseases complicates the healing process.

SKELETAL FIXATION DEVICES

EXTERNAL FIXATION DEVICES

External fixation devices are used to hold bone fragments in normal position. Casts, skeletal and skin traction, braces, and metal pins are examples of these devices.

Skeletal Pin External Fixation

One external fixation technique immobilizes fractures with pins inserted through the bone and attached to a rigid external metal frame (Figure 4-27). This tech-

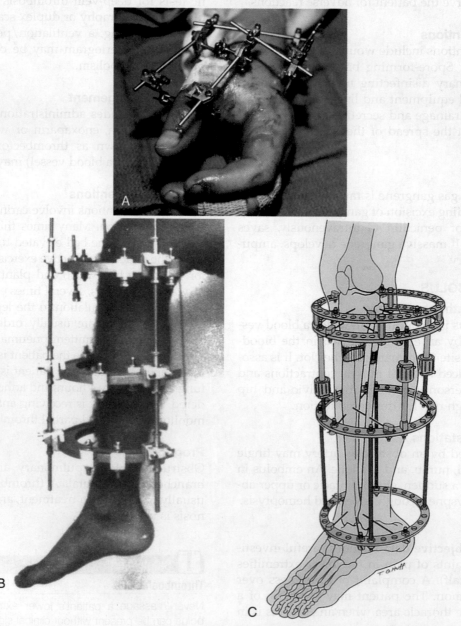

FIGURE 4-27 External fixation apparatuses. **A,** Hoffman. **B,** The Monticello-Spinelli Circular Fixator. **C,** Ilizarov apparatus with corticotomies for lengthening lower leg.

nique is becoming more popular because it provides rigid support of comminuted open fractures, infected nonunions, and infected unstable joints. The patient can use the muscles and joints above and below the fixation. Leaving the fracture open to air has the advantage of visibility of the area and accessibility for wound care.

This procedure is performed with the patient under general anesthesia. Reassure the patient that the pain after the insertion of the pins is minimal. Immediately after the procedure, the extremity is placed in balanced suspension traction to help relieve the edema. Assess the pins that are inserted through the bone at least every 8 hours, with careful observation for signs of infection and loose pins. Remove dried exudate from around the pins once or twice daily with hydrogen peroxide or alcohol, using surgical asepsis. Patients are permitted to ambulate on crutches when soft tissue edema is relieved. They are permitted to shower when the wounds have healed but must avoid salt or chlorinated water to prevent fixator corrosion.

NONSURGICAL INTERVENTIONS FOR MUSCULOSKELETAL DISORDERS

CASTS

Casts are immobilization devices made up of layers of plaster of Paris, fiberglass, or plastic roller bandages. The application is similar to that for an elastic bandage. The type of cast used is indicative of the part of the body immobilized. Examples include (1) short arm cast, which extends from below the elbow to the proximal palmar crease; (2) long leg cast, which extends from the upper thigh to the base of the toes; and (3) spica cast or body cast, which covers the trunk and one or both extremities (Figure 4-28). A cast may be bivalve to relieve pressure. This involves splitting the cast down both sides and securing the pieces so that the extremity is supported (see Skill 4-1, step 8a).

Casts are applied after the physician has properly aligned the bone through either external or internal fixation. Cast application is relatively painless except for the manipulation of the traumatized extremity. The casting procedure involves the application of a piece of stockinette that covers the length of the extremity and area to be casted, followed by sheet wadding (pressed cotton that comes in rolled bandages), followed by the casting material. Most physicians bring the stockinette up and over the distal and proximal edge of the cast. Inspect these edges for rough pieces of casting that may irritate the skin. Superficial burns can occur as the cast begins to set up, especially if the patient is not appropriately padded or too much fiberglass material is used.

Cast Brace

The cast brace is an alternative appliance to the traditional leg cast. It provides the support and stability of

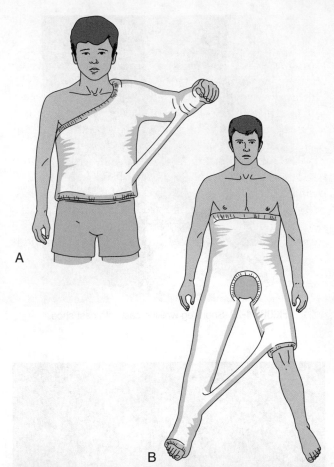

FIGURE 4-28 Spica casts. **A,** Shoulder spica. **B,** One and one-half leg-hip spica.

the plaster cast, with additional support and mobility provided by a hinged brace. The appliance is most effective for fractures of the shaft of the femur and permits early ambulation and weight bearing. It is used approximately 2 to 6 weeks after fracture reduction.

Cast bracing is based on the concept that limited weight bearing helps promote the formation of bone. A problem encountered frequently with cast bracing is edema around the knee. Instruct patients to elevate the leg when sitting to promote venous return. A cast shoe or walking heel incorporated into a lower extremity cast permits weight bearing without damaging the cast (Figure 4-29).

Assessment

Nursing assessment is similar regardless of what kind of casting material is used. Perform a neurovascular assessment, including capillary refill, every 15 to 30 minutes for several hours after casting and every 4 hours the first few days (see Box 4-5). Capillary filling time (capillary refill) is a way to assess arterial flow to the extremities; squeeze the patient's nailbeds to produce blanching and observe for the return of color. With normal arterial capillary perfusion, the color returns to normal within 2 seconds (Figure 4-30). Observe the skin at the cast edges for erythema and irrita-

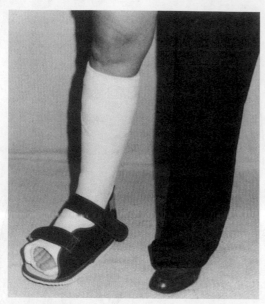

FIGURE 4-29 Short-leg walking cast with cast shoe.

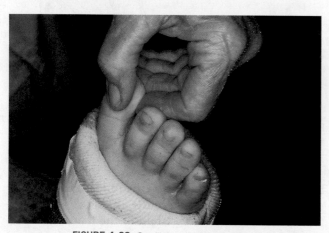

FIGURE 4-30 Capillary refill assessment.

tion. Note any signs of infection, such as odor or drainage coming from under the cast, and document the findings. Assess the patient's ability to use crutches in a three-point gait to establish normal gait and rhythm, and assess crutches for safety by ensuring a proper fit and presence of large, rubber, suction tips on the ends.

Nursing Interventions and Patient Teaching

Nursing interventions for the patient in a cast (Skill 4-1) include patient education on preventing infection, irritation, neurovascular pressure, and misalignment of bone ends. Handle a wet cast gently and support it with the flat of the hand or on pillows to avoid indentations that cause pressure on the skin and lead to skin impairment. Never use the bar in a spica cast as support when turning patient. Turning the patient frequently aids the drying process. If a cast dryer is used, set it on warm, never hot (drying a plaster of Paris cast too quickly from the outside may weaken the cast). Elevating the casted extremity reduces edema (usually elevation is recommended for 24 to 48 hours). Instruct patients using crutches to support their weight on their hands; weight borne on the axillae can damage the brachial plexus nerves (crutch paralysis).

Cast syndrome can occur after the application of a spica (body) cast (see Figure 4-28) and involves acute obstruction of the duodenum. If nausea occurs, place the patient prone to relieve pressure symptoms and alert the charge nurse. Gastric decompression may be necessary, and if conventional measures fail, surgical intervention (duodenojejunostomy—making an opening into the small intestine) may be necessary.

Patient teaching includes information about cleaning around the cast site with a mild soap and rinsing excessive soap so that it does not accumulate around

Skill 4-1   Care of the Patient in a Cast

Nursing Action (Rationale)

1. Patient teaching. *(Ensures patient cooperation; reduces patient anxiety.)*
   a. Explain why the cast is being applied and how it will be applied. *(Sudden movement during procedure could cause injury.)*
   b. Advise the patient that the plaster cast will feel warm as it dries.
   c. Explain the extent of immobilization.
   d. Explain care of the cast and expectations after discharge.
   e. Instruct patient not to insert sharp objects (coat hangers or pencils) under the cast. *(These may abrade the skin and lead to infection.)*
2. Handling the new cast. *(A fiberglass cast dries immediately after application; a plaster extremity cast dries*

in approximately 24 to 48 hours; a plaster spica or body cast dries in 48 to 72 hours [see Figure 4-29].)
   a. Support wet cast with the flat of the hands or on pillows. *(Avoids indentations that will cause pressure on underlying skin.)*
   b. Place cotton blankets or other absorbent material under the cast. *(Aids drying of cast.)*
   c. Expose the cast to air as much as possible. *(Aids drying of cast.)*
   d. Turn the patient frequently. *(Aids drying of cast.)*
   e. Use a cast dryer or hair dryer on a warm (not hot) setting. *(Circulates air over the cast.)*
   f. Do not apply paint, varnish, or shellac to the cast. *(Plaster is a porous material that allows air to circulate to the skin.)*

3. Skin care. *(Decreases the chance of skin irritation or tissue injury.)*
   a. Inspect skin at edges of cast and underlying cast for erythema or skin impairment.
   b. Remove plaster crumbs from skin with a washcloth moistened with warm water.
   c. Use creams and lotions sparingly. *(They may soften the skin and cause the cast to stick to the skin.)*
   d. Apply waterproof material around perineal area. *(Prevents soiling of and damage to cast and prevents skin impairment.)*
   e. Attend to patient's complaint of pain under the cast, particularly over bony prominences. *(This may indicate pressure on the skin.)* If discomfort is not relieved by repositioning, report to physician *(Cast pressure may need to be relieved by windowing or bivalving [cutting into halves].)*
4. Turning: Turning to any position is generally permitted as long as the integrity of the cast is not compromised and the patient is comfortable; do not turn by grasping the abductor bar. *(It is not safe transport.)*
5. Toileting for a long leg or hip spica cast.
   a. Use a fracture pan with blanket roll or padding. *(Provides support under the small of the back.)*
   b. Elevate the head of the bed, if permitted, or place the bed in reverse Trendelenburg position. *(Eases procedure.)*
6. Abdominal discomfort: Cast may be "windowed" (an opening cut into it). *(Provides relief of abdominal distention or a port for checking bladder distention.)*
7. Mobilization.
   a. The physician decides whether and how much weight bearing is allowed.
   b. A cast shoe or a walking heel is incorporated into a lower extremity cast (see Figure 4-30). *(Permits weight bearing without damaging the cast.)*
8. Prevention of neurovascular problems: Establish baseline measurements and assess neurovascular status before cast application; palpate distal pulses; assess color, temperature, and capillary refill of the appropriate fingers or toes; assess neurologic function, including sensation and motion in the affected and unaffected extremity. *(Changes in neurovascular status may occur after casting, possibly further compromising already injured tissues. Note the baseline neurovascular status so that those changes, if they occur, can be readily assessed.)*
   a. Perform neurovascular checks every hour for at least 24 hours after cast application to detect difficulty from edema or pressure of cast on nerves or vessels; notify physician of color changes, alterations in sensation, or motion unrelieved by position change; cast may need to be bivalved to relieve pressure (see illustration below).
   b. Elevate affected extremity on pillows. *(Danger of edema is usually 24 to 48 hours.)*
   c. After mobilization of patient with lower extremity or upper extremity cast, avoid keeping extremity in dependent position for prolonged periods. *(Prevents edema.)*
   d. After lower extremity cast is removed, encourage patient to wear elastic stocking and elevate affected leg while at rest until full mobility is regained. *(After immobilization, the involved joints and muscles will be weak and range of motion may be limited. Activity must be resumed slowly. Elastic stockings enhance deepvein circulation.)*

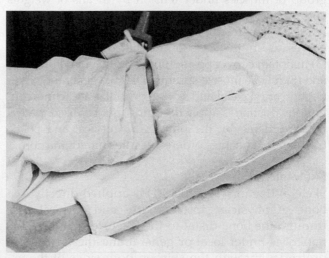

Step **8a**

the cast and impair the skin. A synthetic cast can be flushed with water if it becomes soiled. It must be dried afterward to prevent skin impairment and maceration (softening). A synthetic cast can be dried by blotting it with a towel and then using a blow dryer on cool or warm setting in a sweeping motion across the cast. Proper drying may take as long as 1 hour.

Patients often complain of pruritus (itching) of the skin that is covered by a cast (especially after having the cast for a few weeks). Recommend diversional activities when the pruritus begins. Also advise the patient to gently rub the area below and above the cast to decrease the desire to scratch. Warn patients not to stick sharp objects underneath the cast to relieve the pruritus. This may impair the skin and result in serious complications.

CAST REMOVAL

Casts are removed with an electric vibrating saw rather than a cutting saw. Reassure patients that there is little risk of the saw injuring the skin beneath the cast, even though it is noisy and looks like a cutting saw. Cutting the cast can cause a very fine powder or dust to escape into the air. If this powder is inhaled over a period of time, the plaster deposits can build up in the lungs' small air sacs and cause respiratory distress. It is a safe practice for the nurse, the physician, and the patient to wear masks when casts are removed with a cast cutter.

After removal of a cast, eliminate the buildup of secretions and dead skin on the affected extremity by gently washing and applying lotion or cream to the area. This may take several days, but caution the patient against trying to remove the devitalized material rapidly for fear of causing skin impairment. Muscle atrophy is common, especially if the extremity has been casted for several weeks. Reassure the patient that the muscle will regain strength and size with proper exercise through either physical therapy or home exercise programs.

TRACTION

Traction is the process of putting an extremity, bone, or group of muscles under tension by means of weights and pulleys to (1) align and stabilize a fracture site by reducing the fractured part, (2) relieve pressure on nerves as in the case of herniated disk syndrome, (3) maintain correct positioning, (4) prevent deformities, and (5) relieve muscle spasms. The two general types of traction are skeletal and skin. To stabilize a fracture, continuous traction is applied; it must not be disconnected unless ordered by the physician. Cervical and pelvic traction is sometimes ordered as intermittent traction.

Skeletal Traction

Skeletal traction (Figure 4-31) is applied directly to a bone. A physician inserts wires and surgical pins through the bone distal to the fracture site while the patient is under local or general anesthesia. The pin protrudes through the skin on both sides of the extremity, and traction is applied with weights attached to a rope that is tied to a spreader bar. Skeletal traction can be used for fractures of the femur (see Figure 4-31, *A*), tibia (see Figure 4-31, *B*), humerus, and cervical spine (see Chapter 14).

Skin Traction

Skin traction uses weight that pulls on sponge rubber, moleskin, and elastic bandage with adherent or plastic materials attached to the skin below the site of the fracture, with the pull exerted on the limb. Buck's, Russell's, and Bryant's are types of skin traction.

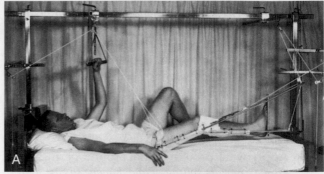

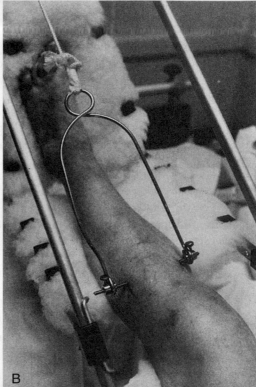

FIGURE 4-31 A, Balanced suspension skeletal traction to the femur. **B,** Tibial pin traction with Steinmann pin used in treatment of distal femoral fracture. The bow attached to the pin provides a place of attachment for the rope that holds the traction weights. The pull exerted by the weight keeps the fracture fragments aligned. Pin sites must be inspected at least daily to detect signs of pin reaction or infection.

Buck's Traction

Buck's traction (Figure 4-32, *C*) is used as a temporary measure to provide support and comfort to a fractured extremity while waiting for more definitive treatment. Traction (pull) is in a horizontal plane with affected extremity. This traction is frequently used to maintain the reduction of a hip fracture before surgery. It can also be used to treat muscle spasms and minor fractures of the lower spine.

Russell's Traction

Russell's traction (Figure 4-32, *B*) is set up similar to Buck's traction. However, a knee sling supports the affected leg. It allows more movement in bed and permits flexion of the knee joint. Russell's traction is commonly used to treat hip and knee fractures.

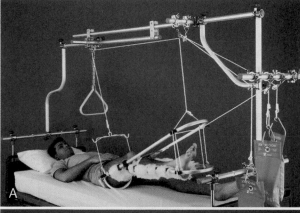

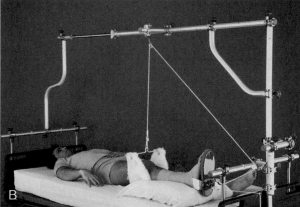

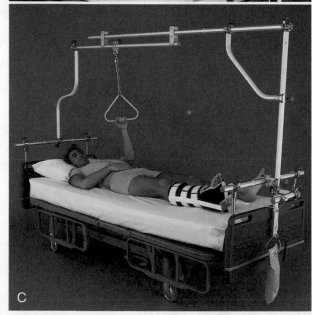

FIGURE 4-32 A, Balanced traction with a Thomas ring and a Pearson attachment. **B,** Russell's traction. **C,** Buck's traction.

Nursing Interventions

Nursing interventions of patients in traction include measures to maintain the body in proper alignment and careful assessment of traction equipment. Care of a patient in skeletal traction involves assessment of the pin sites and application of hydrogen peroxide or normal saline per physician's order. Traction care is summarized in Box 4-6.

Box 4-6	**Nursing Interventions for the Patient in Traction**

- Maintain the patient's body in proper alignment. The force or pull on the extremities should be in alignment with the long axis of the bone.
- Ensure that weights hang freely from the bed and are never removed without a physician's order.
- Question patients as to their understanding of the purpose of the traction, and assess their ability to use a trapeze bar for self-movement. Elevate the foot of the bed to help prevent the patient from sliding down toward the foot of the bed (countertraction).
- Observe the condition of the traction cords, making sure they are not weakened or frayed. All knots used on the rope or cord are to be square knots.
- Center the ropes on the traction pulley.
- Assess, document, and report neurovascular impairment.
- Ensure that weight used is the correct weight as ordered by the physician.
- Carefully observe the skin for signs of impairment. Use sheepskin heel protectors and bed pads to reduce impairment.
- If skeletal traction is used, assess the pin site for signs of infection. Cleanse the pin site every 8 hours with hydrogen peroxide or normal saline, as ordered.
- Assess the distal pulses bilaterally for circulatory integrity of the extremities.
- Inspect for loss of sensation in the dorsal area of the foot with weakness and inversion of the foot (inside surface turned outward).

ORTHOPEDIC DEVICES

Frames can be used for orthopedic patients to assist with turning and positioning while maintaining proper alignment. The **Balkan frame** is a wooden or steel attachment to the hospital bed. It has adjustable pulleys and a trapeze bar attached to an overhead bar.

The **Bradford frame** is made of rectangular steel with two pieces of canvas stretched tightly and laced to the frame. A space is left in the buttocks area for toileting and hygiene.

The **Stryker wedge turning frame** and **Foster bed** are similar and assist in changing the patient's position from supine to prone. Patients may become apprehensive when turned on a frame for fear of falling, so thorough explanations and reassurances are helpful.

The **CircOlectric bed** is a vertical turning bed that can be operated electrically by one person and placed in a variety of positions. Side-to-side movement can be accomplished while maintaining proper positioning if traction is ordered.

The **RotoRest bed** can rock a patient as much as 62 degrees, 17 times per hour. The electric-powered bed can help heal pressure ulcers, prevent venous thrombosis, and reduce kidney stone formation. Orthopedic traction can be attached to the bed, as well as a television set for diversional activity.

Crutch Safety

Crutch safety involves:
- Proper measurement (with weight on hands, not axillae, to avoid brachial plexus paralysis); leave a 2-inch width between the axillary fold and the armpiece on the crutches.
- Rubber tips on the ends of the crutches to prevent slippage.
- Adequate muscle strength in the upper extremities to support the patient's weight.

Splints, crutches, and **braces** are used to immobilize and assist with ambulation. There are numerous types of splints and braces, and it is important that the nurse understand the procedure for proper application for each one.

Safety is the first concern when ambulatory devices such as crutches are used. Encourage the patient to do push-ups by pressing the hands against the mattress and lifting the upper body to gain muscle strength. Types of **crutch walking** depend on the number of points making contact with the floor (Figure 4-33). For

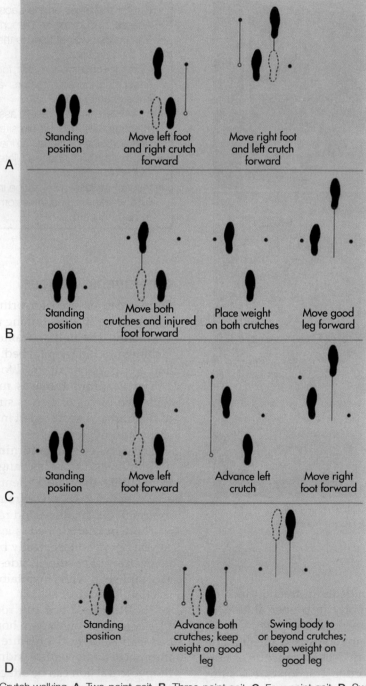

A
| Standing position | Move left foot and right crutch forward | Move right foot and left crutch forward |

B
| Standing position | Move both crutches and injured foot forward | Place weight on both crutches | Move good leg forward |

C
| Standing position | Move left foot forward | Advance left crutch | Move right foot forward |

D
| Standing position | Advance both crutches; keep weight on good leg | Swing body to or beyond crutches; keep weight on good leg |

FIGURE 4-33 Crutch walking. **A,** Two-point gait. **B,** Three-point gait. **C,** Four-point gait. **D,** Swing-through gait.

example, a three-point gait involves two crutch points plus one leg making contact with the floor (patient must have strong arms to support body weight). Instead of a three-point gait, patients may use the four-point gait (slower, but stable) or two-point gait (faster; requires balance). Another type of crutch walking is swing-to or swing-through gait, in which the patient swings the body up to or beyond the two points of the crutch tips. Most crutch walking is taught by a physical therapist (Figure 4-34). However, the nurse monitors the patient's progress.

Older patients are more likely to use **cane walking** for balance and support. Instruct the patient to hold the cane in the opposite hand of the affected extremity and advance the cane at the same time the affected leg moves forward. An effective rubber tip on the point will help prevent slippage (Figure 4-35). Older adults

also use walkers to maintain balance. Safety concerns are the same as those for the cane (Figure 4-36).

The Roll-A-Bout walker is a new gait enhancer designed for patients who have an injury below the knee such as a fractured tibia, fibula, ankle, or foot. The Roll-A-Bout allows the patient to distribute weight evenly by placing the knee of the injured leg on the knee pad and propelling the Roll-A-Bout with the unaffected leg (Figure 4-37).

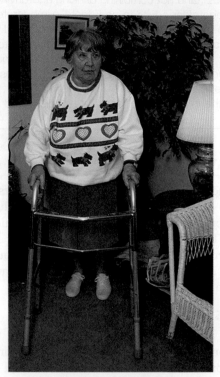

FIGURE 4-36 Patient using a walker.

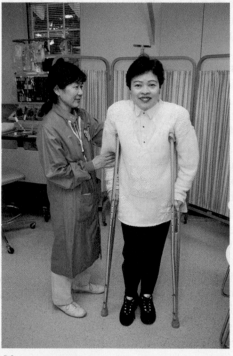

FIGURE 4-34 Assisting the patient with crutch walking. Note how the therapist guards the patient and how the patient's elbows are at no more than 30 degrees of flexion.

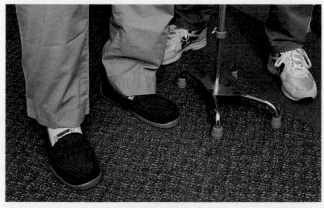

FIGURE 4-35 Quad cane.

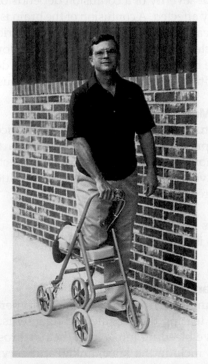

FIGURE 4-37 The Roll-A-Bout walker.

Preventing Musculoskeletal Trauma

- Teach patients and community members to take appropriate safety precautions to prevent injuries while at home, at work, when driving, or when participating in sports.
- Be a vocal advocate for personal actions known to reduce injuries such as regularly using seatbelts, driving within posted speed limits, stretching before exercise, using protective athletic equipment (helmets and knee, wrist, and elbow pads), and not combining drinking and driving.
- Encourage older adults to participate in moderate exercise to aid in the maintenance of muscle strength and balance.
- To reduce falls, examine older adults' living environment to rule out the use of scatter rugs, to ensure adequate footwear and lighting, and to clear paths to bathrooms for night-time use.
- Stress the importance of adequate calcium and vitamin D intake.

TRAUMATIC INJURIES

Traumatic injuries to the musculoskeletal system can occur in all age-groups. However, older adults may have disorders that predispose them to musculoskeletal injuries. The more serious injuries involving fractures are treated in a hospital, whereas the less serious—such as contusions, sprains, or strains—may be treated in an outpatient facility.

CONTUSIONS

Etiology and Pathophysiology

Contusions are the most common soft tissue injury. An injury from a blow or blunt force causes local bleeding under the skin and possibly a hematoma (sac filled with blood). The severity of a contusion depends on the part of the body affected. A contusion of the brain is very serious, whereas a contusion of the arm is less serious. Large areas affected by soft tissue bleeding with slow absorption of the blood have a higher potential of developing into cellulitis (an infection of the subcutaneous tissue).

Medical Management

Most contusions are treated by applying ice bags or cold compresses for 15 to 20 minutes at a time over 12 to 36 hours for the vasoconstricting effects of cold. The involved extremity is elevated to reduce edema and suppress pain.

Prognosis

Prognosis is excellent.

SPRAINS

Etiology and Pathophysiology

Sprains can result from a wrenching or hyperextension of a joint, tearing the capsule and ligaments. A sprain can involve bleeding into a joint (hemarthrosis). Common sites include the knee, ankle, and cervical spine (whiplash). Sprains are often the result of a sudden, twisting injury. Medical management is similar to that for contusions. Treatment usually consists of elevation, compression, ice, and rest of the affected area.

Prognosis

Prognosis is excellent.

WHIPLASH

Etiology, Pathophysiology, and Clinical Manifestations

Injury at the cervical spine, or whiplash, is classified under cervical disk syndrome. Whiplash is caused by an injury that involves hyperextension, which results in compression of the anatomical structures. This type of injury usually occurs as a result of sudden acceleration and deceleration, such as rear-end car collisions that cause violent back-and-forth movements of the head and neck. Symptoms of a whiplash (primarily pain) may not be obvious for a few days or even a week after the injury. Cervical fractures can accompany a whiplash injury.

Assessment

Collection of **subjective data** includes the patient's complaint of pain (the most common symptom), which usually begins in the cervical area but may radiate down the arm to the fingers and increase with cervical motion. The pain may increase sharply with coughing, sneezing, or any radical movement. Other signs and symptoms may be paresthesia (numbness or tingling), headache, blurred vision, decreased skeletal function, and weakened hand grip.

Objective data include edema in the cervical spine region with tightening of the muscles. Vital signs are usually within normal ranges. However, if the assessment findings indicate hypertension with widened pulse pressure and bradycardia, suspect increased intracranial pressure (ICP); report and document the findings immediately. Do a neurologic assessment every 15 to 30 minutes to rule out increased ICP.

Diagnostic Tests

Physical examination and radiographic studies confirm the physician's diagnosis.

Medical Management

Symptoms commonly recur. A medical approach is most often used for treatment of whiplash. Analgesics and muscle relaxants are prescribed, along with intermittent cervical traction. Surgery may be necessary if cervical fracture with displacement occurs. (See Herniation of Intervertebral Disk [Herniated Nucleus Pulposus] later in the chapter.)

Other treatments include special exercises, heat therapy, and administration of mild analgesics as ordered by the physician to control the pain. A soft foam rubber neck brace collar may be used for whiplash injuries to limit head movement.

Nursing Interventions

Nursing interventions include care of the patient with restricted activity to immobilize the cervical vertebrae, decrease irritation, and provide rest for the traumatized area. This is accomplished with cervical traction. If a neck brace is used, carefully inspect the skin around the neck and chin for signs of excoriation.

Prognosis

Prognosis depends on the extent of neurologic involvement. Prognosis is excellent with minor trauma, but because the spinal canal is full of neural tissue in the cervical area, more extensive injury can produce profound disability.

ANKLE SPRAINS

Etiology and Pathophysiology

An ankle sprain is often referred to as a twisted ankle and is caused by a wrenching or twisting of the foot and ankle.

Clinical Manifestations

The ankle area becomes edematous quickly, with spasms of the muscles and pain on passive movement of the joint.

Assessment

Collection of **subjective data** includes assessment of pain and tenderness in the affected ankle that intensifies with movement of the foot or ankle.

Collection of **objective data** includes assessment of the traumatized ankle for signs of edema, limited movement and function of the joint, and ecchymosis of the soft tissue around the ankle.

Diagnostic Tests

A radiographic examination of the injured area is the only accurate way to ensure there is no bone injury.

Medical Management

Surgery may be indicated for severe sprains. The physician sutures torn ligament fibers together. If the ligaments have been torn from the bone, the surgeon reattaches them by drilling small holes in the medial malleolus (rounded bony protrusion on the medial area of the ankle).

Nursing Interventions

The injured area must be elevated and kept at rest. Application of ice for 15 to 20 minutes intermittently for

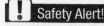 **Safety Alert!**

Strains and Sprains

A strain and a sprain are not the same. Strains are produced by minute muscle tears and overstretching of tendons, whereas sprains are caused by a twisting of the joint

12 to 36 hours—followed after 24 hours by the application of mild heat for 15 to 30 minutes, four times daily—will promote absorption of blood and fluid from the area. Use compressive dressings and splinting to help support the injured area. A neurovascular assessment is necessary to detect impaired tissue perfusion.

Prognosis

Prognosis is generally excellent.

STRAINS

Etiology and Pathophysiology

Strains are characterized by microscopic muscle tears as a result of overstretching muscles and tendons. An acute strain results when the muscles and tendons are overstretched in a forceful movement, such as unaccustomed vigorous exercise.

Assessment

Collection of **subjective data** includes noting the patient's complaint of sudden and severe pain away from the joint, which increases with activity. Chronic muscle strain can occur from repeated muscle overuse, and the pain may not appear for several hours. The patient typically complains of soreness, stiffness, and tenderness in the area.

Collection of **objective data** includes observation of stiffness, ecchymosis, and slight edema over the injury site. The most common sites are calf muscles, hamstrings, quadriceps, and the lumbosacral area. Edema can occur rapidly in the muscle and tendon area.

Diagnostic Tests

A radiographic study is necessary to rule out bone trauma.

Medical Management

Surgical repair is necessary if the muscle is completely ruptured. The physician orders analgesics and muscle relaxants. An exercise program is almost always prescribed if the strain is in the lumbosacral region. The exercises are aimed at strengthening the lower abdominal muscles.

Nursing Interventions

Nursing interventions for a strain are similar to those for a sprain. Ice application helps relieve pain, but some physicians prefer heat application rather than ice. Back strains are among the most common strains. If the symptoms worsen, advise the patient to avoid strenuous activities, use a firm chair with rigid back support, avoid wearing high heels, use a firm mattress for sleep, and never sleep on the abdomen. Encourage the patient to do leg exercises to prevent development of thrombosis.

Prognosis

Prognosis is usually favorable.

DISLOCATIONS

Etiology and Pathophysiology

Dislocations usually involve tearing of the joint capsule; subluxations (partial or incomplete dislocations) involve stretching of the joint capsule. Both are temporary displacements of bones from their normal position within joints. A dislocation may be (1) congenital (e.g., congenital hip displacement), (2) caused by a disease process, or (3) caused by trauma. A dislocation or subluxation can also be accompanied by stretching and tearing of ligaments and tendons and by fractures. The displaced bone may rupture blood vessels. When subluxation occurs, the joint's articulating (movable) surfaces are partially separated.

Clinical Manifestations

Dislocation may or may not be visible. Sometimes a dislocation changes the length of an affected extremity. Pain and loss of function may be similar to those occurring with a fracture. However, dislocation partially immobilizes a joint, whereas a fracture site typically has abnormal free movement. Common dislocation sites include the shoulder, hip, and knee.

Assessment

Subjective data include the patient's description of the injury and pain. For shoulder dislocation, the patient complains of sensation loss and paresthesia.

Collection of **objective data** includes the assessment of any erythema, discoloration, edema, pain, tenderness, limitation of movement, and deformity or shortening of the extremity. Compare both sides for validation. Neurovascular assessment is important to determine whether vascular or nerve injury is present in the affected area. For shoulder dislocation, assess for an absent radial pulse, hypothermia of the hand, and wrist drop.

Diagnostic Tests

The diagnosis is based on complaints of discomfort, physical examination, and diagnostic radiographic examination of the injured site.

Medical Management

The physician may perform a closed reduction, which corrects the deformity through manipulation of the extremity. Surgical intervention to restore joint articulation is sometimes required.

Nursing Interventions and Patient Teaching

Nursing interventions include (1) reduction of edema and discomfort, (2) immobilization of the injured part to promote healing, and (3) patient education. Ice application is recommended for the first 24 hours after trauma. After 24 hours, heat may be used if there are no indications of bleeding. Elevation of the injured extremity on pillows and the application of elastic bandages help relieve edema. Immobilization of joints may involve application of a splint, sling, or elastic bandage. The air cast or air splint brace is an immobilization device. It is inflatable, is lightweight, and conforms to the extremity's size and shape. When immobilization devices are used, perform a neurovascular assessment frequently (see Box 4-5 and Nursing Diagnoses box below). Administer analgesics as prescribed by the physician. Asking the patient to rate the pain on a scale from 0 to 10 is helpful in determining pain severity. For control of extreme pain, the physician may order an opioid, such as morphine. For moderate to mild pain, ibuprofen or acetaminophen (Tylenol) may be prescribed. Positioning and repositioning the injured part can help reduce discomfort.

Nursing diagnoses and interventions for the patient for neurovascular integrity include but are not limited to the following:

Nursing Diagnoses	Nursing Interventions
Ineffective peripheral tissue perfusion, related to: • injury • treatment	Position extremities in alignment; elevate affected extremity. Carefully monitor distal pulses, capillary refill, and temperature of involved area.
Risk for injury, related to neurovascular impairment	Compare affected extremity with unaffected extremity, using same hand for palpation. Test capillary refill (blanching test). Check each digit for sensation and motion. Document location and characteristics of pain. Palpate pedal, tibial, or radial pulses, and compare with unaffected extremity. Assess for edema with pallor, cyanosis, and coldness. Ask patient to describe sensations. Document all findings.

Promoting an accident-free environment is essential. Areas of preventive medicine to explore with patients include the following:

- Grab bars mounted in the bathroom near the toilet or tub and rubber mats or slip guards in the tub and shower help prevent falls.
- Removing throw rugs and obstacles from the floor can prevent falls.
- A gait enhancer, such as a cane, crutches, or a walker, must be used correctly and with attention to safety precautions, such as using rubber tips

on the points that make contact with the floor to prevent slippage.

- Patients in the hospital are at risk of falling out of bed if their disease, condition, or medication results in disorientation. Carefully assess their level of orientation, keep side rails up, and provide safety reminder devices to prevent self-injury.
- Using a safe ladder when climbing can help prevent a fall.
- Wearing protective clothing while engaging in dangerous work or contact sports is recommended.

Appropriate health teaching should be targeted for people at risk for musculoskeletal diseases, such as osteoporosis, which can predispose them to pathologic or nontraumatic fractures.

Prognosis

Prognosis is generally excellent.

AIRBAG INJURIES

Airbag deployment injuries include chemical burns, ocular trauma, cervical injury, soft tissue injury, and upper extremity and chest trauma. Orthopedic injuries tend to involve the upper extremities, especially the wrist, hand, and elbow. Injuries from airbag deployment can be life threatening in the very young. People at increased risk include older adults and small children. Airbag-induced injuries are associated with a rapid, forceful inflation, lasting less than 1 second from inflation to deflation. Research is continuing to develop safer airbag deployment.

CARPAL TUNNEL SYNDROME

Etiology and Pathophysiology

Carpal tunnel syndrome is a painful disorder of the wrist and hand. It is caused by inflammation and edema of the synovial lining of the tendon sheaths in the carpal tunnel of the wrist. As a result, the tunnel space is narrowed, resulting in compression of the median nerve between the inelastic carpal ligament and other structures in the carpal tunnel (Figure 4-38). The

symptoms of **paresthesia** (any subjective sensation such as pricks of pins and needles) and **hypoesthesia** (a decrease in sensation in response to stimulation of the sensory nerves) of the thumb, index, and middle fingers may develop spontaneously or occur as a result of disease or injury.

This condition has a higher incidence in obese, middle-aged women and individuals employed in occupations involving repetitive motions of the fingers and hands (e.g., computing, hairdressing, basket weaving, meat carving, and typing). Carpal tunnel syndrome has become one of the three most common industrial or work-related conditions and is related to increased computer usage. Edema of the tendon sheaths caused by RA can predispose a patient to carpal tunnel syndrome. Curiously, pregnant women may develop the syndrome during their last trimester. The reasons for this are unknown, but it may be related to fluid retention and edema.

Clinical Manifestations

The affected hand has altered ability to grasp or hold small objects. Atrophy of the thenar eminence (the padded area of the palm below the base of the thumb) is noted as the disease progresses. The clinical manifestations also include burning pain, numbness and weakness (especially of the thumb) (Lewis et al., 2007).

Assessment

Subjective data include the patient's description of discomfort, such as burning pain or tingling in the hands relieved by vigorously shaking or exercising the hands. Pain may be intermittent or constant and is often more intense at night. The patient may also complain of numbness (hypoesthesia) of the thumb, index, and ring fingers, especially after prolonged flexion of the wrist; and inability to grasp or hold small objects.

Collection of **objective data** includes assessment of the hand, wrist, or fingers for edema; muscle atrophy; or a depressed appearance of the soft tissue at the base of the thumb on the palmar surface.

Diagnostic Tests

Physical examination reveals deficits in sensory mapping along median nerve innervation pathways; positive Tinel's sign; increased tingling with a gentle tap over the tendon sheath on the ventral surface of the central wrist; edema of the fingers; and thenar surfaces of the palm thinner than normal (wasting). Having the patient hold the wrists against each other in forced palmar flexion for 1 minute can elicit sensory changes of numbness and tingling, which is a positive Phalen's maneuver test (one indication of carpal tunnel syndrome).

An electromyogram shows a weakened muscle response to stimulation. MRI shows compression and flattening of the median nerve, increased signal intensity within the median nerve, and abrupt changes in diameter of the median nerve. A handheld electroneu-

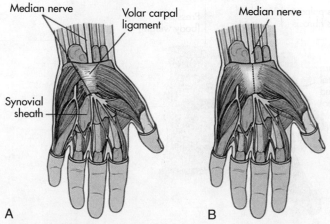

Median nerve Volar carpal ligament   Median nerve

Synovial sheath

A   B

FIGURE 4-38 A, Wrist structures involved in carpal tunnel syndrome. **B,** Decompression of median nerve.

rometer predicts motor latency of the median nerve, which is diagnostic of carpal tunnel syndrome.

Medical Management

If the symptoms are mild and surgery is not a desirable option, an immobilizer such as a splint can be used. Hydrocortisone acetate suspension injected into the carpal tunnel can relieve mild symptoms. Surgery is indicated for severe symptoms with muscle atrophy. The standard surgical treatment is decompression of the median nerve by section of the transverse carpal ligament.

Nursing Interventions and Patient Teaching

Educate the patient about special keyboard pads and mouse devices that may be used to prevent pressure on the medial nerve for computer users. The patient should be encouraged to change body positions and take breaks from activities which promote medial nerve pressure (Lewis et al., 2007).

If surgery is not required, the nurse is involved in the application of an immobilizer to promote comfort. General nursing interventions are use of a wrist cock-up splint to relieve pressure and to lessen wrist flexion, elevation to relieve edema, ROM exercises to lessen sense of clumsiness, and restriction of twisting and turning activities of the wrist.

If surgery is required, postoperative interventions include (1) elevating the hand and arm for 24 hours; (2) implementing and evaluating active thumb and finger motion within limits imposed by the dressing; (3) administering prescribed analgesics as needed; (4) monitoring vital signs (temperature elevation could indicate infection); and (5) checking fingers for circulation, sensation, and movement every 1 to 2 hours for 24 hours.

Encourage patients to use the affected hand in normal activities as soon as 2 to 3 days after surgery.

Prognosis

Mild symptoms of carpal tunnel syndrome are relieved by nonsurgical treatment; severe symptoms require surgical intervention with excellent prognosis. If the patient is pregnant, symptoms are usually relieved after delivery.

HERNIATION OF INTERVERTEBRAL DISK (HERNIATED NUCLEUS PULPOSUS)

Etiology and Pathophysiology

Herniated nucleus pulposus is a rupture of the fibrocartilage surrounding an intervertebral disk, releasing the nucleus pulposus that cushions the vertebrae above and below. This displacement puts pressure on nerve roots. Lumbar and cervical herniations are most common (Figure 4-39). Herniated nucleus pulposus can occur suddenly (from lifting, twisting, or trauma) or gradually (from degenerative changes, as seen with DJD, osteoporosis, aging, and chronic diseases affecting bones). Herniations of the lumbar spine usually affect people 20 to 45 years old; cervical herniations are seen most in people 45 years and older. Men are more prone to this disorder than women.

Clinical Manifestations

Low back pain that occurs with the slightest movement is the most common symptom of lumbar herniation. The pain radiates over the buttock and down the leg, following the sciatic nerve pathway **(radicular pain),** causing numbness and tingling in the affected leg. Neck pain, headache, and neck rigidity are common symptoms of cervical herniations. Complaints of pain in the back radiating down the leg (sciatica) are common. Complaints about activity intolerance and alteration in bowel and bladder elimination (constipation and urinary retention) are significant.

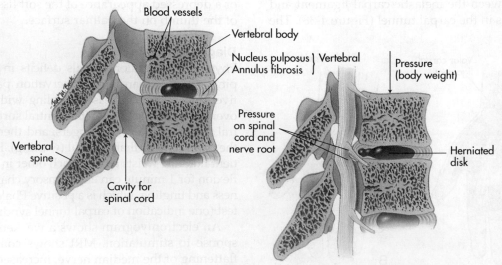

FIGURE 4-39 Sagittal section of vertebrae showing both normal *(left)* and herniated disks.

Assessment

Collection of **subjective data** includes assessing pain and asking patient about measures used for relief and other possible symptoms, such as activity intolerance and altered bowel and bladder function. Pain often gets worse with activity.

Collection of **objective data** includes observing for signs of limited spinal flexibility (limited forward bending) and gait alteration (patient may support weight on one extremity). An ineffective breathing pattern may result from pain and decreased mobility. Assessment includes determination of bowel and bladder elimination and maintenance of traction equipment.

Diagnostic Tests

Obtain a complete history and physical examination. The physician orders radiographic studies, CT, myelography, and electromyelography to determine nerve involvement.

Medical Management

The patient usually follows a 4-week course of conservative therapy such as braces, corset, or belt, local heat or ice, ultrasound and massage, and transcutaneous electrical nerve stimulation (TENS). Drug therapy such as NSAIDs, muscle relaxants, and epidural corticosteroid therapy may be used (Lewis et al., 2007). If the patient demonstrates neurologic deterioration or continued pain, a surgical procedure may be required, such as one of the following:

- **Laminectomy:** Surgical removal of the bony arches or one or more vertebrae performed to relieve compression of the spinal cord caused by bone displacement from an injury or degeneration of a disk or to remove a displaced vertebral disk.
- **Spinal fusion** (arthrodesis; the surgical immobilization of a joint; artificial ankylosis): Removal of the lamina and several herniated nuclei pulposi. A portion of bone taken from the patient's iliac crest or from a bone bank is used as a bone graft in the vertebral spaces.
- **Diskectomy:** Removal of the extruded disk material, often with a microscope. Percutaneous lateral diskectomy—cutting a window around the anulus fibrosus—is performed with the patient under local anesthesia.
- **Artificial disk replacement:** Replacement of a damaged intervertebral disk with an artificial disk called Charité disk. The damaged disk is removed and the Charité disk placed in the spine. The disk allows the natural movement of the spine (U.S. Food & Drug Administration, 2004).
- **Endoscopic spinal microsurgery:** Can be performed with the patient under local anesthesia. Special scopes enable the surgeon to successfully remove herniated disks with minimal damage to surrounding tissues.
- **Chemonucleolysis:** Can be done on patients who have no nerve involvement. The procedure involves administering a local anesthetic agent and then guiding a needle into the nucleus pulposus to inject chymopapain (a drug that dissolves the nucleus pulposus).

Postoperative laminectomy care includes assessing the incision site for signs of infection such as drainage, edema, odor, and temperature elevation. Use of surgical asepsis when changing dressings and handling drainage decreases development of infection. After a chemonucleolysis, carefully assess for signs of allergic reactions to chymopapain, such as urticaria and respiratory difficulties.

Nursing Interventions and Patient Teaching

Nursing interventions are aimed at providing nursing care appropriate for the following nursing diagnoses:

- Anxiety, related to discomfort, fear of unknown, and lifestyle changes
- Pain (back), related to muscle spasms and painful diagnostic tests
- Constipation and impaired urinary elimination, related to pain, analgesics, immobility, and neurologic involvement

Give the patient and family information about procedures and hospital protocol to help reduce their anxiety. Administer the medications prescribed on schedule, and document the effectiveness of the medication. Distraction, heat or ice application (if ordered), and moving (by log-rolling) and positioning the patient every 2 hours (if not contraindicated because of need to maintain traction) can promote patient comfort. Dietary monitoring is important to ensure that the patient maintains a high-protein, iron- and vitamin-enriched diet.

Observe dressing for bleeding or cerebrospinal fluid leakage. Apply antiembolism stockings if ordered. Careful documentation of I&O provides information about bowel and bladder function. Ensure that the patient has voided in the first 8 hours, and use nursing measures to promote voiding before resorting to catheterization. Encourage the patient to sit in a straight, firm chair for no longer than 30 minutes at one time. Monitor the patient for evidence of respiratory distress and paralytic ileus, complications that may occur in laminectomy patients.

Nursing diagnoses and interventions for the patient with herniated disk include but are not limited to the following:

Nursing Diagnoses	Nursing Interventions
Deficient knowledge, related to home care management	Stress importance of rehabilitation plan of activity, rest, and exercise.

Continued

Nursing Diagnoses	Nursing Interventions
Deficient knowledge, related to home care management—cont'd	Provide diet instructions related to type and amount of food and weight maintenance (no gain) if applicable. Discuss medications: name, purpose, schedule, dosage, and side effects. Discuss signs and symptoms to report to physician: severe pain; changes in temperature, color, or sensation in extremity; and malodorous drainage from wound. Encourage follow-up visits with physician.
Powerlessness, related to: • decreased mobility • pain	Use active listening and permit verbalization of anger and helplessness. Assist patient in identifying coping mechanisms that will reduce feeling of powerlessness; use those that have been successful in the past. Offer positive recognition for increased activity level. Assist patient in identifying areas that can be controlled. Involve patient in decision-making process for own care.

The patient may begin activity out of bed as early as 1 day after a simple laminectomy or 2 to 4 days after a laminectomy and fusion. Transfer the patient out of bed with as little time spent in the sitting position as possible. The patient may be permitted to walk as much as tolerated, with assistance if necessary. Braces or corsets, if prescribed, are applied before the patient gets out of bed. Encourage the patient to participate in ADLs within prescribed limits of mobility.

Instruct the patient not to lift or carry anything heavier than 5 pounds (2.25 kg) for at least 8 weeks, not to drive a car until permitted by the surgeon, and to avoid twisting motions of the trunk. Reinforce the importance of follow-up visits to the physician.

Prognosis

With conservative treatment, some patients receive relief of symptoms; if a neurologic pathologic condition develops, surgical intervention is needed. The prognosis is usually favorable.

TUMORS OF THE BONE

Etiology and Pathophysiology

Tumors of the bone may be primary or secondary and may be benign or malignant. As with other types of tumors, the cause of bone tumors is not always known. Carcinoma of the prostate, lung, breast, thyroid, and kidney may metastasize to the bones. **Osteogenic** tumors are primary malignant bone tumors that occur most often in young people.

Osteogenic sarcoma is a fast-growing and aggressive tumor that affects the long bones of the body, particularly the distal femur, the proximal tibia, and the proximal humerus. Osteogenic sarcoma can metastasize to the lungs and to the rest of the body via the bloodstream. It affects males between the ages of 10 and 25 more often than females.

Osteochondroma is the most common benign osteogenic tumor. The incidence is highest in males between 10 and 30 years of age. Osteochondromas can occur as a single tumor or as multiple tumors. They usually affect the humerus, tibia, and femur.

Clinical Manifestations

When healthy bone cells are replaced by cancer cells, the bone's strength is altered and spontaneous fractures can occur. Anemia occurs when cancer invades the long bones and interrupts the manufacture of red blood cells in the bone marrow. Cancerous bone tumors metastasize and invade other bones and lung tissue.

Benign bone tumors can grow large enough to put pressure on blood vessels and nerves. Benign tumors do not spread. However, they may undergo cancerous changes and become malignant.

Assessment

Malignant and benign bone tumors cause pain in the affected bone site. **Subjective data** include complaints of pain, especially with weight bearing. Pain may result from a spontaneous fracture. The patient may also complain of tenderness at the affected site.

Collection of **objective data** includes assessment of the painful part, which may reveal edema and discoloration of the skin.

Diagnostic Tests

Diagnosis is confirmed with radiographic studies, bone scan, bone biopsy, and laboratory studies, such as a CBC (which reveals bone marrow involvement), serum protein levels (elevated in multiple myeloma), and serum alkaline phosphatase level (elevated in osteogenic sarcoma).

Medical Management

The physician evaluates the tumor type, size, and location and plans the treatment accordingly. Larger, symptomatic, benign tumors and malignant tumors require surgical intervention. The surgical procedure depends on the tumor size, location, and extent of tissue involvement. The surgery may involve (1) wide excision or resection, (2) bone curettage, or (3) leg or arm amputation.

Treatment is aimed at destroying or removing the malignant lesion. Amputation of the affected extremity may be necessary. Radiation and chemotherapy may be used before surgery to decrease tumor size or tissue involvement. Limb-salvage surgical procedures in combination with radiation and chemotherapy are being used more frequently for treatment of malignant bone tumors.

Chemotherapy is aimed at destroying cancer cells at both primary and metastatic sites. Patients usually receive chemotherapy in 3- or 4-week cycles. Radiation therapy may be given internally and externally. The nurse must know the safety precautions and side effects of chemotherapy and radiation therapy. (See Chapter 17 for a discussion of care of the patient with cancer.)

Nursing Interventions and Patient Teaching

Preoperatively the patient and family need complete and concise information about procedures and postoperative expectations. Postoperative nursing interventions include (1) performing a neurovascular assessment (see Box 4-5); (2) monitoring vital signs; (3) administering analgesics and evaluating the effectiveness; (4) providing cast care or dressing changes with careful documentation of drainage, odors, and signs of circulation impairment; (5) cooperating with physical and occupational therapists to promote mobility and ADLs; and (6) educating the patient and family about home health care and early detection of tumor recurrence

A nursing diagnosis and interventions for the patient with a bone tumor include but are not limited to the following:

Nursing Diagnosis	Nursing Interventions
Anxiety, related to: • fear of cancer • body image • lifestyle change • possibility of death	Establish therapeutic relationship: acknowledge fear, encourage patient to acknowledge and express feelings. Give accurate information about condition and therapies. Refer patient to other resources when necessary (e.g., social worker, religious counselor).

Prognosis

The prognosis for bone tumors has improved in recent years with the combination of local surgery, chemotherapy, and radiation. Disease-free survival rates for patients whose osteogenic sarcoma is treated with surgery, chemotherapy, and radiation appear to be greater than 50% at 5 years.

AMPUTATION

The amputation of a portion of or an entire extremity may be necessary because of malignant tumors, injuries, impaired circulation (caused by diabetes mellitus or arteriosclerosis), congenital deformities, and infections. Most amputations are elective surgery unless they are related to trauma. Advances in microsurgical techniques enable surgeons to reattach severed extremities. Therefore traumatic amputations can sometimes be reversed by replantation if the severed limb is kept sterile and moist in a plastic bag filled with ice water. (The part should be protected from direct contact with ice; dry ice should not be used.)

Amputation of long bones can result in postoperative anemia. A traumatic or surgical amputation of an extremity can cause serious blood loss. Malignant bone tumors can metastasize via the bloodstream to other body systems.

Preoperative Assessment

Collection of **subjective data** includes questioning the patient about his or her understanding of the injury or disease process. Assess and document complaints of pain and symptoms of neurovascular impairment. Assess the patient's level of orientation, since many amputations occur in the older adult population as a result of impaired circulation.

Collection of **objective data** includes assessment of vital signs (temperature elevation, tachycardia, and tachypnea indicate infection). Assess arterial blood flow by palpation of bilateral pedal pulses and Doppler pressure measurements. Assess wound drainage for color, amount, and presence of odor. Evaluate upper body muscle strength and nutritional status.

Diagnostic Tests

A CBC is done to determine blood dyscrasias, such as anemia and bleeding tendencies, which could increase postoperative complications (such as hemorrhage, delayed wound healing, and disorientation). The physician orders laboratory studies such as BUN, potassium levels, and routine urinalysis. An ECG is performed to detect cardiac dysrhythmias, which are often present in older adult patients.

Medical Management

When the amputation results from traumatic injury to an extremity, the physician's interventions include measures to restore circulating blood volume, control pain, prevent infection in the wound, perform a plastic surgical repair at the amputation site to facilitate the use of a prosthesis, and maintain adequate urinary output.

For elective amputations, the physician assesses the patient's physiologic, psychological, and emotional status. If infection is present in the body (gangrene may occur if circulation is impaired), treatment includes administration of antibiotics, and every attempt is made to control the infection before surgery. The physician discusses the possibility of the patient using a prosthesis. Much of the preoperative preparation focuses on the patient attaining a physical and emotional status conducive to wearing a prosthesis or achieving mobility through the use of a wheelchair or a gait enhancer such as crutches or a walker.

Postoperative Assessment, Nursing Interventions, and Patient Teaching

Collection of **subjective data** includes careful assessment of pain. **Phantom pain** (pain felt in the missing extremity as if it were still present) may occur and be frightening to the patient. Phantom pain occurs because the nerve tracks that register pain in the amputated area continue to send a message to the brain; this is normal.

Collection of **objective data** includes observing for signs of hemorrhage, such as hypotension, tachycardia, tachypnea, pallor, decreased urinary output, restlessness, and progressive loss of consciousness. Monitor and document suction drainage, and assess and protect the remaining extremity. Observe for neurovascular impairment (done hourly in the immediate postoperative period) from tightly applied elastic wraps, dressings, or casts (see Box 4-5).

Nursing intervention is aimed at effective pain management and prevention of deformities (contractures, especially in the joint above the amputation, or abduction deformities are common). Flexion hip contractures can be prevented postoperatively by raising the foot of the bed slightly to elevate the residual extremity (with care taken not to flex the patient's hips by elevating the stump on a pillow), encouraging movement from side to side, and placing the patient in a prone position at least twice a day. This will stretch the flexor muscles. Teach the patient how to strengthen remaining muscles to facilitate mobility and prevent muscle atrophy (push-ups from a prone position and sit-ups from a seated position). Apply elastic wraps to shrink and reshape the residual extremity into a cone and facilitate the proper fit and use of a prosthesis (Figure 4-40). A prosthesis may be fitted as early as 2 or 3 weeks postoperatively. Because many amputations are performed in people between 60 and 70 years of age, observe the patient carefully for pulmonary complications (such as pulmonary embolus) and cardiovascular collapse. Keep suction equipment and oxygen at the bedside.

Patient education concerning phantom-limb sensation, and the fact that it is a normal physiologic response, can help relieve patient fears. The patient may feel pain or other sensations, such as burning, tingling, throbbing, or pruritus in the amputated extremity. These sensations can last for months or decades on a consistent or intermittent basis. Recommend that patients gently rub the residual extremity or take analgesics for relief.

For persistent, severe phantom pain, the following measures may be employed:

- Stump revision with reamputation at a higher level
- Local infiltration of the stump with procaine
- Mechanical percussion by striking the sensitive digital stump against a solid object—believed to shrink neuromas (small tumors that form in the scar tissue of the stump)
- Sympathetic nerve block

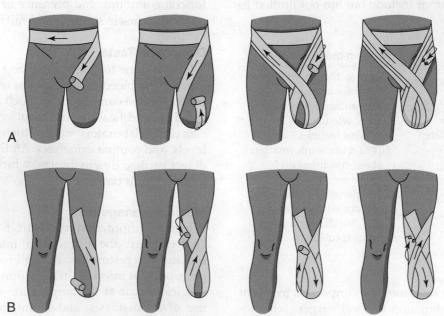

FIGURE 4-40 Correct method of bandaging amputation stump. **A,** Anchor bandage around patient's waist. **B,** Method of bandaging midcalf stump, where bandage need not be anchored around waist.

Encourage the patient to share his or her feelings over the loss of the extremity. Discuss the importance of allowing the grieving process to occur.

Nursing diagnoses and interventions for the patient undergoing an amputation include but are not limited to the following:

Nursing Diagnoses	Nursing Interventions
Disturbed body image, related to loss of limb	Assess effects of amputation on body image.
	Encourage patient to express feelings of mutilation, grief, anger, and loss to aid adaptation processes.
	Encourage patient to help with dressing changes and wrapping of stump as able. Teach family member wrapping techniques if necessary to increase competence and independence.
	Use prescribed pain-management techniques.
	Encourage family members to walk with patient to maintain strength and social contacts.
	Encourage grooming and wearing of personal clothing to maintain individuality and personality.
	Encourage activities for self-care and ambulation to maintain positive outlook and maximum strength.
	Encourage or arrange for social services consultation for economic and employment aid.
	Arrange for follow-up care referral to aid rehabilitation.
Impaired physical mobility, related to loss of limb	Assess ability to use remaining limbs.
	Turn and position on side, back, and abdomen (after 24 hours) to maintain muscle and joint ROM.
	Teach adduction and extension exercises and help patient perform them every 4 hours to prevent abduction and flexion contractures.

Nursing Diagnoses	Nursing Interventions
	Assist with sitting in chair and ambulation with aid as able to maintain muscle strength.
	Prepare patient for physical therapy, transportation for exercises, and stump wrapping, if appropriate.
	Encourage family members to walk with patient during initial ambulation periods, accompanied by health professionals, to increase independence.
	Teach purposes of prone and extension positions to prevent contractures.
	Assist prosthetist with prosthesis measurements and fitting as needed to aid rehabilitation.

Before discharge, teach the patient and family proper positions, exercises, and ambulation techniques. Also demonstrate stump-wrapping techniques to the patient and family (see Figure 4-40). Explain to them that prolonged phantom pain experiences are unusual and should receive medical attention. Discuss skin care with the patient and family so they can take steps to prevent stump irritation or impairment. Also discuss the signs of a wound infection, and instruct them when it is necessary to call the physician.

Prognosis

The prognosis for successful adaptation to an amputation depends on the patient's age, the condition that resulted in amputation, other systemic disorders, emotional health, and support system.

❖ NURSING PROCESS *for the Patient with a Musculoskeletal Disorder*

The role of the licensed practical nurse/licensed vocational nurse (LPN/LVN) in the nursing process as stated is that the LPN/LVN will:

- Participate in planning care for patients based on patient needs
- Review patient's care plan and recommend revisions as needed
- Review and follow defined prioritization for patient care
- Use clinical pathways, care maps, or care plans to guide and review patient care

■ Assessment

The musculoskeletal system provides protection, support, and movement for the body. Proper function of the musculoskeletal system is closely associated with the proper function of the nervous and circulatory systems. Orthopedics is the branch of medicine that deals with the prevention or correction of disorders involving locomotor structures of the body. Permanent disability and crippling will result if patients with musculoskeletal dysfunction do not receive prompt treatment.

Assess orthopedic function for all patients, especially those who are (1) having difficulty with gait; (2) experiencing muscle weakness; (3) suffering from trauma of soft tissue and bone; (4) unable to move and participate in activities for personal, economic, and social fulfillment; (5) experiencing diseases of the musculoskeletal system; or (6) chronically ill.

Assessment of a patient's mobility includes bone integrity, posture, joint function, muscle strength, gait, pain, and neurovascular disturbances related to pressure. Compare body symmetry. For example, assess both legs for same length and diameter size and for comparable muscle strength. Observe the patient's gait for unsteadiness or irregular movements. Difficult ambulation associated with shortness of breath can indicate cardiovascular or respiratory system difficulties.

Assessment of posture and gait simply involves observing the patient walking. Common posture deformities include lateral (or S) curvature of the spine, known as **scoliosis;** a rounding of the thoracic spine (hump-backed appearance), known as **kyphosis;** and an increase in the curve at the lumbar space region that throws the shoulders back, making the "lordly" or "kingly" appearance known as **lordosis** (Figure 4-41). Rigidity of the spine can result from AKS, in which the vertebrae are fused with loss of mobility, producing a rigid gait or "poker spine" appearance.

Assessment of neurologic and circulatory function is important if the patient has experienced a traumatic injury; damaged blood vessels and nerves can cause permanent disabilities.

Assess the skin for signs of coolness, pallor, sensation, or cyanosis to help determine the patient's circulatory status. A faint or absent pulse in an extremity indicates impaired circulation. Palpating the femoral, popliteal, and dorsalis pedis pulses on both extremities provides pertinent data about the lower extremities. If the pulse is not readily palpated with a light touch of the finger, a Doppler instrument can be used to magnify the sound of the pulsation. The absence of a pulse is serious and must be reported to the charge nurse immediately. Assess the brachial and radial pulses to determine circulation in the upper extremities. Palpating a pulse may be difficult if the patient has a cast or bandage. Reach under the cast or bandage if possible. Assess the pulse in the unaffected extremity for comparison.

The **blanching test** (meaning to whiten or pale) is a test of the rate of capillary refill, which signals circulation status. This is also referred to as a **capillary nail refill test.** Compress each fingernail or toenail of the affected extremity (noting the white color as pressure is applied), release the pressure, and note how quickly the pink color returns to the nailbed. The nailbed color should return to normal within 2 or 3 seconds. If the color is slow to return, circulation is impaired and requires prompt attention (see Box 4-5).

Neurovascular assessments are made on patients with musculoskeletal trauma or damage to nerves and blood vessels resulting from surgery, tight bandages, splints, or casts. Impaired circulation resulting in alteration of nerve function can cause loss of the use of an extremity; this impairment is generally seen in the extremities. See Box 4-5 for information concerning neurovascular (circulation) assessment.

▪ Nursing Diagnosis

Nursing assessment establishes the patient's needs regarding mobility. Care of the patient is based on the following nursing diagnoses:

- Impaired physical mobility, related to musculoskeletal impairment
- Impaired bed mobility
- Activity intolerance, related to musculoskeletal impairment
- Ineffective coping
- Anxiety, related to changes in body integrity
- Pain, related to musculoskeletal disorder
- Deficient knowledge regarding therapeutic regimen
- Risk for disuse syndrome

▪ Expected Outcomes and Planning

The plan for facilitating mobility must center on improving and restoring performance and preventing deterioration. Nursing interventions help the patient adapt, reduce, or eliminate activities that cause pain.

Consider the amount of assistance needed for ambulation. Assessment of ROM and muscle strength helps decide whether the patient is able to ambulate

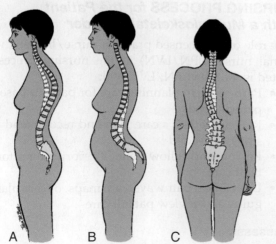

FIGURE 4-41 Abnormal spinal curvatures. **A,** Kyphosis. **B,** Lordosis. **C,** Scoliosis.

safely. Ambulation after surgery often requires physical assistance in addition to the use of mobility aids such as walkers, canes, and crutches.

The care plan focuses on accomplishing individual goals and outcomes that relate to the identified nursing diagnoses. Examples of these include the following:

Goal 1: Patient will demonstrate the use of adaptive devices to increase mobility.

Outcome: Patient demonstrates more independence in mobility by meeting self-care needs.

Goal 2: Patient will demonstrate ambulation and state safety precautions before discharge from health care facility.

Outcome: Patient demonstrates ambulation skills and states correct safety precautions before discharge.

▪ Implementation

Improving the patient's mobility requires awareness of physician's orders specific to ambulation. Check mobility aids for the correct size. Educate patients on safety measures, such as rubber tips in good condition on canes. Shoes that are easy to put on, have nonslip soles, and provide foot and ankle support are safer than bedroom slippers or stockings.

Activities need to be alternated with rest periods. Administer analgesics at least 30 minutes before ambulation for patients experiencing pain. Encourage patients to pace themselves. Patient assistance may be necessary to complete ADLs such as ambulating to the bathroom or to a bedside commode.

Specific principles are involved with mobility:

- Bone loss occurs when patients are confined to bed rest.
- The activities of the human body depend on effective interaction between normal joints and the neuromuscular parts that pilot them.

- Muscles, tendons, ligaments, cartilage, and bones all do their share to ensure smooth function.

Nurses working with patient mobility needs must support physical therapy department activities and goals. Assess a patient's perceptions to help determine his or her motivation for mobility independence. For example, when older adults think they are too fragile to walk, they may be afraid of trying. Use a safety belt when a patient's stability is questionable. The belt encircles the patient's waist; grasp the belt in the middle of the back to help the patient stand, gain balance, and ambulate.

Patients may have difficulty coping with mobility aids and perceive them as a visible sign of weakness. Point out that devices to help mobility are not unlike glasses to help eyesight. Mobility aids increase proficiency of activities and promote joint rest and protection.

▪ Evaluation

Evaluate the success of interventions by noting patient's progress during and after ambulation based on stated goals and outcomes. For example, if the patient is not able to walk to the bathroom, a shorter distance may be more practical. The patient may increase mobility by using a bedside commode. When patients are unable to meet expected outcomes, be ready to revise the care plan to promote success. Examples of goals and their corresponding outcomes include the following:

Goal 1: Patient will demonstrate the use of adaptive devices to increase mobility.

Evaluative measure: Patient ambulates within physical environment.

Goal 2: Patient will understand safety precautions concerning use of mobility aids.

Evaluative measures: Patient checks rubber tips on mobility aid and uses equipment correctly.

Get Ready for the NCLEX® Examination!

Key Points

- The skeletal system has five basic functions: support of the body, protection of internal organs, movement of the body, storage of minerals, and blood cell formation.
- The skeleton is divided into the axial and the appendicular skeletons. The axial skeleton is composed of the skull, vertebral column, and thorax. The appendicular skeleton is composed of the upper extremities, lower extremities, shoulder girdle, and pelvic girdle.
- The three types of joints and their movement are (1) synarthrosis: no movement; (2) amphiarthrosis: slight movement; and (3) diarthrosis: free movement.
- Joints hold the bones together and allow movement and flexibility. Differences in the structure determine the amount of flexibility.

- Some of the more common movements that the body produces are flexion, extension, abduction, adduction, rotation, supination, pronation, dorsiflexion, and plantar flexion.
- The bones and joints provide the framework of the body, but the muscles are necessary for movement. Movement results from contraction and relaxation of the individual muscles.
- An ESR is the most objective laboratory test for determining the severity of RA.
- RA affects a young population (ages 30 to 55) with crippling changes in the synovial membrane of the joints.
- Salicylates and NSAIDs are used to treat RA and osteoarthritis.

- Osteoarthritis is a DJD that affects the population older than 40 years of age and causes articular cartilage degeneration.
- Porous and brittle bones caused by a lack of calcium are one of the physiologic changes noted in osteoporosis.
- Osteoporosis-related fractures occur in one in two women, compared with one in eight men, over the course of a lifetime.
- Vertebroplasty and kyphoplasty are surgical procedures used to relieve pain in women with osteoporosis who do not respond to other pain management programs.
- Arthroplasty procedures (such as hip and knee arthroplasty) are commonly performed on patients suffering from severe arthritis.
- Unicompartmental knee arthroplasty, also referred to as partial knee replacement, is performed on patients who have only one of the compartments of the knee affected by arthritis.
- Nursing intervention specific to the care of a patient suffering from a fractured hip involves maintaining abduction of the affected leg.
- Fractured hip fixation devices—such as hip prosthetic implant, plate and screw fixation, and telescoping nail fixation—require some degree of non–weight bearing for 6 weeks to 3 months.
- The use of antacids and proton pump inhibitors increases a patient's risk of hip fractures.
- A significant postoperative nursing intervention for a patient with an amputation is proper care of the stump to facilitate the use of a prosthetic device.
- Herniated nucleus pulposus is seen most often in the cervical and lumbar spinal regions and can be treated surgically (laminectomy and spinal fusion) or medically (medication, traction, and physical therapy).
- Osteogenic sarcoma is a common primary malignant tumor seen in young people; it can metastasize to the lungs.
- Compartment syndrome, shock, fat embolism, gas gangrene, thromboembolus, and osteomyelitis are complications resulting from a fractured bone.
- Petechiae on the conjunctiva of the eye, the neck, the chest, or the axillary region is a typical sign of a fat embolism.
- External fixation devices such as casts, braces, metal pins, and skeletal and skin traction are used to hold bone fragments in normal position.
- Whether the casting material is plaster of Paris or a synthetic material, proper drying, cleansing, handling, and assessing are required to prevent patient complications.
- The nurse caring for a patient in traction is responsible for knowing (1) the purpose of the traction (traction applied for fractures must be continuous), (2) the equipment needed and appropriate safety measures, (3) the amount of weight ordered, and (4) the patient's understanding of the traction.
- Crutches, canes, walkers, and the Roll-A-Bout are used as gait enhancers for patients with altered mobility.
- Crutch walking involving the three-point gait is most commonly used for patients wearing leg casts.

Additional Learning Resources

 Go to your Companion CD for an audio glossary, animations, video clips, and more.

evolve Be sure to visit the Evolve site at http://evolve.elsevier.com/Christensen/adult/ for additional online resources.

Review Questions for the NCLEX® Examination

1. The bones serve as storage for which two minerals?

   1. Sodium and potassium
   2. Calcium and phosphorus
   3. Copper and iodine
   4. Magnesium and chloride

2. Hematopoiesis takes place in:

   1. the lymph nodes.
   2. the spleen.
   3. the yellow bone marrow.
   4. the red bone marrow.

3. Movement of an extremity away from the midline of the body is called:

   1. adduction.
   2. pronation.
   3. flexion.
   4. abduction.

4. A 65-year-old patient has been diagnosed with rheumatoid arthritis (RA). A diagnostic test used to confirm RA is:

   1. complete blood count.
   2. erythrocyte sedimentation rate.
   3. prothrombin time.
   4. urinary uric acid level.

5. A clinical sign of gouty arthritis is:

   1. Heberden's nodes.
   2. pathologic fractures.
   3. tophi deposits.
   4. Homans' sign.

6. A 55-year-old patient reveals a postmenopausal history of three previous fractures and daily consumption of caffeine. According to her history, she is at increased risk for:

   1. osteomyelitis.
   2. osteoarthritis.
   3. osteogenic sarcoma.
   4. osteoporosis.

7. An appropriate nursing intervention for a patient suffering from a fractured hip with bipolar hip repair is:

   1. release traction weight every 4 to 6 hours.
   2. maintain abduction of the affected extremity.
   3. maintain adduction of the affected extremity.
   4. encourage active range of motion in the affected extremity.

8. The patient is being discharged after a prosthetic hip implant. She asks when she can begin to bear weight on the affected leg. *(Select the most appropriate response.)*

   1. The patient must not bear weight on the affected leg for 6 to 12 months.
   2. Most patients bear weight in 5 days.
   3. The patient must learn to use a gait enhancer and keep the majority of weight off the unaffected leg.
   4. Most patients require some degree of non–weight bearing for 6 weeks to 3 months.

9. A significant postoperative nursing intervention for a patient with an amputation is:

   1. maintaining abduction of the stump.
   2. elevating the stump with no more than two pillows.
   3. proper stump care to facilitate prosthetic use.
   4. leaving the stump open to air to assess suture site.

10. A 75-year-old retired construction worker has been seeing the physician for complaints of osteoarthritis. Today he is discussing concerns over his condition and asks what has caused his osteoarthritis. An appropriate response would be:

    1. You have osteoarthritis because of the difficult construction work you did for so many years.
    2. Everyone your age has arthritis; you are fortunate you are still able to walk.
    3. The cause of osteoarthritis is unknown. However, almost everyone older than 40 years of age has some changes in their joints.
    4. You probably did not exercise as much as you should have, and you should start vigorous exercising now to prevent further complications.

11. An appropriate nursing intervention for a 32-year-old patient in skeletal traction, would be to:

    1. provide cast care.
    2. cleanse pin sites daily with hydrogen peroxide, and observe for signs of infection.
    3. place patient on drainage and secretion precautions.
    4. encourage patient to sit in a straight, firm chair for no longer than 20 minutes each time.

12. After a fracture of the forearm or tibia, complaints of sharp, deep, unrelenting pain in the hand or foot unrelieved by analgesics or elevation of the extremity indicate which complication?

    1. Fat embolism
    2. Compartment syndrome
    3. Gas gangrene
    4. Cast syndrome

13. A 45-year-old patient suffered a knee injury while playing football. He is scheduled for an arthroscopic examination and asks the nurse to explain the procedure. An appropriate response would be:

    1. Your physician will insert a small scope into your knee joint to visualize the joint for damaged tissue.
    2. The test involves the use of magnetism and radio waves to make images of cross-sections of the body.
    3. The radiographic technician will inject your knee joint with an atomic material and take a radiograph of your affected knee.
    4. The physician will insert needle electrodes into the knee muscle to document electrical activity of the knee.

14. A 51-year-old patient with RA asks if there is a cure. An appropriate response would be:

    1. Yes, new drugs offer a cure.
    2. No, but new drugs can interfere with the body's reaction to inflammation and better control the disease process.
    3. Yes, but the patient must take medication for at least 10 years.
    4. No, most patients with RA also develop osteoarthritis.

15. The patient is scheduled for endoscopic spinal microsurgery to correct a herniated disk. Select the most accurate statement concerning this type of surgery.

    1. Endoscopic spinal microsurgery requires a general anesthetic.
    2. Special scopes are placed through small incisions, causing minimal damage to surrounding tissue.
    3. Patients older than 80 years of age are always candidates for endoscopic spinal microsurgery.
    4. Endoscopic spinal microsurgery is limited to the repair of herniated disks.

16. A 45 year-old patient has a history of lactose intolerance, excessive caffeine intake, and excessive cigarette smoking. The physician orders a bone density index test for her. Select the most appropriate statement concerning information about the test.

    1. The test is also called DEXA and is considered an invasive procedure.
    2. The test involves drawing a small amount of blood to determine your blood calcium level.
    3. The test takes about 10 minutes and involves very low amounts of radiation.
    4. The test is always recommended for women older than 30 years of age.

17. A 62-year-old patient has osteoarthritis of the knee and is seeking information about glucosamine supplements. An appropriate response would be:

    1. Glucosamine is a natural substance in the body, and it is not necessary to take a supplement.
    2. Glucosamine supplements are relatively safe in people younger than 40 years of age.
    3. Studies suggest that glucosamine supplements are helpful in maintaining healthy joint function, with minimal side effects unless you are allergic to shellfish.
    4. A healthy lifestyle with high-impact exercise is more important than taking a supplement.

18. Select the most appropriate nursing assessment for the nursing diagnosis of ineffective tissue perfusion, secondary to fractured hip.

    1. Assess for ecchymosis over pelvis and perineum.
    2. Protect patient from cross-contamination.
    3. Assess for adventitious lung sounds.
    4. Assess distal pulses.

19. A 72-year-old patient has just undergone total hip replacement. She asks why she cannot cross her legs when sitting but must do straight leg–raising exercises. An appropriate response would be:

    1. The exercises help strengthen the leg muscles; crossing your legs puts pressure on the joints and could damage the hip prosthesis.
    2. The exercises keep you from getting too tired while you sit; when you want to cross your legs, it is time to rest.
    3. The exercises strengthen the muscles in your upper legs to help you walk.
    4. The doctor ordered these exercises, but did not order you to cross your legs.

20. Which of the following objective data are found in a patient with compartment syndrome?

    1. Hypotension, tachycardia, and tachypnea
    2. Gas bubbles under the skin
    3. Positive Homans' sign
    4. Absence of pulsation in the affected extremity

21. A 77-year-old patient has persistent complaints of severe back pain related to osteoporosis. She walks with a stooped posture and has a noticeable kyphosis. She has been unresponsive to a traditional pain management program. Based on this information, the patient may be a candidate for:

    1. unicompartmental arthroplasty.
    2. complete bed rest.
    3. kyphoplasty.
    4. injections of Forteo.

22. A 47-year-old patient has signs and symptoms of menopause. She recently fell and fractured her wrist. After doing a bone density test, her physician diagnosed her with osteoporosis. She asks about the benefits of taking estrogen. An appropriate response would be:

    1. Estrogen will not help bone density.
    2. Estrogen can cause cancer of the breast.
    3. Estrogen will not correct the condition but will help to prevent fractures and is approved for women at significant risk.
    4. Forteo is a type of estrogen.

23. A 51-year-old patient exercises routinely. He has been noticing pain on the lateral area of his knee for the past 6 months during and after exercise. The patient is scheduled for unicompartmental knee arthroplasty and asks the nurse to explain the surgery. An appropriate response would be:

    1. The procedure involves replacement of the entire knee joint.
    2. You will need to be in the hospital for approximately 5 days.
    3. You will not need an anesthetic.
    4. Minimally invasive knee surgery removes only the most damaged areas of cartilage, and a small plastic disk replaces the worn cartilage, providing a new cushion between the bones.

24. The patient had a compound fracture of his right femur 2 years before the present admission. His physician suspects osteomyelitis and has informed the patient that tests are needed to confirm the diagnosis. The patient wants to know what tests can be ordered to determine osteomyelitis. An appropriate response would be to describe the specific test(s) for osteomyelitis. *(Select all that apply.)*

    1. Goniometer
    2. BMX
    3. Bone scan
    4. Bone biopsy

25. A construction worker suffered a fracture of the femur 48 hours ago. The nurse notices that he has petechiae on the conjunctiva, chest, neck, and axillae. Petechiae in these locations is a typical sign of:

    1. compartment syndrome.
    2. deep-vein thrombosis.
    3. gas gangrene.
    4. fat embolism.

Care of the Patient with a Gastrointestinal Disorder

Barbara Lauritsen Christensen

Objectives

Anatomy and Physiology

1. List in sequence each of the component parts or segments of the alimentary canal and identify the accessory organs of digestion.
2. Discuss the function of each digestive and accessory organ.

Medical-Surgical

3. Discuss the laboratory and diagnostic examinations and give the nursing interventions for patients with disorders of the gastrointestinal tract.
4. Explain the etiology and pathophysiology, clinical manifestations, assessments, diagnostic tests, medical-surgical management, and nursing interventions for the patient with disorders of the mouth, esophagus, stomach, and intestines.
5. Identify nursing interventions for preoperative and postoperative care of the patient who requires gastric surgery.
6. Compare and contrast the inflammatory bowel diseases of ulcerative colitis and Crohn's disease, including etiology and pathophysiology, clinical manifestations, medical management, and nursing interventions.

7. Identify five nursing interventions for the patient with a stoma for fecal diversion.
8. Discuss the etiology and pathophysiology, clinical manifestations, assessment, diagnostic tests, medical management, and nursing interventions for the patient with acute abdominal inflammations (appendicitis, diverticulitis, and peritonitis).
9. Discuss the etiology and pathophysiology, clinical manifestations, assessment, diagnostic tests, medical management, and nursing interventions for the patient with external hernias and hiatal hernia.
10. Differentiate between mechanical and nonmechanical intestinal obstruction, including causes, medical management and nursing interventions.
11. Describe the etiology and pathophysiology, clinical manifestations, assessment, diagnostic tests, medical management, surgical procedures, and nursing interventions for the patient with colorectal cancer.
12. Explain the etiologies, medical management, and nursing interventions for the patient with fecal incontinence.

Key Terms

achalasia (ăk-ăh-LĀ-zē-ă, p. 189)
achlorhydria (ă-chlŏr-HĪ-drē-ă, p. 180)
anastomosis (ă-năs-tŏ-MŌ-sĭs, p. 189)
cachexia (kă-KĔK-sē-ă, p. 221)
carcinoembryonic antigen (CEA) (kăr-sĭn-ō-ĕm-brē-ĂN-ĭk ĂN-tĭ-jĕn, p. 221)
dehiscence (dĕ-HĬS-ĕntz, p. 200)
dumping syndrome (DŬMP-ĭng SĬN-drōm, p. 196)
dysphagia (dĭs-FĀ-jē-ă, p. 188)
evisceration (ĕ-vĭs-ĕr-Ā-shŭn, p. 200)
exacerbations (ĕg-zăs-ĕr-BĀ-shŭnz, p. 205)
hematemesis (hĕ-mă-TĔM-ĕ-sĭs, p. 192)

intussusception (ĭn-tŭs-sŭs-SĔP-shŭn, p. 182)
leukoplakia (lū-kō-PLĀ-kē-ă, p. 185)
lumen (LŪ-mĕn, p. 182)
melena (MĔL-ĕh-nă, p. 192)
occult blood (ŏ-KŬLT, p. 182)
paralytic (adynamic) ileus (p. 218)
pathognomonic (păth-ŏg-nō-MŌN-ĭk, p. 183)
remissions (rĕ-MĬSH-ŭn, p. 205)
steatorrhea (stĕ-ă-tō-RĒ-ă, p. 210)
stoma (STŌ-mă, p. 209)
tenesmus (tĕ-NĔZ-mŭs, p. 202)
volvulus (VŎL-vū-lŭs, p. 218)

ANATOMY AND PHYSIOLOGY OF THE GASTROINTESTINAL SYSTEM

DIGESTIVE SYSTEM

Everyone understands that food is necessary for existence, but not (1) what happens to food once it is chewed and swallowed; (2) how food is prepared for its trip to each individual cell; and (3) the many changes that food undergoes, both chemically and physically. This chapter reviews these changes and their effect on the body.

The digestive tract, or alimentary canal, is a musculomembranous tube extending from the mouth to the anus (Figure 5-1). It is approximately 30 feet long. It consists of the mouth, pharynx, esophagus, small intestine, large intestine, and anus. **Peristalsis** is the coordinated, rhythmic, serial contraction of smooth muscle that forces food through the digestive tract, bile through the bile duct, and urine through the ureter. During peristalsis the tract shortens to approximately 15 feet.

Accessory organs aid in the digestive process but are not considered part of the digestive tract. They release

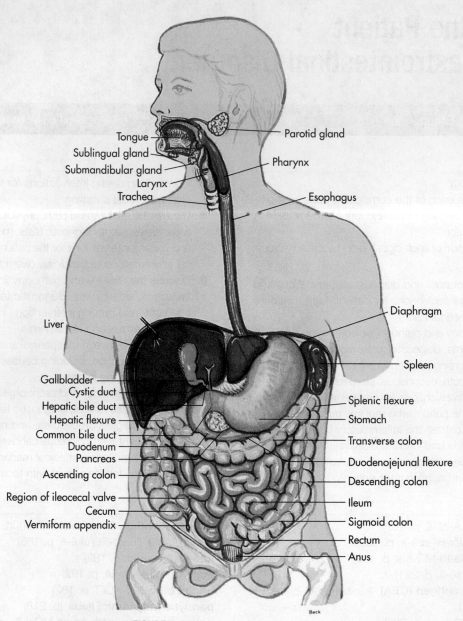

Tongue
Sublingual gland
Submandibular gland
Larynx
Trachea

Parotid gland

Pharynx

Esophagus

Liver

Diaphragm

Spleen

Gallbladder
Cystic duct
Hepatic bile duct
Hepatic flexure
Common bile duct
Duodenum
Pancreas
Ascending colon

Region of ileocecal valve
Cecum
Vermiform appendix

Splenic flexure
Stomach
Transverse colon
Duodenojejunal flexure
Descending colon

Ileum
Sigmoid colon
Rectum
Anus

Beck

FIGURE 5-1 Location of digestive organs.

chemicals into the system through a series of ducts. The teeth, tongue, salivary glands, liver, gallbladder, and pancreas are considered accessory organs.

Organs of the Digestive System and Their Functions

Box 5-1 lists various organs of the digestive system and the accessory organs involved in digestion.

Mouth

The mouth marks the entrance to the digestive system. The floor of the mouth contains a muscular appendage, the tongue. The tongue is involved in chewing, swallowing, and the formation of speech. Tiny elevations, called **papillae,** contain the taste buds. They differentiate between bitter, sweet, sour, and salty sensations.

Digestion begins in the mouth. Here the teeth mechanically shred and grind the food and the enzymes begin the chemical breakdown of carbohydrates.

Teeth

Each tooth is designed to carry out a specific task. In the center of the mouth are the incisors, which are structured for biting and cutting. Posterior to the incisors are the canines, pointed teeth used for tearing and shredding food. The molars are to the rear of the jaw. These teeth have four cusps (points) and are used for mastication (to crush and grind food).

Salivary Glands

The three pairs of salivary glands are the parotid, submandibular, and sublingual glands (see Figure 5-1). They secrete fluid called **saliva,** which is approxi-

Box 5-1 Organs of the Digestive System

ORGANS OF THE ALIMENTARY CANAL
- Mouth
- Pharynx (throat)
- Esophagus (food pipe)
- Stomach
- Small intestine
  —Duodenum
  —Jejunum
  —Ileum
- Large intestine
- Cecum
- Colon
  —Ascending colon
  —Transverse colon
  —Descending colon
  —Sigmoid colon
- Rectum
- Anal canal

ACCESSORY ORGANS
- Teeth and gums
- Tongue
- Liver
- Gallbladder
- Pancreas
- Salivary glands
  —Parotid
  —Submandibular
  —Sublingual

mately 99% water with enzymes and mucus. Normally these glands secrete enough saliva to keep the mucous membranes of the mouth moist. Once food enters the mouth, the secretion increases to lubricate and dissolve the food and to begin the chemical process of digestion. The salivary glands secrete about 1000 to 1500 mL of saliva daily. The major enzyme is salivary amylase (ptyalin), which initiates carbohydrate metabolism. Another enzyme, lysozyme, destroys bacteria and thus protects the mucous membrane from infections and the teeth from decay. After food has been ingested, the salivary glands continue to secrete saliva, which cleanses the mouth.

Esophagus

The esophagus is a muscular, collapsible tube that is approximately 10 inches long, extending from the mouth through the thoracic cavity and the esophageal hiatus to the stomach. Digestion does not take place in the esophagus. Peristalsis moves the bolus (food broken down and mixed with saliva, ready to pass to the stomach) through the esophagus to the stomach in 5 or 6 seconds.

Stomach

The stomach is in the left upper quadrant of the abdomen, directly inferior to the diaphragm (Figure 5-2). A filled stomach is the size of a football and holds approximately 1 L. The stomach entrance is the cardiac sphincter (so named because it is close to the heart); the exit is the pyloric sphincter. As food leaves the esophagus, it enters the stomach through the relaxed cardiac sphincter. The sphincter then contracts, preventing reflux (splashing or return flow), which can be irritating.

Once the bolus has entered the stomach, the muscular layers of the stomach churn and contract to mix and compress the contents with the gastric juices and water. The gastric juices are secretions released by the gastric glands. Digestion of protein begins in the stomach. Hydrochloric acid softens the connective tissue of meats,

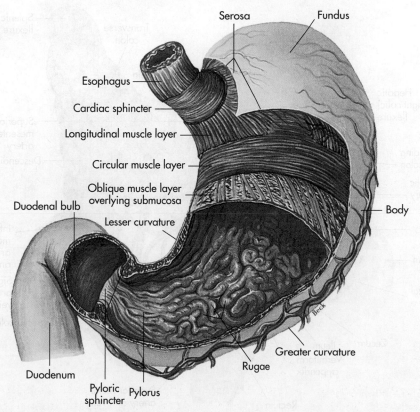

FIGURE 5-2 Stomach. Cut-away sections show muscle layers and interior mucosa thrown into folds called **rugae**.

kills bacteria, and activates pepsin (the chief enzyme of gastric juices that converts proteins into proteoses and peptones). Mucin is released to protect the stomach lining. Intrinsic factor (a substance secreted by the gastric mucosa) is produced to allow absorption of vitamin B_{12}. The stomach breaks the food down into a viscous semi-liquid substance called chyme. The chyme passes through the pyloric sphincter into the duodenum for the next phase of digestion.

Small Intestine
The small intestine (see Figure 5-1) is a tube that is 20 feet long and 1 inch in diameter. It begins at the pyloric sphincter and ends at the ileocecal valve. It is divided into three major sections: **duodenum, jejunum,** and **ileum.** Up to 90% of digestion takes place in the small intestine. The intestinal juices finish the metabolism of carbohydrates and proteins. Bile and pancreatic juices enter the duodenum. Bile from the liver breaks molecules into smaller droplets, which enables the digestive juices to complete their process. Pancreatic juices contain water, protein, inorganic salts, and enzymes. Pancreatic juices are essential in breaking down proteins into their amino acid components, in reducing dietary fats to glycerol and fatty acids, and in converting starch to simple sugars.

The inner surface of the small intestine contains millions of tiny fingerlike projections called **villi,** which are clustered over the entire mucous surface. The villi are responsible for absorbing the products of digestion into the bloodstream. They increase the absorption area of the small intestine 600 times. Inside each villus is a rich capillary bed, along with modified lymph capillaries called lacteals. Lacteals are responsible for the absorption of metabolized fats.

Large Intestine
Once the small intestine has finished its specific tasks, the ileocecal valve opens and releases the contents into the large intestine. The large intestine is a tube that is larger in diameter (2 inches) but shorter (5 feet) than the small intestine. It is composed of the cecum; appendix; ascending, hepatic flexure, transverse, splenic flexure, descending, and sigmoid colons; rectum; and anus (Figure 5-3). This is the terminal portion of the digestive tract, which completes the process of digestion. Basically the large intestine has four major functions: (1) completion of absorption of water, (2) manufacture of certain vitamins, (3) formation of feces, and (4) expulsion of feces.

Just inferior to the ileocecal valve is the cecum, a blind pouch approximately 2 to 3 inches long. The vermiform appendix, a small wormlike, tubular structure, dangles from the cecum. To date, no function for the appendix has been discovered. The open end of the cecum connects to the ascending colon, which continues upward on the right side of the abdomen to the inferior area of the liver. The ascending colon then becomes the transverse colon. It crosses to the left side of the abdomen, where it becomes the descending colon. When the descending colon reaches the level of the iliac crest, the

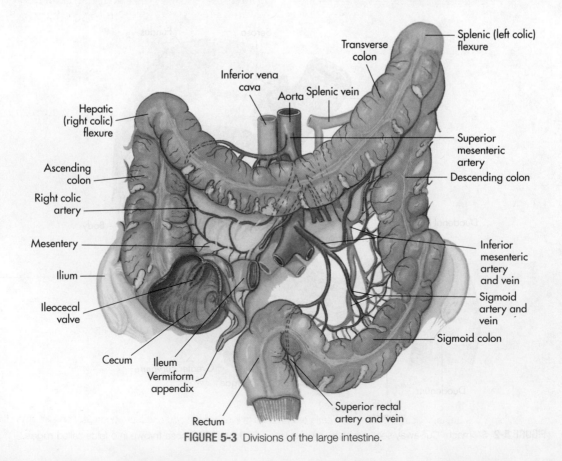

FIGURE 5-3 Divisions of the large intestine.

sigmoid colon begins and continues toward the midline to the level of the third sacral vertebra.

Bacteria in the large intestine change the chyme into fecal material by releasing the remaining nutrients. The bacteria are also responsible for the synthesis of vitamin K, which is needed for normal blood clotting, and the production of some of the B-complex vitamins. As the fecal material continues its journey, the remaining water and vitamins are absorbed into the bloodstream by osmosis.

Rectum

The rectum is the last 8 inches of the intestine, where fecal material is expelled.

ACCESSORY ORGANS OF DIGESTION

Liver

The liver is the largest glandular organ in the body and one of the most complex. In the adult it weighs 3 pounds. It is located just inferior to the diaphragm, covering most of the upper right quadrant and extending into the left epigastrium. It is divided into two lobes. Approximately 1500 mL of blood is delivered to the liver every minute by the portal vein and the hepatic portal artery. The cells of the liver produce a product called **bile,** a yellow-brown or green-brown liquid. Bile is necessary for the emulsification of fats. The liver releases 500 to 1000 mL of bile per day. Bile travels to the gallbladder through hepatic ducts. The gallbladder is a sac about 3 to 4 inches long located on the right inferior surface of the liver. Bile is stored in the gallbladder until needed for fat digestion (Figure 5-4).

In addition to producing bile, the liver's functions include managing blood coagulation; manufacturing cholesterol; manufacturing albumin to maintain normal blood volume; filtering out old red blood cells (RBCs) and bacteria; detoxifying poisons (alcohol, nicotine, drugs); converting ammonia to urea; providing the main source of body heat; storing glycogen for later use; activating vitamin D; and breaking down nitrogenous waste (from protein metabolism) to urea, which the kidneys can excrete as waste from the body.

Pancreas

The pancreas is an elongated gland that lies posterior to the stomach (see Figure 5-4). It is involved in both endocrine and exocrine duties. In this chapter, discussion of the pancreas is limited to its exocrine activities.

Each day the pancreas produces 1000 to 1500 mL of pancreatic juice to aid in digestion. This pancreatic juice contains the digestive enzymes protease (trypsin), lipase (steapsin), and amylase (amylopsin). These enzymes are important because they digest the three major components of chyme: proteins, fats, and carbohydrates. The enzymes are transported through an excretory duct to the duodenum. This pancreatic duct connects to the common bile duct from the liver and gallbladder and empties through a small orifice in the duodenum called the major duodenal papilla, or **papilla of Vater.** In addition, the pancreas contains an alkaline substance, sodium bicarbonate, which neutralizes hydrochloric acid in the gastric juices that enter the small intestine from the stomach.

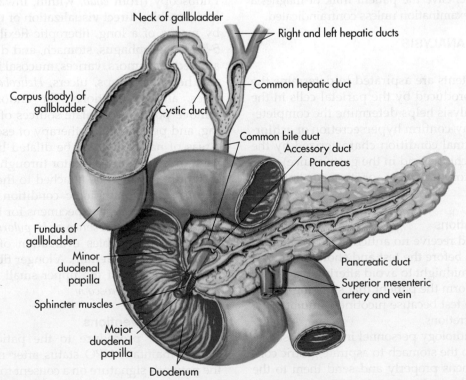

Neck of gallbladder

Right and left hepatic ducts

Common hepatic duct

Corpus (body) of gallbladder

Cystic duct

Common bile duct
Accessory duct
Pancreas

Fundus of gallbladder

Minor duodenal papilla

Pancreatic duct

Superior mesenteric artery and vein

Sphincter muscles

Major duodenal papilla

Duodenum

FIGURE 5-4 Gallbladder and bile ducts. Obstruction of the hepatic or common bile duct by stone or spasm occludes the exit of the bile and prevents matter from being ejected into the duodenum.

REGULATION OF FOOD INTAKE

The hypothalamus, a portion of the brain, contains two centers that have an effect on eating. One center stimulates the individual to eat, and the other signals the individual to stop eating. These centers work in conjunction with the rest of the brain to balance eating habits. However, many other factors also affect eating. For example, distention decreases appetite. Other controls in our bodies, lifestyle, culture, eating habits, emotions, and genetic factors all influence intake of food and individual body build.

LABORATORY AND DIAGNOSTIC EXAMINATIONS

UPPER GASTROINTESTINAL STUDY (UPPER GI SERIES, UGI)

Rationale

The upper gastrointestinal study (UGI) consists of a series of radiographs of the lower esophagus, stomach, and duodenum using barium sulfate as the contrast medium. A UGI series detects any abnormal conditions of the upper gastrointestinal (GI) tract, any tumors, or other ulcerative lesions.

Nursing Interventions

The patient should take nothing by mouth (NPO) and avoid smoking after midnight the night before the study. Explain the importance of rectally expelling all the barium after the examination. Stools will be light colored until all the barium is expelled (up to 72 hours after the test). Eventual absorption of fecal water may cause a hardened barium impaction. Increasing fluid intake is usually effective. Give the patient milk of magnesia (60 mL) after the examination unless contraindicated.

TUBE GASTRIC ANALYSIS

Rationale

The stomach contents are aspirated to determine the amount of acid produced by the parietal cells in the stomach. The analysis helps determine the completeness of a vagotomy, confirm hypersecretion or **achlorhydria** (an abnormal condition characterized by the absence of hydrochloric acid in the gastric juice), estimate acid secretory capacity, or test for intrinsic factor.

Nursing Interventions

The patient should receive no anticholinergic medications for 24 hours before the test and should maintain NPO status after midnight to avoid altering the gastric acid secretion. Inform the patient that smoking is prohibited before the test because nicotine stimulates the flow of gastric secretions.

The nurse or radiology personnel inserts a nasogastric (NG) tube into the stomach to aspirate gastric content. Label specimens properly and send them to the laboratory immediately. Remove the NG tube as soon as specimens are collected. The patient may then eat if indicated.

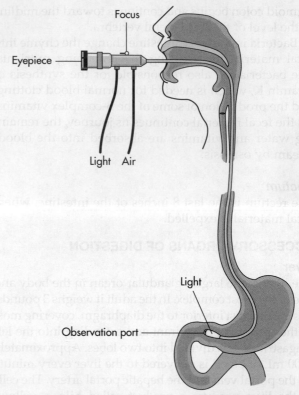

FIGURE 5-5 Fiberoptic endoscopy of the stomach.

ESOPHAGOGASTRODUODENOSCOPY (EGD, UGI ENDOSCOPY, GASTROSCOPY)

Rationale

Endoscopy (from *endo,* within, inward; and *scope,* to look) enables direct visualization of the upper GI tract by means of a long, fiberoptic flexible scope (Figure 5-5). The esophagus, stomach, and duodenum are examined for tumors, varices, mucosal inflammation, hiatal hernias, polyps, ulcers, *Helicobacter pylori,* strictures, and obstructions. The endoscopist can also remove polyps, coagulate sources of active GI bleeding, and perform sclerotherapy of esophageal varices. Areas of narrowing can be dilated by the endoscope itself or by passing a dilator through the scope. Camera equipment can be attached to the viewing lens to photograph a pathologic condition. The endoscope can also obtain tissue specimens for biopsy or culture to determine the presence of *H. pylori.*

Endoscopy enables evaluation of the esophagus, stomach, and duodenum. A longer fiberoptic scope allows evaluation of the upper small intestine. This is referred to as *enteroscopy.*

Nursing Interventions

Explain the procedure to the patient. The patient should maintain NPO status after midnight. Obtain the patient's signature on a consent form and complete a preoperative checklist for the endoscopic examination. The patient is usually given a preprocedure intravenous (IV) sedative such as midazolam (Versed). The patient's pharynx is anesthetized by spraying it with lidocaine hydrochloride (Xylocaine). Therefore do not allow the patient to eat or drink until the gag reflex returns (usually about 2 to 4 hours). Assess for any signs and symptoms of perforation, including abdominal pain and tenderness, guarding, oral bleeding, melena, and hypovolemic shock.

CAPSULE ENDOSCOPY

Rationale
In a capsule endoscopy, the patient swallows a capsule with a camera (approximately the size of a large vitamin) that provides endoscopic evaluation of the GI tract (Figure 5-6). It is commonly used to visualize the small intestine and diagnose diseases (such as Crohn's disease, celiac disease, and malabsorption syndrome). It also helps identify sources of possible GI bleeding in areas not accessible by upper endoscopy or colonoscopy. The camera takes about 57,000 images during an 8-hour examination. The capsule relays images to a data recorder that the patient wears on a belt. After the examination, images are viewed on a monitor.

Nursing Interventions
Dietary preparation is similar to that for colonoscopy. The patient swallows the video capsule and is usually kept NPO until 4 to 6 hours later. The procedure is comfortable for most patients. Eight hours after swallowing the capsule, the patient returns to have the monitoring device removed. Peristalsis causes passage of the disposable capsule with a bowel movement.

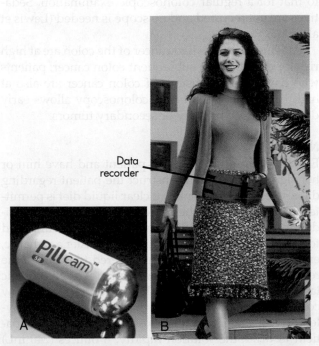

FIGURE 5-6 Capsule endoscopy. **A,** The video capsule has its own camera and light source. After it is swallowed, it travels through the gastrointestinal tract and allows visualization of the small intestine. It sends messages to a data recorder that is worn on a waist belt **B,** During the 8-hour examination, the patient is free to move about. After the test, the images are viewed on a video monitor.

BARIUM SWALLOW AND GASTROGRAFIN STUDIES

Rationale
This barium contrast study is a more thorough study of the esophagus than that provided by most UGI examinations. As in most barium contrast studies, defects in luminal filling and narrowing of the barium column indicate tumor, scarred stricture, or esophageal varices. The barium swallow allows easy recognition of anatomical abnormalities, such as hiatal hernia. Left atrial dilation, aortic aneurysm, and paraesophageal tumors (such as bronchial or mediastinal tumors) may cause extrinsic compression of the barium column within the esophagus.

Diatrizoate meglumine and diatrizoate sodium (Gastrografin) is a product now used in place of barium for patients who are susceptible to bleeding from the GI system and who are being considered for surgery. Gastrografin is water soluble and rapidly absorbed, so it is preferable when a perforation is suspected. Gastrografin facilitates imaging through radiographs, but if the product escapes from the GI tract, it is absorbed by the surrounding tissue. In contrast, if barium leaks from the GI tract, it is not absorbed and can lead to complications.

Nursing Interventions
The patient should maintain NPO status after midnight. Food and fluid in the stomach prevent the barium from accurately outlining the GI tract, and the radiographic results may be misleading. Explain the importance of rectally expelling all barium. Stools will be light colored until this occurs. Eventual absorption of fecal water may cause a hardened barium impaction. Increasing fluid intake is usually effective. Give milk of magnesia (60 mL) after the barium swallow examination unless contraindicated.

ESOPHAGEAL FUNCTION STUDIES (BERNSTEIN TEST)

Rationale
The Bernstein test, an acid-perfusion test, is an attempt to reproduce the symptoms of gastroesophageal reflux. It helps differentiate esophageal pain caused by esophageal reflux from that caused by angina pectoris. If the patient suffers pain with the instillation of hydrochloric acid into the esophagus, the test is positive and indicates reflux esophagitis.

Nursing Interventions
Avoid sedating the patient, since the patient's participation is essential for swallowing the tubes, swallowing during acid clearance, and describing any discomfort during the instillation of hydrochloric acid. The patient is NPO for 8 hours before the examination. Withhold any medications that may interfere with the production of acid, such as antacids and analgesics.

EXAMINATION OF STOOL FOR OCCULT BLOOD

Rationale

Tumors of the large intestine grow into the lumen (the cavity or channel within a tube or tubular organ) and are subject to repeated trauma by the fecal stream. Eventually the tumor ulcerates and bleeding occurs. Usually the bleeding is so slight that gross blood is not seen in the stool. If this occult blood (blood that is obscure or hidden from view) is detected in the stool, suspect a benign or malignant GI tumor. Tests for occult blood are also called guaiac, Hemoccult, and Hematest.

Occult blood in the stool may occur also in ulceration and inflammation of the upper or lower GI system. Other causes include swallowing blood of oral or nasopharyngeal origin.

Stool may be obtained by digital retrieval by the nurse or physician. However, the patient is usually asked to collect stool in an appropriate container. Obtain a specimen for occult blood before barium studies are done.

Nursing Interventions

Instruct the patient to keep the stool specimen free of urine or toilet paper, since either can alter the test results. The nurse or patient should don gloves and use tongue blades to transfer the stool to the proper receptacle. The patient should keep the diet free of organ meat for 24 to 48 hours before a guaiac test.

SIGMOIDOSCOPY (LOWER GI ENDOSCOPY)

Rationale

Endoscopy of the lower GI tract allows visualization and, if indicated, access to obtain biopsy specimens of tumors, polyps, or ulcerations of the anus, rectum, and sigmoid colon. The lower GI tract is difficult to visualize radiographically, but sigmoidoscopy allows direct visualization. Microscopic review of tissue specimens obtained using this procedure lead to diagnoses of many lower bowel disorders.

Nursing Interventions

Explain the procedure to the patient and have him or her sign a consent form. Administer enemas as ordered on the evening before or the morning of the examination to ensure optimum visualization of the lower GI tract. After the examination, observe the patient for evidence of bowel perforation (abdominal pain, tenderness, distention, and bleeding).

BARIUM ENEMA STUDY (LOWER GI SERIES)

Rationale

The barium enema (BE) study consists of a series of radiographs of the colon used to demonstrate the presence and location of polyps, tumors, and diverticula. It can also detect positional abnormalities (such as malrotation). Barium sulfate assists in visualization of mucosal detail. Therapeutically, the BE study may be used to reduce nonstrangulated ileocolic intussusception (infolding of one segment of the intestine into the lumen of another segment) in children.

Nursing Interventions

The evening before the BE, administer cathartics such as magnesium citrate or other cathartics designated by institution policy. Also administer a cleansing enema the evening before or the morning of the BE if directed by physician's order or hospital policy. Milk of magnesia (60 mL) may be ordered after the BE to stimulate evacuation of the barium.

After the BE study, assess the patient for complete evacuation of the barium. Retained barium may cause a hardened impaction. Stool will be light colored until all the barium has been expelled.

COLONOSCOPY

Rationale

The development of the fiberoptic colonoscope has enabled examination of the entire colon—from anus to cecum—in a high percentage of patients. Colonoscopy can detect lesions in the proximal colon, which would not be found by sigmoidoscopy. Benign and malignant neoplasms, mucosal inflammation or ulceration, and sites of active hemorrhage can also be visualized. Biopsy specimens can be obtained and small tumors removed through the scope with the use of cable-activated instruments. Actively bleeding vessels can be coagulated.

A less invasive test than a standard colonoscopy is called virtual colonoscopy. This test uses CT scanning or MRI with computer software to produce images of the colon and rectum. The colon preparation is similar to that for a regular colonoscopic examination. Sedatives are not required and no scope is needed (Lewis et al., 2007).

Patients who have had cancer of the colon are at high risk for developing a subsequent colon cancer; patients who have a family history of colon cancer are also at high risk. For these patients, colonoscopy allows early detection of any primary or secondary tumors.

Nursing Interventions

Explain the procedure to the patient and have him or her sign a consent form. Instruct the patient regarding dietary restrictions: Usually a clear liquid diet is permitted 1 to 3 days before the procedure to decrease the residue in the bowel, and then NPO status is maintained for 8 hours before the procedure. Administer a cathartic, enemas, and premedication as ordered to decrease the residue in the bowel. GoLYTELY, an oral or NG colonic lavage, is an osmotic electrolyte solution that is now commonly used as a cathartic (Box 5-2). It is a polyethylene glycol solution. If it is taken orally, instruct the patient to drink the solution rapidly: 8 ounces (240 mL) every 15 minutes until enough solution has been consumed to make the colonic contents a light yellow liquid. Powdered lemonade may be added to make the oral solution more palatable. If it is given per lavage, it

Box 5-2 GoLYTELY Bowel Preparation

1. Give patient one metoclopramide (Reglan) 10-mg tablet, as prescribed, orally 30 minutes before proceeding with step 2.
2. Administer GoLYTELY solution* (prepared by pharmacy) per physician's orders:
   a. 240 mL orally every 15 minutes *or*
   b. 30 mL/min via nasogastric tube. Use a Travasorb enteral feeding container and a size 10 feeding tube. Administer until stools are clear yellow.
   c. Keep patients warm with heated blankets; they often become chilled after consuming copious amounts of GoLYTELY solution.
   d. Provide a bedside commode for older or weak patients.

*Administer a minimum of 1 gallon of solution over a 2-hour period.

must be given rapidly. Taking the solution slowly will not clean the colon efficiently. Provide warm blankets during the procedure, since many patients experience hypothermia while taking GoLYTELY. Provide a commode at the bedside for older adults and frail patients. Check the patient's stool after the prep to make certain it is light yellow and liquid. A preprocedure IV sedative such as midazolam is often given.

After the colonoscopy, check for evidence of bowel perforation (abdominal pain, guarding, distention, tenderness, excessive rectal bleeding, or blood clots) and examine stools for gross blood. Assess for hypovolemic shock.

STOOL CULTURE
Rationale
The feces (stool) can be examined for the presence of bacteria, ova, and parasites (a plant or animal that lives on or within another living organism and obtains some advantage at its host's expense). The physician may order a stool for culture of bacteria or of ova and parasites (O&P). Many bacteria (such as *Escherichia coli*) are indigenous in the bowel. Bacterial cultures are usually done to detect enteropathogens (such as *Staphylococcus aureus, Salmonella* or *Shigella* organisms, *E. coli* O157:H7, or *Clostridium difficile*).

When a patient is suspected of having a parasitic infection, the stool is examined for O&P. Usually at least three stool specimens are collected on subsequent days. Because culture results are not available for several days, they do not influence initial treatment, but they do guide subsequent treatment if bacterial infection is present.

Nursing Interventions
If an enema must be administered to collect specimens, use only normal saline or tap water. Soapsuds or any other substance could affect the viability of the organisms collected.

Stool samples for O&P are obtained before barium examinations. Instruct the patient not to mix urine with feces. Don gloves to collect the specimen, and ensure the specimen is taken to the laboratory within 30 minutes of collection in specified container.

OBSTRUCTION SERIES (FLAT PLATE OF THE ABDOMEN)
Rationale
The obstruction series is a group of radiographic studies performed on the abdomen of patients who have suspected bowel obstruction, paralytic ileus, perforated viscus (any large interior organ in any of the great body cavities), or abdominal abscess. The series usually consists of at least two radiographic studies. The first is an erect abdominal radiographic study that allows visualization of the diaphragm. Radiographs are examined for evidence of free air under the diaphragm, which is **pathognomonic** (signs or symptoms specific to a disease condition) of a perforated viscus. This radiographic study is used also to detect air-fluid levels within the intestine.

Nursing Interventions
For adequate visualization, ensure that this study is scheduled before any barium studies.

DISORDERS OF THE MOUTH

Common disorders of the mouth and esophagus that interfere with adequate nutrition include poor dental hygiene, infections, inflammation, and cancer.

DENTAL PLAQUE AND CARIES
Etiology and Pathophysiology
Dental decay is an erosive process that results from the action of bacteria on carbohydrates in the mouth, which in turn produce acids that dissolve tooth enamel. Most Americans (95%) experience tooth decay at some time in their life. Dental decay can be caused by several factors:

- Dental plaque, a thin film on the teeth made of mucin and colloidal material found in saliva and often secondarily invaded by bacteria
- The strength of acids and the inability of the saliva to neutralize them
- The length of time the acids are in contact with the teeth
- Susceptibility of the teeth to decay

Medical Management
Dental caries is treated by removal of affected areas of the tooth and replacement with some form of dental material. Treatment of periodontal disease centers on removal of plaque from the teeth. If the disease is advanced, surgical interventions on the gingivae and alveolar bone may be necessary.

Nursing Interventions and Patient Teaching
Proper technique for brushing and flossing the teeth at least twice a day is the primary focus for teaching these patients. Plaque forms continuously and must be

removed periodically through regular visits to the dentist. Stress the importance of prevention through continual care. Because carbohydrates create an environment in which caries develop and plaque accumulates more easily, include proper nutrition in patient teaching. When the patient is ill, the mouth's normal cleansing action is impaired. Illnesses, drugs, and irradiation all interfere with the normal action of saliva. If the patient is unable to manage oral hygiene, the nurse must assume this responsibility.

Nursing diagnoses and interventions for the patient with dental plaque and caries include but are not limited to the following:

Nursing Diagnoses	Nursing Interventions
Deficient knowledge, related to: • inability to prevent dental caries • periodontal disease	Assess and observe the oral cavity for moisture, color, and cleanliness. Stress importance of meticulous oral hygiene. Explain the need to see a dentist at least yearly for an examination.
Noncompliance, related to hygiene and dietary restrictions	Brush teeth twice daily and as needed with toothpaste or powder, baking soda, or mouthwash. Rinse with water or mouthwash. Cleanse mouth with equal parts of hydrogen peroxide and water as needed for halitosis. Teach the patient about oral hygiene.

Prognosis

The prevention and elimination of dental plaque and caries are directly related to oral hygiene, dental care, nutrition, and heredity. All but heredity are controllable factors. The prognosis is more favorable for people who brush, floss, regularly visit the dentist for removal of affected areas, eat low-carbohydrate foods, and drink fluoridated water.

CANDIDIASIS

Etiology and Pathophysiology

Candidiasis is any infection caused by a species of *Candida*, usually *C. albicans*. *Candida* is a fungal organism normally present in the mucous membranes of the mouth, intestinal tract, and vagina; it is also found on the skin of healthy people. This infection is also referred to as **thrush** or **moniliasis.**

This disease appears more commonly in the newborn infant, who becomes infected while passing through the birth canal. In the older individual, candidiasis may be found in patients with leukemia, diabetes mellitus, or alcoholism, and in patients who are

taking antibiotics (chlortetracycline or tetracycline), are undergoing corticosteroid inhalant treatment, or are immunosuppressed (e.g., patients with acquired immunodeficiency syndrome [AIDS] or those receiving chemotherapy or radiation therapy).

Clinical Manifestations

Candidiasis appears as pearly, bluish white "milk-curd" membranous lesions on the mucous membranes of the mouth, tongue, and larynx. One or more lesions may be on the mucosa, depending on the duration of the infection. If the patch or plaque is removed, painful bleeding can occur.

Medical Management

Nystatin or amphotericin B (an oral suspension) or buccal tablets or fluconazole (Diflucan), half-strength hydrogen peroxide and saline mouth rinses may provide some relief.

Nursing Interventions

Use meticulous hand hygiene to prevent spread of infection. The infection may be spread in the nursery by carelessness of nursing personnel. Hand hygiene, care of feeding equipment, and cleanliness of the mother's nipples are important to prevent spread. Cleanse the infant's mouth of any foreign material, rinsing the mouth and lubricating the lips. Inspect the mouth using a flashlight and tongue blade.

For adults, instruct the patient to use a soft-bristled toothbrush and administer a topical anesthetic (lidocaine or benzocaine) to the mouth 1 hour before meals. Give soft or pureed foods and avoid hot, cold, spicy, fried, or citrus foods.

Prognosis

If the host has a strong defense system and medical treatment is initiated early in the course of the disease, the prognosis is good.

CARCINOMA OF THE ORAL CAVITY

Etiology and Pathophysiology

Oral (or oropharyngeal) cancer may occur on the lips, the oral cavity, the tongue, and the pharynx. The tonsils are occasionally involved. Most of these tumors are squamous cell epitheliomas that grow rapidly and metastasize to adjacent structures more quickly than do most malignant tumors of the skin. In the United States, oral cancer accounts for 4% of the cancers in men and 2% in women. An estimated 35,310 new cases and 7590 deaths from oral cavity and pharynx cancer were expected in 2008. Death rates have been decreasing since the 1970s, with rates declining faster in the 2000s (American Cancer Society [ACS], *Cancer facts and figures*, 2008).

Tumors of the salivary glands occur primarily in the parotid gland and are usually benign. Tumors of the submaxillary gland have a high incidence of malignancy. These malignant tumors grow rapidly and may be accompanied by pain and impaired facial function.

Kaposi's sarcoma is a malignant skin tumor that occurs primarily on the legs of men between 50 and 70 years of age. It is seen with increased frequency as a nonsquamous tumor of the oral cavity in patients with AIDS. The lesions are purple and nonulcerated. Irradiation is the treatment of choice.

The tumor seen with cancer of the lip is usually an **epithelioma.** It occurs most frequently as a chronic ulcer of the lower lip in men. The cure rate for cancer of the lip is high because the lesion is apparent to the patient and to others. Metastasis to regional lymph nodes has occurred in only 10% of people when diagnosed. In some instances a lesion may spread rapidly and involve the mandible and the floor of the mouth by direct extension. Occasionally the tumor may be a basal cell lesion that starts in the skin and spreads to the lip.

Cancer of the anterior tongue and floor of the mouth may seem to occur together because their spread to adjacent tissues is so rapid. Because of the tongue's abundant vascular and lymphatic drainage, metastasis to the neck has already occurred in more than 60% of patients when the diagnosis is made. There is a higher incidence of cancers of the mouth and throat among people who are heavy drinkers and have a history of tobacco use (e.g., cigar, cigarette, pipe, chewing tobacco). Also, data show that the mortality rate for males between the ages of 10 and 20 has doubled over the past 30 years as a result of the use of smokeless tobacco (snuff). The combination of high alcohol consumption and smoking or chewing tobacco causes an apparent breakdown in the body's defense mechanism. Predisposing factors include exposure to the sun and wind.

Clinical Manifestations

Leukoplakia (a white, firmly attached patch on the mouth or tongue mucosa) may appear on the lips and buccal mucosa. These nonsloughing lesions cannot be rubbed off by simple mechanical force. They can be benign or malignant. A small percentage develop into squamous cell carcinomas, and biopsy is recommended if the lesions persist for longer than 2 weeks. They occur most frequently between the ages of 50 and 70 years and appear more commonly in men.

Assessment

Collection of **subjective data** includes understanding that malignant lesions of the mouth are usually asymptomatic. The patient may feel only a roughened area with the tongue. As the disease progresses, the first complaints may be (1) difficulty chewing, swallowing, or speaking; (2) edema, numbness, or loss of feeling in any part of the mouth; and (3) earache, facial pain, and toothache, which may become constant. Cancer of the lip is associated with discomfort and irritation caused by a nonhealing lesion, which may be raised or ulcerated. Malignancy at the base of the tongue produces

less obvious symptoms: slight dysphagia, sore throat, and salivation.

Collection of **objective data** includes observing for premalignant lesions, including leukoplakia. Unusual bleeding in the mouth, some blood-tinged sputum, lumps or edema in the neck, and hoarseness may be observed.

Diagnostic Tests

Indirect laryngoscopy is an important diagnostic test for examination of the soft tissue. This procedure is especially important for men 40 years of age or older who have dysphagia and a history of smoking and alcohol ingestion. Radiographic evaluation of the mandibular structures is another essential part of the head and neck examination to rule out cancer. Excisional biopsy is the most accurate method for making a definitive diagnosis. Oral exfoliative cytology is used for screening intraoral lesions. A scraping of the lesion provides cells for cytologic examination. The chance for a false-negative finding is about 26%.

Medical Management

Treatment depends on the location and staging of the malignant tumor. Stage I oral cancers are treated by surgery or radiation. Stages II and III cancers require both surgery and radiation. Chemotherapy may also be used when surgery and radiation therapy fail or as the initial therapy for smaller tumors. Treatment for stage IV cancer is usually palliative. The survival rate for patients with oral cancers averages less than 50%.

Small, accessible tumors can be excised surgically. Surgical options include a glossectomy, removal of the tongue; hemiglossectomy, removal of part of the tongue; mandibulectomy, removal of the mandible; and total or supraglottic laryngectomy, removal of the entire larynx or the portion above the true vocal cords.

Large tumors usually require more extensive and traumatic surgery. In a functional neck dissection of neck cancer with no growth in the lymph nodes, the surgeon removes the lymph nodes but preserves the jugular vein, the sternocleidomastoid muscle, and the spinal accessory nerve. In radical neck dissection, all these structures are removed and reconstructive surgery is necessary after tissue resection. Patients may have drains in the incision sites that are connected to suction to aid healing and reduce hematomas. A tracheostomy may also be performed, depending on the degree of tumor invasion.

Because of the location of the surgery, complications can occur. These include airway obstruction, hemorrhage, tracheal aspiration, facial edema, fistula formation, and necrosis of the skin flaps. If the patient has difficulty swallowing, a percutaneous endoscopic gastrostomy (PEG) tube may be inserted to allow for adequate nutritional intake. Neurologic complications can occur because of nerves being severed and manipulated during surgery.

Radiation therapy may involve (1) external radiation by roentgenograms or other radioactive substances or (2) internal radiation by means of needles or seeds. The purpose of radiation therapy is to shrink the tumor. It can be given preoperatively or postoperatively, depending on the physician's preference and the patient's disease process. In more advanced cases, chemotherapy may be combined with radiation postoperatively to make the patient more comfortable. Other treatment options include laser excision.

Nursing Interventions and Patient Teaching

A holistic approach to patient care includes awareness of the patient's level of knowledge regarding the disease, emotional response and coping abilities, and spiritual needs. Nursing interventions must be individualized to the patient—beginning with the preoperative stage, continuing through the postoperative stage, and ending after the patient's rehabilitation in the home environment. Family members, hospice workers, close friends, social workers, and pastoral care staff may provide information and support during this potentially fatal disease.

Nursing diagnoses and interventions for the patient with oral cancer include but are not limited to the following:

Nursing Diagnoses	Nursing Interventions
Imbalanced nutrition, less than body requirements, related to: • oral pain postoperative tissue loss • oral pain (mucous membranes)	Monitor the patient for changes in the character and quantity of mucus after radiation therapy. Provide meticulous oral hygiene. Observe for temporary or permanent loss of taste and the need for alternative routes for nutrition by monitoring daily weights.
Disturbed body image and personal identity, related to: • disfiguring appearance of an oral lesion • reconstructive surgery	Provide alternative methods for communication if radiation therapy results in dysarthria (difficult, poorly articulated speech, resulting from interference in the control over muscles of speech). Provide information to the patient and family to help with difficult decisions related to surgery, radiation, or chemotherapy. Provide support to the patient and family.

Prevention centers on predisposing factors: avoiding excess exposure to sun and wind on the lips, eliminating smoking or chewing tobacco, and eliminating plaque and caries through good oral and dental care. The incidence of cancer of the mouth bears a high correlation to cirrhosis of the liver associated with alcohol intake. Early detection of oral cancer can increase the

patient's chance of survival. Any person with a mouth lesion that does not heal within 2 to 3 weeks is urged to seek medical care.

Instruct the patient about preoperative and postoperative care, with full explanations regarding speech loss and alternate methods of nutritional intake. Explanation of tracheostomy care and other tubes the patient may have on discharge relieves anxiety and increases the patient's sense of control over the situation.

Prognosis

Staging and biologic characterization of the neoplasm provide prognostic information. The prognosis of carcinoma in the oral cavity is directly related to the size of the primary tumor, the involvement of regional nodes, and the presence or absence of metastasis. The patient's immunologic response and general condition also influence the prognosis and the choice of therapy.

Carcinomas of the lip can be detected early by the patient, the physician, or the dentist during examination, and the prognosis for cure is good. If the carcinoma is difficult to detect, as on the anterior tongue and the floor of the mouth, it will be in a more advanced stage when detected. The prognosis in such cases is bleak. The 5-year survival rate for cancer of the oral cavity and pharynx is 53% for whites and 34% for blacks (ACS, 2009).

DISORDERS OF THE ESOPHAGUS

GASTROESOPHAGEAL REFLUX DISEASE

Etiology and Pathophysiology

Gastroesophageal reflux disease (GERD) is a backward flow of stomach acid up into the esophagus. Symptoms typically include burning and pressure behind the sternum. Most cases are thought to be caused by the inappropriate relaxation of the lower esophageal sphincter (LES) in response to an unknown stimulus. Symptoms of GERD develop when the LES is weak or experiences prolonged or frequent transient relaxation, conditions that allow gastric acids and enzymes to flow into the esophagus. Reflux is much more common in the postprandial state (after meals); more than 60% of reflux sufferers have delayed gastric emptying. GERD occurs in all age-groups and is estimated to affect up to 45% of the population to some degree, which translates to more than 60 million people. GERD is the most common upper GI problem seen in adults.

Clinical Manifestations

The clinical manifestations of GERD are consistent, but vary substantially in severity. The irritation of chronic reflux produces the primary symptom, which is heartburn (pyrosis). The pain is described as a substernal or retrosternal burning sensation that tends to radiate upward and may involve the neck, the jaw, or the back. The pain typically occurs 20 minutes to 2 hours after eating. An atypical pain pattern that closely mimics angina may also occur and must be carefully differentiated from true cardiac disease. The second major symptom of GERD is regurgitation, which is not associated with either eructation or nausea. The individual experiences a feeling of warm fluid moving up the throat. If it reaches the pharynx, a sour or bitter taste is perceived. Water brash, a reflux salivary hypersecretion that does not taste bitter, occurs less commonly.

In severe cases, GERD can produce dysphagia or odynophagia (painful swallowing). Eructation and a feeling of flatulence are other common complaints. Nocturnal cough, wheezing, or hoarseness all may occur with reflux, and it is estimated that more than 80% of adult asthmatics may have reflux. The frequency and severity of reflux episodes usually determine the severity of the symptoms.

Assessment

Subjective data include heartburn, a substernal or retrosternal burning sensation that may radiate to the back or jaw (in some cases the pain may mimic angina); and regurgitation (not associated with nausea or eructation), which causes a sour or bitter taste in the pharynx. Frequent eructation, flatulence, and dysphagia or odynophagia usually occur only in severe cases.

Objective data include nocturnal cough, wheezing, and hoarseness.

Diagnostic Tests

Mild cases of GERD are diagnosed from the classic symptoms, and treatment is initiated based on the presumptive diagnosis. More involved cases may require other screening tools. The gold standard for diagnosis is 24-hour pH monitoring using specially designed probes; such testing accurately records the number, duration, and severity of reflux episodes and is considered to be 85% sensitive. The esophageal motility and Bernstein tests can be performed in conjunction with pH monitoring to evaluate LES competence and the response of the esophagus to acid infusion. The barium swallow with fluoroscopy is widely used to document the presence of hiatal hernia. Endoscopy is routinely performed to evaluate for LES competence, potential scarring and strictures, and the presence and severity of esophagitis, and to rule out malignancy.

Medical Management

In its simplest form, GERD produces mild symptoms that occur infrequently (twice a week or less). In these cases, avoiding problem foods or beverages, stopping smoking, or losing weight may solve the problem. Medication therapy for GERD focuses on improving LES function, increasing esophageal clearance, decreasing volume and acidity of reflux, and protecting the esophageal mucosa. Treatment with antacids or acid-blocking medications called H_2 receptor antagonists—such as cimetidine (Tagamet), ranitidine (Zantac), famotidine (Pepcid), or nizatidine (Axid)—may also be used. More severe and frequent episodes of GERD can trigger asthma attacks, cause severe chest pain, result in bleeding, or promote a

narrowing (stricture) or chronic irritation of the esophagus. In these cases, more powerful inhibitors of stomach acid production called proton pump inhibitors, such as omeprazole (Prilosec), esomeprazole (Nexium), pantoprazole (Protonix), rabeprazole (Aciphex), and lansoprazole (Prevacid), may be added to the treatment prescribed. Sucralfate (Carafate) is an antiulcer drug that may be used in GERD patients for its protective properties by forming a complex that adheres to an ulcer. Metoclopramide (Reglan) is used in moderate to severe cases of GERD. It is in a class of drugs called *promotility agents* that increase peristalsis and therefore promote gastric emptying and reduce the risk of gastric acid reflux.

As a last resort, a surgical procedure called **fundoplication** is performed to strengthen the sphincter. The procedure involves wrapping a layer of the upper stomach wall (fundus) around the sphincter and terminal esophagus to lessen the possibility of acid reflux (see Figure 5-16). If GERD is left untreated, serious pathologic (precancerous) changes in the esophageal lining may develop—a condition called **Barrett's esophagus** (esophageal metaplasia). In Barrett's esophagus the normal squamous epithelium of the esophagus is replaced by columnar epithelium. Because patients with Barrett's esophagus are at higher risk for esophageal cancer, they may need to be monitored regularly (every 1 to 3 years) by endoscopy and biopsy.

Nursing Interventions and Patient Teaching

Nursing interventions involve educating the patient about diet and lifestyle modifications that may alleviate symptoms of GERD.

Dietary instructions include (1) eat four to six small meals daily; (2) follow a low-fat, adequate-protein diet; (3) reduce intake of chocolate, tea, and other foods and beverages that contain caffeine; (4) limit or eliminate alcohol intake; (5) eat slowly, and chew food thoroughly; (6) avoid evening snacking, and do not eat for 2 to 3 hours before bedtime; (7) remain upright for 1 to 2 hours after meals when possible, and never eat in bed; (8) avoid any food that directly produces heartburn; and (9) reduce overall body weight if needed.

Numerous lifestyle changes are also indicated. Encourage patients who smoke to stop. Cigarette smoking has been associated with decreased acid clearance from the lower esophagus. Advise them to avoid constrictive clothing over the abdomen. They should avoid activities that involve straining, heavy lifting, or working in a bent-over position. Also instruct them to never sleep flat in bed. They should elevate the head of the bed at least 6 to 8 inches for sleep, using wooden blocks or a thick foam wedge.

Prognosis

If GERD is not successfully controlled, it can progress to serious and even life-threatening problems. Esophageal ulceration and hemorrhage may result from severe erosion, and chronic nighttime reflux is accompanied by a significant risk of aspiration. Adenocarcinoma can develop from the premalignant tissue (termed *Barrett's epithelium*). Gradual or repeated scarring can permanently damage esophageal tissue and produce stricture.

CARCINOMA OF THE ESOPHAGUS

Etiology and Pathophysiology

Carcinoma of the esophagus is a malignant epithelial neoplasm that has invaded the esophagus and has been diagnosed as a squamous cell carcinoma or an adenocarcinoma. An estimated 30% to 70% of esophageal cancers are adenocarcinomas; the remainder are squamous cell carcinomas. The incidence of squamous cell esophageal cancer is currently decreasing in the United States, whereas the incidence of adenocarcinoma of the distal esophagus is increasing (Lewis et al., 2007). Risk factors for esophageal cancer include alcohol and tobacco use and possibly longstanding achalasia (an abnormal condition characterized by the inability of a muscle to relax, particularly the cardiac sphincter of the stomach). Environmental carcinogens, nutritional deficiencies, chronic irritation, and mucosal damage have all been considered as causes of esophageal cancer. Another risk factor is Barrett's esophagus. It is estimated that 1 of 200 cases of Barrett's esophagus will progress to esophageal adenocarcinoma (see Health Promotion box).

Unfortunately, because of the location, esophageal cancer is usually at a late stage when discovered; treatment is palliative. Carcinoma of the bronchus, stomach, or breast may metastasize to the esophagus. The prevalent age-group for esophageal cancer is 55 to 70 years. It occurs more commonly in men.

Clinical Manifestations

The most common clinical symptom is progressive **dysphagia** (difficulty in swallowing) over a 6-month period. The patient may have a substernal feeling as though food is not passing through the esophagus.

Assessment

Collection of **subjective data** includes noting that initially the patient may have difficulty swallowing when eating bulky foods such as meat; later the difficulty

Health Promotion

Prevention or Early Detection of Esophageal Cancer

- Patients with diagnosed gastroesophageal reflux disease and hiatal hernia need counseling regarding regular follow-up evaluation.
- Health teaching should focus on elimination of smoking and excessive alcohol intake.
- Maintenance of good oral hygiene and dietary habits (intake of fresh fruits and vegetables) may be helpful.
- Patients diagnosed with Barrett's esophagus need to be monitored because this is considered a premalignant condition. Regular endoscopic screening with biopsy is required.
- Encourage patients to seek medical attention for any esophageal problems, especially dysphagia.

occurs with soft foods and finally with liquids and even saliva. Another symptom is odynophagia (painful swallowing). Pain is a late symptom and indicates local extension of the malignancy.

Collection of **objective data** includes observing the patient for regurgitation (backward flowing or casting up of undigested food), vomiting, hoarseness, chronic cough, choking, and iron deficiency anemia. Weight loss may be directly related to the tumor or a side effect of treatment or the inability to swallow. When esophageal stenosis (narrowing) is severe, regurgitation of blood-flecked esophageal contents is common. Hemorrhage occurs if the cancer erodes through the esophagus and into the aorta. Esophageal perforation with fistula formation into the lung or trachea sometimes develops. The tumor may enlarge enough to cause esophageal obstruction. The cancer spreads via the lymph system, with the liver and lung being common sites of metastasis (Lewis et al., 2007).

Diagnostic Tests

A barium swallow examination with fluoroscopy and endoscopy is used to detect esophageal cancer. An endoscopy with biopsy and cytologic examination provides a highly accurate diagnosis. Endoscopic ultrasonography is an important tool used to stage esophageal cancer. Computed tomography (CT) and magnetic resonance imaging also are used to assess the extent of the disease.

Medical Management

The treatment of esophageal cancer depends on the tumor's location and whether invasion or metastasis has occurred. Tumor staging must be determined to guide patient management. In advanced cases, surgery is palliative to relieve dysphagia and restore continuity of the alimentary tract. An aggressive approach provides excellent palliation (therapy designed to relieve or reduce intensity of uncomfortable symptoms but not to produce a cure), increased longevity, and a chance for a cure. Standard resection seems to give as good a result as a radical procedure.

Radiation therapy may be curative or palliative. Problems associated with radiation therapy include the development of an esophagotracheal fistula (an abnormal passage between two internal organs). Aspiration from the fistula and edema from the radiation are common. Chemotherapeutic agents cisplatin (Platinol), paclitaxel (Taxol), and fluorouracil (5-FU) are currently used in combination with radiation before and/or after surgery. If the tumor is in the upper third of the esophagus, radiation is indicated. A tumor in the lower third is usually resected surgically. Because of the extreme toxicity of these drugs, expect the patient to experience side effects of respiratory and liver dysfunction, nausea and vomiting, leukopenia, and sepsis.

The following four types of surgical procedures can be performed:

1. **Esophagogastrectomy:** Resection of a lower esophageal section with a proximal portion of the stomach, followed by **anastomosis** (surgical joining of two ducts, blood vessels, or bowel segments to allow flow from one to the other) of the remaining portions of the esophagus and stomach
2. **Esophagogastrostomy:** Resection of a portion of the esophagus with anastomosis to the stomach
3. **Esophagoenterostomy:** Resection of the esophagus and anastomosis to a portion of the colon
4. **Gastrostomy:** Insertion of a catheter into the stomach and suture to the abdominal wall; performed when the patient cannot take food orally because inoperable cancer of the esophagus interferes with swallowing

Nursing Interventions and Patient Teaching

Nursing diagnoses and interventions for the patient with esophageal carcinoma include but are not limited to the following:

Nursing Diagnoses	Nursing Interventions
Ineffective breathing pattern, related to: • incisional pain • proximity to the diaphragm	Monitor respirations carefully because of proximity of incision to diaphragm and patient's difficulty in carrying out breathing exercises.
Imbalanced nutrition: less than body requirements, related to: • dysphagia • decreased stomach capacity • anorexia	Monitor intake and output (I&O) and daily weights to determine adequate nutritional intake. Assess which foods patient can and cannot swallow to select and prepare edible foods. Administer tube feedings through gastrostomy, if present.

Discuss with the patient and family all aspects of care, including surgery, radiation, and chemotherapy. Psychological adjustment of the patient who cannot ingest food orally, whether temporary or permanent, is difficult. Step-by-step explanations of all diagnostic tests, medications, procedures, and the treatment plan will help relieve the patient's anxiety. Support the patient with this serious diagnosis by allowing time for questions.

Prognosis

In carcinoma of the esophagus, the disease is usually well advanced by the time symptoms appear. The delay between the onset of early symptoms and when the patient seeks medical advice is often 12 to 18 months. High mortality rates among these patients are affected by the following issues: (1) the patient is generally older; (2) the tumor has usually invaded surrounding structures; (3) the malignancy tends to spread to nearby lymph nodes; and (4) the esophagus is close to the heart and lungs, making these organs accessible to tumor extension.

The esophagus has an extensive lymphatic network, which facilitates the rapid spread of malignant cells to varying local and distant sites. Because esophageal cancer is rarely diagnosed in early stages, the 5-year survival rate is less than 20%. The only prognostic variable is the stage of disease (which underlines the importance of early diagnosis).

ACHALASIA

Etiology and Pathophysiology

Achalasia, also called **cardiospasm,** is an abnormal condition characterized by the inability of a muscle to relax, particularly the cardiac sphincter of the stomach. Although the cause is unknown, nerve degeneration, esophageal dilation, and hypertrophy are thought to contribute to the disruption of the esophagus's normal neuromuscular activity. This results in decreased motility and dilation of the lower portion of the esophagus, along with an absence of peristalsis. Thus little or no food can enter the stomach, and in extreme cases the dilated portion of the esophagus holds as much as a liter or more of fluid. This disease may occur in people of any age, but is more prevalent in those between 20 and 50 years.

Clinical Manifestations

The primary symptom of achalasia is dysphagia. The patient has a sensation of food sticking in the lower portion of the esophagus. As the condition progresses, the patient complains of regurgitation of food, which relieves prolonged distention of the esophagus. The patient may also have substernal chest pain.

Assessment

Observe for loss of weight, poor skin turgor, and weakness.

Diagnostic Tests

Radiologic studies show esophageal dilation above the narrowing at the cardioesophageal junction. The diagnosis is confirmed by manometry, which shows the absence of primary peristalsis. Esophagoscopy is also used to confirm the diagnosis.

Medical Management

Conservative treatment of achalasia includes drug therapy and forceful dilation of the narrowed area of the esophagus. Anticholinergics, nitrates, and calcium channel blockers reduce pressure in the lower esophageal sphincter.

Dilation is done by first emptying the esophagus. Then a dilator with a deflated balloon is passed down to the sphincter. The balloon is inflated and remains so for 1 minute; it may need to be reinflated once or twice.

Box 5-3	Nursing Interventions for the Patient Experiencing Esophageal Surgery

PREOPERATIVE NURSING INTERVENTIONS
1. Encourage improved nutritional status.
   a. Offer a high-protein, high-calorie diet if oral diet is possible.
   b. Total parenteral nutrition may be necessary for severe dysphagia or obstruction.
   c. Gastroscopy tube feedings may be indicated.
2. Give meticulous oral hygiene; breath may be malodorous.
3. Give preoperative preparation appropriate for thoracic surgery.
4. Give prescribed antibiotics before esophageal resection or bypass, as ordered.

POSTOPERATIVE NURSING INTERVENTIONS
1. Promote good pulmonary ventilation.
2. Maintain chest drainage system as prescribed.
3. Maintain gastric drainage system.
   a. Small amounts of blood may drain from nasogastric tube for 6 to 12 hours after surgery.
   b. Do not disturb nasogastric tube (to prevent traction on suture line).
4. Maintain nutrition.
   a. Start clear fluids at frequent intervals when oral intake is permitted.
   b. Introduce soft foods gradually, increasing to several small meals of bland foods.
   c. Have patient maintain semi-Fowler's position for 2 hours after eating and while sleeping if heartburn (pyrosis) occurs.

The preferred surgical approach is a cardiomyotomy. The muscular layer is incised longitudinally down to but not through the mucosa. Two thirds of the incision is in the esophagus, and the remaining one third is in the stomach; this permits the mucosa to expand so that food can pass easily into the stomach.

Nursing Interventions and Patient Teaching

Nursing interventions for esophageal surgery are presented in Box 5-3.

Nursing diagnoses and interventions for the patient with achalasia include but are not limited to the following:

Nursing Diagnoses	Nursing Interventions
Imbalanced nutrition: less than body requirements, related to difficulty swallowing both liquids and solids	Encourage fluids with meals to increase lower esophageal sphincter pressure and push food into stomach. Monitor liquid diet for 24 hours after dilation procedure.

Nursing Diagnoses	Nursing Interventions
Anxiety, related to continuous dilation process with threat of complications	Monitor for signs of esophageal perforation (chest pain, shock, dyspnea, fever) after dilation. Provide calm, nonstressful environment. Reinforce physician's explanation of disease process. Encourage verbalization of fears; assist patient with identifying stressors and positive coping behaviors.

Discuss home care and follow-up care in preparation for dismissal. Include a family member or support person if possible, and involve the patient as an active participant in the planning. Explain the need for a high-calorie, high-protein diet, and provide printed material describing same. Explain the need to elevate the head while sleeping and to avoid bending and stooping. Discuss medications if prescribed (including name, dosage, time of administration, purpose, and side effects). Discuss methods of avoiding constipation by using high-fiber foods (if tolerated) and natural laxatives. Explain the importance of follow-up care with the physician. Finally, discuss symptoms of recurrence or progression of disease and the need to report these to the physician.

Prognosis

Surgical separation, in addition to bag dilation, permits the return of normal peristalsis in approximately 10% of patients with achalasia.

DISORDERS OF THE STOMACH

GASTRITIS (ACUTE)

Etiology and Pathophysiology

Gastritis is an inflammation of the lining of the stomach. Acute gastritis is a temporary inflammation associated with alcoholism, smoking, and stressful physical problems, such as burns; major surgery; food allergens; viral, bacterial, or chemical toxins; chemotherapy; or radiation therapy. Changes in the mucosal lining interfere with acid and pepsin secretion. Acute gastritis is often a single incident that resolves when the offending agent is removed.

Clinical Manifestations

If the condition is acute, the patient may experience fever, epigastric pain, nausea, vomiting, headache, coating of the tongue, and loss of appetite. If the condition results from ingestion of contaminated food, the intestines are usually affected and diarrhea may occur. Some patients with gastritis have no symptoms.

Assessment

Collection of **subjective data** includes observing for anorexia, nausea, discomfort after eating, and pain.

Collection of **objective data** includes observing for vomiting, hematemesis, and melena caused by gastric bleeding.

Diagnostic Tests

Diagnosis is based on testing the stools for occult blood, noting white blood cell (WBC) differential increases related to certain bacteria, evaluating serum electrolytes, and observing for elevated hematocrit related to dehydration.

Medical Management

If medical treatment is required, an antiemetic—such as prochlorperazine (Compazine), promethazine (Phenergan), or trimethobenzamide (Tigan)—may be prescribed. Antacids and cimetidine (Tagamet) or ranitidine (Zantac) may be given in combination. Antibiotics are given if the cause is a bacterial agent. IV fluids are used to correct fluid and electrolyte imbalances. Patients who experience GI bleeding from hemorrhagic gastritis require fluid and blood replacement and NG lavage.

Nursing Interventions and Patient Teaching

Record the patient's I&O. Withhold foods and fluids orally as prescribed until signs and symptoms subside. Monitor the patient's tolerance to oral feedings and IV feedings as prescribed. Clear liquids are increased to diet as tolerated.

A nursing diagnosis and interventions for the patient with gastritis include but are not limited to the following:

Nursing Diagnosis	Nursing Interventions
Deficient fluid volume, related to vomiting, diarrhea, and blood loss	Keep patient NPO or on restricted food and fluids as ordered, and advance as tolerated. Monitor laboratory data for fluid and electrolyte imbalance (potassium, magnesium, sodium, and chloride). Maintain IV feedings. Record I&O.

Patient education includes explanations of (1) the effects of stress on the mucosal lining of the stomach; (2) how salicylates, nonsteroidal antiinflammatory drugs (NSAIDs), and particular foods may be irritating; and (3) how lifestyles that include alcohol and tobacco may be harmful. Assist the patient in locating self-help groups in the community to deal with these behaviors.

Prognosis

Because of the many classifications and causes of gastritis, prognosis is variable. Generally, prognosis is good in individuals who are willing to change their lifestyles and follow a medical regimen.

PEPTIC ULCERS

Peptic ulcers are ulcerations of the mucous membrane or deeper structures of the GI tract. They most commonly occur in the stomach and duodenum. The term *peptic ulcer* refers to ulcers resulting from acid and pepsin imbalances. Peptic ulcer disease remains a major health problem and affects more men than women. The disease is increasing among older adults, perhaps as a result of the use of NSAIDs. Symptoms are common between the ages of 25 and 50, with peak occurrence at age 40.

The stomach is normally protected from autodigestion by the gastric mucosal barrier. The GI tract has a high cell turnover rate, and the stomach's surface mucosa is renewed about every 3 days. As a result, the mucosa continuously repairs itself except in extreme instances when the cell breakdown surpasses the cell renewal rate. In such cases, peptic ulcers can occur. Peptic ulcers require the presence of gastric acid and result from four major causes: (1) excess of gastric acid (duodenal ulcers); (2) decrease in the natural ability of the GI mucosa to protect itself from acid and pepsin (gastric ulcers); (3) infection with spiral-shaped bacteria *H. pylori;* and (4) gastric injury from NSAIDs, aspirin, or corticosteroids.

Understanding of the factors that contribute to ulcer formation is developing rapidly. The discovery of the bacterium *H. pylori* provided new insight to ulcer formation. *H. pylori* has been identified in more than 70% of gastric ulcer patients and 95% of those with duodenal ulcers. In Western cultures, half of all people over age 50 harbor *H. pylori,* yet most do not develop peptic ulcer disease. Scientists still have to determine what triggers ulcers in those with *H. pylori.*

A common belief is that people exhibiting certain traits such as tenseness or striving for perfection or success are more likely to develop peptic ulcers. Conclusive evidence to support this belief is lacking.

GASTRIC ULCERS

The most common site of a gastric ulcer is in the distal half of the stomach. The cause of gastric ulcer is not clear, but it is related to factors such as diet; genetic predisposition; ingestion of excessive amounts of salicylates or NSAIDs; the use of tobacco; and *H. pylori.* Once the gastric mucosal barrier is damaged, acid secretion is stimulated. Without intervention, the cells die, erosion occurs, and ulcers develop. Gastric mucosal damage can occur in some individuals within 1 hour after the ingestion of acetylsalicylic acid. Reflux of duodenal contents (bile acids) also causes severe gastric mucosal damage. Gastric ulcers may occur on the surface of a gastric tumor because of interference with the blood supply.

PHYSIOLOGIC STRESS ULCERS

Physiologic stress ulcer or stress-related mucosal disease is an acute ulcer that develops after a major physiologic insult such as trauma or surgery. A stress ulcer is a form of erosive gastritis. It is believed that the gastric mucosa of the stomach undergoes a period of transient ischemia in association with hypotension, severe injury, extensive burns, and complicated surgery. The ischemia is due to decreased capillary blood flow or shunting of blood away from the GI tract so that blood flow bypasses the gastric mucosa. This occurs as a compensatory mechanism in hypotension or shock. The decrease in blood flow produces an imbalance between the destructive properties of hydrochloric acid and pepsin and protective factors of the stomach's mucosal barrier, especially in the fundus portion. Multiple superficial erosions result, and these may bleed. Because of the possibility of development of physiologic stress ulcers and high morbidity, patients at risk receive prophylaxis with antisecretory agents, including H_2 receptor blockers and proton pump inhibitors.

DUODENAL ULCERS

Etiology and Pathophysiology

Duodenal ulcers are a group of disorders that may or may not be caused by hypersecretion. Excessive production or excessive release of gastrin or increased sensitivity to gastrin is found in 40% of people with these ulcers. The other 60% have a normal amount of acid production but may lack the buffering ability in the duodenum. Risk factors include *H. pylori* infection, NSAIDs, cigarette smoking, and coffee. Ulceration occurs when the acid secretion exceeds the buffering factors.

Clinical Manifestations

Both gastric and duodenal ulcers may have similar symptoms but differ in timing, degree, or factors that worsen or alleviate the symptoms. Pain is the characteristic symptom and is described as dull, burning, boring, or gnawing; it is located in the midline of the epigastric region.

Assessment

Collection of **subjective data** requires an awareness that in gastric ulcer patients, the pain is closely associated with food intake and usually does not awaken the patient at night, as does the pain experienced by those with duodenal ulcers. Nausea, eructation, and distention are common complaints; these are termed **dyspepsia.** All these subjective symptoms intensify if perforation and obstruction occur.

Collection of **objective data** includes observing for hemorrhage, a common complication with gastric ul-cers; more gastric ulcers bleed than do duodenal ul-cers. Duodenal ulcers are more likely to have chronic bleeding and are more prone to perforation than gastric ulcers.

When GI bleeding occurs, one sign is vomiting blood **(hematemesis)** that has a coffee-grounds appearance as a result of action of the gastric acid on the hemoglobin molecule. The patient may have **melena** (tarlike, fetid-smelling stool containing undigested blood) that occurs when the blood becomes black and tarry as it passes through the digestive tract. In extreme cases, bright red blood may be passed rectally. Both salicylates and alcohol aggravate bleeding in patients with a history of peptic ulcers.

Bleeding from a gastric ulcer is more difficult to control than bleeding from a duodenal ulcer. Hemorrhage, with accompanying symptoms of shock, occurs when the ulcer erodes into a blood vessel. Surgical intervention is indicated if the patient remains unstable after receiving blood over several hours.

Perforation occurs when the ulcer crater penetrates the entire thickness of the wall of the stomach or duodenum. The release of air, gastric acid, pancreatic enzymes, or bile into the peritoneal cavity causes pain, emesis, fever, hypotension, and hematemesis. Perforation is considered the most lethal complication of peptic ulcer. Bacterial peritonitis may occur within 6 to 12 hours. The severity of the peritonitis is proportional to the amount and duration of the spillage through the perforation.

Gastric outlet obstruction is a complication of peptic ulcer disease that can occur at any time. It occurs more frequently when the ulcer is located close to the pylorus. Symptoms may be relieved by constant NG aspiration of stomach contents. This allows edema and inflammation to subside and permits normal flow of gastric contents through the pylorus.

Diagnostic Tests

Fiberoptic endoscopy can detect both gastric and duodenal ulcers. This is called **esophagogastroduodenoscopy.** Fiberoptic endoscopy is more reliable than barium contrast studies because of the maneuverability of fiberoptic scopes for viewing the entire esophagus and gastric and duodenal mucosa. This procedure also can be used to determine the degree of ulcer healing after treatment. During endoscopy, specimens can be obtained for identification of *H. pylori* or tissue specimens for biopsy. The patient is sedated but remains conscious throughout the endoscopy procedure. Local anesthetics in the throat are used to decrease the gag reflex and minimize pain during the procedure. No liquids or food are allowed for 1 to 2 hours or until the patient can swallow.

In 1996 the U.S. Food and Drug Administration (FDA) approved a breath test to detect *H. pylori.* The test calls for the patient to drink a solution containing carbon 13–enriched urea, a natural, nonradioactive substance. If *H. pylori* infection is present, it breaks down the compound and releases carbon-13 dioxide ($^{13}CO_2$). Thirty minutes after drinking the solution, the patient exhales into a collection bag, which is sent to the manufacturer for analysis. A finding of $^{13}CO_2$ confirms *H. pylori* infection. The test may prove especially useful in determining whether antibiotic therapy eradicated an *H. pylori* infection. Another noninvasive way to confirm *H. pylori* infection is a serum or whole blood antibody test, in particular, immunoglobulin G. This test is approximately 90% to 95% sensitive for *H. pylori* infection but cannot distinguish active from recently treated disease.

Barium contrast studies (UGI) are not as accurate for small lesions but are still commonly used. Testing of feces for occult blood in the intestinal tract is also used for diagnosis.

Medical Management

The physician may order insertion of an NG tube to remove gastric content and blood. Surgery is indicated usually for complications: perforation, penetration, obstruction, or intractability (no longer responding to medical management).

Scar tissue builds up with repeat episodes of ulceration and healing, causing obstruction, particularly at the pylorus. The patient may be seen with gastric dilation, vomiting, and distention. When fluid and electrolyte balance are achieved, surgical intervention is possible.

The primary treatment for peptic ulcers is to reduce signs and symptoms by decreasing or neutralizing normal gastric acidity with drug therapy. The types of drugs most commonly used include the following (Table 5-1).

- **Antacids:** Neutralize or reduce the acidity of stomach contents (e.g., Maalox, Gaviscon, Rolaids, Tums, Mylanta, and Riopan).
- **Histamine (H_2) receptor blockers:** Decrease acid secretions by blocking histamine (H_2) receptors (e.g., cimetidine, ranitidine, famotidine, and nizatidine). Do not give within 2 hours of antacids.
- **Proton pump inhibitors:** Antisecretory agents that inhibit secretion of gastrin by the parietal cells of the stomach (e.g., omeprazole, lansoprazole, pantoprazole, rabeprazole, and esomeprazole).

Table 5-1 Medications for Gastrointestinal Disorders

Generic (Trade)	Action	Side Effects	Nursing Implications
Antacids (aluminum, calcium, and magnesium salts and sodium bicarbonate) (Maalox, Mylanta, Titralac, Alternagel, others)	Neutralizes gastric acid; aluminum and calcium antacids also bind phosphates in renal failure patients	Aluminum: constipation, hypophosphatemia; calcium: constipation, rebound hyperacidity, hypercalcemia; magnesium: diarrhea, hypermagnesemia; sodium bicarbonate: sodium and water retention, alkalosis, rebound hyperacidity	Monitor serum electrolytes with long-term use; do not give antacid simultaneously with other medications because absorption of the other medication may be affected; best to separate administration by 2 hours.
Antispasmodics (including atropine, scopolamine, hyoscyamine, dicyclomine, clidinium) (Donnatal, Bentyl, others)	Anticholinergic agents that decrease GI motility by relaxing GI smooth muscle	Dry mouth and skin, constipation, paralytic ileus, urinary retention, tachycardia, drowsiness, dizziness, confusion, altered vision	Avoid using other CNS depressants or alcohol at the same time; avoid driving or other potentially hazardous tasks until accustomed to sedating effects.
Bismuth subsalicylate (Pepto-Bismol)	Antidiarrheal agent; also used in peptic ulcer disease caused by *Helicobacter pylori*	Fecal impaction, tinnitus	May turn stools dark gray–black; avoid use with aspirin; consult physician if diarrhea is accompanied by high fever or lasts more than 2 days.
Cimetidine (Tagamet)	H_2 receptor antagonist; inhibits gastric acid secretion	Confusion, headache, gynecomastia, bone marrow suppression (rare)	Increases serum levels and clinical effects of oral anticoagulants, theophylline, phenytoin, some benzodiazepines, and propranolol (these medications may require dosage reduction).
Dimenhydrinate (Dramamine, others)	Antiemetic agent; blocks central vomiting center	Drowsiness, dry mouth, constipation	Avoid use with other CNS depressants and alcohol; avoid driving or other hazardous activities until accustomed to sedating effects.

CNS, Central nervous system; *GI,* gastrointestinal;

Continued

Table 5-1 Medications for Gastrointestinal Disorders—cont'd

Generic (Trade)	Action	Side Effects	Nursing Implications
Diphenoxylate with atropine (Lomotil)	Antidiarrheal agent (diphenoxylate: narcotic; atropine: anticholinergic)	Drowsiness, sedation, constipation, dry mouth, urinary retention	Avoid use with other CNS depressants and alcohol; avoid driving or other hazardous activities until accustomed to sedating effects; do not use in infectious diarrhea.
Famotidine (Pepcid)	H$_2$ receptor antagonist; inhibits gastric acid secretion	Headache, dizziness, constipation, thrombocytopenia (rare)	Unlike cimetidine, does not affect serum levels of hepatically metabolized drugs (warfarin, phenytoin, theophylline).
Kaolin-pectin (Kaopectate)	Antidiarrheal agent	Constipation	Shake well before using.
Ketoconazole (Nizoral)	Antifungal agent	Gynecomastia, impotence, hepatotoxicity, abdominal pain	Requires acid environment for absorption; do not use with antacids, H$_2$ receptor blockers, or omeprazole; do not use with terfenadine, astemizole, or loratadine (has caused dysrhythmias and death); monitor liver function tests often; monitor serum levels and clinical effects of warfarin, cyclosporine, and theophylline.
Lansoprazole (Prevacid)	Binds to an enzyme in the presence of acid gastric pH, preventing the final transport of hydrogen ions into the gastric lumen	Drowsiness, abdominal pain, diarrhea, nausea	Sucralfate (Carafate) decreases absorption of lansoprazole (take 30 minutes before sucralfate); administer before meals. Assess patient routinely for epigastric or abdominal pain. May cause abnormal liver function tests.
Loperamide (Imodium)	Antidiarrheal agent	Drowsiness, dry mouth, constipation	Monitor for dehydration; do not use in infectious diarrhea.
Mesalamine (Rowasa, Asacol)	GI antiinflammatory agent	Abdominal cramps and gas, rash, headache, dizziness	Swallow tablets whole; give enema at bedtime, retain 10-15 minutes.
Misoprostol (Cytotec)	Prostaglandin analog that acts as gastric mucosal protectant against NSAID-induced ulcers	Diarrhea, nausea, vomiting, flatulence, uterine cramping	Absolutely contraindicated in pregnant women; women of childbearing age must use reliable contraception.
Nizatidine (Axid)	H$_2$ receptor antagonist, inhibits gastric acid secretion	Drowsiness, headache, dizziness, sweating, thrombocytopenia (rare)	Does not affect serum levels of hepatically metabolized drugs (warfarin, phenytoin, theophylline).
Nystatin (Mycostatin, Nilstat, others)	Antifungal agent, available as oral suspension and topical product	Oral: Nausea, vomiting, diarrhea Topical: Local irritation	Long-term therapy may be needed to clear infection; use for entire course.
Olsalazine (Dipentum)	GI antiinflammatory agent	Diarrhea, abdominal pain and cramps, nausea, allergic reactions, arthralgia, rash, anaphylaxis	Take with food; notify physician if severe diarrhea occurs.
Omeprazole (Prilosec)	Proton pump inhibitor, totally eradicates gastric acid production	Headache, dizziness, abdominal pain, nausea, vomiting, rare bone marrow suppression	Inhibits hepatic metabolism of warfarin, phenytoin, benzodiazepines, and other drugs metabolized by liver; do not crush or chew capsule contents.
Ranitidine (Zantac)	H$_2$ receptor antagonist; inhibits gastric acid secretion	Headache; abdominal discomfort; granulocytopenia and thrombocytopenia (both rare)	Minimal effect on serum levels of hepatically metabolized drugs (phenytoin, warfarin, theophylline).

CBC, Complete blood count; *NSAID,* nonsteroidal antiinflammatory drug.

Table 5-1	Medications for Gastrointestinal Disorders—cont'd		
Generic (Trade)	**Action**	**Side Effects**	**Nursing Implications**
Sucralfate (Carafate)	Gastric mucosal protectant agent; adheres to site of ulcer	Constipation, hypophosphatemia	Do not give with other drugs; coating action may interfere with the absorption of other drugs—separate by 2 hours.
Sulfasalazine (Azulfidine)	GI antiinflammatory agent	Nausea, vomiting, abdominal pain, photosensitivity, rash, Stevens-Johnson syndrome (rare), renal failure, bone marrow suppression (rare), allergic reactions, anaphylaxis	Ensure adequate hydration to prevent crystallization in kidneys; avoid exposure to sunlight; women on oral contraceptives need to use alternative methods because of decreased effectiveness of oral contraceptives; monitor CBC and renal function; take with meals.

- **Mucosal healing agent:** Heals ulcers without antisecretory properties. Sucralfate is a cytoprotective drug. It accelerates ulcer healing, presumably because of the formation of an ulcer-adherent complex that covers the ulcer and protects it from evasion by pepsin, acid, and bile salts.
- **Antisecretory and cytoprotective agent:** Inhibits gastric acid secretion and protects gastric mucosa (misoprostol [Cytotec]). Cytotec is the only drug approved in the United States for the prevention of gastric ulcers induced by NSAIDs and aspirin.

Antibiotic therapy eradicates *H. pylori*. The drugs used include metronidazole (Flagyl), tetracycline, amoxicillin, and clarithromycin (Biaxin). Treatment is typically combined in a therapeutic regimen with other medications, such as bismuth or omeprazole. Another weapon that has entered the battle against *H. pylori* is a combination of bismuth, metronidazole, and tetracycline. Marketed under the brand name Helidac, the medication kit contains a 14-day supply of the three drugs, with each daily dose packaged on a blister card to improve patient compliance.

Among patients whose *H. pylori* is treated with antibiotics, the peptic ulcer recurrence may be as low as 10%. Patients who do not receive antibiotics have a relapse rate of 75% to 90%.

Dietary modification may be necessary to avoid irritating foods and beverages. There is considerable controversy over the therapeutic benefits of a bland diet, since the rationale is not supported by scientific evidence. Therefore it is recommended that the patient eat smaller meals more frequently throughout the day to decrease the degree of gastric motor activity.

Smoking has an irritating effect on the mucosa, increases gastric motility, and delays mucosal healing. Smoking should be eliminated completely or severely reduced. The combination of adequate rest and cessation of smoking accelerates ulcer healing. Because caffeinated and decaffeinated coffee, tobacco, alcohol, and aspirin aggravate the mucosal lining of the stomach and duodenum, educate patients with ulcers about the need for lifestyle change.

Surgical intervention has decreased drastically with more effective diagnosis and medical treatment with antisecretory agents and antibiotics. Approximately 20% of patients with ulcers require surgical intervention. These are patients who are unresponsive to medical management, raising concerns about gastric cancer; patients whose ulcers are drug induced but who cannot be withdrawn from the drugs (e.g., patients with rheumatoid arthritis); or patients who develop complications. Types of surgical procedures include the following:

- **Antrectomy:** Removal of the entire antrum, the gastric-producing portion of the lower stomach, to eliminate the main stimuli to acid production.
- **Gastroduodenostomy (Billroth I)** (Figure 5-7, *A*): Direct anastomosis of the fundus of the stomach to the duodenum; used to remove ulcers or cancer located in the antrum of the stomach.
- **Gastrojejunostomy (Billroth II)** (Figure 5-7, *B*): Closure of the duodenum, and anastomosis of

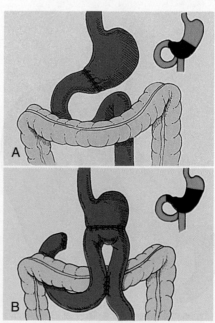

FIGURE 5-7 Types of gastric resections with anastomoses. **A,** Billroth I. **B,** Billroth II.

the fundus of the stomach into the jejunum; used to remove ulcers or cancer located in the body of the fundus.

- **Total gastrectomy:** Removal of the entire stomach; rarely used for patients with gastric cancer.
- **Vagotomy:** Removal of the vagal innervation to the fundus, decreasing acid produced by the parietal cells of the stomach (Figure 5-8); usually done with a Billroth I or II procedure or with a pyloroplasty.
- **Pyloroplasty:** Surgical enlargement of the pyloric sphincter to facilitate passage of contents from the stomach; commonly done after vagotomy or to enlarge an opening that has been constricted from scar tissue. A vagotomy decreases gastric motility and subsequently gastric emptying. A pyloroplasty accompanying vagotomy increases gastric emptying.

The choice of which procedure to use is difficult and depends on physician preference and results of diagnostic testing. Regardless of the procedure selected, postoperative complications are possible. Bleeding may occur up to 7 days after gastric surgery. Abdominal rigidity, abdominal pain, restlessness, elevated temperature, increased pulse, decreased blood pressure, and leukocytosis are all possible indications of postoperative bleeding. Note the amount and type of drainage from the incision. Surgical intervention may be necessary to correct the bleeding.

Dumping syndrome is a rapid gastric emptying causing distention of the duodenum or jejunum produced by a bolus of hypertonic food. Increased intestinal motility and peristalsis and changes in blood glucose levels occur. Patients may report diaphoresis, nausea, vomiting, epigastric pain, explosive diarrhea, borborygmi (noises made from gas passing through the liquid of the small intestine), and dyspepsia. Dumping syndrome is the direct result of surgical removal of a large portion of the stomach and the pyloric sphincter. Approximately one third to one half of patients experience dumping syndrome after peptic ulcer surgery. Treatment includes eating six small meals daily that are high in protein and fat and low in carbohydrates, eating slowly, and avoiding fluids during meals. Treatment also includes (1) anticholinergic agents to decrease stomach motility, and (2) reclining for approximately 1 hour after meals. To increase long-term compliance, reassure patients that following the recommended treatment will decrease symptoms within a few months. The symptoms are self-limiting and often disappear within several months to a year after surgery.

Several other complications after gastric surgery present serious health threats. Diarrhea is common and usually responds to conservative treatment of controlled diet and antidiarrheal agents. Diphenoxylate with atropine (Lomotil), loperamide (Imodium), paregoric, or codeine is often used. Reflux esophagitis and nutritional deficits—including weight loss, malabsorption, anemia, and vitamin deficiency—can also be life threatening.

Pernicious anemia is a serious potential complication for any patient who has had a total gastrectomy or extensive resections. This is caused by a deficiency of the intrinsic factor, produced exclusively by the stomach, which aids intestinal absorption of vitamin B_{12}. Recommend that all patients with a partial gastrectomy have a blood serum vitamin B_{12} level measured every 1 to 2 years so that replacement therapy of vitamin B_{12} via a monthly injection or via nasal route weekly can be instituted before anemia appears.

Nursing Interventions and Patient Teaching

NG or intestinal tube insertion, irrigation, and intermittent suctioning are often performed while a patient is feeling ill and uncomfortable. In addition to being skilled and knowledgeable in performing these procedures, the nurse is responsible for easing the patient's fears and anxieties. Patient cooperation not only makes the procedures easier but also reduces patient discomfort.

Helping patients through the experience of GI intubation requires understanding of the following points:

- For most patients, NG or intestinal tube placement is a new and frightening experience. Convey the rationale for this therapy to the anxious patient and family. Help them understand that the advantages far outweigh the discomfort.
- Inability to chew, taste, and swallow food and liquids may contribute to patient anxiety during GI intubation.

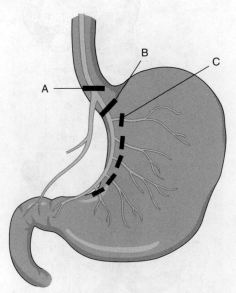

FIGURE 5-8 Types of vagotomies. *A,* Truncal. *B,* Selective. *C,* Proximal or parietal cell.

- A patient with an NG or intestinal tube is usually on NPO status. Occasionally ice chips are allowed.
- An NG or intestinal tube is connected to either continuous or intermittent suctioning, usually at 100 mm Hg for decompression.
- An NG or intestinal tube is a constant irritant to the nasopharynx and nares, requiring frequent care to the mouth and nose.
- A patient with a GI tube may be afraid that moving will dislodge the tube. Implement frequent position changes to enhance tube functioning and prevent complications of immobility.

An NG tube is inserted through the nose, pharynx, and esophagus into the stomach. Various tubes are available, depending on the purpose (Table 5-2).

Nursing interventions depend on the stage of the ulcer disease. The emphasis in patient care should always be on prevention and early detection of pain in the epigastric region, hematemesis, melena, or tenderness and rigidity of the abdomen (see Communication box and Nursing Care Plan 5-1).

Nursing diagnoses and interventions for the specific stages of ulcer care include but are not limited to the following:

Nursing Diagnoses	Nursing Interventions
Deficient knowledge, related to: • medications • diet • signs and symptoms of bleeding, perforation, or gastric outlet obstruction	Provide verbal and written instructions on exact dosage and time intervals for medications and whether medication is taken with or without food. Have dietitian provide instructions on therapeutic diet. Explain that repeat episodes are not uncommon; listen carefully for aggravating factors.
Pain, related to gastric acid on ulceration of gastric or duodenal mucosa	Give prescribed H_2 receptor antagonists (cimetidine, ranitidine, famotidine, or nizatidine) with meals and at bedtime. Give prescribed antacid 1 and 3 hours after meals.

Table 5-2   Purposes of Nasogastric Intubation

PURPOSE	DESCRIPTION	TYPE OF TUBE
Decompression	Removal of secretions and gaseous substances from GI tract; prevention or relief of abdominal distention	Salem sump, Miller-Abbott
Feeding (gavage)	Instillation of liquid nutritional supplements or feedings into stomach for patients unable to swallow fluid	Duo, Dobhoff
Compression	Internal application of pressure by means of inflated balloon to prevent internal GI hemorrhage	Sengstaken-Blakemore
Lavage	Irrigation of stomach in cases of active bleeding, poisoning, gastric dilation, or intestinal obstruction	Ewald, Salem sump

GI, Gastrointestinal.

 Communication

Patient with a GI Bleed

Nurse: You look like you are resting better, Mrs. S. How have you been feeling? *(Reaffirming a relationship that was begun yesterday.)*

Patient: Hello, Mrs. F. My stomach pain is much better. The medicine helped.

Nurse: If you are comfortable, perhaps you and your husband have some questions about why you are here. *(Trying to determine whether the patient is receptive to patient teaching. A knowledge deficit was suspected on admission.)*

Patient: I was scared when I started to vomit blood. It has happened before but not this much. Where does the blood come from?

Nurse: You have a diagnosis of GI bleeding with questionable duodenal ulcer. That means you have bleeding in the gas-

trointestinal system, either in the stomach or in some part of the intestine. Do you understand what I have said so far? *(The nurse begins with the admitting diagnosis and explains one thing at a time, making sure the patient verbalizes understanding before continuing.)*

Patient: Well, I understand where the bleeding is coming from, but why am I bleeding there?

Nurse: We are not sure yet, Mrs. S., but you are scheduled for a procedure that will allow the physician to actually look at the surface of the stomach and a portion of the intestine. It is called an endoscopy, and it will be done tomorrow morning. Did someone explain this to you? *(The nurse answers the patient's question openly and honestly and uses her answer to lead into further patient education.)*

Nursing Care Plan 5-1   The Patient with Gastrointestinal Bleeding

Mr. Dunne, 33 years of age, is admitted with pain in the epigastric region and copious hematemesis. He appears anxious; his skin is pale, cool, and clammy; and he is breathing rapidly. This patient has a history of recurrent episodes of vomiting blood that has a coffee-grounds appearance. He denies passing blood rectally but admits his stools have changed in consistency.

NURSING DIAGNOSIS *Risk for deficient fluid volume, related to hemorrhage, vomiting, and diarrhea*

Patient Goals and Expected Outcomes	Nursing Interventions	Evaluation
Patient will have normal fluid balance as evidence by balanced intake and output (I&O) within 24 hours, including stable weight Blood pressure, pulse, and respiratory rate will be within normal limits Patient will have normal tissue turgor within 24 hours	Monitor IV and blood transfusion therapy as ordered. Accurately record I&O every hour until stable: emesis, urine, and stool. Document fluid losses for possible imbalance; urinary output less than 30 mL/hr may indicate hypovolemia. Monitor for signs and symptoms of dehydration and fluid and electrolyte imbalance (dry mucous membranes, poor skin turgor, thirst, decreased urinary output, and changes in behavior) every 15 minutes until stable, then every 2 hours. Document characteristics of output. Test all emesis and fecal output for presence of blood as ordered. Prepare to assist with inserting a nasogastric (NG) tube and connecting it to wall suction. Irrigate NG tube with saline as ordered to promote clotting; irrigation removes old blood from the stomach.	Patient has urinary output of 1500 mL for prior 24-hour period Patient's blood pressure, pulse, and respiratory rate are within patient's pregastrointestinal bleeding baseline levels. Patient's tissue turgor is normal.

NURSING DIAGNOSIS *Anxiety, related to hospitalization and illness*

Patient Goals and Expected Outcomes	Nursing Interventions	Evaluation
Patient will demonstrate decrease in anxiety as evidenced by ability to sleep or rest at frequent intervals, verbalization of feelings, and blood pressure and pulse within normal limits	Assess physiologic components of anxiety (restlessness, increased pulse and respirations, diaphoresis, and elevated blood pressure) at least every 8 hours. Provide concise explanations for all procedures; prepare patient for surgery if indicated. Develop rapport with patient and family members with each contact.	Patient is sleeping 5 to 6 hours during the night and resting at intervals during the day. Patient verbalizes a feeling of less stress and anxiety. Therapeutic rapport with nurse, patient, and family members is noted.

Critical Thinking Questions

1. Mr. Dunne has an NG tube connected to wall suction that is draining sanguineous fluid. He complains of severe fatigue and epigastric pain. He is pale and drawn, with a hemoglobin level of 5.1 g/dL. Mr. Dunne puts his call light on and requests the nurse to assist him to the bathroom for a bowel movement. What appropriate interventions will ensure Mr. Dunne's safety?
2. During assessment of Mr. Dunne, what signs and symptoms would indicate deficient fluid volume?
3. Mr. Dunne says to the nurse that he fears he may die. He appears anxious and tremulous. What is the most therapeutic approach to help decrease his fears?

Nursing Diagnoses	Nursing Interventions
Pain, related to gastric acid on ulceration of gastric or duodenal mucosa—cont'd	Teach relaxation measures as appropriate. Give prescribed proton pump inhibitors (omeprazole, lansoprazole, pantoprazole, or esomeprazole). Administer antibiotic therapy to eradicate *H. pylori* infections as prescribed. Instruct patient on side effects of antacid drugs (constipation or diarrhea) and importance of contacting physician if this occurs.
Noncompliance, related to: • risk behaviors (use of tobacco or alcohol) • dietary patterns	Assess patient's level of knowledge regarding food and other irritants to mucosal lining. Teach preventive measures, such as quitting smoking. Explain need for small and frequent meals. Caution patient to avoid high-fiber foods, sugar, salt, caffeine, alcohol, and milk. Remind patient to take fluids between meals, not with meals. Explain the need to eat slowly and chew food well. Discuss importance of adequate rest and exercise.
Imbalanced nutrition: less than body requirements, related to preoperative food and fluid restrictions	Maintain NPO status. Connect NG tube to intermittent suction apparatus. Note color and amount of gastric output every 4 hours. Do not reposition tube. Maintain patency of tube by irrigation with measured amounts of saline *only if ordered*. NOTE: After gastrectomy, output is minimal. Monitor parenteral fluids with electrolyte additives as ordered. Measure I&O. When bowel sounds return and flatus is expelled, administer clear liquids as ordered.

Nursing Diagnoses	Nursing Interventions
	Progress to small, frequent meals of soft food as ordered. Avoid milk because it may cause dumping syndrome.

It is necessary to form a trusting relationship with the patient with an ulcer because of the severity of the condition and the need for long-term treatment. Include the family in patient education sessions to increase understanding and support, and involve the patient in goal setting to increase compliance (see Home Care Considerations box).

Instruct the patient to seek medical attention immediately if severe and sudden pain occurs. Assist the patient in describing signs and symptoms of weakness, anorexia, nausea, diarrhea, constipation, anxiety, or restlessness. When medications are prescribed, the patient must fully understand (1) the purpose of taking antibiotic therapy to eradicate *H. pylori;* (2) the importance of taking all medications such as H_2 receptor antagonists, antiulcer drugs, prostaglandin E analog, and proton pump inhibitors as prescribed; (3) why the antacids are taken in large doses (30 mL) seven times daily (1 and 3 hours after a meal and at bedtime) or at the specific times ordered; and (4) the known side effects (diarrhea and constipation). Preventive teaching includes identifying high-risk behaviors, such as the use of tobacco, caffeine, and alcohol. Emphasize that the patient should eat six smaller meals daily and avoid any foods that cause noticeable stomach discomfort.

 Home Care Considerations

Peptic Ulcer Disease

- The patient who has recurrent ulcer disease after initial healing must learn to live with a chronic disease.
- The patient may be angry and frustrated, especially he or she has faithfully followed the prescribed therapy but failed to prevent the recurrence or extension of the disease process.
- Unfortunately, many patients do not comply with the care plan and experience repeated exacerbations.
- Changes in lifestyle are difficult for most people and may be resisted.
- The patient who is instructed to stop smoking or avoid alcohol may resist.
- The goal should be adhering to the prescribed therapeutic regimen, including nutritional management, cessation of smoking, and decreased use of alcohol and caffeine.
- A patient with chronic ulcers needs to be aware of the complications that may result from the disease, the clinical manifestations indicating their presence, and what to do until the physician can be seen.
- Teach the patient to take all medications as prescribed. This includes both antisecretory and antibiotic drugs. Failure to take prescribed medications can result in relapse.

If surgery is required, explain the procedures thoroughly, including the reasons for them. Explain immediate postoperative care, including deep breathing; coughing; position changes; frequent monitoring of vital signs; IV tubing, NG tubing, catheters, and other drainage tubes; and the use of patient-controlled analgesia (PCA) or other medications for pain relief. The patient's ability to eat normally after healing depends on the type of surgery and when peristalsis returns. Help the patient realize that symptoms often recur and he or she should seek medical care if they do.

Prognosis for Peptic Ulcers

Recurrence of an ulcer may happen within 2 years in about one third of all patients. Among patients whose *H. pylori* is treated with antibiotics, the peptic ulcer recurrence drops to 2%. Patients who do not receive antibiotics have a relapse rate of 75% to 90%. The likelihood of recurrence is lessened by eliminating foods that aggravate the condition. If symptoms recur, the prognosis is better in patients who seek immediate medical treatment and comply with the prescribed regimen.

CANCER OF THE STOMACH

Etiology and Pathophysiology

In the 1940s gastric cancer was the most common malignant disease in the United States, but the incidence has declined significantly. The most common neoplasm or malignant growth in the stomach is adenocarcinoma. The primary location is the pyloric area, but the incidence of proximal tumors appears to be rising. Because of the location, the tumor may metastasize to lymph nodes, liver, spleen, pancreas, or esophagus. Gastric cancer is more common in people 50 to 70 years of age.

Many factors have been implicated in the development of stomach cancer, yet no single causative agent has been identified. Stomach carcinogenesis probably begins with a nonspecific mucosal injury as a result of aging; autoimmune disease; or repeated exposure to irritants such as bile, antiinflammatory agents, or smoking. Other factors include history of polyps, pernicious anemia, hypochlorhydria (deficiency of hydrochloride in the stomach's gastric juice), chronic atrophic gastritis, and gastric ulcer. Because the stomach has prolonged contact with food, cancer in this part of the body is associated with diets that are high in salt, smoked and preserved foods (which contain nitrites and nitrates), and carbohydrates, and low in fresh fruits and vegetables. Whole grains and fresh fruits and vegetables are associated with reduced rates of stomach cancer. Infection with *H. pylori*, especially at an early age, is considered a definite risk factor for gastric cancer.

Clinical Manifestations

The patient may be asymptomatic in early stages of the disease. Stomach cancer often spreads to adjacent organs before any distressing symptoms occur. With more advanced disease, the patient may appear pale and lethargic if anemia is present. With a poor appetite and significant weight loss, the patient may appear cachectic.

Assessment

Subjective data include complaints of vague epigastric discomfort or indigestion, early satiety, and postprandial (after meal) fullness. Ten percent of patients complain of an ulcerlike pain that does not respond to therapy. Anorexia and weakness are also common.

Objective data include weight loss, bleeding in the stools, hematemesis, and vomiting after drinking or eating. Anemia is common. It is caused by chronic blood loss as the lesion erodes through the mucosa or as a direct result of pernicious anemia, which develops when intrinsic factor is lost. The presence of ascites is a poor prognostic sign.

Diagnostic Tests

The tumor is diagnosed by radiographic barium studies (GI series). Endoscopic or gastroscopic examinations with biopsy remain the best diagnostic tool. The stomach can be distended with air during the procedure to stretch mucosal folds. Endoscopic ultrasound and CT scans can be used for staging the disease. Stool examination provides evidence of occult or gross bleeding. Carcinoembryonic antigen (CEA) and carbohydrate antigen 19-9 tumor markers are usually elevated in advanced gastric cancer. Serum tumor markers correlate with the degree of invasion, liver metastasis, and cure rate. Laboratory studies of RBCs, hemoglobin, hematocrit, and serum B_{12} assist in the detection of anemia and determination of severity.

Medical Management

The most therapeutic management of stomach cancer is surgical removal. Unfortunately, the surgery may be done as an exploratory celiotomy to determine involvement or to make the patient more comfortable. The surgical intervention used in treating gastric cancer may be the same procedure used for peptic ulcer disease. A partial or total gastric resection is the choice for an extensive lesion. Surgery for advanced gastric cancer carries high morbidity and mortality rates.

Wound healing may be disrupted by **dehiscence** (a partial or complete separation of the wound edges) or by **evisceration** (protrusion of viscera through the disrupted wound). Dehiscence and evisceration may be caused by problems in suturing the wound or by poor tissue integrity. Excessive coughing, straining, malnutrition, obesity, and infection may also increase the chances of dehiscence. Nursing interventions include instructing the patient to remain quiet and to avoid coughing or straining. Keep the patient in a dorsal recumbent position (on back with knees flexed) to remove stress on the wound. If evisceration occurs, keep the patient on bed rest and loosely cover the protruding viscera with a warm sterile saline dressing. Notify the surgeon immediately because treatment consists of reapproximating the wound edges.

Chemotherapy has greater response and longer survival rates than radiation. Because the radiosensitivity of stomach cancer is low, radiation therapy is of little value. However, it may be used as a palliative measure to decrease tumor mass and temporarily relieve obstruction. The combination of chemotherapy and radiation therapy may be used for patients who are at high risk for disease recurrence after surgery. These treatment modalities are often used with surgery.

Nursing Interventions and Patient Teaching

Provide further clarification about the disease and the surgical intervention to the patient and family. The preoperative preparation includes improving the patient's nutritional status by monitoring total parenteral nutrition and providing supplemental feedings. Postoperative teaching is necessary to relieve anxiety and promote understanding of drainage tubes, feeding tubes, dressing changes, weakness, medications, and other routine care.

Nursing diagnoses and interventions for the patient with cancer of the stomach include but are not limited to the following:

Nursing Diagnoses	Nursing Interventions
Ineffective breathing pattern, related to: • pain • exploration of chest and abdominal cavities • abdominal distention	Place the patient in a semi-Fowler's position to aid ventilation. Encourage and assist with gentle turning and repositioning. Encourage the patient to turn, breathe deeply, and cough at least every 2 hours until ambulating well; splint incision before coughing; use incentive spirometer; and ambulate as soon as possible.
Risk for injury, related to: • aspiration • infection • hemorrhage • anastomotic leak into abdominal cavity • anemia or vitamin deficiency	Monitor closely for elevated temperature, bleeding from incision, pallor, dyspnea, cyanosis, tachycardia, increased respirations, and chest pain. Monitor laboratory results and activity tolerance because of possible anemia. Change dressings using sterile technique.

Because care encompasses so many areas, instruction should be (1) planned according to the patient's needs and level of understanding, (2) given when the patient is free of pain and rested, and (3) communi-cated both verbally and in print. Explain surgery, chemotherapy, radiation therapy, continued nutritional needs, pain relief, and support groups for psychosocial needs.

Weight loss indicates the need for additional caloric intake and can be measured by monitoring weight and comparing it with the patient's normal weight before illness. Prevent skin excoriation around the feeding tube. Hypermotility or diarrhea that follows radiation therapy can be treated with medication. The debilitated patient and family may require referral for hospice care.

Prognosis

The prognosis for patients with gastric cancer is usually poor. About 60% have clinical findings at the time of diagnosis, resulting in a low cure rate. Only 10% to 20% of patients develop disease confined to the stomach. For patients with lymph node–negative stomach cancer, surgical treatment alone results in a 75% 5-year survival rate. For patients with lymph node–positive cancer, the 5-year survival rate after surgery is 10% to 30%.

DISORDERS OF THE INTESTINES

INFECTIONS

Etiology and Pathophysiology

Intestinal infections are the invasion of the alimentary canal (both the small and large intestine) by pathogenic microorganisms that reproduce and multiply. The infectious agent can enter the body by several routes. The most common way is through the mouth in contaminated food or water. Some intestinal infections occur as a result of person-to-person contact. Fecal-oral transmission occurs through poor hand hygiene after elimination. In active homosexual males, infectious agents can be introduced by single-cell protozoal infections.

Bacterial flora grow naturally in the intestinal tract and help the immune system combat infection. However, long-term antibiotic therapy can destroy the normal flora. The impaired immune response in some individuals delays the body's attempt to destroy invading pathogens.

Infectious diarrhea causes secretion of fluid into the intestinal lumen. *Clostridia, Salmonella, Shigella,* and *Campylobacter* bacteria are associated with intestinal infections. These bacteria produce toxic substances, and the mucosal cells respond by secreting water and electrolytes, causing an imbalance. The amount of fluid secreted exceeds the ability of the large intestine to reabsorb the fluid into the vascular system.

One strain of *E. coli*—serotype O157:H7—often has a virulent course. Unlike other strains, *E. coli* O157:H7 is not part of the normal flora of the human intestine. Found in the intestines of approximately 1% of food cattle, this strain can, even in small amounts, contaminate a large amount of meat, especially ground beef. It is transmitted in contaminated, undercooked meats such as hamburger, roast beef, ham, and turkey; in produce that has been rinsed with water contaminated by animal or human feces; or by a person who has been handling contaminated food. The bacterium has also been cultured in unpasteurized milk, cheese, and apple juice and can be found in lakes and pools that have been contaminated by fecal matter. Hemorrhagic colitis (which results in bloody diarrhea and severe cramping accompanied by diffuse abdominal tenderness) develops between the second and fourth days. Antidiarrheals should not be given because these medications prevent the intestines from getting rid of the *E. coli* pathogen. Antimotility drugs such as diphenoxylate with atropine or antibiotic therapy is not recommended because they increase the likelihood of developing hemolytic-uremic syndrome, a pathologic condition of the kidney. Poisoning with *E. coli* O157:H7 can be life threatening, particularly in the very young and in older adults. Usually little or no fever is present and the illness resolves in 5 to 10 days. In approximately 2% to 7% of infections, particularly in young children, hemolytic-uremic syndrome occurs and the kidneys fail (Lewis et al., 2007).

Sigmoidoscopic or colonoscopic examination and stool specimens are used to diagnose a type of inflammation or colitis called **antibiotic-associated pseudomembranous colitis** (AAPMC). Immunosuppressed patients and older adults are particularly susceptible. *C. difficile* is a hazardous nosocomial infection because hospitalized patients are often immunosuppressed, antibiotic therapy is common, and the spores can survive for up to 70 days on inanimate objects. *C. difficile* spores have been found on commodes, telephones, thermometers, bedside tables, floors, and other objects in the room, as well as on the hands of health care workers. Health care workers who do not adhere to infection-control precautions can transmit *C. difficile* from patient to patient. Washing hands with soap and water is necessary because antiseptic hand rub does not destroy *C. difficile*. This type of colitis is a complication of treatment with a wide variety of antibiotics, including lincomycin, clindamycin, ampicillin, erythromycin, tetracycline, cephalosporins, and aminoglycosides. A *C. difficile* test is ordered on the stool specimen to aid in the diagnosis of AAPMC in both inpatients and outpatients. Characteristic lesions of AAPMC are identified on tissues obtained through endoscopic examination.

Treatment with antibiotics (especially clindamycin, ampicillin, amoxicillin, and the cephalosporins) inhibits normal bacterial growth in the intestine. This inhibition of normal flora can lead to the overgrowth of other bacteria such as *C. difficile*. Under the right conditions, *C. difficile* produces two toxins, A and B. Both toxins A and B are produced by *C. difficile* at the same time and these toxins cause the tissue damage seen in

AAPMC disease. The incidence of *C. difficile* toxin found in the stool ranges from 1% to 2% in a normal population to 10% in hospital inpatients and up to 85% to 90% in patients with proven AAPMC. The *C. difficile* test alone is not conclusive but does aid in the diagnosis of AAPMC.

Because the level of *C. difficile* antigens associated with the disease state may vary, a negative *C. difficile* test result alone may not rule out the possibility of *C. difficile*–associated colitis. Monitor signs and symptoms of the disease such as the duration and severity of diarrhea. These observations, along with the duration of antibiotic treatment and the presence of colitis or pseudomembranes, are all factors the physician must consider when diagnosing AAPMC disease.

The physician treats a mild case of antibiotic-related *C. difficile*–associated diarrhea by simply discontinuing the antibiotic and providing fluid and electrolyte replacement. In more severe cases the physician discontinues the antibiotic and starts antimicrobial therapy; the drug of choice is metronidazole or, if that is ineffective, vancomycin (Vancocin).

Clinical Manifestations

Diarrhea is the most common manifestation of an intestinal infection. The fecal output has increased water content, and if the intestinal mucosa is directly invaded, the feces may contain blood and mucus.

Assessment

Collection of **subjective data** includes noting complaints of diarrhea, rectal urgency, **tenesmus** (ineffective and painful straining with defecation), nausea, and abdominal cramping.

Objective data include a fever greater than 102° F (38.8° C) and vomiting. History taking provides useful information regarding number and consistency of bowel movements, recent use of antibiotics, recent travel, food intake, and exposure to noninfectious causes of diarrhea. Noninfectious diarrhea may be caused by heavy metal poisoning, shellfish allergy, and ingestion of toxins from mushrooms or fish. Diarrhea from noninfectious causes is usually characterized by a short incubation period (minutes to hours after exposure).

Diagnostic Tests

The key laboratory test for patients with intestinal infections is a stool culture. Stools are examined for blood, mucus, and WBCs. A blood chemistry study to monitor changes in the patient's fluid and electrolyte status may be included.

Medical Management

Usually the treatment of intestinal infections is conservative, letting the body limit the infection. Antibiotics are rarely used to treat acute diarrhea, but may be given in cases of prolonged or severe diarrhea with a stool positive for leukocytes. If fluid and electrolyte replacement is necessary to offset the losses from diarrhea, the oral route is usually sufficient. The IV route is indicated if the patient cannot take sufficient fluids orally.

The use of antidiarrheals and antispasmodic agents may actually increase the severity of the infection by prolonging the contact time of the infectious organism with the intestinal wall. Kaolin and pectin (Kaopectate) may be used to increase stool consistency. Bismuth subsalicylate (Pepto-Bismol) can effectively decrease intestinal secretions and decrease the diarrhea volume. These medications require large doses to be effective (30 to 60 mL every 30 minutes to 1 hour), and their use remains controversial.

Nursing Interventions and Patient Teaching

Do a thorough assessment to determine the seriousness of the intestinal infection. Determining the onset of the disease and the number of people exposed is important, since the majority of GI infections are communicable and represent a community health problem. Also assess for fluid imbalance, including measurement of postural changes in blood pressure, skin turgor, mucous membrane hydration, and urinary output.

Nursing diagnoses and interventions for the patient with intestinal infections include but are not limited to the following:

Nursing Diagnoses	Nursing Interventions
Deficient fluid volume, related to excessive losses from diarrhea and vomiting	If oral intake is tolerated, offer apple juice, clear carbonated beverages, clear broth, plain gelatin, and water. If IV feedings are required to maintain intravascular volume, these fluids should have electrolytes added. Maintain accurate I&O.
Imbalanced nutrition: less than body requirements, related to: • decreased intake • decreased absorption	Monitor for decreasing episodes of diarrhea. Monitor blood pressure, tissue turgor, mucous membranes, and urinary output. Monitor weight loss if symptoms are severe.

Instruct the patient to report the number, color, and consistency of bowel movements; abdominal cramping; and pain. Ensure that the patient and family understand the importance of hand hygiene after bowel movements to interrupt the fecal-oral route of transmission. Inform family members responsible for food preparation about the importance of proper methods of food preparation and storage to reduce the growth of infecting organisms.

Prognosis
Intestinal Infections
The body may be able to successfully defend against the infection without intervention. In severe cases, medications and fluid replacement assist the body, and the cure rate is good.

Antibiotic-Associated Pseudomembranous Colitis
The prognosis of AAPMC is better when the disease is diagnosed early and the antibiotics are changed. This allows the normal growth of bacteria in the intestine to resume.

IRRITABLE BOWEL SYNDROME
Etiology and Pathophysiology
Irritable bowel syndrome (IBS) is a disorder with episodes of altered bowel function and intermittent and recurrent abdominal pain. The American Gastroenterological Association (2009) defines IBS as a combination of chronic and recurrent GI symptoms—mainly intestinal pain and disturbed defecation or abdominal distention—that are not explained by structural or biochemical abnormalities; it is a dysfunction of the intestinal muscles (www.gastro.org/wmspage). The syndrome is now thought to result from hypersensitivity of the bowel wall, which leads to disruption of the normal functioning of the intestinal muscles.

IBS is common, occurring in about 10% to 15% of Western populations. A small number of these people (5%) have severe symptoms that are difficult to manage. The cause of IBS may be a low pain threshold to intestinal distention caused by abnormal intestinal sensory neural circuitry.

The patient with IBS may have associated psychological problems. In patients without psychological problems, the symptoms are attributed to spastic and uncoordinated muscle contractions of the colon, usually related to ingestion of excessively coarse or highly seasoned foods. However, there is also (1) a correlation of panic attacks in patients with IBS, and (2) an association of chronic low abdominal (pelvic) pain and a history of childhood sexual abuse.

Clinical Manifestations
Alterations of bowel function include abdominal pain relieved after a bowel movement; more frequent bowel movements with pain onset; a sense of incomplete evacuation; flatulence; and constipation, diarrhea, or both. Stress increases functional diarrhea; usually weight loss does not occur. The physical examination is generally normal, and nocturnal symptoms are rarely present. The symptoms of IBS are deceptive and are frustrating to manage.

Assessment

Subjective data include complaints of abdominal distress, pain at onset of bowel movements, abdominal pain relieved by defecation, and feelings of incomplete emptying after defecation.

Objective data include mucus in stools, visible abdominal distention, and frequent or unformed stools.

Diagnostic Tests

The key to accurate diagnosis of IBS is a thorough history and physical examination. Emphasize symptoms, health history (including psychosocial aspects such as physical or sexual abuse), family history, and drug and dietary history.

Diagnosis of IBS occurs by exclusion. Patients who see the physician with symptoms of intermittent or chronic abdominal pain and altered bowel motility are screened for pathologic conditions such as Crohn's disease, ulcerative colitis, colorectal cancer, diverticulitis, and infections such as salmonella. When no pathologic or structural abnormality is detected, IBS is a probable diagnosis. Symptom-based criteria for IBS have been standardized and are referred to as the **Rome criteria.** Rome II criteria include abdominal discomfort or pain that lasts at least 12 weeks (not necessarily consecutive) within 12 months and that has at least two of the following characteristics: (1) relieved with defecation, (2) onset associated with a change in stool frequency, and (3) onset associated with a change in stool appearance (Lewis et al., 2007).

Medical Management

Diet and Bulking Agents

Increasing dietary fiber increases stool bulk, frequency of passage, and bloating. Adequate fiber is more reliably provided with bulking agents (e.g., Metamucil) than with diet unless the patient is a strict vegetarian. The bulking agents seem to be most effective in treating constipation-predominant IBS, although they may alleviate mild diarrhea. If the patient's symptoms are consistently exacerbated after certain foods, those should be avoided. Advise the patient whose primary symptoms are abdominal distention and increased flatulence to eliminate common gas-producing foods (e.g., broccoli, cabbage) from the diet and to substitute yogurt for milk products to help determine whether he or she is lactose intolerant.

Medication

Anticholinergic drugs relieve abdominal cramps. Milk of magnesia may be prescribed if constipation does not respond to augmented fiber or if the patient cannot tolerate it. Mineral oil, in sufficient doses, is cheaper, "gasless," and generally effective. Opioids can be effective in diarrhea-predominant IBS. Antianxiety drugs may help patients suffering from panic attacks associated with IBS. Antidepressants may be used sparingly for diarrhea-predominant IBS in patients with severe pain who have not responded to other measures. New drug therapies are in development. Drugs that affect serotonin receptors hold promise in the treatment of IBS. Two serotonergic agents have been approved in select patients with IBS: tegaserod (Zelnorm), and alosteron (Lotronex). Because of its serious side effects (e.g., severe constipation, ischemic colitis), alosteron is available only in a restricted access program for women who have not responded to other therapies and in whom other anatomical and chemical abnormalities have been ruled out (Lewis et al., 2007).

Patients with IBS often report higher levels of psychological distress, including anxiety, panic, and depression, which can amplify symptoms and affect treatment response. Psychological nonpharmacologic treatment may include counseling and cognitive-behavioral interventions such as hypnotherapy and progressive muscle relaxation techniques to reduce stress. A significant proportion of patients with IBS had fewer or less severe symptoms after stress-reduction treatment.

Some patients have reported benefits from the use of complementary therapies such as acupuncture, Chinese herbal therapy, chiropractic techniques, and hatha yoga; patients with IBS are significantly more likely (11%) to use alternative remedies such as herbs than are patients with Crohn's disease (4%) (see Complementary & Alternative Therapies box). Although some studies have examined the use of such therapies in the treatment of IBS, clinical trial data are inadequate to determine their efficacy or to recommend any one as the sole therapy in the treatment of the syndrome.

Nursing Interventions and Patient Teaching

Most patients with IBS learn to cope with their symptoms enough to live in reasonable comfort. It is the nurse's role to assist in identifying the 5% of patients with IBS who need management. The nurse's skill in history taking, listening, nutrition planning, and understanding psychological effects on the body can assist the patient in setting goals to manage the disease. Emphasize the importance of keeping a daily log showing diet; number and type of stools; presence, severity, and duration of pain; side effects of medication; and life stressors that aggravate the disorder. This information assists in the diagnosis and treatment of IBS.

Nursing diagnoses and interventions for the patient with an irritable bowel include but are not limited to the following:

Nursing Diagnoses	Nursing Interventions
Pain, related to diet consumed and bowel evacuation	Have patient log the type of food consumed in terms of fiber content, consistency of stool, degree of pain.

Complementary & Alternative Therapies

Irritable Bowel Syndrome

- Traditional Chinese medicine has long been used to treat a variety of gastrointestinal (GI) complaints. Herbal formulas are chosen according to the specifics of the diagnostic patterns of traditional Chinese medicine. Most of the literature about such usage appears in either Chinese or Japanese journals or in textbooks of Chinese medicine, some of which are now available in English translations.*
- Peppermint oil, an herbal extract, has been studied for its use in irritable bowel syndrome. It resulted in significant improvements in symptoms, but the researchers cautioned that study design flaws make a fully positive conclusion difficult.
- Another promising area of research is biofeedback. Also called "psychophysiologic self-regulation," biofeedback is a relaxation training method that gives individuals a greater degree of awareness and control of physiologic function. Computer-based biofeedback equipment gives immediate feedback to the patient on changes in certain parameters, such as muscle electrical activity and skin temperature.
- Similar interventions have used various psychotherapy, stress management, and relaxation exercises, often in combination.

- Herbs that can cause GI upset include milk thistle (*Silybum marianum*), goldenseal (*Hydrastis canadensis*), ginger (*Zingiber officinale*), kelp (*Fucus vesiculosus*), comfrey (*Symphytum officinale*), chaparral (*Larrea divaricata*), cayenne (capsicum), and alfalfa (*Medicago sativa*).
- Some people find relief from nausea and vomiting through acupuncture or acupressure.
- Some people have found that chiropractic adjustment has improved blood flow to digestive organs and improved digestion.
- Anise has been used to decrease bloating and flatulence and as an antispasmodic. (*Do not confuse with Chinese star anise.*)
- Comfrey is used to treat gastritis.
- Fennel is used to treat mild, spastic disorders of the GI tract, feelings of fullness, and flatulence.
- Queen Anne's lace seeds are used for flatulence, colic, singultus, and dysentery.

Modified from Black, J.M., & Hawks, H.J. (2009). *Medical-surgical nursing: clinical management for positive outcomes.* (8th ed.). Philadelphia: Saunders.
*From Bensoussan, A., Talley N.J., Hing, M. (1998). Treatment of irritable bowel syndrome with Chinese herbal medicine: a randomized controlled trial, *Journal of the American Medical Association, 280*(18):1585.

Nursing Diagnoses	Nursing Interventions
Deficient knowledge, related to the effect of fiber content on spastic bowel	Educate patient regarding the relationship of fiber to both constipation and diarrhea. Teach patient about the use of bulking agents.

IBS involves many personal feelings that the patient must recognize and be comfortable with before a care plan can be established. Therefore it is important to establish a strong relationship with the patient before patient teaching begins. Patient teaching includes diet management and ways to control anxiety in daily living. The goal of patient teaching is to empower the patient to control the disorder. Provide community resources for counseling if psychological problems seem related to increased or decreased elimination accompanied by pain and discomfort.

Prognosis
Approximately 95% of these patients are successfully managed. Compliance with a diet low in residue and a nonstressful daily regimen contributes significantly to a good prognosis.

INFLAMMATORY BOWEL DISEASE

Ulcerative colitis and Crohn's disease are chronic, episodic, inflammatory bowel diseases. These are immunologically related disorders that afflict young adults just beginning their education, careers, and families. These diseases appear more often in women, in the Jewish population, and in the nonwhite population; there seems to be a familial tendency.

The causes of ulcerative colitis and Crohn's disease are unknown. Theories involve both genetic and environmental factors, including bacterial infection, immunologic factors, and psychosomatic disorders. The fact that people with ulcerative colitis commonly have a relative with Crohn's disease and vice versa supports the existence of the common gene. Inflammatory bowel diseases are characterized by **exacerbations** (increases in severity of the disease or any of its symptoms) and **remissions** (decreases in severity of the disease or any of its symptoms).

The two diseases require similar nursing interventions but different surgical interventions and medical treatment. Certain criteria are used to differentiate ulcerative colitis from Crohn's disease (Table 5-3), but the diseases have much in common and cannot be differentiated in about one third of the cases. Patients have been known to have features of both diseases, making a definite diagnosis difficult.

ULCERATIVE COLITIS

Etiology and Pathophysiology
The incidence of ulcerative colitis is twice that of Crohn's disease. Psychosomatic factors may cause, aggravate, or be a result of inflammatory bowel disease. The social isolation and frustration that accompany this chronic illness cause difficulties in effectively coping with daily life.

Ulcerative colitis is confined to the mucosa and submucosa of the colon. The disease can affect segments

Table 5-3	Comparison of Ulcerative Colitis and Crohn's Disease	
FACTOR	**ULCERATIVE COLITIS**	**CROHN'S DISEASE**
Cause of disorder	Unknown; autoimmune; genetic and environment play a role; various bacteria have been proposed	Unknown; possible cause is an altered immune state; autoimmune; various bacteria have been proposed Genetic and environmental factors play a role
Usual age at onset	Teenage years and early adulthood; second peak in sixth decade	Early adolescence; second peak in sixth decade
Area of involvement	Confined to mucosa or submucosa of the colon	Can occur anywhere along the gastrointestinal tract from the mouth to the anus Most common site is terminal ileum
Area of inflammation	Mucosa and submucosa	Transmural (pertaining to the entire thickness of the wall of an organ)
Characteristics of inflammation	Tends to be continuous, starting at the rectum and extending proximally; limited to the mucosal lining	May be continuous or interspersed between areas of normal tissue; may extend through all layers of the bowel
Character of stools	Blood present No fat 15-20 liquid stools daily	No blood present Steatorrhea (fat in stool) 3-4 semisoft stools daily
Major complication	Toxic megacolon, fistulas, and abscesses (rare)	Malabsorption, bowel obstruction, fistulas, tissue abscesses
Major complaints	Rectal bleeding, abdominal cramping	Right lower abdominal pain with mass present
Reason for surgery	Poor response to medical therapy	Complications
Response to surgery	Removal of the colon cures the intestinal disease, but not extraintestinal symptoms, such as inflammation of joints and liver disease	Indicated to remove diseased areas that do not respond to aggressive medical therapy. Surgery does not cure the disease
Cancer potential	Increased risk after 10 years of disease	Small intestine incidence increased; colon incidence increased, but not as much as in ulcerative colitis
Biopsy findings	Architectural changes consistent with chronic inflammation	Architectural changes consistent with chronic inflammation; may show granulomas
Weight loss	Rare	Cobblestoning of mucosa is common; may be severe
Malabsorption and nutritional deficiencies	Minimal incidence	Common; may be severe; frequent

of the entire colon, depending on the staging (phases or periods in the course of the disease). This disease usually starts in the rectum and moves in a continuous pattern toward the cecum. Although sometimes mild inflammation of the terminal ileum occurs, ulcerative colitis is a disease of the colon and rectum. The inflammation and ulcerations occur in the mucosal layer of the bowel wall. Since it does not extend through all bowel wall layers, fistulas and abscesses are rare. Capillaries become friable and bleed, causing the characteristic diarrhea containing pus and blood. Pseudopolyps are common in chronic ulcerative disease and may become cancerous. With healing and the natural formation of scar tissue, the colon may lose elasticity and absorptive capability.

Clinical Manifestations

Pathologic findings differ, but about 90% of patients with ulcerative colitis have mild to moderately severe disease. Patients with severe ulcerative colitis may have as many as 15 to 20 liquid stools per day, containing blood, mucus, and pus. With severe diarrhea, losses of sodium, potassium, bicarbonate, and calcium ions may occur. Abdominal cramps may occur before the bowel movement. The urge to defecate lessens as

scarring within the bowel progresses. This results in involuntary leakage of stool. In mild to moderate ulcerative colitis, diarrhea may consist of two to five stools per day with some blood present.

Complications of ulcerative colitis include toxic megacolon (toxic dilation of the large bowel). This life-threatening complication occurs in less than 5% of patients. The bowel becomes distended and so thin that it could be perforated at any time. Clinical manifestations of toxic megacolon include a temperature of 104° F (40° C) or more and abdominal distention. Among patients who have had chronic ulcerative colitis for 10 to 15 years, 40% to 50% develop carcinoma of the colon with total colonic involvement. Surgical interventions for treatment of this complication are usually necessary.

Assessment

Subjective data include complaints of rectal bleeding and abdominal cramping. Lethargy, a sense of frustration, and loss of control result from painful abdominal cramping and unpredictable bowel movements.

Objective data include weight loss, abdominal distention, fever, tachycardia, leukocytosis, and observation of frequency and characteristics of stools.

Diagnostic Tests

Double-contrast barium enema studies of the intestine, sigmoidoscopy and colonoscopy with biopsy, and stool testing for melena aid the physician in diagnosis. Additional studies include radiologic examination of the abdomen, serum electrolytes and albumin levels, liver function studies, and other hematologic studies.

Medical Management

The medical interventions chosen depend on the phase of the disease and the individual response to therapy. Common treatment modalities include medication, diet intervention, and stress reduction.

Drug Therapy

The four major categories of drugs used are (1) those that affect the inflammatory response, (2) antibacterial drugs, (3) drugs that affect the immune system, and (4) antidiarrheal preparations.

Sulfasalazine (Azulfidine) is the drug of choice for mild chronic ulcerative colitis. Sulfasalazine is broken down by bacteria in the colon into sulfapyridine and 5-aminosalicylic acid (5-ASA). It affects the inflammatory response and provides some antibacterial activity. It is effective in maintaining clinical remission and in treating mild to moderately severe attacks. Newer proportions have been developed to deliver 5-ASA to the terminal ileum and colon (e.g., olsalazine [Dipentum], mesalamine [Pentasa], and balsalazide [Colazal]). These drugs are as effective as sulfasalazine and are better tolerated when administered orally.

Nonsulfa drugs include mesalamine (Rowasa), given by retention enema.

Corticosteroids are antiinflammatory drugs effective in relieving symptoms of moderate and severe colitis; they can be given orally or intravenously if inflammation is severe.

Antidiarrheal agents are recommended over anticholinergic agents because anticholinergic drugs can mask obstruction or contribute to toxic colonic dilation. Loperamide may be used to treat cramping and diarrhea of chronic ulcerative colitis. Azathioprine (Imuran) is also beneficial.

Nutrition Therapy

Diet is an important component in the treatment of inflammatory bowel disease, and a dietitian should be consulted. The goals of diet management are to provide adequate nutrition without making symptoms worse, to correct and prevent malnutrition, to replace fluid and electrolyte losses, and to prevent weight loss. Patients with inflammatory bowel disease must eat a balanced, healthy diet with sufficient calories, protein, and nutrients. Patients can use MyPyramid guidelines to ensure that they get adequate portions from all of the food groups. The diet for each patient is individualized.

Patients with diarrhea often decrease their oral intake to reduce the diarrhea. The anorexia that accompanies inflammation also results in decreases in food intake. Blood loss leads to iron deficiency anemia.

Patients receiving sulfasalazine should receive 1 mg of folate (folic acid) daily, and those receiving corticosteroids need calcium supplements.

Inflammatory bowel disease has no universal food triggers, but patients may find that certain foods initiate diarrhea. A food diary helps them identify problem foods to avoid. Many patients are lactose intolerant and improve when they avoid milk products. High-fat foods also tend to trigger diarrhea. Cold foods and high-fiber foods (cereal with bran, nuts, raw fruit) may increase GI transit. Smoking stimulates the GI tract (increases motility and secretion) and should be avoided. Patients with significant fluid and electrolyte losses or malabsorption may need parenteral nutrition or enteral feedings, such as elemental diets. Elemental diets are high in calories and nutrients, lactose free, and absorbed in the proximal small intestine, which allows the more distal bowel to rest.

Stress Control

Ulcerative colitis is aggravated by stress. Identifying the factors that cause stress is the first step in controlling the disease. Working with the patient to find healthful coping mechanisms is part of the holistic approach in nursing interventions.

Surgical Intervention

If an acute episode does not respond to treatment, if complications occur, or if the risk of cancer becomes greater because of chronic ulcerative colitis, surgical intervention is indicated (Box 5-4). Approximately 25% to 40% of patients with ulcerative colitis need surgery at some time during their illness. Most surgeons prefer a conservative approach, removing only the diseased portion of the colon. The operations of choice may be a single-stage total procto-

---

Box 5-4 **Surgical Interventions for Ulcerative Colitis**

- **Colon resection:** Removal of a portion of the large intestine and anastomosis of the remaining segment
- **Ileostomy:** Surgical formation of an opening of the ileum onto the surface of the abdomen, through which fecal matter is emptied
- **Ileoanal anastomosis:** Removal of the colon and rectum but leaving the anus intact, along with the anal sphincter; anastomosis formed between the lower end of the small intestine and the anus
- **Proctocolectomy:** Removal of anus, rectum, and colon; ileostomy established for the removal of digestive tract wastes
- **Kock pouch (Kock continent ileostomy):** Surgical removal of the rectum and colon (proctocolectomy) with formation of a reservoir by suturing loops of adjacent ileum together to form a pouchlike structure, nipple valve, and stoma

colectomy with construction of an internal reservoir and valve (Kock pouch, or Kock continent ileostomy) (Figure 5-9); total proctocolectomy with ileoanal anastomosis with or without construction of an internal reservoir; and temporary ileostomy. In the case of a poor-risk patient, a subtotal colectomy may be performed with ileostomy (Figure 5-10). After the patient's recovery (approximately 2 to 4 months), removal of the rectum or construction of an internal reservoir can be done.

Today some patients view a permanent ileostomy as worse than the disease itself. Surgical procedures do have some risk, and the patient may want to live with the disease and long-term risk of cancer rather than undergo the procedure.

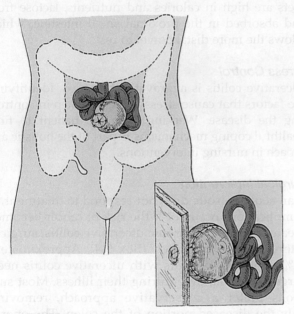

FIGURE 5-9 Kock pouch (Kock continent ileostomy).

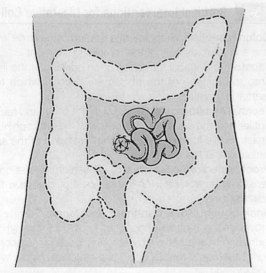

FIGURE 5-10 Ileostomy with absence of resected bowel.

Nursing Interventions

Nursing interventions include a thorough assessment of the patient's bowel elimination, support systems, coping abilities, nutritional status, pain, and understanding of the disease process and treatment required. Patients need a complete understanding of the care plan so they can make informed choices. Prevention of future episodes is a goal for the ulcerative colitis patient.

Preoperative care for these patients includes (1) selecting a stoma site, (2) performing additional diagnostic tests if cancer is suspected, (3) helping the patient accept that previous treatments were unsuccessful in curing the disease, and (4) preparing the bowel for surgery. The bowel is prepared 2 or 3 days preoperatively. A bland to clear liquid diet is ordered, along with a bowel prep of laxatives, GoLYTELY (an oral or NG colonic lavage–electrolyte solution), and enemas (see Box 5-2). Antibiotics, such an erythromycin and neomycin, are given to decrease the number of bacteria in the bowel.

Postoperative nursing interventions depend on the type of procedure performed and the individual's response. Areas of concern are bowel and urinary elimination; fluid and electrolyte balance; tissue perfusion; comfort and pain; nutrition; gas exchange; infection; and, in the case of ostomy construction, assessment of the ileostomy and peristomal skin integrity.

Nursing diagnoses and interventions for the patient with chronic inflammatory bowel disease include but are not limited to the following:

Nursing Diagnoses	Nursing Interventions
Imbalanced nutrition: less than body requirements, related to: • bowel hypermotility • decreased absorption	Provide small frequent meals, which will help patient with poor appetite or intolerance to consume larger amounts. Eliminate foods that aggravate condition.
Powerlessness, related to loss of control of body function	Assist weakened patient with activities of daily living (bathing, oral hygiene, shaving, and other grooming needs). Offer choices to patient, when possible, to provide a sense of control.

Nursing diagnoses for the surgical patient include *risk for ineffective coping, situational low self-esteem*, and *disturbed body image*. Nursing interventions include reinforcing the physician's explanation of the surgical procedure and expected outcomes. Providing reading material and demonstrating the care of an ostomy pouch when the patient seems ready will reduce anxiety. A visitor from the United Ostomy Association can provide hope, as a recovered and productive role model. But do not expect immediate patient accep-

---

Box 5-5	Postoperative Nursing Interventions for Ulcerative Colitis

1. Monitor nasogastric (NG) suction for patency until bowel function is resumed. Maintain correct wall suctioning. Accurately record color and amount of output. Irrigate NG tube as needed. Apply water-soluble lubricant to nares. Assess bowel sounds, being certain to turn off NG suction during auscultation.
2. Initiate ostomy care and teaching when bowel activity begins. Be sensitive to patient's pain level and readiness for teaching of ostomy care.
3. Observe **stoma** (an artificial opening of an internal organ on the body's surface) for color and size (should be erythematous and slightly edematous). Document assessment (e.g., "stoma pink and viable").
4. Select appropriate pouching system that has skin-protective barrier, accordion flange to ease pressure applied to new incisional site, adhesive backing, and pouch opening no more than $\frac{1}{16}$ inch larger than the stoma. Stomas change in size over time and should be measured before new supplies are ordered.
5. Empty pouch when it is approximately one third full to prevent breaking the seal, resulting in pouch leakage.
6. Explain that initial dark green liquid will change to yellow-brown as patient is allowed to eat.
7. Teach patient to care for the stoma; this includes having patient look at stoma and gradually assist with emptying, cleaning, and changing pouch. Teach patient that normal grieving occurs after loss of rectal function. Be supportive of patient's concerns.
8. Promote independence and self-care to decrease state of denial.
9. Instruct on follow-up home care, including changing skin barrier (a piece of pectin-based or Karaya wafer with measurable thickness and hydrocolloid adhesive properties) every 5 to 7 days. Using antacids, skin protective paste, and liquid skin barrier may be appropriate if skin excoriation is observed.
10. Patient may shower or bathe with or without pouch on.
11. Patient should avoid lifting objects heavier than 10 pounds until physician says it is allowed.
12. A special diet is not necessary, but patients should drink 8 to 10 glasses of water a day, chew food well, and limit or avoid certain gas-forming foods.
13. Sexual relationships can be resumed when physician feels it is not harmful to the surgical area. Counseling may be appropriate if patient has fear of resuming this activity.

---

tance of the stoma; acceptance will be gradual. Be supportive and encourage the patient to share fears. Box 5-5 lists postoperative nursing interventions.

Peristomal Area Integrity

Assess the peristomal skin for impaired integrity. Four primary factors contributing to loss of peristomal skin integrity are allergies, mechanical trauma, chemical reactions, and infection.

Allergies to pouches, adhesives, skin barriers, powders and paste, or belts are evident at areas of contact. The skin may appear erythematous, eroded, weeping, and bleeding. Changing the type of pouch, tape, or adhesive may resolve the problem.

Mechanical trauma caused by pressure, friction, or stripping of adhesives and skin barriers can be avoided by changing the pouch less frequently, using adhesive tape sparingly, and wearing a belt only when the patient feels it is necessary. The skin must be protected when the pouch is removed.

The most common chemical irritant is the stool from the stoma. Protect the skin from these digestive enzymes by using skin barriers before applying the pouch. Skin barriers include adhesives (Stomahesive), powders (Stomahesive power), liquid skin barriers (Skin Prep), and caulking paste (Stomahesive paste).

A common cause of infection of the peristomal skin is *Candida albicans*. People who have been taking antibiotics for 5 or more days may be prone to this problem. Treatment is application of nystatin powder or cream, by physician order. Apply a skin barrier over the medicated area to ensure the adhesive sticks.

Patient Teaching

Teach the patient or significant other the appropriate care of the ileostomy or colostomy to foster independence. This includes pouch change, cleansing, irrigation, and skin care. Provide a list of foods that are known to commonly cause constipation, diarrhea, blockage, odors, and flatus. Also, before discharge, give the patient a list of resource people, phone numbers, supplies, and where to obtain them.

Prognosis

The prognosis for patients with chronic ulcerative colitis is directly related to the number of years they have had the disease. The incidence of carcinoma increases when the colon is extensively involved over time. The disease carries a higher mortality rate in patients who have the disease 15 to 20 years.

CROHN'S DISEASE

Etiology and Pathophysiology

Crohn's disease, although not as prevalent as ulcerative colitis, is increasing in incidence. Crohn's disease is characterized by inflammation of segments of the GI tract. It was once thought to be a disease specific to the small intestine and was called regional enteritis. The cause of the disease is not known, but there seems to be a strong association between Crohn's disease and altered immune mechanisms. Both genetic and environmental factors seem to play a role. It commonly occurs during adolescence and early adulthood with a second peak in the sixth decade (Lewis et al., 2007). Crohn's disease can occur anywhere in the GI tract from the mouth to the anus, but occurs most commonly in the terminal ileum and colon. The inflammation involves all layers of the bowel wall. It may involve only one segment of the bowel, or segments of diseased tissue may alternate with healthy tissue. In the early stages of the disease, tiny ulcers form on various parts of the intestinal wall. Over time, horizontal rows of these ulcers fuse with vertical rows, giving the mucosa a cobblestone appearance. Inflammation, fibrosis, and scarring often involving the entire thickness of the intestine are characteristics of Crohn's disease. Patients with Crohn's disease are likely to have a bowel obstruction, fistulas, fissures, and abscesses. In some patients the disease may involve the colon without any changes in the small intestine.

Malabsorption is the major problem when the small intestine is involved, and this contributes to nutritional problems. Megaloblastic (pernicious) anemia results from decreased absorption of vitamin B_{12} in the small intestine. Fluid and electrolyte disturbances with acid-base imbalances can occur, particularly with depletion of sodium or potassium associated with diarrhea or with excessive small intestine drainage through fistulas associated with the pathologic process.

Clinical Manifestations

The manifestations depend largely on the anatomical site of involvement, extent of the disease process, and presence of complications. The onset of Crohn's disease is usually insidious, with nonspecific complaints such as diarrhea, fatigue, abdominal pain, weight loss, and fever. As the disease progresses, the patient experiences weight loss, malnutrition, dehydration, electrolyte imbalance, anemia, and increased peristalsis.

Assessment

Collection of **subjective data** for the patient with Crohn's disease includes noting the patient's list of vague complaints, including weakness, loss of appetite, abdominal pain and cramps, intermittent low-grade fever, sleeplessness caused by diarrhea, and stress. Right-lower-quadrant abdominal pain is characteristic of the disease and may be accompanied by a tender mass of thickened intestines in the same area.

Objective data include complaints of diarrhea—three or four semisolid stools daily, containing mucus and pus but no blood. **Steatorrhea** (excess fat in the feces) may also be present if the ulceration extends high in the small intestine. With small intestine involvement, weight loss occurs from malabsorption. Scar tissue from the inflammation narrows the lumen of the intestine and may cause strictures and obstruction, a frequent complication. Intestinal fistulas are a cardinal feature and may develop between segments of bowel. Cutaneous fistulas, common in the perianal area, and rectovaginal fistulas may occur. Fistulas communicating with the urinary tract may cause urinary tract infections. Poor absorption of bile salts by the ileum may lead to watery stools. Fever and unexplained anemia may also occur.

Diagnostic Tests

A small bowel barium enema is preferred over an upper GI roentgenographic series; small bowel follow-through detects defining mucosal abnormalities such as cobblestoning of the mucosa, fistulas, and strictures of the ileum. The most definitive test to differentiate Crohn's disease from ulcerative colitis is colonoscopy with multiple biopsies of the colon and terminal ileum. The appearance of the mucosa in Crohn's disease can range from normal to severely inflamed, and areas of inflammation may be continuous or interspersed with areas that appear normal. Granulomas in the biopsy specimen confirm the diagnosis of Crohn's disease, but their absence does not rule it out. In contrast, biopsies from a patient with ulcerative colitis show chronic inflammatory changes with no granulomas. Blood tests for anemia may also be ordered. Since an endoscope can enter little of the small intestine, it has not been possible to get a direct view of the ileal inflammation of Crohn's disease. Capsule endoscopy (see Figure 5-6) is used in the diagnosis of small intestine diseases. Thus far, it has been shown to have greater sensitivity than radiography when diagnosing Crohn's disease (Lewis et al., 2007).

Medical Management

Treatment is individualized depending on the patient's age, the location and severity of the disease, and any complications present. Once Crohn's disease has been diagnosed, the patient is started on drug therapy to try to get the disease in remission. Those with mild to moderate disease usually take antiinflammatory agents such as sulfasalazine, mesalamine, olsalazine, or balsalazide. When inflammation is severe, corticosteroids such as prednisone may be prescribed. Patients are weaned off steroids as soon as possible to prevent dependency and long-term complications. Multivitamins and B_{12} injections are often recommended to correct deficiencies.

If first-line therapy fails, treatment with more toxic, second-line drugs becomes necessary. These include immunosuppressive agents such as azathioprine; cyclosporine (Neoral, Sandimmune); methotrexate, or MTX (Folex, Mexate, Rheumatrex); and IV immunoglobin. The FDA approved the use of infliximab (Remicade) for Crohn's disease. It is a monoclonal antibody drug given as a single IV infusion except to those with fistulizing disease, in which case the patient needs two additional infusions. Infliximab works by neutralizing tumor necrosis factor, a protein that causes much of the intestinal inflammation. Infliximab is the only medication specifically indicated for the treatment of Crohn's disease.

Diet intervention, stress reduction, and surgery are also used to manage Crohn's disease.

Diet

Minimize bowel symptoms and diarrhea by excluding from the diet (1) lactose-containing foods in patients suspected of having lactose intolerance; (2) brassica vegetables (cauliflower, broccoli, asparagus, cabbage, and brussels sprouts); (3) caffeine, beer, monosodium glutamate, and sugarless (sorbitol-containing) gum and mints; and (4) highly seasoned foods, concentrated fruit juices, carbonated beverages, and fatty foods.

Diets high in protein (100 g/day) are recommended for patients with hypoproteinemia caused by mucosal loss, malabsorption, maldigestion, or malnutrition. Elemental diets have been shown to induce remission in 90% of patients. Free elemental diets may help patients with diarrhea because they require minimal digestion and reduce stool volume. Such elemental dietary preparations include Criticare, Travasorb HN, and Precision High Nitrogen. Total parenteral nutrition has been shown to be more effective in patients with Crohn's disease than in those with ulcerative colitis.

Medications

Corticosteroids are the preferred medical treatment of active Crohn's disease when the small intestine is involved. Sulfasalazine, olsalazine, mesalamine, and balsalazide are effective in active Crohn's disease, especially when there is colonic involvement. Antibiotics may be used, although no specific infectious agent has been discovered. Metronidazole, ciproflaxin (Cipro), and clarithromycin have been used successfully. Antidiarrheal agents (diphenoxylate with atropine and loperamide) and antispasmodics (Donnatal [atropine, hyoscyamine, phenobarbital, and scopolamine]; and dicyclomine [Bentyl]) have proven effective but are used with caution because of side effects. Biologic drug therapies include monoclonal antibodies to tumor necrosis factor–alpha (infliximab) and to a leukocyte adhesion molecule (natalizumab [Antegren]). Infliximab has been shown to reduce the degree of inflammation; however, not all patients with Crohn's disease respond to infliximab. Natalizumab, on the other hand, works by interrupting the movement of lymphocytes into the endothelial layer of the gut wall and thus decreasing the inflammatory process. Problems with inadequate vitamin B_{12} absorption result when the terminal ileum is resected; lifelong replacement of vitamin B_{12} is then necessary.

Complications of inflammation with fibrous scarring, obstruction, fistula formation in the small intestine, abscesses, and perforation are indications for surgical excision and anastomosis. Resection is the preferred surgery because bypass has a greater failure rate.

Surgical Treatment

About 75% of patients with Crohn's disease eventually require surgery. Although surgery produces remission, recurrence rates are high. Surgical removal of large segments of the small intestine can lead to short-bowel syndrome, a condition in which the absorption surface is inadequate to maintain life and parenteral nutrition is used. Surgery is reserved for emergency situations (excessive bleeding, obstruction, peritonitis) or when medical treatment has failed. The principal surgical technique for Crohn's disease is stricture-plasty to widen areas of narrowed bowel. It is sometimes necessary to resect the diseased bowel and anastomose the ends. Unfortunately, the disease commonly recurs at the area of anastomosis. Emergency surgery is necessary when perforation allows bowel contents to drain into the abdominal cavity. In this situation, the purulent exudate is drained, the abdomen is washed out, and the patient has a temporary ostomy. An abscess that is walled off may be surgically drained (Lewis et al., 2007).

Nursing Interventions

In caring for the patient with Crohn's disease, consider nutrition, fluid balance, elimination, medications, psychological aspects, and sexuality. Total parenteral nutrition may be ordered in cases of severe disease and marked weight loss. Tube feedings that allow rapid absorption in the upper GI tract are begun, and then oral intake of a low-residue, high-protein, high-calorie diet is gradually introduced. Vitamin supplements are frequently necessary, and vitamin B_{12} is given when there is a marked loss of ileum. When anemia is present, iron dextran (DexFerrum) is given by Z-track injection because oral intake of iron is ineffective due to intestinal ulceration.

Oral diets of 2500 mL/day to replace fluids and electrolytes lost from diarrhea are not uncommon. Monitor weight for losses or gains. Monitor skin condition and all fluid I&O daily. A urinary output of at least 1500 mL/day is desired.

When a patient is hospitalized, a bedside commode or a bedpan must be accessible at all times because of the urgency and frequency of stools. Emptying the bedpan immediately and deodorizing the room maintain an aesthetic environment. The anal region may become excoriated from frequent stools. Examine the anal area regularly and keep it clean using medicated wipes (Tucks) and sitz baths. These nursing interventions promote comfort and hygiene for the patient.

Most patients with Crohn's disease require emotional support from nurses, physicians, aides, stomal therapists, and others. The onset of the disease (often at 10 to 15 years of age) often occurs before the person has the emotional development and maturity to cope. The support groups sponsored by the Crohn's and Colitis Foundation of America (formerly the National Foundation of Ileitis and Colitis) can play a major role in helping patients. Tranquilizers, antidepressants, and psychology or psychiatry services may be required when managing the disease. Current evidence suggests that Crohn's disease is not caused by psychological stress but that psychiatric disturbances are the result of the disease's symptoms and chronicity.

Nursing diagnoses and interventions for patients with Crohn's disease include but are not limited to the following:

Nursing Diagnoses	Nursing Interventions
Powerlessness, related to exacerbations and remissions	Explore with patient factors that aggravate the disease. Assist patient in listing factors that can be controlled: diet, stressors, medication compliance, self-monitoring of symptoms.
Imbalanced nutrition: less than body requirements, related to: • bowel hypermotility • decreased absorption	Emphasize the importance of weighing daily, following special diets, and assessing energy levels.

Nursing Interventions and Patient Teaching

The patient must understand how diarrhea and rapid emptying of the small intestine affects the body's nutritional needs. This will lead to acceptance of special diets and the ability to retain some personal control of the disease. The patient must also understand the relationship of emotional feelings to Crohn's disease. Identifying resources for emotional support in the family and community and among health professionals will promote coping skills and mental hygiene.

Prognosis

Crohn's disease is a chronic disorder; it has a high rate of recurrence, especially in patients under 25 years of age. The rate of recurrence after surgery is 50% for the first 5 years and 75% in 10 years. Prognosis depends on the extent of involvement, duration of illness, and success of medical interventions. No known therapy will maintain a patient with Crohn's disease in remission.

ACUTE ABDOMINAL INFLAMMATIONS

APPENDICITIS

Etiology and Pathophysiology

Appendicitis is the inflammation of the vermiform appendix, usually acute, which if undiagnosed leads rapidly to perforation and peritonitis. Appendicitis is most likely to occur in teenagers and young adults and is more common in men.

The vermiform appendix is a small tube in the right lower quadrant of the abdomen. The lumen of the proximal end is shared with that of the cecum, whereas the distal end is closed. The appendix fills and empties regularly in the same way as the cecum. However, the lumen is tiny and easily obstructed. The most common causes of appendicitis are obstruction of the lumen by a fecalith (accumulated feces), foreign bodies, and tumor of the cecum or appendix. If it becomes obstructed and inflamed, pathogenic bacteria (*E. coli*) begin to multiply in the appendix and cause an infection with the formation of pus. If distention and infection are severe enough, the appendix may rupture, releasing its contents into the abdomen. The infection may be contained within an appendiceal abscess or may spread to the abdominal cavity, causing generalized peritonitis.

Clinical Manifestations

Light palpation of the abdomen elicits rebound tenderness in the right lower quadrant. The abdomen musculature overlying the right lower quadrant may feel tense as a result of voluntary rigidity. The patient often lies on the back or side with knees flexed in an attempt to decrease muscular strain on the abdominal wall.

Assessment

Subjective data include the most common complaint of constant pain in the right lower quadrant of the abdomen around McBurney's point (halfway between the umbilicus and the crest of the right ileum). The pain may be accompanied by nausea and anorexia.

Objective data include vomiting, a low-grade fever (99° to 102° F [37.2° to 38.8° C]), an elevated WBC count, rebound tenderness, a rigid abdomen, and decreased or absent bowel sounds.

Diagnostic Tests

The physician orders a WBC count with differential. Approximately 90% of patients have a WBC level above 10,000/mm^3 (normal range is 5000 to 10,000/mm^3). Approximately 75% have a neutrophil count greater than 75% (normal range is 60% to 70%). An abdominal CT scan and abdominal ultrasound are excellent diagnostic tools. NeutroSpec imaging is a new technique to diagnose appendicitis. It uses an injection of technetium-labeled anti-CD15 monoclonal antibody that selectively binds to neutrophils at the infection site, labeling these cells with technetium. As a result, physicians can rapidly detect an infection using a gamma camera that records radioactivity. NeutroSpec's advantage over the current standard of care is in vivo labeling of WBCs and a diagnosis in less than 1 hour (Lewis et al., 2007).

Medical Management

Emergency surgical intervention is the treatment of choice for acute appendicitis, or surgery may be performed when a patient is having another abdominal surgical procedure. Because mortality correlates with perforation and peritonitis, and perforation correlates with duration of symptoms, early diagnosis and appendectomy are essential. Antibiotic therapy is given when perforation is likely. Complications include infection, intraabdominal abscess, and mechanical small bowel obstruction (see Safety Alert box).

Nursing Interventions and Patient Teaching

Nursing interventions include following general preoperative procedure. Explain diagnostic tests and possible surgical procedures to relieve anxiety. Maintain

Appendicitis

- Encourage the patient with abdominal pain to see a health care provider and to avoid self-treatment, particularly the use of laxatives and enemas.
- The increased peristalsis of laxatives and enemas may cause perforation of the appendix.
- Until the patient is seen by a health care provider, he or she should remain NPO to ensure the stomach is empty in case surgery is needed.
- An ice bag may be applied to the right lower quadrant to decrease the flow of blood to the area and impede the inflammatory process.
- *Heat is never used* because it could cause the appendix to rupture.
- Surgery is usually performed as soon as a diagnosis is made.

bed rest and NPO status, provide comfort measures for pain relief so that symptoms are not masked by medication, and replace fluids and electrolytes. Monitor the temperature, blood pressure, pulse, and respirations and document these every hour because of the threat of perforation with peritonitis.

Administer prescribed opioids after the physician has assessed the patient. Opioids can mask symptoms of acute appendicitis. In some cases an ice bag to relieve pain is given; no heat is applied because this increases circulation to the appendix and could lead to rupture. A cleansing enema is not ordered because of the danger of rupture. General postoperative care is performed.

Nursing diagnoses and interventions for the patient with appendicitis include but are not limited to the following:

Nursing Diagnoses	Nursing Interventions
Deficient fluid volume, related to vomiting	Monitor patient for signs of dehydration and fluid and electrolyte imbalance (poor skin turgor; flushed dry skin; coated tongue; oliguria; confusion; and abnormal sodium, potassium, and chloride levels).
Pain, related to inflammation	Support the patient and the family by listening and by explaining tests and procedures. Administer opioids as soon as indicated after the physician assesses the patient. Monitor for increases in pain, rebound tenderness, and abdominal rigidity. Take vital signs frequently (every 15 minutes).

Patient teaching may include the reason for IV fluids with gradual advancement of the diet from clear liquids to regular diet as peristalsis returns. If antibiotics or oral

medications are continued postoperatively, make certain the patient understands the name, purpose, and side effects of each medication. If complications occur, necessitating an NG tube or drainage tubes, tell the patient the reason for these interventions.

Prognosis

The rate of cure through surgical intervention is high in patients with appendicitis. The patient's prognosis is altered if peritonitis complicates this diagnosis.

DIVERTICULOSIS AND DIVERTICULITIS

Etiology and Pathophysiology

Diverticular disease has two clinical forms: **diverticulosis** and **diverticulitis**. Diverticulosis is the presence of pouchlike herniations through the circular smooth muscle of the colon, particularly the sigmoid colon (Figure 5-11). Diverticulitis is the inflammation of one or more of the diverticular sacs.

The incidence of diverticulosis in people older than 50 years of age is increasing, possibly as a result of high luminal pressures from a deficiency of dietary fiber intake and an increase in refined carbohydrates combined with a loss of muscle mass and collagen with the aging process. Penetration of fecal matter through the thin-walled diverticula causes inflammation and abscess formation in the tissues surrounding the colon. With repeated inflammation, the lumen of the colon narrows and may become obstructed. When one or more diverticula become inflamed, diverticulitis results, which is a complication of diverticulosis. This inflammation can lead to perforation, abscess, peritonitis, obstruction, and hemorrhage. Diverticulitis is the most common cause of lower GI hemorrhage.

Clinical Manifestations

When diverticula perforate and diverticulitis develops, the patient complains of mild to severe pain in the left lower quadrant of the abdomen, has a fever, and has an elevated WBC count and sedimentation rate. If the condition goes untreated, septicemia and septic shock can develop. This patient is hypotensive and has

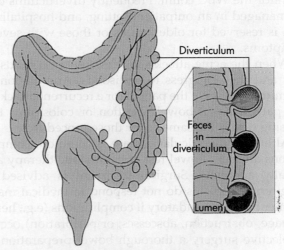

FIGURE 5-11 Diverticulosis.

a rapid pulse. Intestinal obstruction can occur, causing abdominal distention, nausea, and vomiting.

Assessment

Collection of **subjective data** includes an awareness that the patient with diverticulosis may not display any problematic symptoms. Complaints of constipation and diarrhea accompanied by pain in the left lower quadrant are common. Other common symptoms include increased flatus and chronic constipation alternating with diarrhea, anorexia, and nausea.

Objective data include abdominal distention, low-grade fever, leukocytosis, vomiting, blood in the stool, and sometimes a palpable abdominal mass.

Diagnostic Tests

Ultrasound and CT scan with oral contrast are used to confirm the diagnosis and evaluate the severity of the disease. A CBC, urinalysis, and fecal occult blood test should be performed. A barium enema is used to determine narrowing or obstruction of the colonic lumen. Colonoscopy may help rule out polyps or a malignancy. A patient with acute diverticulitis should not have a barium enema or colonoscopy because of the possibility of perforation and peritonitis.

Medical Management

A diet high in fiber, mainly from fresh fruits and vegetables, and decreased intake of fat and red meat are recommended for preventing diverticular disease. High levels of physical activity also seem to decrease the risk.

Weight reduction is important for the obese person. Patients should avoid increased intraabdominal pressure, which may precipitate an attack. Factors that increase intraabdominal pressure are straining at stool; vomiting; bending; lifting; and tight, restrictive clothing.

In acute diverticulitis, the goal of treatment is to allow the colon to rest and the inflammation to subside. Observe the patient for signs of possible peritonitis. Administer broad-spectrum antibiotics as ordered. Monitor the WBC count. Frequently diverticulitis can be managed in an outpatient setting, and hospitalization is reserved for older adults or those with severe symptoms.

When the acute attack subsides, give oral fluids at first and then progress to semisolids. Ambulation is permitted. Observe the patient for a recurrent attack. If the patient has a bowel resection or colostomy, the nursing care is the same as for those procedures.

Although diverticular disease is common, complications are rare. Bowel rest and antibiotic therapy are usually adequate. Surgical treatment is advised if long-term problems do not respond to medical management and is mandatory if complications (e.g., hemorrhage, obstruction, abscesses, or perforation) occur. In elective surgery a thorough bowel preparation is

most important. Laxatives, enemas, or intestinal lavage by GoLYTELY (see Box 5-2) are given to cleanse the bowel, depending on the surgeon's preference. Antibiotics are given orally and parenterally.

In cases of perforation, abscess, peritonitis, or fistula, resection of the bowel with a temporary colostomy is needed. Either the one-stage procedure (resection of the affected bowel with anastomosis and no diverting colostomy) or the two-stage procedure (resection of the diseased bowel with diverting colostomy) is performed.

The bowel diversion can be accomplished by Hartmann's procedure (Figure 5-12), in which the descending colon is resected, the proximal end is brought to the abdominal wall surface, and the distal bowel is sealed off for later anastomosis. Other procedures are the double-barrel colostomy, in which the bowel is brought up through the abdominal surface (Figure 5-13), and transverse loop colostomy, in which a loop is formed and the bowel is held in place with a glass rod or a plastic butterfly between the bowel and the abdomen (Figure 5-14). The bowel can be opened at the time of surgery or postoperatively.

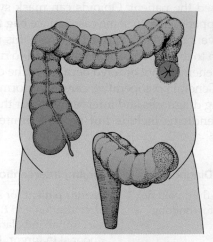

FIGURE 5-12 Hartmann's pouch.

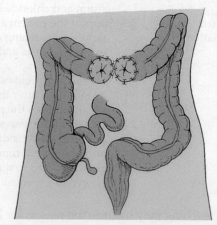

FIGURE 5-13 Double-barrel transverse colostomy.

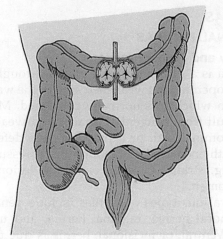

FIGURE 5-14 Transverse loop colostomy with rod or butterfly.

Removal of the affected bowel segment and reanastomosis of the bowel are done during the initial procedure.

Closure of the temporary colostomy is the desired goal in the case of diverticular disease. Usually this takes place 6 weeks to 3 months after the initial surgical procedure. Again, the bowel must be prepared for closure by a liquid diet; laxatives; antibiotics; intestinal lavage as mentioned; and a cleansing colostomy irrigation of the proximal and, in the case of the loop or double-barrel colostomy, distal end of the stoma.

Nursing Interventions and Patient Teaching
Remember that when the distal loop is irrigated, irrigating solution and bowel contents usually return from both the distal opening and rectum, so place the patient on the toilet or bedpan during the procedure.

The return of bowel activity after closure may take several days. The patient will have IV fluids and an NG tube for the first few days postoperatively.

Nursing interventions include patient teaching of the disease process and surgery, if planned. Assess the nutritional status and reinforce the prescribed diet. Determine the nature of the pain the patient is having so that comfort measures or medication can be administered. Include the patient and the family in setting goals for the teaching plan.

Nursing diagnoses and interventions for the patient with diverticular disease include but are not limited to the following:

Nursing Diagnoses	Nursing Interventions
Deficient knowledge, related to disease process and treatment	Instruct patient and family in disease process and signs and symptoms of acute diverticulitis attack.

Nursing Diagnoses	Nursing Interventions
Imbalanced nutrition: less than body requirements, related to decreased oral intake	Instruct patient about dietary fiber (for prevention) or bland, low-residue diet (for inflammatory phase). Assess daily weights, calorie counts, and I&O. Monitor serum protein and albumin.

When a colostomy is performed, have the patient or family member verbalize and demonstrate understanding of the ostomy care. Do not rush the teaching of colostomy care; wait until the patient is free of pain and receptive to learning. A family member may be taught to help until the patient is able to assume self-care, keeping in mind that the ultimate goal is patient independence. A home care referral may be needed so that the teaching process can continue after discharge.

Prognosis
With diverticulosis, the prognosis is good. Most patients have few symptoms except for occasional bleeding from the rectum. Diverticulitis has a good prognosis, with 30% of patients needing bowel resection of the affected part in acute cases to reduce mortality and morbidity.

PERITONITIS
Etiology and Pathophysiology
Peritonitis is an inflammation of the abdominal peritoneum. This condition occurs after fecal matter seeps from a rupture site, causing bacterial contamination of the peritoneal cavity. Some examples are diverticular abscess and rupture, acute appendicitis with rupture, and strangulated hernia. Peritonitis can also be caused by chemical irritants, such as blood, bile, necrotic tissue, pancreatic enzymes (pancreatitis), and foreign bodies. Ascites that occurs with cirrhosis of the liver provides an excellent liquid environment for bacteria to flourish. Patients who use continuous ambulatory peritoneal dialysis are also at high risk. No matter what the cause, the resulting inflammation response leads to massive fluid shifts (peritoneal edema and adhesions as the body attempts to wall off the infection).

Clinical Manifestations
Generalized peritonitis is an extremely serious condition characterized by severe abdominal pain. The patient usually lies on the back with the knees flexed to relax the abdominal muscles; any movement is painful. Rebound tenderness, muscular rigidity, and spasm are major symptoms of irritation of the peritoneum. The abdomen is usually tympanic and extremely tender to the touch.

Assessment
Collection of **subjective data** includes observing for severe abdominal pain. Nausea and vomiting occur, and as peristalsis ceases, constipation occurs with no passage

of flatus. Chills, weakness, and abdominal tenderness (local and diffuse, often rebound) are also manifested.

Collection of **objective data** includes noting a weak and rapid pulse, fever, and lowered blood pressure. Leukocytosis and marked dehydration occur, and the patient can collapse and die.

Diagnostic Tests

A flat plate of the abdomen is ordered to find out whether free air is present under the diaphragm as a result of visceral perforation. A CBC with differential is ordered to determine the degree of leukocytosis. A blood chemistry profile to determine renal perfusion and electrolyte balance is done. Peritoneal aspiration may be performed and the fluid analyzed for blood, bile, pus, bacteria, or fungus. Ultrasound and CT scans may be useful in identifying ascites and abscesses.

Medical Management

Aggressive therapy includes correction of the contamination or removal of the chemical irritant by surgery, and parenteral antibiotics. NG intubation is ordered to prevent GI distention. IV fluids and electrolytes prevent or correct imbalances. Analgesics are provided intravenously via PCA pump. The patient may be placed on total parenteral nutrition because of increased nutritional requirements. Early treatment to prevent severe shock from the loss of fluid into the peritoneal space is essential.

Nursing Interventions and Patient Teaching

Nursing interventions for the patient with peritonitis include the following:

- Place patient on bed rest in semi-Fowler's position to help localize purulent exudate in lower abdomen or pelvis.
- Give oral hygiene to prevent drying of mucous membranes and cracking of lips from dehydration.
- Monitor fluid and electrolyte replacement.
- Encourage deep-breathing exercises; patient tends to have shallow respirations as a result of abdominal pain or distention.
- Use measures to reduce anxiety.
- Use meticulous surgical asepsis for wound care.

Instruct the patient about the importance of ambulation, coughing, deep breathing, use of an incentive spirometer, and leg exercises. If the patient has a draining wound at discharge, teach surgical asepsis for dressing changes. Encourage a nutritious diet. Instruct the patient not to lift more than 10 pounds until the physician approves it. Stress the importance of keeping physician follow-up appointments.

Prognosis

The mortality rate of generalized peritonitis is 40% with the use of antibiotics and intensive support systems. Age, etiology of the peritonitis, and ineffective tissue perfusion negatively affect the prognosis.

HERNIAS
EXTERNAL HERNIAS
Etiology and Pathophysiology

A hernia is a protrusion of a viscus through an abnormal opening or a weakened area in the wall of the cavity in which it is normally contained. Most hernias result from congenital or acquired weakness of the abdominal wall or a postoperative defect, coupled with increased intraabdominal pressure from coughing, straining, or an enlarging lesion within the abdomen.

The various types of hernias include ventral hernia, femoral hernia, inguinal hernia, and umbilical hernia. Ventral, or incisional, hernia is due to weakness of the abdominal wall at the site of a previous incision. It is found most commonly in patients who are obese, who have had multiple surgical procedures in the same area, and who have inadequate wound healing because of poor nutrition or infection. A femoral, or inguinal, hernia is caused by a weakness in the lower abdominal wall opening through which the spermatic cord emerges in men and the round ligament emerges in women.

A hernia may be reducible (able to be returned to its original position by manipulation) or irreducible (or incarcerated; unable to be returned to its body cavity). When the hernia is irreducible, it may obstruct intestinal flow. The hernia is strangulated when it occludes blood supply and intestinal flow. To prevent anaerobic infection in the area, immediate surgical intervention is performed when a hernia strangulates.

Factors such as age, wound infection, malnutrition, obesity, increased intraabdominal pressure, or abdominal distention affect formation of hernias after surgical incisions. Fewer hernias occur with transverse incisions than with longitudinal incisions. Also, upper abdominal incisions are associated with fewer hernias than lower abdominal incisions.

Assessment

Collection of **subjective data** includes palpation of the hernia area, revealing the contents of the sac as soft and nodular (omentum) or smooth and fluctuant (bowel). Never attempt to reduce the sac in the ring because this can lead to complications such as rupture of the strangulated contents.

Both subjective and objective signs and symptoms depend on where the hernia occurs. With an inguinal hernia, the patient may complain of pain, urgency, and a mass in the groin region.

Objective data include a visible protruding mass or bulge around the umbilicus, in the inguinal area, or near an incision; this is the most common objective sign. If complications such as incarceration or strangulation follow, the patient may have bowel obstruction, vomiting, and abdominal distention.

Diagnostic Tests

The diagnosis is aided by palpation of the weakened wall. Radiographs of the suspected area may be ordered.

Medical Management

Hernias that cause no discomfort can be left unrepaired unless strangulation or obstruction follows. Teach the patient to seek medical advice promptly if abdominal pain, distention, changing bowel habits, temperature elevation, nausea, or vomiting occurs. If the hernia can be reduced manually, a truss or firm pad placed over the patient's hernia site and held in place with a belt prevents the hernia from protruding and holds the abdominal contents in place.

Elective surgery for hernia repair may be done because of inconvenience to the patient or constant risk of strangulation. A procedure to close the hernia defect by approximating adjacent muscles or using a synthetic mesh is done on either an inpatient or outpatient basis.

Nursing Interventions and Patient Teaching

Nursing interventions for external hernia require observation of the hernia's location and size and tissue perfusion to the area. The patient may be limited in activity and the type of clothing worn.

Open abdominal surgery may be necessary for the patient with a strangulated hernia. Prepare the patient for a long hospitalization, which may include NG suctioning, IV antibiotics, fluid and electrolyte replacement, and parenteral analgesics until peristalsis returns.

Postoperatively monitor the patient for urinary retention; wound infection at the incision site; and, with inguinal hernia repair, scrotal edema. If scrotal edema is present, elevate the scrotum on a rolled pad, apply an ice pack, and provide a supportive garment (jockstrap or briefs). The patient should deep breathe every 2 hours, but many physicians discourage coughing. Verify the postoperative orders. Teach the patient how to support the incision by splinting the area with pillow or pad. This support, along with analgesics, will help relieve pain.

Nursing diagnoses and interventions for the patient with a hernia include but are not limited to the following:

Nursing Diagnoses	Nursing Interventions
Deficient knowledge, related to disease process	Instruct patient to observe and report hernias that become irreducible or edematous. Instruct patient to report increased pain, abdominal distention, or change in bowel habits. Explain reason to avoid prolonged standing, lifting, or straining.
Ineffective tissue perfusion, related to strangulation or incarceration of hernia	Instruct patient to support weakened area by use of truss or manually as needed (as when coughing). Monitor patient for increased pain, distention, changing bowel habits, abnormal bowel sounds, temperature elevation, nausea, and vomiting. Report changes in appearance and signs and symptoms to physician.

Follow-up care includes teaching the patient to limit activities and avoid lifting heavy objects or straining with bowel movements for 5 to 6 weeks. Also the patient should immediately report to the physician any erythema or edema of the surgical area or increased pain or drainage.

HIATAL HERNIA

A hiatal hernia (esophageal hernia or diaphragmatic hernia) results from a weakness of the diaphragm. Hiatal hernia is a protrusion of the stomach and other abdominal viscera through an opening, or hiatus, in the diaphragm (Figure 5-15). A hiatal hernia is the most common problem of the diaphragm that affects the alimentary tract. It is an anatomical condition, not a disease. This condition occurs in about 40% of the population; most people display few, if any, symp-

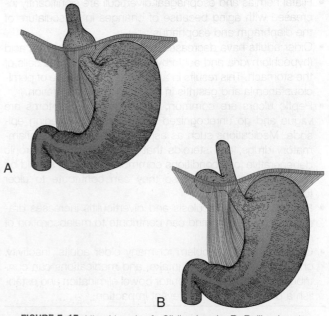

FIGURE 5-15 Hiatal hernia. **A,** Sliding hernia. **B,** Rolling hernia.

toms. The major difficulty in symptomatic patients is gastroesophageal reflux, manifested as pyrosis (heartburn) after overeating. Complications of strangulation, infarction, or ulceration of the herniated stomach are serious and require surgical intervention. Factors contributing to the development of these hernias include obesity, trauma, and a general weakening of the supporting structures as a result of aging (see Life Span Considerations box).

Medical Management

The physician may perform (1) a posterior gastropexy, in which the stomach is returned to the abdomen and sutured in place; or (2) a laparoscopically performed Nissen fundoplication, in which the fundus is wrapped around the lower part of the esophagus and sutured in place (Figure 5-16). The use of laparoscopic techniques has reduced the overall morbidity, complications, and the cost of hospitalization associated with a thoracic or open abdominal approach. However, a thoracic or open abdominal approach may be used in selected cases.

Nursing Interventions

Nursing care of the patient after surgery is similar to that after gastric surgery or thoracic surgery, depending on the procedure performed.

Life Span Considerations

Older Adults

Gastrointestinal Disorders

- Loss of teeth and resultant use of dentures can interfere with chewing and lead to digestive complaints.
- Dysphagia is commonly seen in the older adult population and may be caused by changes in the esophageal musculature or by neurologic conditions.
- Hiatal hernias and esophageal diverticuli are significantly increased with aging because of changes in musculature of the diaphragm and esophagus.
- Older adults have decreased secretion of hydrochloric acid (hypochlorhydria and achlorhydria) from the parietal cells of the stomach. This results in an increased incidence of pernicious anemia and gastritis in the older adult population.
- Peptic ulcers are common, but often the symptoms are vague and go unrecognized until there is a bleeding episode. Medications such as aspirin, nonsteroidal antiinflammatory drugs, and steroids that are taken for the chronic degenerative joint conditions common with aging should be used with caution because they can contribute to ulcer formation.
- Frequency of diverticulosis and diverticulitis increases dramatically with aging and can contribute to malabsorption of nutrients.
- Constipation is a problem for many older adults. Inactivity, changes in diet and fluid intake, and medications can contribute to this problem. Monitor bowel elimination and establish a bowel regimen to prevent impaction.

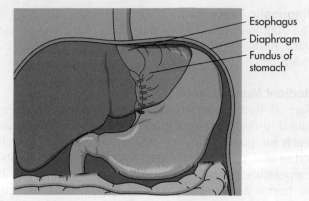

FIGURE 5-16 Nissen fundoplication for hiatal hernia showing fundus of stomach wrapped around distal esophagus and sutured to itself.

Prognosis

The prognosis for hernias is good because surgical intervention is usually successful. The result can be altered if the patient is a poor surgical risk or has other complications.

INTESTINAL OBSTRUCTION

Etiology and Pathophysiology

Intestinal obstruction occurs when intestinal contents cannot pass through the GI tract; it requires prompt treatment. The obstruction may be partial or complete. The causes of intestinal obstruction are classified as mechanical or nonmechanical.

Mechanical Obstruction

Mechanical obstruction may be caused by an occlusion of the lumen of the intestinal tract. Most obstructions occur in the ileum, which is the narrowest segment of the small intestine. Mechanical obstructions account for 90% of all intestinal obstructions. Mechanical obstructions include adhesions (Figure 5-17, *A*) or incarcerated hernias. Adhesions can develop after abdominal surgery. Other causes include impacted feces, diverticular disease, tumor of the bowel, intussusceptions, **volvulus** (Figure 5-17, *B*) (a twisting of bowel onto itself), or the strictures of inflammatory bowel disease. Residues from foods high in fiber, such as raw coconut or fruit pulp, can also obstruct the small bowel.

Nonmechanical Obstruction

Nonmechanical obstruction may result from a neuromuscular or vascular disorder. The cause is something that decreases the muscle action of the bowel and affects the ability of fecal matter and fluid to move through the intestines (Kent, 2007). **Paralytic (adynamic) ileus** (lack of intestinal peristalsis and bowel sounds) is the most common form of nonmechanical obstruction. It occurs to some degree after any abdominal surgery. Other causes include inflammatory responses (e.g., acute pancreatitis, acute appendicitis), electrolyte abnormalities (especially hypokalemia), and thoracic or lumbar spinal

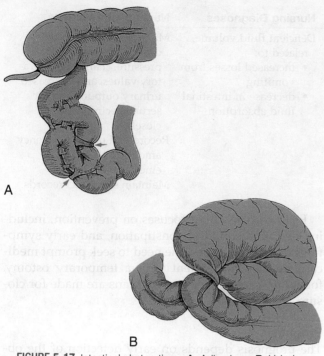

A

B

FIGURE 5-17 Intestinal obstructions. **A,** Adhesions. **B,** Volvulus.

trauma from either fractures or surgical intervention. Vascular obstructions are rare and are due to an interference with the blood supply to a portion of the intestines. The most common causes are emboli and atherosclerosis of the mesenteric arteries. The celiac, inferior, and superior mesenteric arteries supply blood to the bowel. Emboli may originate from thrombi in patients with chronic atrial fibrillation, diseased heart valves, and prosthetic valves.

When the small intestine becomes obstructed, it interrupts the normal process of secretion and reabsorption of 6 to 8 L of electrolyte-rich fluid. Large amounts of fluid, bacteria, and swallowed air build up in the bowel proximal to the obstruction. Water and salts shift from the circulatory system to the intestinal lumen, causing distention and further interfering with absorption. As the fluid increases, so does the pressure in the lumen of the bowel. The increased pressure leads to an increase in capillary permeability and extravasation of fluids and electrolytes into the peritoneal cavity. Edema, congestion, and necrosis from impaired blood supply and possible rupture of the bowel may occur. The retention of fluid in the intestine and peritoneal cavity can lead to a severe reduction in circulating blood volume and result in hypotension and hypovolemic shock.

Clinical Manifestations

The signs and symptoms of intestinal obstruction vary with the site and degree of obstruction. During partial or early phases of mechanical obstruction, auscultation of the abdomen reveals loud, frequent, high-pitched

sounds. However, when smooth muscle atony (weak, lacking normal tone) occurs, bowel sounds are absent.

Assessment

Subjective data include the pattern of the patient's pain, including onset, frequency, and characteristics. Nausea and the inability to pass flatus are common symptoms. Early complaints of obstruction of the small intestine include spasms of cramping abdominal pain as peristaltic activity increases proximal to the obstruction. As the obstruction progresses, the intestine becomes fatigued, with periods of decreased or absent bowel sounds and increased abdominal pain. Note any history of previous bowel disorders or abdominal surgeries and changes in bowel elimination.

Collection of **objective data** begins with assessing the abdominal surface for evidence of distention, hernias, scars indicating previous surgeries, or visible peristaltic waves. The increased peristaltic activity produces an increase in auscultated bowel sounds. Other objective data include vomiting; signs of dehydration caused by the fluid shift; abdominal distention, tenderness, and muscle guarding; and decreased blood pressure.

Obstruction of the colon causes less severe pain than obstruction of the small intestine, marked abdominal distention, and constipation. The patient may continue to have bowel movements, since the colon distal to the obstruction continues to empty.

Diagnostic Tests

Abdominal x-rays are the most useful diagnostic aids. Flat, upright, and lateral x-rays show gas and fluid in the intestines. Intraperitoneal air (sometimes referred to as free air under the diaphragm) indicates perforation. Radiographic examination reveals the level of obstruction and its cause. Sigmoidoscopy or colonoscopy may provide direct visualization of an obstruction in the colon. CT scans may also be used in diagnosis. Monitor the fluid and electrolyte balance through laboratory test results. Elevated blood urea nitrogen and decreased serum sodium, chloride, potassium, and magnesium are common. The patient's hemoglobin and hematocrit levels may increase because of hemoconcentration associated with the fluid volume deficit.

Medical Management

Treatment is directed toward decompression of the intestine by removal of gas and fluid, correction and maintenance of fluid and electrolyte balance, and relief or removal of the obstruction. Treatment may include the evacuation of intestinal contents by means of an intestinal tube. An NG or nasojejunal tube is inserted and connected to wall suction to decompress the intestine. A long intestinal tube (10 feet [300 cm]) (e.g., Miller-Abbott) may be used instead of an NG tube to decompress the bowel; however, its use is controversial and limited because it is more difficult and time consuming to insert and may not be more effective than an NG tube. Surgical repair is necessary to relieve mechanical obstructions caused by adhesions, volvulus, and strangulated hernias. Restore fluid and electrolyte balance by carefully monitoring IV infusion. Nonopioid analgesics are usually prescribed to avoid the decrease in intestinal motility that often accompanies the administration of opioid analgesics.

Nursing Interventions and Patient Teaching

Unless surgery is indicated, nursing interventions include careful monitoring of fluids and electrolytes, measuring the patient's urinary output, observing the function of tubes used to decompress and relieve distention, and administering analgesics.

For the patient with intestinal obstruction undergoing surgery, preoperative preparation includes explaining the procedure at a level the patient can understand. Provide emotional support for the patient because he or she is experiencing the stressors of pain and vomiting plus the added stressor of emergency surgery.

Postoperative nursing interventions are similar to those for any patient who has had abdominal surgery. Place the patient in a Fowler's position for greater diaphragm expansion. Encourage the patient to breathe through the nose and not swallow air, which would increase distention and discomfort. Encourage deep breathing and coughing. Continue nasointestinal suctioning until bowel activity returns. Assess for bowel sounds and abdominal girth and expulsion of flatus and stool to help determine the return of peristalsis. When the patient is ready to eat, usually within 24 to 48 hours after surgery or at the first sounds of peristalsis, provide a progressive diet as tolerated. Some patients require temporary bowel diversion via a double-barrel or loop colostomy to manage the obstruction.

To manage pain, administer all medications as prescribed. Medications may include opioids or opioid derivatives (note that morphine increases nausea and vomiting and causes constipation [Kent, 2007]).

Nursing diagnoses and interventions for the patient with an intestinal obstruction include but are not limited to the following:

Nursing Diagnoses	Nursing Interventions
Acute pain, related to increased peristalsis	Reposition patient frequently to help intestinal tube advance. Irrigate suction tubing with 30 mL sterile saline to keep tube patent. Explain purpose of all procedures. Provide comfort measures. Administer analgesics as ordered.

Nursing Diagnoses	Nursing Interventions
Deficient fluid volume, related to: • increased losses from vomiting • decrease in intestinal fluid absorption	Monitor for signs of dehydration, decreased blood pressure, change in laboratory values, and decreased urinary output. Monitor serum electrolyte levels closely. Record and report frequency, amount, and nature of emesis. Maintain strict I&O records.

Follow-up teaching focuses on prevention, including diet, prevention of constipation, and early symptoms of recurrence and the need to seek prompt medical care. For the patient with a temporary ostomy, follow-up care is necessary as plans are made for closure of the stoma.

Prognosis

The prognosis depends on early detection of the obstruction and the type and cause of the obstruction, as well as the success of medical interventions. The prognosis is poorer in patients who develop complications such as hypovolemic shock.

COLORECTAL CANCER

Etiology and Pathophysiology

Malignant neoplasms that invade the epithelium and surrounding tissue of the colon and rectum are the third most prevalent internal cancers in the United States and the second leading cause of cancer deaths.

In the colon, 45% of growths are seen in the sigmoid and rectal areas; 25% in the cecum and ascending colon; and the remaining 30% in the transverse splenic flexure, hepatic flexure, and descending colon. Cancer occurs with the same frequency in men and women, with the highest incidence in people 60 years and older.

The cause of colorectal cancer remains unknown, but certain conditions appear to make patients more susceptible to malignant changes. These conditions are termed *predisposing* or *risk factors*. Fortunately, about 85% of colorectal cancers arise from adenomatous polyps, which can be detected and removed from the rectum and sigmoid colon by sigmoidoscopy or colonoscopy. Some diseases, including ulcerative colitis and diverticulosis, increase the risk of colorectal cancer over time. Recent research has isolated a gene that causes colon cancer in certain families. Hereditary diseases (e.g., familial adenomatous polyposis) account for about 5% to 10% of colorectal cancer cases. Hereditary nonpolyposis colorectal cancer syndrome, also called Lynch syndrome, is the most common inherited form of hereditary colorectal cancer. History taking and regular checkups are important preventive measures.

Other factors implicated in colorectal cancer include lack of bulk in the diet, high fat intake, and high bacterial counts in the colon. It is theorized that carcinogens are formed from degraded bile salts, and the stool that remains in the large bowel for a longer period as a result of too little fiber to stimulate its passage may overexpose the bowel to these carcinogens. Another theory is that the increased transit time for low-fiber foods to pass through the intestine is related to malignancy. These factors have led to diet changes; decreased animal fat, reduced red meat, and increased high dietary fiber found in fruits, vegetables, and bran may have a protective effect and act as a primary preventive measure. Cruciferous vegetables such as cauliflower, broccoli, brussels sprouts, and cabbage may help protect against the malignancy. NSAIDs (e.g., aspirin) also seem to reduce the risk.

Clinical Manifestations

Signs and symptoms of cancer of the colon vary with the location of the growth. During the early stages, most patients are asymptomatic. Clinical manifestations are usually nonspecific or do not appear until the disease is advanced.

Assessment

Subjective data include changes in bowel habits alternating between constipation and diarrhea, excessive flatus, and cramps. Constipation is more likely with descending colon cancer, whereas ascending colon cancer may produce no change in bowel habits. Another complaint may be rectal bleeding (the most common sign of colorectal cancer), with the color varying from dark to bright red, depending on the location of the neoplasm. Later stages of colon cancer may involve subjective symptoms of abdominal pain, nausea, and **cachexia** (weakness and emaciation associated with general ill health and malnutrition).

Collection of **objective data** includes observing for vomiting, weight loss, abdominal distention or ascites, and test results that are compatible with the diagnosis. The most common clinical manifestations are chronic blood loss and anemia.

Diagnostic Tests

Early diagnosis of the tumor, including identification of the type of cells involved, is the most important factor in treating the disease. Digital examination can identify 15% of colorectal cancers. Since half of all cases are found in areas of the colon that are inaccessible by sigmoidoscopy, colonoscopy is considered the gold standard for colorectal cancer screening and the detection and removal of precancerous polyps. Other procedures include endorectal ultrasonography and CT scan of the abdomen and pelvis to localize the lesion or determine its size.

A baseline colonoscopy before age 50 should be performed on those who have a family history of colon cancer. Individuals with known gene mutations need to be monitored with colonoscopy every year.

Routine physical examinations should include a digital rectal examination because rectal polyps and cancer can be reached with a finger. The American Cancer Society recommends that a person with no established risk factors receive a fecal occult blood test yearly, a double-contrast enema every 5 years, a sigmoidoscopy every 5 years, or a colonoscopy every 10 years starting at age 50. All positive tests are followed up with colonoscopy (see Health Promotion box). Other laboratory and diagnostic studies include a UGI series, radiologic abdominal series, and barium enema. Hemoglobin, hematocrit, and electrolyte levels are examined, and a blood test is done for **carcinoembryonic antigen (CEA)** (an oncofetal glycoprotein found in colonic adenocarcinoma and other cancers and in nonmalignant conditions) when cancer and metastasis are suspected. Antibodies to this antigen are measured. Because the CEA level can be elevated in benign and malignant diseases, it is not considered a specific test for colorectal cancer. Its use is limited to determining the prognosis and monitoring the patient's response to antineoplastic therapy.

Medical Management

Medical treatment includes radiation, chemotherapy, and surgery. Radiation therapy is often used before surgery to decrease the chance of cancer cell implantation at the time of resection. Radiation can both reduce the size of the tumor and decrease the rate of lymphatic involvement. Radiation before surgery has few side effects but some complications.

Postoperatively those patients at high risk for recurrence or people whose disease has progressed may receive radiation administered over 4 to 6 weeks.

Chemotherapy is given (1) to patients with systemic disease that is incurable by surgery or radiation alone; (2) to patients in whom metastasis is suspected (e.g., when a patient has positive lymph node involvement at the time of surgery); or (3) for palliative therapy to reduce tumor size or relieve symptoms of the disease, such as obstruction or pain. Physician opinion and individual patient response vary regarding use of chemotherapy for colorectal cancer.

Surgical interventions depend on the tumor's location, presence of obstruction or perforation of the bowel, possible metastasis, the patient's health status, and the surgeon's preferences. When obstruction has not occurred, a portion of the bowel on either side of the tumor is removed and an end-to-end anastomosis (EEA) is done between the divided ends. When obstruction of the bowel occurs, the commonly used procedures are as follows:

- One-stage resection with anastomosis.
- Two-stage resection with (1) the ends of the bowel brought to the surface and creation of a temporary colostomy and mucus fistula or Hartmann's pouch (see Figure 5-12); (2) a double-barrel colostomy (see Figure 5-13); or (3) a temporary loop colostomy (see Figure 5-14), for closure later.

Surgical procedures for colorectal cancer include the following:

- **Right hemicolectomy:** Resection of ascending colon and hepatic flexure (Figure 5-18, *A*); ileum anastomosed to transverse colon
- **Left hemicolectomy:** Resection of splenic flexure, descending colon, and sigmoid colon (Figure 5-18, *B*); transverse colon anastomosed to rectum
- **Anterior rectosigmoid resection:** Resection of part of descending colon, the sigmoid colon, and upper rectum (Figure 5-18, *C*); descending colon anastomosed to remaining rectum

In carcinoma of the rectum, the surgeon makes every effort to preserve the sphincter, often with an EEA. The use of EEA staplers allows lower and more secure anastomosis. The stapler is passed through the anus, where the colon is stapled to the rectum. This technique makes it possible to resect lesions as low as 5 cm from the anus. If the surgeon is unable to do an anastomosis, an abdominoperineal resection may be done.

In the abdominoperineal resection, an abdominal incision is made and the proximal sigmoid is brought through the abdominal wall in a permanent colostomy. The distal sigmoid, rectum, and anus are removed

through a perineal incision (Figure 5-19). The perineal wound may be closed around a drain or left open with packing to allow healing by granulation. Possible complications are delayed wound healing, hemorrhage, persistent perineal sinus tracts, infections, and urinary tract and sexual dysfunction.

Nutritional status is important because of the threat of infection and a compromised postoperative healing process as a result of constipation, diarrhea, nausea, vomiting, and possible obstruction.

Nursing Interventions and Patient Teaching

Nursing interventions include assessment of bowel and urinary elimination, fluid and electrolyte balance, tissue perfusion, nutrition, pain, gas exchange, infection, and peristomal skin integrity, as discussed previously.

Preoperative Care

The patient has some type of bowel preparation, which usually includes 2 or 3 days of liquid diets; a combination of laxatives, GoLYTELY, or enemas; and oral antibiotics to sterilize the bowel. The antibiotic of choice may be neomycin, kanamycin, or erythromycin; each suppresses anaerobic and aerobic organisms in the colon.

Before surgery, provide instruction in turning, coughing, and deep breathing; use of incentive spi-

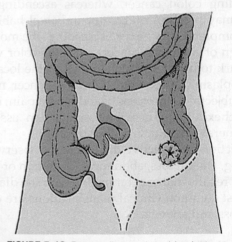

FIGURE 5-19 Descending or sigmoid colostomy.

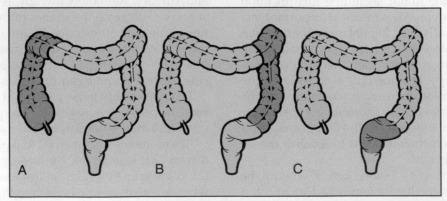

FIGURE 5-18 Bowel resection. **A,** Right hemicolectomy. **B,** Left hemicolectomy. **C,** Anterior rectosigmoid resection.

rometer; wound splinting; and leg exercises. Inform the patient that that he or she will have IV lines, a Foley catheter, possibly an NG tube, a Davol drain, and abdominal dressings after surgery.

If a stoma is planned, the enterostomal therapist should be notified so that the stoma site can be marked before surgery. The stoma should be placed at the best site for the patient.

Postoperative Care

Assess the patient for stable vital signs and return of bowel sounds. Check the dressings for drainage or bleeding and change them as needed per the physician's order. Monitor the NG tube, the Davol drain, and the Foley catheter for flow, amount, and color of output. Keep accurate I&O records to maintain the fluid and electrolyte balance. Other postoperative care includes coughing, deep breathing, early ambulation, adequate nutrition, pain control, and meticulous wound and stoma care.

Paralytic ileus, a common complication of abdominal surgery, produces the classic signs of increased abdominal girth, distention, nausea, and vomiting. Interventions include decompression of the bowel with an NG tube connected to wall suction, NPO status, and increased patient activity.

Long-term complications of abdominal resection with permanent colostomy are urinary retention or incontinence, pelvic abscess, failure of perineal wound healing or wound infection, and sexual dysfunction.

In addition to monitoring the stoma for color, size, location, and the condition of the peristomal skin, watch for possible complications, including necrosis and abscess. Necrosis results from a compromised blood flow to the stoma; the stoma appears pale and dusky to black. Abscess caused by stoma placement too close to the wound, retention sutures, and drains must be assessed promptly. Report all complications promptly to the surgeon and document them in the medical record.

Nursing diagnoses and interventions for the patient with cancer of the colon include but are not limited to the following:

Nursing Diagnoses	Nursing Interventions
Imbalanced nutrition: less than body requirements, related to: • vomiting or anorexia • surgical intervention • depression	Maintain NPO status as ordered. Monitor parenteral fluids. Monitor patency and function of NG tube. Measure I&O. Monitor vital signs and serum electrolytes, hematocrit, and hemoglobin. Provide high-protein, high-carbohydrate, high-calorie, low-residue diet as allowed and tolerated.

Nursing Diagnoses	Nursing Interventions
Disturbed body image, related to loss of normal body function (colostomy)	Allow time for grieving. Assist patient and family in accepting ostomy. Allow time for and encourage verbalization. Observe for signs of denial, grief, or anger. Answer all questions, and explain treatment and procedure. Provide care in positive manner; always avoid facial expressions connoting distaste. Provide privacy and a safe environment. Encourage self-care and independence when patient demonstrates readiness. Facilitate contact with individuals with similar changes in body image to provide realistic experiences of having ostomy.

The patient with a permanent end colostomy can be taught two forms of colostomy management: (1) emptying and cleansing the pouch as needed and (2) managing colostomy irrigation. In planning patient teaching, consider past bowel habits; location of the colostomy; and the patient's age, general health, and personal preference.

Nerves that control the bladder may be damaged when a large amount of tissue is removed in the abdominoperineal resection. When the Foley catheter is removed after surgery, the patient may be unable to void or empty the bladder completely. If the problem does not resolve, the patient may need a Foley catheter and a urology consultation.

When a large amount of tissue is removed, as in the abdominoperineal resection, the cavity left is a sanctuary for bacteria, increasing the risk of infection. Monitor the drain site for increased pain, erythema, and purulent drainage, and monitor for elevated body temperature. The perineal wound may be closed in one of three ways. The closed wound with a drain to suction has a high risk for abscess formation. The semiclosed wound has either a Davol or Penrose drain left in place, with the drain shortened over time by the physician or nurse. The open wound (in which packing is used and later removed) may need irrigation and sitz baths to facilitate healing. Report to the physician any changes in exudate color and odor and temperature elevation.

Sexual dysfunction of both men and women is related to removal of the rectum. Contributing factors may be partial to complete disruption of the nerve's supply to the genital organs, psychological factors, or decreased activity associated with age. When the nurse and the patient have a comfortable relationship, it is easier to introduce the topic of sex. Exploring the patient's and the partner's fears and providing information on penile prosthesis surgery and simple suggestions to both partners will help decrease anxiety concerning intercourse. Counseling may be necessary if the patient's and the partner's perceptions of body image have been altered. Support groups are available to the cancer patient in most communities. Above all, the nurse's silent communication of touch and eye contact can give the patient a message that he or she is accepted and valued.

Prognosis
The 5-year survival rate is 90% for patients with early localized colorectal cancer and 64% for cancer that has spread to adjacent organs and lymph nodes. Only distant metastases prevent the possibility of a cure.

HEMORRHOIDS
Etiology and Pathophysiology
Hemorrhoids are varicosities (dilated veins) that may occur outside the anal sphincter as external hemorrhoids or inside the sphincter as internal hemorrhoids. This is one of the most common health problems seen in humans, with the greatest incidence from ages 20 to 50 years. Etiologic factors include straining at stool with increased intraabdominal and hemorrhoidal venous pressures. With repeated increased pressure and obstructed blood flow, permanent dilation occurs. Hemorrhoids may be caused by constipation, diarrhea, pregnancy, congestive heart failure, portal hypertension, and prolonged sitting and standing.

Clinical Manifestations
The most common symptoms associated with enlarged, abnormal hemorrhoids are prolapse and bleeding. The bright red bleeding and prolapse usually occur at time of defecation.

Assessment
Subjective data include complaints of constipation, pruritus, severe pain when dilated veins become thrombosed, and bleeding from the rectum that is not mixed with feces.

Collection of **objective data** includes observing external hemorrhoids and palpating internal hemorrhoids. Because bleeding and constipation are signs of cancer of the rectum, all patients with these symptoms should have a thorough examination to rule out cancer.

Diagnostic Tests
Internal hemorrhoids are diagnosed by digital examination, anoscopy, and sigmoidoscopy. External hemorrhoids can be diagnosed by visual inspection and digital examination.

Medical Management
Therapy is directed toward the causes and the patient's symptoms. A high-fiber diet and increased fluid intake prevent constipation and reduce straining, which allows engorgement of the veins to subside. Conservative interventions include the use of bulk stool softeners—such as Metamucil, bran, and natural food fibers—to relieve straining. Topical creams with hydrocortisone relieve pruritus and inflammation, and analgesic ointments, such as dibucaine (Nupercainal), relieve pain. Sitz baths are usually given to relieve pain and edema and promote healing.

Rubber band ligation is a popular and easy method of treatment (Figure 5-20). Tight bands are applied with a special instrument in the physician's office, causing constriction and necrosis. The destroyed tissue sloughs off in about 1 week, and discomfort is minimal. Sclerotherapy (with a sclerosing agent injected at the apex of the hemorrhoid column), cryotherapy (tissue destruction by freezing), infrared photocoagulation (destruction of tissue by creation of a small burn), laser excision, and operative hemorrhoidectomy are additional interventions.

Hemorrhoidectomy, the surgical removal of hemorrhoids, can be performed if other interventions fail to relieve the distressing signs and symptoms. Surgery is indicated for patients with prolapse, excessive pain or bleeding, or large hemorrhoids. In general, hemorrhoidectomy is reserved for patients with severe symptoms related to multiple thrombosed hem-

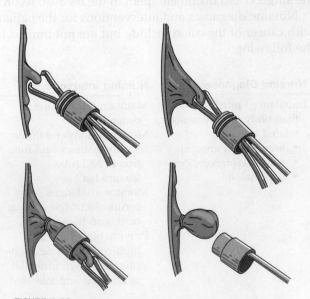

FIGURE 5-20 Rubber band ligation of an internal hemorrhoid.

orrhoids or marked protrusion. Surgical removal may be done by cautery, clamp, or excision. After removal of the hemorrhoid, wounds can be left open or closed, although closed wounds are reported to heal faster. Hemorrhoidectomy is not considered a major procedure, but pain may be acute, requiring opioids and analgesic ointments. Complications include hemorrhage, local infection, pain, urinary retention, and abscess.

Nursing Interventions and Patient Teaching

Rectal conditions can be embarrassing to the patient, and the nurse's direct but concerned attitude can decrease this embarrassment. Assess the knowledge level by asking patients about their condition, what they have been told about treatment, and what treatments have been done before surgery and why.

Observe the patient with a prolapsed hemorrhoid for edema, thrombosis, and ischemia. Ischemic tissue will be dark red to necrotic (black). Explain that a low-bulk diet can produce chronic constipation (see Evidence-Based Practice box).

For the surgical patient, take vital signs frequently for the first 24 hours to rule out internal bleeding. Sitz baths are given several times daily. Early ambulation and a soft diet facilitate bowel elimination. The patient may have a great deal of anxiety concerning the first defecation; open a discussion on this and provide an analgesic before the bowel movement to reduce discomfort. A stool softener such as docusate (Colace) is usually ordered for the first few postoperative days.

Nursing diagnoses and interventions for the patient with hemorrhoids include but are not limited to the following:

Nursing Diagnoses	Nursing Interventions
Pain, related to edema, prolapse, and surgical interventions	Instruct patient to wash anal area after defecation and pat dry.
	Sitz baths or local heat applied to site may be soothing.
	Use of local anesthetics (dibucaine ointment or Tucks pads) may give relief.
	Reinforce need for high-residue diet.
	Instruct patient on manual reduction of external hemorrhoids.
	Apply ice packs to hemorrhoids if thrombosed to prevent edema and pain.
	Use cushion for sitting postoperatively.
Anxiety, related to:	Establish a supportive relationship with patient.
• previous experiences	Explain need for high-residue diet.
• fear of first bowel movement postoperatively	Administer laxatives and oil-retention enema as ordered.
• lack of knowledge regarding diet	Give analgesics before first bowel movement and a sitz bath for pain relief.

Evidence-Based Practice | Treatment of Chronic Constipation in Older Adults

Evidence Summary

The combined effect of decreased activity, change in diet, multiple diseases, and multiple drugs all put older adults at increased risk for constipation. Constipation is diagnosed when a person has two of the following criteria for 12 weeks during the past year: straining, pelletlike stools, sensation of incomplete evacuation, sensation of anal blockage, or using manual maneuvers, all for more than 25% of bowel movements; or having fewer than three bowel movements per week. Data are too limited in the older adult population to recommend one treatment over another. Because constipation in older adults is more likely to be a result of multiple physical and pathologic conditions, there is no consensus that fits all older adults. From a pharmacologic perspective, the ideal drug is selected in terms of effectiveness, tolerance, adverse effects, drug interactions, and cost-effectiveness.

Application to Nursing Practice

• When possible, replace a medication causing constipation with a substitute.
• Encourage older adults to increase physical activity when feasible.

• Give attention to the potential risk of fluid overload in older adult clients with congestive heart failure or renal failure.
• Encourage fiber intake of 20 g/day of wheat bran to start. Observe for bloating and flatulence in older adults.
• Stool softeners are no longer recommended for constipation.
• Fiber and bulk-forming laxatives are the first step in treating constipation in older adults.
• Osmotic laxatives are effective in the treatment of constipation in older adults because they are well tolerated and have no known interactions with other drugs.
• Stimulant laxatives are more effective than placebo, but concern remains regarding their adverse effects on older adults.
• Older adults who have mobility problems often need enemas to avoid an impaction. The tap water enema is the safest for regular use. Glycerol suppositories trigger the defecatory reflex and are sometimes useful in treating older adults.

From Potter, P.A., & Perry, A.G. (2009). *Fundamentals of nursing: concepts, process, and practice.* (7th ed.) St. Louis: Mosby. Adapted from Bosshard, W., Dreher, R., Schnegg, J.F., (2004). The treatment of chronic constipation in elderly people: an update, *Drugs Aging, 21*(14), 911-930.

Advise the patient to include bulk-forming foods in the diet, such as fresh fruits, vegetables, and bran cereals, as well as 8 to 10 glasses of fluid a day unless contraindicated. If the patient is anemic, discuss foods high in iron, such as red meats, liver, and dark green leafy vegetables. Sitz baths are recommended for 1 to 2 weeks postoperatively. Emphasize the need for moderate exercise and a routine time for a daily bowel movement. Also instruct the patient to report any signs of infection or delayed healing.

Prognosis

There are several preferred methods of treatment for hemorrhoids. Both conservative modes of treatment and surgical intervention for hemorrhoids have good prognostic rates.

ANAL FISSURE AND FISTULA

Anal fissure is a linear ulceration or laceration of the skin of the anus. Usually it is the result of trauma caused by hard stool that overstretches the anal lining. The fissure is aggravated by defecation, which initiates spasm of the anal sphincter; pain; and, at times, slight bleeding. If the lesion does not heal spontaneously, the tract is excised surgically.

An anal fistula is an abnormal opening on the cutaneous surface near the anus. Usually this is from a local crypt abscess; it is also common in Crohn's disease. A perianal fistula may or may not communicate with the rectum. It results from rupture or drainage of an anal abscess. This chronic condition is treated by a fistulectomy (removal) or fistulotomy (opening of the fistula tract).

The postoperative care required for repair of an anal fissure or fistula is similar to that for the patient who has had a hemorrhoidectomy.

Prognosis

The prognosis for anal fissures and fistulas is good, whether the patient is treated with conservative measures or with surgical intervention.

FECAL INCONTINENCE

Etiology and Pathophysiology

Fecal incontinence is a complex problem that has a variety of causes. The external anal sphincter may be relaxed, the voluntary control of defecation may be interrupted in the central nervous system, or messages may not be transmitted to the brain because of a lesion within or external pressure on the spinal cord. The disorders that cause breakdown of conscious control of defecation include cortical clouding or lesions, spinal cord lesions or trauma, and trauma to the anal sphincter (e.g., from fistula, abscess, or surgery). Perineal relaxation and actual damage to the anal sphincter are often caused by injury from perineal surgery, childbirth, or anal intercourse. Relaxation of the sphincter usually occurs with the general loss of muscle tone in aging. The normal changes

that occur with aging are usually not significant enough to cause incontinence, however, unless concurrent health problems predispose the patient to the disorder.

Normally the contents of the bowel are moved by mass peristaltic movements toward the rectum. The rectum then stores the stool until defecation occurs. Distention of the rectum initiates nerve signals that are transmitted to the spinal cord and then back to the descending colon, initiating peristaltic waves that force more feces into the rectum. The internal anal sphincter relaxes, and if the external sphincter is also relaxed, defecation results. Defecation is a reflex response to the distention of the rectal musculature, but this reflex can be voluntarily inhibited. Voluntary inhibition of defecation is learned in early childhood, and control typically lasts throughout life. The rectum is emptied when the external anal sphincter (under cortical control) relaxes, and the abdominal and pelvic muscles contract.

Reflex defecation continues to occur even in the presence of most upper or lower motor neuron lesions, since the musculature of the bowel contains its own nerve centers that respond to distention through peristalsis. Therefore, even when the patient has motor paralysis, reflex defecation often persists or can be stimulated. Defecation occurs primarily in response to mass peristaltic movements that follow meals or distention of the rectum. Any physical, mental, or social problem that disrupts any aspect of this complex learned behavior can result in incontinence.

Medical Management and Nursing Interventions

Biofeedback training is the cornerstone of therapy for patients who have motility disorders or sphincter damage that causes fecal incontinence. The patient learns to tighten the external sphincter in response to manometric measurement of responses to rectal distention. This technique has been proven effective with alert, motivated patients.

Bowel training is the major approach used with patients who have cognitive and neurologic problems resulting from stroke or other chronic diseases. If a person can sit on a toilet, he or she may be able to defecate automatically given a pattern of consistent timing, familiar surroundings, and controlled diet and fluid intake. This approach allows many patients to defecate predictably and remain continent throughout the day. Surgical correction is possible for a small group of patients whose incontinence is related to structural problems of the rectum and anus.

Patient Teaching

Bowel training requires significant amounts of time and effort on the part of the nursing staff, family, and patient. Incontinence is a major issue in home care and frequently is cited as the most common reason for older adults to be admitted to nursing homes.

To plan the most effective approach, gather specific information concerning the person's general physical and cognitive condition, ability to contract the abdominal and perineal muscles on command, and awareness of the need or urge to defecate. Also collect data about the nature and frequency of the incontinence problem, particularly its relationship to meals or other regular activities.

Teach the family about the training program and how they can assist and support the effort. This includes the importance of providing a high-fiber diet and ensuring that the patient consumes at least 2500 mL of fluid daily. Evaluate the need for a regular stool softener or bulk former. When an optimal time for defecation has been established, usually after breakfast, a glycerin suppository may be inserted to stimulate defecation.

Despite efforts by family members, staff, and patient, fecal incontinence may remain uncontrolled. Efforts then shift to odor control, prevention of skin impairment, and support for the patient's psychological integrity. Commercially available protective briefs are expensive, but they can substantially reduce the burden of care for the family and provide the patient with a sense of security and dignity.

❖NURSING PROCESS *for the Patient with a Gastrointestinal Disorder*

The role of the licensed practical nurse/licensed vocational nurse (LPN/LVN) in the nursing process as stated is that the LPN/LVN will:

- Participate in planning care for patients based on patient needs
- Review patient care plan and recommend revisions as needed
- Review and follow defined prioritization for patient care
- Use clinical pathways, care maps, or care plans to guide and review patient care

■ Assessment

In caring for the patient admitted with a GI disorder, a thorough, immediate, and accurate nursing assessment is an essential first step. The assessment includes the patient's level of consciousness; vital signs; skin color; edema; appetite; weight loss; nausea; vomiting; and bowel habits, including color and consistency of stools. Assess the abdomen for distention, guarding, and peristalsis. Also obtain a past history of smoking or alcohol use, medications, epigastric or abdominal pain, and acute or chronic stressors and coping–stress tolerance.

■ Nursing Diagnosis

Assessment provides the data for identifying the patient's problems, strengths, potential complications, and learning needs. Once the diagnoses are defined, assist in formulating a care plan that meets the pa-

tient's needs and prioritizing nursing interventions. Possible nursing diagnoses that should be considered for the patient with a GI disorder include but are not limited to the following:

- Activity intolerance
- Anxiety
- Disturbed body image
- Constipation
- Ineffective coping
- Diarrhea
- Fear
- Risk for deficient fluid volume
- Impaired home maintenance
- Ineffective management of therapeutic regimen
- Imbalanced nutrition: less than body requirements
- Pain
- Risk for impaired skin integrity
- Disturbed sleep pattern
- Social isolation
- Ineffective tissue perfusion

■ Expected Outcomes and Planning

Care planning for the patient with a GI disorder involves looking at the nursing diagnoses and establishing nursing interventions to assist in eliminating the problems. Include the patient in planning to promote compliance with the nursing interventions.

The care plan may be based on one or more of the following goals:

Goal 1: Patient will have no evidence of excoriation around stomal area.

Goal 2: Patient will begin to adjust to disturbed body image.

■ Implementation

Nursing interventions for the patient with a GI disorder may be simple or complex. Interventions include assessment, monitoring nutritional status, administering medications, promoting health, relieving pain, maintaining skin integrity, managing fluid and electrolyte imbalance, promoting normal bowel elimination patterns, preventing wound infection, health counseling to focus on elimination of smoking and excessive alcohol intake, and patient teaching for enterostomal

---

🌐 **Cultural Considerations**

Gastrointestinal Disorders

- Inflammatory bowel disease (Crohn's disease and ulcerative colitis) is more common among whites than blacks and Asian Americans.
- Inflammatory bowel disease is more common among Jewish people and those of Central European origin.
- The incidence of colorectal cancer is higher in the United States and Canada than in Japan, Finland, or Africa.
- The incidence of colorectal cancer is declining in the United States except among black men.

therapy. Cultural considerations are a vital part of nursing interventions for the patient with a GI disorder (see Cultural Considerations box).

■ Evaluation

Determining the outcomes of the nursing interventions is an ongoing process that helps the nurse establish the most effective care plan. The nurse and the patient evaluate the goals to see whether the criteria for assessment have been met.

Goal 1: Patient will have no evidence of excoriation around stomal area.

Evaluative measure: There is no impairment of skin integrity around stoma.

Goal 2: Patient will begin to adjust to disturbed body image.

Evaluative measures: Patient demonstrates adjustment to disturbed body image by expressing feelings about stoma and is beginning to assume some stoma and pouch care.

Get Ready for the NCLEX® Examination!

Key Points

- The digestive tract begins with the mouth, extends through the thoracic and abdominal cavities, and ends with the anus.
- The major processes of digestion and absorption take place in the small intestine.
- The large intestine is responsible for the preparation and evacuation of the waste products: feces.
- Diet therapy has an important role in the treatment of GI disorders.
- Treatment of esophageal disorders often involves providing the patient with a means of eating, in addition to treating the disorder.
- Common causes of gastric disorders are alcohol, tobacco, aspirin, and antiinflammatory agents.
- Duodenal ulcers are the most common type of peptic ulcer disease.
- A relatively new diagnostic examination is a capsule endoscopy in which the patient swallows a capsule with a camera to visualize the small intestine and diagnose diseases such as Crohn's disease.
- Surgical procedures are available as alternatives to the traditional ileostomy and colostomy.
- A nursing goal for the patient with an ileostomy or a colostomy is fostering patient independence in daily care when the patient demonstrates readiness.
- Keeping the surgical area free of contamination is of primary importance after rectal surgery.
- The approximate location of GI bleeding may be determined by the characteristics of the emesis or the fecal material.
- Explain the purpose of any diagnostic procedure, how the procedure is performed, and the preparation necessary for the procedure, and help the patient understand the results.
- *H. pylori* has been identified in more than 70% of gastric ulcer patients and 95% of those with duodenal ulcers.
- Individuals with inflammatory bowel disease have a greater risk of developing cancer of the bowel.
- Early detection of cancer in the GI system facilitates early treatment and a better prognosis.
- An NG tube is inserted to keep the stomach empty until peristalsis resumes after a general anesthetic or any condition that interferes with peristalsis.
- Effective postoperative care begins with patient teaching during the preoperative period.

Additional Learning Resources

 Go to your Companion CD for an audio glossary, animations, video clips, and more.

evolve Be sure to visit the Evolve site at http://evolve.elsevier.com/Christensen/adult/ for additional online resources.

Review Questions for the NCLEX® Examination

1. Because the small intestine needs bile only a few times a day, bile is stored and concentrated in the:
   1. pancreas.
   2. gallbladder.
   3. liver.
   4. small intestine.

2. Although food is digested throughout the alimentary canal, up to 90% of digestion is accomplished in the:
   1. gallbladder.
   2. mouth.
   3. small intestine.
   4. large intestine.

3. The exit from the stomach is called the:
   1. cardiac sphincter.
   2. pyloric sphincter.
   3. lesser curvature.
   4. greater curvature.

4. The intrinsic factor is a gastric secretion necessary for the intestinal absorption of vitamin:
   1. B_1.
   2. B_{12}.
   3. C.
   4. K.

5. Which organ manufactures heparin, prothrombin, and fibrinogen?
   1. Gallbladder
   2. Liver
   3. Pancreas
   4. Salivary gland

6. Paralytic (adynamic) ileus is a functional intestinal obstruction that may result from:

1. impacted feces, tumor of the colon, or pancreatitis.
2. electrolyte imbalance, postabdominal surgery, or acute inflammatory reactions.
3. adhesions or a strangulated hernia.
4. volvulus, intussusceptions, or electrolyte imbalances.

7. To prepare the patient for endoscopic examination of the upper GI tract, the patient's pharynx is anesthetized with lidocaine (Xylocaine). Nursing interventions for postendoscopic examination include:

1. allowing fluids up to 4 hours before examination.
2. withholding anticholinergic medications.
3. prohibiting smoking before the test.
4. keeping the patient NPO until the gag reflex returns.

8. A 35-year-old man has been admitted with a diagnosis of peptic ulcers. Which drugs are most commonly used in these patients to decrease acid secretions?

1. Maalox and Kayexalate
2. Tagamet and Zantac
3. Erythromycin and Flagyl
4. Dyazide and Carafate

9. A patient is scheduled in the morning for a hemicolectomy for removal of a cancerous tumor of the ascending colon. The physician has ordered intestinal antibiotics for her preoperatively to:

1. decrease the bulk of colon contents.
2. reduce the bacteria content of the colon.
3. soften the stool.
4. prevent pneumonia.

10. A 78-year-old woman was admitted during the evening shift with a tentative diagnosis of cancer of the esophagus. The nurse in her initial assessment finds the patient's major complaint is:

1. dysphagia.
2. malnutrition.
3. pain.
4. regurgitation of food.

11. Deficient knowledge is a commonly used nursing diagnosis when patients need information regarding their conditions and diagnostic tests. Before a gastroscopy, the nurse should inform the patient that:

1. fasting for 6 to 8 hours is necessary before the examination.
2. a general anesthetic will be used.
3. after gastroscopy, the patient may eat or drink immediately.
4. admission to the hospital is necessary.

12. In evaluating the care of a young executive admitted with bleeding peptic ulcer, the nurse focuses on nursing interventions. A nursing intervention associated with this type of patient is:

1. checking the blood pressure and pulse rates each shift.
2. frequently monitoring arterial blood levels.

3. observing vomitus for color, consistency, and volume.
4. checking the patient's low-residue diet.

13. The staff nurse on the surgical floor is aware of pulmonary complications that frequently follow upper abdominal incisions. These are most frequently related to:

1. aspiration.
2. pneumothorax if the chest cavity has been entered.
3. shallow respirations to minimize pain.
4. not forcing fluids.

14. Which tests can distinguish between peptic ulcer disease and gastric malignancy?

1. Radiographic GI series
2. Breath test for *H. pylori*
3. Serum test for *H. pylori* antibodies
4. Endoscopy with biopsy

15. A recently approved medication for the treatment of Crohn's disease, infliximab (Remicade), is classified as which type of drug?

1. Enzyme
2. Antimetabolite
3. Alkylating agent
4. Monoclonal antibody

16. During assessment of the patient with esophageal achalasia, the nurse would expect the patient to report:

1. a history of alcohol use.
2. a sore throat and hoarseness.
3. dysphagia, especially with liquids.
4. relief of pyrosis with the use of antacids.

17. A nursing intervention that is most appropriate to decrease postoperative edema and pain in the male patient following an inguinal herniorrhaphy is:

1. applying a truss to the hernial site.
2. allowing the patient to stand to void.
3. elevating the scrotum with a support or small pillow.
4. supporting the incision during routine coughing and deep breathing.

18. The use of nonabsorbable antibiotics as preparation for bowel surgery is done primarily to:

1. reduce bacterial flora in the colon.
2. prevent additional formation of ammonia.
3. prevent postoperative formation of intestinal gas.
4. stimulate bowel bacteria to increase production of vitamin K.

19. In planning care for the patient with ulcerative colitis, the nurse recognizes that a major difference between ulcerative colitis and Crohn's disease is that ulcerative colitis:

1. causes more nutritional deficiencies than does Crohn's disease.
2. causes more abdominal pain and cramping than does Crohn's disease.
3. is curable with a colectomy, whereas Crohn's disease often recurs after surgery.
4. is more highly associated with a familial relationship than is Crohn's disease.

20. Which group of medications should be avoided in patients with *E. coli* O157:H7?

    1. Antiemetics
    2. Antimotility drugs
    3. Antilipidemic agents
    4. Beta blockers

21. What should a patient be taught after a hemorrhoidectomy?

    1. Do not use the Valsalva maneuver.
    2. Eat a low-fiber diet to rest the colon.
    3. Administer an oil-retention enema to empty the colon.
    4. Use a prescribed analgesic before a bowel movement.

22. The medication of choice to treat *Clostridium difficile* intestinal infection is:

    1. erythromycin.
    2. neomycin.
    3. Flagyl.
    4. Ancef.

23. It is believed that the gastric mucosa of the body of the stomach undergoes a period of transient ischemia in association with hypotension, severe injury, extensive burns, or complicated surgery. This results in the development of what disorder?

    1. Crohn's disease
    2. Ulcerative colitis
    3. Volvulus
    4. Stress ulcers

24. In Crohn's disease, major complications that develop due to the granulomatous cobblestone lesions of the small intestine include:

    1. malabsorption of nutrients.
    2. severe diarrhea of 15 to 20 stools per day.
    3. a high probability of developing intestinal cancer.
    4. an inability of the body to absorb water.

25. A severe intestinal infection caused by contaminated undercooked beef such as hamburger from a specific pathogenic bacteria present in some cattle is called:

    1. *Escherichia coli* O157:H7 intestinal infection.
    2. *Clostridium difficile* intestinal infection.
    3. *Salmonella* intestinal infection.
    4. *Staphylococcus aureus* infection.

26. After a transverse loop colostomy, the nurse inspects the patient's stoma. The stoma appears mostly pink with some dusky discoloration at the lower border. An appropriate action would be to:

    1. clean the area around the stoma and record the observation in the nurses' notes.
    2. carefully place a clean pouch over the stoma to prevent any further tissue loss.
    3. cover the stoma with a petroleum gauze dressing to prevent any further irritation to the stoma.
    4. clean the area around the stoma, apply a clean pouch, and notify the physician about the discoloration.

27. The nurse is teaching a postgastrectomy patient about dumping syndrome. The patient would indicate the need for further instruction if she made which statement?

    1. I will lie down after eating a meal.
    2. I will eat smaller portions of food, more frequently.
    3. I will not drink liquids when I eat.
    4. I will avoid fats and increase carbohydrates.

28. The primary medical management for a patient with duodenal ulcers is:

    1. gastric resection.
    2. antacids, histamine (H$_2$) receptor blockers, proton pump inhibitors, mucosal healing agents, antibiotic therapy.
    3. a diet low in fat and carbohydrates, Rowasa, Imodium.
    4. a diet high in protein and milk products, Azulfidine, Dipentum.

29. An 84-year-old patient has a history of a large ventral hernia. He is complaining of nausea, vomiting, abdominal distention, and abdominal pain. A serious complication of a hernia in which the blood supply to the tissue becomes occluded is called a(n):

    1. strangulated hernia.
    2. hiatal hernia.
    3. incarcerated hernia.
    4. sliding hernia.

30. Peptic ulcers result from *(Select all that apply.)*:

    1. excess of gastric acid or a decrease in the natural ability of the GI mucosa to protect itself from acid and pepsin.
    2. invasion of the stomach and/or duodenum by *Helicobacter pylori*.
    3. viral infection, allergies to certain foods, immunologic factors, and psychosomatic factors.
    4. taking certain drugs, including corticosteroids and antiinflammatory medications.

Care of the Patient with a Gallbladder, Liver, Biliary Tract, or Exocrine Pancreatic Disorder

Barbara Lauritsen Christensen

Objectives

1. Discuss nursing interventions for the diagnostic examinations of patients with disorders of the gallbladder, liver, biliary tract, and exocrine pancreas.
2. Explain the etiology, pathophysiology, clinical manifestations, assessment, diagnostic tests, medical management, and nursing interventions for the patient with cirrhosis of the liver, carcinoma of the liver, hepatitis, liver abscesses, cholecystitis, cholelithiasis, pancreatitis, and cancer of the pancreas.
3. Discuss specific complications and teaching content for the patient with cirrhosis of the liver.
4. Define jaundice and describe signs and symptoms that may occur with jaundice.
5. State the six types of viral hepatitis, including their modes of transmission.
6. List the subjective and objective data for the patient with viral hepatitis.
7. Discuss the indicators for liver transplantation and the immunosuppressant drugs to reduce rejection.
8. Discuss the two methods of surgical treatment for cholecystitis and cholelithiasis.

Key Terms

ascites (ă-SĪ-tēz, p. 236)
asterixis (ăs-tĕr-ĬK-sĭs, p. 240)
esophageal varices (ĕ-sŏf-ă-JĔ-ăl VĂR-ĭ-sēz, p. 238)
flatulence (FLĂT-ū-lĕns, p. 249)
hepatic encephalopathy (hĕ-PĂT-ĭk ĕn-sĕf-ĕ-LŎP-ĕ-thē, p. 240)
hepatitis (hĕ-pă-TĪ-tĭs, p. 234)

jaundice (JĂWN-dĭs, p. 237)
occlusion (ŏ-KLŪ-zhŭn, p. 253)
paracentesis (păr-ă-sĕn-TĒ-sĭs, p. 237)
parenchyma (pă-rĕng-KĪ-mă, p. 236)
spider telangiectases (SPĪ-dĕr tĕl-ăn-jē-ĔK-tĕ-sēz, p. 236)
steatorrhea (stē-ă-tō-RĒ-ă, p. 249)

This chapter discusses disorders of the accessory organs of digestion—namely the liver, the gallbladder, and the exocrine pancreas. These organs assist in digestion in various ways. See Chapter 5 for a review of the anatomy and physiology of the liver, the biliary tract, the gallbladder, and the pancreas.

LABORATORY AND DIAGNOSTIC EXAMINATIONS IN THE ASSESSMENT OF THE HEPATOBILIARY AND PANCREATIC SYSTEMS

SERUM BILIRUBIN TEST

Normal values are as follows:
 Direct bilirubin: 0.1 to 0.3 mg/dL
 Indirect bilirubin: 0.2 to 0.8 mg/dL
 Total bilirubin: 0.3 to 1 mg/dL

Rationale

Total serum bilirubin determination measures both direct, or conjugated (water-soluble), and indirect, or unconjugated (water-insoluble), bilirubin. Total serum bilirubin level is the sum of the direct and indirect bilirubin levels. Testing for bilirubin in the blood provides valuable information for diagnosis and evaluation of liver disease, biliary obstruction, and hemolytic anemia. Jaundice, the discoloration of body tissues caused by abnormally high blood levels of bilirubin, is visible when the total serum bilirubin exceeds 2.5 mg/dL.

Nursing Interventions

Keep the patient on nothing by mouth (NPO) status until after the blood specimen is drawn.

LIVER ENZYME TESTS

The normal values are as follows:

- **AST (aspartate aminotransferase; formerly serum glutamic oxaloacetic transaminase [SGOT]):** Adult: 0 to 35 units/L. AST level is elevated in myocardial infarction, hepatitis, cirrhosis, hepatic necrosis, hepatic tumor, acute pancreatitis, and acute hemolytic anemia.
- **ALT (alanine aminotransferase; formerly serum glutamic pyruvic transaminase [SGPT]):** Adult or child: 4 to 36 units/L. ALT level is elevated in hepatitis, cirrhosis, hepatic necrosis, and hepatic tumors and by hepatotoxic drugs.

- **LDH (lactic dehydrogenase):** Adult: 100 to 190 units/L. Values are increased in myocardial infarction, pulmonary infarction, hepatic disease (e.g., hepatitis, active cirrhosis, neoplasm), pancreatitis, and skeletal muscle disease.
- **Alkaline phosphatase:** Adult: 30 to 120 units/L. Alkaline phosphatase level is elevated in obstructive disorders of the biliary tract, hepatic tumors, cirrhosis, hepatitis, primary and metastatic tumors, hyperparathyroidism, metastatic tumor in bones, and healing fractures.
- **Gamma GT (gamma glutamyl transferase):** Male and female older than age 45: 8 to 38 units/L; female younger than age 45: 5 to 27 units/L. Levels are elevated in liver cell dysfunction such as hepatitis and cirrhosis; in hepatic tumors; with the use of hepatotoxic drugs; in jaundice; and in myocardial infarction (4 to 10 days after), heart failure, alcohol ingestion, pancreatitis, and cancer of the pancreas.

Rationale

The liver is a storehouse of many enzymes. Injury or diseases affecting the liver cause release of these intracellular enzymes into the bloodstream, and their levels become elevated. Some of these enzymes are also produced in other organs, and injury or disease affecting these organs will raise the serum level. Therefore, although elevation of these serum enzymes is found in pathologic liver conditions, the test is not specific for liver diseases alone.

Nursing Interventions

Assess the venipuncture site for bleeding.

SERUM PROTEIN TEST

The normal values are as follows:
Total protein: 6.4 to 8.3 g/dL
Albumin: 3.5 to 5 g/dL
Globulin: 2.3 to 3.4 g/dL
Albumin/globulin (A/G ratio): 1.2 to 2.2 g/dL

Rationale

One way to assess the liver's functional status is to measure the products it synthesizes. One of these products is protein, especially albumin. When disease affects the liver cell, the hepatocyte loses its ability to synthesize albumin and the serum albumin level is markedly decreased. Low serum albumin levels may also result from excessive loss of albumin into urine (as in nephrotic syndrome) or into third-space volumes (as in ascites), liver disease, increased capillary permeability, or protein-caloric malnutrition.

Nursing Interventions

Assess the venipuncture site for bleeding.

ORAL CHOLECYSTOGRAPHY
Rationale

The oral cholecystogram (OCG) provides roentgenographic visualization of the gallbladder after the oral ingestion of a radiopaque, iodinated dye. Adequate visualization requires concentration of the dye within the gallbladder. An OCG (also called a gallbladder [or GB] series) is less accurate than a gallbladder ultrasound and is less commonly used for visualizing the biliary tree. OCG will not visualize the biliary tree in the jaundiced patient. Adequate dye concentration depends on the following factors:

- The patient's ingestion of the correct number of dye tablets the evening before the examination
- Adequate absorption of the dye from the gastrointestinal (GI) tract; vomiting or diarrhea preclude absorption of the dye
- Abstinence from food (especially a fatty meal) on the morning of the test
- Uptake from the portal system and excretion of the dye by the liver
- Patency of the cystic duct
- Concentration of the dye within the gallbladder

Nursing Interventions

Before administering the dye, make certain the patient is not allergic to iodine to prevent adverse or allergic reaction. This rarely occurs because the dye is not administered intravenously. If the patient is not allergic to iodine, administer six tablets orally (e.g., iopanoic acid (Telepaque), iodalphionic acid (Priodax), or iprodate (Oragrafin), one every 5 minutes, beginning after the evening meal. The patient is on NPO status from midnight. The patient may be given a high-fat meal or beverage to stimulate emptying of the gallbladder after the test has begun. No other food or fluids are allowed until after the examination.

INTRAVENOUS CHOLANGIOGRAPHY
Rationale

In intravenous cholangiography, intravenously administered radiographic dye is concentrated by the liver and secreted into the bile duct. The intravenous cholangiogram (IVC) allows visualization of the hepatic and common bile ducts and also the gallbladder if the cystic duct is patent. IVC is used to demonstrate stones, strictures, or tumors of the hepatic duct, common bile duct, and gallbladder. IVC is a less commonly used method of visualizing the biliary tree and will not do so in a jaundiced patient.

OPERATIVE CHOLANGIOGRAPHY
Rationale

In operative cholangiography the common bile duct is directly injected with radiopaque dye. Stones appear as radiolucent shadows, and tumors cause partial or total obstruction of the flow of dye into the duodenum. Visualization of the biliary duct structures provides the surgeon with a "road map" of a difficult anatomical area. This reduces the possibility of inadvertently injuring the common duct.

If common duct stones are suspected, a cholecystectomy as well as a common duct exploration (CDE) must be performed. When intraoperative cholangiography is used routinely, CDE is performed only on those with positive cholangiograms.

T-TUBE CHOLANGIOGRAPHY

Rationale

T-tube cholangiography (postoperative cholangiography) is performed to diagnose retained ductal stones postoperatively in the patient who has had a cholecystectomy and a common bile duct (CBD) exploration to demonstrate good flow of contrast into the duodenum. The test is performed through a T-shaped rubber tube that the surgeon places in the bile duct during the operation. The end of the T-tube exits through the abdominal wall, where dye is injected and radiographic films taken.

Nursing Interventions

Protect the patient from sepsis by connecting the T-tube (if left in place) to a sterile closed-drainage system. If the T-tube is removed, cover the T-tube tract site with a sterile dressing to prevent bacteria from entering the ductal system.

Before administering the dye, ensure that the patient is not allergic to iodine. Preparation of the patient also includes NPO status after midnight and until the examination is completed. Administer a cleansing enema on the morning of the examination, if ordered.

ULTRASONOGRAPHY OF THE LIVER, THE GALLBLADDER, AND THE BILIARY SYSTEM

Rationale

Ultrasonography (ultrasound, echogram) is an imaging technique that visualizes deep structures of the body by recording the reflections (echoes) of ultrasonic waves directed into the tissues. This diagnostic test is not effective in examining all tissue because ultrasound waves do not pass through structures that contain air, such as the lungs, the colon, or the stomach. Although fasting is preferred, it is not necessary for ultrasonography. Because ultrasound requires no contrast material and has no associated radiation, it is especially useful for patients who are allergic to contrast media or are pregnant. Ultrasound is used with increasing frequency to corroborate data already obtained by "questionable positive" cholangiograms, liver scans, and OCGs.

Nursing Interventions

The patient is on NPO status from midnight. If the patient had recent barium contrast studies, request an order for cathartics. Ultrasound cannot penetrate barium, and the study will not be adequate.

GALLBLADDER SCANNING

Rationale

The biliary tract can be evaluated safely, accurately, and noninvasively with the use of intravenous (IV) injection of technetium (^{99}Tc; technetium99m), and positioning the patient under a camera to record distribution of tracer in the liver, the biliary tree, the gallbladder, and the proximal small bowel. The primary use of this study is in the diagnosis of acute cholecystitis. This procedure is superior to oral cholecystography, ultrasonography, and computed tomography (CT) scanning of the abdomen for the detection of acute cholecystitis. Hepatobiliary iminodiacetic acid (HIDA) scanning is also useful for identifying diffuse hepatic disease (such as cirrhosis or neoplasm).

Nursing Interventions

Reassure the patient that exposure to radioactivity is minimal because only a trace dose of the radioisotope is used. The patient is on NPO status from midnight until the examination is complete.

NEEDLE LIVER BIOPSY

Rationale

Needle liver biopsy is a safe, simple, and valuable method of diagnosing pathologic liver conditions. A specially designed needle is inserted through the skin, between the sixth and seventh or eighth and ninth intercostal spaces, and into the liver. The patient lies supine with the right arm over the head. The patient is instructed to exhale fully and not breathe while the needle is inserted. This procedure is often done using ultrasound or CT guidance. A piece of hepatic tissue is removed for microscopic examination. The tissue sample is placed into a labeled specimen bottle containing formalin and sent to the pathology department. Percutaneous liver biopsy is used in the diagnosis of various liver disorders, such as cirrhosis, hepatitis, drug-related reactions, granuloma, and tumor.

Nursing Interventions

Explain the procedure to the patient and obtain the patient's signature on a consent form. Ensure that measurements of platelets, clotting or bleeding time, prothrombin time, and International Normalized Ratio (INR) have been ordered; report any abnormal values to the physician. After the procedure observe the patient for symptoms of bleeding. Monitor vital signs every 15 minutes (two times), then every 30 minutes (four times), and then every hour (four times).

Some pain is common. When leakage involves a large quantity of blood or bile, the peritoneal reaction is great and the resulting pain severe. Assess the patient for pneumothorax (collapsed lung) caused by improper placement of the biopsy needle into the adjacent chest cavity or for bile peritonitis. Immediately report to the physician signs and symptoms of pneumothorax such as shortness of breath, change in respiratory and cardiac rate, or decreased breath sounds on the affected side. Keep the patient lying on the right side for at least 2 hours to splint the puncture site. In this position, the liver capsule is compressed against the chest wall, decreasing the risk of hemorrhage or bile leak.

RADIOISOTOPE LIVER SCANNING

Rationale
This radionuclide procedure is used to outline and detect structural changes of the liver. A radionuclide is given intravenously. Later, a gamma-ray detecting device (Geiger counter) is passed over the patient's abdomen. This records the distribution of the radioactive particles in the liver. The spleen can also be visualized by the detector when technetium 99m sulfur is used.

Nursing Interventions
The patient is on NPO status from midnight. Assure patients that they will not be exposed to a large amount of radioactivity, since only trace doses of isotopes are used.

SERUM AMMONIA TEST
Normal value is 10 to 80 mcg/dL.

Rationale
Ammonia is a by-product of protein metabolism. Most of the ammonia is made by bacteria acting on proteins in the intestine. By way of the portal vein, ammonia goes to the liver, where it is normally converted into urea and then excreted by the kidneys. When the patient has severe liver dysfunction or altered blood flow to the liver, ammonia cannot be catabolized, the serum ammonia level rises, and the blood urea nitrogen level decreases. The serum ammonia level is primarily used as an aid in diagnosing hepatic encephalopathy and hepatic coma. Elevated serum ammonia levels suggest liver dysfunction as the cause of these signs and symptoms.

Nursing Interventions
On the laboratory requisition, list any antibiotics the patient is currently taking. Certain broad-spectrum antibiotics such as neomycin can cause a decreased ammonia level, thus giving inaccurate test results.

HEPATITIS VIRUS STUDIES
A normal laboratory test result will be negative for hepatitis-associated antigen.

Rationale
Hepatitis is an inflammation of the liver caused by viruses, bacteria, and noninfectious causes of liver inflammation. Six viruses, designated A through G, can cause this disease. Hepatitis A and B viruses have been recognized for years, but hepatitis C, D, E, and G viruses were

identified more recently (so-called hepatitis F virus was eventually found to be a mutation of hepatitis C virus [HCV]). Hepatitis A, B, and C viruses are the most common viruses that cause hepatitis. Hepatitis D virus is carried by the hepatitis B virus (HBV). Both hepatitis D and E viruses are seen less frequently in the United States than the hepatitis A, B, or C viruses (Pagana & Pagana, 2008). The individual hepatitis viruses can be detected by different antigen and antibody levels, and different incubation periods must be considered.

Nursing Interventions
Use standard precautions and handle the serum specimen as if it were capable of transmitting viral hepatitis. Don gloves when handling any blood or body fluids, and wash hands carefully after handling equipment.

SERUM AMYLASE TEST
Normal value is 60 to 120 Somogyi units/dL, or 30 to 220 units/L (SI units).

Rationale
The serum amylase test is an easily and rapidly performed test for pancreatitis. Damage to pancreatic cells (as in pancreatitis) or obstruction to the pancreatic ductal flow (as in pancreatic carcinoma) causes an outpouring of this enzyme into the intrapancreatic lymph system and the free peritoneum. Blood vessels draining the free peritoneum and absorbing the lymph pick up this excess amylase. An abnormal rise in the serum level of amylase occurs within 2 hours of the onset of pancreatic disease. Because amylase is rapidly cleared by the kidney, serum levels may return to normal within 36 hours. Persistent pancreatitis, duct obstruction, or pancreatic duct leak (e.g., pseudocysts) cause persistent elevated serum levels.

Nursing Interventions
Note on the laboratory requisition whether the patient is receiving intravenous dextrose or any medications, since these can cause a false-negative result.

URINE AMYLASE TEST
The normal value for this study is up to 5000 Somogyi units/24 hr, or 6.5 to 48.1 units/hr.

Rationale
Levels of amylase in the urine remain elevated for 7 to 10 days after the onset of disease. Urine amylase is particularly useful in detecting pancreatitis late in the disease course. This fact is important for diagnosing pancreatitis in patients who have had symptoms for 3 days or longer.

Nursing Interventions
Record the exact time at the beginning and end of the collection period. A 2-hour spot urine or 6-hour, 12-hour, or 24-hour collection can be performed, depending on

the physician's order. The collection begins after the patient empties the bladder and discards that specimen. All subsequent urine is collected, including the voiding at the end of the collection period. Keep the specimen on ice or refrigerated until it is sent to the laboratory.

SERUM LIPASE TEST

The normal value is 10 to 140 units/L.

Rationale

Like serum amylase, serum lipase is elevated in acute pancreatitis and is a helpful complementary test because other disorders (e.g., mumps, cerebral trauma, renal transplantation) may also cause an increase in serum amylase. Lipase appears in the bloodstream after damage to the pancreas. The lipase levels rise a little later than amylase levels (4 to 48 hours after the onset of pancreatitis), peak around 24 hours, and remain elevated for at least 14 days. Because lipase peaks later and remains elevated longer than amylase, it is more useful in the diagnosis of acute pancreatitis later in the course of the disease.

Nursing Interventions

Instruct the patient to remain on NPO status from midnight, except for water.

ULTRASONOGRAPHY OF THE PANCREAS

Rationale

With the use of reflected sound waves, ultrasonography of the pancreas provides diagnostic information of this inaccessible abdominal organ. Ultrasound examination of the pancreas is mainly used to diagnose carcinoma, pseudocyst, pancreatitis, and pancreatic abscess. Because abnormalities seen on ultrasound persist from several days to weeks, it can support the diagnosis of pancreatitis even after the serum amylase and lipase levels have returned to normal. Furthermore, follow-up ultrasound study is used to monitor the resolution of pancreatic inflammation and a tumor's response to therapy.

Nursing Interventions

Fluids and food are withheld for 8 hours before the examination, but fasting is not mandatory to obtain accurate results. If the patient's abdomen is distended with gas or if the patient has had a recent barium examination, postpone this study, since gas or barium interferes with sound wave transmission.

COMPUTED TOMOGRAPHY OF THE ABDOMEN

Rationale

CT scan of the abdomen is a noninvasive, accurate radiographic procedure used to diagnose pathologic pancreatic conditions such as inflammation, tumors, pseudocyst formation, ascites, aneurysms, cirrhosis, abscesses, trauma, cysts, and anatomical abnormalities. The recognizable cross-sectional image produced

by a CT scan is especially important for studying the pancreas, since this organ is well hidden by the overlying peritoneal organs.

Nursing Interventions

Fluids and food are withheld from midnight until the examination is complete; however, this test can be performed on an emergency basis on patients who have recently eaten. If possible, show the patient a picture of the machine and encourage the patient to verbalize fears because some patients suffer claustrophobia when enclosed in the machine.

ENDOSCOPIC RETROGRADE CHOLANGIOPANCREATOGRAPHY OF THE PANCREATIC DUCT

Rationale

Endoscopic retrograde cholangiopancreatography (ERCP) enables visualization not only of the biliary system but also of the pancreatic duct. The test involves inserting a fiberoptic duodenoscope through the oral pharynx, through the esophagus and the stomach, and into the duodenum (Figure 6-1). Dye is injected for radiographic visualization of the common bile duct and pancreatic duct. ERCP of the pancreas is a sensitive and reliable procedure for detecting clinically significant degrees of pancreatic dysfunction. It can also be used to evaluate obstructive jaundice, remove common bile duct stones, and place biliary and pancreatic duct stents to bypass obstruction. Localized pancreatic duct narrowing indicates tumor. Chronic pancreatitis is demonstrated by multiple areas of ductal narrowing, which can be visualized by ERCP.

Nursing Interventions

Withhold food and fluids for 8 hours before the examination, and obtain the patient's signature on a consent form. Assess prothrombin time and INR before the

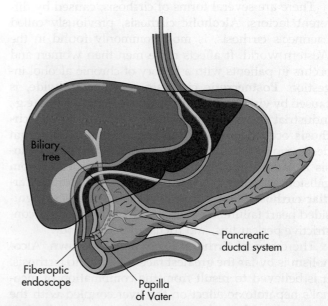

FIGURE 6-1 Endoscopic retrograde cholangiopancreatography (ERCP).

procedure. Tell patients that the test takes approximately 1 to 2 hours, during which time they must lie completely motionless on a hard x-ray table, which may be uncomfortable. After the procedure, keep the patient on NPO status until the gag reflex returns; assess for abdominal pain, tenderness, and guarding. Assess for signs and symptoms of pancreatitis (the most common ERCP complication), including increasingly intense abdominal pain, nausea, fever, chills, vomiting, and diminished or absent bowel sounds. Assess for hypovolemic shock.

DISORDERS OF THE LIVER, BILIARY TRACT, GALLBLADDER, AND EXOCRINE PANCREAS

The liver, the gallbladder, and the exocrine pancreas are all organs that assist with digestion. Review anatomy and physiology of accessory organs of digestion (see Chapter 5) and hepatic portal circulation.

CIRRHOSIS

Etiology and Pathophysiology

Cirrhosis is a chronic, degenerative disease of the liver in which the lobes are covered with fibrous tissue, the parenchyma (tissue of an organ, as opposed to supporting or connective tissue) degenerates, and the lobules are infiltrated with fat. The liver tries unsuccessfully to regenerate and, as a result, forms abnormal blood vessels and biliary duct abnormalities (Lewis et al., 2007). The overgrowth of new and fibrous (scar) tissue restricts the flow of blood to the organ, which contributes to its destruction. Hepatomegaly (enlargement of the liver) and, later, liver contraction cause loss of the organ's function.

Cirrhosis is ranked as the ninth leading cause of death in the United States and fourth leading cause of death in people between ages 35 and 54. The highest incidence occurs between ages 40 and 60.

There are several forms of cirrhosis, caused by different factors. **Alcoholic cirrhosis,** previously called Laennec's cirrhosis, is most commonly found in the Western world. It affects more men than women and occurs in patients with a history of chronic alcohol ingestion. **Postnecrotic cirrhosis,** found worldwide, is caused by viral hepatitis, exposure to hepatotoxins (e.g., industrial chemicals), or infection. **Primary biliary cirrhosis** occurs more often in women and results from destruction of the bile ducts. **Secondary biliary cirrhosis** is caused by chronic biliary tree obstruction from gallstones, a tumor, or biliary atresia in children. **Cardiac cirrhosis** results from longstanding, severe right-sided heart failure in patients with cor pulmonale, constrictive pericarditis, and tricuspid insufficiency.

The cause of cirrhosis is not always known. Alcoholism is by far the greatest factor leading to cirrhosis. It is believed to result from the combination of alcohol's hepatotoxic effect on the liver coupled with the common problem of protein malnutrition seen in alcoholics. Cirrhosis of the liver from severe malnutrition without alcoholism has also occurred. Patients with a diagnosis of chronic hepatitis B and C have a 10% to 20% chance of developing cirrhosis of the liver (Lewis et al., 2007).

With repeated insults, the liver progresses through the following stages: destruction, inflammation, fibrotic regeneration, and hepatic insufficiency. Although liver cells have a great potential for regeneration, repeated scarring decreases their ability to be replaced. As the blood supply continues to diminish and scar tissue increases, the organ atrophies.

Functions of the liver are altered in several ways. The liver's ability to synthesize albumin is reduced as a result of liver cell damage. Obstruction of the portal vein as it enters the liver results in portal hypertension—increased venous pressure in the portal circulation caused by compression or by occlusion in the portal or hepatic vascular system. In most instances, portal hypertension that is caused by cirrhosis is irreversible.

This increased pressure causes ascites (an accumulation of fluid and albumin in the peritoneal cavity). The damaged liver cannot metabolize protein in the usual manner; therefore protein intake may result in an elevation of blood ammonia levels. Reduced synthesis of protein and the leaking of existing protein result in hypoalbuminemia (reduced protein or albumin level in the blood), which reduces the blood's ability to regain fluids through osmosis. Protein must be present in adequate amounts to create colloidal osmotic pressure and "attract" the fluid to pass back into the blood vessels after it escapes in the capillaries. As fluid leaves the blood and the circulating volume decreases, the receptors in the brain signal the adrenal cortex to increase secretion of aldosterone to stimulate the kidneys to retain sodium and water. The normal liver inactivates the hormone aldosterone, but the damaged liver allows its effect to continue (hyperaldosteronism). Retention of fluid and sodium results in increased pressure in blood vessels and lymphatic channels, resulting in portal hypertension. Ascites is thus a result of portal hypertension, hypoalbuminemia, and hyperaldosteronism.

Hepatic insufficiency gradually causes distention in veins in the upper part of the body, including the esophageal vein. Esophageal varicosities develop and may rupture, causing severe hemorrhage.

Clinical Manifestations

Clinical manifestations of cirrhosis of the liver differ, depending on the stage of the disease. In the early stages the liver is firm and therefore easier to palpate, and abdominal pain may be present because rapid enlargement produces tension on the organ's fibrous covering. Later stages of the disease are characterized by dyspepsia, changes in bowel habits, gradual weight loss, ascites, enlarged spleen, malaise, nausea, jaundice, ecchymosis, and **spider telangiectases** (small, dilated blood vessels with a bright red center point and spiderlike branches). Spider telangiectases occur on the nose, cheeks, upper trunk, neck, and shoulders. These later manifestations are the result of scarring of liver tissue that produces chronic failure of liver function and also fibrotic changes that cause obstruction of the portal circulation.

When enough cells of the liver become involved to interfere with its function and obstruct its circulation, the GI organs and the spleen become congested and cannot function properly. Anemia occurs because of the body's decreased ability to produce red blood cells (RBCs). The cirrhotic liver cannot absorb vitamin K or produce the clotting factors VII, IX, and X. Thus the patient with cirrhosis develops bleeding tendencies.

Assessment
Subjective data in the **early stages** includes the patient's description of flulike symptoms, including loss of appetite, nausea and vomiting, general weakness, fatigue, indigestion, abnormal bowel function (either constipation or diarrhea), flatulence, and abdominal discomfort. The anatomical area most commonly affected is in the epigastric region or the right upper quadrant of the abdomen.

Collection of **subjective data** in the **later stages** includes noting those subjective symptoms listed under early stages, although they are more intense in later stages. The patient may complain of dyspnea, pruritus, and severe fatigue that interfere with the ability to carry out routine activities. Pruritus is a result of an accumulation of bile salts under the skin from the jaundice.

Collection of **objective data** in the **early stages** includes observing low hemoglobin, fever, **jaundice** (yellow discoloration of the skin, mucous membranes, and sclerae of the eyes [scleral icterus], caused by greater than normal amounts of bilirubin in the serum), and weight loss.

Collection of **objective data** in the **later stages** includes noting epistaxis, purpura, hematuria, spider angiomas (telangiectasis), and bleeding gums. Late symptoms are ascites, hematologic disorders, splenic enlargement, and hemorrhage from esophageal varices or other distended GI veins. The patient may also appear mentally disoriented and display abnormal behaviors and speech patterns. Any prolonged interference with gas exchange leads to hypoxia, coma, and ultimately death.

Diagnostic Tests
Many diagnostic tests aid in the diagnosis of cirrhosis. Poor liver functioning may be manifested in abnormal electrolyte values; elevated serum bilirubin, AST, ALT, LDH, and gamma GT; decreased total protein and serum albumin; elevated ammonia; low blood glucose (hypoglycemia) from impaired gluconeogenesis; prolonged prothrombin time, increased INR; and de-

creased cholesterol levels. Visualization through ERCP (to detect common bile duct obstruction), esophagoscopy with barium esophagography to visualize esophageal varices, scans and biopsy of the liver, and ultrasonography are used to diagnose cirrhosis. **Paracentesis** (a procedure in which fluid is withdrawn from the abdominal cavity) relieves ascites and also provides fluid for laboratory examination.

Medical Management
When possible causes have been identified, the initial treatment is to eliminate these causes, decrease the buildup of fluids in the body, prevent further damage to the liver, and provide individual supportive care. Eliminating alcohol, hepatotoxins (e.g., acetaminophen [Tylenol]), or environmental exposure to harmful chemicals is essential to prevent further damage to the liver. Diet therapy is aimed at correcting malnutrition, promoting the regeneration of functional liver tissue, and compensating for the liver's inability to store vitamins, while avoiding fluid retention and hepatic encephalopathy. A diet that is well balanced, high in calories (2500 to 3000 calories/day), moderately high in protein (75 g of high-quality protein per day), low in fat, low in sodium (1000 to 2000 mg/day), and with additional vitamins and folic acid will usually meet the needs of the patient with cirrhosis and improve deficiencies. A protein-restricted diet may be prescribed for a patient recovering from an acute episode of hepatic encephalopathy.

Antiemetics may be prescribed to control nausea or vomiting. Monitor the patient closely for toxicity, which develops quickly when the poorly functioning liver cannot clear these drugs from the system. Diphenhydramine (Benadryl) or dimenhydrinate (Dramamine) may be given, whereas prochlorperazine maleate (Compazine), hydroxyzine pamoate (Vistaril), or hydroxyzine hydrochloride (Atarax) are contraindicated in severe liver dysfunction.

Later manifestations may be severe and result from liver failure and portal hypertension. Jaundice, peripheral edema, esophageal varices, hepatic encephalopathy, and ascites develop gradually (Figure 6-2).

Complications and Treatment
Ascites is the presence of excessive fluid in the peritoneal cavity. The severity of fluid retention determines the treatment. Initially the patient is placed on bed rest with accurate monitoring of intake and output (I&O). Restrictions are placed on the amount of fluid (500 to 1000 mL) and sodium (1000 to 2000 mg). Diuretic therapy may be added if the diet does not control the ascites and edema. Spironolactone (Aldactone) 300 to 1,000 mg/day may be used to obtain the desired diuresis. Other diuretics may be added, including furosemide (Lasix) or hydrochlorothiazide (HydroDIURIL). Vitamin supplements include vitamin K, vitamin C, and folic acid. Salt-poor albumin

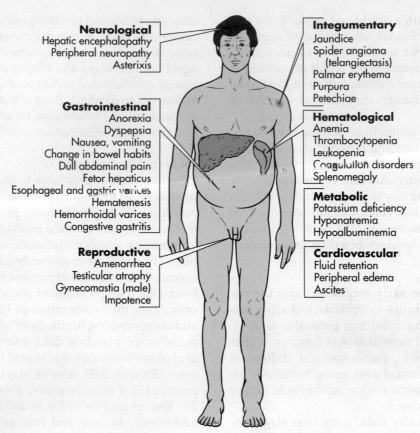

Neurological
Hepatic encephalopathy
Peripheral neuropathy
Asterixis

Gastrointestinal
Anorexia
Dyspepsia
Nausea, vomiting
Change in bowel habits
Dull abdominal pain
Fetor hepaticus
Esophageal and gastric varices
Hematemesis
Hemorrhoidal varices
Congestive gastritis

Reproductive
Amenorrhea
Testicular atrophy
Gynecomastia (male)
Impotence

Integumentary
Jaundice
Spider angioma
  (telangiectasis)
Palmar erythema
Purpura
Petechiae

Hematological
Anemia
Thrombocytopenia
Leukopenia
Coagulation disorders
Splenomegaly

Metabolic
Potassium deficiency
Hyponatremia
Hypoalbuminemia

Cardiovascular
Fluid retention
Peripheral edema
Ascites

FIGURE 6-2 Systemic clinical manifestations of liver cirrhosis.

may be administered in an attempt to restore plasma volume if the intravascular volume is decreased significantly. Complications of diuretic therapy include plasma volume deficit, decreased renal function, and electrolyte imbalance.

Another method of treatment for ascites and edema is the LeVeen continuous peritoneal jugular shunt (Figure 6-3). This procedure allows the continuous shunting of ascitic fluid from the abdominal cavity through a one-way, pressure-sensitive valve into a silicone tube that empties into the superior vena cava. Monitor the patient carefully for complications, which include congestive heart failure, leakage of ascitic fluid, infection at the insertion sites, peritonitis, septicemia, and shunt thrombosis.

Paracentesis is a temporary method of removing fluid by withdrawing it from the abdominal cavity by either gravity or vacuum. Have the patient void immediately before the procedure to prevent puncture of the bladder. The patient should sit on the side of the bed or be placed in high Fowler's position. An incision is made in the skin, and a hollow trocar, cannula, or catheter is passed through the incision and into the cavity. The fluid is removed over a period of 30 to 90 minutes to prevent sudden changes in blood pressure, which could lead to syncope. Monitor the patient closely for signs of hypovolemia and electrolyte imbalances. Apply a dressing over the insertion site, and observe for bleeding and drainage.

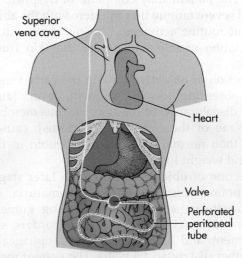

Superior
vena cava

Heart

Valve

Perforated
peritoneal
tube

FIGURE 6-3 LeVeen continuous peritoneal jugular shunt.

Esophageal varices (a complex of longitudinal, tortuous veins at the lower end of the esophagus) enlarge and become edematous as the result of portal hypertension. They are susceptible to ulceration and hemorrhage; avoiding this is a main goal of treatment. For patients who have not bled from esophageal varices, prophylactic treatment with nonselective beta blockers (e.g., propranolol [Inderal]) has been shown to reduce the risk of bleeding and bleeding-related deaths. Varices can rupture as a result of anything that increases abdominal venous pressure, such as coughing, sneezing, vomiting, or the Valsalva maneuver. Rupture may occur slowly over several days or suddenly and without pain. An endoscopy may be performed to identify the varices or to rule out bleeding from other sources. Endoscopic therapies include sclerotherapy and ligation of varices.

Therapeutic management of a ruptured esophageal varix is a medical emergency. The patient's airway must be maintained, the bleeding varix controlled, and IV lines established for fluids and blood replacement as needed. The hormone vasopressin (VP), administered intravenously or directly into the superior vena cava, is used to decrease or stop the hemorrhaging. VP produces vasoconstriction of the vessels, decreases portal blood flow, and decreases portal hypertension. Current drug therapy in some institutions is a combination of VP and nitroglycerin (NTG). The NTG reduces the detrimental effects of VP, which are decreased coronary blood flow and increased blood pressure. VP should be avoided or used cautiously in the older adult because of the risk of cardiac ischemia. If the VP drip does not stop or control bleeding, a Sengstaken-Blakemore tube with openings at the tip may be inserted. This triple-lumen tube has a lumen for inflating the esophageal balloon, one for inflating the gastric balloon, and one for gastric lavage (Figure

6-4). The tube is passed through the nose, and the balloon in the stomach, the one in the esophagus, or both are inflated to press against the bleeding vessels and control the hemorrhage. The gastric aspiration is attached to low, intermittent suction. When either balloon is inflated, a Levin tube is passed into the esophagus through the mouth and attached to low suction to drain the saliva that cannot drain into the stomach. The balloon must be deflated periodically to prevent necrosis. Give the patient nothing by mouth and elevate the head of the bed 30 to 45 degrees to help prevent aspiration of stomach contents and help the patient breathe.

Gastric lavage is performed to remove any swallowed blood from the stomach. Some facilities use iced isotonic saline solutions for the lavage to facilitate vasoconstriction. Endoscopic sclerotherapy may also be used to control the bleeding.

Patients suffering from portal hypertension and esophageal varices may benefit from surgical shunting procedures that divert blood from the portal system to the venous system. The portacaval shunt diverts blood from the portal vein to the inferior vena cava. The splenorenal shunt requires the removal of the spleen, and the splenic vein is anastomosed to the left renal vein. The mesocaval shunt involves anastomosis of the

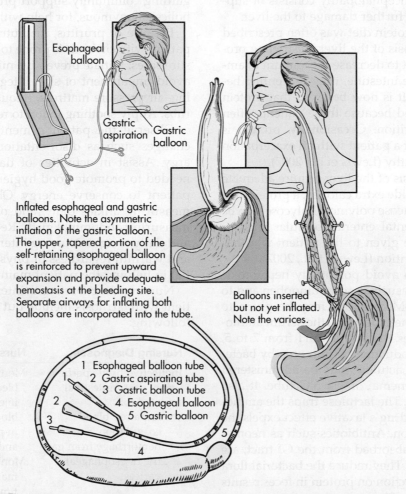

Esophageal balloon

Gastric aspiration   Gastric balloon

Inflated esophageal and gastric balloons. Note the asymmetric inflation of the gastric balloon. The upper, tapered portion of the self-retaining esophageal balloon is reinforced to prevent upward expansion and provide adequate hemostasis at the bleeding site. Separate airways for inflating both balloons are incorporated into the tube.

Balloons inserted but not yet inflated. Note the varices.

1 Esophageal balloon tube
2 Gastric aspirating tube
3 Gastric balloon tube
4 Esophageal balloon
5 Gastric balloon

FIGURE 6-4 Esophageal tamponade accomplished with Sengstaken-Blakemore tube.

superior mesenteric vein to the inferior vena cava. These procedures are associated with a high mortality rate. They may be performed in an emergency to control acute esophageal varix bleeding or in a therapeutic situation when a patient has already bled. Complications of surgical shunting procedures are hepatic encephalopathy, GI bleeding, ascites, and liver failure.

Care of the patient who has hemorrhaged from an esophageal varix includes maintenance of oxygen content levels within the blood and administration of fresh frozen plasma and packed RBCs, vitamin K (AquaMEPHYTON), histamine (H_2) receptor blockers such as cimetidine (Tagamet), and electrolyte replacements as needed without fluid overload. Avoid ammonia buildup with the use of cathartics (e.g., lactulose [Chronulac]) and neomycin. Preventing ammonia buildup keeps hepatic encephalopathy from breaking down blood and releasing ammonia in the intestine.

Hepatic encephalopathy is a type of brain damage caused by liver disease and consequent ammonia intoxication. It is thought to result from a damaged liver being unable to metabolize substances that can be toxic to the brain, such as ammonia. The patient's signs and symptoms progress from inappropriate behavior, disorientation, flapping tremors, and twitching of the extremities to stupor and coma. Treatment of the patient with hepatic encephalopathy consists of supportive care to prevent further damage to the liver.

In the past, a low-protein diet was often prescribed for patients with cirrhosis of the liver. Restricting protein intake was thought to decrease the amount of ammonia produced in the intestine, thus preventing hepatic encephalopathy. It is now believed that protein should not be restricted because these patients often have existing malnutrition. Occasionally, protein is decreased in the diet of a patient with an exacerbation of hepatic encephalopathy (Lewis et al., 2007).

Patients with cirrhosis of the liver require adequate carbohydrates. To provide extra calories, a protein-free supplement such as glucose polymer (Polycose) can be used. Other supplemental enteral formulas such as Hepatic-Aid II may be given to the patient who has protein-calorie malnutrition (Lewis et al., 2007).

Teach the patient to avoid potentially hepatotoxic over-the-counter drugs such as acetaminophen and to abstain from alcohol. Medications may be given to cleanse the bowel and help decrease the serum ammonia. Lactulose decreases the bowel's pH from 7 to 5, thus decreasing the production of ammonia by bacteria within the bowel. Lactulose may be administered orally, as a retention enema, or via NG tube. It also functions as a cathartic. The lactulose traps the ammonia in the gut, and the drug's laxative effect expels the ammonia from the colon. Antibiotics such as neomycin, which are poorly absorbed from the GI tract, are given orally or rectally. They reduce the bacterial flora of the colon. Bacterial action on protein in feces results in ammonia production. Because neomycin may cause

renal toxicity and hearing impairment, lactulose is frequently preferred.

Asterixis is a hand-flapping tremor in which the patient stretches out an arm and hyperextends the wrist with the fingers separated, relaxed, and extended. A rapid, irregular flexion and extension (flapping) of the wrist occurs in the patient who is acutely ill.

Nursing Interventions and Patient Teaching

Check vital signs every 4 hours, or more often if evidence of hemorrhage is present. Observe the patient for GI hemorrhage as evidenced by hematemesis, melena, anxiety, and restlessness.

Most patients require a well-balanced, moderate, high-protein, high-carbohydrate diet with adequate vitamins. With impending liver failure, protein and fluids are restricted. Sodium restriction is frequently necessary, which can make providing a palatable diet more difficult. Provide frequent oral hygiene and a pleasant environment to help the patient increase food intake.

A major nursing focus for many patients is helping them deal with alcoholism. This requires establishing trust that the health team is interested in the patient's well-being. Patients must admit that they have a drinking problem. Confrontation is sometimes used to help patients accept the problem. Provide information regarding community support programs, such as Alcoholics Anonymous, for help with alcohol abuse.

Because of pruritus, malnutrition, and edema, the patient with cirrhosis is prone to skin lesions and pressure sores. Initiate preventive nursing interventions to avoid impairment of skin integrity, such as alternating–air pressure mattress, frequent turning, and back rubs. Apply soothing lotion to relieve pruritus.

Observe the patient's mental status and report changes such as disorientation, headache, or lethargy. Assist in activities of daily living (ADLs) as needed to promote good hygiene while allowing the patient to conserve energy. Observe for edema by measuring ankles daily, and observe for ascites by measuring abdominal girth. Record an accurate I&O and daily weight. Nursing intervention with concern and warmth regardless of physical changes is essential in helping the patient maintain self-esteem.

Nursing diagnoses and interventions for the patient with cirrhosis include but are not limited to the following:

Nursing Diagnoses	Nursing Interventions
Ineffective tissue perfusion, gastrointestinal, related to: • impaired blood coagulation • hemorrhage from gastric or esophageal varices	Monitor patient for signs of bleeding in the gums and injection sites, decrease in blood pressure, increase in pulse, hematemesis, and melena. Monitor hemoglobin, hematocrit, prothrombin time, and INR.

Nursing Diagnoses	Nursing Interventions
Ineffective tissue perfusion, gastrointestinal, related to: • impaired blood coagulation • hemorrhage from gastric or esophageal varices—cont'd	Monitor parenteral fluids and blood transfusions. Administer vitamin K and neomycin as ordered. Instruct patient to avoid straining with stools and to avoid vigorous tooth brushing. Monitor gastric output (color and consistency).
Acute confusion, related to potential increase of serum ammonia and hepatic coma	Observe frequently for changes in mental status such as lethargy, drowsiness, and confusion. Monitor neurologic status for decreased motor ability. Encourage fluids (if not restricted). Give lactulose as ordered to decrease production of ammonia. Provide a safe environment: side rails up, bed in low position, and safety reminder devices if necessary. Avoid use of sedatives, tranquilizers, and opioids. Occasionally a low-protein diet is ordered until signs and symptoms of hepatic encephalopathy disappear, since ammonia (a breakdown product of protein) is responsible for mental changes (Lewis et al., 2007). Protein is not restricted for prolonged periods because of patient having malnutrition.

The patient with cirrhosis must understand the need for getting adequate rest and avoiding infections. Plan activity around complete bed rest until strength is regained. Turning the patient at least every 2 hours and providing range-of-motion exercises will help avoid infection and prevent thrombophlebitis. Instruct the patient to use a soft-bristled toothbrush, use an electric razor, blow nose cautiously, and avoid straining at stools to prevent bleeding as a result of a lack of vitamin K and certain clotting factors. Avoid soap, perfumed lotion, and rubbing alcohol because they will further dry the skin. For pruritus and dry skin, administer diphenhydramine (Benadryl). Explain the relationship of the therapeutic diet to the diagnosis and the liver's ability to function.

Help the patient and family identify community resources for home health care and alcohol rehabilitation to help them deal with problems that arise after discharge. Because of the seriousness of the disease, the patient and the family need understanding and support throughout the treatment (see Home Care Considerations box).

Prognosis

The prognosis for cirrhosis of the liver is related to the cause of the disease, the patient's general health status, and the extent of the involvement. Fibrosis of the cirrhotic liver cannot be cured, but its progression may be halted or slowed by proper management by the physician, the nurse, the patient, and family members (Nursing Care Plan 6-1). For patients who have recurring problems of hepatic encephalopathy or who are in the late stages of cirrhosis, a liver transplant may be an option (Lewis et al., 2007).

LIVER CANCER

Etiology and Pathophysiology

Primary liver cancer is the seventh most common cancer in men and the ninth most common in women. The type of primary liver cancer seen most frequently is hepatocellular carcinoma; the other primary tumors are cholangiomas or biliary duct carcinomas. Cirrhosis of the liver and infection with hepatitis C or hepatitis B are high-risk factors in primary liver cancer. The increase in cases of primary liver cancer stems from the increased incidence of hepatitis C. In the United States, liver cancer usually occurs in people over 40 years of age.

Metastatic carcinoma of the liver occurs more often than primary liver cancer because of the portal vein circulation with its high rate of blood flow and extensive capillary structure. Malignant cells from other areas of the body migrate to the liver by means of the portal vein (Lewis et al., 2007). Cancer cells often cause hepatomegaly. The tumors can also invade nearby organs and structures such as the gallbladder, the peritoneum, the diaphragm, or the lungs (Lewis et al., 2007).

Home Care Considerations

Cirrhosis of the Liver

- The patient and the family need to understand the importance of continual health care and medical supervision.
- Encourage measures to achieve and maintain remission. These include proper diet, rest, avoidance of potentially hepatotoxic over-the-counter drugs (e.g., acetaminophen [Tylenol]), and abstinence from alcohol.
- Provide information regarding community support programs, such as Alcoholics Anonymous, for help with alcohol abuse.
- Help the patient maintain the highest level of wellness possible and initiate and maintain necessary lifestyle changes.

Nursing Care Plan 6-1   The Patient with Cirrhosis of the Liver

Mr. Kaplan, 49 years of age, is admitted with loss of appetite, generalized edema, pruritus, flappy tremors of the hands, ascites, and lethargy. He appears disoriented. His skin has areas of excoriation caused by scratching and a sallow appearance. His wife states that he has been unable to concentrate, appears confused and listless, and has been eating poorly. Mr. Kaplan has been an alcoholic for the past 18 years. His total bilirubin is 4.5 mg/dL, gamma GT is 65 units/L, total protein is 4.8 g/dL, albumin is 2.8 g/dL, and blood ammonia is 160 mcg/dL. He is demonstrating signs and symptoms of hepatic encephalopathy.

NURSING DIAGNOSIS *Imbalanced nutrition: less than body requirements, related to anorexia, nausea, and impaired utilization and storage of nutrients, as manifested by lack of interest in food, aversion to eating, inadequate food intake*

Patient Goals and Expected Outcomes	Nursing Interventions	Evaluation/Rationale
Patient will eat 50% of meal Patient will maintain baseline body weight	Monitor weight to determine whether weight loss occurs. Provide oral care before meals to remove foul taste and improve taste of food. Administer antiemetics as ordered to relieve nausea and vomiting. Provide small, frequent meals at times the patient can best tolerate them to prevent feeling of fullness and to maintain nutritional status. Determine food preferences and allow these whenever possible to increase appeal of food for patient.	Patient is eating 50% to 75% of his meals. Patient has no weight loss indicating maintaining satisfactory nutritional balance.

NURSING DIAGNOSIS *Acute confusion, related to increased formation of ammonia as manifested by inability to concentrate, lethargy, disorientation, and flappy tremors of the hands*

Patient Goals and Expected Outcomes	Nursing Interventions	Evaluation
Patient will be oriented to person, place, time, and purpose	Monitor for hepatic encephalopathy by assessing patient's general behavior, orientation to time and place, speech, and ammonia levels, since liver is unable to convert accumulating ammonia to urea for renal excretion. Encourage fluids (if not restricted), and give laxatives and enemas as ordered to decrease ammonia production. Provide prescribed protein-restricted diet until acute clinical signs and symptoms of hepatic encephalopathy are decreased. Administer lactulose (Chronulac) or neomycin (Mycifradin) as prescribed. Limit physical activity because exercise produces ammonia as a by-product of metabolism. Control factors known to precipitate hepatic coma.	Patient responds appropriately to assessment of person, place, time, and purpose.

Critical Thinking Questions

1. Mr. Kaplan is thrashing about in his bed and has attempted to climb over the side rails. He is disoriented to time and place. What appropriate nursing interventions will ensure Mr. Kaplan's safety?
2. Mrs. Kaplan notes that her husband has a low-protein diet. She confides to the nurse that she thinks he needs more meat, eggs, and cottage cheese to improve his nutrition. What is the most appropriate response?

Clinical Manifestations and Diagnostic Tests

Diagnosing carcinoma of the liver is difficult. In its early stages many of the clinical manifestations (e.g., hepatomegaly, weight loss, peripheral edema, ascites, portal hypertension) are similar to those of cirrhosis of the liver. Other common manifestations include dull abdominal pain in the epigastric or right upper quadrant region, jaundice, anorexia, nausea and vomiting, and extreme weakness. Palpation may reveal an enlarged, nodular liver. Patients frequently have pulmonary emboli. Tests to assist in the diagnosis are a liver scan, ultrasound, CT scan, magnetic resonance imaging, hepatic arteriography, ERCP, and liver biopsy needle. The test for alpha-fetoprotein (AFP) may be positive in hepatocellular carcinoma. AFP helps distinguish primary cancer from metastatic cancer.

Medical Management and Nursing Interventions

Treatment of cancer of the liver is largely palliative. Surgical excision (lobectomy) is sometimes performed if the tumor is localized to one portion of the liver. Only 5% of patients have surgically resectable disease.

usually the cancer is too advanced for surgery when it is detected. Surgical excision or transplant offers the only chance for cure. Medical management is similar to that for cirrhosis of the liver. Chemotherapy may be used, but the response is usually poor. Portal vein or hepatic artery perfusion with 5-fluorouracil (5-FU) may be attempted.

Nursing interventions for the patient with liver carcinoma focus on keeping the patient as comfortable as possible. Because the problems are the same as with advanced liver disease, the nursing interventions discussed for cirrhosis of the liver apply.

Prognosis

The prognosis for cancer of the liver is poor. The cancer grows rapidly, and death may occur within 4 to 7 months as a result of hepatic encephalopathy or massive blood loss from GI bleeding.

HEPATITIS

Etiology and Pathophysiology

Hepatitis is an inflammation of the liver resulting from several types of viral agents or exposure to toxic substances. Rarely, hepatitis is caused by bacteria, such as streptococci, salmonellae, or *Escherichia coli*.

The six types of viral hepatitis are caused by distinct but similar viruses that produce almost identical signs and symptoms but vary in their incubation period, mode of transmission, and prognosis. Hepatitis A (formerly called infectious hepatitis) is the most common form today and is a short-incubation virus (10 to 40 days). Hepatitis B (formerly called serum hepatitis) is a long-incubation virus (28 to 160 days). Hepatitis C has an incubation period of 2 weeks to 6 months (commonly 6 to 9 weeks). Hepatitis D (also called delta virus) causes hepatitis as a coinfection with hepatitis B and may progress to cirrhosis and chronic hepatitis. The incubation period is 2 to 10 weeks. Hepatitis E (also called enteric non-A–non-B hepatitis) is transmitted through fecal contamination of water, primarily in developing countries. It is rare in the United States. The incubation period is 15 to 64 days. Recently hepatitis G virus has been discovered. Hepatitis G virus has been found in blood donors and can be transmitted by transfusion. It frequently coexists with other hepatitis viruses, such as hepatitis C.

Health officials are required by law to report all cases of viral hepatitis to the Centers for Disease Control and Prevention (CDC) in Atlanta. Modes of transmission for the different types of hepatitis are listed in Box 6-1.

 Safety Alert!

Prevention of Acute Viral Hepatitis

HEPATITIS A
- Wash your hands. Hepatitis A virus (HAV) is transmitted when people put something in their mouths that is contaminated with fecal material (called "fecal-oral transmission"). Teach patients the importance of good hand hygiene after using the bathroom or changing a diaper, as well as proper food preparation, to prevent the spread of HAV.
- The best protection against HAV transmission is the two-dose HAV vaccine.

HEPATITIS B
- Wash your hands.
- One of the best preventive measures against hepatitis B virus (HBV) is the HBV vaccine.
- Children younger than 18 years of age are routinely vaccinated today.
- People who are at risk for the virus, such as health care workers, should be vaccinated.
- People who play or work in inner-city parks and playgrounds are at risk for exposure to HBV from litter containers and used needles and syringes. They should be vaccinated, as should men who have sex with men, individuals who use illicit IV drugs, and those who travel to areas with a high infection rate.
- People who are positive for HBV should not donate blood, organs, or tissue.
- Ensure proper disposal of needles.
- Use Standard Precautions when handling blood products.
- Use needleless IV access devices if available.

HEPATITIS C
- Wash your hands.
- Hepatitis C virus is transmitted by needle sharing among illicit IV drug users.
- Other significant risk factors include receipt of clotting factor made before 1987, hemodialysis, receipt of blood or solid organs donated before 1992, maternal-fetal transmission, and multiple or infected sex partners.
- Ensure proper disposal of needles.
- Use standard precautions when handling blood products.
- Use needleless IV access devices if available.

HEPATITIS D
- Modes of hepatitis D virus (HDV) transmission are similar to those of HBV. Sexual transmission of HDV is less efficient than for HBV. Educate patients regarding risky behavior.

HEPATITIS E
- Educate patients to avoid drinking water or beverages with ice in areas with uncertain water quality. They should refrain from eating raw shellfish and avoid raw produce unless it is prepared with purified water.
- Hepatitis E is most often seen in southeastern and central Asia, the Middle East, Africa, and Mexico.

HEPATITIS G
- Hepatitis G has been detected in blood samples in Europe, Asia, and Australia.
- Transmission of hepatitis G virus occurs when tainted injectable drugs are used; tainted blood, organs, or tissues are received through hemodialysis; or unsafe methods are used for tattooing or body piercing.

| Box 6-1 | Modes of Transmission of the Six Types of Viral Hepatitis |

- Hepatitis A spreads by direct contact through the oral-fecal route, usually by food or water contaminated with feces. Up to 50% of all people in the United States have been infected by the time they reach adulthood; most suffer minimal symptoms or none at all. Two or more weeks before symptoms appear, the virus can be found in the bile, blood, and stool. Patients are rarely infectious once they develop jaundice (Durston, 2004).
- Hepatitis B is transmitted by contaminated serum via blood transfusion, contaminated needles and instruments, needlesticks, illicit intravenous (IV) drug use, and dialysis, and by direct contact with body fluids from infected people, such as breast milk and sexual contact. An ever-increasing risk comes from improper disposal of used needles and syringes. Sharing toothbrushes, razor blades, or personal items with an infected person may also lead to exposure.
- Hepatitis C (HCV) is transmitted through needlesticks, blood transfusions, illicit IV drug use, and unidentified

means. HCV can also be transmitted by sharing contaminated straws used for snorting cocaine. In the past, hepatitis C could not be detected in banked blood, so it was more easily transmitted through transfusion. The advent of routine blood screening in 1992 greatly reduced the number of cases of transfusion-related hepatitis C.
- Hepatitis D is transmitted the same way as hepatitis B; it appears as a coinfection of hepatitis B.
- Hepatitis E is transmitted by the oral-fecal route; it spreads through the fecal contamination of water.
- Hepatitis G is frequently seen as a coinfection with hepatitis C; it spreads through bloodborne exposure. Hepatitis G has been found in some blood donors and can be transmitted by transfusion. Transmission occurs through contaminated injectable drugs; contaminated blood, organs, or tissues; hemodialysis; or unsafe methods of tattooing or body piercing.

The basic pathologic findings in the six forms of viral hepatitis are identical. A diffuse inflammatory reaction occurs, liver cells begin to degenerate and die, and the liver's normal functions slow down. The outcome may be affected by the virulence of the virus, the liver's preexisting condition, the health care given when the disease is diagnosed, and patient compliance with treatment.

Clinical Manifestations

The clinical manifestations for viral hepatitis vary greatly; some patients are asymptomatic, whereas others develop hepatic failure or hepatic encephalopathy.

Assessment

Subjective data include patients' reports of general malaise, aching muscles, photophobia, lassitude, headaches, and chills. Abdominal pain, dyspepsia, nausea, diarrhea, and constipation are reported also. The patient may complain of pruritus from bile on the skin. The patient complains of tenderness in the liver and remains fatigued for several weeks.

Collection of **objective data** includes observing hepatomegaly, enlarged lymph nodes, weight loss, and rhinitis. Jaundice appears because of the damaged liver's inability to metabolize bilirubin; the resultant signs are yellowish skin, discoloration of the sclera (scleral icterus) and mucous membrane (Figure 6-5), dark tea-colored urine, and clay-colored stools. Relapses are common in the convalescent stage.

Diagnostic Tests

Changes in the liver caused by viral hepatitis result in elevated direct bilirubin, gamma GT, AST, ALT, LDH, and alkaline phosphatase levels; a prolonged prothrombin time and increased INR; and, in severe hepatitis, decreased serum albumin. Leukopenia is com-

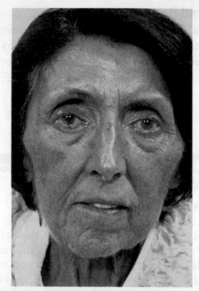

FIGURE 6-5 Severe jaundice.

mon in these patients, with a transient neutropenia and lymphopenia, followed by lymphocytosis. Hypoglycemia is present in approximately 50% of patients with hepatitis. Serum is examined for the presence of hepatitis-associated antigen A, B, C, D, or G. A CT of the abdomen reveals hepatomegaly.

Medical Management

Providing supportive therapy for existing signs and symptoms and preventing transmission of the disease are important aspects of treatment of the patient with viral hepatitis. Hospitalization is an option for patients whose bilirubin concentrations in the blood are more than 10 mg/dL and for those with a prolonged prothrombin time and increased INR, but usually patients are cared for at home. Bed rest for several weeks is commonly prescribed.

Drug therapy for chronic hepatitis B focuses on decreasing the viral load, decreasing the rate of disease progression, and monitoring for detection of drug-resistant HBV. At present, several drugs are useful in suppressing viral activity and decreasing viral load in patients with HBV. However, the percentage of patients seroconverting (developing antibodies against the virus) remains relatively low. Lamivudine (Epivir, 3TC), interferon-α, and adefovir dipivoxil (Hepsera) are three drugs being used in the treatment of chronic hepatitis B. Telbivudine (Tyzeka) is a new drug used to treat chronic HBV infection. Telbivudine has been shown to decrease the viral load more effectively than lamivudine and adefovir (Hussar, 2007).

In chronic hepatitis C, drug therapy is also directed at reducing the viral load, decreasing progression of the disease, and promoting seroconversion. Treatment options for HCV are interferon alfa-2b (Intron A), ribavirin (Rebetol), and pegylated interferon alfa-2a (Pegasys). This combination therapy eradicates the virus more effectively than monotherapy. Another treatment option is liver transplantation. In fact half of all liver recipients are HCV positive. Most transplanted livers eventually become infected with HCV, but recipients can increase both quantity and quality of life by avoiding risky behaviors (Durston, 2004).

The patient is not allowed alcohol for at least 1 year and may need supportive care from the community to comply. Most patients tolerate small, frequent meals of a low-fat, high-carbohydrate diet. If the patient is dehydrated, IV fluids are given with addition of vitamin C for healing, vitamin B complex to assist the damaged liver's inability to absorb fat-soluble vitamins, and vitamin K to combat prolonged coagulation time. Avoid all unnecessary medications, particularly sedatives.

Give gamma globulin or immune serum globulin as soon as possible to people who have been in direct contact with a person with hepatitis A during the infectious period (2 weeks before and 1 week after onset of symptoms). The dosage of 0.02 mL/kg of body weight, given intramuscularly, is effective in preventing hepatitis A in 80% to 90% of cases. Currently three vaccines are used to prevent hepatitis A: Havrix, Vaqta, and Avaxim.

Primary immunization consists of a single dose administered intramuscularly in the deltoid muscle. A booster is recommended between 6 and 12 months after the primary dose to ensure adequate antibody titers and long-term protection. However, primary immunization provides immunity within 30 days after a single dose.

Until routine vaccination of children is feasible, people who are at risk for infection should be vaccinated for hepatitis A. This includes people traveling to countries where hepatitis A is endemic; sexually active homosexual and bisexual men; patients with chronic liver disease; injecting drug users; and people at risk for occupational infection, such as those who work with hepatitis A in research laboratory settings.

Individuals who have been exposed to HBV via a needle puncture or sexual contact should be protected with hepatitis B immune globulin. A dose of 0.06 mL/kg of body weight is administered intramuscularly as quickly after exposure as possible. This dose is repeated 1 month later. People identified as being at high risk for developing hepatitis B should be vaccinated if they are not already immune. These people include the following:

- All health care personnel (especially emergency department, operating room, intensive care unit [ICU], and dialysis personnel; phlebotomists; and laboratory technicians)
- People with high-risk lifestyles (drug users, tattoo recipients, homosexual men, and prostitutes)
- Infants born to mothers who are hepatitis B surface antigen positive
- Hemodialysis patients
- Individuals sharing a household with an infected person

The CDC Immunization Practices Advisory Committee (2009) recommends making hepatitis B vaccine a part of routine vaccination schedules for all newborns and adolescents. The protection program consists of three vaccinations: an initial vaccination, a vaccination 1 month later, and a third vaccination 6 months after the first injection. The hepatitis B vaccine has been shown to provide protection for 3 to 5 years in approximately 90% of the people treated. It is hoped that universal vaccination will lead to eventual prevention and control of hepatitis B.

Hepatitis B, C, D, and G are spread through blood transfusions. The blood used should be screened for elevated ALT and anti–hepatitis B core, anti–hepatitis C, anti–hepatitis D, and anti–hepatitis G.

Liver Transplantation

The first human liver transplant was performed in 1963. Liver transplantation has become a practical therapeutic option for many people with end-stage liver disease, generally improving their quality of life. Indications for liver transplantation include congenital biliary abnormalities, inborn errors of metabolism, hepatic malignancy (confined to the liver), sclerosing cholangitis, and chronic end-stage liver disease. Liver disease related to chronic viral hepatitis is the leading indication for liver transplantation. Liver transplants are not recommended for the patient with widespread malignant disease. There are approximately 17,000 people waiting for liver transplants; however, only 6000 transplants are performed annually (Verna & Brown, n.d.; McCaughan et al., 2005).

The major postoperative complications are rejection and infection. Liver transplant candidates must go through a rigorous presurgery screening. However, the liver seems to be less susceptible to rejection than the kidney.

The source of a liver used for transplantation may be a deceased (cadaver) donor or a live donor. The live donor donates only a portion of his or her liver to the recipient. The donor faces potential risks, however, such as biliary problems, hepatic artery thrombosis, wound infection, postoperative paralytic ileus, and pneumothorax (Lewis et al., 2007).

The use of cyclosporine, an effective immunosuppressant drug, has been a major factor in the success rates of liver transplantation. It does not cause bone marrow suppression and does not impede wound healing. Other immunosuppressants used include azathioprine (Imuran), corticosteroids, tacrolimus (Prograf) and mycophenolate mofetil (Cellcept), New agents, including the interleukin-2 receptor antagonists basiliximab (Simulect) and daclizumab (Zenapax), are being used in combination with other immunosuppressive agents to reduce rejection. Other factors in the improved success rate are advances in surgical techniques, better selection of potential recipients, and improved management of the underlying liver disease before surgery.

Patients who have liver disease secondary to viral hepatitis often experience reinfection of the transplanted liver with hepatitis B or C. HCV recurrence as evidenced by histologic damage is almost universal after transplant. Approximately 20% to 30% of patients develop cirrhosis of the transplanted liver by the fifth year posttransplant. Antiviral therapy for HCV initiated posttransplant, even before the development of histologic evidence of recurrence, has failed to alter this recurrence pattern. Approximately 75% of patients survive more than 3 years following transplants (Lewis et al., 2007).

Nursing Interventions and Patient Teaching

The patient who has a liver transplant requires competent and highly skilled nursing interventions, in either an ICU or another specialized unit. Postoperative nursing care includes assessing neurologic status; monitoring for signs of hemorrhage; preventing pulmonary complications; monitoring drainage, electrolyte levels, and urinary output; and monitoring for signs and symptoms of infection and rejection. Common respiratory problems are pneumonia, atelectasis, and pleural effusions. Have the patient use measures such as coughing, deep breathing, incentive spirometry, and repositioning to prevent these complications. Measure and record drainage from the Jackson-Pratt drain, NG tube suctioning, and T-tube, and note the color and consistency of drainage. A critical aspect of nursing interventions after liver transplantation is monitoring for infection. The first 2 months after the surgery are critical. Infection can be viral, fungal, or bacterial. Fever may be the only sign of infection. Emotional support and teaching the patient and family are essential.

The care of the patient with viral hepatitis includes ensuring rest, maintaining adequate nutrition, providing adequate fluids, and caring for the skin. The care of the patient with hepatitis continues over time, and support and patient education are necessary throughout the entire illness.

Preventing transmission of the disease is of primary importance in caring for the patient with viral hepatitis. The patient, family, and health care providers must be knowledgeable about routes of transmission of the virus and take steps to avoid such transmission. Proper personal hygiene and good sanitation, as well as hepatitis A vaccine, will help prevent the spread of hepatitis A. Give patients a thorough explanation of the reasons for the precautions, and instruct them in the proper handling of their own secretions and body wastes and in thorough methods of hand hygiene. Wear gown and gloves when handling excreta, giving enemas, taking rectal temperatures, handling food waste, handling needles, disposing of urine, or carrying out any other procedure or hygiene measure that involves direct contact with the patient's body fluids.

When a patient has hepatitis B, take utmost care in handling syringes, needles, and other instruments that are contaminated with the patient's serum. Use disposable equipment and dishes and take isolation precautions. Maintaining standard precautions while exposed to blood and body fluids such as saliva, semen, and vaginal secretions is essential to prevent the transmission of hepatitis B. Use enteric precautions for 7 days after onset of hepatitis A. Use standard precautions for all patients.

Nursing diagnoses and interventions for the patient with hepatitis include but are not limited to the following:

Nursing Diagnoses	Nursing Interventions
Risk for injury, related to: • poor nutrition • prolonged clotting times	Pad side rails if necessary. Assist weakened patient with activities. Encourage use of electric razor and soft toothbrush.
Imbalanced nutrition: less than body requirements, related to: • anorexia • nausea • vomiting • altered metabolism of nutrients by the liver	Provide diet high in carbohydrates and low in fats, and encourage total fluid intake of 2500 to 3000 mL daily. Monitor I&O. Monitor daily weight. Note color and consistency of stool and color and amount of urine. Administer antiemetics as ordered. Offer support and understanding. Promote adequate rest.

For the patient with viral hepatitis being cared for at home, teach the family necessary precautions. Patients should avoid sexual activity during the acute stage of hepatitis B, C, and D. Patients with hepatitis must wash hands thoroughly after toileting, must disinfect articles soiled with feces (boil 1 minute), and must not prepare foods for others while symptomatic. If possible, the patient should use separate bathroom facilities. Personal care items and drinking glasses should not be shared. The patient's clothes should be laundered separately in hot water. Contaminated items should be disposed of properly.

Inform the patient and family about signs and symptoms associated with hepatitis, including light-colored stools, dark-colored urine, jaundice, fever, GI disturbances, unusual bleeding that might be indicative of a prolonged prothrombin time and increased INR, and tenderness or pain in the abdomen. The danger of alcohol use and its effect on the liver should be clearly understood.

Prognosis

The prognosis of hepatitis differs with the causative agent. Recovery from hepatitis A is high, with a mortality rate of 0.5%. Mortality from hepatitis B has been reported to be as high as 10%. Hepatitis B is a very serious form of hepatitis, often progressing to cirrhosis, chronic hepatitis, liver cancer, and death. Hepatitis C often progresses to chronic hepatitis, cirrhosis, liver cancer, and death. There is a greater risk for hepatitis C infection becoming chronic compared with hepatitis B. Approximately 75% to 80% of patients who acquire HCV go on to develop chronic infection, and 20% develop liver failure. The prognosis of chronic hepatitis C infection has greatly increased the demand for liver transplants. Hepatitis D may progress to cirrhosis and chronic hepatitis. It has a high mortality rate. Hepatitis E has a 10% mortality rate in pregnant women; otherwise it is not believed to be fatal. Hepatitis G infections frequently coexist with other hepatitis infections, such as hepatitis C. However, most hepatitis G infections are not associated with chronic hepatitis; thus hepatitis G virus's association with liver disease is, at this time, uncertain.

Recovery from acute toxic hepatitis is rapid if the hepatotoxin is identified early and removed or if exposure to the agent has been limited. However, the prognosis is poor if the period between exposure and the onset of signs and symptoms is prolonged, since there are no effective antidotes.

LIVER ABSCESSES

If an infection develops anywhere along the GI tract, there is danger of the infecting organisms reaching the liver through the biliary system, portal venous system, or hepatic arterial or lymphatic systems. Most bacteria are promptly destroyed, but occasionally some gain a foothold. If the disease progresses, it can become life threatening. In the past the mortality rate with liver abscesses was 100% because of the vague clinical symptoms, inadequate diagnostic tools, and inadequate surgical drainage. Today medical management is more successful.

Etiology and Pathophysiology

If the body is not successful in destroying bacteria, the bacterial toxins attack neighboring liver cells, and the necrotic tissue produced serves as a protective wall for the organism. Meanwhile, leukocytes migrate into the infected area. The result is an abscess cavity full of a liquid containing living and dead leukocytes and bacteria. Pyogenic (pus-producing) abscesses of this type may be single or multiple.

Clinical Manifestations

Patients with liver abscess are seen with vague signs and symptoms. Fever accompanied by chills, abdominal pain, and tenderness in the right upper quadrant of the abdomen are common complaints.

Assessment

Subjective data include chills, complaints of dull abdominal pain, abdominal tenderness, and discomfort.

Objective data include fever, hepatomegaly, jaundice, and anemia.

Diagnostic Tests

The diagnosis is established by demonstrating a space-occupying lesion in the liver radiographically (radiograph, ultrasound, CT, and liver scan). Amebic (microscopic, single-celled parasite) liver abscess can also be confirmed by amebic serologic examination (laboratory examination of antigen-antibody reaction of amebae in serum).

Medical Management

Usually liver abscesses are managed by medical therapy. Treatment includes IV antibiotic therapy that is specific to the organism identified.

Percutaneous (performed through the skin) drainage of a liver abscess is reserved for patients who do not respond to medical therapy or are at high risk for rupture. Open surgical drainage has been the standard in patients whose liver abscesses have ruptured into the peritoneal space, but some of these patients are now being managed with percutaneous drainage. All patients require a full course of antibiotic therapy.

Nursing Interventions and Patient Teaching

Continuous monitoring and supportive care are indicated because of the seriousness of the patient's condition. Monitoring objective and subjective symptoms is important. Notify the physician if signs and symptoms increase in depth and severity.

The patient's response to drug therapy is determined by a decrease in fever, tenderness and rigidity of the abdomen, chills, and discomfort. If percutaneous or open surgical drainage is instituted, observe the drainage for amount, color, and consistency.

Nursing diagnoses and interventions for the patient with a liver abscess include but are not limited to the following:

Nursing Diagnoses	Nursing Interventions
Risk for imbalanced body temperature, related to infectious state	Check temperature as ordered by physician or as indicated by the patient's worsening condition, and report findings to physician. Encourage fluids to prevent dehydration. Monitor IV fluids. Explain how fever and drainage can deplete fluids in the body. Record I&O. Monitor oral mucous membranes and skin turgor.
Deficient knowledge, related to relationship of infection to nutritional needs	Explain the body's need for added calories and protein to fight infection. Weigh patient daily for weight gain or loss to determine adequate nutritional intake.

In addition to the relationship of infection and nutrition, teach preoperative and postoperative procedures if the patient requires percutaneous or open surgical drainage. A thorough explanation and assessment for the patient's understanding are necessary. The seriously ill patient becomes less anxious as the knowledge base increases and the patient feels more in control of the situation.

Prognosis

The prognosis for patients with liver abscesses was very poor in the past, with a mortality rate of 100%. The prognosis today is much improved because of advanced diagnostic tests, including CT and liver scans, and aggressive medical and nursing interventions.

CHOLECYSTITIS AND CHOLELITHIASIS

Etiology and Pathophysiology

Disorders of the biliary system are common in the United States and are responsible for the hospitalization of more than a half million people a year. The two most common conditions are cholecystitis (inflammation of the gallbladder) and cholelithiasis (presence of gallstones in the gallbladder) (Box 6-2). These two diseases are seen more commonly in women than men; in Native Americans and whites than in Asian Americans

Box 6-2	Definitions

chole- pertaining to bile
cholang- pertaining to bile ducts
cholangiography radiographic examination of bile ducts
cholangitis inflammation of bile duct
cholecyst- pertaining to gallbladder
cholecystectomy removal of gallbladder
cholecystitis inflammation of gallbladder
cholecystography radiographic examination of gallbladder
cholecystostomy incision into the gallbladder (usually for drainage)
choledocho- pertaining to common bile duct
choledocholithiasis stones in common bile duct
choledochostomy exploration of common bile duct
cholelith- gallstone
cholelithiasis presence of gallstones

and blacks; and in obese people, pregnant women, multiparous women, women who use birth control pills, and people with diabetes.

Cholecystitis can be caused by an obstruction, a gallstone, or a tumor. More than 90% of cases are caused by gallstones. The exact cause of stone formation in the gallbladder and the common bile duct is not known. However, an alteration in lipid metabolism and the role of female sex hormones are related to the disease. The stones usually occur in multiples but can occur singly (Figure 6-6).

When an obstruction, gallstone, or tumor prevents bile from leaving the gallbladder, the trapped bile acts as an irritant, causing cellular infiltration of the gallbladder wall after 3 to 4 days. A typical inflammatory response occurs, and the gallbladder becomes enlarged and edematous. The vascular occlusion along with bile

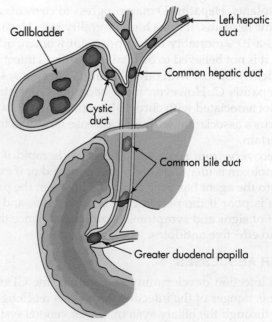

FIGURE 6-6 Common sites of gallstones.

stasis causes the mucosal lining of the gallbladder to become necrotic. Initially the bile in the gallbladder is sterile. The bacterial growth is caused by the ischemia and occurs usually within a few days. The gallbladder is in danger of rupturing and spreading infection to the hepatic duct and liver. When the disease is severe enough to interfere with the blood supply, the gallbladder wall may become gangrenous.

Clinical Manifestations

The condition may be acute, with a sudden onset of indigestion; nausea and vomiting; and severe, colicky pain in the right upper quadrant of the abdomen. The pain may be referred to the right shoulder and scapula. If the condition is chronic, the patient usually has had several milder attacks of pain and a history of fat intolerance. Many patients with gallstones are asymptomatic, and the gallstones are discovered only during an examination for another problem. The patient complains of more severe pain if the gallstones are mobile and moving through the biliary ducts. A gallstone occluding a biliary duct or a stone passing through the ducts may trigger a biliary spasm (Lewis et al., 2007).

Assessment

Subjective data include complaints of indigestion after eating foods high in fat. The pain of acute cholecystitis is abrupt in onset, reaches peak intensity quickly, and remains at that level for 2 to 4 hours. It localizes in the right upper quadrant epigastric region. The pain radiates around the midtorso to the right scapular area. Anorexia, nausea, vomiting, and **flatulence** (excess formation of gases in the stomach or intestine) are also noted. Patients may experience increased heart and respiratory rates and become diaphoretic, leading them to think they are having a heart attack. These symptoms are decreased or absent in patients with chronic cholecystitis.

Objective data include a low-grade fever, increased pulse and respirations, nausea, vomiting, an elevated leukocyte count, mild jaundice, stools that contain fat (**steatorrhea**), and clay-colored stools caused by a lack of bile in the intestinal tract. The urine may be dark amber to tea colored and contain urobilinogen as the kidneys try to remove the excess bilirubin from the bloodstream.

Diagnostic Tests

A number of diagnostic studies are performed to confirm a diagnosis of cholecystitis and cholelithiasis. Fecal studies, serum bilirubin tests, ultrasound of the gallbladder and biliary system, HIDA scan, and OCG may be done. Ultrasound of the gallbladder is 90% to 95% accurate in diagnosing cholelithiasis. HIDA scanning is helpful in assessing the patency of the cystic and common bile ducts. Operative cholangiography—

in which the common bile duct is directly injected with radiopaque dye—is frequently done at the time of gallbladder surgery.

Medical Management

If the attack of cholelithiasis is mild, the patient is treated conservatively. Bed rest is prescribed, an NG tube is inserted and connected to low suction, and the patient is placed on NPO status. This allows the GI tract and thus the gallbladder to rest. IV fluids are given to rehydrate the patient and replace drainage from the NG tube.

Antispasmodic and analgesic drugs may be given to decrease pain. Meperidine (Demerol) is commonly used, since it decreases the incidence of spasms of the sphincter of Oddi. Morphine may be used for pain management. Antibiotics may be given (1) prophylactically to prevent infection; (2) to treat an existing infection; and (3) after perforation, should it occur. A diet that is low in fat and cholesterol may be prescribed. Avoidance of spicy foods is also suggested (see Complementary & Alternative Therapies box).

Lithotripsy

Extracorporeal shock wave lithotripsy is used to treat a patient who has mild or moderate symptoms caused by a few stones. The machine discharges a series of shock waves through water or a cushion that breaks the stone into fragments. The natural flow of bile car-

---

Complementary & Alternative Therapies

Gallbladder, Biliary, and Pancreatic Disorders

- Fresh black root is used as an emetic. The dried root has a gentler action and is used to treat constipation and liver and gallbladder disease and to increase bile flow. Caution patients with gallstones or bile duct obstruction to avoid using it because it may worsen these diseases.
- Blessed thistle is used orally to treat digestive problems such as liver and gallbladder diseases.
- Dandelion is traditionally used as a bile stimulator to treat gallbladder ailments.
- Onion is used as a gallbladder stimulant. It increases the risk of hypoglycemia, so monitor diabetic patients closely.
- Autumn crocus (active ingredient: colchicine) has been used to treat hepatic cirrhosis and primary biliary cirrhosis. Because of the plant's toxicity, internal use is not recommended.
- Papaya (pawpaw) is used to treat pancreatic insufficiency. Patients with a history of Crohn's disease and chronic gastritis should avoid this herb.
- Royal jelly (bee pollen complex) is used in treating liver disease and pancreatitis. Do not confuse royal jelly with bee pollen and honeybee venom. (Royal jelly should be used with extreme caution by patients with asthma because allergic reactions to royal jelly have led to asthma attacks, anaphylaxis, and death.)

ries the stone fragments out of the gallbladder into the intestine for eventual excretion. Nursing intervention after the procedure is similar to that for patients undergoing liver biopsy.

Surgical Intervention

The treatment of choice is cholecystectomy (removal of the gallbladder) with ligation of the cystic duct, vein, and artery. A laparoscopic cholecystectomy and open abdominal cholecystectomy are the two surgical procedures. (See Figure 6-7 for stone retrieval.) A Jackson-Pratt, Penrose, or Davol drain (which promotes drainage and prevents pressure and fluid accumulation under the diaphragm) may be inserted if an open cholecystectomy is performed. If the stones are in the common bile duct and edema is present, a biliary drainage tube, or T-tube, is inserted to keep the duct open and allow drainage of the bile until the edema resolves. The short end of the tube is placed in the common bile duct, and the longer end is brought to the surface through a stab wound (Figure 6-8). The long end is attached to a closed drainage system (bile bag) that is placed below the level of the common bile duct.

The T-tube also provides a route for postoperative cholangiography if desired (T-tube cholangiogram) to

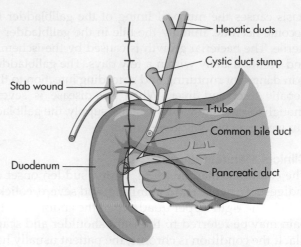

FIGURE 6-8 T-tube in common bile duct.

assess the patency of the common bile duct. The T-tube is removed 24 hours after the cholangiogram if the edema is resolved and the common bile duct appears normal. The 24-hour period allows the dye to drain out of the common bile duct. If the edema does not resolve in this time, the patient may be discharged with the T-tube in place.

The most common treatment for cholecystitis and cholelithiasis is done by an endoscopic technique called **laparoscopic cholecystectomy,** which uses a laser or cautery to remove the gallbladder. This procedure replaces the open surgical procedure 80% to 85% of the time. It involves removing the gallbladder through one of four small punctures in the abdomen (a comparatively minor procedure). During surgery, the abdominal cavity is inflated with 3 to 4 L of carbon dioxide to improve visibility. A laparoscope, which has a camera attached, is inserted into the abdomen. The surgeon removes the deflated gallbladder through a laparoscope. If the organ contains so much bile or gallstones that it cannot be collapsed, its contents will be aspirated first. Laparoscopic cholecystectomy offers several advantages over the common open abdominal cholecystectomy, including the following:

- It is less invasive (and thus there is less chance of wound infection or respiratory impairment) and has a shorter healing time and a shorter recuperative time.
- There is no unsightly scar.
- There is less pain and thus more rapid return to normal activities.

When a medical history, physical examination, and blood studies are complete, an ultrasound is done to locate gallstones and detect any dilation of the hepatic bile ducts. If **choledocholithiasis** (stones in common bile duct) is confirmed, a sphincterotomy and stone extraction (see Figure 6-7) are performed before laparoscopic surgery.

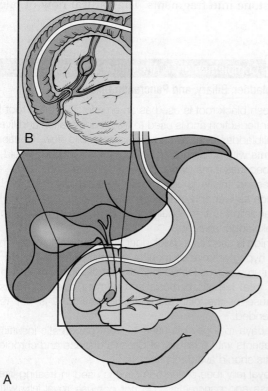

FIGURE 6-7 A, During endoscopic sphincterotomy, a flexible endoscope is advanced through the mouth and the stomach until its tip sits in the duodenum opposite the common bile duct. **B,** After widening the duct mouth by incising the sphincter muscle, the physician advances a basket attachment into the duct and retrieves the stone.

It is important to obtain informed consent for endoscopic and open cholecystectomy in case converting from one procedure to the other is necessary. The conversion may be necessary if extensive adhesions, gallstones within the common bile duct, unusual vascular or ductal anatomy, unsuspected pathologic condition of the abdomen, or excessive bleeding complicates the endoscopic procedure.

Postoperative Care for Laparoscopic Cholecystectomy

A small number of patients report minor discomfort at the laparoscopic insertion site or mild shoulder or neck pain resulting from diaphragmatic irritation secondary to abdominal stretching or residual carbon dioxide. Oral analgesics or antiinflammatory agents relieve these symptoms.

Oral liquids and a light meal are given the first night after surgery. The patient has four bandages at the puncture site on the abdomen. Assess vital signs routinely. The patient is ambulatory the first postoperative night.

One out of six patients is discharged the day of surgery. Most patients are discharged the next day. Patients are usually able to resume moderate activity within 48 to 72 hours.

Patient Teaching

Before discharge, patients should be able to eat without difficulty and walk and should have no abdominal distention, evidence of bleeding, or bile leakage. Instruct them to immediately report to the health care provider any severe pain, tenderness in the right upper quadrant, increase in abdominal girth, leakage of bile-colored drainage from the puncture site, increase in pulse, or symptoms of low blood pressure. Patients are usually able to return to work in 3 days and resume full activity after 1 week.

Although there are contraindications for endoscopic cholecystectomies, most patients are treated with this less painful, less expensive procedure.

Nursing Interventions and Patient Teaching

Nursing interventions begin with careful assessment of the characteristics of pain (if it is present) and any signs of jaundice of the skin, sclera, and mucous membrane. Observe the patient's urine and stool for alterations in the presence of bilirubin.

When the patient is treated conservatively, nursing interventions center on keeping the patient comfortable by carefully administering the medications prescribed and monitoring the patient's response to the medication. The patient is on NPO status or on clear liquids. Administer antiemetics if nausea is present. Observe IV infusions for patency, correct rates, and entry sites that are free from erythema and edema. Measure I&O and describe carefully.

Preoperative care includes teaching the patient to turn, cough, and deep breathe and to use an incentive spirometer to facilitate air movement in and out of the lungs to prevent pneumonia and atelectasis. To enable the patient to follow postoperative instructions more easily, teach him or her how to splint the abdomen with the hands, small pillow, or rolled bath blanket before attempting a cough; practice repositioning in the hospital bed; and assume a sitting position from a standing or lying position. If an open cholecystectomy is anticipated, explaining the IV tubing and urinary catheter and their functions will help relieve patient anxiety. The patient should be familiar with any medications that may be used to relieve pain and nausea and should understand that vitamin K and antibiotics may be given preoperatively to prevent hemorrhage and infection.

Postoperative care for open cholecystectomy includes monitoring vital signs and observing dressings frequently and carefully for exudate or hemorrhage. The dressings usually require reinforcement at the drain site. Place the patient in semi-Fowler's position to facilitate drainage. Monitor the Jackson-Pratt, Penrose, or Davol drain for patency. Initially there should be less than 50 mL of serosanguineous exudate during an 8-hour period. Notify the surgeon if the drainage is excessive, contains bile, or is bright red.

The patient needs encouragement to perform deep breathing, cough, and use the incentive spirometer because of the location of the incision. Provide analgesics frequently in the early postoperative period to facilitate movement and deep breathing. Help the patient to dangle the night of surgery and ambulate the first postoperative day. Monitor the patient's neurologic status by checking ability to be aroused easily, orientation to the environment and family, and ability to move extremities equally on command.

Maintain fluid balance with IV therapy; potassium is usually added to compensate for loss from surgery. Check the physician's order before giving ice or clear liquids to the patient, and allow the patient to rinse the mouth frequently.

The nurse is responsible for the care of the T-tube if one is placed. The drainage bag for the T-tube is placed below the level of the common bile duct to prevent the reflux of bile. Position the bag so the tube is not kinked and bile cannot drain from the liver. Frequently check the position of the bag and tube and the color and amount of exudate during the first 24 hours and record the results. Place a gauze roll under the tube, anchoring it to the patient's abdomen and preventing tension and pull on the tube from the weight of the bag. The T-tube drains as much as 500 mL during the first 24 hours. The amount should decrease as the edema resolves and bile begins flowing through the common bile duct. Be careful not to dislodge the T-tube when changing the patient's dressings, as prescribed by the physician.

After oral intake is resumed, the physician may order the T-tube clamped for 1 to 2 hours before meals and unclamped 1 to 2 hours after the patient eats, to aid in the digestion of fat. While the T-tube is clamped, the patient may show signs of distress, including abdominal pain, nausea, vomiting, light brown urine, and clay-colored stools. If distress occurs, unclamp the tube immediately. Increase the time that the T-tube remains clamped as the patient tolerates the procedure. The tube may be left in place for as long as 10 days. The physician removes the tube when the common bile duct is patent for drainage of bile.

Check bowel sounds every 8 hours for the return of peristalsis. Other indicators of the return of peristalsis include expelling flatus, return of appetite, and absence of nausea or vomiting (Madsen et al., 2005). A clear liquid diet is usually ordered immediately or within the first 24 hours postoperatively and increased as tolerated. When solid food is started, it will usually be low in fat. Flatulence or nausea after eating certain foods may persist after surgery; instruct the patient to experiment with different foods.

The patient who undergoes a cholecystectomy must be observed for complications. These include jaundice (from an occluded common duct) and hemorrhage (indicated by decreased blood pressure, increased pulse, and increased exudate at the dressing site). An elevated temperature could indicate peritonitis or wound infection. Pancreatitis may occur after cholecystectomy.

Patients at high risk of not surviving a cholecystectomy may need a cholecystostomy (forming an opening into the gallbladder through the abdominal wall). This can be done using a local anesthetic. The opening provides a means of removing purulent exudate and possibly the stone. It also allows drainage of bile.

Nursing diagnoses and interventions for the patient with open cholecystectomy or cholecystostomy include but are not limited to the following:

Nursing Diagnoses	Nursing Interventions
Ineffective breathing pattern, related to: • pain of high abdominal incision • failure to splint area with coughing and movement	Encourage use of incentive spirometer. Help patient cough and to take 10 deep breaths hourly. Instruct patient on splinting techniques. Turn every 2 hours. Administer analgesics as ordered to facilitate deep breathing and movement. Ambulate as early as possible.

Nursing Diagnoses	Nursing Interventions
Risk for impaired skin integrity, related to: • wound drainage • accidental obstruction of bile drainage	Maintain patency and prevent tension on T-tube. Promote drainage of T-tube by placing patient in low Fowler's to semi-Fowler's position. Observe, describe, and record amount and character of drainage from T-tube at least every 8 hours. Empty bile bag when half full. Clamp T-tube as ordered by physician 3 to 4 days postoperatively. Reinforce primary dressing and observe exudates; change and apply sterile, dry dressing as ordered; use Montgomery straps to secure if drainage is profuse. Cleanse skin thoroughly at insertion site before applying sterile dressing. Apply skin barriers as needed for added protection.

Dietary teaching is necessary for the patient who is treated conservatively for cholecystitis, as well as the patient who undergoes surgery. The patient who is treated conservatively must continue to avoid fatty foods, including fried foods, cream, whole milk, butter, margarine, peanut butter, nuts, chocolate, pastries, and gravies. For the postsurgical patient, provide instructions to try small amounts of foods that previously caused discomfort and gradually eliminate those that continue to do so. The patient can usually resume a normal diet without difficulty.

The patient should understand that stones may recur elsewhere in the biliary system. Teach the patient to identify the signs of complications that should be reported. These include jaundice caused by occlusion or stricture of a duct, hemorrhage or leakage of bile, elevated temperature, pain, and dietary intolerance associated with another attack. The patient should also be able to demonstrate care of the T-tube, if present on discharge; identify activity restrictions; and identify a date for a return visit to the physician.

Prognosis

To prevent complications from cholecystitis or cholelithiasis, assess the patient for signs and symptoms of gangrenous cholecystitis, subphrenic abscess, pancreatitis, cholangitis, biliary cirrhosis, fistulas, and rupture of the gallbladder with bile peritonitis. A stone occluding the common bile duct (choledocholithiasis) may cause obstructive jaundice (Lewis et al., 2007).

Life Span Considerations

Older Adults

Gallbladder, Liver, Biliary Tract, or Exocrine Pancreatic Disorder

- The incidence of cholelithiasis increases with aging. Closely observe older adults with histories of this disease for changes in the color of urine and stool or other signs and symptoms of gallbladder problems.
- As the body ages, the number and size of hepatic cells decreases, which results in an overall reduced size and weight of the liver. The liver also has decreased ability to regenerate after injury or from hepatotoxic injury. Also, a transplanted liver takes longer to regenerate in the older patient (Lewis et al., 2007).
- Older adults have a decrease in protein synthesis in the liver and possible changes in the production of enzymes that assist in the metabolism of drugs, particularly anticonvulsants, psychotropics, and oral anticoagulants.
- Be alert to the signs and symptoms of drug toxicity, even when the drugs are administered in normal doses, because the decreased metabolism in the liver can cause an accumulation of the drug.
- The pancreas exhibits ductal hyperplasia and fibrosis with aging, but these changes are not necessarily associated with altered functioning. The output of pancreatic secretions steadily declines after age 40, but related problems with absorption cannot be documented.

With prompt treatment of cholecystitis and cholelithiasis, the prognosis is excellent. Laparoscopic surgery has further decreased the number of complications. The prognosis is not as favorable in patients who develop pancreatitis (see Life Span Considerations box).

PANCREATITIS

Etiology and Pathophysiology

Pancreatitis is an inflammatory condition of the pancreas that may be acute or chronic. The degree of inflammation varies from mild edema to severe hemorrhagic necrosis. Although the exact cause of pancreatitis remains unknown, many predisposing factors have been identified. Acute or chronic pancreatitis is generally the result of damage to the biliary tract (most common in women), alcohol consumption (most common in men), trauma, infectious disease, or certain drugs. Alcoholism and biliary tract disease are the two factors most commonly associated with pancreatitis. Pancreatitis can develop as a postoperative complication in patients who have had surgery of the pancreas, stomach, duodenum, or biliary tract. Pancreatitis can also occur after undergoing ERCP (see Figure 6-1).

In the pathophysiologic process of pancreatitis, the enzymes cannot flow out of the pancreas because of **occlusion** (an obstruction or closing off) of the pancreatic duct (duct of Wirsung) by edema, stones, or scar tissue. The pancreatic enzymes build up and increase pressure within the duct. The duct ruptures, releasing enzymes that begin digesting the pancreas (autodiges-

tion). In chronic pancreatitis, atrophy of the acinar tissue allows replacement of fibrotic tissue, and the pancreas becomes necrotic.

The development of pseudocysts or abscesses in pancreatic tissue is a serious complication. After autodigestion occurs, the pancreas and occasionally surrounding organs form walls around cystic fluid, including pancreatic enzymes, and necrotic debris. These pseudocysts can develop into an abscess.

Clinical Manifestations

Manifestations include severe abdominal pain radiating to the back. The pain is usually located in the left upper quadrant. The pain is sometimes relieved by leaning forward, taking the stomach weight off the pancreas. Jaundice may be noted if the common bile duct is obstructed.

Assessment

Collection of **subjective data** may include noting that patients exhibit extreme symptoms or none at all. It is difficult to distinguish the symptoms of pancreatitis from those of other abdominal disorders. The most specific complaint is abdominal pain (often excruciating) that radiates to the back (Lewis et al., 2007). The pain is caused by the enlargement of the pancreatic capsule, an obstruction, or chemical irritation from enzymes. The pain is usually decreased by flexing the trunk, leaning forward from a sitting position, or by assuming the fetal position. It is increased by eating or lying down. Other complaints include anorexia, nausea, malaise, and restlessness.

Collection of **objective data** includes noting the presence of low-grade fever, leukocytosis, hypotension, vomiting (in 70% to 90% of patients), jaundice if the common bile duct is obstructed, weight loss, steatorrhea, and tachycardia. Bowel sounds may be decreased or absent. Ileus may occur, causing marked abdominal distention. The lungs are frequently involved, with crackles present (Lewis et al., 2007).

Diagnostic Tests

Both acute and chronic pancreatitis are diagnosed by radiologic studies (abdominal CT scan and ultrasound of the pancreas), endoscopy, and laboratory analysis of the pancreatic enzymes in the serum and urine. Laboratory tests reveal an increased level of serum amylase and lipase during the first few days and increased urine amylase thereafter. In acute pancreatitis the level of serum amylase may become elevated early, within 2 to 36 hours. However, the amylase level is not a specific indicator for pancreatitis; abnormal levels also can be seen in cases of perforated peptic ulcer, perforated bowel, and diabetic ketoacidosis. The level of lipase is more specific for diagnosing acute pancreatitis. The lipase level rises in 4 to 8 hours, peaks at 24 hours, and may remain elevated for 14 days. Amylase and lipase levels may be elevated to 5 to 40 times normal (Holcomb, 2007). Leukocytosis, an elevated hematocrit level, hypocalcemia, hypoalbuminemia, and hyperglycemia may also be present. Pancreatic insulin production may be diminished if the islets of Langerhans become infected, and some patients develop diabetes mellitus.

Medical Management

Treatment is medical unless the precipitating cause is biliary tract disease; then surgery may be indicated. Food and fluids are withheld to avoid stimulating pancreatic activity, and IV fluids are administered. The patient is on NPO status, and an NG tube is inserted to decrease pancreatic stimulation, treat or prevent nausea and vomiting, and decrease abdominal distention. A common complaint is constant, severe pain; morphine is used because of its effective control of pain. Meperidine is no longer the drug of choice because of its toxic metabolite, normeperidine, which can cause seizures; all opioids may cause some spasm of the sphincter of Oddi (Holcomb, 2007). Analgesics may be combined with an antispasmodic.

Parenteral anticholinergic medication, such as atropine or propantheline (Pro-Banthine), helps decrease pancreatic activity. This medication is contraindicated in paralytic ileus. Antacids or antihistamine H_2 receptor antagonists, such as cimetidine, may be given to prevent stress ulcers caused by decreased gastric pH. Some physicians prescribe antibiotics to treat secondary infections.

Enteral feeding is begun 24 to 48 hours after the onset of acute pancreatitis and is administered via the jejunum to prevent the release of pancreatic enzymes. Enteral feeding is preferred to the IV route because it is more nutritionally sound, is less costly, and has fewer complications. However, if enteral feeding is not tolerated in 5 to 7 days, the patient may need to be switched to IV feeding.

A clear liquid diet with gradual progression may be started once the patient's pain is under control for at least 24 hours. Notify the health care provider if the patient does not tolerate oral feedings. If pain returns after oral feeding, again place the patient on NPO status for 24 hours or until the pain has ceased (Holcomb, 2007). The diet must be free of alcohol and gastric stimulants, such as coffee. Oral hypoglycemic agents or insulin may be needed if there is destruction of the islets of Langerhans.

Nursing Interventions and Patient Teaching

Determine the presence and location of pain, as well as what aggravates or relieves the pain. Keep the patient as comfortable as possible through proper administration of analgesic medications. The patient is usually on bed rest with bathroom privileges to decrease the flow of pancreatic enzymes. Nutritional needs are met by enteral feeding via the jejunum as long as necessary. If enteral feedings fail, the patient may need parenteral feedings. The patient who is addicted to alcohol may go through withdrawal while in the hospital. Be prepared

to protect the patient from injury and provide supportive care to the patient and the family. Carefully monitor all replacement fluids and medications for proper administration.

Nursing diagnoses and interventions for the patient with pancreatitis include but are not limited to the following:

Nursing Diagnoses	Nursing Interventions
Pain, related to stimulation of nerve endings caused by enlargement of pancreatic capsule, obstruction, or chemical irritation from enzymes	Administer medications as prescribed and monitor the response. Restrict diet as necessary to prevent aggravation of pain (eliminate fats, alcohol, caffeine). Use alternative comfort measures: repositioning, positive imagery, and time for listening. Monitor NG tube to wall suction for functioning to prevent abdominal distention.
Imbalanced nutrition: less than body requirements, related to: • anorexia • nausea • vomiting • loss of enzymes necessary for the digestive process	Administer enteral feeding via jejunum as ordered. Weigh patient daily at same time and using same scale. Record I&O, including NG tube suctioning output. Administer antacids and antiemetics as prescribed. Instruct patient to follow a diet that is low in fat and high in protein and carbohydrates when tolerated.
Deficient fluid volume, related to: • decreased oral intake • vomiting • diarrhea • NG suctioning • hemorrhage	Monitor I&O; weigh patient daily. Assess hemodynamic stability: pulse, blood pressure. Assess for signs and symptoms of fluid volume deficit: decreased level of consciousness; poor skin turgor; cool, dry, or clammy skin; and weak peripheral pulses. Assess for signs and symptoms of hemorrhage; assess abdominal girth; monitor NG aspirate for occult or frank bleeding. Monitor for the administration of fluid volume replacement.

The patient remains on a low-fat, high-calorie, high-carbohydrate diet after discharge. Alcohol and beverages or foods containing caffeine are not allowed if full recovery is desired. Ensure that the patient understands the disease process and the severity of the disease and related complications.

Prognosis

The prognosis of pancreatitis depends on the course of the disease and complications, including pseudocysts and abscesses. In most patients, acute pancreatitis is mild, requiring less than 1 week of hospitalization. However, 5% to 25% of patients have a more compli-

cated course. The severity of the disease varies according to the extent of pancreatic destruction. Some patients recover completely; others have recurring attacks. Interestingly, complications can occur with mild, acute, chronic, or severe pancreatitis. Mortality rates for acute necrotizing pancreatitis range from 10% to 50% (Table 6-1).

CANCER OF THE PANCREAS

Although once considered relatively rare, pancreatic cancer is now the fourth leading cause of cancer death in the United States and Canada. According to the American Cancer Society, more than 37,000 Americans

Table 6-1   Medications for Disorders of the Gallbladder, Liver, Biliary Tract, and Exocrine Pancreas

Generic (Trade)	Action	Side Effects	Nursing Implications
Gemcitabine hydrochloride (Gemzar)	Exhibits antitumor activity; indicated as first-line treatment of locally advanced or metastatic adenocarcinoma of the pancreas	Myelosuppression; nausea and vomiting, macular papular pruritic rash	Monitor CBC. Provide antiemetic to control nausea and vomiting. Provide relief measures to control pruritus.
Lactulose (Chronulac, Cephulac)	Acidifies colonic contents, thus decreasing absorption of ammonia from gut; also has cathartic laxative properties; primarily used in hepatic encephalopathy	Nausea, vomiting, diarrhea	Titrate dose to 3-4 loose stools per day; monitor for dehydration; monitor for serum ammonia levels and improved mental status.
Spironolactone (Aldactone)	Competes with aldosterone at receptor sites in distal tubule, resulting in excretion of sodium chloride and water and retention of potassium and phosphate; used in cirrhosis of the liver with ascites	Headache, confusion, diarrhea, bleeding, dysrhythmias, impotence, hypokalemia	Assess electrolytes, sodium, chloride, potassium, BUN, serum creatinine. Weigh daily; monitor I&O. Administer in AM to avoid interference with sleep.
Meperidine (Demerol)	Binds to opiate receptors in CNS; alters perception of and response to painful stimuli, while producing generalized CNS depression; used for biliary pain because morphine may cause spasms of the sphincter of Oddi	Sedation, confusion, respiratory depression, hypotension, bradycardia, nausea, vomiting, urinary retention	Assess type, location, intensity of pain before and 1 hour after administration. If respiratory rate is <10 breaths/min, assess level of sedation.
Propantheline (Pro-Banthine)	Antisecretory and antispasmodic agent; slows GI motility through anticholinergic activity; decreases pancreatic activity	Drowsiness, confusion, dry mouth, constipation, urinary retention, tachycardia, blurred vision	Avoid use with other CNS depressants or alcohol; avoid driving or other activities until accustomed to effects; may cause hypotension when given IV; do not use in patients with Parkinson's disease.
Vasopressin (Pitressin)	Synthetic pituitary agent; antidiuretic effects on kidney; a potent vasoconstrictor; used to treat bleeding esophageal varices	Hypertension; ischemia to heart, mesenteric organs, and kidneys; angina; myocardial infarction; water retention; hyponatremia	Use with caution in older adults and in patients with known coronary artery disease or known CHF; discontinue if chest pain develops; monitor urinary output and serum sodium.
Neomycin (Mycifradin, Myciguent)	Inhibits protein synthesis in bacteria at the level of the 30S ribosome; decreases the number of ammonia-producing bacteria in the gut as part of management of hepatic encephalopathy	Ototoxicity; local stinging, burning; nephrotoxicity	Monitor neurologic status and renal function.

BUN, Blood urea nitrogen; *CBC,* complete blood count; *CHF,* congestive heart failure; *CNS,* central nervous system; *GI,* gastrointestinal; *I&O,* intake and output; *IV,* intravenously.

Table 6-1	Medications for Disorders of the Gallbladder, Liver, Biliary Tract, and Exocrine Pancreas—cont'd			
Generic (Trade)	**Action**	**Side Effects**	**Nursing Implications**
Cholestyramine (Questran)	Binds bile acids in the GI tract, forming an insoluble complex; relief of pruritus associated with elevated levels of bile acids	Nausea, constipation, abdominal discomfort	Assess severity of pruritus and skin integrity.
Pancrelipase (Pancrease, Cotazym)	Increased digestion of fats, carbohydrate, and proteins in the GI tract; treatment of pancreatic insufficiency associated with chronic pancreatitis, pancreatectomy	Diarrhea, nausea, stomach cramps, abdominal pain	Assess patient's nutritional status; monitor stools for high fat content; assess patient for allergy to pork; administer immediately before meals or with meals.

were diagnosed with pancreatic cancer during 2007 and approximately 33,000 Americans died of the disease (American Cancer Society, *Facts and figures*, 2007). A major factor in the high death rate from pancreatic cancer is the difficulty in diagnosing it at an early curable stage. The disease usually occurs after middle age. The risk increases with age, with peak incidence occurring between 65 and 80 years of age.

Etiology and Pathophysiology

The cause of pancreatic cancer is unknown, but it is diagnosed more often in cigarette smokers; people exposed to chemical carcinogens; and people with diabetes mellitus, cirrhosis, and pancreatitis. Diets high in red meat and pork (especially processed meat such as bacon), fat, and coffee are also linked to pancreatic cancer. Obese people are 20% more likely to develop pancreatic cancer (Riehl, 2007).

The cancer may originate in the pancreas or be the result of metastasis from cancer of the lung, the stomach, the duodenum, or the common bile duct. Most often the head of the pancreas is involved and causes jaundice by compressing and obstructing the common bile duct. As the cancer spreads, it may invade the posterior wall of the stomach, the duodenal wall, the colon, and the common bile duct. Biliary obstruction and gallbladder dilation are subsequent complications. It is not uncommon for the tumor to grow rapidly and invade the vascular and lymphatic systems. Many patients live only 4 to 8 months after diagnosis.

Clinical Manifestations

The insidious onset of the disease with initially vague symptoms generally accounts for delays in diagnosis. Abdominal pain occurs in about 85% of the patients. About half the patients develop diabetes mellitus if islet cells are involved.

Assessment

A psychosocial history during patient assessment may reveal at-risk populations such as engineers, coal- and gas-plant employees, chemists, and workers exposed to beta-naphthol and benzidine. **Subjective data** include anorexia; fatigue; nausea; flatulence; a change in stools; and steady, dull, and aching pain in the epigastrium or referred to the back. The pain is usually worse at night.

Objective data include weight loss, often gradual and progressive, which is one of the earliest signs. Jaundice usually is progressive and may occur late. Pruritus accompanies the jaundice. Many patients have recent onset of diabetes mellitus.

Diagnostic Tests

Diagnosis of pancreatic cancer is based on the patient's history, signs and symptoms, and diagnostic studies. Better diagnostic measures are needed for detection of pancreatic cancer because most of the current methods detect only advanced stages. Diagnostic studies include transabdominal ultrasound and CT, duodenal endoscopy to obtain specimens for cytologic examination, ERCP, and pancreatic scans. ERCP is the gold standard for visualization of the pancreatic duct and biliary system. With ERCP, pancreatic secretions and tissues can be collected for analysis of different tumor markers (see Figure 6-1).

The level of the tumor marker cancer-associated antigen CA 19-9 is elevated in patients with pancreatic cancer. It is the most commonly used tumor marker to diagnose pancreatic adenocarcinoma and to monitor the patient's response to treatment. However, CA 19-9 can be elevated in other diseases such as cancer of the gallbladder or in nonmalignant conditions such as acute and chronic pancreatitis, hepatitis, and biliary duct obstruction (Riehl, 2007).

Medical Management

Often, malignant tumors of the pancreas are inoperable by the time they are diagnosed. Treatment of pancreatic cancer is primarily surgical and has been associated with a high mortality rate. Cancer of the head of the pancreas is usually treated by pancreatoduodenectomy; the Whipple procedure involves resection of the antrum of the stomach, the gallbladder, the duodenum, and varying amounts of the pancreas. Anastomoses are constructed between the stomach, the common bile duct and the pancreatic ducts, and the jejunum (Figure 6-9). In most cases, this procedure is performed by surgeons who are specially trained and experienced.

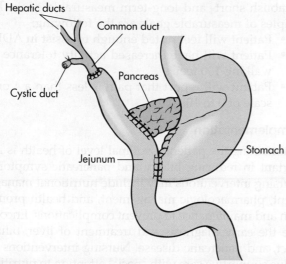

FIGURE 6-9 Whipple procedure, or radical pancreaticoduodenectomy. This surgical procedure involves resection of the proximal pancreas, adjoining duodenum, distal portion of the stomach, and distal portion of the common bile duct. The pancreatic duct, common bile ducts, and stomach are anastomosed to the jejunum.

Another procedure is total pancreatectomy with resection of parts of the GI tract. Subtotal pancreatic resection has complications of postoperative pancreatic fistulas and is not recommended.

Combinations of drugs such as fluorouracil and gemcitabine (Gemzar) may produce a better response than a single chemotherapeutic agent. Gemcitabine is a main treatment for pancreatic cancer that has metastasized. The current role of chemotherapy in pancreatic cancer is limited. Adjuvant therapy—using surgical resection, radiation, and chemotherapy—is believed by some to be the most effective way to manage the almost always fatal cancer of the pancreas.

Nursing Interventions and Patient Teaching

Pancreatic surgery is radical and requires critical care nursing. Postoperative care focuses on maintaining fluid and electrolyte balance, preventing hemorrhage, preventing respiratory complications, and monitoring endocrine and exocrine functions of the pancreas.

Patients with pancreatic cancer may have acute and chronic pain. The patient may receive long-acting opioid analgesics for chronic pain, supplemented by quick-acting opioids for breakthrough pain. A method for providing effective temporary pain relief is to inject corticosteroids and analgesics via a celiac plexus nerve block (Riehl, 2007).

The health care provider caring for the patient with pancreatic cancer must offer compassionate physical and emotional assistance. Refer the patient and the family to social services and support groups. When the patient stops active therapy for the cancer, provide the patient and the family with information about hospice care (Riehl, 2007).

Nursing diagnoses and interventions for patients with cancer of the pancreas include but are not limited to the following:

Nursing Diagnoses	Nursing Interventions
Risk for deficient fluid volume, related to possible hemorrhage and drainage	Maintain patency of GI tubes to relieve distention and compression at the surgical site. Measure I&O and weigh daily. Monitor IV fluid replacement. Assess for signs and symptoms of dehydration (dry mucous membranes, poor skin turgor, oliguria).
Risk for impaired skin integrity, related to drainage from wound	Monitor for excoriation and infection; use skin barriers and disposable postoperative pouches and appliances to prevent enzymatic contact with the skin and to aid in the accurate collection and measurement of pancreatic drainage.

The patient is facing a life-threatening illness, and family members and close friends are important for the patient's well-being. If the patient has an inadequate support system, it is important to use the resources that are available. The hospital chaplain or a personal minister, the social worker, the dietitian, the physician, and the nurse can become a support system. These members of the health care team can provide active listening and a caring attitude for this patient.

Prognosis

The prognosis for patients with cancer of the pancreas is very poor. Median survival after diagnosis is only 5 to 12 months. The 5-year survival rate remains less than 10%. Resection of the tumor improves median survival to 17 to 20 months. Prognosis is related to the tumor's location.

❖NURSING PROCESS *for the Patient with Gallbladder, Liver, Biliary Tract, or Exocrine Pancreatic Disorder*

The role of the licensed practical nurse/licensed vocational nurse (LPN/LVN) in the nursing process as stated is that the LPN/LVN will:

- Participate in planning care for patients based on patient needs
- Review patient's care plan and recommend revisions as needed
- Review and follow defined prioritization for patient care
- Use clinical pathways, care maps, or care plans to guide and review patient care

▪ Assessment

Nursing assessment of the patient with a gallbladder, liver, biliary tract, or exocrine pancreatic disorder must be performed accurately. Perform a head-to-toe assessment. Also assess the patient's knowledge of the disease process, nutritional status, pain, discomfort, current health problems, and signs and symptoms. Note changes in appetite and weight. Measure vital signs, noting any alterations from normal, such as hyperthermia, hypotension, hypertension, tachycardia, or tachypnea. Observe the skin, the sclerae, the mucous membranes, the urine, and the stool for alterations in the presence of bilirubin. Inspect, auscultate, and palpate the abdomen. Document any abdominal tenderness, pain, or abnormal bowel sounds.

▪ Nursing Diagnosis

Assessment provides data for identifying the patient's problems, strengths, potential complications, and learning needs. Nursing diagnoses for patients with disorders of the liver, biliary tract, or exocrine pancreas include but are not limited to the following:

- Activity intolerance
- Ineffective breathing pattern
- Deficient fluid volume
- Impaired home maintenance
- Risk for injury
- Deficient knowledge
- Noncompliance
- Imbalanced nutrition: less than body requirements
- Acute pain
- Chronic pain
- Powerlessness
- Impaired skin integrity
- Acute confusion

▪ Expected Outcomes and Planning

When planning care, look at the nursing diagnosis and establish the cause of the nursing problem. The overall goals for patients with disorders of the gallbladder, liver, biliary tract, and exocrine pancreas include (1) relief of pain and discomfort; (2) stabilization of fluid and electrolyte balance; (3) minimal to no complications; (4) ability to resume normal activities; (5) a return, if possible, to normal pancreatic and liver function without complications; and (6) a return to as normal a lifestyle as possible.

Planning includes the development of realistic goals and outcomes from the identified nursing diagnoses.

Establish short- and long-term measurable goals. Examples of measurable goals are the following:

- Patient will feel rested enough to assist in ADLs.
- Patient will have increased activity tolerance by walking 100 feet.
- Patient will report that pain is less than a 4 on a scale of 0 to 10.

▪ Implementation

Maintaining the patient's optimal level of health is important in reducing biliary and pancreatic symptoms. Nursing interventions may include nutritional management, pharmacologic management, and health promotion and maintenance to prevent complications. Encourage the early diagnosis and treatment of liver, biliary tract, and pancreatic disease. Nursing interventions involve supportive care with special attention to nutrition, hydration, skin care, and pain relief.

▪ Evaluation

During and after the planned nursing interventions, determine the outcomes of the interventions. This is an ongoing process of continually trying to establish the most effective care plan.

Evaluation involves determining whether the established goals have been met. Involve the patient in evaluating the goals to see whether the criteria for measurement have been met. Goals and evaluative measures for disorders of the liver, biliary tract, and exocrine pancreas may include the following:

Goal 1: Patient achieves improved activity tolerance.
Evaluative measure: Observe patient exercise.
Goal 2: Patient remains free of bodily injury.
Evaluative measure: Ask patient to list factors that increase the risk of injury.
See Cultural Considerations box.

 Cultural Considerations

Gallbladder, Liver, Biliary Tract, or Exocrine Pancreatic Disorder

- Mortality from cirrhosis occurs more frequently among blacks than in other ethnic groups.
- Primary hepatic cancer has a higher incidence among blacks, Asian Americans, and Inuit (Eskimos) than among whites.
- Pancreatic cancer occurs more frequently among blacks and Asian Americans than among whites.
- Whites and Native Americans have a higher incidence of gallbladder disease than blacks and Asian Americans.

Get Ready for the NCLEX® Examination!

Key Points

- Planned nursing interventions must be individualized according to each patient's and family's unique needs.
- The most common cause of cirrhosis of the liver is alcohol ingestion.
- Clinical manifestations of cirrhosis of the liver differ, depending on whether the patient is in the early or later stages of the disease.
- An important aspect of nursing interventions in patients with hepatitis and cirrhosis of the liver is the relief of pruritus.
- Prevention of the spread of viral hepatitis is a primary concern of health care professionals.
- Vaccine is now available to prevent the development of hepatitis A and hepatitis B.
- If an infection develops anywhere along the GI tract, there is danger that the infecting organism may reach the liver through the biliary system, portal venous system, or hepatic arterial or lymphatic system and result in a liver abscess.
- Cholecystectomy (removal of the gallbladder by means of laparoscopic or open abdominal procedure) is one of the most commonly performed surgical procedures.
- Pancreatic disorders may cause diabetes mellitus because of interference with insulin production.
- Clinical manifestations of acute pancreatitis include severe abdominal pain radiating to the back; the pain is sometimes relieved when the patient leans forward, taking the weight of the stomach off the pancreas.
- Tumor markers are used both for establishing the diagnosis of pancreatic adenocarcinoma and monitoring the response to treatment of cancer; CA 19-9 is elevated in pancreatic cancer and is the most commonly used tumor marker.

Additional Learning Resources

Go to your Companion CD for an audio glossary, animations, video clips, and more.

evolve Be sure to visit the Evolve site at http://evolve.elsevier.com/Christensen/adult/ for additional online resources.

Review Questions for the NCLEX® Examination

1. Nurses, as well as other health care providers, are at risk for hepatitis B. For prophylaxis to be most effective in these workers:

   1. prophylaxis must be instituted before exposure.
   2. prophylaxis can be instituted either before or after exposure.
   3. prophylaxis must be instituted after exposure.
   4. prophylaxis instituted before or after exposure is effective forever.

2. Liver needle biopsy is a safe method of diagnosing pathologic liver conditions. However, the nurse must anticipate possible complications, including which nursing diagnosis?

   1. Pain, related to leakage of blood and bile into the peritoneal cavity
   2. Noncompliance of medications, related to testing procedure
   3. Social isolation, related to tissue sample removal for biopsy
   4. Disturbed sleep pattern, related to lack of information on hospital protocol

3. A 78-year-old patient is admitted with common bile duct obstruction related to cancer of the pancreas. Which clinical manifestations would the nurse expect to find? (Select all that apply.)

   1. Brown feces
   2. Scleral icterus
   3. Dark, tea-colored urine
   4. Jaundice

4. It is especially important for the patient to cough and breathe deeply postoperatively following an open cholecystectomy because:

   1. the patient is often obese.
   2. the patient usually smokes.
   3. the patient is on bed rest for a prolonged period.
   4. the patient tends to take shallow breaths due to the placement of the incision.

5. In hepatic encephalopathy, when the nurse requests that the patient stretch out the arm and hyperextend the wrist with fingers separated, relaxed, and extended to see whether rapid, irregular flexion and extension (flapping) of the wrist occur, the nurse is assessing for the presence of:

   1. varices.
   2. asterixis.
   3. pruritus.
   4. bacterial toxins.

6. The patient has advanced cirrhosis of the liver with an acute exacerbation of hepatic encephalopathy. What type of food might be limited in his diet?

   1. Fruits
   2. Vegetables
   3. Meats
   4. Carbohydrates

7. Patients with liver abscess are seen with vague signs and symptoms, which are often:

   1. asterixis, ascites, and esophageal varices.
   2. fever accompanied by chills, abdominal pain, and tenderness in the right upper quadrant.
   3. enlarged spleen and spider telangiectases.
   4. constipation; left quadrant abdominal cramping; and loud, high-pitched abdominal sounds on auscultation.

8. A small number of patients who have had a laparoscopic cholecystectomy report mild shoulder pain resulting from:
   1. paralytic ileus with mesenteric irritation.
   2. incision along the rectus abdominis muscle.
   3. diaphragmatic irritation secondary to residual carbon dioxide.
   4. spasm of the duct of Wirsung.

9. The patient has been admitted with right upper quadrant pain and has been placed on a low-fat diet. Which of the following trays would be acceptable for her?
   1. Whole milk, veal, rice, and pastry
   2. Liver, fried potatoes, gelatin, and avocado
   3. Skim milk, lean fish, tapioca pudding, and fruit
   4. Ham, mashed potatoes, creamed peas, and gelatin

10. Hepatitis types B, C, D, and G are spread mainly through the following: *(Select all that apply.)*
    1. Blood transfusions
    2. Contaminated needles and instruments
    3. Direct contact with body fluids from infected people, such as through breast milk and sexual contact
    4. Oral-fecal route

11. In patients with acute pancreatitis, the analgesic meperidine is no longer the opioid of choice because of:
    1. paralytic ileus.
    2. increased possibility of addiction.
    3. urinary retention.
    4. its toxic metabolite, normeperidine, which can cause seizures.

12. A patient is scheduled for surgery for a common bile duct exploration. The nurse would expect the patient to return from surgery with:
    1. an underwater-seal drainage.
    2. a T-tube connected to gravity drainage.
    3. a Penrose drain.
    4. a nephrostomy tube.

13. Which types of hepatitis now have vaccines for prevention?
    1. B only
    2. B and D
    3. A and B
    4. A, B, C, D, E, and G

14. Nursing interventions for the patient with cholecystitis associated with cholelithiasis are based on the knowledge that:
    1. the disorder can be successfully treated with oral bile salts that dissolve gallstones.
    2. analgesics are usually not necessary to relieve the pain of bile duct spasms during an acute attack.
    3. a heavy meal with a high fat content may precipitate the signs and symptoms of the disease.
    4. a low-cholesterol diet is indicated to reduce the availability of cholesterol for gallstone formation.

15. Teaching in relation to home management following a laparoscopic cholecystectomy should include:
    1. keeping the bandages on the puncture sites for 48 hours.
    2. reporting any bile-colored drainage or pus from any incision.
    3. using over-the-counter antiemetics if nausea and vomiting occur.
    4. emptying and measuring the contents of the bile bag from the T-tube every day.

16. A patient with advanced cirrhosis asks the nurse why his abdomen is so swollen. The nurse's response is based on the knowledge that:
    1. a lack of clotting factors promotes the collection of blood in the abdominal cavity.
    2. portal hypertension and hypoalbuminemia cause a fluid shift into the peritoneal space.
    3. decreased peristalsis in the GI tract contributes to gas formation and bowel distention.
    4. bile salts in the blood irritate the peritoneal membranes, causing edema and pocketing of fluid.

17. When caring for a patient with acute exacerbation of hepatic encephalopathy, the nurse may give a lactulose enema, provide a low-protein diet, and limit physical activity. These measures are done to:
    1. promote fluid loss.
    2. eliminate potassium ions.
    3. decrease portal pressure.
    4. decrease ammonia production.

18. In planning care for a patient with metastatic cancer of the liver, the nurse includes interventions that:
    1. focus primarily on symptomatic and comfort measures.
    2. reassure the patient that chemotherapy offers a good prognosis for recovery.
    3. promote the patient's confidence that surgical excision of the tumor will be successful.
    4. provide information necessary for the patient to make decisions regarding liver transplantation.

19. Patients who receive a liver transplant secondary to viral B or C hepatitis often experience
    _____ or _____
    of the transplanted liver.

20. If a patient is scheduled for an ultrasound of the pancreas, which two situations would cause the examination to be postponed?
    1. Technetium-99m injected into biliary tract, low serum albumin
    2. CT of abdomen, elevated amylase
    3. ERCP examination, elevated LDH
    4. Abdomen distended with gas, recent barium enema examination

21. The surgical procedure for cancer of the pancreas involves resection of the antrum of the stomach, the gallbladder, the duodenum, and varying amounts of the pancreas. Anastomoses are constructed between the stomach, the common bile and pancreatic ducts, and the jejunum. This procedure is called:

   1. Whipple procedure.
   2. pancreatectomy.
   3. Billroth I.
   4. Billroth II.

22. A major factor in the high death rate from pancreatic cancer is: *(Select all that apply.)*

   1. difficulty in diagnosing it at an early curable stage.
   2. denial on the part of the patient.
   3. the majority of cancers have metastasized at the time of diagnosis.
   4. tumors starting in the body or tail often remain silent until their growth is advanced.

23. The patient with cirrhosis has bleeding tendencies because the cirrhotic liver cannot:

   1. produce RBCs and vitamin K.
   2. produce prothrombin; fibrinogen; and clotting factors VII, IX, and X, or absorb vitamin K.
   3. produce erythropoietin, reticulocytes, and fibrin.
   4. manufacture vitamins E, C, A, and K.

24. Monitoring the color of stools of a patient with hepatitis A is important. The nurse caring for such a patient would expect the stools to be:

   1. dark brown.
   2. black.
   3. clay colored (acholic).
   4. green.

25. Laboratory values that are often abnormal in a patient with liver disease include: *(Select all that apply.)*

   1. gamma GT.
   2. alkaline phosphatase.
   3. total bilirubin.
   4. CEA, AST.
   5. CA 125.

26. A 56-year-old patient has cirrhosis of the liver. He has an accumulation of serous fluid in the abdominal cavity called ascites. The nurse is assisting the physician in the procedure to remove this fluid from his abdominal cavity. This procedure is called an:

   1. abdominal paracephalus.
   2. abdominal paracentesis.
   3. abdominal thoracentesis.
   4. abdominal perimetrium.

27. The patient has acute pancreatitis. The diagnostic examination that would probably be ordered would include: *(Select all that apply.)*

   1. serum amylase and lipase, ultrasound of pancreas.
   2. fecal studies, prothrombin time.
   3. CEA, CBC.
   4. urine, amylase.

28. The patient was scheduled for a laparoscopic cholecystectomy. Complications developed during surgery, and he underwent an open cholecystectomy with a T-tube inserted into the common bile duct. The purposes of the T-tube are to:

   1. decrease abdominal distention and increase peristalsis.
   2. improve diaphragmatic expansion and prevent atelectasis.
   3. shorten postoperative recovery and hasten healing process.
   4. keep the common bile duct open until edema resolves, and allow drainage of bile into drainage bag.

29. The patient has a history of cholelithiasis. He has excruciating pain in the right upper quadrant radiating to the scapula, and severe nausea and vomiting; within a few hours he develops early signs of jaundice. The physician suspects:

   1. obstruction choledocholithiasis.
   2. cirrhosis of the liver.
   3. cancer of the pancreas.
   4. asterixis.

Care of the Patient with a Blood or Lymphatic Disorder

Objectives

Anatomy and Physiology

1. Describe the components of blood.
2. Differentiate between the functions of erythrocytes, leukocytes, and thrombocytes.
3. Discuss factors necessary for the formation of erythrocytes.
4. Define the white blood cell differential.
5. Describe the blood clotting process.
6. List the basic blood groups.
7. Describe the generalized functions of the lymphatic system and list the primary lymphatic structures.

Medical-Surgical

8. List common diagnostic tests for evaluation of blood and lymph disorders, and discuss the significance of the results.
9. Compare and contrast the different types of anemia in terms of etiology and pathophysiology, clinical manifestations, assessment, diagnostic tests, medical management, nursing interventions, patient teaching, and prognosis.
10. List six signs and symptoms associated with hypovolemic shock.

11. Discuss important issues to cover in patient teaching and home care planning for the patient with pernicious anemia.
12. Discuss the etiology and pathophysiology, clinical manifestations, assessment, diagnostic tests, medical management, nursing interventions, patient teaching, and prognosis for patients with acute and chronic leukemia.
13. Compare and contrast the disorders of coagulation (thrombocytopenia, hemophilia, disseminated intravascular coagulation) in terms of etiology and pathophysiology, clinical manifestations, assessment, diagnostic tests, medical management, nursing interventions, and prognosis.
14. Discuss the etiology and pathophysiology, clinical manifestations, assessment, diagnostic tests, medical management, nursing interventions, patient teaching, and prognosis for the patient with multiple myeloma, malignant lymphoma, and Hodgkin's lymphoma.
15. Discuss the primary goal of nursing interventions for the patient with lymphedema.
16. Apply the nursing process to the care of the patient with disorders of the hematological and lymphatic systems.

KEY TERMS

anemia (ă-NĒ-mē-ă, p. 269)

aplasia (ă-PLĀ-zhă, p. 273)

disseminated intravascular coagulation (DIC) (dĭ-SĔM-ĭ-nāt-ĕd, p. 289)

erythrocytosis (ĕ-rĭth-rō-sī-TŌ-sĭs, p. 279)

erythropoiesis (ĕ-rĭth-rō-pō-Ē-sĭs, p. 265)

hemarthrosis (hē-măr-THRŌ-sĭs, p. 287)

hemophilia A (hē-mō-FĒL-ē-ă, p. 287)

heterozygous (hĕt-ĕr-ō-ZĪ-gŭs, p. 277)

homozygous (hō-mō-ZĪ-gŭs, p. 276)

idiopathic (ĭd-ē-ō-PĂTH-ĭk, p. 273)

leukemia (lū-kĒ-mē-ă, p. 282)

leukopenia (lū-kō-PĒ-nē-ă, p. 281)

lymphangitis (lĭm-făn-GĪ-tĭs, p. 292)

lymphedema (lĭm-fĕ-DĒ-mă, p. 293)

multiple myeloma (MŬL-tĭ-pŭl mī-ĕ-LŌ-mă, p. 291)

myeloproliferative (mī-ĕ-lō-prō-LĬF-ĕr-ă-tĭv, p. 279)

pancytopenic (păn-sī-tō-PĔN-ĭc, p. 273)

pernicious (pĕr-NĬSH-ŭs, p. 272)

Reed-Sternberg cells (rēd-STĔRN-bĕrg, p. 294)

thrombocytopenia (thrŏm-bō-sīt-ō-PĒ-nē-ă, p. 286)

ANATOMY AND PHYSIOLOGY OF THE HEMATOLOGIC AND LYMPHATIC SYSTEMS

Transportation and protection are two of the body's most important functions. Without transportation and protection for the cells, the body's homeostasis would be threatened. The systems that provide these vital services for the body are the circulatory and lymphatic systems. This chapter discusses the primary transportation fluid—blood—and presents an overview of the lymphatic system. Blood not only performs vital transportation ser-

vices, but also provides much of the protection necessary to withstand foreign invaders. The lymphatic system helps maintain fluid balance, and lymphoid tissues help protect the internal environment.

CHARACTERISTICS OF BLOOD

In ancient times, blood was referred to as the "river of life" or "fluid of life." Some people believed it had magical properties. All knew it was necessary to maintain life.

Blood is a viscous (thick), red fluid that contains red blood cells (RBCs), white blood cells (WBCs), and platelets, which are suspended in a light yellow fluid called **plasma**. Plasma constitutes 55% of the blood's volume; the remaining 45% is composed of the blood cells and platelets (Figure 7-1). Blood is slightly alka-line, with a pH range of 7.35 to 7.45. It has a sodium chloride concentration of 0.9%. The average adult blood volume is 5 to 6 L (10½ to 12½ pints).

The blood performs three critical functions. First, it transports oxygen and nutrition to the cells and waste products away from the cells, and it transports hormones from endocrine glands to tissues and cells. Second, it regulates the acid-base balance (pH) with buffers, helps regulate body temperature because of its water content, and controls the water content of its cells as a result of dissolved sodium ions. Third, it protects the body against infection with special cells and prevents blood loss with special clotting mechanisms.

The following sections discuss individual components of the blood.

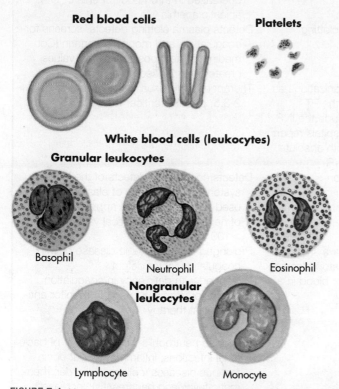

FIGURE 7-1 Human blood cells. There are approximately 30 trillion blood cells in an adult. Each cubic millimeter of blood contains from 4.5 million to 5 million red blood cells, 5000 to 10,000 white blood cells, and 150,000 to 400,000 platelets.

Red Blood Cells

Erythrocytes (RBCs) give blood its rich color. In men, RBCs average approximately 5.5 million/mm^3 of blood; in women, they average approximately 4.8 million/mm^3 (Table 7-1). A mature RBC contains cytoplasm and the red pigment hemoglobin, a compound in the blood that carries oxygen from the lungs to the cells and carbon dioxide away from the cells to the lungs. Erythrocytes are classified according to size, shape, and color. Hemoglobin content is expressed as normochromic or hypochromic anemia, whereas RBC size is usually expressed as macrocytic, microcytic, or normocytic. The normal hemoglobin level is 14 to 18 g/dL for men and 12 to 16 g/dL for women. The average life span of an RBC is 120 days. An erythrocyte is the major cellular element of the circulating blood; its principal function is to transport oxygen and carbon dioxide. Erythrocytes are continuously produced in the red bone marrow,

Table 7-1 | Diagnostic Blood Studies

BLOOD TEST	NORMAL VALUES	DESCRIPTION	CLINICAL SIGNIFICANCE
Red blood cells (RBCs)	Males: 4.7-6.1 million/mm^3 Females: 4.2-5.4 million/mm^3	Actual cell count	Increased in dehydration, with polycythemia, at high altitudes, and with hypoxia; decreased in anemia, leukemia, and posthemorrhage
Hemoglobin	Males: 14-18 g/dL Females: 12-16 g/dL	Measure of total amount of hemoglobin (Hgb) in peripheral blood	Increased in polycythemia, dehydration, chronic obstructive lung disease; decreased in anemia and after hemorrhage
Hematocrit	Males: 42%-52% Females: 37%-47%	Measure of the percentage of the total blood volume that is made up by the RBCs	Increased with severe burns, shock, severe dehydration, and polycythemia; decreased with severe blood loss, leukemia, and anemia
Erythrocyte sedimentation rate (ESR)	Male: 0-15 mm/hr Female: 0-20 mm/hr	Rate at which RBCs settle out of a tube of unclotted blood in 1 hour	Increased in tissue destruction; indicates infection when results are compared with elevation in WBC count; a fairly reliable indicator of the course of disease and therefore used to monitor disease therapy, especially for inflammatory autoimmune diseases

Continued

Table 7-1	Diagnostic Blood Studies—cont'd		
BLOOD TEST	**NORMAL VALUES**	**DESCRIPTION**	**CLINICAL SIGNIFICANCE**
Reticulocyte count	0.5%-2%	Number of reticulocytes in whole blood	Increased in bone marrow hyperactivity and hemorrhage; decreased in hemolytic disease
Platelet count	150,000-400,000/mm³	Actual cell count	Increased in granulocytic leukemia; decreased in thrombocytopenia or aplastic anemia
Prothrombin time (PT)	11-12.5 seconds	Rapidity of blood clotting	Detects plasma clotting defects, screens for coagulation, and monitors warfarin (Coumadin) therapy; possible critical values greater than 20 seconds
International Normalized Ratio (INR)	0.7-1.8	World Health Organization has recommended the PT results now include the INR value; many hospitals report PT results in both absolute numbers and INR	Therapeutic INR usually considered to be 2-3.5; possible critical values >3.5
Partial thromboplastin time (PTT)	60-70 seconds	Fibrin clot formation	Detects coagulation defects of the intrinsic system and deficiency of plasma clotting; used for monitoring the appropriate dose of heparin; possible critical values >100 seconds
Bleeding time	1-9 minutes (Ivy method)	Amount of time for a small stab wound to stop bleeding	Prolonged in hemorrhagic disease or with coagulation factor defect
Clotting time	3-9 minutes	Amount of time for blood in a tube to clot	Prolonged with deficiency in coagulation factors or vitamin K; used to monitor anticoagulant therapy
WHITE BLOOD CELLS (WBCs) COUNT WITH DIFFERENTIAL			
WBC	5000-10,000/mm³	Actual cell count	Increased neutrophils with a number of bacterial infections, inflammatory but noninfectious diseases (collagen disorder, rheumatic fever, and pancreatitis); increased with infectious diseases (usually of bacterial origin) and with trauma or leukemia; decreased by chemotherapy, radiation, aplastic anemia, and agranulocytosis
Neutrophils	60%-70%* 3000-7000/mm³†		Increased with burns, crushing injuries, diabetic acidosis, and infections; decreased in bone marrow failure following antineoplastic chemotherapy or radiation therapy or in agranulocytosis, dietary deficiencies, and autoimmune diseases
Eosinophils	1%-4%* 50-400/mm³†		Increased with allergic and parasitic disorders
Basophils	0.5%-1%* 25-100/mm³†		Increases uncommon; found with some forms of acute leukemia
Lymphocytes	20%-40%* 1000-4000/mm³†		Increased in infectious mononucleosis, measles, certain viruses, infectious hepatitis, and lymphocytic leukemia; decreased in AIDS, lupus erythematosus, and Hodgkin's disease
Monocytes	2%-6%* 100-600/mm³†		Increased in the recovery phase of bacterial infections and chronic inflammatory conditions

AIDS, Acquired immunodeficiency syndrome.
*Relative values: expressed as percentage of total WBC.
†Absolute values: expressed in actual numbers × 10⁹/mm³.

principally in the vertebrae, ribs, sternum, and proximal ends of the humerus and femur.

Erythropoiesis (the process of RBC production) depends on several factors, among them healthy conditions of the bone marrow; dietary substances such as iron and copper, plus essential amino acids; and certain vitamins, especially vitamin B_{12}, folic acid, riboflavin (vitamin B_2), and pyridoxine (vitamin B_6). When the amount of oxygen delivered to the tissues by RBCs is decreased, it triggers the release of an enzyme, the renal erythropoietic factor, in the kidneys. Erythropoietin is carried to the bone marrow, where it initiates the development of mature RBCs. The increased number of RBCs allows more oxygen to be delivered to the tissues, and as a result shuts off the signal to increase RBC production.

A common laboratory test called the **hematocrit** (a measure of the packed cell volume of RBCs, expressed as a percentage of the total blood volume) can tell a great deal about the volume of RBCs in a blood sample. Normally about 42% to 52% of the blood volume in men and 37% to 47% in women consists of RBCs.

If hemoglobin falls below the normal level, as it does in anemia, an unhealthy chain reaction begins: less hemoglobin means less oxygen transported to cells, a slower breakdown and use of nutrients by cells, less energy produced by cells, and decreased cellular function. Understanding the relationship between hemoglobin and energy makes it clear why an anemic person complains of feeling "tired all the time."

White Blood Cells

Unlike erythrocytes, **leukocytes** (WBCs) have nuclei, are colorless, and live from a few days to several years. They are primarily involved in body defenses, such as destruction of bacteria and viruses. They number 5000 to 10,000/mm³ of blood. Some WBCs can actually leave the bloodstream and move through tissue spaces to fight foreign invaders, such as bacteria. WBCs have two broad categories: granulocytes and nongranulocytes. The three types of granulocytes are neutrophils, eosinophils, and basophils. The nongranulocytes include lymphocytes and monocytes. A **differential white blood cell count** is an examination in which the different kinds of WBCs are counted and reported as percentages of the total examined. They also may be reported as absolute (actual number) (see Figure 7-1).

Because leukocytes respond predictably to symptoms of infection and recovery, they are a reliable gauge of the state of the body's defenses. That is why the differential WBC is such a common blood test. Although the differential WBC cannot, by itself, be used to diagnose a disease or to discriminate between a bacterial and viral infection, it reveals activity that points to occult (hidden) infection or that signals the intensity of chemotherapy.

The granulocytes develop from the red bone marrow and contain granules in their cytoplasm. The granules are demonstrated when the cells are stained with Wright's stain (a chemical solution). **Neutrophils** (granular circulating leukocytes essential for **phagocytosis**— the process by which bacteria, cellular debris, and solid particles are destroyed and removed) ingest bacteria and dispose of dead tissue. Neutrophils are the primary phagocytic cells involved in acute inflammatory response. A mature neutrophil is called a segmental neutrophil, or "seg," because the nucleus is segmented into two to five lobes connected by strands. They also release lysozyme, an enzyme that destroys certain bacteria. The normal value of neutrophils is 60% to 70%.

Mature neutrophils have a short life span (approximately 7 hours), after which they die, along with the bacteria and debris they have engulfed. Bone marrow thus needs to manufacture neutrophils constantly; normally it stores approximately a 6-day supply. Because neutrophils respond in proportion to the severity of the infection, an overwhelming infection may deplete marrow reserves. When this happens, the marrow releases polymorphonuclear leukocytes ("polys") that are in the final stages of development. These immature neutrophils are called bands. When the band count exceeds 8% of the total number of polys, the marrow has used up its reserve. In the differential white count, an increase in the number of band neutrophils is called **bandemia**. Bandemia is seen in patients with serious bacterial infections. The presence of excess bands in the peripheral blood was traditionally called "a shift to the left." This term originated when laboratory reports were handwritten with the immature neutrophils recorded on the left side of paper. This term is still used in some areas (McCarron, 2004).

Eosinophils are WBCs that play a role in allergic reactions and are effective against certain parasitic worms. Normal values of eosinophils are 1% to 4%.

Basophils are WBCs that are essential to the non-specific immune response to inflammation because they release histamine (vasodilator) during tissue damage or invasion. They have cytoplasmic granules that contain heparin, serotonin, and histamine. If a basophil is stimulated by an antigen or by tissue injury, it releases substances within the granules. This is part of the response seen in allergic and inflammatory reactions. Normal values of basophils are 0.5% to 1%.

Monocytes are WBCs that function like neutrophils; they circulate in the bloodstream and move into tissue, where they engulf foreign antigens and cell debris. Monocytes are the second type of WBC to arrive at the scene of an injury. They are useful in removing dead bacteria and cells in the recovery stage of acute bacterial infections. Normal values of monocytes are 2% to 6%.

Lymphocytes are WBCs that form antibody, a special protein that combats foreign invaders, or antigens. They set up the antigen-antibody process, which protects the body. Lymphocytes have two groups: B cells and T cells. B cells search out, identify, and bind with specific antigens. T cells, when exposed to an antigen, divide rapidly and produce large numbers of new

T cells that are sensitized to that antigen. T cells work together with the B cells to destroy the foreign antigen. Normal values of lymphocytes are 20% to 40%.

Thrombocytes (Platelets)

Thrombocytes, or platelets, are the smallest cells in the blood. They are circular cell fragments that do not contain nuclei. They have a life span of 5 to 9 days and number 150,000 to 400,000/mm³ of blood (see Figure 7-1). They are produced in the red bone marrow and have a role in the process of hemostasis (the prevention of blood loss). They assist in forming clots, which seal off a break in the continuity of the walls of the blood vessels (Figure 7-2).

Hemostasis

Hemostasis is a body process that arrests the flow of blood and prevents hemorrhage. Three actions take place: (1) vessel spasm, (2) platelet plug formation, and (3) clot formation. When a vessel has a tear or rupture, the smooth muscle in the walls of the vessel causes it to contract. Platelets rush in and attempt to seal the area, which is effective in small vessel tears. The third process, clot formation, is more detailed and occurs in larger injuries. This process can be summarized as follows (see Figure 7-2):

1. Injury
2. Hemorrhage
3. Grouping platelets
4. Thromboplastin released (reacts along with calcium ions)
5. Converts prothrombin to thrombin
6. Links with fibrinogen
7. Formation of fibrin
8. Traps RBCs and platelets
9. Forms clot

Blood Types (Groups)

A person's blood group or type is genetically determined and is inherited from his or her parents. Blood types are determined by the presence or absence of specific antigens on the outer surface of the RBCs. In certain types of blood, the antigens on the RBCs are accompanied by antibodies found in the blood plasma. In the ABO system, every person's blood is one of the following types: type **A**, type **B**, type **AB**, or type **O**.

Forty-one percent of Americans have type A blood. The letter *A* stands for a certain type of antigen in the plasma membrane of the RBCs at birth. A person who is born with type A antigen does not form antibodies to react with it. In other words, this person's blood plasma contains no anti-A antibodies; it does, however, contain anti-B antibodies. For some unknown reason, these antibodies are present naturally in type A blood plasma. The body did not form them in response to the presence of B antigen. In summary, then, in type A blood the RBCs contain type A antigen and the plasma contains anti-B antibodies.

Correspondingly, in type B blood, the RBCs contain type B antigen and the plasma contains anti-A antibodies. In type AB, as its name indicates, the RBCs contain both type A and B antigens, and the plasma contains neither anti-A nor anti-B antibodies. The opposite is true of type O blood: its RBCs contain neither type A nor type B antigens, and the plasma contains both anti-A and anti-B antibodies.

Harmful effects or even death can result from a blood transfusion if antibodies in the recipient's plasma react to the donor's blood and the RBCs become agglutinated. If the donor's blood is type O, and therefore its RBCs do not contain any A or B antigen, the blood cannot be clumped by anti-A or anti-B antibodies. For this reason type O blood is known as **universal**

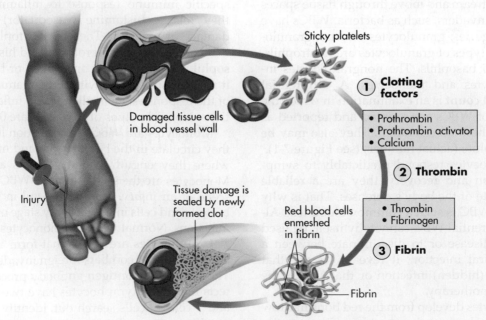

Sticky platelets

1 Clotting factors
- Prothrombin
- Prothrombin activator
- Calcium

2 Thrombin
- Thrombin
- Fibrinogen

3 Fibrin

Damaged tissue cells in blood vessel wall

Injury

Tissue damage is sealed by newly formed clot

Red blood cells enmeshed in fibrin

Fibrin

FIGURE 7-2 Blood clotting. The extremely complex clotting mechanism can be distilled into three basic steps: *1*, release of clotting factors from both injured tissue cells and sticky platelets at the injury site; *2*, formation of thrombin; and *3*, formation of fibrin and trapping of red blood cells to form a clot.

donor blood; it can be used in an emergency as donor blood, no matter what the recipient's blood type. Similarly, blood type AB has been called the **universal recipient** blood because it contains neither anti-A nor anti-B antibodies in its plasma. Therefore it does not clump any donor's RBCs containing A or B antigens. In a normal clinical setting, however, all blood intended for transfusion is typed and crossmatched carefully to the blood of the recipient for a variety of factors. Figure 7-3 shows the results of combinations of donor and recipient blood.

Two types of reactions can occur: agglutination and hemolyzation. In agglutination the donor cells clump together because of the antibodies; this occludes arteries and can result in death. In hemolyzation the antibodies cause the RBCs of the recipient to rupture and release their cell contents; this can also lead to death.

Rh Factor

Rh factor is located on the surface of the RBCs. People who have Rh factor are said to be Rh positive; people who do not have Rh factor are said to be Rh negative. Eighty-five percent of humans have Rh factor; 15% do not. Normally, human plasma does not contain Rh antibodies; these develop in response to an individual's receiving the wrong type of blood (i.e., if an Rh-negative person receives Rh-positive blood). Within approximately 2 weeks, Rh antibodies are produced and remain in the blood. If the Rh-negative person then receives more Rh-positive blood, a severe reaction occurs because the Rh-positive antibodies react with the donor blood. The antibodies hemolyze the donor RBCs, causing them to rupture and lose their contents.

Rh incompatibility is seen most commonly in pregnancy. Fortunately, this incompatibility can be prevented. The mother's blood is tested for antibodies, and if they are present, she can receive an intramuscular dose of Rh$_o$(D) immune globulin (RhoGAM)—a desensitization drug. This enables her to carry the next infant without the potential complications associated with Rh incompatibility.

LYMPHATIC SYSTEM

The lymphatic system is a subdivision of the cardiovascular system. It consists of lymphatic vessels, the lymph fluid, and the lymph tissue. The system has three basic functions: (1) maintenance of fluid balance, (2) production of lymphocytes, and (3) absorption and transportation of lipids from the intestine to the bloodstream.

Lymph and Lymph Vessels

The constancy of the fluid around each body cell can be maintained only if numerous homeostatic mechanisms function together in a controlled and integrated response to changing conditions. The circulatory system plays a key role in bringing many needed substances to cells and then removing the waste products that accumulate as a result of metabolism. This exchange of substances between blood and tissue fluid occurs in capillary beds. Many other substances that cannot enter or return through the capillary walls, including excess fluid and protein molecules, are returned to the blood as lymph.

Lymph is a specialized fluid formed in the tissue spaces and transported by way of lymphatic vessels to eventually reenter the circulatory system. In addition

Recipient's blood		Reaction with donor's blood			
RBC antigens	Plasma antibodies	Donor type O	Donor type A	Donor type B	Donor type AB
None (Type O)	Anti-A Anti-B				
A (Type A)	Anti-B				
B (Type B)	Anti-A				
AB (Type AB)	(none)				

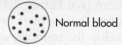 Normal blood   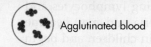 Agglutinated blood

FIGURE 7-3 Results of different combinations of donor and recipient blood. The left columns show the recipient's blood characteristics, and the top row shows the donor's blood type.

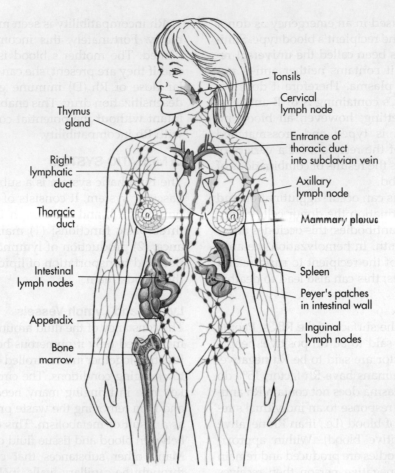

Tonsils

Cervical lymph node

Entrance of thoracic duct into subclavian vein

Axillary lymph node

Mammary plexus

Spleen

Peyer's patches in intestinal wall

Inguinal lymph nodes

Thymus gland

Right lymphatic duct

Thoracic duct

Intestinal lymph nodes

Appendix

Bone marrow

FIGURE 7-4 Principal organs of the lymphatic system.

to lymph and the lymphatic vessels, the lymphatic system includes lymph nodes and lymphatic organs such as the thymus and the spleen (Figure 7-4).

Lymphatic Tissue
Lymph Nodes
Lymph nodes (glands) have two functions: (1) to filter impurities from the lymph (much like an oil filter in a car) and (2) to produce lymphocytes (WBCs). The body contains 500 to 600 lymph nodes. They are small bean-shaped structures, usually appearing in groups. They range from 0.04 to 1 inch (1 to 25 mm) in length. Lymph nodes are most numerous in the axilla, the groin, the abdomen, the thorax, and the cervical regions (see Figure 7-4). The structure of the lymph nodes makes it possible for them to perform two functions: defense and WBC production.

Tonsils
The tonsils are masses of lymphoid tissue embedded in the mucous membrane of the oral cavity and the pharynx. The tonsils protect the body against invasion of foreign substances by producing lymphocytes and antibodies. They also trap bacteria and may become enlarged. The tonsils are larger in children and begin to atrophy (shrink) at about age 7.

Spleen
The spleen is a soft, roughly ovoid, highly vascularized organ located in the left upper quadrant of the abdominal cavity, just below the diaphragm (see Figure 7-4). The spleen is 5 to 6 inches (12.7 to 15.2 cm) long and 2 to 3 inches (5 to 7.6 cm) wide. It contains lymphatic nodules.

The spleen stores 1 pint of blood, which can be released during emergencies, such as hemorrhage, in less than 60 seconds. This large amount of blood gives the spleen its deep purple color. The main functions of the spleen are (1) to serve as a reservoir for blood; (2) to form lymphocytes, monocytes, and plasma cells; (3) to destroy worn-out RBCs; (4) to remove bacteria by phagocytosis (engulfing and digesting); and (5) to produce RBCs before birth (the spleen is believed to produce RBCs after birth only in cases of extreme hemolytic anemia).

Thymus
The thymus is located in the upper thorax posterior to the sternum and between the lungs in the mediastinum (see Figure 7-4). The thymus gland functions in utero (before birth) and a few months after birth to develop the immune system. The thymus is responsible for the development of T lymphocytes in the cell-

mediated immune response before they migrate to the lymph nodes and the spleen. At puberty the thymus gland atrophies; it is eventually replaced by fat and connective tissue.

LABORATORY AND DIAGNOSTIC TESTS

Complete Blood Count
The complete blood count (CBC) is an important part of routine screening and hospital admission. It involves several tests, each of which assesses the three major cells formed in the bone marrow. The CBC detects many disorders of the hematological system and provides data for diagnosing and evaluating disorders in other body systems. A CBC includes red and white cell counts, hematocrit and hemoglobin levels, erythrocyte indexes, differential white cell count, and examination of the peripheral blood cells (see Table 7-1). Prepare the patient by explaining that a blood sample will be taken from the hand or arm and evaluated for indicators of infection or anemia in the body.

Erythrocyte Indexes
Erythrocyte indexes are measurements of the size and hemoglobin content of RBCs. This measurement provides information about the average volume or size of a single RBC (mean corpuscular volume [MCV]). Mean corpuscular hemoglobin (MCH) is a measure of the average amount (weight) of hemoglobin within an RBC. Mean corpuscular hemoglobin concentration (MCHC) is a measure of the average concentration or the percentage of hemoglobin within an RBC.

Peripheral Smear
A peripheral smear along with the differential WBC count allows examination of the size, shape, and structure of individual RBCs and platelets. This information is useful in differentiating various forms of anemias and blood dyscrasias. All three hematological cell lines (RBCs, WBCs, platelets) can be examined. When adequately prepared and examined microscopically by an experienced technologist, a smear of peripheral blood is the most informative of all hematological tests.

Schilling Test and Megaloblastic Anemia Profile
The Schilling test is a laboratory blood test for diagnosing pernicious anemia. The test measures the absorption of radioactive vitamin B_{12}, before and after parenteral injection of the intrinsic factor, by examination of the urinary excretion of vitamin B_{12}. Normal findings are excretion of 8% to 40% of radioactive vitamin B_{12} within 24 hours. The Schilling test for pernicious anemia is being replaced by a serum test called **megaloblastic anemia profile,** which measures vitamin B_{12}, methylmalonic acid, and homocysteine levels.

Gastric Analysis
Gastric analysis is an older test for determining pernicious anemia. In pernicious anemia the gastric secretions are minimal and the pH remains elevated, even after injection of histamine.

Radiologic Studies
Radiologic studies for the hematological system involve primarily the use of computed tomography (CT) or magnetic resonance imaging (MRI) for evaluating the spleen, the liver, and the lymph nodes. In the past, lymphangiography with contrast dye was a common procedure for evaluating deep lymph nodes. CT is now the preferred method (Lewis et al., 2007).

Bone Marrow Aspiration or Biopsy
When the diagnosis is not clearly established by peripheral blood smears or further information is needed, bone marrow aspiration or biopsy helps establish the diagnosis and assess treatment response. The most common site for this procedure is the posterior iliac crest. The sternum can also be used, but generally only for aspiration. Normal bone marrow is soft and semifluid and can be removed by aspiration through a needle. Bone marrow aspiration is most commonly performed in people with marked anemia, neutropenia (decreased number of WBCs), acute leukemia, and thrombocytopenia (decreased number of platelets). Cell types, numbers, and maturation are examined. Although complications of bone marrow aspiration are minimal, there is a possibility of penetrating the bone and underlying structures. This hazard is greatest in an aspiration procedure involving the sternum.

DISORDERS OF THE HEMATOLOGIC AND LYMPHATIC SYSTEMS

The hematologic and lymphatic systems include the blood and the organs of blood production—the bone marrow and lymphatic tissue. Disorders of blood production, bone marrow, or lymphatic tissues affect virtually all body systems. Disturbances in this delicate balance can produce life-threatening signs and symptoms, severe pain, and incapacitation.

DISORDERS ASSOCIATED WITH ERYTHROCYTES
ANEMIA
Anemia is a disorder characterized by levels of RBCs, hemoglobin, and hematocrit that are below normal range. In hemolytic anemia, increased RBC destruction also occurs. In persons with anemia, insufficient amounts of oxygen are delivered to tissues and cells.

Etiology and Pathophysiology
Anemia can be caused by many factors, including blood loss (hemorrhage), impaired production of RBCs (bone marrow depression), increased destruction of RBCs (hemolysis), or nutritional deficiencies (long-term iron deficiency). Hemorrhage or blood

loss accounts for temporary anemia, whereas nutritional deficit can cause long-term iron deficiency anemia. Marrow failure is linked to a disease process, toxic exposure, tumor, or unknown causes. A decrease in RBC production or increased destruction results in a lower number of circulating RBCs. Bone marrow hematopoietic function is unable to produce the needed quantity.

Loss of the oxygen-carrying element in the blood results in a supply/demand imbalance in vital organs. Peripheral circulation compensates by shunting blood to vital organs, thus causing hypoxia in other areas of the body. Rapid hematopoietic effort causes blood cell irregularities (immature RBCs) and inability to produce RBCs, with a resultant decrease in the RBC count.

Clinical Manifestations

Most adults do not experience symptoms until the hemoglobin level is less than 8 g/dL. Older adults, however, may show symptoms with a hemoglobin concentration of less than 10 g/dL. Although each type of anemia has specific signs and symptoms, the decreased oxygen-carrying capacity leads to signs and symptoms that are common in all anemias. These include anorexia, cardiac dilation, disorientation, dizziness, dyspepsia, dyspnea, exertional dyspnea, fatigue, headache, insomnia, pallor (mucous membranes and skin), palpitations, shortness of breath, systolic murmur, tachycardia, and vertigo.

Assessment

Subjective data commonly include expressions of weakness, dyspnea, fatigue, and vertigo. Anorexia and dyspepsia may accompany headache and insomnia, but the patient generally does not link these complaints to the condition unless questioned. In older adult patients with impaired cardiopulmonary reserves, be alert to complaints of chest pain, dyspnea on exertion, palpitations, and dizziness.

Collection of **objective data** includes observing signs of bleeding or shock (hypovolemic anemia). Laboratory values will show a low RBC count and hematocrit and hemoglobin levels. Skin and mucous membranes are pale, and cardiac symptoms are related to anemia. With long-term anemia, the patient may have ulcerations of the extremities.

Diagnostic Tests

Blood studies show RBC count and hemoglobin and hematocrit levels to be below normal. Serum iron, total iron-binding capacity, and serum ferritin levels are below normal. Reticulocyte count is increased because of immaturity of RBCs. A bone marrow study shows a deviation from normal findings. Peripheral blood smears enable identification of abnormalities of shape and color of cells. A megaloblastic anemia profile reveals decreased levels of vitamin B$_{12}$.

 Cultural Considerations

Jehovah's Witness Opposition to Blood Transfusion

The nurse who provides culturally appropriate nursing interventions to a Jehovah's Witness has a number of factors to consider. The paramount concern is that Jehovah's Witnesses are opposed to homologous blood transfusion (blood obtained from a blood bank or through donations). Jehovah's Witnesses believe that receiving blood products from another person carries eternal consequences. However, many (but not all) Jehovah's Witnesses will submit to certain types of autologous blood transfusions (autotransfusion). One type of autologous transfusion that might be acceptable is blood retrieved through induced hemodilution at the start of surgery (blood that is directed to storage bags outside the patient's body).

In addition, some Jehovah's Witnesses permit the use of certain blood volume expanders. Many Jehovah's Witnesses carry a card with the types of blood volume expanders permitted. Ask the patient for this card or, if the patient is unconscious, examine the patient's personal belongings to find this extremely important card.

The consensus of the U.S. Supreme Court has been that a person of adult majority age has the right to refuse treatment but not to withhold a potentially life-saving treatment from a minor child.

Medical Management

Intervention depends on the cause. Correction of the disease process may correct or lessen the anemic condition. Transfusion is appropriate for blood loss; iron and vitamin B$_{12}$ are replaced if these are deficient. Treatment is often specific to the particular anemia (see Cultural Considerations box).

Nursing Interventions and Patient Teaching

Nursing diagnoses and interventions for the patient with anemia include but are not limited to the following:

Nursing Diagnoses	Nursing Interventions
Ineffective tissue perfusion (cardiovascular), related to reduction of cellular components necessary for delivery of oxygen to the cells	Monitor changes in vital signs and in mental alertness. Monitor cardiac rhythms. Monitor hemoglobin, hematocrit, and RBCs. Assess baseline arterial blood gases and electrolytes. Note presence and degree of dyspnea, cyanosis, hemoptysis.
Impaired gas exchange, related to deficient: • RBCs • hemoglobin • hematocrit	Evaluate ability to manage activities of daily living (ADLs), related to oxygen decrease. Assess activity response, dyspnea, and heart rate.

Nursing Diagnoses	Nursing Interventions
Impaired gas exchange, related to deficient: • RBCs • hemoglobin • hematocrit	Observe for cyanosis, hypoxia, and hypercapnia. Maintain bed rest as necessary and provide range-of-motion (ROM) exercise. Monitor oxygen saturations frequently per pulse oximetry. Administer oxygen as ordered. Explain activity-oxygen deficit relationship.
Activity intolerance, related to: • oxygen deficit • secondary to decreased hemoglobin and hematocrit	Plan care to provide optimum rest. Limit environmental stimuli to reduce demands placed on the patient. Assist in identifying factors causing intolerance. Assess ability to perform ADLs, ambulation, and exercise. Assess potential for injury caused by mobility impairment. Teach patient to perform at own rate of ability, to reduce energy expenditure. Monitor hemoglobin and hematocrit levels.

Tailor patient education to the individual conditions and needs.

Hypovolemic Anemia (Blood Loss Anemia)

Etiology and Pathophysiology

Secondary anemia is when deficiencies in RBCs and other components are caused by an abnormally low circulating blood volume from hemorrhage. Blood loss of 1000 mL or more in an adult can be severe. Such a loss is usually related to internal or external hemorrhage caused by a surgical procedure, gastrointestinal (GI) bleeding, menorrhagia, trauma, or severe burns.

Loss of blood decreases the amount of circulating fluid and hemoglobin and thus decreases the amount of oxygen carried to the body tissues. The tissues must have oxygen to survive. The average adult has an approximate total blood volume of 6000 mL (6 L [12 pints]) and can tolerate a loss of up to 500 mL. If the loss approaches 1000 mL, acute complications, such as hypovolemic shock, may occur. The rapidity of blood loss is related to the severity and number of signs and symptoms. The sudden reduction in the total blood volume can lead to hypovolemic shock. RBC count and the hematocrit level drop to half the normal range.

Clinical Manifestations

Signs and symptoms include restlessness; a subtle rise in respiratory rate; weakness; stupor; irritability; and pale, cool, moist skin. Excessive blood loss results in shock. Shock occurs when there is a deprivation of oxygen and nutrients to organs. Hemorrhagic blood loss results in a decrease in blood volume. In shock, vasoconstriction occurs in blood vessels to noncritical organs such as skin, muscles, and intestines. This decreases the blood flow to these organs and shunts blood to the vital organs such as the heart and the brain.

The amount of blood loss affects the heart rate and the blood pressure. In the early stages of shock, when 750 to 1000 mL of blood has been lost, the heart rate is less than 100 bpm with a normal blood pressure. As the blood loss increases to 1000 to 1500 mL, the pulse increases to more than 100 bpm and the patient has orthostatic blood pressure. When the blood loss is 1500 to 2600 mL (about 30% to 40% of the blood volume), the systolic blood pressure decreases to less than 90 mm Hg and the pulse increases to more than 120 bpm. With a blood loss of 1500 to 2000 mL, irreversible end-organ damage can result (Beattie, 2007a).

The patient's clinical signs and symptoms are more important than the laboratory values. Be alert to the patient's expression of pain. Internal hemorrhage may cause pain because of tissue distention, organ displacement, and nerve compression. Pain may be localized or referred. Decreased RBC, hemoglobin, and hematocrit levels may not be evident until several days after severe blood loss has occurred. The severity of the patient's signs and symptoms correlates with the severity of the blood loss.

Assessment

Subjective data commonly include complaints of thirst, weakness, irritability, and restlessness.

Objective data include decreased blood pressure; rapid, weak, thready pulse; and rapid respirations. Cold, clammy skin with pallor is noted. Oliguria is often evident. Mental disorientation and physical collapse with prostration can occur.

Diagnostic Tests

When blood loss is sudden, plasma volume has not yet had a chance to increase, the loss of RBCs is not reflected in laboratory data, and values may seem normal or high for 2 to 3 days. However, once the plasma is replaced, the RBC mass is less concentrated. RBC, hemoglobin, and hematocrit levels are severely decreased, often to half the normal values.

Medical Management

In the case of massive hemorrhage, measures are taken to stop the blood loss and treat for shock and lost volume. Severe hemorrhaging often results in the need for mechanical ventilation. Oxygen therapy restores oxygen that is less available because of decreased hemoglobin in the blood. To replace fluid volume, intravenous (IV) saline is used. In severe fluid volume depletion, a bolus of 2 L of normal saline is given. If hypotension continues or if the hemoglobin is below 6 g/dL, packed RBCs are usually given. It is now recommended to keep the hemoglobin over 7 g/dL. Often platelets, fresh frozen plasma (FFP), or cryoprecipitate is included in the treatment to control hemorrhage (Beattie, 2007a).

Monitor the hemoglobin level to note the effectiveness of the treatment. Be aware that one unit of packed RBCs should increase the hemoglobin by 1 g/dL (Beattie, 2007a). The patient may also need supplemental iron because the availability of iron affects the marrow production of erythrocytes. Oral or parenteral iron preparations are often administered.

Nursing Interventions and Patient Teaching
Monitor blood and fluid restoration and identify blood loss sites to control the bleeding. Keep patients flat and warm. Take vital signs at frequent intervals. Take precautions to prevent injury to a restless or disoriented patient. Measure intake and output (I&O), with careful monitoring of urinary output for oliguria caused by decreased renal perfusion. The decrease in urinary output correlates to the amount of blood lost. If a patient has a blood loss of 1000 to 1500 mL, the urinary output is 20 to 30 mL/hr; with a blood loss of 1500 to 2000 mL, the urinary output is less than 20 mL/hr; and a blood loss of 2000 mL or more would result in anuria (very low urinary output) (Beattie, 2007a).

If hemorrhage is caused by a chronic problem, teach the patient to monitor bleeding amounts and associated factors and to report to the physician immediately for treatment.

Prognosis
Without treatment, death will result. With aggressive treatment, the prognosis is favorable.

Pernicious Anemia
Etiology and Pathophysiology
A **pernicious** disease is one that is capable of causing great injury, destruction, or death. Without treatment, pernicious anemia would be fatal. This type of anemia is the result of a metabolic defect: the absence of a glycoprotein intrinsic factor secreted by the gastric mucosa. Intrinsic secretion fails because of gastric mucosal atrophy. Pernicious anemia is an autoimmune disease in which antibodies in the parietal walls of the stomach prevent the production of the intrinsic factor (Lewis et al., 2007). It is a progressive, megaloblastic, macrocytic anemia primarily affecting older adults. The intrinsic factor is essential for absorption of vitamin B_{12} (cyanocobalamin).

The intrinsic factor is not available to combine with vitamin B_{12}, preventing transport of this necessary vitamin to the ileum (vitamin B_{12} is normally absorbed in the distal ileum). Deficiency of the vitamin affects growth and maturity of all body cells, including RBCs in the marrow. The erythrocyte membrane becomes fragile and ruptures easily. This vitamin is related to nerve myelination; its absence leads to progressive demyelination and degeneration of nerves and white matter.

Clinical Manifestations
Extreme weakness is noted with dyspnea, fever, and hypoxia. As the condition progresses, weight loss is apparent, as is slight icterus (jaundice) with pallor. The skin color may appear a pale lemon-yellow because of the excessive destruction of the RBCs, which causes the bile pigments to increase in the blood serum. The patient experiences edema of the legs, intermittent constipation, and diarrhea.

Assessment
Subjective data include the patient's complaints of palpitations, nausea, flatulence, and indigestion. The tongue is sore and burning. Weakness and difficulty swallowing (dysphagia) may occur. Neurologic symptoms include tingling of the hands and feet and loss of the sense of body position (impaired proprioception).

Collection of **objective data** includes observation of a smooth and erythematous tongue, with infection about the teeth and gums. Cerebral signs include mental disorientation, personality changes, and behavior problems. Severe neurologic impairments can result, including partial or total paralysis from destruction of the nerve fibers of the spinal cord.

Diagnostic Tests
The Schilling test shows malabsorption of vitamin B_{12}. This test is being replaced by the serum megaloblastic anemia profile, which reveals decreased serum levels of vitamin B_{12}, serum methylmalonic acid, and homocysteine. Bone marrow aspiration reveals abnormal RBC development.

The erythrocytes appear large (macrocytic) and have abnormal shapes; serum cyanocobalamin (B_{12}) levels are reduced. A gastric analysis may be done to determine the cause of the vitamin B_{12} deficiency. Pernicious anemia is caused by an absence of intrinsic factor, from either gastric mucosal atrophy or autoimmune destruction of parietal cells of the stomach. This results in a decrease of hydrochloric acid secretion by the stomach. An acidic environment in the stomach is required for the secretion of intrinsic factor.

Medical Management
Oral vitamin B_{12} is ineffective if there is an absence of the intrinsic factor in the stomach or a malabsorption problem in the ileum (Lewis et al., 2007). Cyanocobalamin injections, folic acid supplement, and iron replacement are ordered. If the anemia is severe, the patient may be transfused with packed RBCs. The standard treatment includes initiating vitamin B_{12} re-

placement therapy; without it, these individuals will die in 1 to 3 years. Treatment is 1,000 units of vitamin B_{12} administered intramuscularly daily for 2 weeks, then weekly until the hematocrit is normal, and finally monthly for life. An intranasal form of cyanocobalamin (Nascobal) is self-administered once weekly. The patient's blood values should return to normal within 2 months of B_{12} therapy. A CBC is necessary every 3 to 6 months to monitor the long-term success of treatment.

Nursing Interventions and Patient Teaching

The nursing interventions depend to some extent on the stage of the disease. A symptomatic approach is appropriate. When the patient is confined to the hospital, check vital signs every 4 hours. Perform special mouth care several times daily. The diet should be high in protein, vitamins, and minerals. Anemic patients are especially sensitive to cold, so additional lightweight, warm blankets may be needed. Interventions should conserve energy and prevent injury.

Nursing diagnoses and interventions for the patient with pernicious anemia include but are not limited to the following:

Nursing Diagnoses	Nursing Interventions
Risk for injury, related to: • sensory and motor losses • alteration in mental status	Use bed rest, with side rails up as needed, to prevent patient fatigue and falls caused by weakness. Assist with ambulation to avoid falls. Use bed cradle or footboard to prevent pressure on lower extremities. Apply heat with extreme caution to avoid burning the skin. If heat therapy is required, evaluate the patient's skin at frequent intervals to detect erythema. Support patient with patience and reassurance to reduce irritability and depression.
Imbalanced nutrition: less than body requirements, related to: • sore mouth and tongue • diarrhea • constipation	Administer vitamin B_{12} and other medications prescribed to promote production of erythrocytes. Encourage diet high in vitamins, iron, and protein to promote production of healthy erythrocytes.

Nursing Diagnoses	Nursing Interventions
Imbalanced nutrition: less than body requirements, related to: • sore mouth and tongue • diarrhea • constipation	Provide meticulous and frequent oral hygiene to promote improved appetite and prevent infection. Offer small, frequent feedings to prevent digestive overload. Observe for diarrhea or constipation and treat as prescribed to avoid fluid and electrolyte imbalance and discomfort.

To control the disease, the patient must understand the disease process and the importance of lifetime therapy of vitamin B_{12}. Discuss the importance of a diet high in vitamin B_{12}. Adjusting activities when signs and symptoms are present may lessen the patient's stress. The need for assistance with ADLs and for frequent rest periods should be impressed on the patient and significant people involved in the care.

Prognosis

This condition, if untreated, can be considered terminal in 1 to 3 years. With treatment the patient may be asymptomatic. Because the potential for gastric carcinoma is increased in pernicious anemia, the patient should have frequent and careful evaluation for this problem.

Aplastic Anemia
Etiology and Pathophysiology

Aplastic anemia, or **aplasia** (a hematological term for a failure of the normal process of cell generation and development), has two etiologic classifications: **congenital** and **acquired.** Approximately 30% of aplastic anemias that appear in childhood are inherited, caused by chromosomal alterations. Acquired aplastic anemia is directly related to exposure to viral invasion, medications, chemicals (e.g., benzene, insecticides, arsenic, alcohol), radiation, or chemotherapy, in which the hematopoietic tissue is replaced by fatty marrow, causing a defect in RBC production. The causes of 70% of acquired cases of aplastic anemia are **idiopathic** (cause unknown). Aplastic anemia is probably an immune-mediated disease.

Depression of erythrocyte production results in lowered hemoglobin and RBCs. Leukopenia and thrombocytopenia may develop. People with aplastic anemia are usually **pancytopenic**; that is, all three major blood elements (red cells, white cells, and platelets) from the bone marrow are reduced or absent. The incidence of aplastic anemia is low, affecting approximately 4 of every 1 million people.

Clinical Manifestations

The signs and symptoms of aplastic anemia may have an acute onset or develop slowly over several weeks to months. With suppression of all three major blood elements, the patient may have signs and symptoms related to each. For example, suppression of WBCs may result in infection, suppression of RBCs may lead to anemia, or suppression of thrombocytes may cause petechiae (Lewis et al., 2007). Repeated infections with high fevers may occur, along with fatigue, weakness, general malaise, dyspnea, and palpitations. Mortality is high from complications of infection and hemorrhage. Bleeding tendencies are reported: petechiae, ecchymoses, bleeding gums, epistaxis, and GI and genitourinary system bleeding.

Assessment

Subjective data include a history of exposure to chemicals such as insecticides and drugs in addition to a family history of aplastic anemia. Ask the patient about the ability to carry out ADLs without fatigue.

Collection of **objective data** includes monitoring the patient for pallor, signs of infection, and bleeding tendencies. Also, dyspnea and tachycardia may be noted.

Diagnostic Tests

A bone marrow study (aspiration biopsy) shows hypoplastic or aplastic fatty deposits, a decrease in cellular elements with increased yellow marrow (fat content), and depressed hematopoietic activity. The diagnostic findings are especially important because the marrow is hypocellular, with increased yellow marrow, a finding termed *dry tap.* Peripheral blood smears show that blood cells may be normocytic and normochromic.

Medical Management

The cause of aplastic anemia must be identified promptly and removed or discontinued. Bone marrow suppression is expected with certain antineoplastic medications or radiation therapy, and laboratory values should be monitored frequently to maintain control.

Avoid blood transfusions, if possible, to prevent iron overloading and the development of antibodies to tissue antigens. Platelet transfusions that are human lymphocyte antigen (HLA) matched are used to treat serious bleeding in a thrombocytopenic patient. Blood transfusions are used cautiously to minimize the risk of rejection for a bone marrow transplant candidate.

A splenectomy may be required in patients with hypersplenism that is destroying normal platelets. Steroids and androgens are sometimes used to stimulate the bone marrow. Immunosuppressive therapy with antithymocyte globulin and cyclosporine or high-dose cyclophosphamide (Cytoxan) has become important for patients who are not candidates for bone marrow transplantation or hematopoietic stem cell transplant (SCT). Bone marrow transplantation or hematopoietic SCT is the treatment of choice in patients younger than the age of 45 who have a compatible donor. Granulocyte-macrophage colony-stimulating factor (GM-CSF) is used as biologic response modifier treatment for aplastic anemia.

Bone marrow transplant. A bone marrow transplant is indicated in certain cases such as immunodeficient states, cancer, leukemia, and recurrent aplastic anemia. A matched donor and recipient are essential to avoid rejection or complications. Specimens from twins, siblings, or self (autologous) while in remission are preferred.

After emotional and physical preparation of the patient, perform blood studies to set baselines and assess the patient's status. Establish a pathogen-free environment, with the immunocompromised patient placed on reverse isolation (neutropenic precautions). Monitor for fever or infection. The medication therapy used in this preparation may include immunosuppressants, antibiotics, and antianxiety agents.

Bone marrow transplants are used increasingly in hematological malignancies after large doses of chemotherapy or radiation therapy. A limited amount of chemotherapy or radiation can ordinarily be administered because of its toxicity to the bone marrow. When bone marrow is transplanted after these therapeutic modes, much larger therapeutic doses are possible.

Bone marrow is obtained by multiple marrow aspirations under general or spinal anesthesia, usually yielding 500 to 800 mL of marrow. The marrow is cryopreserved (frozen) until it is used. Shortly after chemotherapy (with or without radiation therapy) is completed, the patient receives the donated marrow through an IV catheter. This infusion of marrow is called the **rescue process.** The marrow travels through the bloodstream to the bone marrow, where it begins to manufacture new leukocytes, erythrocytes, and thrombocytes. The infused marrow repopulates the patient's marrow after several weeks. The patient runs a great risk of toxicity, including infections, marrow rejection, and graft-versus-host disease. Medications supporting graft acceptance include cyclosporine (immunosuppressant) and chemotherapy (to prevent graft-versus-host complications).

Splenectomy. Surgical excision of the spleen may be performed to treat blood dyscrasias with splenomegaly, to treat trauma to the spleen, or to remove a diseased spleen. Preoperative assessment includes cardiovascular observation, respiratory function determination, and GI evaluation. Postoperatively, compare these observations with the patient's baseline evaluations, and observe the patient for infection or inflammation. Potential complications include infection, hemorrhage, shock, and paralytic ileus. Maintain parenteral therapy. Use nasogastric (NG) suction if a paralytic ileus develops. Address the patient's postoperative pain. Also maintain movement and use positioning to prevent infection or postoperative pneumonia.

Nursing Interventions and Patient Teaching

Proper observation and care after bone marrow study are essential. Patients with aplastic anemia are highly susceptible to infection; thus nursing interventions should be directed toward prevention. Adhere to strict aseptic techniques for dressing changes and IV site care. To prevent impaired skin and mucous membranes, avoid intramuscular injections and rectal medications or rectal temperatures. Use protective devices, such as an air mattress. In the presence of thrombocytopenia, observe carefully for any signs of bleeding and prevent even the slightest trauma. Monitor the patient's urine and stool for occult or gross blood.

Nursing diagnoses and interventions for the patient with aplastic anemia include but are not limited to the following:

Nursing Diagnoses	Nursing Interventions
Activity intolerance, related to inadequate tissue oxygenation	For hypoxia, place the patient in a sitting position; observe respiration rate, pulse, and dyspnea; observe skin color and temperature; assist with care; plan rest periods; administer oxygen as needed; monitor laboratory values to improve gas exchange. Monitor pulse oximetry levels carefully. Assist with ADLs as needed. Encourage patient to engage in activities on a progressive basis as fatigue decreases in response to therapy. Help patient explore feelings associated with fatigue.
Risk for infection, related to increased susceptibility	Maintain reverse isolation to avoid exposure to pathogen. Observe for increase in temperature, pulse, and respirations as signs of infection. Observe the patient for "sniffles," sore throat, anorexia, and pain on urination. Administer antibiotics as ordered to combat specific pathogens. Encourage mobility, turning, coughing, deep breathing, and increased fluids to reduce susceptibility to infection.

Everyone with aplastic anemia needs to know how to protect themselves from excessive bleeding. Help the patient maintain a balance between rest and activity. Discuss with the patient how to avoid infection, especially of the respiratory or urinary tract (see Safety Alert box).

Prognosis

The prognosis of untreated aplastic anemia is poor (approximately 75% fatal). However, advances in medical management have improved outcomes significantly in aggressively treated patients. The object of care is to produce remission and prolong survival.

Iron Deficiency Anemia
Etiology and Pathophysiology

Iron deficiency anemia is a condition in which the RBCs contain decreased levels of hemoglobin. The most common cause of iron deficiency anemia is excessive iron loss. In adults the most common source is chronic intestinal or uterine bleeding; however, iron deficiency anemia can also be caused by bleeding from gastric or duodenal ulcers, esophageal varices, hiatal hernias, colonic diverticula, and tumors. The major sources of chronic blood loss are from the GI and genitourinary systems (Box 7-1).

GI bleeding is often not apparent and may exist for a considerable time before being identified. Loss of 50 to 75 mL of blood from the upper GI tract is required for stools to appear as black or melenic. The color results from the iron in the RBCs. Blood losses related to men-

| Box 7-1 | Causes of Iron Deficiency Anemia |

- Iron deficiency may develop from inadequate dietary intake, malabsorption, blood loss, or hemolysis (breakdown of red blood cells).
- Daily iron intake from food and dietary supplements is adequate to meet the needs of men and older women, but it may be inadequate for those with higher iron needs (e.g., menstruating or pregnant women).
- Malabsorption of iron may occur after certain types of gastrointestinal (GI) surgery and in malabsorption syndromes. Iron absorption occurs in the duodenum. Malabsorption of iron may involve disease of the duodenum in which the absorption surface is altered or destroyed.
- Blood loss is a major cause of iron deficiency in adults. The major sources of chronic blood loss are from the GI and genitourinary systems. Common causes of GI blood loss are peptic ulcers, gastritis, esophagitis, diverticulitis, hemorrhoids, and neoplasms. The average monthly menstrual blood loss is about 45 mL and causes the loss of 22 mg of iron.

struation or pregnancy are common causes of iron deficiency anemia in young women. Rarely, excessive losses occur through microhemorrhages into lung tissue or from intestinal parasites. Even without excessive blood loss, iron deficiency anemia can result when the body's demand for iron exceeds its absorption, which commonly occurs in infants, young adolescents, and pregnant women. Less commonly, iron deficiency anemia results from malabsorption of iron caused by diseases such as celiac disease and sprue. Subtotal gastrectomy may lead to iron deficiency caused by **achlorhydria** (loss of hydrochloric acid), occult bleeding, and decreased iron in postgastrectomy diets. Deficiency caused by poor dietary intake is rare in middle-age adults.

Approximately 1 mg of every 10 to 20 mg (5% to 10%) of iron ingested is absorbed in the duodenum. This amount of dietary iron meets the needs of men and older women, but it may be inadequate for people who have higher iron needs (e.g., children, pregnant and lactating women).

Clinical Manifestations

The most common symptoms of iron deficiency anemia are (in order) pallor and glossitis (inflammation of the tongue). Fatigue, weakness, and shortness of breath also often occur. Signs and symptoms typical of angina and heart failure may also occur.

Assessment

Collection of **subjective data** includes noting GI symptoms such as glossitis (manifested by inflammation and soreness of the tongue) and **pagophagia** (the desire to eat ice, clay, or starches). The patient may complain of headache, paresthesia, and a burning sensation of the tongue, all of which are caused by lack of iron in the tissues.

Collection of **objective data** includes noting the signs, including pallor and tachycardia. Fingernails may be fragile and shaped like the head of a spoon with a central depression and raised borders. Mucous membranes of the mouth may be inflamed (stomatitis), and lips may be erythemic with cracking at the angles.

Diagnostic Tests

The peripheral blood counts show that RBC, hemoglobin levels, and hematocrit are decreased; serum iron levels are low.

Medical Management

Administer iron salts such as ferrous sulfate. In 3 weeks the hematocrit level should rise 5% to 15%, and the hemoglobin level should rise to 2 to 5 g/dL. For the body to incorporate 100 mg of iron per day, administer 900 mg/day. Iron is administered orally or by injection. Ascorbic acid has been shown to enhance iron absorption. Food sources of iron include meat, fish, poultry, eggs, green leafy vegetables, whole grains, and dried beans (Box 7-2).

When the patient cannot tolerate oral preparations of iron, parenteral iron therapy is used. The Z-track method of giving iron dextran (DexFerrum) intramuscularly is preferable to prevent skin staining. Iron sucrose (Venofer) is an IV drug frequently used for treatment of iron deficiency anemia.

Nursing Interventions and Patient Teaching

Because treatment is directed toward diagnosis and alleviation of the cause, the patient interview is important. Medication therapy for iron replacement is initiated as ordered. Plan for rest periods when fatigue is present. Education about nutritional needs relative to the condition may prevent this anemia (see Box 7-2).

Explanation of the side effects of iron therapy is essential to alleviate distress and to extend the therapy for the necessary time (see Health Promotion box). The patient must know which signs and symptoms are significant and need to be reported to the physician. Diarrhea or nausea is significant, but black, tarry stools are not (these are to be expected with iron therapy).

Prognosis

The prognosis is usually good with correction of the underlying cause and compliance with the medical treatment.

Sickle Cell Anemia

Etiology and Pathophysiology

Sickle cell anemia is the most common genetic disorder in the United States, predominantly affecting the black population. A sickle cell is an abnormal, crescent-shaped RBC containing hemoglobin S (Hg-S), a defective hemoglobin molecule. This anemia is a severe, chronic, incurable condition that occurs in people **homozygous** (having two identical genes inherited from each parent for a

Box 7-2   Food Sources of Nutrients Needed for Erythropoiesis

IRON
- Organ meats: liver, kidney, heart, and tongue
- Muscle meats, especially dark meat from poultry
- Eggs
- Shellfish
- Whole-grain breads and cereals
- Iron-enriched or iron-fortified breads and cereal
- Dark green vegetables: spinach, Swiss chard, kale, greens (dandelion, beet, and turnip)
- Dried fruits: apricots, dates, figs, prunes, and raisins
- Legumes and nuts

FOLIC ACID
- Green leafy vegetables
- Asparagus, broccoli
- Organ meats: liver
- Meat
- Whole-grain breads and cereals
- Enriched and fortified breads and cereals
- Fish
- Legumes

VITAMIN B$_{12}$
- Organ meats: liver and kidney
- Muscle meats
- Milk and cheese
- Eggs

AMINO ACIDS
- Eggs
- Meat
- Milk and milk products (cheese, ice cream)
- Poultry
- Fish
- Legumes
- Nuts

VITAMIN C
- Citrus fruits
- Leafy green vegetables
- Strawberries
- Cantaloupe

Health Promotion

Iron Administration

- Iron preparations supplement the body's natural iron stores.
- Dosages are determined by the elemental iron content of the preparation.
- Iron supplements may be contraindicated in peptic ulcer disease.
- Side effects include gastrointestinal (GI) upset (nausea, vomiting), constipation or diarrhea, and green to black stools. Elixir may stain teeth.
- Iron is absorbed best from the duodenum and proximal jejunum. Therefore enteric-coated or sustained-release capsules, which release iron farther down in the GI tract, are counterproductive; they are also more expensive.
- If side effects develop, the dose and type of iron supplement may be adjusted. Some people cannot tolerate ferrous sulfate because of the effects of the sulfate base. Ferrous gluconate may be an acceptable substitute.
- Iron is best absorbed in an acidic environment. To avoid binding the iron with food, iron should be taken about an hour before meals, when the duodenal mucosa is most acidic. Taking iron with vitamin C (ascorbic acid) or orange juice, which contains ascorbic acid, also enhances iron absorption. Gastric side effects, however, may necessitate ingesting iron with meals.
- Do not administer with antacids.
- If a dose is missed, continue with schedule; do not double a dose.
- Iron may interfere with absorption of oral tetracycline antibiotics. Do not take within 2 hours of each other.
- Dilute liquid iron preparations in juice or water, and administer with a straw to avoid staining teeth. Provide oral hygiene after taking.
- Check for constipation or diarrhea. Record color (iron turns stools green to black) and amount of stool.
- Iron is toxic, and caution must be taken to store iron preparations out of a child's reach.

given hereditary characteristic) for Hg-S. Sickle cell crisis is an episode of acute "sickling" of RBCs, which causes occlusion and ischemia in distal blood vessels. Sickling leads to clumping, or aggregation, of these misshapen RBCs, which lodge in small vessels. Sickle cell trait is the **heterozygous** (having two different genes) form of sickle cell anemia whereby the individual has both Hg-S and hemoglobin A (Hg-A) in the RBCs. Patients with sickle cell trait do not have signs or symptoms, but risk passing the disorder on to their children.

Approximately 81% of black Americans have sickle cell trait (about 2 million in the United States), and approximately 1 of every 600 (about 80,000 individuals in the United States) has sickle cell anemia (Lewis et al., 2007). Tissue hypoxia and ischemia occur, causing pain and edema as a result of inflammation. Compared with a normal life span of about 120 days, an RBC affected by sickle cell disease has a life span of only 10 to 20 days (Lewis et al., 2007). Destruction of fragile RBCs thus inhibits the oxygen-carrying function.

Clinical Manifestations

Usually the newborn with sickle cell anemia is asymptomatic for the first 10 to 12 weeks of age, until most of the fetal hemoglobin (Hb-F) has been replaced by Hb-S. However, periods of crisis then occur, accelerating the signs and symptoms. Many people with sickle cell anemia are in reasonably good health the majority of the time. The typical patient is anemic but asymptomatic except during painful episodes. Physical and probably emotional factors (stress) precipitate a painful episode. Physical factors include events that cause dehydration or change the oxygen tension in the body, such as infection, overexertion, weather changes (cold), ingestion of alcohol, and smoking.

Infections are a major complication of sickle cell anemia. Pneumonia, meningitis, influenza, and hepatitis may occur. Loss of appetite and irritability with weakness follow minor infections. Abdominal enlargement with pooling of blood in the liver, spleen, and other organs may accompany jaundice. Joint and back pain is noted, as is edema of the extremities. Complications include multisystem failure, infarctions, hemorrhage, and retinal damage leading to blindness.

Assessment

Collection of **subjective data** begins with assessing the patient's knowledge and feelings about the disease and factors that appear to precipitate crisis or exacerbate signs and symptoms. Fatigue may be reported when anemia is severe. The primary symptom associated with sickling is pain. During the sickle cell crisis, the pain is severe due to tissue ischemia. Aching joints, especially those of the hands and feet, are common complaints. The pain associated with these attacks is often described as deep, gnawing, and throbbing.

Collection of **objective data** includes observing for abdominal enlargement and jaundice, edema of the extremities, and signs of hemorrhage. As a result of the accelerated RBC breakdown, the patient has a characteristic clinical finding of hemolysis (jaundice, elevated serum bilirubin levels).

Diagnostic Tests

Electrophoresis of hemoglobin in a patient with sickle cell anemia is specific for detecting sickle cell crisis or anemia. More than 80% of hemoglobin as shown by electrophoresis is Hg-S, not Hg-A. A stained blood smear detects anemia only. Hematocrit and hemoglobin levels are below normal values. WBCs are increased with infection. Skeletal roentgenograms demonstrate bone and joint deformities and flattening. MRI may be used to diagnose a stroke caused by occluded cerebral vessels from sickled cells.

Medical Management

Sickle cell anemia has no specific treatment. Therapy is usually directed toward alleviating the symptoms that result from complications. For example, chronic leg ulcers may be treated with bed rest, antibiotics, warm saline soaks, mechanical or enzyme debridement, and dressings. Serious infections, such as meningitis, pneumonia, sepsis, and osteomyelitis, must be aggressively treated to prevent death (Lewis at al., 2007). *Haemophilus influenzae*, pneumococcal-conjugated, meningococcal, and hepatitis immunizations should be administered.

Sickle cell crisis may require hospitalization. Oxygen may be administered to alter hypoxia and control sickling. Encourage rest and administer fluids and electrolytes intravenously to reduce blood viscosity and maintain renal function. Use analgesics to treat pain. Sickle cell crisis pain is often undertreated. The nurse needs a clear understanding of the disease process and of current approaches to pain management.

According to pain experts, parenteral morphine and hydromorphone are the preferred opioid analgesics for acute sickle cell crisis pain. Large doses of continuous (rather than prn) opioid analgesics are the mainstay of pain management during the acute phase. Patient-controlled analgesia may be used during an acute crisis. After discharge, patients often continue taking oral opioid analgesics. Health care personnel must overcome their fears of opioid addiction to treat pain optimally and to avoid prolonging its duration. Blood transfusions of packed RBCs should be used cautiously to treat a crisis. Packed RBCs have little role, if any, in treating patients between crises. These patients have an increased need for folic acid, so it is important for them to take daily supplements. Iron therapy generally is not suggested.

Hydroxyurea therapy significantly boosts the production of Hg-F, reduces hemolysis, increases hemoglobin concentration, and decreases sickled cells. An oral antifungal medication is in clinical trials for patients with sickle cell anemia to see if it will decrease sickling and keep the RBCs hydrated by preventing potassium loss (Platt, 2007).

Hematapoietic stem cell transplantation (HSCT) is the only therapy that can cure selected patients with sickle cell anemia. The use of HSCT is limited because of scarcity of appropriate donors, selection of appropriate recipients, and the risks as well as cost effectiveness (Lewis et al., 2007).

Nursing Interventions and Patient Teaching

Supportive treatment depends on signs and symptoms presentation: hydration and analgesia during crises, and dilution of blood with increased fluid intake to reverse sickling. Monitoring the transfusion therapy for evidence of transfusion reaction is vital. Attention to fever and infection is important. Genetic counseling is indicated.

Nursing diagnoses and interventions for the patient with sickle cell anemia include but are not limited to the following:

Nursing Diagnoses	Nursing Interventions
Pain, related to thrombotic crisis	Place patient in proper anatomic alignment, and protect joints. Position patient by slow, gentle handling. Apply warmth with soaks or compresses to relieve discomfort. Give analgesics on a fixed time schedule to maintain a steady serum drug level, which improves pain control, minimizes complications, and decreases anxiety. (A patient-controlled analgesic infusion pump provides a constant, low-dose infusion of an opioid for excellent pain control.)

Nursing Diagnoses	Nursing Interventions
Impaired skin integrity, related to altered circulation to tissues, resulting in hypoxia and inadequate nutrition	Remove constrictive clothing to enhance circulation. Maintain room and body warmth to avoid discomfort or chilling. Initiate ROM exercises; support joints at rest and with movement to stimulate circulation. Palpate for arterial pulses to assess patency of arterial circulation. Monitor blood studies for gas exchange and hematological indicators of adequate tissue perfusion. Place patient on bed rest to decrease resistance to peripheral circulation. Elevate affected parts to enhance venous return. Implement cleaning procedure (use hydrogen peroxide or normal saline solution) to remove drainage and necrotic tissue. Apply sterile dressing or expose affected area to air to promote healing. Apply heat with lamp or cradle as ordered to enhance circulation and healing. Observe response to evaluate effectiveness of therapy. Cut patient's nails and discourage scratching to avoid injury.

Alert the patient to the need for family testing to determine the presence of Hg-S; genetic counseling is available for carriers. Explain how to avoid sickle cell crises: avoid high altitudes, flying in unpressurized planes, dehydration, extreme temperatures, iced liquids, and vigorous exercise; use stress-reduction methods. Patients should not smoke and should protect extremities from injury because of impaired circulation. Patients with sickle cell disease have frequent problems with infections. It is important for the patient to remain current with vaccinations and take prophylactic antibiotics to protect against these infections. Explain that young pregnant women have a high risk for developing pulmonary and/or renal complications. Alert the patient to the signs and symptoms of increased intracranial pressure and to the need to blow the nose gently, avoid coughing, and avoid straining on elimination.

Practice ROM exercises with the patient and encourage regular physical activity to prevent bone demineralization. Explain the need for a balance between rest (physical and mental) and activity, such as ROM

and isometric exercises. Also discuss the principles of good nutrition, such as the importance of protein, calcium, vitamins, and adequate fluids. Demonstrate to the patient how to monitor oral intake, urinary output, and urine protein.

Prognosis
Earlier detection, improved treatments, and greater use of immunizations help patients with sickle cell disease live longer, more productive lives (Platt, 2007). Still, the prognosis is guarded. In addition to hemolytic anemia, painful crises with multiple infarctions of most organ systems can occur. With repeated episodes of sickling, there is gradual involvement of all body systems, especially the spleen, the lungs, the kidneys, and the brain. Bone marrow grafts from HLA-identical siblings are providing hope for sickle cell patients.

Polycythemia (Erythrocytosis)
Etiology and Pathophysiology
Two types of polycythemia are **primary polycythemia (polycythemia vera)** and **secondary polycythemia.** Their etiologies and pathophysiology differ, although their complications and clinical manifestations are similar.

Polycythemia vera is a **myeloproliferative** (characterized by excessive bone marrow production) disorder with hyperplasia of bone marrow; it manifests with an increase in circulating erythrocytes (**erythrocytosis**), granulocytes, and platelets. The condition is a stem cell abnormality of unknown cause. Polycythemia vera develops gradually and is a chronic disease. The average age for the patient is 60 years. It occurs slightly more frequently in men. The patient has blood that is relatively thick and flows more slowly than usual (Lewis et al., 2007). There is also an elevated WBC count with basophilia. Secondary polycythemia is caused by hypoxia rather than by a defect in the development of the RBC. Hypoxia stimulates erythropoietin in the kidneys, which in turn stimulates erythrocyte production. The need for increased oxygen may result from high altitude, pulmonary disease, cardiovascular disease, or tissue hypoxia. Secondary polycythemia is not a pathologic response, but a physiologic response in which the body tries to compensate for a hypoxic problem. In polycythemia vera the pathologic response is a malignancy of the blood cells.

Multiorgan system disease is affected by hyperplastic bone marrow elements. Because of the increased erythrocyte mass, hypervolemia and hyperviscosity (stickiness) of the blood result in congestion of tissues and organs. The sluggish circulatory process results in hypercoagulopathies that predispose patients to infarctions of vital organs.

Clinical Manifestations
Patients with polycythemia vera have increased blood volume and viscosity, which can result in hypertension, angina pectoris, heart failure, and thrombophlebitis

(Platt, 2007). Venous distention and platelet dysfunction cause esophageal varices, epistaxis, GI bleeding, and petechiae. Hepatomegaly and splenomegaly from organ engorgement may contribute to patient complaints of satiety and fullness.

Assessment

Subjective data include patient complaints of sensitivity to hot and cold. Generalized pruritus (often exacerbated by a hot bath) may be a striking symptom and is related to histamine release from an increased number of basophils. Headaches, vertigo, tinnitus, blurred vision, and painful burning of the hands and feet are often present.

Objective data include eczema and dermatologic changes. The skin may develop an erythemic appearance (plethora). Elevated blood pressure accompanies left ventricular hypertrophy and angina.

Diagnostic Tests

Plasma and RBC volume are increased. Elevations are seen in hemoglobin and hematocrit levels, reticulocyte and erythrocyte counts, platelets (thrombocytes), and WBC count with basophilia. Elevated alkaline phosphatase, uric acid, and histamine levels are noted. Bone marrow examination in polycythemia vera shows hypercellularity of RBCs, WBCs, and platelets. The basal metabolic rate (BMR) is increased without thyroid function alteration. Splenomegaly is found in 90% of patients with primary polycythemia but does not accompany secondary polycythemia.

Medical Management

Blood viscosity is decreased by repeated phlebotomy—removal of 500 to 2000 mL of blood until the hematocrit level is maintained at 45% to 48%. The procedure is repeated if hematocrit rises to more than 50%. Once the diagnosis of polycythemia vera is made, treatment is directed toward reducing blood volume and viscosity and bone marrow activity. Myelosuppressive agents such as busulfan (Myleran), hydroxyurea (Hydrea), melphalan (Alkeran), and radioactive phosphorus are often given to inhibit bone marrow activity. Allopurinol may reduce the number of acute gouty attacks.

Nursing Interventions and Patient Teaching

Polycythemia vera is not preventable. However, because secondary polycythemia is generated by any source of hypoxia, problems may be prevented by maintaining adequate oxygenation. Therefore controlling chronic pulmonary disease, stopping smoking, and avoiding high altitudes may be important.

When acute exacerbations of polycythemia vera develop, the nurse has several responsibilities. Judiciously evaluate fluid I&O during hydration therapy to avoid fluid overload (which further complicates the circulatory congestion) and dehydration (which can cause the blood to become even more viscous). If myelosuppressive agents are used, administer the drugs as ordered, observe the patient, and teach the patient about medication side effects.

Assess the patient's nutritional status with the dietitian if necessary to offset the inadequate food intake that can result from GI symptoms of fullness, pain, and dyspepsia. Institute activities, such as active or passive leg exercises and ambulation, to decrease the risk of thrombus formation.

Because of its chronic nature, polycythemia vera requires ongoing evaluation. Phlebotomy may need to be performed every 2 to 3 months, reducing the blood volume by about 500 mL each time. Evaluate the patient for the development of complications.

Nursing diagnoses and interventions for the patient with polycythemia vera include but are not limited to the following:

Nursing Diagnoses	Nursing Interventions
Ineffective tissue perfusion (cardiopulmonary, cerebral, GI, and peripheral), related to: • hyperviscosity of fluid • potential bleeding	Have patient maintain comfortable position. When patient is on bed rest, do not raise knee gatch. Provide active or passive ROM exercises every 2 to 4 hours. Check peripheral pulses and color and temperature of extremities every 4 to 6 hours. Report early signs or symptoms of thrombosis or bleeding to physician. If patient has bleeding tendency, avoid invasive procedures when possible. Avoid trauma; provide soft-bristled toothbrush.
Activity intolerance, related to ischemia	Encourage avoidance of sodium-rich foods to reduce fluid retention. Encourage adequate exercise and mobility to prevent stasis. Explain disease course and signs and symptoms expected.

Educate the patient about this condition if necessary. Emphasize the importance of compliance with the medical and nutritional regimen. Dietary teaching should emphasize avoiding foods that contain iron while increasing the intake of calories and protein (because of BMR increase).

Emphasize that certain signs and symptoms (such as pain, edema, or erythema associated with thrombosis) require medical supervision. Because this is a chronic illness, emotional support is imperative.

Prognosis

Polycythemia vera is a chronic, life-shortening disorder. Although the incidence is small, leukemia and lymphomas develop in some patients with polycythemia vera. This may occur as a result of the chemotherapeutic drugs used to treat the disease or may be secondary to a disorder in the stem cells that progresses to leukemia. The major cause of morbidity and mortality from polycythemia vera is thrombosis. Permanent cure cannot be achieved today, but remission of many years can be produced.

DISORDERS ASSOCIATED WITH LEUKOCYTES

AGRANULOCYTOSIS

Etiology and Pathophysiology

Agranulocytosis is a potentially fatal condition of the blood characterized by a severe reduction in the number of granulocytes (basophils, eosinophils, and neutrophils). The WBC count is extremely low (**leukopenia**), as is the differential neutrophil count (less than 200/mm³ [neutropenia]). Normal neutrophil value is 3000 to 7000/mm³.

Adverse medication reaction or toxicity is the primary cause of agranulocytosis. However, neoplastic disease, chemotherapy, and radiation therapy are often cited as causative. Viral and bacterial infections are possible causes of the condition. Heredity is also considered.

Suppression of the bone marrow by the causative agent reduces the number and production of WBCs. Leukocytes, formed in the bone marrow, provide body protection against microorganisms. This protection is ineffective when bone marrow suppression has occurred.

Clinical Manifestations

Fever, chills, headache, and fatigue are symptoms associated with infection and the inflammatory process. Ulcerations of mucous membranes—mouth, nose, pharynx, vagina, and rectum—are also found. Bronchial pneumonia and urinary tract infections are complications that occur in the later stages.

Assessment

Subjective data include common complaints of fever, extreme fatigue, and prostration. All medications taken, whether prescription or over-the-counter, are considered as possible causes of the condition.

Objective data include fever over 100.6° F (38.1° C). Erythema and pain from ulcerations may occur. Ulcerations are cultured for microorganisms. Lung and bronchial auscultation reveals crackles and rhonchi because of trapped exudates.

Possible causative chemical agents are antibiotics (chloramphenicol, penicillin derivatives, cephalosporins), antiepileptics (phenytoin), antihistamines, antineoplastic drugs (vincristine [Oncovin]), antithyroid drugs (propylthiouracil), diuretics, phenothiazides (chlorpromazine [Thorazine], fluphenazine [Prolixin], promazine [Sparine], prochlorperazine [Compazine]), and sulfonamides and derivatives.

Diagnostic Tests

The levels of leukocytes with neutrophils differential are below normal. A bone marrow study shows depression of activity.

Medical Management

The main objective of treatment is to alleviate the factors responsible for bone marrow depression and prevent or treat infection. Blood cultures may be performed when fever is elevated, and cultures may be ordered if ulceration occurs. Transfusions of packed RBCs are often ordered. Granulocyte colony-stimulating factor (G-CSF) (filgrastim [Neupogen]), pegfilgrastim (Neulasta), and GM-CSF (sargramostin [Leukine, Prokine]) given subcutaneously or intravenously can be used to treat a neutropenic patient. Immunocompromised (neutropenic) precautions may also be instituted.

Nursing Interventions and Patient Teaching

A patient with a compromised WBC system is highly susceptible to life-threatening infections. Nursing interventions are directed toward protecting the patient from potential sources of infection. Monitor the patient conscientiously to detect the earliest signs of infection so that therapy may be initiated promptly. Meticulous hand hygiene by medical and nursing personnel and strict asepsis are mandatory.

A nursing diagnosis and interventions for the patient with agranulocytosis include but are not limited to the following:

Nursing Diagnosis	Nursing Interventions
Risk for infection, related to depressed WBC (leukocyte) production	Maintain scrupulously clean patient environment.
	Be certain no person with any type of infection is allowed in contact with the patient.
	Observe for signs and symptoms of infection, such as elevated temperature and chills.
	Wash hands meticulously and use strict asepsis for procedures.
	Enforce protective isolation to protect patient from pathogens.
	Provide high-protein, high-vitamin, high-calorie diet to maintain nutritional status.

Nursing Diagnosis	Nursing Interventions
Risk for infection, related to depressed WBC (leukocyte) production—cont'd	Avoid raw foods, such as sushi, Caesar salad dressing (may have raw eggs), blue cheese, and fruits that cannot be peeled or vegetables that cannot be well cleaned. Encourage patient to take fluids to promote hydration. Monitor heart rate, respirations, blood pressure, and temperature to assess for signs of infection. Observe the patient for extreme fatigue, sore throat or mouth, and fever as signs of infection. Monitor WBC count. Use cooling measures (cooling blanket and tepid baths) to reduce fever if present. Administer antibiotics as ordered to combat specific pathogens. Have patient bathe or shower daily. Provide perineal care to maintain hygiene and prevent infection.

In patient teaching, discuss the use of frequent, thorough oral hygiene to treat or prevent mouth and pharyngeal infection. Explain the need to avoid crowds, people with infectious diseases, and cold or hot environments; also teach signs and symptoms of infection and appropriate interventions. Explain the need for a soft, bland diet high in protein, vitamins, and calories. And encourage a balance between rest and activity to prevent fatigue and generalized weakness.

Prognosis
Agranulocytosis is a potentially fatal condition because of the possibility of a life-threatening bacterial infection.

LEUKEMIA
Etiology and Pathophysiology
Leukemia is a malignant disorder of the hematopoietic system in which an excess of leukocytes accumulates in the bone marrow and lymph nodes. The cause, although unknown, is attributed to genetic origin, a virus, people previously treated with radiation, or chemotherapeutic agents that are toxic to bone marrow. A viral cause for human leukemia has been established only for some patients with adult T-cell leukemia (Lewis et al., 2007).

Bone marrow is replaced by rapidly developing white cells with abnormal numbers and forms of immature cells found in the circulation and infiltrated into the lymph nodes, the spleen, and the liver. The increased numbers of WBCs can lead to infiltration and damage to the bone marrow; the lymph nodes; the spleen; and organs, including those of the central nervous system. Leukemic infiltration leads to problems such as hepatomegaly, splenomegaly, lymphadenopathy, bone pain, meningeal irritation, and oral lesions. Hematopoietic function is disturbed by incompetent bone marrow. Increased susceptibility to infection results.

Classification
Leukemias are classified by identifying the type of leukocyte involved, whether it is of myelogenous or lymphocytic origin. Specific leukemia types are further categorized by combining the acute and chronic conditions with the cell type involved. Thus the four major types of leukemia are acute lymphocytic leukemia (ALL), acute myelogenous leukemia (AML), chronic myelogenous (granulocytic) leukemia (CML), and chronic lymphocytic leukemia (CLL). The peak incidence for ALL is between 2 and 9 years of age and in older adults. In AML the peak incidence is around 4 to 5 years of age, in CLL it is between 50 and 70 years of age, and in CML, it is between 25 and 60 years of age (Lewis et al., 2007).

Clinical Manifestations
The clinical manifestations of leukemia vary. Essentially they relate to problems caused by bone marrow failure and the formation of leukemic infiltrates. Bone marrow failure results from (1) bone marrow overcrowding by abnormal cells and (2) inadequate production of normal marrow elements. The patient is predisposed to anemia and thrombocytopenia.

As leukemia progresses, fewer normal blood cells are produced. The abnormal WBCs continue to accumulate. The leukemic cells infiltrate the patient's organs, leading to problems such as splenomegaly, hepatomegaly, lymphadenopathy, bone pain, meningeal irritation, and oral lesions. Enlarged lymph nodes and painless splenomegaly may be the first signs of the disease in some people.

Diagnostic Tests
The WBC count is low, elevated, or excessively elevated. Anemia and thrombocytopenia are noted. Bone marrow biopsy shows immature leukocytes. Chest radiographic examination may show mediastinal node and lung involvement and bone changes. Lymph node biopsy reveals excessive blasts (immature cells). Peripheral blood evaluation and bone marrow examination are the primary methods of diagnosing and classifying the type of leukemia. Further studies such as lumbar puncture and CT scan can be performed to determine the presence of leukemic cells outside of the blood and bone marrow.

Assessment

Subjective data include patient complaints regarding symptoms that may seem unrelated at first. Patients often have pain in bones or joints, fatigue, malaise, decreased activity tolerance, and irritability.

Objective data include those signs listed in clinical manifestations. Infections are common. Occult blood is detected in laboratory specimens of urine and stool. Abnormalities of skin (petechiae, ecchymoses) and mucous membranes (bleeding) may be present.

Medical Management

The goal of treatment is to achieve remission or to control the symptoms. Treatment is aimed at eradicating the leukemia with chemotherapy or bone marrow transplant. Combination chemotherapy is the mainstay for treating leukemia. Multiple drugs are used to (1) decrease drug resistance, (2) minimize the drug toxicity by using multiple drugs with varying toxicities (with lower dosages of each), and (3) interrupt cell growth at multiple points in the cell cycle. Observation for drug toxicity is imperative (Table 7-2).

Table 7-2 Medications for Blood and Lymphatic Disorders

Generic (Trade)	Action	Side Effects	Nursing Implications
Cyanocobalamin (Cobex, vitamin B₁₂)	Needed for adequate nerve functioning, protein and carbohydrate metabolism, normal growth, RBC development, and cell reproduction	Flushing, diarrhea, itching, rash, hypokalemia	Assess GI functions and potassium levels at beginning of treatment; stress need for patients with pernicious anemia to return for monthly injections; give intramuscularly only.
Folic acid (B complex vitamin) (Folvite)	Needed for erythropoiesis; increases RBC, WBC, and platelet formation in megaloblastic anemias	Pruritus, rash, general malaise, bronchospasm, slight flushing	Drug may be administered by deep intramuscular, subcutaneous, or intravenous routes; do not mix with other medications in same syringe for intramuscular injections.
Ferrous sulfate (Feosol, Fer-In-Sol)	Replaces iron stores needed for RBC development	Nausea, constipation, epigastric pain, black and red tarry stools, vomiting, diarrhea, discolored urine, staining of teeth	Between-meal dosing is preferable but can be given with some foods, although absorption may be decreased; give tablets with orange juice to promote iron absorption; to avoid staining teeth, give elixir iron preparations through straw; oral iron may turn stools black.
Iron dextran (DexFerrum)	Released into the plasma and carried by transferring to the bone marrow, where it is incorporated into hemoglobin	Stained skin at site of injection, fever, chills, headache, sweating, discolored urine, diarrhea	Administer 0.5-mL test dose by preferred route before therapy; wait at least 1 hour before giving remaining portion.
Desmopressin acetate (DDAVP, Concentraid)	Promotes reabsorption of water by kidneys and increase in plasma factor VIII levels, which increases platelet aggregation, resulting in vasopressor effect	Nasal irritation, congestion, drowsiness, headache, flushing, nausea, abdominal cramps, heartburn, vulval pain, hypertension	Avoid overhydration; assess pulse and blood pressure when giving drug subcutaneously; monitor factor VIII antigen levels and aPTT.
Filgrastim (G-CSF) (Neupogen)	Stimulates proliferation and differentiation of neutrophils	Fever, alopecia, skeletal pain, nausea, vomiting, diarrhea, mucositis, anorexia	Monitor CBC and platelet count before treatment and twice weekly; refrigerate but do not freeze; avoid shaking; store at room temperature for at least 6 hours; discard any vial that has been at room temperature for more than 6 hours.

aPTT, Activated partial thromboplastin time; *CBC,* complete blood count; *G-CSF,* granulocyte colony-stimulating factor; *GI,* gastrointestinal; *RBC,* red blood cell; *WBC,* white blood cell.

Tremendous progress in the treatment of leukemia has been made in recent years with the use of a complex combination of chemotherapeutic drugs and radiation therapy. Bone marrow transplant and HSCT may be the treatment of choice in patients with suitable donors and initial remission of the acute leukemia (see Chapter 17). Before the transplant, the patient's bone marrow cells and leukemic cells must be killed by massive chemotherapy and total body irradiation. The patient may succumb to infection, hemorrhage, or graft-versus-host disease.

In chronic leukemia, which occurs almost exclusively in adults and develops slowly, the desired objectives of treatment depend on the kind of cells involved. Medications commonly used include chlorambucil (Leukeran), hydroxyurea, corticosteroids, and cyclophosphamide. Lymph nodes are often irradiated, and blood transfusion may be given if anemia is severe. Although medications are not curative in chronic leukemia, they help to prolong life (see Table 7-2).

Nursing Interventions and Patient Teaching

Prevent infection by teaching patients about immunocompromised (neutropenic) precautions and the avoidance of infectious agents. Leukopenia (an abnormal decrease in the number of WBCs to less than 5000 cells/mm^3) can be fatal. The usual inflammatory process to control infection is decreased; thus frequent observation for signs and symptoms of infection is necessary. Thrombocytopenia-induced hemorrhage may be life threatening; prevent this condition through safe, gentle care. Control pain through analgesia as ordered and by comfort measures. Coping mechanisms may be strained because of pain, complexities of treatment, side effects and toxicities, change of body image, or fear of death. Support the patient and family by developing a positive nurse-patient-family relationship and referring them to community support groups.

Nurses have contact with a patient 24 hours a day and can reduce feelings of abandonment and loneliness by balancing the demanding technical needs with a humanistic, caring approach. Therefore a nurse faces a special challenge in learning how to meet the intense psychosocial needs of a patient with leukemia while continuing to offer the complex physical care that is usually required. Consult with other health professionals (e.g., psychiatric clinical specialists, oncology clinical specialists, social workers) to help develop the skills required to meet the many needs of a patient with leukemia.

From a physical care perspective, it is challenging to make astute assessments and plan care to help the patient survive the severe side effects of chemotherapy. The life-threatening results of bone marrow suppression (anemia, thrombocytopenia, neutropenia) require aggressive nursing interventions. Additional complications of chemotherapy may affect the patient's GI tract, nutritional status, skin and mucosa, cardiopulmonary status, liver, kidneys, and neurologic system.

Be informed about all drugs being administered, including mechanism of action, purpose, routes of administration, usual doses, potential side effects, safe handling considerations, and toxic effects. In addition, know how to assess laboratory data reflecting the effects of the drugs. Patient survival and comfort during aggressive chemotherapy are significantly affected by the quality of nursing intervention.

Discuss procedures, meaning of treatments, and care plans with the patient and family. Be certain to cover the nature of the disease and previous information given the patient. Community resources for support and information are invaluable for educating the patient and the family. Examine expectations of physical abilities, remission, and future plans. Encourage continuation of the medical regimen and avoidance of situations in which infection can be transmitted. Most patients should receive the pneumococcal vaccine (Pneumovax) at diagnosis and every 5 years and an annual influenza vaccine (Lewis et al., 2007). Medication and diet information is important.

Prognosis

Perhaps more dramatically than in any other malignant disorder, chemotherapy has improved the prognosis of children with ALL. Untreated patients have a median survival time of 4 to 6 months. With current therapy of vincristine and prednisone, plus an anthracycline drug (daunorubicin or doxorubicin [Adriamycin]), the median survival rate is about 5 years, and approximately 50% of children with ALL can now be cured. In AML, remission can be achieved in up to 75% of cases; however, relapse eventually occurs in most cases. Only about 20% to 25% of adults with AML experience a 5-year remission. Overall survival for CLL is variable. When diagnosed in early stages, median survival rate ranges from 10 to 12½ years; when diagnosed in advanced stages, survival is approximately 18 months (Nursing Care Plan 7-1).

DISORDERS OF COAGULATION

Etiology and Pathophysiology

Release of blood from the vascular system results from trauma or vessel damage, vessel inadequacy, disturbance of the function of platelets or clotting factors, or liver disease (impaired clotting mechanisms).

The clotting mechanism is a hemostatic chain reaction. Vasoconstriction inhibits capillary leakage; hematoma compression provides pressure. The body reacts by lowering arterial blood pressure. Any manifestation that alters this process predisposes the body to hemorrhage. The affected mechanism may be vascular, platelet dysfunction, or an alteration in plasma coagulation factor. The disorder may be congenital or acquired, possibly secondary to another disease or to medication toxicity.

Nursing Care Plan 7-1   The Patient with Leukemia

Ms. May is a 26-year-old patient diagnosed with acute lymphocytic leukemia. She is married and the mother of a 3-year-old daughter. Ms. May has been receiving chemotherapy and is immunocompromised, with a differential white blood cell (WBC) count revealing a neutrophil count of 22%. Her hemoglobin is 8.8 g/dL, and her platelets are 55,000/mm³. Her mouth appears edematous, and she complains of oral tenderness.

NURSING DIAGNOSIS *Risk for infection, related to leukopenia*

Patient Goals and Expected Outcomes	Nursing Intervention	Evaluation/Rationale
Patient or caregiver will identify measures to prevent or control infection	Inspect all body sites for infection at least daily; note and report fever, sore throat, purulent exudate, chills, cough, burning with urination, erythema, edema, tenderness, and pain.	Patient will remain free of infection.
Patient or caregiver will verbalize and report signs and symptoms of infection	Monitor vital signs. Obtain cultures as ordered. Monitor WBC counts and culture reports. Administer antibiotics on time as ordered. Promote and maintain hygiene integrity of skin and mucous membranes. Use aseptic technique in treatments. Teach the patient and family: • Necessity of avoiding crowds or people with infections while WBC count is <1000/mm³ • Personal hygiene measures • Signs and symptoms of infection	Patient demonstrates no signs or symptoms of infection; temperature and WBC count are within normal range.

NURSING DIAGNOSIS *Ineffective coping, related to diagnosis and disease process*

Patient Goals and Expected Outcomes	Nursing Intervention	Evaluation
Patient and family will demonstrate measures to effectively cope by verbalizing role of family, significant others, and support groups in therapeutic coping	Assess coping capabilities of patient and significant others. Discuss disease process and expectations. Alleviate knowledge deficit. Encourage questions and self-expression: listen actively, demonstrate compassion, reassure with touch and personal contact. Assess fear of threat of death: allow time for personal expression and provide one-on-one discussion opportunity.	Patient and family express factors that are causing anxiety and powerlessness.

Critical Thinking Questions

1. What should the nurse do if a visitor with an obvious upper respiratory tract infection is seen approaching Ms. May's room?
2. What nursing interventions would be most appropriate in providing therapeutic oral hygiene for Ms. May?
3. What kind of a bath and activities of daily living would be most beneficial for Ms. May?

Clinical Manifestations

Skin and mucous membrane manifestations include petechiae and ecchymoses. Epistaxis and gingival bleeding are common. Circulatory hypovolemia is noted through hypotension; pallor; cool, clammy skin; and tachycardia. GI tract bleeding is common, with abdominal flank pain caused by internal bleeding. CNS involvement ranges from altered response and malaise to loss of consciousness or affected speech.

Assessment

Subjective data include a history of bleeding after surgical or dental procedures. Exposure to toxic or hazardous agents or to radiation may be revealed.

Complaint of headache, extremity pain, and numbness is noted. Medications taken (e.g., aspirin) may lead to suspicion of toxicity.

Collection of **objective data** involves observation of pain on pressure to the abdomen, revealing liver and spleen tenderness and perhaps enlargement. Skin and mucous membranes may have petechiae, ecchymoses, and occasionally hematoma. Emesis and stool may show signs of bleeding. Joint examination reveals motion pain.

Diagnostic Tests

The platelet count is low. The RBC count is low with a decreased hemoglobin level. Coagulation time is altered. Bone marrow studies show abnormal cells.

Medical Management

The underlying cause is assessed and corrected, and replacement transfusions may be ordered. Heparin therapy or medication toxicity is considered as a possible cause. Infections and complications are treated or prevented.

Nursing Interventions

Medical intervention often depends on accurate reporting of signs and symptoms and nursing observations. In coagulation disorders, monitor vital signs to note any signs of hypovolemic shock. Move the patient gently to prevent trauma to the tissues. Monitor IV infusions and transfusions as ordered.

DISORDERS ASSOCIATED WITH PLATELETS

THROMBOCYTOPENIA

Etiology and Pathophysiology

A deficiency of the number of circulating platelets or change in the function of platelets alters the process of coagulation. Thrombocytopenia is an abnormal hematological condition in which the number of platelets is reduced to fewer than 150,000/mm³. Decreased production occurs in aplastic anemia, leukemia, tumors, and chemotherapy. Decreased platelet survival occurs when there is antibody destruction, infection, or viral invasion. Increased platelet destruction is caused by disseminated intravascular coagulation (DIC). Splenomegaly results from entrapment of blood in the spleen.

The most common cause of increased destruction of platelets is thrombocytopenic purpura, which may be drug-induced or immune thrombocytopenic purpura. This is the most common acquired thrombocytopenia. It is a syndrome of abnormal destruction of circulating platelets termed *immune thrombocytopenic purpura* (ITP). It was originally termed *idiopathic* (cause unknown) *thrombocytopenic purpura*. However, it is now known that ITP is an autoimmune disease. In ITP, platelets are coated with antibodies. Although these platelets function normally, when they reach the spleen, the antibody-coated platelets are recognized as foreign and are destroyed by macrophages in the spleen. Normal platelets survive 8 to 10 days, but with ITP, platelet survival is an average of 1 to 3 days. If thrombocytopenia is medication induced (Box 7-3), the patient's platelet counts usually return to normal 1 to 2 weeks after the medication is withdrawn. The acute form of ITP is found mostly in children, whereas the chronic form is found among patients of all ages but is more common in 20- to 40-year-old women. It is an autoimmune process caused by the production of an autoantibody (immunoglobulin G) directed against a platelet antigen.

Clinical Manifestations

The major signs of thrombocytopenia that are observable by physical examination are petechiae and ecchymoses on the skin. Petechiae occur only in platelet disorders. The severity of signs and symptoms correlates

---

Box 7-3	Medications with Thrombocytopenic Effects

- Aspirin
- Digitalis derivatives
- Furosemide
- Nonsteroidal antiinflammatory agents (azathioprine, D-penicillamine, phenylbutazone, ibuprofen, indomethacin)
- Oral hypoglycemics
- Penicillins
- Quinidine
- Rifampicin
- Sulfonamides
- Thiazides

---

with the platelet count. As the level drops to less than 100,000/mm³, the risk for bleeding from mucous membranes and in cutaneous sites and internal organs increases. Significant risk for serious bleeding occurs once the count is less than 20,000/mm³. When the platelet count is less than 5000/mm³, spontaneous, potentially fatal CNS or GI hemorrhage can occur.

Assessment

Collection of subjective data includes questioning the patient about recent viral infections (which may produce a transient thrombocytopenia), medications in current use, and the extent of alcohol ingestion.

Collection of objective data includes observing the patient's skin for petechiae and ecchymoses. Epistaxis and gingival bleeding may be noted. Signs of increased intracranial pressure caused by cerebral hemorrhage may be detected.

Diagnostic Tests

To ascertain the characteristics of all blood cells, laboratory studies include platelet count, peripheral blood smear, and bleeding time. In addition, a bone marrow analysis is performed to determine the presence of immature platelets. Examination also reveals the presence or absence of primary bone marrow abnormalities, such as neoplastic invasion or aplastic anemia.

Medical Management

Usually, no therapy is needed if the patient has a platelet count of 30,000/mm³ or greater (Lewis et al., 2007). The primary treatments are corticosteroid therapy to suppress the phagocytic response of splenic macrophages. Corticosteroid therapy also increases the life span of the platelets (Lewis et al., 2007). If the patient does not respond initially to prednisone or requires unacceptably high doses to uphold an adequate platelet count, splenectomy is indicated.

Other treatments may include IV immunoglobulin in the patient who is unresponsive to corticosteroids or splenectomy. Transfusion with platelet concentration may be used in people with thrombocytopenic bleeding. Platelet transfusions are generally not recommended until the count is below 10,000/mm^3 unless the patient is actively bleeding. Each platelet transfusion can be expected to increase a patient's platelets by 10,000/mm^3 (Lewis et al., 2007). Plasmapheresis is used to treat ITP by removing antibodies produced by the autoimmune process.

Immunosuppressive therapy used in refractory cases includes ritaximab (Rituxan), azathioprine (Imuran), cyclosporine, and mycophenolate mofetil (CellCept) (Lewis et al., 2007).

Nursing Interventions and Patient Teaching

Support the medical treatment regimen, using specific interventions for specific disease causes. If medication toxicity is the cause, the medication is discontinued. Prevent infections by meticulous asepsis and gentle handling of the patient. Closely monitor plasma and platelet infusion and whole-blood transfusions for reaction and effects on patients' conditions.

Nursing diagnoses and interventions for the patient with thrombocytopenia include but are not limited to the following:

Nursing Diagnoses	Nursing Interventions
Ineffective tissue perfusion (cerebral, cardiopulmonary, renal, GI, peripheral), related to bleeding	Monitor vital signs and neurologic status. Monitor platelet count. Assess for bleeding and fluid imbalance. Check patient's urine, stool, and emesis for blood. Monitor invasive diagnostic procedure sites for bleeding. Maintain comfort measures and bed rest. Avoid trauma and infection. Monitor patient receiving parenteral fluids and blood components for untoward signs. Monitor potential sites of hemorrhage.
Pain, related to hemorrhage	Assess discomfort and pain level. Assess patient's ability to cope and response to pain. Administer analgesia as ordered and note patient response. Provide education.

The patient must understand the disease process and causative agents to provide self-care and prevent trauma or infection. Provide instructions on signs, symptoms, and preventive measures: avoid trauma, use stool softeners, maintain a high-fiber diet to prevent constipation, check for presence of blood, use a soft toothbrush, and blow nose gently. Stress the importance of notifying the physician of signs and symptoms of bleeding.

Prognosis

The prognosis is variable, depending on the underlying cause. In ITP, treatment may need to be administered for 3 to 4 weeks before a complete response is seen. In chronic ITP, transient remissions occur. Approximately 80% of patients benefit from splenectomy, resulting in a complete or partial remission.

CLOTTING FACTOR DEFECTS

HEMOPHILIA

Etiology and Pathophysiology

Hemophilia, a hereditary coagulation disorder, is characterized by a disturbance of the clotting factors. In hemophilia A, the more common type (representing 80% of the total incidence), antihemophilic factor VIII is absent. This factor is essential for conversion of prothrombin to thrombin through thromboplastin component. A decrease in the formation of prothrombin activators occurs as a result of the decrease in clotting factors. Hemophilia B (Christmas disease) exhibits a deficiency of factor IX with an absence of plasma thromboplastin component (a plasma protein), resulting in nonformation of thromboplastin.

Hemophilia is an X-linked hereditary trait that affects mainly males; females are carriers.

In the past the patient with hemophilia was at high risk for being infected with human immunodeficiency virus (HIV) and later developing acquired immunodeficiency syndrome because of the need for cryoprecipitate concentrates, which were potentially contaminated with HIV. Unfortunately, the HIV contamination of blood products caused the majority of hemophilia deaths in the late 1980s (Lewis et al., 2007). Now with viral-detecting processes, donor screening, and heat treatment of factor VIII concentrates (which destroys HIV), the risk of contracting HIV and hepatitis B and C through transfusions is greatly reduced. The use of recombinant replacement factors also is improving long-term survival rates.

Clinical Manifestations

Internal or external hemorrhage occurs with large ecchymoses into tissue—especially muscles, which may show deformity; and joints, which become ankylosed. Hemarthrosis, or bleeding into a joint space, is a hallmark of severe disease and usually occurs in the knees, the ankles, the elbows, the shoulders, and the hips. Pain, edema, erythema, and fever accompany hemarthrosis. Small cuts can prove fatal; blood loss from simple dental procedures may be significant.

Assessment

Subjective data include reports by patient and family of incidents of ecchymoses and hemorrhage from even the slightest trauma. Pain is associated with joint motion.

Collection of **objective data** includes noting blood in subcutaneous tissues, urine, or stool and noting edematous or immobile joints.

Diagnostic Tests

Factors VIII and IX are absent or deficient. Coagulation profiles reveal a normal platelet count, bleeding time, prothrombin time, and International Normalized Ratio. The partial thromboplastin time is prolonged. Notify laboratory personnel of the patient's disorder to alleviate further incidents of trauma as a result of diagnostic procedures (e.g., venipuncture).

Medical Management

Care focuses on preventing and treating bleeding and relieving pain. Transfusions and administration of factor VIII or IX concentrate may be prophylactic or used to stop the hemorrhage. Two different clotting factor concentrates made from human plasma can be used. One, cryoprecipitate, is a clotting factor concentrate rich in factor VIII. Its use is waning because of the associated risk, although small, of viral disease transmission. Additionally, home administration of cryoprecipitate is difficult because it must be stored at low temperatures. The second human-derived product, factor VIII concentrate, is most typically used. A wide variety of these products are available; all are freeze-dried concentrates of factor VIII prepared from pooled plasma from thousands of donors. These products are specially treated to inactivate any viral contamination (such as HIV or hepatitis viruses). Factor IX concentrates are prepared in a similar fashion.

Because human plasma products still carry a slight risk of infection transmission and require human donors, scientists have used genetic engineering to manufacture factor VIII. This product, recombinant factor VIII, is advantageous because of viral safety, unlimited supply, and lower cost. Recombinant replacement factor VIII is now commercially available for widespread use.

Nursing Interventions and Patient Teaching

Control hemorrhages in emergency situations by applying pressure and cold to the site. Support and reassurance are imperative. Educate the patient and the entire family because many people may be involved in the patient care. Monitor transfusions of factor VIII concentrate. Supportive care measures include pain management and genetic counseling. Do not give hemophilia patients aspirin because it can further complicate the bleeding tendency.

Nursing diagnoses and interventions for the patient with hemophilia include but are not limited to the following:

Nursing Diagnoses	Nursing Interventions
Ineffective tissue perfusion, related to blood loss from coagulation deficit	Assess for extent of hemorrhage. Prevent further hemorrhage or extension. Monitor vital signs and laboratory reports. Apply cold compresses to bleeding areas. Assess for anxiety, shock, disorientation, and decreased urinary output. Teach safety precautions to prevent trauma. Administer analgesia as ordered. Move patient gently and slowly, supporting joints. Prevent deformity through support, splints, and physical therapy.
Ineffective coping, related to long-term illness	Discuss disease process, altered lifestyle, and acceptance. Suggest genetic counseling. Encourage independence. Encourage compliance with medical regimen. Be an active listener.
Deficient fluid volume, related to bleeding	Monitor vital signs and level of consciousness for evidence of acute hemorrhage. Monitor blood component therapy as ordered to control bleeding. Monitor I&O. Apply ice pack to affected joint or traumatized area to control bleeding. Administer analgesics to relieve joint pain. Assess amount, consistency, and frequency of bleeding: • Nose • Joints • Skin • Stool and urine • Pad counts Monitor laboratory tests to assess degree of blood loss. Avoid trauma, such as falls, bumps, or injections.

Discuss with the patient ways to avoid injury and control bleeding. Also discuss physical activity within limits. Encourage the patient to wear a medical-alert tag. Emergency care teaching includes immobilizing the affected part, applying ice, and notifying the physician. Discuss diet to prevent obesity, which puts excess pressure on joints. Regular dental care and preventive dental and medical measures are important aspects. Overprotection is sometimes a factor to discuss. No aspirin or any other medication should be taken except with the physician's knowledge (Home Care Considerations box).

Prognosis

Before the appearance of the HIV virus, the average life span for a person with hemophilia was near normal. After HIV appeared, the majority of severe hemophiliacs who received clotting factor concentrate before 1984 became seropositive for HIV. Now, with the development of methods to heat-inactivate the virus, the risk of contracting HIV from clotting factor concentrates is almost nil. With the methods to control HIV and hepatitis B and C transmission and the use of recombinant re-

 Home Care Considerations

Hemophilia

- Home management is a primary consideration for a patient with hemophilia because the disease follows a chronic, progressive course.
- The quantity and length of life may be significantly affected by the patient's knowledge of the illness and understanding of how to live with it.
- Refer the patient and family to the local chapter of the National Hemophilia Foundation to encourage association with other individuals who are dealing with the problems associated with hemophilia.
- Teach the patient with hemophilia to recognize disease-related problems and to learn which problems can be resolved at home and which require hospitalization.
- Immediate medical attention is required for severe pain or edema of a muscle or joint that restricts movement or inhibits sleep and for a head injury, edema in the neck or mouth, abdominal pain, hematuria, melena, and skin wounds in need of suturing.
- Daily oral hygiene must be performed without trauma.
- Aspirin should not be taken because it decreases platelet aggregation.
- Understanding how to prevent injuries is an important consideration. The patient can learn to participate in noncontact sports (e.g., golf) and wear gloves when doing household chores to prevent cuts or abrasions from knives, hammers, and other tools.
- The patient should wear a medical-alert tag to ensure that health care providers know about the hemophilia in case of an accident.
- A person with hemophilia who is mature enough or a family member can be taught to administer some of the factor replacement therapies at home.

placement factors, the average life span for a person with hemophilia is once again near normal.

VON WILLEBRAND'S DISEASE

Etiology and Pathophysiology

von Willebrand's disease is an inherited bleeding disorder characterized by abnormally slow coagulation of blood and spontaneous episodes of GI bleeding, epistaxis, and gingival bleeding caused by a mild deficiency of factor VIII. It is common during postpartum periods, as menorrhagia, and after surgery or trauma. Although similar to hemophilia, its incidence is not limited to males.

Treatment includes administration of cryoprecipitate containing factor VIII, fibrinogen, or fresh plasma. Desmopressin (DDAVP) is becoming the treatment of choice for patients who have a mild form of hemophilia. This drug is a synthetic of the human antidiuretic hormone, vasopressin. It causes an increase in factor VIII release from storage sites in the body. Desmopressin is often administered prophylactically to patients with mild hemophilia who require surgery or dental extractions. Observation and nursing interventions for hemophilia A and B can easily be adapted to von Willebrand's disease.

Prognosis

The prognosis is usually good.

DISSEMINATED INTRAVASCULAR COAGULATION

Etiology and Pathophysiology

Disseminated intravascular coagulation (DIC) is a grave coagulopathy resulting from the overstimulation of clotting and anticlotting processes in response to disease or injury, including septicemia, obstetric complication, malignancies, tissue trauma, transfusion reaction, burns, shock, and snake bites (Box 7-4). Plasma clotting factors are depleted during widespread clotting within small vessels. This in turn leads to a bleeding disorder and thrombosis. The primary disorder initiates generalized intravascular clotting, which in turn overstimulates fibrinolytic mechanisms. As a result, the initial hypercoagulability is followed by a deficiency in clotting factors with subsequent hypocoagulability and hemorrhaging.

Clinical Manifestations

Bleeding is noted in mucous membranes, venipuncture or surgical sites, GI and urinary tracts, and generally from all orifices. Bleeding ranges from occult to profuse. Dyspnea; hemoptysis (blood-tinged sputum); and diaphoresis with cold, mottled digits are observed.

Assessment

Subjective data include patient complaints of bone and joint pain. Changes in vision occur.

Collection of **objective data** includes observing for occult or obvious bleeding. Purpura on the chest and abdomen, reflecting fibrin deposits in capillaries, is a

| Box 7-4 | Precipitating Causes of Disseminated Intravascular Coagulation |

OBSTETRIC
- Abruptio placentae
- Acute fatty liver of pregnancy
- Amniotic fluid embolism
- Hydatidiform mole (intrauterine mass of grapelike chorionic villi)
- Retained dead fetus
- Retained placenta
- Toxemia

NEOPLASTIC
- Acute leukemias
- Adenocarcinomas
- Carcinomas
- Pheochromocytoma (a vascular tumor of the adrenal medulla)
- Polycythemia vera
- Sarcomas

HEMATOLOGICAL
- Blood transfusion reaction
- Sickle cell crisis
- Thalassemia major (genetic hemolytic anemia; occurs in people of Mediterranean origin)

TRAUMA
- Aspirin poisoning
- Burns
- Fat emboli
- Heatstroke
- Multiple injuries
- Snake bite
- Surgery, particularly if extracorporeal circulation (heart-lung machine) was used
- Transplant rejection

OTHER
- Acute infectious process or sepsis
- Anaphylaxis
- Cirrhosis
- Glomerulonephritis
- Hepatitis
- Necrotizing enterocolitis
- Purpura
- Shock
- Systemic lupus erythematosus

From Young, L.M. (1990). DIC: the insidious killer. *Critical Care Nurse*, *10*(9):27. Reprinted with permission of *Critical Care Nurse*.

common first sign of DIC. Note the color of skin and mucosa and the presence of petechiae. Abdominal tenderness may be present. GI bleeding, hematuria, pulmonary edema, pulmonary embolism, hypotension, tachycardia, absence of peripheral pulses, decreased blood pressure, restlessness, confusion, seizures, or coma may be present.

Diagnostic Tests
The coagulation profile shows prolonged clotting. The platelet count shows marked thrombocytopenia. Other tests show hypofibrinogenemia and deficits of factors V, VII, VIII, X, and XII.

D-dimer test results are elevated. D-dimer reveals the breakdown of fibrin and is a specific marker for the degree of fibrinolysis in the serum.

Medical Management
In keeping with the medical therapeutic approach, the underlying cause is addressed and corrected and transfusion replacement and cryoprecipitate are ordered. Heparin therapy blocks the subsequent formation of microemboli by inhibiting thrombin activity. It has no effect, however, on existing clots. The goal of administering heparin is to stop the rapid overproduction of microemboli and thus allow for reperfusion of vital organs and replenishment of clotting factor supplies. However, the use of heparin in treating DIC remains controversial. Fibrinolytic inhibitors should be given to adults. This may be dangerous if the thrombotic process has not been previously treated with

heparin. Packed RBC transfusion should be initiated to reestablish normal hemostatic potential if the thrombosis is blocked by heparin. FFP is administered to replace other coagulation factors.

Nursing Interventions and Patient Teaching
Protection from bleeding and trauma and pressure to sites of hemorrhage are essential nursing measures. Support and reassurance of the patient may aid in relieving high stress levels. Monitor the patient in a quiet, nonstressful environment. Use padded side rails and foam or cotton swabs for mouth care. Monitor vital signs and administer heparin, blood and FFP transfusions, and cryoprecipitate. Use the blood pressure cuff infrequently to avoid subcutaneous bleeding.

A nursing diagnosis and interventions for the patient with DIC include but are not limited to the following:

Nursing Diagnosis	Nursing Interventions
Risk for injury, bleeding, and fluid deficit, related to: • depleted coagulation factors • adverse effect of heparin (excess heparin, insufficient heparin)	Monitor hematocrit and hemoglobin. Examine skin surface for signs of bleeding; note petechiae; purpura; hematomas; oozing of blood from IV sites, drains, and wounds; and bleeding from mucous membranes.

Nursing Diagnosis	Nursing Interventions
Risk for injury, bleeding, and fluid deficit, related to: • depleted coagulation factors • adverse effect of heparin (excess heparin, insufficient heparin)	Observe for signs of bleeding from GI and genitourinary tracts. Note any hemoptysis or blood obtained during suctioning. Observe for changes in mental status; institute neurologic checklist (mental status changes may occur with the decreased fluid volume or with decreasing hemoglobin). Monitor vital signs. Observe for signs of orthostatic hypotension (drop of greater than 15 mm Hg when changing from supine to sitting position indicates reduced circulating fluids). Avoid intramuscular injections; any needlestick is a potential bleeding site. Apply pressure to oozing site. Prevent trauma to catheter and tubes by proper taping, minimum pulling.

Discuss with the patient and family the signs and symptoms of DIC, and have them repeat this information to the nurse or physician. Teach the patient to self-administer heparin therapy subcutaneously if prescribed. Instruct the patient and family to avoid mechanical trauma, such as from a hard toothbrush, blade razor, rough nose blowing, or contact sports.

Prognosis

Mortality rates from DIC vary, depending on severity. Death is usually a result of either uncontrolled hemorrhage, irreversible end-organ damage, or both.

DISORDER OF PLASMA CELLS

MULTIPLE MYELOMA

Etiology and Pathophysiology

Multiple myeloma, or plasma cell myeloma, is a malignant neoplastic immunodeficiency disease of the bone marrow. Neoplastic plasma cells infiltrate the bone marrow. The tumor destroys osseous tissue, especially in flat bones, causing pain, fractures, and skeletal deformities.

The specific immunoglobulin produced by the myeloma cells is present in the blood and/or urine and is referred to as the monoclonal protein. This protein is a helpful marker to monitor the extent of the disease

and the patient's response to treatment. It is measured by serum or urine protein electrophoresis.

Be alert to an older adult patient whose chief complaint is back pain and who has an elevated total serum protein. Evaluate these patients for possible multiple myeloma. It most frequently occurs in patients older than age 40, with a peak incidence around 65 years of age, and affects twice as many men as women. Onset is gradual and insidious; the disease often goes unrecognized for years while the individual experiences frequent, recurrent bacterial infections. This increased susceptibility to infection follows disturbances of antibody formation by abnormal plasma cells. Suppression of normal antibody levels is seen in this plasma cell tumor disease. The incidence of multiple myeloma has increased and now approaches that of Hodgkin's disease.

Clinical Manifestations

The disease process shows a proliferation of malignant plasma cells and development of single or multiple bone marrow tumors. This is followed by bone destruction with dissemination into lymph nodes, liver, spleen, and kidneys.

The skeletal system symptoms typically involve the ribs, the spine, and the pelvis. Osteolytic lesions are seen in the skull, the vertebrae, and the ribs. Vertebral destruction can lead to collapse of vertebrae with ensuing compression of the spinal cord. Patients complain of bone pain that increases with movement. About 30% develop pathologic fractures accompanied by severe pain.

In an individual with multiple myeloma, production of erythrocytes, platelets, and leukocytes is disrupted because the marrow is crowded by the abnormal proliferation of plasma cells. This leads to infection, anemia, and increased potential for bleeding. Calcium and phosphorus drain from bones, leading to hypercalcemia and renal problems. In addition, cell destruction contributes to the development of hyperuricemia, which, along with the high protein levels caused by the myeloma protein, can result in renal failure.

Assessment

Collection of **subjective data** includes assessment of the patient's complaints of pain, especially skeletal pain in the pelvis, the spine, and the ribs.

Collection of **objective data** includes assessing the patient's facial expression for signs of increased pain with movement, the ability to perform ADLs, increased body temperature, increased potential for bleeding, changes in urine characteristics, and effectiveness of medication administration.

Diagnostic Tests

Diagnosis of multiple myeloma is made with radiographic skeletal studies, bone marrow biopsy, and laboratory examination of blood and urine. A monoclonal

(M) antibody protein may be present, as evidenced in serum or urine electrophoresis. Bony degeneration also causes loss of calcium in the bones, eventually causing hypercalcemia. Pancytopenia, hypercalcemia, hyperuricemia, and elevated creatinine may be found. In addition, an abnormal globulin known as Bence Jones protein is found in the urine and can result in renal failure.

Radiographic skeletal examinations reveal widespread demineralization, lytic lesions, and osteoporosis. Lytic lesions may be seen on bone roentgenograms but are not well visualized on bone scans. Bone marrow studies reveal large numbers of immature plasma cells, which normally account for only 5% of marrow population.

Medical Management

Treatment is symptomatic, since multiple myeloma is not curable. Radiation and chemotherapy are initiated to reduce tumor size, impede tumor growth, and produce remission. Radiation is used in small doses. The antineoplastic drugs of choice are the alkylating agents, such as melphalan, cyclophosphamide, chlorambucil, and carmustine (BiCNU). Vincristine, doxorubicin (Adriamycin), and dexamethasone can be added for patients who do not respond to alkylating agents. Bone marrow depression occurs as a side effect; therefore the CBC is monitored during treatment.

Hypercalcemia and pain also should be addressed. Analgesics, orthopedic supports, and localized radiation help reduce the skeletal pain. Hospitalization to administer chemotherapy, corticosteroids, and fluids may be required.

Nursing Interventions and Patient Teaching

Care of the patient with multiple myeloma focuses on relieving pain, preventing infection and bone injury, administrating chemotherapy and radiation, and maintaining hydration. Use ambulation and adequate hydration to treat hypercalcemia, dehydration, and potential renal damage. Fluid intake of 3 to 4 L/day is encouraged to prevent dehydration and maintain a urinary output of 1.5 to 2 L/day. Patients with multiple myeloma with high tumor burdens who receive chemotherapy will have an increased cell lysis and release of uric acid, resulting in hyperuricemia. Adequate hydration and allopurinal (Zyloprim) will help treat hyperuricemia (Lewis et al., 2007). Weight bearing helps the bones reabsorb some calcium, and fluids dilute calcium and prevent protein precipitates from causing renal tubular obstruction.

Because of the potential for pathologic fractures, be careful when moving and ambulating the patient. A slight twist or strain in the wrong area (e.g., a weak area in the patient's bones) may be sufficient to cause a fracture. Attention to the psychosocial, emotional, and spiritual needs is also extremely important.

Nursing diagnoses and interventions for the patient with multiple myeloma include but are not limited to the following:

Nursing Diagnoses	Nursing Interventions
Risk for injury, related to: • osteoporosis • lytic lesions	Protect from bone injury; use log-roll, turning sheet.
Pain, related to disease process	Administer analgesics as ordered (such as nonsteroidal antiinflammatory drugs, acetaminophen, or an acetaminophen-opioid combination). Combination drugs may be more effective than opioids alone in diminishing bone pain. Provide comfort measures. Assess contributing factors.
Deficient fluid volume, related to impaired renal function	Increase fluid intake to 3 to 4 L/day. Maintain I&O records.

Teach the patient to avoid traumatic bone injury and infection. Discuss the importance of adequate hydration and review the pain control modalities available. It is also important to identify spiritual resources. Address the patient's understanding of the disease, verbalization of discouragement and hopelessness, and desires for emotional and spiritual support.

Prognosis

This disease is usually progressive and generally fatal. A patient usually lives for approximately 2 years if untreated. With proper therapeutic treatment, the chronic phase of multiple myeloma may last for more than 10 years. Multiple myeloma is seldom cured, but treatment can relieve symptoms, produce remissions, and prolong life.

DISORDERS OF THE LYMPHATIC SYSTEM

LYMPHANGITIS

Etiology and Pathophysiology

Lymphangitis is an inflammation of one or more lymphatic vessels or channels that usually results from an acute streptococcal or staphylococcal infection in an extremity.

Clinical Manifestations

Lymphangitis is characterized by fine red streaks from the affected area in the groin or axilla. The infection is usually not localized, and edema is diffuse. Chills, fever, and local pain accompany headache and myalgia. Septicemia may occur; lymph nodes enlarge.

Medical Management

Administration of penicillin or other antimicrobial drugs controls the infection. Hot, moist heat (soaks or packs) brings comfort.

Nursing Interventions

Aseptic technique promotes healing. Rest and extremity elevation may relieve the pressure.

Prognosis

With treatment, the prognosis is usually good.

LYMPHEDEMA

Etiology and Pathophysiology

Lymphedema is a primary or secondary disorder characterized by the accumulation of lymph in soft tissue and edema. The accumulation of lymph in soft tissue is caused by obstruction, an increase in the amount of lymph, or removal of the lymph channels and nodes. The condition may be hereditary.

If the lymphatic drainage function is disturbed, an inflammatory process may result.

Clinical Manifestations

Massive edema and tightness cause pressure and pain in the affected extremities. It progresses toward the trunk and is aggravated by standing; pressure, as with pregnancy or premenstruation; obesity; and warm, humid environments.

Assessment and Diagnostic Test

Subjective data include complaints of pain and pressure. Medical history of varicosities, pregnancy, or modified radical mastectomy is important.

Collection of objective data includes observation of the extremities for edema and palpation of pedal pulses. Lymphangiography is used to differentiate lymphedema from venous disorders.

Medical Management

Diuretics are not prescribed because they remove water from the interstitial spaces and leave the protein. The proteins concentrated in the interstitial spaces then draw the fluid back into the affected area (Holcomb, 2006). Mechanical management includes special massage techniques, compression bandaging, compression pumps, and elastic sleeves or stockings on the affected limb. Diet restrictions include limiting sodium and avoiding spicy foods, which would precipitate thirst. Encourage the patient to consume a healthy diet, maintain a normal body weight, and exercise regularly.

Nursing Interventions and Patient Teaching

The primary goal of care is to increase lymphatic drainage and avoid trauma. Elevation of the extremities while asleep and periodically during the day facilitates drainage. Massage toward the trunk followed by active exercise (e.g., walking) decreases the edema.

Advise patients to avoid constrictive clothing, shoes, or stockings (except elastic stockings). Patients with lymphedema are susceptible to infection, so maintain meticulous skin care and make every effort to prevent infections. Discuss precautions they should take to protect the affected area (Holcomb, 2006).

Emotional support for the patient is also important. Address body image disturbance related to the appearance of the lymphedematous extremity. Emphasize that lymphedema need not prevent the individual from engaging in routine activity.

A nursing diagnosis and interventions for the patient with lymphedema include but are not limited to the following:

Nursing Diagnosis	Nursing Interventions
Impaired skin integrity, related to impaired lymphatic drainage	Protect engorged tissues. Consider physical therapy or ROM exercises (aids lymphatic flow). Examine skin for impaired skin integrity. Gently handle affected parts. Apply skin-protecting moisturizers or emollients. Teach application of supportive stockings or elastic sleeves.

Make certain the patient is aware of the condition's progression and cause. If the disorder is long term and ongoing, discuss how to cope with its effects. Explain the rationale behind nursing interventions to enhance the ongoing medical regimen. Encourage the patient to socialize to enhance feelings of well-being.

Prognosis

The prognosis is better when the patient begins treatment early in the course of the disorder (Damsky, 2006). The patient should be referred to a physiatrist (physician specializing in physical medicine and rehabilitation) or another physician experienced in lymphedema diagnosis and treatment and to a physical or occupational therapist or nurse certified by the Lymphology Association of North America (Damsky, 2006).

Lymphedema has no cure, but signs and symptoms can be controlled by compliance with treatment.

HODGKIN'S LYMPHOMA

Etiology and Pathophysiology

Hodgkin's lymphoma, also called Hodgkin's disease, is a malignant disorder characterized by painless, progressive enlargement of lymphoid tissue. It affects males twice as frequently as females, and the age incidence curve is bimodal (two separate populations), with a peak early in life at 15 to 35 years, and a peak later in life at 50 years. The two peaks in incidence may represent separate diseases. The first incident peak suggests a viral cause. Beginning as an inflammatory or infectious process, it develops into a neoplasm. The exact cause is unknown, but Hodgkin's lymphoma is thought to be an immune disorder (T-cell disease).

Hodgkin's lymphoma has no major risk factors, but the disease occurs more frequently in people who have had mononucleosis (an infection caused by the Epstein-Barr virus), have acquired or congenital immunodeficiency syndromes, are taking immunosuppressive drugs after organ transplantation, have been exposed to occupational toxins, or have a genetic predisposition. The presence of HIV increases the incidence of Hodgkin's lymphoma.

Lymphoid tissue enlargement is usually first noticed in the cervical nodes and is characterized by abnormal or atypical cells. **Reed-Sternberg cells** are atypical histiocytes consisting of large, abnormal, multinucleated cells in the lymph nodes found in Hodgkin's lymphoma. These cells increase in number, replacing normal cells. The main diagnostic feature of Hodgkin's lymphoma is the presence of Reed-Sternberg cells in lymph node biopsy specimens.

The disease is believed to arise in a single location (the lymph nodes in 90% of patients) and then spread along adjacent lymphatics. It eventually infiltrates other organs, especially the lungs, the spleen, and the liver. In approximately two thirds of patients, the cervical lymph nodes are affected first. Unless they exert pressure on adjacent nerves, the enlarged nodes are not painful. When the disease begins above the diaphragm, it remains confined to lymph nodes for a variable period. Disease originating below the diaphragm frequently spreads to extralymphoid sites such as the liver.

Clinical Manifestations
Enlargement of the cervical, axillary, or inguinal lymph nodes is most often the initial development. The next most common location is a mediastinal node mass. Anorexia, weight loss, fever, night sweats, malaise, and extreme pruritus are complaints associated with this condition. Night sweats, weight loss, and fever, which are referred to as "B" symptoms, are associated with a worse prognosis (Box 7-5). Low-grade fever may occur. Anemia and leukocytosis follow, with development of respiratory tract infections.

Assessment
Subjective data include the common complaints of malaise and appetite loss. Pruritus is often severe. After the ingestion of even small amounts of alcohol, individuals with Hodgkin's lymphoma may complain of a rapid onset of pain at the site of the disease. The cause for the alcohol-induced pain is unknown. Bone pain occurs later in the disease's course.

Collection of **objective data** includes palpating enlarged cervical and supraclavicular lymph nodes. Splenomegaly, hepatomegaly, and abdominal tenderness are found. Excoriation of skin and evidence of scratching from pruritus are noted. Clinical signs and symptoms vary depending on where the enlarged lymph nodes are located. Involvement in the thoracic area may lead to superior vena cava syndrome with edema of the face, neck, and arms (Lewis et al., 2007).

The patient may develop palpable abdominal masses or interference with renal function as a result of enlarged retroperitoneal nodes. Spinal cord compression causing paraplegia can occur with extradural involvement. If the patient has liver involvement, jaundice may occur (Lewis et al., 2007).

Diagnostic Tests
Peripheral blood studies show anemia (normocytic, normochromic), WBC increase, and an abnormal erythrocyte sedimentation rate. Other blood studies may show hypoferremia caused by excessive iron intake by the liver and the spleen, elevated leukocyte alkaline phosphatase from liver and bone involvement, hypercalcemia from bone involvement, and hypoalbuminemia from liver involvement. Chest radiographic examination may reveal a mediastinal

---

Box 7-5 | **Clinical Staging System for Hodgkin's Disease***

STAGE I
- Abnormal single lymph nodes
- Regional or single extranodal site

STAGE II
- Two or more abnormal lymph nodes on the same side of diaphragm
- Localized involvement of extranodal site and one or more lymph node regions on the same side of diaphragm

STAGE III
- Abnormal lymph node regions on both sides of diaphragm
- May be accompanied by spleen involvement
- Now subdivided into lymphatic involvement of the upper abdomen in the spleen (splenic, celiac, and portal nodes) (stage III$_1$) and the lower abdominal nodes in the periaortic, mesenteric, and iliac regions (stage III$_2$)

STAGE IV
- Diffuse and disseminated involvement of one or more extralymphatic tissues and/or organs—with or without lymph node involvement; the extranodal site is identified as *H*, hepatic; *L*, lung; *P*, pleural; *M*, marrow; *D*, dermal; *O*, osseous

*Nomenclature used in staging uses a roman numeral (*I* to *IV*) that reflects the location and extent of the disease. *A* and *B* are added after the stage, depending on whether symptoms are present when disease is found. If there are no symptoms at time of diagnosis, add A after staging. If symptoms of night sweats, fever, and weight loss are present, add B after staging (From Lewis, S.L., et al. (2007). *Medical-surgical nursing: assessment and management of clinical problems* (7th ed.). St. Louis: Mosby.

mass. CT or MRI can detect retroperitoneal node involvement. Lymph node biopsy that includes laparoscopy for retroperitoneal nodes is performed. Bone marrow biopsy is an important aspect of staging. A CT scan and an ultrasound examination can indicate an enlarged spleen or liver. The presence of Reed-Sternberg cells remains a hallmark of the presence of Hodgkin's lymphoma.

Positron emission tomography (PET) with or without CT scans is used to assess the response to therapy. PET or CT scans are helpful to note the patient's response to treatment such as observing mediastinal lymphadenopathy; abdominal lymph node enlargement; and liver, spleen, bone, and brain disease (Lewis et al., 2007).

Medical Management

Treatment depends on the staging process (see Box 7-5). The stage of Hodgkin's lymphoma must be established before selecting an appropriate treatment plan. Figure 7-5 illustrates nodal involvement, by stage, in Hodgkin's lymphoma.

Combination chemotherapy is used in some early stages in patients believed to have resistant disease or be at high risk for relapse. Chemotherapy and radiation therapy are used against the generalized forms (stages III and IV). Advances in treatment now enable some stage IIIB and stage IV diseases to be cured with high-dose chemotherapy and bone marrow or peripheral SCT. The site of the disease and the amount of resistant disease after chemotherapy determine the role of radiation in supplementing chemotherapy.

Treatment for Hodgkin's lymphoma involves several drugs. An aggressive treatment approach is required (Lewis et al., 2007). Until recently, a traditional regimen for Hodgkin's disease had been MOPP: mechlorethamine (Mustargen), vincristine, procarbazine (Matulane), and prednisone. Mechlorethamine (also called nitrogen mustard) is one of a group of drugs known as alkylating agents. These can cause serious long-term side effects, such as leukemia, particularly when combined with radiation therapy. Instead of MOPP, oncologists are now choosing a regimen known as ABVD, or they're replacing mechlorethamine with cyclophosphamide to de-

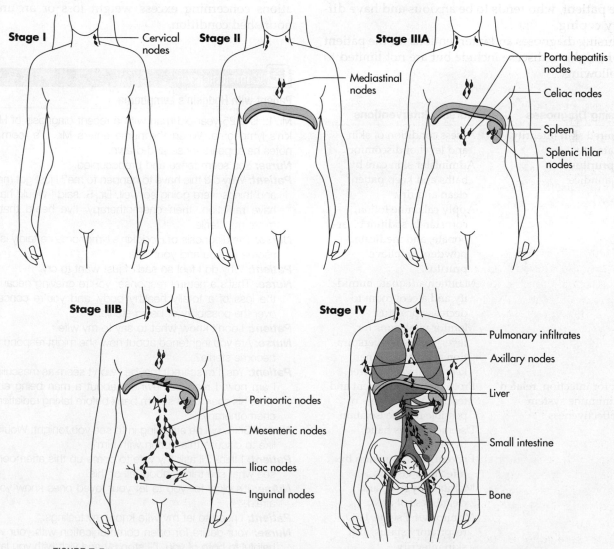

FIGURE 7-5 Nodal involvement by stage in Hodgkin's disease (based on modified Ann Arbor Staging System).

crease the likelihood of long-term complications. ABVD includes doxorubicin, bleomycin (Blenoxane), vinblastine (Velban), and dacarbazine (DTIC-Dome) (Lewis et al., 2007). A biologic response modifier (filgrastim) that stimulates proliferation and differentiation of neutrophils is a treatment option. Filgrastim is used to decrease infection in patients receiving antineoplastics that suppress neutrophil production.

Nursing Interventions and Patient Teaching

Plan care according to the staging level. Awareness of side effects of radiation therapy or chemotherapy is important in preparing the patient to deal effectively with the treatment. Because the survival of patients with Hodgkin's lymphoma depends on their response to treatment, helping the patient deal with the consequences of treatment is extremely important. Comfort measures focus on skin integrity. Soothing baths with an antipruritic medication (as ordered) can be effective. Control fever and perspiration with medication (with attention to increased fluid intake) plus linen changes as necessary to prevent further skin problems. Explain extensive tests to the patient, who tends to be anxious and have difficulty coping.

Nursing diagnoses and interventions for the patient with Hodgkin's disease include but are not limited to the following:

Nursing Diagnoses	Nursing Interventions
Impaired skin integrity, related to: • pruritus • jaundice	Assess condition of skin and level of discomfort. Administer skin care by baths and keep patient clean and dry. Apply calamine lotion, cornstarch, sodium bicarbonate, and medicated powders to relieve pruritus. Maintain adequate humidity and a cool room to decrease pruritus. Monitor vital signs for fever; assess for perspiration and change linen, keeping it wrinkle free.
Risk for infection, related to immune system ineffectiveness	Protect the environment and teach the importance of possible reverse isolation. Use meticulous hand hygiene. Prevent contamination by infectious visitors. Maintain hygiene and cleanliness of area. Monitor vital signs, I&O, respiratory status, and skin integrity.

Nursing Diagnoses	Nursing Interventions
Anxiety and fear, related to unknown outcome	Instruct patient on symptoms, disease progression, and treatment regimen. Encourage open communication and venting of feelings. Encourage questions and problem solving.

Understanding the disease is important for the patient to perform self-care and retain independence. Fertility issues may be of particular concern because this disease is frequently seen in adolescents and young adults. Help ensure that these issues are addressed soon after diagnosis (Communication box). The effect on the patient's life, as well as on significant others, is a prime consideration in patient attitude and adjustment. Realistic approaches to the illness and therapies are imperative. Referrals for patients seeking counseling for stress management can be helpful. Discuss special nutritional considerations concerning excess weight loss or an undernourished condition.

 Communication

Patient with Hodgkin's Lymphoma

Mr. L. is a 25-year-old man with a recent diagnosis of Hodgkin's lymphoma. When the nurse enters Mr. L.'s room, she notes he appears tense and drawn.

Nurse: You seem tense and preoccupied.

Patient: Why did this have to happen to me? I just got married and things were going so well. Dr. S. said I would have to have radiation, then chemotherapy. I've heard that can make me sterile.

Nurse: The diagnosis of Hodgkin's lymphoma certainly is worrisome for you and your wife.

Patient: Why do I feel so sad? I just want to cry.

Nurse: That's a natural response; you're grieving because of the loss of a totally healthy body, and you're concerned over the possibility of being sterile.

Patient: I don't know what to say to my wife.

Nurse: Are you frightened about how she might respond if you become sterile?

Patient: Yes, I'm scared; maybe I won't seem as masculine as I am now. I read somewhere about a man being able to store his sperm in a sperm bank before taking radiation and chemotherapy.

Nurse: Dr. S. will be stopping in to see you tonight. Would you like to discuss this option with him?

Patient: I think I'll ask my wife to come up this afternoon and see what she thinks about all of this.

Nurse: It's okay for you to let your loved ones know you are afraid.

Patient: I need to let my wife know my feelings.

Nurse: Your desire for open communication with your wife is helpful to both of you. I'll stop by and visit with you later.

Prognosis

The prognosis is steadily improving but depends on the stage of the disease. Those diagnosed and treated in stage I or II have a 10-year survival rate near 90%, whereas those in stage III or IV have a 10-year survival rate of more than 50% (Lewis et al., 2007). A serious consequence of the treatment for Hodgkin's lymphoma is the later development of secondary malignancies. The estimated risk of a secondary cancer is approximately 18% at 15 years after treatment for Hodgkin's disease. The most common secondary malignancies are AML, non-Hodgkin's lymphoma (NHL), and solid tumors.

NON-HODGKIN'S LYMPHOMA

Etiology and Pathophysiology

NHLs are a group of malignant neoplasms of primarily B- or T-cell origin affecting all ages. B-cell lymphomas constitute about 90% of NHLs. The condition is starting to be characterized as a neoplasm of the immune system. The cause is unknown, but a herpeslike viral source is suspected. The neoplasms are classified according to different cellular and lymph node characteristics. Patients who receive immunosuppressive agents have a greater chance of developing NHL, probably because the immunosuppressive agents activate tumor viruses. NHL is more common in men older than 60 years of age, whites, and those of Jewish ancestry.

A variety of clinical presentations and courses are recognized, from slowly developing to rapidly progressive disease. Common names for different types of lymphoma include Burkitt's lymphoma, diffuse large B-cell lymphoma, lymphoblastic lymphoma, and follicular lymphoma. Thus NHL comprises a large group of different lymphoid malignancies (Lewis et al., 2007). There is no hallmark pathologic feature in NHL that parallels the Reed-Sternberg cell of Hodgkin's disease. However, all NHLs involve lymphocytes arrested in various stages of development. Tumors usually start in lymph nodes and spread to lymphoid tissue in the spleen, the liver, the GI tract, and the bone marrow. Involvement of lymphoid tissue also results in malabsorption and bone lesions.

NHL is the most commonly occurring hematological cancer and the fifth leading cause of cancer death (Lewis et al., 2007). Each year, approximately 54,000 new cases of NHL are diagnosed and approximately 25,000 deaths occur. As the population ages, the incidence of NHL has increased 2% to 3% per year for at least the past 30 years.

Clinical Manifestations

The method of spread can be unpredictable when NHLs originate outside the lymph nodes. At the time of diagnosis, most patients have widely scattered disease. Painless, enlarged lymph nodes and fever, weight loss, night sweats, anemia, pruritus, and susceptibility to infection may develop. Pressure symptoms in the involved areas are noted. Pleural effusion, bone fractures, and paralysis are complications. Because the disease is usually disseminated when it is diagnosed, other symptoms are present, depending on where the disease has spread (e.g., hepatomegaly with liver involvement).

Assessment

Subjective data include frequent patient complaints of fatigue, malaise, and anorexia.

Collection of **objective data** includes examination of the abdomen for splenomegaly. Enlarged lymph nodes are also evident. Fever, night sweats, and weight loss are usually present.

Diagnostic Tests

A bone scan may reveal fractures, lesions, and tumor infiltration. Blood studies show hypercalcemia and anemia; leukocytosis; and elevated sedimentation rate, platelet count, and alkaline phosphatase level. A Coombs' test yields a positive result for antiglobulin. The patient needs a chest roentgenogram; CT scans of the chest, abdomen, and pelvis; a gallium scan; and possibly a lymphangiogram. Biopsies of lymph nodes, liver, and bone marrow are performed to establish the cell type and pattern. Diagnostic studies used for NHL resemble those used for Hodgkin's disease. Staging, as described for Hodgkin's disease, is used to guide therapy. The International Working Formulation is a useful system for classifying NHL. This system divides each subtype of lymphoma into indolent (low grade), aggressive (intermediate grade), and very aggressive (high grade).

Medical Management

Once the diagnosis is made, the extent of the disease (staging) is determined. Accurate staging is crucial to determine the treatment regimen. The therapeutic regimen for NHLs includes chemotherapy and radiation. Indolent lymphomas have a naturally long course, but are difficult to treat effectively. In contrast, more aggressive lymphomas are more likely to be cured, since they are more responsive to treatment. Some chemotherapy agents used are cyclophosphamide, vincristine, prednisone, doxorubicin, bleomycin, and methotrexate. The monoclonal antibody rituximab (Rituxan) was approved for the treatment of follicular lymphoma. Ibritumomab (Zevalin) is another monoclonal antibody that can be used in patients who are refractory to rituximab or in conjunction with it. Conventional chemotherapy used to treat patients with relapsed, aggressive NHL, who are still responding to salvage chemotherapy, is not as effective as high-dose chemotherapy with autologous (tissue derived from the same individual) hematopoietic stem cells (HSCT).

Patients with lymphoma commonly receive radiation to the chest wall, mediastinum, axillae, and neck—the region known as the "mantle field." Some patients also need radiation to the abdomen; paraaortic area; spleen; and, less commonly, the pelvis.

Chemotherapy is the mainstay of treatment of NHLs that are not localized. High-dose chemotherapy with peripheral blood stem cell or bone marrow transplantation may be indicated. Tumor necrosis factor is being used; it has direct cell toxicity and stimulates the immune system. Interferon is being investigated as a treatment option. Older patients have difficulty tolerating the aggressive chemotherapy treatments. This population is increasing in number, and new approaches are being examined.

Nursing Interventions and Patient Teaching

Supportive care of the patient during radiation and chemotherapy is primary in nursing management. Observation for complications follows. Further intervention is similar to that for Hodgkin's disease.

Explanations of the extensive diagnostic workup and its importance for staging the disease and determining the treatment plan are an important focus of patient teaching during the diagnostic period.

Prognosis

The prognosis is influenced by the staging classification. The prognosis for NHL is generally not as good as that for Hodgkin's disease.

❖NURSING PROCESS for the Patient with a Blood or Lymphatic Disorder

The role of the licensed practical nurse/licensed vocational nurse (LPN/LVN) in the nursing process as stated is that the LPN/LVN will:

- Participate in planning care for patients based on patient needs
- Review patient's care plan and recommend revisions as needed
- Review and follow defined prioritization for patient care
- Use clinical pathways, care maps, or care plans to guide and review patient care

■ Assessment

Collect data from diverse sources: patient and family observation, physical examination, and diagnostic evaluation results (see Table 7-1).

The **subjective data** collected at the onset of the disease process are generally vague and nonspecific: malaise, fatigue, and weakness. The patient may relate a history of illness, easy bruising, bleeding tendencies with petechiae, and ecchymosis. Integumentary changes (including pruritus, nonhealing cuts and bruises, draining lesions, jaundice, and palpable subcutaneous nodules) may be reported. Edema and tenderness in lymph node regions may be accompanied by pain, sometimes severe. GI complaints are noted, as well as cardiovascular and respiratory changes. Neurologic complaints include headache,

 Life Span Considerations

Older Adults

Blood or Lymphatic Disorder

- The subjective symptoms of hematological disorders (e.g., fatigue, weakness, dizziness, and dyspnea) may be mistaken for normal changes of aging or attributed to other disease processes commonly seen in older adults.
- The most common blood disorders are forms of anemia.
- Decreased production of the intrinsic factor in an aging gastric mucosa results in increased incidence of pernicious anemia.
- Many older adults suffer from conditions such as colonic diverticula, hiatal hernia, or ulcerations that can cause occult bleeding. Older adults with these conditions should be observed for iron deficiency anemia.
- Age-related problems such as altered dentition, limited financial resources, difficulty in food preparation, and poor appetite resulting from emotional upset or depression can cause an increased incidence of iron deficiency anemia.
- Severe or persistent anemia can place additional stress on the aging or diseased heart.
- Administer blood products with caution because older adults are at increased risk of developing congestive heart failure. Careful assessment of cardiopulmonary function and intake and output is essential.
- Oral administration of iron preparations increases the risk of gastrointestinal (GI) irritation and constipation in older adults.
- Ingestion of large amounts of aspirin and other antiinflammatory medications commonly taken by older adults increases the risk of GI bleeding and can lead to alteration in clotting.
- Chronic lymphocytic leukemia is the most common form seen among older patients. This form of leukemia usually progresses slowly in older adults and is rarely treated.

numbness, tingling, paresthesias, and behavioral alteration (Life Span Considerations box).

Collection of **objective data** follows a system-by-system approach to confirm patient complaints. Manipulation of joints can reveal stiffness and hematoma and may produce pain. Examination of the oral cavity can reveal lesions, ulcers, signs of bleeding, or gingivitis. Cardiovascular and respiratory assessments include breath and heart sound variations and pain or dyspneic positioning. Note any patient anxiety, and observe for diminished comprehension. Listening and an unhurried interview may reveal many symptoms not previously mentioned.

■ Nursing Diagnosis

Nursing diagnoses are determined from the assessment, which provides data for identifying the patient's problems, strengths, potential complications, and learning needs. Nursing diagnoses for the patient with a blood or lymphatic disorder include but are not limited to the following:

- Risk for infection
- Injury (trauma), risk for (bleeding, falls)
- Fatigue

- Deficient knowledge
- Acute pain
- Chronic pain
- Ineffective tissue perfusion
- Impaired gas exchange
- Activity intolerance
- Ineffective coping
- Impaired skin integrity

▪ Expected Outcomes and Planning

Most patients have more than one nursing diagnosis. Therefore the planning step in the nursing process involves determining the priority for nursing interventions from the list of nursing diagnoses. Use Maslow's hierarchy of needs; that is, assign the highest priority to immediate problems that may be life threatening. For example, impaired gas exchange would have a higher priority than ineffective coping.

Planning includes developing realistic goals and outcomes that stem from the identified nursing diagnosis. Examples of expected patient outcomes for the patient with a blood or lymphatic disorder may include but are not limited to the following:

Goal 1: Patient is free of signs and symptoms of an infection.

Goal 2: Patient has no evidence of bleeding (any bleeding is quickly controlled).

▪ Implementation

The implementation of the nursing process is the actual initiation of the nursing care plan. Patient outcomes and goals are achieved by performance of the nursing interventions. Nursing interventions for the patient with a blood or lymphatic disorder may include the following:

- Place patient in private room; avoid contact with visitors or staff members who have an infection (in the immunocompromised patient).
- Stress careful hand hygiene to patient, significant others, and all caregivers.
- Assist in planning daily activities to include rest periods to decrease fatigue and weakness.
- Provide oxygen for dyspnea or excessive fatigue with exertion.
- Explain the disease process, and stress the importance of continued medical follow-up. Most important is the patient's ability to identify the body's signals that blood abnormalities are present. Petechiae, ecchymoses, and gingival bleeding are the warning signs that one should seek medical attention promptly.

▪ Evaluation

To evaluate the effectiveness of nursing interventions, compare the patient's behaviors with those stated in the expected patient outcomes. Successful achievement of patient outcomes for the patient with a blood or lymphatic disorder is indicated by the following evaluative measures:

- Patient shows no sign of infection; temperature and WBC count are within normal limits.
- Patient has not fallen.
- Patient shows no signs of bleeding (e.g., petechiae, hemorrhage); any bleeding is quickly controlled.
- Patient is able to bathe self in 30 minutes without becoming fatigued.
- Patient is able to correctly explain measures to prevent infection by good hand hygiene techniques and avoidance of people with infectious conditions.
- Patient is able to explain measures to prevent hemorrhage by avoiding traumatic injury and intramuscular injections.
- Patient reports no shortness of breath with activity.

Get Ready for the NCLEX® Examination!

Key Points

- Blood is a thick, red fluid composed of plasma, a light yellow fluid; RBCs; WBCs; and platelets, which are suspended in plasma.
- The blood performs several critical functions: It transports oxygen and nutrients to the cells and waste products away from the cells; it regulates acid-base balance (pH) with buffers; and it protects the body against infection and prevents blood loss with special clotting mechanisms.
- Every person's blood is one of the following blood types in the ABO system of typing: type A, type B, type AB, or type O.

- The lymphatic system is a vast, complex network of capillaries, thin vessels, valves, ducts, nodes, and organs that helps to protect and maintain the internal fluid environment of the entire body by producing, filtering, and conveying lymph and by producing various blood cells.
- The tonsils are composed of lymphoid tissue and are responsible for filtering bacteria.
- The thymus gland is composed of lymphoid tissue in utero (before birth) and the early years of life. It aids in the development of the immune system.
- The spleen is also composed of lymphoid tissue and has many functions, such as filtering out old RBCs, storing a pint of blood, producing antibodies, and phagocytosing bacteria.

- Anemia may be caused by blood loss, impaired RBC production, increased RBC destruction, or nutritional deficiency.
- Shock occurs when organs are deprived of oxygen and nutrients.
- Hypotension, defined as systolic blood pressure of less than 90 mm Hg and tachycardia of more than 120 bpm, occurs with blood loss of 1500 to 2000 mL. By the time blood pressure reaches this point, about 30% to 40% of blood volume may have been lost and end-organ damage may be irreversible.
- Weakness and fatigue are major symptoms of anemia. They result from decreased oxygenation from decreased levels of hemoglobin and increased energy needs required by increased RBC production.
- Ingestion of iron compounds or intramuscular Z-track administration of iron dextran is part of the therapy for iron deficiency anemia.
- Sickle cell anemia is a hemolytic anemia with a genetic basis; a sickle cell crisis occurs when the RBCs become deoxygenated and sickle shaped, thus causing stasis and obstruction of the microvasculature, leading to organ infarction and necrosis.
- Polycythemia vera is characterized by excessive bone marrow production that manifests with an increase in circulating erythrocytes, granulocytes, and platelets. Secondary polycythemia is caused by hypoxia rather than a defect in the development of the RBC.
- Thrombocytopenia is a decrease in the number of circulating platelets and leads to bleeding; people with thrombocytopenia need to learn how to prevent injury and hemorrhage.
- Hemophilia is a hereditary coagulation disorder; hemophilia A is a lack of coagulation factor VIII, and hemophilia B is a lack of factor IX. Maintenance therapy consists of blood factor replacement therapy and prevention of injury.
- DIC is a coagulation disorder characterized initially by clotting and secondarily by hemorrhage. It results from an alteration in the balance between clotting factors and fibrinolytic factors; the person is usually critically ill.
- People with alterations of WBCs are at high risk of infection because leukocytes are a major factor in the body's defense against invading microorganisms.
- The leukemias are malignant disorders characterized by uncontrolled proliferation of WBCs and their precursors; the cause is unknown, but several theories have been proposed.
- Leukemias may be lymphocytic, or myelogenous, and acute or chronic. Acute leukemias have a rapid onset and a short course, if untreated; chronic leukemias have a more insidious onset and longer course. The major therapies for leukemias are chemotherapy and bone marrow transplantation.
- Multiple myeloma is a malignant neoplastic immunodeficiency disease of the bone marrow that affects the plasma cells. The specific immunoglobulin produced by the myeloma cells is present in the blood and urine and is referred to as the monoclonal protein.
- Lymphomas are malignant disorders of the lymphatic system. People with Hodgkin's lymphoma have defec-

tive cellular immunity and are therefore at high risk for infection. NHL is a group of lymphoid malignancies. Chemotherapy and radiation are the primary medical treatment for lymphomas.

Additional Learning Resources

 Go to your Companion CD for an audio glossary, animations, video clips, and more.

🕮volve Be sure to visit the Evolve site at http://evolve.elsevier.com/Christensen/adult/ for additional online resources.

Review Questions for the NCLEX® Examination

1. Another name for a red blood cell is:
   1. leukocyte.
   2. monocyte.
   3. erythrocyte.
   4. platelet.

2. The test for a measure of the packed cell volume of red cells expressed as a percentage of the total blood volume is:
   1. hematocrit.
   2. erythrocyte sedimentation rate.
   3. reticulocyte.
   4. differential.

3. The gland that plays a role in the development of the body's immune system is the:
   1. tonsils.
   2. thymus.
   3. spleen.
   4. liver.

4. The compound in the blood that carries oxygen to the cells from the lungs and carbon dioxide away from the cells to the lungs is:
   1. leukocyte.
   2. thrombocyte.
   3. hemoglobin.
   4. erythrocyte.

5. The type of blood that is called the universal donor blood is:
   1. type A.
   2. type B.
   3. type AB.
   4. type O.

6. The spleen is located in which quadrant of the abdominal cavity?
   1. Upper right
   2. Upper left
   3. Lower left
   4. Lower right

7. A patient is immunosuppressed by chemotherapy. She has a WBC count of 1500/mm³, with neutrophils of 20%. Which statement indicates she understands

home care instructions relating to her immune system?

1. Take antibiotics prophylactically.
2. Take large doses of vitamins.
3. Avoid individuals with infections.
4. Use only sterile bed linens.

8. A patient's platelets have decreased to 18,000/mm³. The most appropriate nursing intervention is to:

1. provide oral hygiene four times per day.
2. institute bleeding precautions.
3. order a high-protein diet.
4. request an order for oxygen per nasal cannula.

9. A patient's spouse tells the nurse that her husband, who has been admitted to the hospital with advanced leukemia, is talking about dying and expresses fears of death. She asks for suggestions for helping her husband. Which response is best?

1. "Your husband will probably die of another disease before he dies of leukemia."
2. "Your husband is expressing a readiness to be admitted to a hospice."
3. "Talk of death is natural at this time but will diminish as he feels better."
4. "It's normal to want to talk about death; what we can do is be supportive by listening."

10. A 28-year-old man is admitted with fatigue; discomfort; enlarged, painless cervical lymph nodes; and pruritus. A lymph node biopsy leads to the diagnosis of Hodgkin's lymphoma. The abnormal cells noted by the pathologist in Hodgkin's lymphoma are called:

1. Rodem-Lee cells.
2. Bullus-Frendelenburg cells.
3. Reed-Sternberg cells.
4. Stevens-Jorgens cells.

11. A 27-year-old housewife and mother of two children is being seen by the nurse at the health maintenance organization for signs of fatigue. She has a history of iron deficiency anemia. What data from the nursing history indicate that the anemia is not currently managed effectively?

1. Pallor
2. Poor skin turgor
3. Heart rate 68 bpm, weak pulse
4. Respirations 18 breaths/min and regular

12. An important nursing intervention goal to establish for a patient who has iron deficiency anemia is:

1. use birth control to avoid pregnancy.
2. increase fluids to stimulate erythropoiesis.
3. decrease fluids to prevent sickling of RBCs.
4. alternate periods of rest and activity to balance oxygen supply and demand.

13. The nurse instructs a patient about foods rich in iron. Which foods should be included in the diet?

1. Fresh fruit and milk
2. Cheeses and processed lunch meats
3. Dark green leafy vegetables and organ meats
4. Fruit juices and cornmeal bread

14. Which statement by the patient with pernicious anemia would indicate that she understood the teaching?

1. "I'll be glad when I can stop the injections and take only oral medicine."
2. "I'll have to take B₁₂ shots for the rest of my life."
3. "After a while I'll no longer need to take shots, just the pills."
4. "I was glad to hear that pills are available to treat me."

15. A patient is admitted with polycythemia vera. He has a hemoglobin value of 20 g/dL. A probable treatment that will be ordered is:

1. whole blood transfusion.
2. platelet transfusion.
3. phlebotomy with removal of 800 mL of blood.
4. vitamin B₁₂ injection.

16. Which laboratory finding is a strong indicator of disseminated intravascular coagulation (DIC)?

1. An elevated platelet count
2. An elevated D-dimer test
3. A normal prothrombin time
4. An elevated fibrinogen level

17. In teaching the patient with pernicious anemia about the disease, the nurse explains that it results from a lack of:

1. folic acid.
2. intrinsic factor.
3. extrinsic factor.
4. an RBC enzyme.

18. In addition to the general symptoms of anemia, the patient with pernicious anemia also manifests:

1. neurologic symptoms.
2. coagulation deficiencies.
3. cardiovascular disturbances.
4. a decreased immunologic response.

19. A patient with sickle cell anemia asks the nurse why the sickling crisis does not stop when oxygen therapy is started. The nurse explains that:

1. sickling occurs in response to decreased blood viscosity, which is not affected by oxygen therapy.
2. when red cells sickle, they occlude small vessels, which causes more local hypoxia and more sickling.
3. the primary problem during a sickle cell crisis is destruction of the abnormal cells, resulting in fewer RBCs to carry oxygen.
4. oxygen therapy does not alter the shape of the abnormal erythrocytes but only allows for increased oxygen concentration in hemoglobin.

20. A nursing intervention that is indicated for the patient during a sickle cell crisis is:

1. frequent ambulation.
2. application of antiembolism hose.
3. restriction of sodium and oral fluids.
4. administration of therapeutic doses of continuous opioid analgesics.

21. Hodgkin's lymphoma occurs more frequently in individuals who have:

    1. a history of cancer treated with radiation.
    2. been exposed to nuclear explosions.
    3. had an infection caused by the Epstein-Barr virus.
    4. had an infection of *Helicobacter pylori*.

22. Which statement concerning Hodgkin's lymphoma is correct?

    1. The 10-year survival rate for stage I or II Hodgkin's lymphoma is more than 90%.
    2. The incidence of Hodgkin's lymphoma has increased over the past 20 years.
    3. Hodgkin's lymphoma is considered a difficult form of cancer to treat.
    4. The incidence of Hodgkin's lymphoma in the older adult has increased.

23. A patient with hemophilia is hospitalized with acute knee pain and edema. Nursing interventions include:

    1. wrapping the knee with an elastic bandage.
    2. placing the patient on bed rest and applying ice to the joint.
    3. gently performing ROM exercises to the knee to prevent adhesions.
    4. administering nonsteroidal antiinflammatory drugs as needed for pain.

24. During physical assessment of a patient with thrombocytopenia, the nurse would expect to find:

    1. petechiae and purpura.
    2. jaundiced sclera and skin.
    3. tender, enlarged lymph nodes.
    4. splenomegaly.

25. Which nursing interventions are necessary when caring for a patient who has a WBC of 1800/mm^3? *(Select all that apply.)*

    1. Prevent patient contact with people who have respiratory tract infections or influenza.
    2. Wash hands frequently before and after patient contact.
    3. Report temperature elevation.
    4. Monitor hemoglobin.

26. Which are necessary for the maturation of a red blood cell? *(Select all that apply.)*

    1. Vitamin B$_{12}$
    2. Folic acid
    3. Renal erythropoietic factor
    4. Capric acid
    5. Iron

27. Choose the correct medical management for the patient with DIC: *(Select all that apply.)*

    1. Addressing and correcting underlying cause
    2. Transfusion replacement
    3. Cryoprecipitate
    4. Administering colony-stimulating factor (filgrastim [Neupogen])
    5. Heparin therapy

28. A young adult with hemophilia A is admitted with uncontrolled bleeding in the left knee joint as a result of a fall from his motorcycle. Which are appropriate nursing interventions and medical management? *(Select all that apply.)*

    1. Applying pressure
    2. Cold applications
    3. Administering cyclophosphamide (Cytoxan)
    4. RBC transfusions
    5. Administering factor VIII concentrate

29. The nurse anticipates that an older adult patient with severe iron deficiency anemia will require which blood product?

    1. Whole blood
    2. Packed red blood cells
    3. Fresh frozen plasma
    4. Frozen red blood cells

30. Acute blood loss can have several serious effects on the body. Serious consequences result when the loss is:

    1. 100 mL.
    2. 300 mL.
    3. 500 mL.
    4. 1000 mL.

31. What is the most important measure in preventing transmission of harmful pathogens to a patient with depressed bone marrow function?

    1. Strict and frequent hand hygiene by all persons having contact with the patient
    2. Placement of the patient in a private room with high-efficiency particulate air filtration
    3. Administration of combinations of prophylactic antibiotics
    4. Creation of a "sterile" environment for the patient with the use of laminar airflow rooms

32. A patient is chronically hypoxic and has an RBC count of 7 million/mm^3, hemoglobin of 20 g/dL, and hematocrit of 50%; his condition would be classified as:

    1. primary polycythemia.
    2. secondary polycythemia.
    3. autoimmune thrombocytopenia.
    4. purpura splenomegaly.

33. The vital signs of a patient who has a blood loss of 1500 to 2000 mL would be: *(Select all that apply.)*

    1. Pulse >120 bpm
    2. Pulse >100 bpm
    3. Blood pressure normal
    4. Blood pressure <90 mm Hg

34. One unit of packed RBCs is expected to raise the hemoglobin level by how many grams per deciliter?

    1. 2 g/dL
    2. 1 g/dL
    3. 0.5 g/dL
    4. 3 g/dL

Care of the Patient with a Cardiovascular or a Peripheral Vascular Disorder

Barbara Lauritsen Christensen

Objectives

Anatomy and Physiology

1. Discuss the location, size, and position of the heart.
2. Identify the chambers of the heart and their functions.
3. Identify the valves of the heart and their locations.
4. Discuss the electrical conduction system that causes the cardiac muscle fibers to contract.
5. Explain what produces the two main heart sounds.
6. Trace the path of blood through the coronary circulation.

Medical-Surgical

7. List diagnostic tests used to evaluate cardiovascular function.
8. For coronary artery disease, compare nonmodifiable risk factors with factors that are modifiable in lifestyle and health management.
9. Describe five cardiac dysrhythmias.
10. Compare the etiology and pathophysiology, clinical manifestations, assessment, diagnostic tests, medical management, nursing interventions, and prognosis for patients with angina pectoris, myocardial infarction, or heart failure.
11. Specify patient teaching for patients with cardiac dysrhythmias, angina pectoris, myocardial infarction, heart failure, and valvular heart disease.
12. Discuss the purposes of cardiac rehabilitation.
13. Discuss the etiology and pathophysiology, clinical manifestations, assessment, diagnostic tests, medical management, nursing interventions, and prognosis for the patient with pulmonary edema.
14. Compare and contrast the etiology and pathophysiology, clinical manifestations, assessment, diagnostic tests, medical management, nursing interventions, and prognosis for the patient with rheumatic heart disease, pericarditis, and endocarditis.

15. Identify 10 conditions which may result in the development of secondary cardiomyopathy.
16. Discuss the indications and contraindications for cardiac transplant.
17. Describe the effects of aging on the peripheral vascular system.
18. Identify risk factors associated with peripheral vascular disorders.
19. Compare and contrast signs and symptoms associated with arterial and venous disorders.
20. Discuss nursing interventions for arterial and venous disorders.
21. Compare essential (primary) hypertension, secondary hypertension, and malignant hypertension.
22. Discuss the etiology and pathophysiology, clinical manifestations, assessment, diagnostic tests, medical management, and nursing interventions for the patient with hypertension.
23. Discuss the importance of patient education for hypertension.
24. Compare and contrast the etiology and pathophysiology, clinical manifestations, assessment, diagnostic tests, medical management, nursing interventions, and prognosis for patients with arterial aneurysm, Buerger's disease, and Raynaud's disease.
25. Discuss the etiology and pathophysiology, clinical manifestations, assessment, diagnostic tests, medical management, nursing interventions, and prognosis for patients with thrombophlebitis, varicose veins, and stasis ulcer.
26. Discuss appropriate patient education for thrombophlebitis.

Key Terms

aneurysm (ĂN-ŭr-ĭ-zĭm, p. 359)
angina pectoris (ăn-JĪ-nă PĔK-tŏr-ĭs, p. 321)
arteriosclerosis (ăr-tē-rē-ō-sklĕ-RŌ-sĭs, p. 355)
atherosclerosis (ăth-ĕr-ō-sklĕ-RŌ-sĭs, p. 320)
bradycardia (brăd-ĕ-KĂR-dē-ă, p. 315)
B-type natriuretic peptide (BNP) (nā'trĕ-yū-rĕt-ĭk, p. 311)
cardioversion (kăr-dē-ō-VĔR-zhŭn, p. 310)
coronary artery disease (CAD) (p. 320)
defibrillation (dē-fīb-rĭ-LĀ-shŭn, p. 317)
dysrhythmia (dĭs-RĬTH-mē-ă, p. 314)
embolus (ĔM-bō-lŭs, p. 326)
endarterectomy (ĕnd-ăr-tĕr-ĔK-tō-mē, p. 358)
heart failure (p. 332)

hypoxemia (hī-pŏk-SĒ-mē-ă, p. 310)
intermittent claudication (klăw-dĕ-KĀ-shŭn, p. 349)
ischemia (ĭs-KĒ-mē-ă, p. 321)
myocardial infarction (MI) (mī-ō-KĂR-dē-ăl ĭn-FĂRK-shŭn, p. 326)
occlusion (ō-KLŪ-zhŭn, p. 326)
orthopnea (ŏr-thŏp-NĒ-ă, p. 334)
peripheral (pĕ-RĬF-ĕr-ăl, p. 348)
pleural effusion (PLŪR-ăl ĕ-FŪ-zhŭn, p. 333)
polycythemia (pŏl-ē-sī-THĒ-mē-ă, p. 310)
pulmonary edema (PŬL-mō-nă-rē ĕ-DĒ-mă, p. 340)
tachycardia (tăk-ē-KĂR-dē-ă, p. 314)

ANATOMY AND PHYSIOLOGY OF THE CARDIOVASCULAR SYSTEM

The cardiovascular (circulatory) system is the transportation system of the body. It delivers oxygen and nutrients to the cells to support their individual activities and transports the cells' waste products to the appropriate organs for disposal. This chapter discusses the structure and function of the blood vessels and the heart.

HEART

The heart is a remarkable organ, not much bigger than a fist (Figure 8-1). It is responsible for pumping 1000 gallons of blood every day through the closed circuit of blood vessels. It beats 100,000 times a day and transports the blood 60,000 miles through a network of blood vessels. The heart is a hollow organ composed mainly of muscle tissue with a series of one-way valves.

The heart is located in the chest cavity between the lungs in a region called the **mediastinum** (the mass of organs and tissues separating the lungs; in addition to the heart and its greater vessels, the mediastinum contains the trachea and the esophagus). Two thirds of the heart lies left of the midline. The wider **base** of the heart lies superior and beneath the second rib. The **apex,** or narrow part, of the heart lies inferiorly, slightly to the left between the fifth and sixth ribs near the diaphragm.

Heart Wall

The heart is composed of three layers: **pericardium, myocardium,** and **endocardium.** The pericardium is a two-layered, serous membrane that covers the entire structure. Between the two thin membranes is a serous fluid that allows friction-free movement of the heart as it contracts and relaxes. The pericardium is the outermost layer of the heart. The myocardium forms the bulk of the heart wall and is the thickest and strongest layer of the heart. It is composed of cardiac muscle tissue. Contraction of this tissue is responsible for pumping blood. The endocardium (innermost layer) is composed of a thin layer of connective tissue. This structure lines the interior of the heart, the valves, and the larger vessels of the heart.

Heart Chambers

The heart is divided into a right and left half by a muscular partition called the **septum** (Figure 8-2). The heart has the following four chambers:

1. The **right atrium** is the upper right chamber. It receives deoxygenated blood from the entire body. The superior vena cava returns blood from the head, the neck, and the arms. The inferior vena cava returns blood from the lower body. The coronary vein returns it from the heart muscle to the coronary sinus.
2. The **right ventricle** is the lower right chamber. It receives deoxygenated blood from the right atrium. The right ventricle pumps blood to the lungs via the **pulmonary artery** to release carbon dioxide and receive oxygen.
3. The **left atrium** is the upper left chamber. It receives oxygenated blood from the lungs via the **pulmonary veins.**
4. The **left ventricle** is the lower left chamber. It receives oxygenated blood from the left atrium. It is the thickest, most muscular section of the heart and pumps the oxygenated blood out through the aorta to all parts of the body.

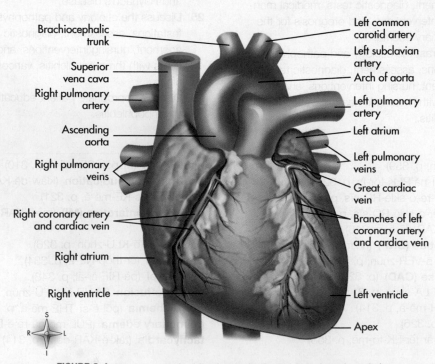

Brachiocephalic trunk
Superior vena cava
Right pulmonary artery
Ascending aorta
Right pulmonary veins
Right coronary artery and cardiac vein
Right atrium
Right ventricle

Left common carotid artery
Left subclavian artery
Arch of aorta
Left pulmonary artery
Left atrium
Left pulmonary veins
Great cardiac vein
Branches of left coronary artery and cardiac vein
Left ventricle
Apex

FIGURE 8-1 Heart and major blood vessels viewed from front (anterior).

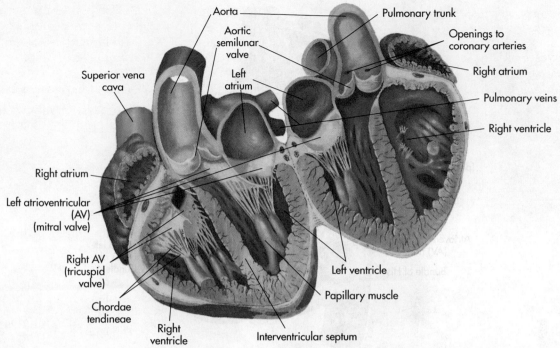

FIGURE 8-2 Interior of the heart. This illustration shows the heart as it would appear if it were cut along a frontal plane and opened like a book. The front portion of the heart lies to the reader's right; the back portion of the heart lies to the reader's left. The four chambers of the heart—two atria and two ventricles—are easily seen.

The heart actually functions as two separate pumps: (1) the right side receives deoxygenated blood and pumps it to the lungs, and (2) the left side receives oxygenated blood from the lungs and pumps it throughout the body.

Heart Valves

Located within the heart are four valves that keep the blood moving forward and prevent backflow. The heart has two **atrioventricular (AV) valves.** They are located between the atrium and the ventricles. The right AV valve, located between the right atrium and the right ventricle, is called the **tricuspid valve** because it contains three flaps, or cusps. The left AV valve is composed of two cusps (bicuspid) and is commonly called the **mitral valve.** It is located between the left atrium and the left ventricle. Both of these valves rapidly close to prevent backflow of blood. Small cordlike structures, **chordae tendineae,** connect the AV valves to the walls of the heart and work with the **papillary muscles** located in the walls of the ventricles to make a tight seal to prevent backflow when the ventricles contract.

The two remaining valves, the **semilunar valves,** are located at the points where the blood exits the ventricles. The **pulmonary semilunar valve** is located between the right ventricle and the pulmonary artery. Blood is pushed out of the right ventricle and travels to the lung via the pulmonary artery. The **aortic semilunar valve** is located between the left ventricle and the aorta. When the left ventricle contracts, the blood is forced into the aorta and the aortic semilunar valve closes. Both of the semilunar valves have three cusps that resemble a half moon, hence the name **semilunar** (see Figure 8-2).

Electrical Conduction System

Heart muscle tissue contains an inherent ability to contract in a rhythmic pattern. This ability is called **automaticity.** If heart muscle cells are removed and placed under a microscope, they continue to beat. In addition, they can respond to a stimulus in the same way that nerve cells do. This unique property is called **irritability.** Automaticity and irritability are two characteristics that affect the functions of the conduction system. Hormones, ion concentration, and changes in body temperature also affect the conduction of messages around the heart, initiation of heartbeat, and coordination of beating patterns between the atria and the ventricles.

The heartbeat is initiated in the **sinoatrial (SA) node,** which is located in the upper part of the right atrium, just beneath the opening of the superior vena cava (Figure 8-3). Because it regulates the heartbeat, the SA node is known as the **pacemaker.** Impulses are passed to the AV node, which is located in the base of the right atrium. The AV node slows the impulses to allow the atrium to complete contraction and to allow the ventricles to fill. The impulses then pass to a group of conduction fibers called the **bundle of His** and divides into right and left branches of AV bundle to travel to smaller branches called the **Purkinje fibers,**

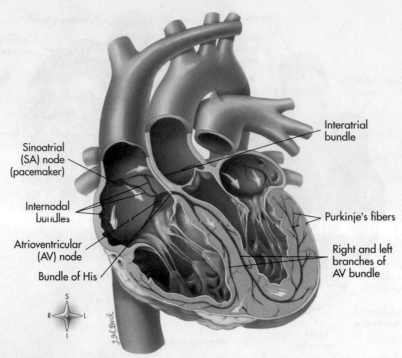

FIGURE 8-3 Conduction system of the heart. Specialized cardiac muscle cells in the wall of the heart rapidly initiate or conduct an electrical impulse throughout the myocardium. The signal is initiated by the SA node (pacemaker) and spreads to the rest of the right atrial myocardium directly, to the left atrial myocardium by way of the bundle of interatrial conducting fibers, and to the AV node by way of the three internodal bundles. The AV node then initiates a signal that is conducted through conduction fibers called the bundle of His and breaks into the right and left branches to travel to smaller branches called the Purkinje fibers, which surround the ventricles.

which surround the ventricles. The message travels rapidly through the ventricles and causes contractions, which empty the ventricles.

IMPULSE PATTERN: SA node → AV node → bundle of His → right and left bundle branches of AV bundle → Purkinje fibers

Cardiac Cycle

The cardiac cycle refers to a complete heartbeat. The two atria contract while the two ventricles relax. When the ventricles contract, the two atria relax. The phase of contraction is called **systole** (Figure 8-4), and the phase of relaxation is called **diastole** (the period between contraction of the atria or the ventricles during which blood enters the relaxed chambers from the systemic circulation and the lungs [Figure 8-5]). Complete diastole and systole of both atria and ventricles constitute a cardiac cycle; this takes an average of 0.8 second.

The heart sounds, **lubb** and **dubb**, are produced by closure of the valves. The first sound, **lubb** (long duration and low pitch), is heard when the AV valves close. The second sound, **dubb** (short duration, sharp sound), is heard when the semilunar valves close. Occasionally a murmur (swishing sound) can be heard. This can be a normal functional phenomenon produced by rapid filling of the ventricles, or it can be an abnormal condition produced by ineffective closure of the valves.

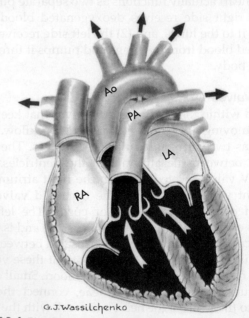

FIGURE 8-4 Blood flow during systole. *Ao,* Aorta; *LA,* left atrium; *LV,* left ventricle; *PA,* pulmonary artery; *RA,* right atrium; *RV,* right ventricle.

BLOOD VESSELS

Three main types of blood vessels are organized to carry blood to and from the heart. **Capillaries** (tiny blood vessels joining arterioles and venules) connect the **arteries** (large vessels carrying blood away from the heart) to the **veins** (vessels that convey blood from the capillaries and return it to the heart). The heart de-

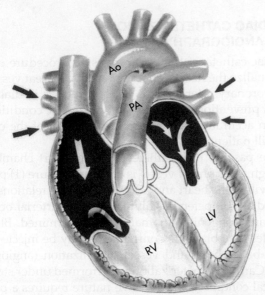

FIGURE 8-5 Blood flow during diastole. *Ao*, Aorta; *LA*, left atrium; *LV*, left ventricle; *PA*, pulmonary artery; *RA*, right atrium; *RV*, right ventricle.

livers the blood to the arteries, which branch into tiny vessels called **arterioles** (blood vessels of the smallest branch of the arterial circulation), which deliver the blood to the tissues. Within the tissues, microscopic vessels (capillaries) form an extensive (50,000 miles) network that allows exchanges of products and by-products between the tissues and blood. The capillaries then join with tiny veins, or **venules,** that link with the larger veins and return to the heart. The pattern is as follows:

Artery → arteriole → capillary → venule → vein

CIRCULATION

CORONARY BLOOD SUPPLY

To sustain life, the heart must pump blood throughout the body on a continuous basis. As a result, the heart muscle (or myocardium) requires a constant supply of blood containing nutrients and oxygen to function effectively. The delivery of oxygen and nutrient-rich arterial blood to cardiac muscle tissue and the return of oxygen-poor blood from this active tissue to the venous system are called the **coronary circulation** (Figure 8-6).

Blood flows into the heart muscle by way of two small vessels, the right and left coronary arteries, which are the best known of all the blood vessels. The coronary arteries form a crown around the myocardium (see Figures 8-1 and 8-6). The openings into these vessels lie behind the flaps of the aortic semilunar valves (see Figure 8-6). The coronary arteries bring oxygen and nutrition to the myocardium. Once the circulation is completed and the carbon dioxide and waste products have been collected, the blood flows into a large coronary vein and finally into the coronary sinus, which empties into the right atrium. These two main arteries have many tiny branches that serve the heart muscle. If an artery becomes occluded, these branches provide collateral circulation (alternate routes) to nourish the heart muscle. If the occlusion is severe, surgery and other procedures may be needed. These treatments are discussed later in this chapter.

SYSTEMIC CIRCULATION

Systemic circulation occurs when blood is pumped from the left ventricle of the heart through all parts of the body and returns to the right atrium. When the oxygenated blood leaves the left ventricle, it enters the largest artery (1 inch [2.5 cm] in diameter) of the body, the **aorta.** This is the main trunk of the systemic arterial circulation and is composed of four parts: the ascending aorta, the arch, the thoracic portion of the descending aorta, and the abdominal portion of the descending aorta. As the blood flows through the artery branches, the branches become smaller in diameter (arterioles). The blood continues to flow into the capillaries. The capillaries surround the cells and exchange oxygen, nutrients, carbon dioxide, and other waste products. The blood proceeds to the tiny venules, then to the larger veins, and finally returns to the right atrium via the largest vein, the **vena cava** (one of two large veins returning blood from the peripheral circulation to the right atrium of the heart).

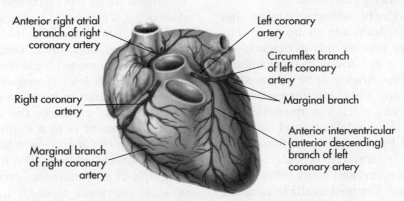

FIGURE 8-6 Arterial coronary circulation (anterior).

The blood is now deoxygenated and needs to be replenished with oxygen. Note that the upper portion of the vena cava (superior vena cava) returns deoxygenated blood from the head, neck, chest, and upper extremities. The inferior vena cava returns deoxygenated blood from parts of the body below the diaphragm.

PULMONARY CIRCULATION

The deoxygenated blood now passes through the pulmonary circulation to pick up the needed oxygen. Blood is pumped from the right atrium to the right ventricle, where it leaves the heart to travel via the pulmonary artery to the lungs. Once the blood reaches the lungs, it travels through arterioles to the capillaries. The microscopic capillaries surround the **alveoli** (air sacs), where oxygen diffuses into the bloodstream. The capillaries then connect with the venules and finally with the four pulmonary veins, which return the oxygenated blood to the left atrium of the heart. It is then pumped to the left ventricle and to the aorta, and systemic circulation is then repeated. The blood circulation pattern is as follows:

Superior or inferior vena cava → right atrium → tricuspid valve → right ventricle → pulmonary semilunar valve → pulmonary artery → capillaries in the lungs → pulmonary veins → left atrium → bicuspid valve → left ventricle → aortic semilunar valve → aorta

LABORATORY AND DIAGNOSTIC EXAMINATIONS

A number of diagnostic tests are used to evaluate cardiovascular function. The nursing responsibilities are to physically prepare the patient for diagnostic procedures and to explain the examination to the patient.

DIAGNOSTIC IMAGING

Radiographic examination of the chest provides a film record of heart size, shape, and position and outline of shadows. Lung congestion is also shown, indicating heart failure (HF), perhaps in the earliest stages. Pleural effusion may be noted in left-sided HF.

Fluoroscopy, the action-picture radiograph, allows observation of movement. It is invaluable in pacemaker or intracardial catheter placement.

An **angiogram** is a series of radiographs taken after injection of a contrast medium into an artery or vein. Picturing the circulatory process aids in diagnosis of vessel occlusion, pooling in various heart chambers, and congenital anomalies. Angiography allows x-ray visualization of the heart, aorta, inferior vena cava, pulmonary artery and vein, and coronary arteries.

In an **aortogram,** the abdominal aorta and the major leg arteries are viewed by x-ray visualization after a contrast medium is injected through the femoral artery and into the aorta. Aneurysms and many other abnormalities can be diagnosed. Contrast media to visualize the aortic arch and branches may also be used.

CARDIAC CATHETERIZATION AND ANGIOGRAPHY

Cardiac catheterization is an invasive procedure used to visualize the heart's chambers, valves, great vessels, and coronary arteries. This procedure aids in diagnosis, in prevention of progression of cardiac conditions, and in accurate evaluation and treatment of the critically ill patient.

The passage of a catheter into the heart chambers through a peripheral vessel is used to measure (1) pressure within the heart and (2) blood-volume relationship to cardiac competence. Valvular defects, arterial occlusion, and congenital anomalies are determined. Blood samples are obtained. Contrast dye may be injected to allow better heart and vessel visualization (angiography). Cardiac catheterization is performed under sterile surgical conditions; its invasive nature requires a prior signed consent. Because iodine is in the contrast medium, determine sensitivity to iodine before injection to avoid an allergic reaction. After the procedure, assess circulation to the extremity used for catheter insertion. Check peripheral pulses, color, and sensation of the extremity every 15 minutes for 1 hour and then with decreasing frequency. Observe the puncture site for hematoma and bleeding. Monitor vital signs. Assess for abnormal heart rate, dysrhythmias, and signs of pulmonary emboli (respiratory difficulty). The patient lies supine for a designated period with a compression device over the pressure dressing at the insertion site to prevent hemorrhage.

ELECTROCARDIOGRAPHY

The electrocardiogram (ECG, or EKG) is a graphic study of the electrical activities of the myocardium to determine transmission of cardiac impulses through the muscles and conduction tissue. Each ECG has three distinct waves, or deflections: the **P wave,** the QRS complex, and the **T wave.** When the heart contracts, the electrical activity is called **depolarization.** **Repolarization** is the relaxation phase. The P wave represents the depolarization of the atria. The QRS complex represents the depolarization of the ventricles. The T wave represents the repolarization of the ventricles. Atrial repolarization is not represented but does occur; it is covered by the large QRS complex and cannot be seen on the ECG tracing.

A standard ECG has 12 electrodes attached to the skin surface to measure the total electrical activity of the heart. Each lead records the electrical potential between the limbs or between the heart and limbs. A conductive gel enhances the contact and transmission. The patient is in a supine position. However, ambulatory ECGs and exercise stress test ECGs require position variation. The machine, an electrocardiograph or galvanometer, records the energy wave of each heartbeat through a vibrating needle on graph paper, which feeds through the machine at a

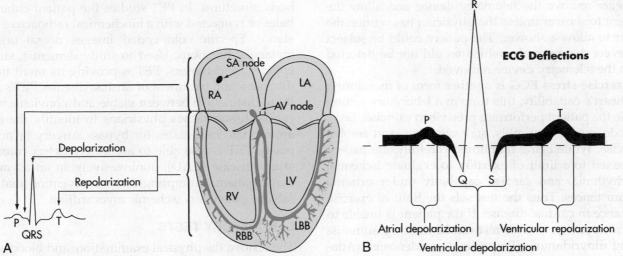

FIGURE 8-7 Normal electrocardiographic (ECG) deflections. **A,** P wave. **B,** Relationship of ECG to cardiac muscle activity. *AV,* Atrioventricular; *LA,* left atrium; *LBB,* left bundle block; *LV,* left ventricle; *RA,* right atrium; *RBB,* right bundle block; *RV,* right ventricle; *SA,* sinoatrial.

standard rate. Each ECG waveform represents a single electrical impulse as it travels through the heart (Figure 8-7).

The ECG tracing is read or interpreted by a cardiac specialist (cardiologist) or by internal medicine specialists, family practitioners, pediatricians, and emergency department practitioners. The reading can also be displayed on the fluorescent screen (oscilloscope) of a cardiac monitor. A graphic tracing may be printed out by the monitor.

Ambulatory ECGs can be used to monitor heart rhythm over prolonged periods—12, 24, or 48 hours—and compared with various activities or symptoms recorded in a diary kept by the patient. A Holter monitor (small portable recorder) is attached to the patient by leads, with a 2-pound tape recorder carried on a belt or shoulder strap. The monitor operates continuously to record the patterns and rhythms of the patient's heartbeat. In conjunction with the diary, the physician can note various events, times, and medication peaks that affect or precipitate dysrhythmias. An ambulatory ECG is particularly useful for patients whose clinical symptoms indicate heart disorders but who may have normal ECG tracings on a resting test.

CARDIAC MONITORS

It is common practice to continuously assess the cardiac electrical activity of patients who are known or suspected to have dysrhythmias or who are prone to develop dysrhythmias or acute cardiovascular symptoms. A cardiac monitor displays information on the electrical activity of the heart transferred via conductive electrodes placed on the chest.

Most monitors provide a visual display of cardiac electrical activity and the correct heart rate. Preset alarms warn of heart rates that exceed or drop below limits considered acceptable for each patient and also warn of dysrhythmias.

Ambulatory patients are increasingly monitored by battery-powered ECG transmitters that do not directly connect the patient to the oscilloscope. This monitoring is called **telemetry,** which is the electronic transmission of data to a distant location. The electrodes placed on the patient's chest are attached to a transmitter the patient carries in a pocket or pouch. The transmitter sends a radio signal to a receiver, usually located at the nurse's station.

Patients need telemetry monitoring for various reasons, including a history of cardiac disease, angina pectoris, suspected dysrhythmias, a change in medications, an electrolyte abnormality, or unexplained syncope. Many of these patients are monitored in a centralized area such as an intermediate care or step-down unit (with monitors at the nurse's station). Remote telemetry means the patient is on a medical-surgical unit and is monitored at a separate location, called the **home unit,** which is usually on a critical care unit. Remote telemetry patients are usually stable. But even a stable patient's condition can change rapidly, and telemetry allows continuous heart monitoring to detect abnormalities.

Attachment to a cardiac monitor does not change a patient's need for nursing interventions. Because the monitoring electrodes are on the anterior thorax (chest) rather than the extremities, the patient is relatively free to carry on usual activities. Pay special attention to the electrode site to ensure a constant tight seal between the electrode and the skin and to note the development of any skin impairment. The conduction gel dries out, even if the pad is sealed; changing electrodes regularly is recommended. Also check the telemetry pack for integrity of the lead wires and test the monitoring device's battery with a battery tester. Inform the monitoring area whenever the patient is moved off the unit for a diagnostic test, since the patient may go outside the monitor's range. Another important safety measure is to *never* remove the telemetry device and allow the patient to shower unless the physician has written the order to allow a shower. The patient could be subject to severe dysrhythmia, which would not be detected with the telemetry device removed.

Exercise-stress ECG is another form of monitoring the heart's capability, this time in a laboratory setting while the patient performs a prescribed exercise. Tasks include use of treadmills, stair climbing, and aerobic exercise. While being monitored carefully, the patient is coaxed to a limit of exertion to evaluate ischemia, dysrhythmia, and cardiac capability under extreme circumstances. Thus the test sets the limit of exercise tolerance in cardiac disease. If the patient is unable to tolerate activity, a stress test can be done by administering dipyridamole (Persantine) or adenosine (Adenocard), which mimics the patient's heart under stress or activity.

THALLIUM SCANNING

Thallium 201 is an intracellular ion that is actively transported into normal cells. If the cell is ischemic or infarcted, the thallium will not be picked up. Because the thallium concentrates in tissue with normal blood flow, tissue with inadequate perfusion appears as dark areas on scanning—a "cold spot." The radioisotope is injected intravenously while the patient exercises on a treadmill. Breast tissue in the female can produce artifact, leading to a false-positive result. Using technetium 99m sestamibi instead of thallium can help minimize artifact and thus improve accuracy. In patients who cannot tolerate physical exercise, dipyridamole is given before the thallium to physiologically simulate exercise-induced stress.

ECHOCARDIOGRAPHY

Echocardiography uses high-frequency ultrasound directed at the heart. The echo, or reflected sound, is graphically recorded, outlining size, shape, and position of cardiac structures. This test is used to detect pericardial effusion (collection of blood or other fluid in the pericardial sac), ventricular function, cardiac chamber size and contents, ventricular muscle and septal motion and thickness, cardiac output (ejection fraction), cardiac tumors, valvular function, and congenital heart disorder.

Ejection fraction (EF) of ventricles as demonstrated by an echocardiogram is as follows:

- Normal: greater than 60%
- Moderate HF: 40% to 60%
- Moderate to severe HF: 20% to 40%
- Severe HF (candidate for heart transplant): less than 20%

POSITRON EMISSION TOMOGRAPHY

Positron emission tomography (PET) is a computerized radiographic technique that uses radioactive substances to examine the metabolic activity of various body structures. In PET studies the patient either inhales or is injected with a biochemical radioactive substance. Specific color-coded images reveal organs' metabolic functions. Used to study dementia, stroke, epilepsy, and tumors, PET is proving its merit in the diagnosis and treatment of cardiac disease. PET's ability to distinguish between viable and nonviable myocardial tissue allows physicians to identify the most appropriate candidates for bypass surgery or angioplasty. PET is also able to accurately detect coronary artery disease (CAD), noninvasively, in an asymptomatic patient, prompting early intervention that can salvage potentially ischemic myocardium.

LABORATORY TESTS

The history, the physical examination, and blood studies aid the health care provider in diagnosing and monitoring the cardiovascular disease process. The nurse's responsibility is to prepare the patient by explaining the tests and the preparation required for each test.

Blood cultures to detect growth of bacteria in the blood are crucial to the diagnosis of infective endocarditis.

A **complete blood count** (CBC) is a determination of the number of red and white blood cells per cubic millimeter, as well as the white blood cell differential, platelets, hemoglobin, and hematocrit. Low hemoglobin indicates decreased ability to carry oxygen to the cells and anemia; an elevated white blood cell (leukocyte) count indicates infection or inflammation; and an elevated red blood cell (erythrocyte) count indicates that the body is compensating for chronic **hypoxemia** (an abnormal deficiency of oxygen in the arterial blood) by stimulating red blood cell production by the bone marrow, leading to secondary **polycythemia** (abnormal increase in the number of red blood cells in the blood). Chronic hypoxemia is often noted in HF.

Coagulation studies are useful in monitoring the patient receiving anticoagulant drug therapy, which is prescribed for patients with myocardial infarction (MI). Coagulation studies are also important in patients who have chronic atrial fibrillation or patients with atrial fibrillation who are undergoing **cardioversion** (the restoration of the heart's normal sinus rhythm by delivery of a synchronized electric shock through two metal paddles placed on the patient's chest). Coagulation studies are needed if an MI is diagnosed in case fibrinolytics are needed to dissolve the thrombus. These studies include prothrombin time (PT), International Normalized Ratio (INR), and partial thromboplastin time (PTT).

Erythrocyte sedimentation rate (ESR) is used to monitor or rule out inflammatory infective conditions. The ESR is elevated with MI and infective endocarditis and decreases when healing begins. The ESR also indicates the extent of inflammation and infection in rheumatic fever.

Serum electrolyte tests focus on the body's balance of sodium, potassium, calcium, and magnesium, which are necessary for myocardial muscle function. Sodium (Na^+) helps maintain fluid balance. Potassium (K^+) is required for relaxation of cardiac muscle, and calcium (Ca^{++}) is necessary for contraction of cardiac muscle. Magnesium (Mg^{++}) helps maintain the correct level of electric excitability in the nerves and the muscles, including the myocardium and the cardiac conduction system. The health care provider compares serum electrolyte levels with ECG changes.

Serum lipids are associated with vascular disease, particularly CAD. Cholesterol and triglycerides bound to plasma proteins are found in the blood as lipoproteins. Density levels vary according to the protein-fat ratio. An elevated high-density lipoprotein (HDL) is desired, but low-density lipoprotein (LDL) or very-low-density lipoprotein (VLDL) increases the risk for cardiovascular disease (see Box 8-1, p. 313).

Arterial blood gases are measured to monitor oxygenation (Pao_2, $Paco_2$) and acid-base balance (pH). This test is useful in patients with unstable cardiac conditions to determine the blood oxygenation process and in evaluation of patients in cardiac failure.

Serum cardiac markers are certain proteins that are released into the blood in large quantities from necrotic heart muscle after an MI. These markers, specifically cardiac serum enzymes and troponin I, are important screening diagnostic criteria for an acute MI. The cardiac enzyme creatine kinase (CK) and its isoenzyme, creatine phosphokinase (CK-MB), have been the gold standard for years. However, CK-MB is also found in skeletal muscle and can be elevated by surgery, muscle trauma, and muscular diseases, so it is not a specific indicator for MI. CK and CK-MB start to rise within 2 to 3 hours after the beginning of an MI, peak in 24 hours, and return to normal within 24 to 40 hours (Nagle, 2002). When cardiac cells die, their cellular enzymes are released into circulation. The increase in serum enzymes that occurs after cell death can demonstrate whether cardiac damage is present and the approximate extent of the damage. Other causes of increased serum enzymes may make the differential diagnosis more difficult.

Troponin I is a myocardial muscle protein released into circulation after a myocardial injury. In the heart there are two subtypes: cardiac-specific troponin T and troponin I. These are sensitive markers that identify very small amounts of myocardial damage. Troponin T appears in the blood 3 to 5 hours after an MI and may remain elevated for up to 21 days. Like CK-MB, troponin T is affected by skeletal muscle injury and renal disease. Troponin I is a sensitive and specific cardiac marker, not influenced by skeletal muscle trauma or renal failure. Troponin I rises 3 hours after MI, peaks at 14 to 18 hours, and returns to normal in 5 to 7 days. Troponin I is useful in diagnosing an MI (Nagle, 2002). The recent ability to measure myocardial contractile proteins (troponins) in serum is a milestone in the diagnosis of acute MI and acute myocardial damage resulting from other causes.

Myoglobin is released into circulation within a few hours after an MI. Although it is one of the first serum cardiac markers that increase after an MI, myoglobin is also present in skeletal muscle, so an increase can be associated with noncardiac causes. In addition, it is rapidly excreted in urine so that blood levels return to normal range within 24 hours after an MI.

B-type natriuretic peptide (BNP) is a neurohormone secreted by the heart in response to ventricular expansion. An elevated BNP of greater than 100 pg/mL indicates HF. BNP is present in the ventricle of the heart and correlates well to left ventricular pressure. The greater the BNP level, the more severe the HF (Pagana & Pagana, 2007).

Homocysteine is an amino acid produced during protein digestion. Normal values range from 4 to 14 μmol/L. Elevated blood levels of homocysteine may act as an independent risk factor for ischemic heart disease, cerebrovascular disease, peripheral arterial disease (PAD), and venous thrombosis. Homocysteine appears to promote the progression of atherosclerosis by causing endothelial damage, promoting LDL deposits, and promoting vascular smooth muscle growth. Homocysteine is an amino acid that plays an important role in blood clotting. An elevated level results in increased platelet aggregation. Screening for elevated homocysteine levels (more than 14 μmol/L) should be considered in patients who have progressive and unexplained atherosclerosis despite normal lipoproteins and who have no other risk factors. It is also recommended in patients with an unusual family history of atherosclerosis, especially at a young age.

Dietary deficiency of vitamins B_6, B_{12}, or folate is the most common cause of elevated homocysteine. Some researchers believe that elevated levels of homocysteine can be treated by administration of vitamins B_6, B_{12}, and folate. Whether this treatment will reduce the incidence of MI remains to be seen (Pagana & Pagana, 2007).

The liver produces **C-reactive protein (CRP)** during periods of acute inflammation. The presence of CRP is a predictor of cardiac events and is emerging as an independent risk factor for CAD. Persons who have diabetes mellitus are already at high risk for developing cardiovascular disease. If a patient has both an elevated CRP and diabetes, his or her risk for a cardiovascular disorder becomes even greater (Pagana & Pagana, 2007).

DISORDERS OF THE CARDIOVASCULAR SYSTEM

Cardiovascular disorders are a major health care problem in the United States. Public awareness, modifications in lifestyles, and improvements in medical treatment have contributed to a decline in overall deaths. The nurse's role in caring for patients with cardiovascular disorders includes being aware of the prevalence of cardiac disease, risk factors, and the disease process; implementing nursing interventions; and patient teaching.

NORMAL AGING PATTERNS

By the time an individual reaches the age of 65 years, physiologic changes have reduced the efficiency of the heart as a pump. Yet the heart still is capable of functioning adequately unless there is underlying cardiac disease (see Life Span Considerations box).

RISK FACTORS

Research has identified risk factors that indicate predispositions to developing cardiovascular disease. The presence of more than one risk factor is associated with an increasing risk of developing cardiovascular disease. Risk factors are classified as those that are nonmodifiable and those that are modifiable.

Nonmodifiable Factors

An important aspect of caring for the patient with a cardiovascular disorder is understanding the risk factors for cardiovascular disease and incorporating them

Life Span Considerations
Older Adults

Cardiac Disease

- Changes in the cardiac musculature lead to reduced efficiency and strength, resulting in decreased cardiac output.
- Disorientation, syncope, and decreased tissue perfusion to organs and other body tissues can occur as a result of decreased cardiac output.
- Aging causes sclerotic changes in blood vessels and leads to decreased elasticity and narrowing of the lumen. Arterial disease resulting from the aging process causes hypertension because of the increased cardiac effort needed to pump blood through the circulatory system.
- Progressive coronary artery changes can lead to the development of collateral coronary circulation. This can modify the severity of signs and symptoms seen in MI. Angina symptoms may be less pronounced, and dyspnea may replace angina as a key symptom of acute infarction.
- Heart failure can result from rapid intravenous infusion.
- Edema secondary to heart failure may cause tissue impairment in the immobile older adult. Immobility leads to venous stasis, venous ulcer, and poor wound healing. It also increases the risk of venous thrombosis and embolus formation.
- Older adults with cardiac disease often receive several medications, which are often prescribed at lower doses than for younger adults. Even with lower doses of medications, observe the older adult closely for signs of toxicity, since the rate of drug metabolism and excretion decreases with age.
- Independent older adults with cardiac conditions should receive adequate teaching regarding medication, diet, and warning signs of complications. Encourage them to maintain regular contact with the physician and to seek care at the first sign of problems.

into patient teaching. The nonmodifiable risk factors associated with cardiovascular disorders include the following.

Family History

A family member such as a parent or sibling who has a cardiovascular problem before 50 years of age places the patient at greater risk for developing cardiovascular disease.

Age

Normal physiologic changes that occur with aging and past lifestyle habits increase the patient's risk for developing cardiovascular disease with advancing age. CAD and MI occur most frequently among white, middle-aged men.

Gender

Middle-aged men are at a greater risk of developing cardiovascular disease than women. Although the incidence in men and women equalizes after age 65, cardiovascular disease is a greater cause of death in women than in men. Women develop CAD about 10 years later than men because natural estrogen is believed to have a cardioprotective effect before menopause. The incidence of cardiovascular disease in women 50 years of age and older is increasing. Factors believed to be responsible are increased social and economic pressures on women and changes in lifestyle. Ten times more women die from heart disease than die from breast cancer. The mortality rate for women with CAD has remained relatively constant even though cardiovascular disease remains the leading cause of death. Despite this statistic, only 15% of women consider CAD their greatest health risk. Recent research on CAD has shown that women often do not have the classic signs and symptoms of an acute coronary event (Lewis et al., 2007).

Cultural and Ethnic Considerations

Black men have a higher incidence of hypertension than do white men. Black women have a higher incidence of CAD, with greater severity and higher death rates, than white women (Lewis et al., 2007).

Modifiable Factors
Smoking

Individuals who smoke have a two to three times greater risk of developing cardiovascular disease than nonsmokers. The degree of risk is proportional to the number of cigarettes smoked. Individuals who quit smoking decrease their risk. Tobacco smoke contains nicotine, which causes catecholamine (i.e., epinephrine, norepinephrine) release. Catecholamine release causes tachycardia, hypertension, and vasoconstriction of the peripheral arteries, which in turn increase the work of the heart and result in greater myocardial oxygen consumption (Lewis et al., 2007). Nicotine also increases platelet adhesion, which results in increased risk of embolism (Lewis et al., 2007). The nicotine content of cigarettes causes the production of carbon monoxide, which places a greater demand on the heart and interferes with oxygen supply.

Hyperlipidemia

Hyperlipidemia is elevated concentrations of any or all lipids in the plasma. The ratio of HDL to LDL is the best predictor for the development of cardiovascular disease. Density levels vary according to the protein-fat ratio:

- VLDL contains more fat than protein (primarily triglycerides); triglycerides are the main storage form of lipids and constitute approximately 95% of fatty tissue.
- LDL contains an equal amount of fat and protein (approximately 50%) with moderate amounts of phospholipid cholesterol.

Less than 100 mg/dL	Optimal
100 to 129 mg/dL	Near optimal to above optimal
130 to 159 mg/dL	Borderline high
160 to 189 mg/dL	High
More than 190 mg/dL	Very high

- HDL contains more protein than fat (which serves a protective function, removing cholesterol from tissues). It is suspected that HDL also removes cholesterol from the peripheral tissues and transports it to the liver for excretion. Also, HDL may have a protective effect by preventing cellular uptake of cholesterol and lipids. Low levels (less than 40 mg/dL) are believed to increase a person's risk for CAD, whereas high levels (more than 60 mg/dL) are considered protective (Box 8-1).

A diet high in saturated fat, cholesterol, and calories contributes to hyperlipidemia. Therefore dietary control is an important factor in modifying this risk factor. An overall serum cholesterol level of less than 200 mg/dL is desirable, 200 to 239 mg/dL is borderline high, and more than 239 mg/dL is high.

Change in diet is probably the most important method of lowering cholesterol level. Weight reduction, in overweight patients with abnormal lipid profiles, is an essential element of the dietary intervention. In addition to lowering LDL levels, weight reduction leads to decreases in triglyceride level and blood pressure. A combination of weight reduction and physical exercise improves the lipid profile, with a decrease in

---

Box 8-1   Cholesterol Numbers: What Do They Mean?

YOUR TOTAL CHOLESTEROL NUMBER
A total cholesterol level less than 200 is considered desirable.

HDL CHOLESTEROL NUMBER
The higher the HDL cholesterol level, the better, because this means that there are more good lipoproteins to remove adhered cholesterol from the arteries.

LDL CHOLESTEROL NUMBER
The higher the number of bad lipoproteins, or LDLs, in the blood, the more likely it is that cholesterol is beginning to adhere to the arteries. Monitor risk factors to assess for probability of development of heart disease.

TOTAL CHOLESTEROL
Desirable: Less than 200
Borderline: 200 to 239
High: 240 or greater

HDL CHOLESTEROL
Low: Less than 40
High: Greater than 60

LDL CHOLESTEROL
Optimal: Less than 100
Near to above optimal: 100-129
Borderline high: 130-159
High: 160-189
Very high: Greater than 190

SET LDL CHOLESTEROL GOAL
Once the LDL cholesterol number is known, one can change the diet to help lower the amount of cholesterol in the blood. The table below shows the target LDL cholesterol goal. Reducing the risk factors is important too, so health care providers must make recommendations to assist the patient in maintaining acceptable cholesterol levels.

Risk Factors	Start Diet Treatment If LDL Cholesterol Is:	The LDL Goal Is:
No heart disease and fewer than two risk factors other than high LDL cholesterol	**160** or more	Less than **160**
No heart disease but two or more risk factors other than high LDL cholesterol	**130** or more	**100** or less
Definite heart disease or arterial disease	**100** or more	Less than **130**

Modified from Third Report of National Cholesterol Education Program (NCEP) Expert Panel on Detection, Evaluation, and Treatment of High Blood Cholesterol in Adults, 2001.
HDL, High-density lipoprotein; *LDL,* low-density lipoprotein.

LDL level, an increase in HDL level, and a decrease in triglyceride levels. Low HDL levels are often familial and only somewhat modifiable.

Cholesterol-lowering drugs are often included in treatment of hyperlipidemia. Cholesterol-lowering drugs are divided into six classes: (1) bile acid sequestrants; (2) nicotinic acid (niacin); (3) statins such as simvastatin (Zocor), pravastatin (Pravachol), and rosuvastatin (Crestor); (4) fibric acid derivatives such as gemfibrozil (Lopid) and probucol (Lorelco); (5) the cholesterol absorption inhibitor ezetimibe [Zetia]; and (6) combination drugs such as ezetimibe and simvastatin (Vytorin) (Cuddy, 2006). Pravastatin reduces the risk of a first MI by about one third in hypercholesterolemic patients with no history of coronary disease. Simvastatin is now allowed by the U.S. Food and Drug Administration (FDA) to add a label statement that the drug can reduce deaths by lowering cholesterol.

Hypertension
Hypertension is blood pressure higher than 140/90 mm Hg, which increases an individual's risk of developing cardiovascular disease. Adhering to medical therapy for control of elevated blood pressure helps to modify the individual's risk.

Diabetes Mellitus
Cardiac disease has been found to be more prevalent in individuals with diabetes mellitus. Diabetes mellitus poses a greater risk than other factors. This is thought to be related to elevated blood glucose levels, which damage the arterial intima and contribute to atherosclerosis. Diabetic patients also have alterations in lipid metabolism and tend to have high cholesterol and triglyceride levels. Medical therapy for regulating blood glucose levels helps to modify the individual's risk.

Obesity
Excess body weight increases the workload of the heart. It also contributes to the severity of other risk factors. A weight-reduction program and maintenance of an ideal body weight help to modify the individual's risk.

Sedentary Lifestyle
Lack of regular exercise has been correlated with increased risk of developing cardiovascular disease. Regular aerobic exercise can improve the heart's efficiency and help lower blood glucose levels, improving the ratio of HDLs to LDLs, reducing weight, lowering the blood pressure, reducing stress, and improving overall feelings of well-being. Some practitioners define regular physical exercise as exercising at least three to five times a week for at least 30 minutes, causing perspiration and an increase in heart rate by 30 to 50 bpm. Walking is one of the best forms of exercise.

Stress
The body's stress response releases catecholamines that increase the heart rate. Catecholamines also affect myocardial cells and may result in cellular damage. The vasoconstriction that occurs may contribute to development of cardiovascular disease. Stress reduction measures may be important in modifying an individual's risk.

Psychosocial Factors
People who develop CAD are more likely to have the coronary-prone, or type A, personality. Type A personality traits include aggressiveness, competitiveness, perfectionism, compulsiveness, and an urgent sense of time. When the type A personality is combined with other risk factors such as age, high lipid levels, and smoking, the risk of heart disease increases.

CARDIAC DYSRHYTHMIAS
A **dysrhythmia** (or arrhythmia) refers to any cardiac rhythm that deviates from normal sinus rhythm. Normal sinus rhythm originates in the SA node and is characterized by the following:
- Rate: 60 to 100 bpm
- P waves: precede each QRS complex (atrial depolarization)
- P-R interval: interval between atrial and ventricular repolarization
- QRS complex: ventricular depolarization
- T wave: ventricular repolarization
- Rhythm: regular

A dysrhythmia is the result of an alteration in the formation of impulses through the SA node to the rest of the myocardium. It also results from irritability of myocardial cells that generate impulses, which is independent of the conduction system. Signs and symptoms of dysrhythmia vary, as does treatment, depending on the type and severity of the dysrhythmia. A short overview of each dysrhythmia follows.

Types of Cardiac Dysrhythmias
Sinus Tachycardia
Sinus **tachycardia** is a rapid, regular rhythm originating in the SA node. It is characterized by a heartbeat of 100 to 150 bpm or more.

Causes of sinus tachycardia include exercise, anxiety, fever, shock, medications, HF, excessive caffeine, recreational drugs, and tobacco use. Tachycardia increases the amount of oxygen delivered to the cells by increasing the amount of blood circulated through the vessels.

Clinical manifestations include occasional palpitations. Many patients are asymptomatic. Other signs and symptoms may include hypotension and angina, if cardiovascular disease is also present.

Medical management is directed at the primary cause. This is a normal rhythm and is not usually caused by a cardiac problem.

Sinus Bradycardia

Sinus bradycardia is a slow rhythm originating in the SA node. It is characterized by a pulse rate of less than 60 bpm (or even less than 50 bpm, according to some sources). Causes of sinus bradycardia include sleep, vomiting, intracranial tumors, MI, drugs (especially digitalis toxicity), carotid sinus massage, vagal stimulation, endocrine disturbances, increased intracranial pressure, and hypothermia. When found in association with MI, it is a beneficial rhythm because it reduces myocardial oxygen demand. This may be a normal rate and rhythm for an athlete.

Clinical manifestations include fatigue, lightheadedness, and syncope. Some patients are asymptomatic.

Medical management is directed toward the primary cause of the problem and maintaining cardiac output. Atropine may be prescribed to increase the heart rate. A temporary or permanent implantable pacemaker is sometimes necessary (Figures 8-8 and 8-9).

Supraventricular Tachycardia

Supraventricular tachycardia (SVT) is the sudden onset of a rapid heartbeat. It originates in the atria. It is characterized by a pulse rate of 150 to 250 bpm.

Causes of SVT include drugs, alcohol, mitral valve prolapse, emotional stress, smoking, and hormone imbalance. The cause is typically not associated with heart disease.

Clinical manifestations include palpitations, lightheadedness, dyspnea, and anginal pain.

Medical management first looks at how well the patient tolerates the dysrhythmia and at the overall clinical picture. Then the focus is aimed at decreasing the heart rate and eliminating the underlying cause. Specific treatments may include carotid sinus pressure, adenosine, digoxin (Lanoxin), calcium channel blockers (e.g., diltiazem [Cardizem]), beta-adrenergic blockers, propranolol (Inderal), antidysrhythmics, amiodarone (Cordarone), and cardioversion. Persistent, recurring SVT may ultimately be treated with radiofrequency catheter ablation of the accessory pathway.

Atrial Fibrillation

In atrial fibrillation, electrical activity in the atria is disorganized, causing the atria to fibrillate, or quiver, rather than contract as a unit. Atrial fibrillation is a very rapid production of atrial impulses. The atria beat chaotically and are not contracting properly. It is char-

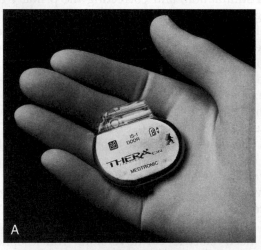

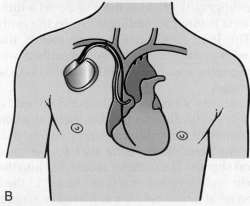

FIGURE 8-8 A, Ventricular pacing. Impulses are initiated in ventricle. **B,** Atrial pacing. Impulses are initiated in atrium and travel to ventricles by normal conduction system through the atrioventricular *(AV)* node. *LV,* Left ventricle; *PA,* pulmonary artery; *RA,* right atrium; *RV,* right ventricle.

FIGURE 8-9 A, A dual-chamber, rate-responsive pacemaker (shown here actual size) from Medtronic, Inc., is designed to detect body movement and automatically increase or decrease paced heart rates based on the level of physical activity. **B,** Cardiac leads, in both the atrium and the ventricle, enable a dual-chamber pacemaker to sense and pace in both heart chambers.

acterized by an atrial rate of 350 to 600 bpm. If untreated, the ventricular response rate may be 100 to 180 bpm.

Causes of atrial fibrillation include cardiac surgery, longstanding hypertension, pulmonary embolism, atherosclerosis, mitral valve disease, HF, cardiomyopathy, congenital abnormalities, chronic obstructive pulmonary disease, and thyrotoxicosis. Clinical manifestations include pulse deficit, palpitations, dyspnea, angina, lightheadedness, syncope, fatigue, change in level of consciousness, and pulmonary edema. Because of ventricular rhythm irregularity and ineffective atrial contractions, decreased cardiac output may be noted, resulting in HF, angina, and shock. Thrombi may form in the atria as a result of ineffective atrial contraction and cause emboli, thus affecting the lungs or periphery (away from the center of the body). An embolized clot may pass to the brain, causing a stroke. Risk of stroke increases fivefold with atrial fibrillation. Risk of stroke is even higher in patients who have structural heart disease, hypertension, and an age over 65 years.

Medical management focuses on treating the irritability of the atria, slowing the ventricular response to atrial stimulation, and correcting the primary cause. The goal of therapy is to prevent atrial thrombi from developing and becoming emboli in the body, such as in the lungs or periphery. Specific treatments for pharmacologic cardioversion may include (1) digitalis; (2) calcium channel blockers such as intravenous (IV) diltiazem (Cardizem) and verapamil (Calan, Isoptin); (3) antidysrhythmics such as procainamide (Procan SR, Pronestyl), amiodarone (Cordarone), dofetilide (Tikosyn), flecainide (Tambocor), or propafenone (Rythmol) (Benz, 2006); and anticoagulants such as heparin or warfarin (Coumadin). Outpatients typically take oral warfarin to maintain anticoagulation. The goal of anticoagulation is to maintain an INR between 2 and 3. If pharmacologic cardioversion fails, the patient may need electric cardioversion. Transesophogeal echocardiography (TEE) is used to detect a thrombus in the atria before proceeding with electric cardioversion. The Joint Commission recommends that patients with atrial fibrillation be prescribed warfarin and long-term antidysrhythmic medication therapy at discharge.

For patients who do not respond to medication therapy or electrical conversion, catheter ablation (cutting or removal) with radiofrequency energy is used to destroy the areas in the atria that trigger abnormal electrical signals. The catheter is inserted into the femoral vein and threaded via fluoroscopy to the heart. The special ablation catheter is placed in strategic areas, and bursts of radiofrequency energy destroy the irritable area (Rocca, 2007; Benz, 2006).

Catheter ablation to treat atrial fibrillation is usually performed on younger patients because of a better response rate and fewer complications than in the older adult. After the catheter ablation procedure, perform neurovascular assessment checks at the peripheral sites distal to the catheter insertion site (Rocca, 2007).

Atrioventricular Block

AV block occurs when a defect in the AV junction slows or impairs conduction of impulses from the SA node to the ventricles. Three types of blocks are seen: first degree, second degree, and third degree. The third-degree block indicates a worsening of the impairment in the AV junction and a complete heart block.

Common causes of AV block include atherosclerotic heart disease (ASHD), MI, and heart failure (HF). Other causes may be digitalis toxicity, congenital abnormality, drugs, and hypokalemia.

Clinical manifestations include no symptoms for first-degree block; vertigo, weakness, and irregular pulse for second-degree block; and hypotension, angina, bradycardia, heart rate often in the 30s, and HF for third-degree block.

Medical management involves evaluating the patient's response and determining the cause of the dysrhythmia. Atropine and isoproterenol may be prescribed. A pacemaker frequently is needed with third-degree block (see Figure 8-8).

Premature Ventricular Contractions

Premature ventricular contractions (PVCs) are abnormal heartbeats that arise from the right or left ventricle. PVCs are early ventricular beats that occur in conjunction with the underlying rhythm, which is unchanged except for the PVC itself.

PVCs may originate from more than one location in the ventricles and be caused by irritability of the ventricular musculature, exercise, stress, electrolyte imbalance, digitalis toxicity, hypoxia, and MI.

Clinical manifestations depend on the frequency of PVCs and their effect on the heart's ability to pump blood effectively. Some patients are asymptomatic; others may experience palpitations, weakness, and lightheadedness. Other symptoms are associated with decreased cardiac output.

Medical management focuses on treating the underlying heart condition. Symptomatic PVCs can be treated with beta-adrenergic blockers such as carvedilol (Coreg), antianginals, propranolol (Inderal), and antidysrhythmics such as procainamide, amiodarone, or lidocaine (Xylocaine).

PVC may be a single event or may occur several times in a minute or in pairs or strings. PVCs that last long enough to cause ventricular tachycardia (VT) may lead to death.

Ventricular Tachycardia

VT occurs when three or more successive PVCs occur. The ventricular rate is greater than 100 bpm (usually 140 to 240 bpm). The rhythm is regular or slightly irregular. Conditions that favor its occurrence include hypoxemia, drug toxicity such as digitalis or quinidine, electrolyte imbalance (e.g., potassium, magnesium), and bradycardia. Repeated and prolonged episodes of VT in the second week after MI may be a warning of ventricular fibrillation and require aggressive evaluation and treatment.

Medical management focuses on intravenously administered procainamide or amiodarone. These drugs depress excitability of cardiac muscle to electrical stimulation and slow conduction in the atria, bundle of His, and ventricles. Lidocaine is used only if acute myocardial ischemia or MI is considered to be the cause of VT. If pharmacologic measures are unsuccessful, the alternative is cardioversion. Catheter ablation can be helpful. Ongoing VT suppression is obtained with oral beta-adrenergic blockers or calcium channel blockers.

Ventricular Fibrillation

Ventricular fibrillation occurs when the ventricular musculature of the heart is quivering. This medical emergency is characterized by rapid and disorganized ventricle pulsation.

The cause is usually myocardial ischemia or infarction. Other causes are untreated VT, electrolyte imbalances, digitalis or quinidine toxicity, and hypothermia. It may also occur with coronary reperfusion after thrombolytic therapy.

Clinical manifestations are the result of no cardiac output and include loss of consciousness, lack of a pulse, decreases in blood pressure and respirations, possible seizures, and sudden death if untreated.

Medical management focuses on providing emergency treatment, including cardiopulmonary resuscitation (CPR), defibrillation (the termination of ventricular fibrillation by delivering a direct electrical countershock to the patient's precordium), and medications such as lidocaine or procainamide. Defibrillation is the most effective method of ending ventricular fibrillation and should ideally be performed within 15 to 20 seconds of onset to avoid brain damage from the lack of blood flow.

Assessment

Subjective data for the patient with a cardiac dysrhythmia include the patient's report of symptoms associated with the specific dysrhythmia. Symptoms may include palpitations, skipped beats, nausea, lightheadedness, vertigo, anxiety, dyspnea, fatigue, and chest discomfort.

Collection of **objective data** includes immediate visual observation of the patient when ECG monitoring indicates a dysrhythmia. Signs may include syncope, irregular pulse, tachycardia, and tachypnea. Noting the patient's response to the dysrhythmia is important to plan and implement appropriate nursing interventions. Monitor vital signs and observe for signs of decreased cardiac output.

Diagnostic Tests

ECG monitoring, telemetry, and Holter monitoring are commonly used to confirm the diagnosis of cardiac dysrhythmias.

Medical Management

Treatment varies according to the type of cardiac dysrhythmia (Table 8-1).

Nursing Interventions and Patient Teaching

Nursing interventions focus on symptomatic relief, promotion of comfort, relief of anxiety, emergency action as needed, and patient teaching.

Assess the apical (*not* radial) pulse to obtain an accurate pulse rate when dysrhythmias are present. Because the rhythm is irregular, take the apical pulse for 1 minute. Assess the patient's anxiety and degree of understanding, noting both verbal and nonverbal expressions regarding diagnosis, procedures, and treatments.

Explain the diagnostic and monitoring devices in use. Monitor heart rate and rhythm. Administer antidysrhythmic agents as ordered and monitor response. Maintain a quiet environment; administer sedation or analgesic medication as ordered. Administer oxygen per protocol.

Nursing diagnoses and interventions for the patient with a cardiac dysrhythmia include but are not limited to the following:

Nursing Diagnoses	Nursing Interventions
Pain, related to ischemia	Administer medications as ordered.
	Teach relaxation techniques.
	Institute position change and support.
	Administer prescribed oxygen.
Decreased cardiac output, related to cardiac insufficiency	Monitor heart rate and rhythm.
	Reduce cardiac workload by encouraging bed rest.
	Elevate head of bed 30 to 45 degrees for comfort.
	Restrict activities as ordered; plan care to avoid fatigue.
	Administer antidysrhythmic agents as ordered.
	Monitor for signs of drug toxicity.
Ineffective coping, related to fear of and uncertainty about disease process	Assist patient in identifying strengths and coping skills.
	Supply emotional support.
	Teach relaxation techniques.
	Assess coping ability and level of family support.
	Explain purpose of care as related to specific dysrhythmia.

Table 8-1 Medications for Cardiac Dysrhythmias

Generic (Trade)	Action	Nursing Interventions
CARDIOGLYCOSIDE		
Digoxin (Lanoxin)	Used to control rapid ventricular rate in atrial fibrillation and to convert paroxysmal supraventricular tachycardia to normal sinus rhythm Increases cardiac force and efficiency, slows heart rate, increases cardiac output	Monitor apical pulse to ensure rate above 60 bpm (call physician if digoxin held). Monitor for digitalis toxicity (nausea, vomiting, anorexia, dysrhythmias, bradycardia, tachycardia, headache, fatigue, visual disturbance).
ANTIDYSRHYTHMIC		
Procainamide (Pronestyl, Procan SR)	IV solutions given for severe ventricular dysrhythmias Depresses excitability of cardiac muscle to electrical stimulation and slows conduction in atrium, bundle of His, and ventricle, thus increasing refractory period	Observe for new dysrhythmias, dry mouth, blurred vision, bradycardia, hypotension, nausea, anorexia, dizziness, visual disturbances.
Lidocaine (IV)	Suppresses the impulse that triggers dysrhythmias	Monitor heart rate and BP closely.
Disopyramide (Norpace CR)	Provides long-term treatment of premature ventricular contractions, ventricular tachycardia, and atrial fibrillation	Monitor BP and apical pulse.
Adenosine (Adenocard)	Slows conduction through AV node, can interrupt reentry pathways through AV node, and can restore normal sinus rhythm in patients with paroxysmal supraventricular tachycardia (PSVT)	Monitor BP, pulse rate, and respirations. Assess patient for headache, dizziness, gastrointestinal complaints, new dysrhythmias. Do not give caffeine within 4-6 hours of adenosine because caffeine inhibits the effect of the drug.
Amiodarone (Cordarone, Pacerone)	Prolongs duration of action potential and effective refractory period; provides noncompetitive alpha- and beta-adrenergic inhibition; increases P-R and Q-T intervals; decreases sinus rate; decreases peripheral vascular resistance. Used for severe ventricular tachycardia, supraventricular tachycardia, atrial fibrillation, ventricular fibrillation not controlled by first-line agents, cardiac arrest	Observe for headache, dizziness, hypotension, bradycardia, sinus arrest, heart failure, dysrhythmia. Assess BP continuously for hypotension or hypertension. Report dysrhythmia or bradycardia. Monitor for dyspnea, chest pain.
Mexiletine HCl (Mexitil) Propafenone HCl (Rythmol)	Decreases excitability of cardiac muscle	Monitor pulse, BP. Monitor for diarrhea, visual disturbances, respiratory distress.
Tocainide HCl (Tonocard)	Suppresses automaticity of conduction tissue	Notify health care provider if cough, wheezing, or shortness of breath occurs.
BETA-ADRENERGIC BLOCKERS		
Propranolol (Inderal) Sotalol HCl (Betapace) Acebutolol HCl (Sectral) Esmolol HCl (Brevibloc) Metoprolol (Lopressor) Carvedilol (Coreg)	Used to treat supraventricular and ventricular dysrhythmias, persistent sinus tachycardia Decreases myocardial oxygen demand, decreases workload of the heart, decreases heart rate	Monitor heart rate and BP carefully. Use caution with patient with bronchospastic disease. Monitor for bradycardia, hypotension, new dysrhythmias, dizziness, headache, nausea, diarrhea, sleep disturbances.

AV, Atrioventricular; *BP*, blood pressure; *CHF*, congestive heart failure; *HCl*, hydrochloride; *IV*, intravenous.

Table 8-1	Medications for Cardiac Dysrhythmias—cont'd	
Generic (Trade)	**Action**	**Nursing Interventions**
CALCIUM CHANNEL BLOCKERS		
Verapamil (Calan, Isoptin)	Treat supraventricular tachycardia and control rapid rates in atrial tachycardia	Use caution in patients with CHF.
Diltiazem HCl (Cardizem)	Produce relaxation of coronary vascular smooth muscle, dilate coronary arteries	Monitor apical pulse and BP. Watch for fatigue, headache, dizziness, peripheral edema, nausea, tachycardia. Both verapamil and diltiazem increase the toxicity of digoxin.
INOTROPIC AGENT		
Dobutamine (Dobutrex) (IV)	Used in severe CHF with pulmonary edema	Monitor BP, heart rate, and urinary output continuously during the administration.
Dopamine (Intropin) (IV)	Increases myocardial contractility Increases cardiac output, increases BP, and improves renal blood flow	Palpate peripheral pulses; notify physician if extremities become cold or mottled.
ANTICOAGULANT		
Warfarin (Coumadin)	Used in treatment of atrial fibrillation with embolization to prevent complication of stroke	Assess patient for signs of bleeding and hemorrhage. Monitor prothrombin time and International Normalized Ratio (PT/INR) frequently during therapy. Review foods high in vitamin K. Patient should have consistently limited intake of these foods because these foods will cause levels to fluctuate.

Explain the importance of avoiding or stopping smoking or use of nicotine products. Teach the patient about medication therapy and its purposes, desired effects, and dosage and the side effects to report to the physician. Explain the reason for and method of taking pulse rate and rhythm. Explain the need to avoid exercising beyond the tolerance level, to avoid strenuous or isometric activity, and to check with the physician regarding limitations and allowances. Instruct the patient regarding conserving energy for activities of daily living (ADLs): taking regular rest periods between activities and for 1 hour after meals; when possible, sitting rather than standing while performing a task; and stopping an activity or task if symptoms such as fatigue, dyspnea, or palpitations begin. Stress management is important to promote healing and prevent further cardiac events.

CARDIAC ARREST

The sudden cessation of cardiac output and circulatory process is termed **cardiac arrest.** Conditions leading to cardiac arrest are severe VT, ventricular fibrillation, and ventricular asystole. The absence of an oxygen–carbon dioxide exchange leads to symptoms of anaerobic tissue cell metabolism and respiratory and metabolic acidosis. Thus immediate CPR is necessary to prevent major organ damage. Signs and symptoms of cardiac arrest include abrupt loss of consciousness with no response to stimuli, gasping respirations followed by apnea, absence of pulse (radial, carotid, femoral, and apical), absence of blood pressure, pupil dilation, and pallor and cyanosis.

CPR is initiated by the first person to discover the condition. The aim is to reestablish circulation and ventilation. Prevention of severe damage to the brain, the heart, the liver, and the kidneys as a result of anoxia is of primary concern. Remember the *ABCs* of CPR: **A,** open *A*irway; **B,** restore *B*reathing; and **C,** restore Circulation. Resuscitation measures are divided into two components: basic cardiac life support in the form of CPR and advanced cardiac life support (ACLS).

ACLS is a systematic approach to provide early treatment of cardiac emergencies. ACLS includes (1) basic life support, (2) the use of adjunctive equipment and special techniques for establishing and maintaining effective ventilation and circulation, (3) ECG monitoring and dysrhythmia recognition, (4) therapies for emergency treatment of patient with cardiac or respiratory arrest, and (5) treatment of patient with suspected acute MI.

Artificial Cardiac Pacemakers

A pacemaker is made of titanium with computer circuits that control the pacing system; one or more leads are placed into the heart and a lithium battery is used (Sunderlin, 2006). It initiates and controls the heart rate by delivering an electrical impulse via an electrode to the myocardium. These catheter-like electrodes are placed within the area to be paced: right atrium, right ventricle, or both (see Figures 8-8 and 8-9). A permanent pacemaker power source is placed subcutaneously, usually over the pectoral muscle on the patient's nondominant side (Lewis et al., 2007). Most are demand pacemakers, which send electrical stimuli to pace the heart when the heartbeat decreases below a preset rate. Some pacemakers have a single-chamber device with one lead that paces the right atrium or right ventricle; other pacemakers are dual chamber with separate leads that connect to both the right atrium and the right ventricle (Sunderlin, 2006).

Another pacemaker, the biventricular pacemaker, has three leads, one lead for each ventricle and one lead for the right atrium. This device restores normal simultaneous contraction of the ventricles. A biventricular pacemaker significantly improves left ventricular ejection fraction and exercise tolerance. It improves the quality of life for patients with worsening HF (Sunderlin, 2006).

A pacemaker maintains a regular cardiac rhythm by electrically stimulating the heart muscle. It is used when patients experience adverse symptoms because of dysrhythmias that cannot be managed by medications alone. These include second- and third-degree AV block, **bradydysrhythmias** (slow and/or irregular heartbeat), and **tachydysrhythmias** (rapid heartbeat that can be regular or irregular).

An external pacemaker is used in emergency situations on a short-term basis. Temporary pacemakers are used for cardiac support after some MIs or open-heart surgery. A permanent pacemaker is placed when other measures have failed to convert the dysrhythmia or conduction problem. The batteries used in permanent pacemakers today are small, weighing less than 1 ounce, and can last 15 years or more.

Nursing Interventions and Patient Teaching

After placement of a pacemaker, closely monitor heart rate and rhythm by apical pulse and by ECG patterns. Check vital signs and level of consciousness frequently until stable. Observe the insertion site for erythema, edema, and tenderness, which could indicate infection. The patient may be on bed rest with the arm on the pacemaker side immobilized for the first few hours. Discharge teaching includes instructions not to lift the arm on the surgical side over the head for 6 to 8 weeks. The patient needs to refrain from swimming, golfing, and weight lifting until given permission by the health care provider (Sunderlin, 2006).

Inform the patient of the necessity to continue medical management, and advise that he or she wear medical-alert identification and carry pacemaker information. Emphasize the importance of reporting signs and symptoms of pacemaker failure: weakness, vertigo, chest pain, and pulse changes.

Teach the patient to avoid potentially hazardous situations. Each pacemaker manufacturer can provide a list of devices that patients with pacemakers should avoid, such as proximity to high-output electrical generators or large magnets such as an MRI scanner. This may cause interference, placing the pacemaker in a fixed mode and interfering with its functioning. Instruct the patient to move away from any device that may cause untoward symptoms such as vertigo.

The heart rate of the pulse generator for the pacemaker is set according to the patient's clinical condition and the desired therapeutic goal. With rare exceptions, the rate is set between 70 and 80 bpm. If the heart rate falls below the preset level, notify the physician.

Teach the patient how and when to take a radial pulse. The pulse should be taken at the same time each day and when symptoms of vertigo or weakness occur. During patient education, remember to (1) list symptoms to expect and to report to physician, (2) promote understanding of medication administration, (3) explain treatment outcomes, (4) explain importance of maintaining prescribed diet and fluid amounts, and (5) explain importance of not smoking.

Prognosis

The patient can expect to lead a reasonably normal life with full resumption of most activities as prescribed by the physician.

DISORDERS OF THE HEART

CORONARY ATHEROSCLEROTIC HEART DISEASE

The coronary arteries arise from the base of the aorta just below the semilunar valves (see Figure 8-6). These arteries curve and angle to adequately supply the heart muscle with oxygen and nutrients. The shapes, contours, and arrangements of the vessels allow for easy entrapment of substances that interfere with blood flow.

Coronary artery disease (CAD) is the term used to describe a variety of conditions that obstruct blood flow in the coronary arteries. **Atherosclerosis** (a common arterial disorder characterized by yellowish plaques of cholesterol, lipids, and cellular debris in the inner layers of the walls of large and medium-size arteries) is the primary cause of ASHD. The **lumen** (a cavity or channel within any organ of the body) of the vessel narrows as the disease progresses. Blood flow to the heart is obstructed when this process occurs in the coronary arteries.

Atherosclerosis, the basic underlying disease affecting coronary lumen size, is characterized by changes in the intimal lining (the innermost layer) of the arteries. The severity of the disease is measured by the degree of obstruction within each artery and by the number of vessels involved. Obstructions exceeding 75% of the lumen of one or more of the three coronary arteries increase the risk of death.

The basic physiologic changes of the atherosclerotic process result in problems with myocardial oxygen

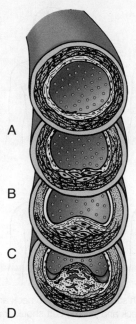

FIGURE 8-10 Progressive development of coronary atherosclerosis. **A,** Injury to intimal wall. **B,** Lipoprotein invasion of smooth muscle cells. **C,** Development of fatty streak and fibrous plaque. **D,** Development of complicated lesion.

 Cultural Considerations

Cardiovascular Disorder

- White, middle-aged men have the highest incidence of coronary artery disease (CAD).
- Blacks, Puerto Ricans, Cubans, and Mexican Americans have a higher incidence of hypertension than white Americans.
- Blacks have an early age of onset of CAD.
- Black women have a higher incidence of CAD than white women.
- Native Americans younger than 35 years of age have a heart disease mortality rate twice as high as that of other Americans.
- Hispanics have a lower death rate from heart disease than non-Hispanics.
- Major modifiable cardiovascular risk factors for Native Americans are obesity and diabetes mellitus.

supply and demand. When the myocardial oxygen demand exceeds the supply delivered by the coronary arteries, ischemia results (Figure 8-10). The artery walls also become less elastic and less responsive to blood flow (see Cultural Considerations box).

ANGINA PECTORIS

Etiology and Pathophysiology

Angina means a spasmodic, cramplike, choking feeling. *Pectoris* refers to the breast or chest area. **Angina pectoris** refers to the paroxysmal (severe, usually episodic, increase in symptoms) thoracic pain and choking feeling caused by decreased oxygen or anoxia (lack of oxygen) of the myocardium.

Angina pectoris occurs when the cardiac muscle is deprived of oxygen. Atherosclerosis of the coronary arteries is the most common cause. The narrowed lumina of the coronary arteries are unable to deliver enough oxygen-rich blood to the myocardium. When the myocardial oxygen demand exceeds the supply, **ischemia** (decreased blood supply to a body organ or part, often marked by pain and organ dysfunction) of the heart muscle occurs, resulting in chest pain or angina. Typically angina occurs with an increased cardiac workload brought on by exposure to intense cold, exercise, unusually heavy meals, emotional stress, or any other strenuous activity.

CAD is the nation's number one killer. Many people who die from the disease, however, experience several episodes of unstable angina first. If unstable angina were accurately diagnosed and promptly managed, many deaths and much of the disability associated with CAD could be avoided.

Unstable angina is defined as an unpredictable and transient episode of severe and prolonged discomfort that appears at rest, has never been experienced before, or is considerably worse than previous episodes. It mimics an MI in that the discomfort it causes is often described as tightness or a crushing sensation in the chest, arms, back, neck, or jaw. For some patients, unstable angina is a red flag that an MI will occur.

Clinical Manifestations

Pain is the outstanding characteristic of angina pectoris (Figure 8-11). The patient usually describes the pain as a heaviness or tightness of the chest. At times it is thought to be indigestion. The pain is often substernal (below the sternum) or retrosternal (behind the sternum). Pain may radiate to other sites, or it may occur in only one site. The pain often radiates down the left inner arm to the little finger and also upward to the shoulder and jaw. Patients may also describe it as a pressure or a squeezing sensation, but usually not as a sharp pain. Sometimes a patient experiences posterior thoracic or jaw pain only. The chest pain may be accompanied by other signs and symptoms such as dyspnea, anxiety, apprehension, diaphoresis, and nausea. Symptoms of CAD in women vary and may be more subtle or generalized than in men. Women often report heaviness, squeezing, or pain in the left side of the chest, or pain in the abdomen, arm, mid-back, or scapular region. Women may also complain of palpitations and chest discomfort during rest, during sleep, or with exertion (Cheek, 2008).

The signs and symptoms of angina are often similar to those of MI. Anginal pain is believed to be caused by a temporary lack of oxygen and blood supply to the heart. It is often relieved by rest or medication such as nitroglycerin, which dilates the coronary arteries and increases the flow of oxygenated blood to the myocardium. Nitroglycerin administered sublingually usually relieves angina symptoms but does not relieve the pain from an MI. This is often used as a preliminary diagnostic tool to quickly differentiate angina from an MI.

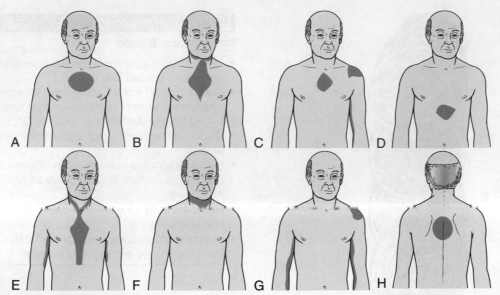

FIGURE 8-11 Sites to which ischemic myocardial pain may be referred. **A,** Upper chest. **B,** Beneath sternum radiating to neck and jaw. **C,** Beneath sternum radiating down left arm. **D,** Epigastric. **E,** Epigastric radiating to neck, jaw, and arms. **F,** Neck and jaw. **G,** Left shoulder and inner aspect of both arms. **H,** Intrascapular.

Assessment

Subjective data include the patient's statements regarding the location, intensity, radiation, and duration of pain. The patient may express a feeling of impending death. Assess precipitating factors that led to the development of symptoms. Determine what relief measures have been used. Identify whether the symptoms have changed in frequency or severity, indicating a worsening of the ischemia.

Collection of **objective data** includes noting the patient's behavior, such as rubbing the left arm or pressing a fist against the sternum. Monitor vital signs and note changes or abnormalities. Increases in pulse rate, blood pressure, and respiratory rate may be noted. Identify the presence of diaphoresis or anxiety.

Diagnostic Tests

The diagnosis of angina pectoris is frequently based on the patient's history. The ECG may reveal ischemia and rhythm changes. Holter monitoring correlates activity with precipitating factors. The exercise stress test determines ischemic changes in a controlled environment. Thallium 201 scanning and PET are used to diagnose ischemic heart disease. Coronary angiography may be done to determine the extent of CAD.

Medical Management

The focus of medical management is to control symptoms by reducing cardiac ischemia. Cardiovascular risk factors are identified and corrected if possible. Precipitating factors—such as exposure to intense cold, strenuous exercise, smoking, heavy meals, and emotional stress—are identified and avoided. Antiplatelet aggregation therapy is a first-line treatment of angina. Aspirin (ASA) is the drug of choice. Low-dose aspirin is indicated for people at risk for CAD who have a calculated

10-year CAD risk of less than 10%. (American Heart Association, 2005). Aspirin, even in low doses (81 mg), is effective in inhibiting platelet aggregation. For patients unable to tolerate aspirin, ticlopidine (Ticlid) or clopidogrel (Plavix) may be given (Lewis et al., 2007). Medication therapy to dilate coronary arteries and decrease the workload of the heart consists of vasodilators (nitrates, especially nitroglycerin); beta-adrenergic blocking agents such as propranolol, metoprolol (Lopressor), nadolol (Corgard), atenolol (Tenormin), and timolol (Blocadren); and calcium channel blockers such as nifedipine (Procardia), verapamil, diltiazem, and nicardipine (Cardene). Give nitroglycerin sublingually for angina. Repeat dose in 5 minutes if pain does not subside. Repeat two or three times at 5-minute intervals. Call physician if pain has not subsided after third nitroglycerin tablet. High-risk, unstable angina patients should be given supplemental oxygen.

Surgical Interventions

Coronary artery bypass graft. Surgical management of the patient with ASHD or CAD may consist of performing a coronary artery bypass graft (CABG) after diagnosis by cardiac catheterization. Any number of grafts can be done, depending on the areas of occlusion in the coronary arteries. Blood flows to the myocardium through the grafts, which bypass the occluded coronary arteries. The grafts are usually taken from sections of the saphenous veins in the legs, or the internal mammary (breast) artery is used.

When the saphenous vein is used for the graft, one end is sutured to the aorta and the other end is sutured to the coronary artery distal to the occlusion. When an internal mammary artery is used, the distal end of this vessel is freed from the anterior chest wall and sutured in place distal to the occlusion in the coronary artery.

Internal mammary arteries are the preferred blood vessels for bypass surgery. A typical procedure involves one or two mammary arteries and saphenous vein grafts. Internal mammary arteries usually last more than 15 years, whereas saphenous vein grafts last an average of 5 to 10 years. Researchers continue to search for alternative blood vessels for CABG surgery (Figures 8-12 and 8-13).

Percutaneous transluminal coronary angioplasty. Another surgical procedure for management of the patient with CAD is percutaneous transluminal coronary angioplasty (PTCA). PTCA is an invasive procedure performed in the cardiac catheterization laboratory. The technique widens the narrowing in a coronary artery without open-heart surgery. *Percutaneous* indicates that the procedure is performed through the skin; *transluminal* means that it is within the lumen of the artery. Patients undergoing PTCA are required to sign a surgical permit for a CABG because of the possibility of complications developing during the procedure that require immediate surgical intervention. Fluoroscopy is used to guide a catheter from the femoral or brachial artery to the coronary arteries to be treated. A balloon is inflated in the catheter once it is positioned (Figure 8-14). The outward push of the balloon against the narrowing wall of the coronary artery reduces the constriction until it no longer interferes with blood flow to the heart muscle. Vessel patency is reestablished by angioplasty (vessel repair). This procedure may take 1 to 2 hours, with the patient usually awake but mildly sedated.

Postprocedure nursing interventions are to continually monitor the patient, as with any surgical recovery. Observe the area of catheter insertion for hemorrhage potential. Monitor the patient in the cardiac care unit, usually for 1 day before dismissal to the medical-surgical unit. The total hospitalization stay is 1 to

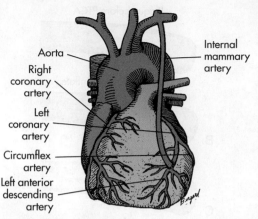

FIGURE 8-13 Coronary artery bypass graft. Internal mammary artery is used; the distal end of this vessel is freed from the anterior chest wall and sutured in place distal to the occlusion in the coronary artery.

3 days compared with the 4- to 6-day stay after open-heart surgery with a CABG; thus PTCA reduces hospital costs. Patients return to work rapidly (approximately 5 to 7 days after PTCA) rather than requiring the 2- to 8-week convalescence common after CABG.

Stent placement. Stents are used to treat abrupt or threatened vessel closure after PTCA. Stents are expandable, meshlike structures designed to maintain vessel patency by compressing the arterial walls and resisting vasoconstriction (Figure 8-15). Stents are carefully placed over the angioplasty site to hold the vessel open. Because stents are thrombogenic, the patient must take anticoagulants for at least 3 months. The primary complications from stent placement are hemorrhage and vascular injury. Less common complications are stent thrombosis, acute MI, emergency CABG, and coronary spasms. The possibility of dysrhythmias is always present.

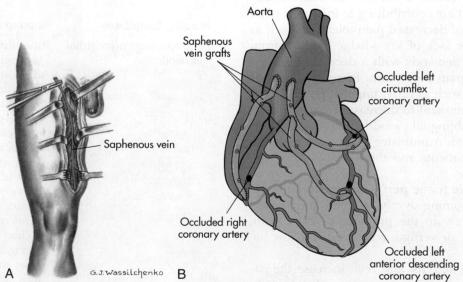

FIGURE 8-12 A, Saphenous vein. **B,** Saphenous aortocoronary artery bypass or revascularization involves taking a piece of saphenous vein from the leg and creating a conduit for blood from the aorta to the area below the blockage in the coronary artery. A triple bypass is illustrated.

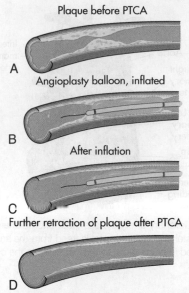

FIGURE 8-14 Percutaneous transluminal coronary angioplasty (PTCA). **A,** Plaque before PTCA. **B,** Inflation of angioplasty balloon. **C,** Plaque after PTCA. **D,** Plaque has retracted even further 6 months after PTCA.

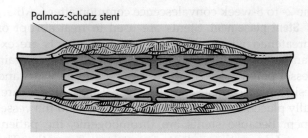

FIGURE 8-15 Palmaz-Schatz stent, an articulated stainless steel mesh deployed by balloon inflation.

Nursing Interventions and Patient Teaching

Nursing interventions are based on the patient's individual needs. They focus on achievement of five major patient outcomes.

First, **promote comfort.** Reduce or remove any known factors that are contributing to increased pain. Assess for causes of decreased pain tolerance, such as anxiety, fatigue, or lack of knowledge. Fatigue from increased oxygen demands with a decreased oxygen supply increases pain perception. Promote measures to reduce fatigue, such as providing rest periods. Provide a calm environment to decrease stress and anxiety. Administer sublingual vasodilators, such as nitroglycerin, as ordered. Administer oxygen for high-risk unstable angina patients and those with cyanosis or respiratory distress.

Second, **promote tissue perfusion.** Instruct the patient to avoid becoming overly fatigued and to stop activity immediately in the presence of chest pain, dyspnea, syncope, or vertigo, which indicate low tissue perfusion.

Third, **promote activity and rest.** Increase the patient's activity tolerance by encouraging slower activity or shorter periods of activity with more rest peri-

ods. Most people with angina pectoris are able to tolerate mild exercise such as walking or playing golf, but exertion such as running or climbing stairs rapidly causes pain. Nitroglycerin may be used prophylactically to prevent pain from strenuous activities. Isosorbide mononitrate (Imdur) or isosorbide dinitrate (Isordil) are nitrates that are used for acute treatment of angina attacks (sublingual only) or orally for prophylactic management of angina pectoris. Anginal pain occurs more easily in cold weather. The key is to avoid overexertion.

Fourth, **promote relief of anxiety and a feeling of well-being.** Help the patient reduce the level of anxiety. The patient should minimize emotional outbursts, worry, and tension. People with angina may need continuing help in accepting situations. Supportive family members, a spiritual adviser, business associates, and friends can sometimes be of assistance. Relaxation techniques and music therapy may be beneficial. Peer support groups and behavioral change programs are available. An optimistic outlook helps to relieve the work of the heart. Many people who learn to live within their limitations live out their expected life span despite the disease.

Finally, **teach the patient and the family.** Delay teaching until the patient is ready (see Communication box). The patient needs to be relatively free of pain and anxiety to learn. Promote a positive attitude and active participation of patient and family to encourage compliance. The teaching plan should include information on medications, ways to minimize the events that trigger angina pectoris, effects of exercise on reduction of myocardial oxygen needs, the need to stop smoking because of the vasoconstriction of nicotine, and the need for regular medical follow-up (see Patient Teaching box).

Nursing diagnoses and interventions for the patient with angina pectoris include but are not limited to the following:

Nursing Diagnoses	Nursing Interventions
Pain, related to myocardial ischemia	Administer oxygen as ordered.
	Administer prescribed nitroglycerin. Repeat every 5 minutes, three times. If pain is unrelieved, notify physician.
	Monitor blood pressure and pulse before and after administration of nitroglycerin.
	Promote rest.
	Maintain diet as ordered; if chest pain occurs while eating or immediately after, advise small feedings rather than two or three large meals.

Communication

Methods to Decrease Angina Pectoris Attacks

Mrs. M., a patient with angina, has been admitted for further care, diagnosis, and treatment. After the initial nursing assessment, Nurse G. interviews the patient about the course of her anginal episodes. With the data she gathers, Nurse G. will participate in the development of a program to educate Mrs. M. to minimize or control the attacks.

Nurse: I would like to ask you some questions, Mrs. M., about the anginal pain you are experiencing.

Patient: I already told Dr. T. all about those attacks when I visited his office. His nurse, Miss N., has all those records.

Nurse: Yes, I know. Your physician has asked us to help you plan a program for preventing or minimizing these attacks. With the information we gather, we can set goals for your care. We can also identify how angina relates to some of your activities.

Patient: OK, Mrs. G., I would like to understand it better. Perhaps I would be less frightened when it happens. My friend J. told me about her aunt who had angina—she died. That really worries me.

Nurse: We hope to decrease some of your fears, Mrs. M., by helping you understand. First, when do your attacks usually occur?

Patient: Oh, mostly after a real busy day, you know—shopping or gardening or housecleaning. But a few times, I had problems after my sister-in-law visited. She and my husband always seem to get into upsetting discussions. They never got along well. She upsets us both—she criticizes everything!

Nurse: Have you noticed if a big meal is related to the pain?

Patient: No, not really . . . well, only when my sister-in-law is there. We hardly ever eat big meals anymore, except when she comes. She expects to be fed well. My husband and I have cut down a lot. Big meals upset our systems—and then her, that harping on old problems and how she thinks we should run our lives! She upsets me so!

Nurse: Mrs. M., I think we must talk more on how to handle stressful situations like your sister-in-law. But first, could you describe the pain for me? Does it come on suddenly? How long does it last? What does it feel like?

Patient: Oh, no, not all of a sudden. It is just dull at times, like an upset stomach. But then, it travels up in my chest and gets really heavy, like pressure. Sometimes, it makes my face and teeth hurt; and my arm, too—this one [left]—all the way down to my little finger. If it's a really bad attack, I sometimes feel like I am going to vomit.

Nurse: On a scale of 0 to 10, how would you rate most of your angina attacks?

Patient: Probably 5 to 6 would be the average, but sometimes it's a 10.

Nurse: Does your heart beat faster?

Patient: Oh, yes, and I just have to sit down and be quiet or I can't catch my breath. That's when I take the nitroglycerin. I carry it with me all the time now, in this special little container.

Nurse: I see. And how long does it take for the pain to stop after you take the medicine?

Patient: I used to think it took forever, but my husband—he times it for me—says it lasts about 15 to 20 minutes. I relax a little, and it passes.

Nurse: What about the weather, Mrs. M.? Have you noticed that it affects your attacks in any way?

Patient: I don't know if it is all those clothes or the weather, but I get more pains if I get out in the cold.

Nurse: Do you or your husband smoke?

Patient: Not anymore. I gave up cigarettes when this angina started on me. I noticed the difference, too. Now, I can't even stay in a room if people are smoking. I also cut down on coffee when I retired. Dr. T. said that too much caffeine isn't good for the angina. All the good things, they have to go when you get old!

Nurse: Maybe with some understanding of how certain activities and other factors affect your condition, you can find new "good things" that you'll enjoy just as much. We'll talk again soon. There are some effective coping methods to decrease your stress when your sister-in-law visits that we can explore.

Nursing Diagnoses	Nursing Interventions
Pain, related to myocardial ischemia—cont'd	Balance rest with activity. Instruct patient to stop activity at the first sign of chest pain or other symptoms of cardiac ischemia.
Ineffective tissue perfusion, cardiovascular, related to narrowing of coronary arteries	Administer prescribed oxygen. Instruct patient that nitroglycerin may need to be taken before exercise and sexual activity to prevent cardiac ischemia. Encourage less strenuous or shorter periods of activity interspersed with rest.

Nursing Diagnoses	Nursing Interventions
	Avoid exercise in cold weather. Take prescribed nitroglycerin before activities that will increase the workload of the heart.

Prognosis

The prognosis for the patient with angina pectoris may be grave. Attacks may be intermittent. With early and aggressive management of angina, mortality rate can be reduced and the disorder can be managed.

Patient Teaching

Angina Pectoris

USING NITRATE MEDICATIONS

- Use nitroglycerin prophylactically to avoid pain known to occur with certain activities.
- Burning sensation on tongue indicates nitroglycerin is activated.
- Throbbing sensation in head and flushing may occur.
- Sit and stand slowly after taking nitroglycerin. Postural hypotension is a side effect of nitroglycerin.
- Place nitroglycerin tablets under the tongue at the onset of anginal pain; second tablet can be taken after 5 minutes and third tablet after another 5 minutes if pain is unrelieved.
- Call physician if pain does not subside after third nitroglycerin tablet; go to nearest emergency department; do not drive yourself.
- Always carry nitroglycerin on your person.
- Store nitroglycerin in a dark bottle and keep in a dry place.
- Replenish nitroglycerin supply every 6 months or before expiration date.
- Remove all old nitrate ointment before application of new cream.
- Place nitroglycerin patches on skin in the morning and remove at bedtime. This prevents development of tolerance and maintains effectiveness.

MINIMIZING PRECIPITATING EVENTS

- Be careful in using medications for erectile dysfunction when using nitrate medications; they could cause severe hypotension.
- Avoid overexertion. Take nitroglycerin before exercise.
- Try to reduce stress and anxiety, which cause blood vessels to constrict.
- Avoid overeating because it places an increased workload on the heart.
- Avoid cold weather (constricts coronary vessels to conserve body heat; hence anginal pain can develop more easily).
- Dress warmly in cold weather.
- Avoid hot, humid conditions (increases workload on the heart).
- Walk downhill and with wind, since walking uphill and against wind increases workload on the heart.
- Stopping smoking is a necessity because of vasoconstriction of arteries from nicotine.

EXERCISING TO REDUCE MYOCARDIAL OXYGEN NEEDS

- Engage in a regular exercise program to improve collateral circulation.
- Exercise conditions heart muscle and can decrease oxygen demand during exertion.
- Space exercise period with rest periods.
- Take nitroglycerin before exertion.

MYOCARDIAL INFARCTION

Etiology and Pathophysiology

Myocardial infarction (MI) is an occlusion of a major coronary artery or one of its branches with subsequent necrosis of myocardium caused by atherosclerosis or an embolus (a foreign object, a quantity of air or gas, a bit of tissue, or a piece of a thrombus that circulates in the bloodstream until it becomes lodged in a vessel). An obstruction by atherosclerotic process or an embolus may interrupt the blood supply. Coronary occlusion (an obstruction or closing off in a canal, vessel, or passage of the body) is the general term for occlusion of a coronary artery. The occlusion may also be caused by the formation of a thrombus. Eighty percent to 90% of all acute MIs are secondary to thrombus formation. (Lewis et al., 2007). This is generally referred to as a coronary thrombosis. The occlusion leads to tissue ischemia. Ischemia to the myocardium lasting more than 35 to 45 minutes produces cellular damage and necrosis. The ability of the cardiac muscle to contract and pump blood is impaired. The extent of damage to the surrounding tissues depends on the ability to develop collateral circulation. Collateral circulation refers to the development of new vessels in the heart that compensate for the loss of circulation from the occluded artery. The location of the occlusion and the extent of tissue damage affect the patient's response to the injury (Figure 8-16).

The body's response to cell death is the inflammatory process. Within 24 hours, leukocytes infiltrate the area. Enzymes are released from the dead cardiac cells

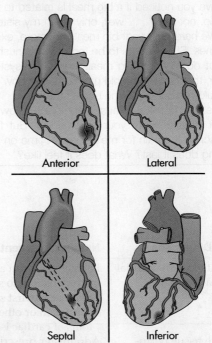

FIGURE 8-16 Four common locations where myocardial infarctions occur.

and are important diagnostic indicators. (See the discussion on serum cardiac markers, p. 311.) Phagocytes (neutrophils and monocytes) clear the necrotic debris from the injured area, and by 6 weeks after an MI, scar tissue has replaced necrotic tissue.

Clinical Manifestations

An asymptomatic MI may occur. This is referred to as a *silent MI*. Many of the symptoms of MI are associated with irreversible ischemia, but they are similar to the signs and symptoms of angina pectoris. The symptoms of an MI are more severe and last longer than those of an angina attack. Pain is the foremost symptom of MI (Table 8-2).

The pain location and radiation to other sites are depicted in Figure 8-11. It is often described as crushing or viselike, an oppressive sensation as though a heavy object is sitting on the chest. The pain is retrosternal (behind the sternum) and in the heart region. It of-ten radiates down the left arm and to the neck, jaws, teeth, and epigastric area. It may occur suddenly, or it may build up over a few minutes. It may occur in conjunction with intense emotion, during exertion, or at rest. The pain is prolonged and more intense than anginal pain. It lasts 30 minutes to several hours or longer. It is not relieved by changes in body position, nitroglycerin, or rest. Physicians often tell patients who call complaining of chest pain to take an aspirin (chewable if they have it) and report to the emergency department. Other signs and symptoms that may occur in conjunction with the pain include nausea, dyspnea, dizziness, weakness, diaphoresis, pallor, ashen color, and a sense of impending doom. Early signs and symptoms of an acute MI in women are unusual fatigue, sleep disturbances, shortness of breath, weakness, indigestion, and anxiety. Frequently acute chest pain is not present. With these signs and symptoms, an acute MI can commonly be misdiagnosed as indigestion, gallbladder disease, depression, or anxiety (Sherrod et al., 2007). Table 8-3 provides a comparison of signs and symptoms and the medical management of angina pectoris and MI.

Assessment

Subjective data include the onset, location, quality, duration, and radiation of pain. The patient may complain of shortness of breath, dizziness, weakness, anxiety, fear, or unusual fatigue. Identify precipitating factors. Inquire about measures the patient has tried to relieve the pain.

Table 8-2	Signs and Symptoms of Myocardial Infarction
SUBJECTIVE DATA (SYMPTOMS)	**OBJECTIVE DATA (SIGNS)**
Heavy pressure or squeezing in center of chest behind sternum	Pallor
	Erratic behavior
	Hypotension, shock
Pain, retrosternal and in heart region, often radiating down the left arm and to the neck, jaw, and teeth	Cardiac rhythm changes
	Vomiting
	Fever
	Diaphoresis
Anxiety	
Dyspnea	
Weakness, faintness	
Nausea	

Table 8-3	Coronary Artery Disorders	
SIGNS AND SYMPTOMS		**MEDICAL MANAGEMENT**
ANGINA PECTORIS		
Chest pain (substernal, retrosternal), may radiate to neck, jaw, left arm, and shoulder; great anxiety, fear of approaching death; face pale, ashen; pulse variable, usually tense and quick; blood pressure elevated during an attack; usually brought on by exertion, emotional upsets; relieved by rest, nitroglycerin		Avoidance of precipitating factors
		Reduction of modifiable risk factors
		Medications: nitrates, beta blockers, calcium channel blockers
		Oxygen therapy
		ECG monitoring
		Aspirin for unstable angina
MYOCARDIAL INFARCTION		
Severe, crushing chest pain; prolonged heavy pressure or squeezing pain in center of chest; may spread to shoulder, neck, arm, fourth and fifth fingers on left hand, teeth, and jaw; may radiate as with angina; not relieved with rest or nitroglycerin; may be associated with dyspnea, diaphoresis, apprehension, nausea, and vomiting; signs and symptoms of cardiogenic shock may develop; the pain is prolonged and more intense than anginal pain		Relief of pain (oxygen), morphine, and other analgesics
		ECG monitoring
		Thrombolytic therapy to dissolve clot
		Reduction of oxygen demand (rest)
		Prevention of complications (through use of stool softeners, anticoagulants)
		Treatment of complications (dysrhythmias, HF)
		Anticoagulants to prevent further clotting
In women, these classic symptoms are far less common; most frequent early warning symptoms: unusual fatigue, sleep disturbances, shortness of breath, weakness, indigestion, and anxiety; in one study, only 30% of women reported chest pain, and acute chest pain was absent in 43% (Sherrod et al., 2007).		

ECG, Electrocardiogram; *HF,* heart failure.

Collection of **objective data** includes observation of the patient's behavior to detect apprehension and anxiety. Typical vital signs reveal hypotension, pulse abnormalities such as tachycardia or a barely perceptible pulse, and early temperature elevation. Note the presence of diaphoresis; vomiting; ashen color; cool, clammy skin; labored respirations; and cardiac dysrhythmias. If possible, find out about risk factors. A respiratory assessment should also be done.

Diagnostic Tests

Diagnostic tests are used to confirm the diagnosis of MI. Serum tests are initially obtained. Serum cardiac markers (e.g., CK-MB, myoglobin) are released into the vascular system when infarcted myocardial muscle cells die. A sensitive cardiac marker present in serum called **troponin I** has proven useful in detecting ischemic myocardial injury. Troponin I is cardiac specific and therefore a highly specific indicator of an MI. (See the discussion of serum cardiac markers on p. 311.) An elevated white blood cell count of 12,000 to 15,000/mm^3 is associated with severe infarcts. The increase begins a few hours after the onset of pain and lasts for 3 to 7 days. The ESR rises during the first week and may remain elevated for several weeks.

Twelve-lead ECG findings that indicate MI include ST-segment elevation and the development of Q waves. In time the ST segment returns to normal and the T wave inverts. These ECG changes are important in confirming the diagnosis of MI. Significantly, ECG findings are different for men and women. A woman experiencing an MI is far less likely than a man to have concurrent ST-segment elevation (Cheek, 2008). Thus, she may be misdiagnosed and not receive correct treatment (Cheek, 2008). A chest radiograph is done to note size and configuration of the heart. More complex tests are occasionally done, including cardiac fluoroscopy, myocardial imaging (thallium scan), echocardiogram, PET, and multigated acquisition scanning (MUGA). These tests may be done in conjunction with other tests to diagnose MI and determine the severity of CAD.

Medical Management

Medical management focuses on preventing further tissue injury and limiting the size of the infarction. It is extremely important that a patient with a suspected MI is rapidly diagnosed and treated to preserve cardiac muscle. Intervention is designed to restore cardiac tissue perfusion and reduce the workload of the heart. Promoting tissue oxygenation, relieving pain, preventing complications, improving tissue perfusion, and preventing further tissue damage are all important medical considerations.

Medications such as morphine and diazepam (Valium) are used to alleviate pain and anxiety. A continuous IV infusion of amiodarone may be given to the patient who has frequent PVCs, which may precede ventricular fibrillation. Prophylactic lidocaine is not recommended by the American College of Cardiology practice guidelines for the treatment of acute MI (Singh, 2002). However, lidocaine may be a treatment option for the patient who has sustained VT or ventricular fibrillation. The use of beta-adrenergic blockers such as atenolol, metoprolol, propranolol, nadolol, and carvedilol (Coreg) early in the acute phase of an MI and during a 1-year follow-up regimen can decrease morbidity and mortality. Angiotensin-converting enzyme (ACE) inhibitors may be used after MIs. Their use can help to prevent or slow the progression of HF (Table 8-4). Calcium channel blockers or longer acting nitrates can be added if the patient is already on adequate doses of beta-adrenergic blockers or cannot tolerate beta-adrenergic blockers. Examples of calcium channel blockers are amlodipine (Norvasc), diltiazem, nifedipine, and verapamil. An example of a long-acting nitrate is isosorbide dinitrate (Antman et al., 2004). Oxygen is prescribed to facilitate cardiac tissue perfusion. Attention is given to respiratory difficulties, fluid overload, and cardiac dysrhythmias.

Medical therapy is also directed toward limiting the size and extent of injury by attempting to reperfuse (reinstitute blood flow to an area that was ischemic) the occluded coronary artery. Fibrinolytic agents such as streptokinase (Streptase), anistreplase, and a tissue plasminogen activator (TPA) such as alteplase are currently used to attempt reperfusion. Thrombolytic therapy is the standard practice in the treatment of acute MI. Thrombolytics salvage heart muscle by minimizing infarct size and maximizing heart function. They lyse (decompose or dissolve) the clot in the occluded coronary artery, reopening the vessel and allowing perfusion of the heart muscle.

Remember the adage, "Time is muscle." Fast action to restore myocardial blood flow limits infarct size, preserves heart tissue, and improves the patient's chance of survival and recovery. To be effective, reperfusion must occur 3 to 5 hours after the onset of symptoms. Myocardial cells do not die instantly. In most patients, it takes approximately 4 to 6 hours for the entire thickness of the muscle to become necrosed. Mortality and infarction size can be significantly reduced if thrombolytic therapy starts within 30 to 60 minutes of symptom onset. Before a thrombolytic is administered, obtain a thorough history. Thrombolytics are not used for patients with active internal bleeding, suspected aortic dissecting aneurysm, recent head trauma, history of hemorrhagic stroke within the past year, or surgery within the past 10 days.

PTCA may be used instead of thrombolytic therapy as a primary treatment in some cases. This involves advancing a balloon-tipped catheter into the lumen of the obstructed coronary artery. The balloon is inflated

Table 8-4 Medications for Myocardial Infarction

Classification	Generic (Trade)	Action
Vasopressors	Dopamine (Intropin)	Raise systemic arterial pressure and cardiac output
Anticoagulants	Heparin Warfarin (Coumadin)	Reduce incidence of clotting
Antiplatelets	Ticlopidine (Ticlid) Aspirin (ASA)	Decrease platelet release of thromboxane, so that vasoconstriction and platelet aggregation are decreased Decrease platelet aggregation
Analgesics	Morphine	Control pain; reduce myocardial oxygen demand
Tranquilizers	Diazepam (Valium)	Decrease anxiety and restlessness
Thrombolytic agents	Streptokinase (Streptase)	Thrombolytic (pertaining to dissolution of blood clots) agents used when acute MI symptoms are less than 6 hours, preferably 30 minutes to 1 hour duration; restore blood flow and therefore limit infarct size in certain patients
Tissue plasminogen activator	Alteplase, recombinant Activase	
Nitrates	Nitroglycerin Isosorbide Atenolol (Tenormin)	Dilate blood vessels by reducing coronary artery spasm, increase coronary artery blood supply, and decrease oxygen demands
Beta-adrenergic blockers	Propranolol (Inderal) Nadolol (Corgard) Metoprolol (Lopressor) Carvedilol (Coreg)	Block beta-adrenergic stimulation and decrease myocardial oxygen demands, thus decreasing myocardial damage; decreases mortality rate
Calcium channel blockers	Nifedipine (Procardia) Diltiazem (Cardizem) Verapamil (Calan, Isoptin) Amlodipine (Norvasc)	Dilate blood vessels, increase coronary artery blood supply, and decrease myocardial oxygen demands
Angiotensin-converting enzyme (ACE) inhibitors	Captopril (Capoten) Enalapril (Vasotec)	Can help prevent ventricular remodeling and prevent or slow the progression of HF Prevent conversion of angiotensin I to angiotensin II Decrease endothelial dysfunction
Salicylates	Aspirin	Decrease platelet adhesion and thus decrease thrombosis formation
Antidysrhythmics	Lidocaine (Xylocaine) IV	Treat ventricular dysrhythmias (rarely used except for ventricular tachycardia)
Stool softeners	Surfak Colace	Reduce straining at stool; prevent constipation produced by decreased mobility and use of constipating narcotics
Diuretics	Furosemide (Lasix)	Control edema
Electrolyte replacement	Slow-K	May be necessary when diuretics are used
Inotropic agents	Digoxin (Lanoxin) Amrinone (Inocor) IV Dobutamine (Dobutrex)	Increase the heart's pumping action (contractility) Indicated when left ventricle failure is present

HF, Heart failure; *MI,* myocardial infarction.

intermittently to dilate the artery and improve blood flow (see Figure 8-14). Along with balloon compression, stents may be used to prevent acute closure and restenosis (see Figure 8-15).

CABG surgery may be considered for patients with multiple vessel disease and when less invasive interventions, such as thrombolysis and PTCA, have failed (see Figures 8-12 and 8-13).

Complications commonly associated with MI include ventricular fibrillation, cardiogenic shock (Table 8-5), HF, and dysrhythmias. Cardiogenic shock, often referred to as pump failure, is characterized by low cardiac output and peripheral vascular system collapse. Left ventricular function is severely decreased, resulting in an inadequate blood supply to the vital organs. Immediate detection and treatment are necessary to prevent irreversible shock and death. Cardiogenic shock proves fatal in 50% to 80% of cases. Other possible complications include ventricular aneurysm, pericarditis, and embolism.

Table 8-5 | **Cardiogenic Shock**

CLINICAL MANIFESTATIONS	SIGNS AND SYMPTOMS	MEDICAL MANAGEMENT	NURSING INTERVENTIONS
Decreased cardiac output	Dysrhythmias, chest pain	Recognition and control of life-threatening signs and symptoms	Monitor vital signs every 5 minutes during acute stage and every 1 hour when stabilized.
Myocardial ischemia	Anxiety, agitation, restlessness, disorientation		
Cerebral hypoxia		Oxygenation to promote tissue perfusion	
Impaired tissue perfusion	Urinary output diminished or absent		Administer oxygen as ordered.
Renal circulation decreased	Lactic acid accumulation in blood	Parenteral fluid as a volume expander	Maintain bed rest to reduce myocardial workload and increase oxygenation.
Anaerobic metabolism with lactic acidosis	Tachycardia, thready pulse, tachypnea	Drug therapy:	
Peripheral vascular system collapse	Decreased blood pressure	• Vasopressors: raise arterial blood pressure	Monitor acid-base balance.
Shock	Narrowed pulse pressure	• Inotropic, cardiac glycoside: (digoxin, Lanoxin) increases cardiac contraction and strengthens and corrects dysrhythmias	Monitor urinary output hourly to determine adequate kidney perfusion.
	Cyanosis; cold, moist, pale, clammy skin		Allow nothing by mouth.
	Decreased peripheral pulses		Initiate bed rest to minimize energy expenditure.
	Capillary refill time decreased	• Adrenergic drugs: dopamine (Intropin) at therapeutic levels increases cardiac output and blood pressure	Administer medications as ordered.
	Hypoactive bowel sounds		Provide comfort measures.
		• Sodium bicarbonate: combats lactic acidosis (given sparingly because it causes fluid retention)	

Nursing Interventions and Patient Teaching

Administer oxygen per protocol for 24 to 48 hours or longer if pain, hypotension, dyspnea, or dysrhythmias persist. Administer medications as prescribed:

- IV morphine sulfate for relief of pain and anxiety and to produce vasodilation. Morphine also decreases myocardial oxygen demands, reduces contractility, and slows the heart rate. Provisions for comfort and rest are essential to reduce stress and increase myocardial oxygen perfusion.
- Heparin therapy or unfractionated or low-molecular-weight heparin such as enoxaparin (Lovenox) or dalteparin (Fragmin) to inhibit further clotting and prevent reocclusion of the coronary artery after the thrombolytic therapy opens the vessel.
- Antiplatelet agents such as aspirin and ticlopidine to decrease platelet release of thromboxane. These drugs are platelet aggregation inhibitors. Ticlopidine can be ordered for patients allergic to aspirin and should be administered immediately. Clopidogrel inhibits platelet aggregation and is an alternative for patients who cannot use aspirin.
- IV nitroglycerin may help patients with left-ventricular infarctions. It reduces cardiac oxygen demand by relaxing vascular smooth muscle and dilating peripheral vessels; it also dilates coronary vessels, improving blood flow to the heart. Administer beta-adrenergic blockers to inhibit cardiotoxicity of catecholamines.
- Administer lipid-lowering agents such as simvastatin, atorvastatin (Lipitor), or rosuvastatin to prevent elevated cholesterol levels.
- Stool softener as prescribed to prevent rectal straining. The Valsalva maneuver may cause severe changes in blood pressure and heart rate, which may trigger ischemia, dysrhythmias, or cardiac arrest.

To help the post-MI patient minimize straining, offer the use of a bedside commode or nearby bathroom whenever possible. Teach mouth breathing to help decrease the severity of straining to prevent use of the Valsalva maneuver, which is contraindicated in the patient with an MI.

Instruct the patient to avoid excessive fatigue and to stop activity immediately in the presence of chest pain, dyspnea, or faintness. Plan nursing interventions to promote rest and minimize disturbances. Monitor vital signs; document rate and rhythm of pulse.

The patient is usually placed on bed rest with commode privileges for 24 to 48 hours. Assist with ADLs. During this period, sedation with diazepam or an equivalent may be prescribed to relieve anxiety and restlessness and to promote sleep. After the first 24 to 48 hours, encourage the patient to increase activity gradually, depending on the size of the infarction. Continually monitor the patient for signs of dysrhythmias, cardiac pain, and changes in vital signs.

Diet is usually withheld until the patient is stabilized. This is important because of the possible need for cardiac catheterization, PTCA, or a CABG procedure. Liquid diet is progressed as tolerated to regular diet with modifications. A low-fat, low-sodium, easily digested diet is desirable.

Prevention of complications is a primary objective. Antiembolic stockings are used. Continue to assess and report cardiac status, dyspneic condition, and pulse change (rate, rhythm, and volume).

During hospitalization, many patients experience denial, depression, and anxiety. Anxiety varies in intensity, depending on the severity of the perceived threat and the patient's success in coping.

Nursing diagnoses and interventions for the patient with an MI include but are not limited to the following:

Nursing Diagnoses	Nursing Interventions
Acute chest pain, related to myocardial ischemia	Assess original pain and location, duration, radiation, and onset of new symptoms.
	Administer prescribed analgesics (usually morphine sulfate, which relieves pain, reduces anxiety, causes vasodilation of vascular smooth muscle, and reduces myocardial workload).
	Maintain bed rest and reduced patient activity.
	Administer oxygen as prescribed.
	Record patient's response to pain relief measures.
	Employ alternative methods of pain relief.
	Provide calm, restful environment.
Anxiety, related to: • change in health status • fear of death	Assess for signs and verbal expressions of anxiety and coping mechanisms used.
	Promote restful sleep patterns.
	Reassure patient by providing education, enlisting family support, and allowing positive and negative expression of feelings.
	Remain with patient during periods of highest anxiety; offer reassurance; use calm, but concerned voice.
	Administer antianxiety agents as needed, per physician's order.
	Initiate relaxation techniques (deep breathing, visual imagery, soft rhythmic music).
	Encourage participation in cardiac rehabilitation program.

Nursing Diagnoses	Nursing Interventions
Decreased cardiac output, related to conduction defects (dysrhythmias) and decreased myocardial pumping action	Assess and monitor vital signs every 4 hours.
	Maintain bed rest with head of bed elevated 30 degrees for first 24 to 48 hours to reduce myocardial oxygen demand.
	Monitor IV feedings; infuse according to physician's order.
	Administer prescribed medications such as antidysrhythmics, nitrates, and beta blockers.
	Auscultate breath sounds and heart rate every 4 hours; increase activity level as prescribed.
	Palpate for pedal pulses, assess capillary refill, auscultate bowel sounds, assess for pedal or dependent edema every 4 hours, and strictly monitor intake and output (I&O).

Patients and their family members need to be reassured of recovery. More than 85% of patients with an uncomplicated MI return to work. Provide information on the resumption of sexual activities. Once patients with an uncomplicated MI are able to climb two flights of stairs without difficulty, they are usually able to resume sexual activities. Approximately 80% of all postcoronary patients resume sexual activity without serious risks. The other 20% need not abstain totally, but should limit their sexual activity according to their cardiac capacity.

Cardiac Rehabilitation

Before discharge from the hospital, discuss participation in a cardiac rehabilitation program. A monitored exercise program and continuing education are provided with outpatient cardiac rehabilitation. The physician may prescribe cardiac rehabilitation during the inpatient and outpatient phase of recovery after an MI.

Cardiac rehabilitation services are designed to help patients with heart disease recover faster and return to full and productive lives. Cardiac rehabilitation has two major parts:

1. Exercise training to help the patient learn how to exercise safely, strengthen muscles, and improve stamina. The exercise plan is based on the individual's ability, needs, and interests.
2. Education, counseling, and training to help the patient understand his or her heart condition and find ways to reduce the risk of future heart problems. The cardiac rehabilitation team assists the patient in adjusting to a new lifestyle and

dealing with fears about the future. Cardiac rehabilitation may last 6 weeks, 6 months, or longer. Cardiac rehabilitation has lifelong favorable effects (see Health Promotion and Home Care Considerations boxes).

Prognosis

It is imperative that medical care be instituted without delay. Many MI patients not treated before reaching the hospital die. The prognosis also depends on the area and extent of the damage and the presence or absence of complications.

HEART FAILURE

Etiology and Pathophysiology

When the heart is no longer able to pump enough blood to sustain the body's metabolic needs, it is referred to as heart failure or cardiac insufficiency. **Heart failure (HF)** is a syndrome traditionally defined as circulatory congestion as a result of the heart's inability to act as an effective pump. Because many patients suffer pulmonary or systemic congestion with HF, the

 Home Care Considerations

Exercise Program after Myocardial Infarction

- During posthospitalization convalescent period, many patients are encouraged to begin a 2- to 12-week walking program. This is a structured program designed to have the patient walking 2 miles in less than 60 minutes by the end of 12 weeks.
- Encourage patients to work through this program at their own rate until they achieve a pace below a slow jog and their heart rate is below the prescribed rate set by the cardiologist.
- Not all postinfarction patients are physiologically capable of participating in a rigorous exercise program.
- Eventually, most patients are encouraged to participate in a maintenance (lifetime), unsupervised, home-based exercise program designed specifically for them.
- Almost everyone can benefit from some type of cardiac rehabilitation.

syndrome was once called **congestive HF** (CHF). However, this term has lost favor because it excludes patients who do not experience congestion. The most recent definition is that HF should be viewed as a neurohormonal problem that progresses as a result of

 Health Promotion

Myocardial Infarction

- Teach the effects of myocardial infarction (MI), the healing process, and the treatment regimen.
- Teach the effect of medications in the treatment of MI.
- Teach the association between risk factors and coronary artery disease (CAD).
- Teach the patient to identify nonmodifiable risk factors.
- Teach the patient to identify modifiable risk factors (especially cigarette smoking and stress). The patient should stop smoking and encourage family and significant others to stop.
- Teach the effect of dietary restrictions on atherosclerotic heart disease or CAD. Recommended daily intake is 2 g sodium, 1500 calories, low cholesterol, and fluid restrictions.
- Limit total fat intake to 25% to 35% of total calories each day. Limit intake of saturated fats to less than 7% of total fat intake. Teach the patient that saturated fats (e.g., shortening, lard, or butter) are solid at room temperature; better sources of fat include vegetable, olive, and fish oils.
- Teach the patient to avoid foods high in sodium, saturated fats, and triglycerides. Review alternative ways of seasoning foods to avoid cooking with salt. Explain the need to limit intake of eggs, cream, butter, and foods high in animal fat. Teach the patient and family how to read labels on foods.
- Teach the patient to eat 20 to 30 g of soluble fiber every day. Foods such as bran, beans, and peas help lower bad cholesterol (low-density lipoprotein).
- Teach the effect of activity on the heart and the need to participate in a progressive activity plan.
- Refer the patient to social support groups as indicated.
- Stress the importance of participating in cardiac rehabilitation services.
- Explain cardiac warning symptoms. Patients and their partners are often unsure which symptoms must be reported. If

the patient has a prescription for nitroglycerin, advise him or her to take it when experiencing chest pain and to notify the physician if pain is not relieved within 15 minutes. Other signs to report include shortness of breath, rapid heart rate, dizziness, insomnia, a persistent increase in heart rate or blood pressure, and extreme fatigue after sexual activity.

- Advise the patient on when to resume sexual activity (if appropriate). Explain what is safe and when. The joint guidelines of the American College of Cardiology and the American Heart Association recommend that after an "uncomplicated MI" (meaning that the patient was stable and experienced no complications), sexual intercourse can be resumed in a week to 10 days. However, previous studies have found that patients tend to resume sexual activity more gradually than this. A "complicated MI" means that the patient required cardiopulmonary resuscitation or had hypotension, serious dysrhythmia, or heart failure while hospitalized. Patients with complicated MIs must resume sexual activity more gradually, depending on their tolerance for exercise and activity. Encourage patients to talk to their physicians about resuming sexual activity; the type and extent of damage from the MI might influence recommendations. Most patients have concerns about resuming sexual activity after an MI but may not express them to their nurses. Therefore initiating the conversation is the nurse's responsibility.
- Teach the importance of taking prescribed medications such as beta blockers. The patient who uses beta-adrenergic blockers in the treatment of an acute MI for 1 year after the infarction has a decreased chance of reinfarction and increased survival. Continue with taking lipid-lowering agents such as simvastatin (Zocor), atorvastatin (Lipitor), lovastatin (Mevacor), pravastatin (Pravachol), or rosuvastatin (Crestor).

chronic release in the body of substances such as catecholamines (epinephrine and norepinephrine). Epinephrine and norepinephrine are hormones of the sympathetic nervous system and produce negative effects on the failing heart and circulatory system.

Circulatory congestion and compensatory mechanisms may occur. HF may develop after an MI, in response to prolonged hypertension or diabetes mellitus, or in relation to valvular or inflammatory heart disease. Other factors associated with HF include infection, stress, hyperthyroidism, anemia, and fluid replacement therapy. HF is the most common diagnosis for the hospitalized patient over 65 years of age. HF affects about 5 million Americans and accounts for 200,000 deaths annually. The increasing prevalence and incidence of HF result from people (1) living longer and (2) being more likely to survive cardiovascular disease.

Because the left ventricle is most often affected by coronary atherosclerosis and hypertension, HF usually begins there. If untreated, the condition progresses to right-sided failure. Right ventricular failure can occur separately from left ventricular failure, but its appearance is more often a consequence of left-sided failure. The signs and symptoms of HF are the result of decreased cardiac output from impaired cardiac pumping power and congestion that involves the pulmonary and/or venous systems (Box 8-2).

Left Ventricular Failure

When the left ventricle is unable to pump enough blood to meet the body's demands, major consequences occur. The first consequences are the signs and symptoms of decreased cardiac output. The second is pulmonary congestion. Increased pressure in the left side of the heart backs up into the pulmonary system, and the lungs become congested with fluid. Fluid leaks through the engorged capillaries and permeates air spaces in the lungs. If during each heartbeat the right ventricle pumps out just one more drop of blood than the left, then within only 3 hours the pulmonary blood volume will have expanded by 500 mL. Pulmonary edema and **pleural effusion** (an abnormal accumulation of fluid in the thoracic cavity between the visceral and parietal pleurae) occur. Signs and symptoms of this condition include dyspnea; orthopnea; pulmonary crackles; wheezing; pink, frothy sputum; and cough.

Right Ventricular Failure

Right ventricular failure occurs when the right ventricle is unable to pump effectively against increased pressure in the pulmonary circulation. Most often the increased pressure is the result of blood backing up from a failing left ventricle, but right ventricular failure can also be a result of chronic pulmonary disease (cor pulmonale) and pulmonary hypertension. The right ventricle's inability to pump blood forward into the lungs results in peripheral congestion and an inability to accommodate all the venous blood that is normally returned to the right side of the heart. Venous blood is reflected backward into the systemic circulation. Increased venous volume and pressure force fluid out of the vasculature into interstitial tissue (peripheral edema). Edema appears in dependent areas of the body such as the sa-

---

Box 8-2 Classifying and Staging Heart Failure

NEW YORK HEART ASSOCIATION HEART FAILURE CLASSIFICATION

The New York Heart Association classification is a universal gauge of heart failure severity based on physical limitations.

Class I: Minimal
- No limitations.
- Ordinary physical activity does not cause undue fatigue, dyspnea, palpitations, or angina.

Class II: Mild
- Slightly limited physical activity.
- Comfortable at rest.
- Ordinary physical activity results in fatigue, palpitations, dyspnea, or angina.

Class III: Moderate
- Markedly limited physical activity.
- Comfortable at rest.
- Less than ordinary activity causes fatigue, palpitations, dyspnea, or anginal pain.

Class IV: Severe
- Patient unable to perform any physical activity without discomfort.
- Angina or symptoms of cardiac inefficiency may develop at rest. Physical activity increases discomfort.

AMERICAN COLLEGE OF CARDIOLOGY AND AMERICAN HEART ASSOCIATION (ACC/AHA) HEART FAILURE STAGES

Stage A Patient is at high risk for developing heart failure but has no structural disorder of the heart. The patient has a primary condition that is strongly associated with heart failure (such as diabetes mellitus, hypertension, substance abuse, or history of rheumatic fever) but no signs or symptoms of heart failure.

Stage B Patient has a structural disorder of the heart, such as left ventricular remodeling, left ventricular hypertrophy, valvular heart disease, or previous myocardial infarction, but has never developed symptoms of heart failure.

Stage C Patient has past or current symptoms of heart failure associated with underlying structural disease. The patient may display signs of dyspnea or fatigue, but is responding to therapy.

Stage D Patient has end-stage disease and requires specialized treatment strategies that may include mechanical circulatory support, continuous inotropic infusions, heart transplant, or hospice care. These patients are frequently hospitalized and cannot be discharged without symptom recurrence.

The New York Heart Association (NYHA) classification system. Available at www.hearthealthywomen.org. American College of Cardiology and American Heart Association. (ACC/AHA). Heart failure: classification and stages. The AHA/ACC stages of heart failure.

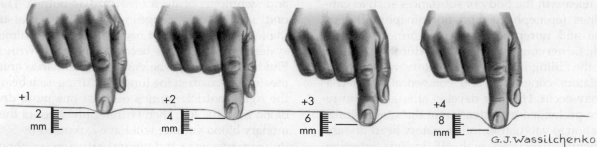

FIGURE 8-17 Scale for pitting edema depth.

Table 8-6	Pitting Edema Scale	
SCALE	**DEGREE**	**RESPONSE**
1+ Trace	2 mm (0-1/16 inch)	Rapid
2+ Mild	4 mm (0-1/4 inch)	10-15 seconds
3+ Moderate	6 mm (1/4-1/2 inch)	1-2 minutes
4+ Severe	8 mm (1/2-1 inch)	2-5 minutes

crum when supine and the feet and ankles while in an upright position. As right ventricular failure continues, edema may progress to pitting edema and move up the legs into the thighs, external genitalia, and lower trunk. To check for edema, press down on the tissue for several seconds and lift the finger. If the depression does not fill almost immediately, pitting edema is present (Figure 8-17; Table 8-6).

One liter of fluid equals 1 kg (2.2 pounds); a weight gain of 2.2 pounds signifies a gain of 1 L of body fluid. The liver may become congested, and fluid can accumulate in the abdomen (ascites). Distended neck veins may be observed when the patient is sitting.

Clinical Manifestations

Manifestations of HF are those associated with decreased cardiac output, left ventricular failure, and right ventricular failure (Box 8-3).

Assessment

Subjective data include complaints of dyspnea, **orthopnea** (an abnormal condition in which a person must sit or stand to breathe deeply or comfortably) or paroxysmal nocturnal dyspnea (sudden awakening from sleep because of shortness of breath), and cough. The patient may report fatigue, anxiety, weight gain from fluid retention, and edema. Physical symptoms and impaired physical function cause psychosocial stress. Patients with New York Heart Association (NYHA) class III or IV HF are at very high risk for major depression (Artinian, 2003). Document any pain (anginal or abdominal) and the patient's stated ability to perform ADLs.

Collection of **objective data** includes noting presence of respiratory distress, the number of pillows required to breath comfortably while attempting to rest (orthopnea), edema (site, degree of pitting), abdominal distention secondary to ascites, weight gain, adventi-

---

Box 8-3 Signs and Symptoms of Heart Failure

DECREASED CARDIAC OUTPUT
- Fatigue
- Anginal pain
- Anxiety
- Oliguria
- Decreased gastrointestinal motility
- Pale, cool skin
- Weight gain
- Restlessness

LEFT VENTRICULAR FAILURE
- Dyspnea
- Paroxysmal nocturnal dyspnea
- Cough
- Frothy, blood-tinged sputum
- Orthopnea
- Pulmonary crackles (moist popping and cracking sounds heard most often at the end of inspiration)
- Radiographic evidence of pulmonary vascular congestion with pleural effusion

RIGHT VENTRICULAR FAILURE
- Distended jugular veins
- Anorexia, nausea, and abdominal distention
- Liver enlargement with right upper quadrant pain
- Ascites
- Edema in feet, ankles, sacrum; may progress up the legs into thighs, external genitalia, and lower trunk

---

tious breath sounds, abnormal heart sounds (gallop and murmurs), activity intolerance, and jugular vein distention. Blood flow to the kidneys is diminished, resulting in oliguria. Oxygen deficit in tissues results in cyanosis and general debilitation.

Diagnostic Tests

Diagnosis is based on presenting signs and symptoms of HF and is confirmed by various diagnostic tests. A chest radiograph reveals pulmonary vascular congestion, pleural effusion, and cardiomegaly (cardiac enlargement). ECG reveals cardiac dysrhythmias. The most noninvasive diagnostic tool for evaluating a patient with HF is an echocardiogram. Echocardiography is done to determine valvular heart disease, presence of pericardial fluid, HF (the percentage of end-diastolic blood volume ejected during systole), and ejection fraction. Pulmonary artery catheterization is done to assess right and left ventricular function.

Exercise stress testing is done to determine activity tolerance and severity of underlying ischemic cardiovascular disease. **Cardiac catheterization** may be performed to detect cardiac abnormalities and underlying cardiovascular disease. **MUGA scanning** is ordered to evaluate cardiac function, ejection fraction, and wall motion abnormalities.

Laboratory tests include electrolytes, sodium, calcium, magnesium, and potassium levels. Blood chemistry will reveal elevated blood urea nitrogen (BUN) and creatinine resulting from decreased glomerular filtration; liver function values (alanine aminotransferase, aspartate transaminase, gamma glutamyltransferase, alkaline phosphatase) will be mildly elevated. **BNP** is a neurohormone secreted by the heart in response to expansion of ventricular volume and pressure overload. With a normal BNP level of less than 100 pg/mL, the patient does not have HF; a level greater than 100 pg/mL is suggestive of HF. Levels greater than 700 pg/mL indicate decompensated HF. A higher level of BNP correlates with an increase in the patient's signs and symptoms of HF. BNP is useful in monitoring chronic HF. Arterial blood gases may reveal hypoxemia and acid-base imbalance.

Medical Management

The objectives of medical management include increasing cardiac efficiency with digoxin and vasodilators (nitroglycerin, isosorbide) for expanded output. Digoxin, a digitalis glycoside that was once the cornerstone of HF treatment, is now used less often and at lower doses. ACE inhibitors such as captopril (Capoten), enalapril (Vasotec), ramipril (Altace), benazepril (Lotensin), lisinopril (Prinivil, Zestril), quinapril (Accupril), and fosinopril (Monopril) decrease peripheral vascular resistance, improve cardiac output, and have proven to extend the lives of patients with HF and lengthen the time between admissions. In January 1999, the Advisory Council to Improve Outcomes Nationwide in Heart Failure (ACTION-HF) recommended that all patients with stable class II or III NYHA HF (see Box 8-2), or stage C or D American College of Cardiology and American Heart Association HF due to left ventricular dysfunction receive a beta blocker to prevent cardiac remodeling. (Remodeling occurs when the left ventricle dilates, hypertrophies, and develops a more spherical shape. The shape change stresses the ventricle walls, increases the magnitude of regurgitation through the mitral valve, and depresses mechanical performance.) Two beta blockers that the FDA has approved to treat HF are carvedilol (an alpha, nonselective beta blocker) and metoprolol. Beta blockers inhibit chronic activation of the sympathetic nervous system. Beta blockers have been so effective at reducing symptoms, improving clinical status, and reducing mortality and hospitalizations that the guidelines identify them as the most significant medications for HF management (Lewis et al., 2007). Angiotensin II receptor blockers such as irbesartan (Avapro), losartan (Cozaar), and valsartan (Diovan) selectively and competitively block the vasoconstrictive and aldosterone-secreting effects of angiotensin, leading to vasodilation. Research for their use in HF is in progress. Angiotensin II receptor blockers are not a substitute for ACE inhibitors unless an ACE inhibitor is clearly not tolerated. In 2001 the FDA approved nesiritide (Natrecor) for the IV treatment of patients with acutely decompensated HF who have shortness of breath (i.e., dyspnea) at rest or with minimal activity. Nesiritide is the first of the drug class called human BNPs. It reduces pulmonary capillary pressure, helps improve breathing, and causes vasodilation with increase in stroke volume and cardiac output (Riggs, 2004).

An additional goal of therapeutic management is to lower oxygen requirements of the body systems; this is accomplished by elevating the head of the bed to 45 degrees or having the patient sit on the edge of the bed with arms resting on the overbed table to reduce myocardial oxygen demand and decrease circulating volume returning to the heart. Oxygen therapy provides oxygen to the tissues if the patient is hypoxic.

Edema and pulmonary congestion are treated with diuretics, a sodium-restricted diet, and restriction of fluid intake. Weigh the patient daily to monitor fluid retention.

Once the workload of the heart is decreased and diuresis of engorged tissues and organs is achieved, the patient's activity level will increase. These objectives are achieved by medication therapy and activity per a physician's orders. Medication therapy with digoxin, ACE inhibitors, thiazide, and loop diuretics is a common initial treatment (Table 8-7).

A biventricular pacemaker can improve symptoms and function, improve quality of life, and decrease hospitalization for patients with HF who also have conduction system disease (Chojnowski, 2007).

The use of an implantable cardioverter-defibrillator can decrease the risk for sudden cardiac death for patients with a family history of sudden cardiac death, life-threatening dysrhythmias, or mild to moderate HF who have an ejection fraction of less than 30% (Chojnowski, 2007).

In acute HF, administration of oxygen and medication should be of first concern. Decreasing oxygen requirements through rest will slow the heart rate and increase cardiac and respiratory reserves. Anxiety produced from the signs and symptoms and the fear of a life-threatening situation can be allayed by reassurance and explanation. Accurate interventions, observation, and reporting reduce the threat of complications such as embolus, thrombophlebitis, MI, and pulmonary edema.

Nursing Interventions

Nursing interventions include measures to prevent disease progression and complications. Monitor vital signs for changes. Note any signs of respiratory distress or pulmonary edema. Carefully monitor signs and symptoms of left-sided versus right-sided HF. Urinary output is typically low, and edema is soft and pitting; legs are elevated to decrease edema.

Also note an increase in abdominal girth and total body weight as indicators of fluid retention, which is common in HF. Auscultate the lung fields to detect presence of crackles and wheezes; also note coughing and complaints of dyspnea. Restful sleep may be possible only in the sitting position or with the aid of extra pillows. Activity intolerance is accompanied by extreme fatigue and anxiety. Assess patients for depression. Explain to patients with HF and depression that the depression is readily treatable and that several approaches to treatment can be used separately or in combination, including pharmacologic therapy, psychosocial and psychotherapeutic interventions, and cardiac rehabilitation.

Table 8-7 Medications for Heart Failure

Generic (Trade)	Action	Nursing Interventions
CARDIAC GLYCOSIDES		
Digitalis preparations, such as digoxin (Lanoxin)	Strengthen cardiac force and efficiency Slow heart rate Increase circulation, effecting diuresis	Monitor apical pulse to ensure rate greater than 60 bpm; monitor for toxicity (nausea, vomiting, anorexia, dysrhythmia, bradycardia, tachycardia, headache, fatigue, and blurred or colored vision).
DIURETICS		
Thiazides, such as chlorothiazide (Diuril), hydrochlorothiazide (Esidrix, Hydrodiuril)	Increase renal secretion of sodium Are safe for long-term use Block sodium and water reabsorption in kidney tubules	Monitor electrolyte depletion; weigh daily to ascertain fluid loss.
Sulfonamides (loop diuretic), such as furosemide (Lasix), bumetanide (Bumex)	Act rapidly for less responsive edema	Administer in AM to prevent nocturia. Monitor for electrolyte depletion. Consider sulfa allergy (furosemide).
Aldosterone antagonist (potassium-sparing), such as spironolactone (Aldactone)	Relieves edema and ascites that do not respond to usual diuretics Blocks sodium-retaining and potassium-excreting properties of aldosterone	Monitor for gastrointestinal irritation and hyperkalemia.
POTASSIUM SUPPLEMENTS		
Potassium (K-Lyte)	Restores electrolyte loss	Monitor blood potassium levels.
SEDATIVES AND ANALGESICS		
Temazepam (Restoril)	Promotes rest and comfort	Monitor rest and sleep benefits.
Morphine	Relieves chest and abdominal pain, reduces anxiety, and decreases myocardial oxygen demands Lessens dyspnea	
NITRATES		
Nitroglycerin (Cardabid)	Dilates arteries, improves blood flow Reduces blood pressure	Monitor blood pressure for hypotension. Monitor for headache and flushing.
ACE INHIBITORS		
Captopril (Capoten) Enalapril (Vasotec) Vamipril (Altace) Benazepril (Lotensin) Lisinopril (Prinivil; Zestril) Quinapril (Accupril) Fosinopril (Monopril) Moexipril (Univasc) Perindopril (Aceon) Trandolapril (Mavik)	Act as antihypertensives and reduce peripheral arterial resistance and improve cardiac output	Observe patient closely for a precipitous drop in blood pressure within 3 hours of initial dose; monitor blood pressure closely. Monitor blood potassium levels.

ACE, Angiotensin-converting enzyme; *CHF,* congestive heart failure; *HF,* heart failure; *I&O,* intake and output.

Table 8-7   Medications for Heart Failure—cont'd

Generic (Trade)	Action	Nursing Interventions
BETA-ADRENERGIC BLOCKERS		
Carvedilol (Coreg)	Directly blocks the sympathetic nervous system's negative effects on the failing heart.	Start at low dose, increasing the dosage slowly every 2 weeks as tolerated by the patient. Monitor blood pressure and notify prescriber of significant change. Monitor pulse: if <50 bpm, hold drug, call prescriber.
Metoprolol (Toprol-XL)	Blocks beta$_2$-adrenergic receptors in bronchial and vascular smooth muscle. Lowers blood pressure by beta blocking effects; reduces elevated rennin plasma levels.	Monitor I&O, weigh daily. Monitor apical or radial pulse before administration. Notify prescriber of any significant changes or pulse <50 bpm.
INOTROPIC AGENTS		
Dobutamine (Dobutrex IV) Dopamine HCl (Intropin IV)	Low-dose dobutamine and low-dose dopamine relatively safe on medical-surgical units; in low doses, dilate renal blood vessels, stimulating renal blood flow and glomerular filtration rate, which in turn promotes sodium excretion, often helping CHF patients improve	Make certain patient is not taking monoamine oxidase (MAO) inhibitors, tricyclic antidepressants, phenytoin (Dilantin), or haloperidol (Haldol). Record accurate I&O; assess for dizziness, nausea, vomiting, headache. Assess vital signs carefully every 15 minutes for first 2 hours, then every 2 hours for following 4 hours, and finally once a shift. Observe carefully for extravasation, tachycardia, bradycardia, angina, palpitations, hypotension, hypertension, azotemia, and anxiety.
HUMAN B-TYPE NATRIURETIC PEPTIDES		
Nesiritide (Natrecor)	New class of synthetic HF drugs; causes arterial and venous dilation, thereby decreasing systemic vascular resistance and pulmonary arterial pressures; decreases blood pressure, promotes better left ventricle ejection, and increases cardiac output; may also promote diuresis; an IV treatment for patients with acutely compensated CHF.	Observe carefully for hypotension. Natrecor should not be used for patients with cardiogenic shock or with a systolic blood pressure <90 mm Hg.

Key Components of Care

The Institute for Healthcare Improvement recommends these components of care for all patients with HF (unless patient cannot tolerate them or unless contraindicated):

- Assess left ventricular systolic function.
- At discharge from hospital (when left ventricular ejection fraction is less than 40%, indicating systolic dysfunction), administer ACE inhibitor or angiotensin.
- At discharge, administer an anticoagulant if the patient has chronic or recurrent atrial fibrillation.
- Encourage smoking cessation.
- Instruct the patient at discharge regarding activity, diet, medication, follow-up appointment, weight monitoring, and what to do if symptoms worsen.

- Provide influenza and pneumococcal immunization.
- At discharge, institute optional beta blocker therapy for stabilized patients with left ventricular systolic dysfunction who have no contraindications.

The new guidelines also advocate a discussion of end-of-life decisions with the patient and the family. Patients should talk with their health care providers about treatment preferences, advance directives, living wills, power of attorney for health care, and life-support issues. Because HF is progressive, patients should make these decisions while they are capable of expressing choices. Hospice services, originally developed to assist cancer patients, are appropriate for the patient with end-stage HF (Nursing Care Plan 8-1; Box 8-4; and Patient Teaching box).

⭐ **Nursing Care Plan 8-1** **The Patient with Heart Failure**

Mr. Domrose is a 61-year-old clinical administrator. He was admitted to the hospital with the diagnosis of heart failure. He has a history of hypertension and coronary artery disease. Six months ago he had a myocardial infarction. He has felt tired for the past 3 weeks and has been experiencing increased dyspnea. He has noticed some edema in his ankles and is concerned about gaining 5 pounds in the past week and having an increasing intolerance to exertion. The nursing admission history revealed:

- Mr. Domrose has not been taking his antihypertensive medication regularly. He did not like the side effects and stopped taking the medication, but he was too embarrassed to call his physician.
- Vital signs revealed an elevated blood pressure.
- He has shortness of breath during activities and when lying down.
- Pitting edema is seen on both ankles.
- Crackles are heard bilaterally in the lungs.

NURSING DIAGNOSIS *Decreased cardiac output, related to cardiac insufficiency*

Patient Goals and Expected Outcomes	Nursing Intervention	Evaluation
Patient will have decreased dyspnea with activities and when lying in bed within 24 hours Patient will have decreased adventitious lung sounds Patient will have oxygen saturations at 91% with prescribed oxygen within 24 hours Patient will have vital signs within acceptable levels within 72 hours Patient will have decreased edema and weight loss of 5 pounds within 72 hours	Maintain initial bed rest with stress-free environment. Maintain semi-Fowler's to high Fowler's position. Explain and encourage gradual increases in activity to prevent a sudden increase in cardiac workload. Monitor respirations, lung sounds, heart sounds, and vital signs every 4 hours. Palpate pedal pulses, and assess capillary refill every 8 hours. Administer digitalis, diuretics, angiotensin-converting enzyme inhibitors, vasodilators, beta blockers, and antihypertensive medication as prescribed. Monitor intake and output and weigh daily. Monitor oxygen saturation with pulse oximetry every 4 hours. Administer prescribed oxygen.	Patient has decreased crackles in lung fields within 24 hours of admission. Patient has an oximetry reading of 91% oxygen saturation with oxygen prescribed within 24 hours of admission. Patient has a heart rate of 80 bpm, respiratory rate of 22 breaths/min, and blood pressure of 148/86 mm Hg within 72 hours of admission. Patient has a weight loss of 5 pounds within 72 hours of admission. Patient has pedal pitting edema decreased to 1+ within 2 days of admission.

NURSING DIAGNOSIS *Anxiety, related to change in health status, lifestyle changes, fear of death, or threats to self-concept.*

Patient Goals and Expected Outcomes	Nursing Intervention	Evaluation
Patient will verbalize anxieties within 48 hours of admission Patient will demonstrate reduction of anxiety by enjoying periods of rest and sleep undisturbed for 6 hours within 48 hours of admission	Identify coping techniques. Provide information to decrease fears. Identify support systems. Provide calm, relaxing environment. Administer antianxiety medications per physician's orders as needed. Help patient cope with lifestyle changes. He may feel anxious due to changes in body image, family and social roles, and finances. Focus on progress patient is making in managing his condition. Encourage patient to participate in health care decisions, and allow him to release anger and frustration. Allow patient to sleep undisturbed for 6 hours when vital signs are stable.	Patient is verbalizing anger and frustration over current medical conditions within 48 hours of admission. Patient is sleeping 5 to 6 hours per night within 48 hours of admission.

⭐ Nursing Care Plan 8-1   The Patient with Heart Failure—cont'd

Critical Thinking Questions

1. Mr. Domrose is experiencing severe dyspnea, with the presence of crackles bilaterally in all lung fields. His pulse is 108 bpm, and respirations are 33 breaths/min. When performing his morning activities of daily living, what nursing interventions would be most beneficial?
2. On assessing Mr. Domrose's skin, the nurse notes 4+ pitting edema in his lower extremities. A weight gain of 6 pounds in the past 24 hours is also noted. For therapeutic diuresis to occur, what would the medical management include?
3. Mr. Domrose puts his call light on to request assistance to ambulate. The nurse notes subclavicular retractions and cyanosis of his nailbeds. What would be the most appropriate nursing actions?

Box 8-4   Guidelines for Nursing Interventions for the Patient with Heart Failure

- Provide oxygenation.
- Administer oxygen by nasal cannula per protocol as prescribed for dyspnea.
- Patient should be well supported in semi-Fowler's or high Fowler's position.
- Reinforce importance of conservation of energy and planning for activities that avoid fatigue.
- Encourage activity within prescribed restrictions; monitor for intolerance to activity (dyspnea, fatigue, increased pulse rate that does not stabilize).
- Assist with activities of daily living as necessary; encourage independence within patient's limitations.
- Provide diversionary activity that will assist in conservation of energy.
- Monitor for signs of fluid and potassium imbalance; record daily weights, intake and output.

- Provide skin care, particularly over edematous areas; use prophylactic measures to prevent skin impairment.
- Assist in maintaining an adequate nutritional intake while observing prescribed dietary modifications (sodium restrictions).
- Monitor for constipation; give prescribed stool softeners.
- Give prescribed medications:
  —Digitalis (take apical pulse before administration)
  —Diuretics (assess for hypokalemia)
  —Vasodilators, angiotensin-converting enzyme inhibitors, beta blockers
  —Medications to reduce anxiety and promote sleep
- Provide the patient and the family opportunities to discuss their concerns.
- Teach patient about the disorder and self-care.

👥 Patient Teaching

Heart Failure

- Monitor for signs and symptoms of recurring heart failure and report them to the physician or clinic:
  —Weight gain of 2 to 3 pounds (1 to 1.5 kg) over a short period (about 2 days)
  —Shortness of breath
  —Orthopnea
  —Swelling of ankles, feet, or abdomen
  —Persistent cough
  —Frequent nighttime urination
- Avoid fatigue and plan activity to allow for rest periods.
- Plan and eat meals within prescribed sodium restrictions. Avoid salty foods.
- Avoid drugs with high sodium content (e.g., some laxatives and antacids, Alka-Seltzer); read the labels. Ideally, limit sodium intake to 2 g/day.
- Maintain low-fat diet, with fat intake less than 30% of total calories.
- Eat several small meals rather than three large meals per day.
- Take medications as prescribed.

- If several medications are prescribed, develop a method to facilitate accurate administration.
- When taking digoxin, check own pulse rate daily; report a rate of less than 60 bpm to the physician. Do not take digoxin if pulse is less than 60 bpm.
- Take diuretics as prescribed.
- Weigh self daily at same time.
- Eat foods high in potassium and low in sodium (such as oranges and bananas).
- Take all prescribed medications.
- Report signs of hypotension (lightheadedness, rapid pulse, syncope) to the physician.
- Avoid alcohol when taking vasodilators.
- Reinforce the importance of regular exercise once heart failure is stabilized. Thorough treatment regimen may allow the patient to increase activity level over time. The physician may ultimately recommend 30 to 45 minutes of aerobic exercise three or four times a week to improve patient's well-being.
- Report to the physician for follow-up as directed.

Prognosis

Approximately 10% of patients diagnosed with HF die in the first year, and 50% within 5 years. HF is a chronic condition. With treatment advances, many people now survive for years with damaged hearts. With the advent of ACE inhibitors and new research on the benefits of prescribed exercise, improvement in the quality of life for HF patients is being seen.

PULMONARY EDEMA

Etiology and Pathophysiology

Pulmonary edema (the accumulation of extravascular fluid in lung tissues and alveoli, most often caused by HF) is an acute and extensive, life-threatening complication of HF caused by severe left ventricular dysfunction. Fluid from the left side of the heart backs up into the pulmonary vasculature and results in extravascular fluid accumulation in the interstitial space and alveoli. This causes the patient to "drown" in the secretions.

Clinical Manifestations

The patient exhibits signs of severe respiratory distress when pulmonary edema occurs. Frothy sputum is produced from air mixing with the fluid in the alveoli; the sputum is blood-tinged from blood cells that have exuded into the alveoli.

Assessment

See Box 8-5 for signs and symptoms of pulmonary edema.

Diagnostic Tests

Diagnosis is made by observing signs and symptoms and is supported by chest radiograph and arterial blood gas studies. Pao_2 and $Paco_2$ may reveal respiratory alkalosis or acidosis.

Medical Management

Medical management involves simultaneous interventions to promote oxygenation, improve cardiac output, and reduce pulmonary congestion. Without emergency treatment, respiratory failure may occur (Table 8-8).

Box 8-5	Signs and Symptoms of Pulmonary Edema

- Restlessness
- Vague uneasiness
- Agitation
- Disorientation
- Diaphoresis
- Severe dyspnea
- Tachypnea
- Tachycardia
- Pallor or cyanosis
- Cough production of large quantities of blood-tinged, frothy sputum
- Audible wheezing, crackles
- Cold extremities

Nursing Interventions

Interventions include administering oxygen. Place the patient upright with legs in a dependent position to decrease venous return to the heart, relieving pulmonary congestion and dyspnea. Monitor arterial blood gases and administer drugs as ordered. Auscultate lung sounds often. Provide emotional support; remain with patient. Explain all procedures. Monitor vital signs, fluid I&O, and serum electrolytes.

Nursing diagnoses and interventions for the patient with pulmonary edema include but are not limited to the following:

Nursing Diagnoses	Nursing Interventions
Excess fluid volume, related to fluid accumulation in pulmonary vessels	Administer medications as ordered. Carefully monitor I&O. Weigh patient at same time each day. Assess for edema.
Impaired gas exchange, related to fluid in lungs	Assess for signs of hypoxia, such as restlessness, disorientation, and irritability. Monitor arterial blood gases per physician's order. Administer oxygen per physician's order. Position patient in high Fowler's position with legs in dependent position, or sitting and leaning forward on overbed table to facilitate breathing.
Anxiety, related to fear of suffocation and death	Promote optimal air exchange to decrease anxiety. Assess level of anxiety and coping mechanisms. Deliver nursing interventions in a supportive, kind, and proficient manner. Assess support systems available to patient and mobilize resources.

Prognosis

Pulmonary edema is a grave, life-threatening condition that is usually responsive to aggressive interventions.

VALVULAR HEART DISEASE

Etiology and Pathophysiology

Normal heart valves function to maintain the direction of blood flow through the right atrium, right ventricle, lungs, left atrium, and left ventricle and to the rest of the body. Heart valves operate by passively opening

Table 8-8   Medical Management for Acute Pulmonary Edema

INTERVENTION	RATIONALE
Patient in high Fowler's position or over side of bed with arms supported on bedside table	Promotes expansion of lungs; legs in dependent position causes venous pooling and reduction in venous return (preload)
Morphine sulfate, 10-15 mg IV; titrated	Decreases patient anxiety; relieves pain; slows respirations; reduces venous return; decreases oxygen demand; dilates the pulmonary and systemic blood vessels
Oxygen at 40%-100%; nonrebreather face mask; intubation as needed	Promotes oxygenation; increased tidal volume also promotes removal of secretions from alveoli
Administer sublingual nitroglycerin	Increases myocardial blood flow
Diuretics: furosemide (Lasix), bumetanide (Bumex) (IV)	Reduce pulmonary edema by decreasing the fluid in the lungs and increasing excretion through the kidneys
Insert Foley catheter	Allows patient to rest and conserve energy; monitors urinary output after IV furosemide has been administered.
Inotropic agents: dobutamine (Dobutrex), amrinone (Inocor)	Increase myocardial contractility without increasing oxygen consumption Increase peripheral vasodilation Increase cardiac output
Nitroprusside (Nitropress)	A potent vasodilator; improves myocardial contraction and reduces pulmonary congestion

and closing in response to pressure changes in the heart. The tricuspid valve is located between the right atrium and the right ventricle. The pulmonary semilunar valve allows blood to flow through the pulmonary artery into the lungs. The mitral (bicuspid) valve is located between the left atrium and the left ventricle. The aortic semilunar valve allows blood to flow from the left ventricle into the aorta. Valvular disease occurs when the valves are compromised and do not open and close properly. Two valvular problems are **stenosis,** which is a thickening of the valve tissue, causing the valve to narrow, and **insufficiency,** which occurs when the valve is unable to close completely. Valvular heart disorders include mitral stenosis, mitral insufficiency, aortic insufficiency, aortic stenosis, tricuspid insufficiency, tricuspid stenosis, pulmonary insufficiency, and pulmonary stenosis.

Valvular disorders occur in children, adolescents, and adults, primarily from congenital conditions. Another prominent factor in the development of valvular disease is a history of rheumatic fever. Clinical symptoms of valvular heart disease tend to occur 10 to 40 years after an episode of rheumatic fever. Because the blood volume and workload of the heart are greater on the left than on the right, the mitral and aortic valves are affected more frequently.

Clinical Manifestations

Signs and symptoms seen in valvular disorders are related to decreased cardiac output (Table 8-9).

Assessment

Subjective data include the patient's statement of a history of rheumatic fever and of an inability to perform activities and ADLs without fatigue or weakness. Ask the patient about his or her chest pain, including its quality, duration, onset, precipitating factors, and measures that provide relief. The patient may complain of heart palpitations, lightheadedness, dizziness, or fainting. The history may include a patient statement of weight gain. Dyspnea, exertional dyspnea, nocturnal (nighttime) dyspnea, and orthopnea are often reported, depending on the degree of HF.

Collection of **objective data** includes observing for a heart murmur and noting the character and the presence of any adventitious breath sounds (crackles, wheezes) and edema (pitting or nonpitting).

Diagnostic Tests

The diagnostic tests used to confirm valvular heart disease are chest radiograph, ECG, echocardiogram, and cardiac catheterization.

Medical Management

Medical management includes activity limitations, sodium-restricted diet, diuretics, digoxin, and antidysrhythmics.

When medical therapy no longer alleviates clinical symptoms or when diagnostic evidence exists of progressive myocardial failure, surgery is often performed. The surgery may include the following:

- **Open mitral commissurotomy:** A surgical splitting of the fused mitral valve leaflet for treating stenosis of the mitral valve.
- **Valve replacement:** Replacement of the stenosed or incompetent valve with a bioprosthetic or mechanical valve. Commonly used valves include tilting disks, porcine (pig) heterografts (tissue taken from one species and grafted onto another), homografts (a graft of tissue obtained from a member of the same species as the individual receiving it), and ball-in-cage valves.

Table 8-9	Clinical Manifestations of Valvular Heart Diseases	
NURSING DIAGNOSES	**CLINICAL MANIFESTATIONS**
Mitral valve stenosis	Dyspnea on exertion, hemoptysis; fatigue; palpitations; loud, accentuated S_1; low-pitched, rumbling diastolic murmur; atrial fibrillation on ECG
Mitral valve regurgitation	**Acute:** Generally poorly tolerated, with fulminating pulmonary edema and shock developing rapidly; new systolic murmur
	Chronic: Weakness, fatigue, exertional dyspnea, palpitations; an S_3 gallop
Mitral valve prolapse	Palpitations, dyspnea, chest pain, activity intolerance, syncope,; midsystolic click
Aortic valve stenosis	Angina, syncope, dyspnea on exertion, heart failure; normal or soft S_1, diminished or absent S_2
Aortic valve regurgitation	**Acute:** Abrupt onset of profound dyspnea, chest pain, left ventricular failure, and shock
	Chronic: Fatigue, exertional dyspnea, orthopnea, paroxysmal nocturnal dyspnea; water-hammer pulse; heaving precordial impulse; diminished or absent S_1, S_3, or S_4
Tricuspid and pulmonic stenosis	**Tricuspid:** Peripheral edema, ascites, hepatomegaly; diastolic low-pitched murmur
	Pulmonic: Fatigue, loud midsystolic murmur

From Lewis, S.L., et al. (2007). *Medical-surgical nursing: Assessment and management of clinical problems.* (7th ed.). St. Louis: Mosby.
ECG, Electrocardiogram.

Nursing Interventions and Patient Teaching

Nursing interventions focus on assisting with ADLs, relieving specific symptoms associated with decreased cardiac output, and promoting comfort. Administer the prescribed medications (diuretics, digoxin, and antidysrhythmics). Also record I&O, daily weight, respiratory rate and rhythm, auscultation of breath sounds, heart sounds, and blood pressure. Check for capillary perfusion, pedal pulses, and presence of edema. Have the patient consume a sodium-restricted diet for control of edema. Maintain oxygen therapy as prescribed. Discuss with the patient a plan for rest periods, and identify those ADLs that produce fatigue and require assistance.

Nursing diagnoses and interventions for the patient with valvular heart disease include but are not limited to the following:

Nursing Diagnoses	Nursing Interventions
Activity intolerance, related to: • weakness • fatigue • dyspnea	Balance activities with rest periods. Identify fatiguing activities and obtain assistance as needed. Use oxygen as prescribed by physician.
Excess fluid volume, related to decreased cardiac output	Administer prescribed oxygen, digoxin, diuretics, and antidysrhythmics. Monitor I&O. Weigh patient daily. Perform respiratory assessment. Perform cardiovascular assessment. Inspect for presence of edema. Obtain vital signs routinely. Maintain sodium-restricted diet.

Patient teaching focuses on medications, dietary management, activity limitations, diagnostic tests, surgical interventions, and postoperative care as appropriate. Discuss with the patient the disease process and associated symptoms to report to the physician. Explain antibiotic prophylaxis to prevent infective endocarditis. Explain the importance of notifying the dentist, urologist, and gynecologist of valvular heart disease. Patient must remain on higher dosages of warfarin after valve replacement surgery. Carefully monitor PT and INR. Discuss with the patient the need to maintain good oral hygiene and make regular visits to the dentist.

Prognosis

The prognosis for valvular heart disease varies, depending on the specific disease. The prognosis after surgery is fair to good with amelioration (improvement) of signs and symptoms but often without resolution of all abnormalities.

INFLAMMATORY HEART DISORDERS

All cardiac tissues are susceptible to inflammation, and HF can be a serious and rapid result of the inflammatory process.

RHEUMATIC HEART DISEASE

Etiology and Pathophysiology

Rheumatic heart disease, is the result of rheumatic fever and the clinical manifestation of carditis resulting from an inadequately treated childhood pharyngeal or upper respiratory tract infection (group A β-hemolytic streptococci). By the 1980s rheumatic fever had almost disappeared in developed countries such as the United States. However, it remained common and severe in most developing countries. Antibiotics, especially penicillin, are responsible for the decline in rheumatic fever. A great deal of interest has been generated by a number of "mini-epidemics," with 10 to 75 cases of acute rheumatic fever in a single region. In searching for the cause of the reappearance, researchers have isolated highly virulent strains of the same types of group A streptococci that were prevalent in epidemic rheumatic fever more than 30 years ago (Lewis et al., 2007).

Ineffective treatment of infection results in delayed reaction and inflammation of the cardiac tissues and the central nervous system, joints, skin, and subcutaneous tissues. Ninety percent of patients with rheumatic fever are between 5 and 15 years of age. The onset of rheumatic fever is usually sudden, often occurring in from 1 to 5 symptom-free weeks after recovery from pharyngitis (sore throat) or from scarlet fever. However, rheumatic fever may progress with symptoms and go undiagnosed and untreated. Years later the patient may develop clinical manifestations of valvular heart disease.

Rheumatic heart disease can affect the pericardium, myocardium, or endocardium. The affected tissue develops small areas of necrosis, which heal, leaving scar tissue. The heart valves are typically the most affected by Aschoff's nodules (vegetative growth) and become fibrous and incompetent. With healing, the valves become thickened and deformed. These changes result in valvular stenosis and insufficiency, varying in extent and severity.

Clinical Manifestations
Fever, increased pulse, epistaxis, anemia, joint involvement, and nodules on joints and subcutaneous tissue may be noted. Carditis can develop. When valvular involvement occurs, signs and symptoms are specific to each condition.

Assessment
Collection of **subjective data** may reveal joint pain (polyarthritis) and chest pain. Lethargy and fatigue are also present.

Objective data include skin manifestations of small erythematous circles and wavy lines on the trunk and abdomen that appear and disappear rapidly (erythema marginatum). The nurse may observe involuntary, purposeless movement of the muscles if Sydenham's chorea (St. Vitus' dance), a disorder of the central nervous system, is present. Heart murmur may be auscultated if the patient has carditis with valve involvement. Rheumatic heart disease is characterized by heart murmurs resulting from stenosis or insufficiency of the valves.

Diagnostic Tests
Diagnosis is made through signs and symptoms and supported by laboratory study results. An echocardiogram is done to determine the extent of damage to the valves and myocardium. An ECG shows cardiac dysrhythmia. Cardiac murmurs or friction rub can be heard. No specific diagnostic test exists for rheumatic fever. Sedimentation rate and leukocyte count are elevated. The development of serum antibodies against the streptococci (measured by antistreptolysin-O titer)

may occur. CRP, elevated in a specimen of blood, is abnormally high.

Medical Management
Preventive measures are the most effective interventions. Rapid treatment for pharyngeal infection, usually with prolonged antibiotic therapy, is desired. Penicillin is the preferred antibiotic. Prolonged periods of bed rest were recommended, but now the patient without carditis may be ambulatory as soon as acute symptoms have subsided. When carditis is present, ambulation is postponed until HF is controlled. Symptomatic treatment and care are given. Nonsteroidal antiinflammatory drugs (NSAIDs) for joint pain and inflammation are accompanied by application of gentle heat. A well-balanced diet, following the personalized daily food choices and number of servings recommended by the U.S. Department of Agriculture's MyPyramid food planning tool, is supplemented by vitamins B and C and high-volume fluid intake. In some patients, surgical commissurotomy or valve replacement is necessary.

Nursing Interventions and Patient Teaching
Signs and symptoms largely determine the type of nursing interventions. Bed rest during the acute phase is recommended when carditis is present. If the patient has polyarthritis, minimize joint pain by proper positioning. After the acute stage, the child or the adult is treated at home. Review a schedule of daily events with the patient and the parents.

Carry out nursing interventions quickly and skillfully to minimize discomfort and avoid tiring the patient. Throughout the course of the disease, the patient and the family benefit from emotional support and appropriate diversions. Teaching focuses on increasing understanding of the disease process, signs and symptoms, and gradually increasing activity levels. Emphasize the importance of eating a nutritional diet and keeping appointments for medical checkups. Patients with a history of rheumatic fever or evidence of rheumatic heart disease should receive daily prophylactic penicillin by mouth or monthly intramuscular injections of penicillin to prevent streptococcal infection, at least during childhood and adolescence. Patients with evidence of deformed heart valves should be given prophylactic antibiotics before surgery and all dental procedures.

Prognosis
Prognosis depends on involvement of the heart; carditis can result in a serious heart disease, including valvular disease.

PERICARDITIS
Etiology and Pathophysiology
Pericarditis is inflammation of the membranous sac surrounding the heart. It may be an acute or a chronic condition. Bacterial, viral, or fungal infection is associated

with acute pericarditis. It may occur as a complication of noninfectious conditions such as azotemia; acute MI; neoplasms such as lung cancer, breast cancer, leukemia, Hodgkin's disease, and lymphoma; scleroderma; trauma after thoracic surgery; systemic lupus erythematosus; radiation; and drug reactions (e.g., from procainamide and hydralazine [Apresoline]). Fibrosis of the pericardial sac develops in the chronic form.

Fibrous constriction and thickening of the pericardium occur gradually, causing compression severe enough to prevent normal filling during diastole. Surgical removal of the pericardium may be necessary to restore normal cardiac output.

Clinical Manifestations
Pericarditis differs clinically from other inflammatory conditions of the heart in that patients often have debilitating pain, much like that of MI. The pain is aggravated by lying supine, deep breathing, coughing, swallowing, and moving the trunk and is alleviated by sitting up and leaning forward. Dyspnea, fever, chills, diaphoresis, and leukocytosis are observed. The hallmark finding in acute pericarditis is pericardial friction rub; grating, scratching, and leathery sounds are detected, although this appears in only about half of cases.

Decreased heart function to the level of cardiac failure can occur when the heart is compressed by excess fluid in the pericardial sac. Normally 15 to 50 mL of fluid are found in the pericardial sac, but with pericarditis 150 to 200 mL or more may develop.

Assessment
Subjective data include the patient's description of muscle aches, fatigue, and dyspnea. Excruciating chest pain is said to originate precordially and radiate to the neck and shoulders with severe and sudden onset.

Collection of **objective data** includes noting expressed substernal chest pain that radiates to the shoulder and neck; such pain is evidenced by orthopneic positioning and facial grimace on inspiration. Elevated temperature accompanies chills and may be followed by diaphoresis. A nonproductive cough is often present. Patients commonly verbalize anxiety, anticipation of danger, or uneasiness. Vital sign changes include a rapid and forcible pulse and rapid, shallow breathing. Pericardial friction rub heart sounds become muffled, and the physician may note a dysrhythmia.

Diagnostic Tests
ECG changes (dysrhythmia) are noted. Echocardiography shows pericardial effusion or cardiac tamponade. Laboratory studies show leukocytosis (10,000 to 20,000/mm^3), and the sedimentation rate is elevated. Blood cultures may be ordered to identify the specific pathogen present. To rule out an MI, cardiac enzyme levels are done. A CRP test used to diagnose

bacterial infectious disease and inflammatory disorder may be ordered (Holcomb, 2006). Chest radiographic findings are generally normal or nonspecific in acute pericarditis unless the patient has a large pericardial effusion.

Medical Management
Analgesia for comfort and relief of pain reassures the anxious patient. Oxygen and parenteral fluids are usually given. Antibiotics are used to treat bacterial pericarditis. The physician prescribes salicylates for increased temperature and antiinflammatory agents (e.g., indomethacin) and corticosteroids for a persistent inflammatory process. These medicines require nursing knowledge of troublesome effects and nursing implications for control of this condition. When pericardial effusion restricts heart movement (**cardiac tamponade**), a pericardial tap (**pericardiocentesis**) may be performed to remove excess fluid and restore normal heart function. Surgical intervention—pericardial fenestration (pericardial window) or pericardiocentesis (pericardial tap)—may be performed to provide continuous drainage of pericardial fluid and restore normal heart function. Complications include atelectasis and introduction of infectious agents.

Nursing Interventions
Carefully evaluate vital signs and auscultate lung and heart sounds. Provide supportive measures and observe for complications. Maintain bed rest to promote healing and decrease the cardiac workload. Elevate the head of the bed to 45 degrees to decrease dyspnea. Hypothermia treatment may be necessary to reduce elevated temperature. Remain with the patient if he or she is anxious. Explain all procedures thoroughly.

Nursing diagnoses and interventions for the patient with inflammatory heart conditions include but are not limited to the following:

Nursing Diagnoses	Nursing Interventions
Decreased cardiac output, related to inflammatory process	Maintain bed rest with head of bed elevated to 45 degrees. Assess vital signs every 2 to 4 hours as indicated by patient's condition. Administer medications as ordered. Monitor I&O. Provide planned rest periods.
Pain, related to inflammatory process	Assess and record pain type and quality. Administer analgesics according to need, as ordered. (Pain is what the patient says it is.)

Nursing Diagnoses	Nursing Interventions
Pain, related to inflammatory process—cont'd	Maintain the patient on bed rest with the head of the bed elevated to 45 degrees and provide a padded overbed table for the patient to rest the arms. Use comfort measures to provide physical and emotional support.
Excess fluid volume, related to ineffective myocardial pumping action	Restrict sodium in diet as prescribed; monitor I&O. Weigh daily; compare values. Administer diuretic therapy as ordered; monitor electrolyte values. Observe respiration and pulse quality. Assess for dyspnea and peripheral edema.

Prognosis

The prognosis is fair in early stages but extremely grave if purulent and fibrinous stages develop.

ENDOCARDITIS

Etiology and Pathophysiology

Endocarditis is an infection or inflammation of the inner membranous lining of the heart, particularly the heart valves. Classified on the basis of cause, it may result from invasion of an organism (**infective endocarditis**) or from injury to the lining. The term **bacterial endocarditis** has been replaced by **infective endocarditis** because causative organisms include fungi, chlamydiae, rickettsiae, viruses, and bacteria. The causative organisms—most commonly *Streptococcus viridans*, *Streptococcus pyogenes*, *Staphylococcus aureus*, *Staphylococcus epidermidis*, and enterococci—are deposited on the heart lining or valves. As the organism embeds into the tissue, a vegetative growth perforates the chambers or valve leaflets. Fibrin and calciferous growths of the vegetation may ulcerate and scar the valves; or the growths may break away, causing emboli, infection, or abscess in organs where they lodge. The loss of portions of vegetative lesions into the circulation results in embolization. Systemic embolization occurs from left-sided heart vegetation, progressing to infarction of an organ (particularly the brain, the kidneys, and the spleen) and limb. Right-sided heart lesions embolize to the lungs. Endocarditis may develop after cardiac surgery, which in itself is traumatic.

People at risk include patients with rheumatic, congestive, or degenerative heart disease. With the increasing use of valve replacement, the incidence of prosthetic valve endocarditis continues to rise. In some cases endocarditis occurs after intrusive procedures such as dental procedures, minor surgery, gynecologic examinations, or insertion of indwelling urinary catheters. People at high risk include those who use illegal IV drugs, which can cause bacteremia from contaminated needles and syringes. Conditions predisposing people to infective endocarditis have changed because of decreasing incidence of rheumatic heart disease, increased recognition and treatment of mitral valve prolapse, the aging population with degenerative heart disease, and IV drug abuse (Lewis et al., 2007).

Clinical Manifestations

Endocarditis occurs in acute or subacute forms. Signs and symptoms progress either rapidly; in dangerous sequence during the acute phase; or gradually in the subacute phase, with damage occurring over a long period.

Assessment

Subjective data include patient complaints of influenza-like symptoms with recurrent fever, undue fatigue, chest pain, headaches, joint pain, and chills.

Collection of **objective data** may reveal the significant signs of petechiae in the conjunctiva, oral mucosa, neck, anterior chest, abdomen, and legs. Splinter hemorrhages (black longitudinal streaks) may occur in the nailbeds. Other signs are nontender macula on the palms and soles, plus tender erythematous, elevated nodules on the pads of the fingers and toes. Microemboli, vasculitis, and embolism are responsible for the development of these signs. They also have the potential to cause serious complications such as stroke and renal or splenic infarction (Holcomb, 2006). Weight loss may occur. Pulse is rapid. Infective endocarditis may cause a murmur, with the aortic and mitral valves most commonly affected.

Diagnostic Tests

ECG changes and chest radiographic examination reveal evidence of HF and cardiomegaly. TEE and digital imaging using two-dimensional transthoracic echograms can detect vegetation or thrombi and abscesses on valves. Laboratory findings indicate leukocytosis, increased ESR, anemia, and hyperglobulinemia. Blood cultures determine the causative organism, and sensitivity tests indicate the antibiotic needed for medical management.

Medical Management

The medical management of the patient with endocarditis includes support of cardiac function, destruction of the pathogen, and prevention of complications.

Embolization, a serious and common complication, can occur. An emboli may go to the brain, the lungs, the coronary arteries, the spleen, the bowel, and the extremities, with catastrophic results. The most frequent embolic events usually occur during the first

2 weeks of acute infective endocarditis. Anticoagulation is not recommended because of the risk of an intracerebral hemorrhage. A patient who was receiving anticoagulation therapy before developing endocarditis may continue therapy as long as neurologic function is carefully monitored (Holcomb, 2006).

Management relies on rest to decrease the heart's workload. Complete bed rest is usually not indicated unless the temperature remains elevated and there are signs of HF. After the blood cultures, massive doses of antibiotics are administered, usually parenterally, to combat the organism. Antibiotic therapy continues often as long as 1 to 2 months. Traditionally this has required a prolonged hospitalization for most patients, but with newer, more versatile antibiotics (and growing economic concerns), outpatient treatment of patients with infective endocarditis is more common.

Prophylactic antibiotic treatment is recommended for individuals who are considered at high risk for developing infective endocarditis. Patients at risk include those with previous valve surgery, preexisting valvular heart disease, or congenital abnormalities. Infective endocarditis precautions involve antibiotic therapy as prescribed by the physician before any invasive procedure such as dental work or minor surgery.

Surgical repair of diseased valves or prosthetic valve replacement may be necessary if the patient's condition is severe. Valve replacement has become an important adjunct procedure in the management of endocarditis. It is used in more than 25% of cases.

Nursing Interventions and Patient Teaching

The nursing interventions are based primarily on the signs and symptoms. Observe for petechiae, location of pain, vomiting, and fever, and report these signs and symptoms if observed.

During the acute phase, maintain the patient on decreased activity and provide a calm, quiet environment. Take vital signs, including apical pulse, every 4 hours. When increased activity or ambulation begins, assess pulse before and after to determine the effects on the heart muscle.

Ensuring adequate nutrition is important. Frequently patients have a decreased appetite because of the disease process. Provide attractive meals with supplemental between-meal nourishment. Promote rest and comfort and prevent further inflammation and infection during hospitalization.

Patient teaching focuses on identifying causes, infective endocarditis precautions, dietary requirements, and gradually increasing activity levels. Also advise the patient on the need for prophylactic antibiotics before any invasive procedure if the patient has preexisting valvular heart disease. Instruct the patient about signs and symptoms that may indicate recurrent infections such as fever, fatigue, malaise, and chills and the need to report any of these signs and symptoms to the physician.

Prognosis

Before the advent of antibiotics, patients with infective endocarditis could be expected to live approximately 1 year; prompt treatment with intensive antibiotic therapy will now cure about 90% of patients with this condition.

MYOCARDITIS

Acute myocarditis is relatively rare. Inflammation of the myocardium may originate from rheumatic heart disease; viral, bacterial, or fungal infection; or endocarditis or pericarditis. In the United States, most significant cases of acute myocarditis are caused by coxsackievirus type B (Holcomb, 2006). However, sometimes the cause may be unknown.

Signs and symptoms vary. The patient may have upper respiratory tract symptoms such as fever, chills, and sore throat; abdominal pain and nausea; vomiting; diarrhea; and myalgia. These generally occur up to 6 weeks before the patient has signs and symptoms of myocarditis, such as chest pain and overt HF with dyspnea (Holcomb, 2006). Cardiac enlargement, murmur, gallop, and tachycardia are typically seen in myocarditis. Cardiomyopathy may develop as a complication. Enlargement of the myocardium may result in dysrhythmias.

Useful tests to help diagnose myocarditis are chest x-ray, ECG, echocardiography, and endomyocardial biopsy (Holcomb, 2006).

Therapy is symptomatic and primarily follows the same approach as that of endocarditis: bed rest, oxygen, antibiotics, antiinflammatory agents, careful assessments, and correction of dysrhythmias.

The goals of treatment are to preserve myocardial function and to prevent HF and other serious complications such as dilated cardiomyopathy. Patients may recover, but may later develop cardiomyopathy. As a result, the disease may have a long, benign course, or it may result in sudden death during exercise.

CARDIOMYOPATHY

Etiology and Pathophysiology

Cardiomyopathy is a term used to describe a group of heart muscle diseases that primarily affect the structural or functional ability of the myocardium. This primary dysfunction is not associated with CAD, hypertension, vascular disease, or pulmonary disease.

When cardiomyopathies are classified by cause, two forms are recognized: primary and secondary. Primary cardiomyopathy consists of heart muscle disease of unknown cause and is classified as dilated, hypertrophic, or restrictive. **Dilated cardiomyopathy,** characterized by ventricular dilation, is the most common type of primary cardiomyopathy. **Hypertrophic cardiomyopathy** results in increased size and mass of the heart because of increased muscle thickness (especially of the septal wall) and decreased ventricular size. In **restrictive cardiomyopathy** the ventricular walls are rigid, thus limiting the ventricles' ability to expand and resulting in impaired diastolic filling (Chojnowski, 2004). Secondary cardiomyopathy has a number of types: (1) infective (viral, bacterial, fungal, or protozoal myocarditis); (2) metabolic; (3) severe nutritional deprivation; (4) alcohol (large quantities consumed over many years leading to dilated cardiomyopathy); (5) peripartum (unexplained cause; may develop in last month of pregnancy or within first few months after delivery); (6) drugs (doxorubicin [Adriamycin] or other medications); (7) radiation therapy; (8) systemic lupus erythematosus; (9) rheumatoid arthritis; and (10) "crack" heart, caused by cocaine abuse.

Cardiomyopathy caused by cocaine abuse is seen more frequently now than ever before. Cocaine causes intense vasoconstriction of the coronary arteries and peripheral vasoconstriction, resulting in hypertension. This can result in increased myocardial oxygen needs and decreased oxygen supply to the myocardium and can lead to acute MI or ischemic cardiomyopathy. Cocaine also causes high circulating levels of catecholamines, which may further damage myocardial cells, leading to ischemic or dilated cardiomyopathy. The cardiomyopathy produced is difficult to treat. Interventions deal mainly with the HF that ensues (Lewis et al., 2007). The prognosis is poor.

Clinical Manifestations

Angina, syncope, fatigue, and dyspnea on exertion are common signs and symptoms. The most common symptom is severe exercise intolerance. The patient may have signs and symptoms of both left-sided and right-sided HF, including dyspnea, peripheral edema, ascites, and hepatic dysfunction.

Diagnostic Tests

Diagnosis of cardiomyopathy is made by the patient's clinical manifestations and noninvasive and invasive cardiac procedures to rule out other causes of dysfunction. Diagnostic studies include ECG, chest radiograph, echocardiogram, CT scan, nuclear imaging studies, MUGA scanning, cardiac catheterization, and endomyocardial biopsy.

Medical Management

Medical management consists of treatment of underlying cause and HF management to slow the progression of the disease and symptoms. Medications may include diuretics, ACE inhibitors, antidysrhythmics, and beta-adrenergic blockers. An automatic internal defibrillator is occasionally implanted. In patients with advanced disease that is not responding to medical treatment, cardiac transplantation should be considered. Educate the patient about avoiding strenuous exercise because of the risk of sudden death.

Cardiac Transplantation

The first heart transplant was performed in 1967. Since that time, heart transplantation has become the treatment of choice for patients with end-stage heart disease who are unlikely to survive the next 6 to 12 months. Patients with cardiomyopathy account for more than 50% of cardiac transplant recipients. Dilated cardiomyopathy is the most common type of cardiomyopathy requiring transplantation. Inoperable CAD is the second most common indication for transplantation, accounting for 40% of candidates (Box 8-6).

Once a patient meets the criteria for cardiac transplantation, the goal of the evaluation process is to identify patients who would most benefit from a new heart. In addition to the physical examination, psychological assessment of candidates is valuable. A complete history of coping abilities, family support system, and motivation to follow through with the transplant and the rigorous transplantation regimen is essential. The complexity of the transplant process may be overwhelming to a patient with inadequate support systems and a poor understanding of the lifestyle changes required after transplant.

Once potential recipients are placed on the transplant list, they may wait at home and receive ongoing medical care if their medical condition is stable. If their condition is not stable, they may require hospitalization for more intensive therapy. Unfortunately, the overall waiting period for a transplant is long, and many patients die while waiting for a transplant.

Donor and recipient matching is based on body and heart size and ABO type. Tissue crossmatching between donor and recipient is generally not done because of difficulty in obtaining good matches and lack of correlation between match and outcome.

Most donor hearts are obtained at locations distant from the institution performing the transplant. The

---

Box 8-6   Indications and Contraindications for Cardiac Transplantation

INDICATIONS

- Suitable physiologic and chronologic age
- End-stage heart disease that is not responding to medical therapy
- Dilated cardiomyopathy
- Inoperable coronary artery disease
- Vigorous and healthy individual (except for end-stage cardiac disease) who would benefit from procedure
- Compliance with medical regimens
- Demonstrated emotional stability and social support system
- Financial resources available

CONTRAINDICATIONS

- Systemic disease with poor prognosis
- Active infection
- Active or recent malignancy
- Diabetes mellitus type 1, with end-organ damage
- Recent or unresolved pulmonary infarction
- Severe pulmonary hypertension unrelieved with medication
- Severe cerebrovascular or peripheral vascular disease
- Irreversible renal or hepatic dysfunction
- Active peptic ulcer disease
- Severe osteoporosis
- Severe obesity
- History of drug or alcohol abuse or mental illness

maximum acceptable ischemic time for cardiac transplant is 4 to 6 hours.

The recipient is prepared for surgery, and cardiopulmonary bypass is used. The usual surgical procedure involves removing the recipient's heart, except for the posterior right and left atrial walls and their venous connections. The recipient's heart is then replaced with the donor heart, which has been trimmed to match. Care is taken to preserve the integrity of the donor SA node so that a sinus rhythm can be achieved postoperatively.

Immunosuppressive therapy usually begins in the operating room. Regimens vary but usually include azathioprine (Imuran), corticosteroids, and cyclosporine. Cyclosporine was first used in heart transplantation in 1980. Currently it is used with corticosteroids for maintenance immunosuppression. Its use has reduced rejection and also slowed the rejection process so that early treatment can be instituted.

The postoperative care is similar to that of other open-heart surgeries. Endomyocardial biopsies via the right internal jugular vein are performed periodically to detect rejection. In addition, peripheral blood T-lymphocyte monitoring is done to assess the recipient's immune status.

Because the patient is immunosuppressed, nursing interventions involve prevention of infection, which is the leading cause of death in this population. Many deaths from infection occur during augmented immunosuppressive therapy for acute rejection episodes. Provide a great deal of emotional support and teaching for both the patient and the family, since transplantation is a last resort. In addition, the patient is often a long distance from home and significant others.

Advances in surgical technique and postoperative care have improved early survival rates after cardiac transplantation. Attention is directed toward improvements in immunosuppression and management of long-term complications. Nursing management focuses on promoting patient adaptation to the transplant process, monitoring, managing lifestyle changes, and educating the patient and the family. Ongoing data collection and research continue in regard to quality of life, functional level, and rehabilitation of the cardiac transplant recipient (Lewis et al., 2007).

Nursing Interventions and Patient Teaching
Nursing interventions focus on relieving symptoms, observing for and preventing complications, and providing emotional and psychological support. Monitor the response to medications and monitor for dysrhythmias. Teach patients to adjust their lifestyle to avoid strenuous activity and dehydration. Instruct patients to space activities and allow for rest periods.

Prognosis
Most patients have a severe, progressively deteriorating course, and the majority (particularly those older than 55 years of age) die within 2 years of the onset of signs and symptoms. However, improvement or stabilization occurs in a minority of patients. Death is due to either HF or ventricular dysrhythmia. Sudden death resulting from dysrhythmia is a constant threat.

DISORDERS OF THE PERIPHERAL VASCULAR SYSTEM

Peripheral vascular disease is any abnormal condition that affects the blood vessels outside the heart and the lymphatic vessels. The word peripheral means pertaining to the outside, surface, or surrounding area. The peripheral vascular system consists of arteries, capillaries, and veins. This system supplies oxygen-rich blood to the upper and lower extremities of the body, and returns blood and carbon dioxide from those areas to the heart and lungs. Disorders of the peripheral vascular system occur when circulation to the upper and lower extremities is compromised.

NORMAL AGING PATTERNS
Degenerative changes occur in the vascular system as part of the normal aging process. These changes affect the walls of the blood vessels and lead to problems in the transport of blood and nutrients to the tissues. The inner walls of the blood vessels (tunica interna) become thick and less compliant. The middle walls of the blood vessels (tunica media) become less elastic. With marked decreases in the elasticity and flexibility of the vessels, peripheral vascular resistance increases, causing a rise in blood pressure and increasing a person's susceptibility to peripheral vascular disease (see Life Span Considerations box).

RISK FACTORS
Risk factors for peripheral vascular disorders are similar to those for cardiovascular disorders. An important aspect of caring for the patient with a peripheral vascular disorder is understanding the risk factors and incorporating them into patient teaching.

Nonmodifiable Factors
Age
As a person ages, arteriosclerotic changes in the peripheral vascular system lead to increased peripheral vascular resistance and decreased blood flow to the tissues.

Gender
Men are more susceptible than women to arteriosclerotic changes. This gender difference decreases after menopause, when the effects of estrogen are no longer present.

Family History
A family history of atherosclerosis increases an individual's risk.

Modifiable Factors

Smoking

Smoking is one of the major contributing factors in the development of peripheral vascular problems. The nicotine in cigarettes causes vasoconstriction and spasms of the arteries, elevates blood pressure, and reduces circulation to the extremities. The carbon monoxide inhaled in cigarette smoke reduces oxygen transport to the tissues.

Hypertension

Increased blood pressure causes wear and damage to the inner arterial walls, resulting in a buildup of fibrous tissue. This in turn leads to further narrowing of the vessel and increased resistance to blood flow.

Hyperlipidemia

An elevation in serum cholesterol and triglycerides contributes to the buildup of plaque inside the blood vessels. The patient should maintain a diet with decreased saturated fat and cholesterol. If serum cholesterol remains elevated, drug therapy must be considered.

Obesity

Excessive body weight and body fat contribute to the severity of other risk factors. Extra weight in relation to bone structure and height places an increased workload on the heart and blood vessels and may contribute to congestion in the venous system.

Lack of Exercise

Decreased activity may compromise the peripheral vascular system because of a lack of muscle tone. The contraction and relaxation of muscles facilitate the return of blood in the veins to the heart and the lungs. A sedentary person does not realize the benefits of regular physical activity, such as weight and stress reduction and improved vascular tone.

Emotional Stress

Stress contributes to increased blood pressure, increased production of cholesterol, and increased vasoconstriction of the blood vessels.

Diabetes Mellitus

Uncontrolled elevated serum glucose levels contribute to the atherosclerotic process, although the exact mechanism by which diabetes mellitus leads to peripheral vascular disorders is unknown. Elevated serum glucose levels result in circulatory disorders.

ASSESSMENT

Arterial Assessment

The first symptom of decreased arterial circulation is pain from arterial insufficiency and ischemia. Arterial insufficiency occurs when not enough blood is available or able to flow through the arteries to body tissues. Ischemia occurs when the tissue does not receive enough oxygen-rich blood to function normally. Ischemic pain in the lower extremities is usually a dull ache in the calf muscles. It is often accompanied by leg fatigue and cramping. The pain is brought on by exercise and relieved by rest. It is referred to as **intermittent claudication** (a weakness of the legs accompanied by cramplike pains in the calves caused by poor circulation of the arterial blood to the leg muscles). Pain may also be felt in the thighs and buttocks. As arterial disease progresses and becomes chronic, pain occurs even at rest. Burning, tingling, and numbness of the legs may occur at night while the patient is lying down.

Other nursing assessments include palpating and comparing pulses in the extremities. Pulses may be weak, thready, or absent in the affected extremity because of decreased blood flow. Several scales are used to measure pulses. To ensure that the patient's pulses are graded the same way each time, all the nurses should use the same scale, such as the following:

0 Absent

+1 Barely palpable, intermittent

+2 Weak, possibly thready, but constantly palpable and with consistent quality

+3 Normal strength and quality

+4 Bounding, easily palpable, may be visible

A Doppler ultrasound device may be needed to check the patient's pulses if pulmonary vascular disease (PVD), low blood pressure, edema, or large amounts of subcutaneous tissue impede the assessment. If a Doppler device is used, record pulsation as **present** or **absent** rather than using the numeric scale. For future reference, use a skin marker to indicate where the pulse is present (Willis, 2001). Check the affected extremity and compare it with the unaffected extremity for color, temperature, skin characteristics, and capillary refill time (Box 8-7).

For a uniform assessment and documentation technique for **veins** and **arteries,** the following mnemonic device, PATCHES, is helpful (Willis, 2001):

P for **pulses:** Assess the patient's affected extremity first. Then assess the apical pulse and bilateral temporal, carotid, brachial, radial, femoral, popliteal, posterior tibial, and dorsalis pedis pulses. Absence of pulses is generally a medical emergency that requires immediate treatment, but in some cases it may be normal. Compare the find-

---

Box 8-7	Capillary Refill Time

1. Apply pressure to a toenail or fingernail for several seconds until it blanches (the area loses its color).
2. Relieve the pressure.
3. Note the amount of time it takes for the color to return.
   —The color should return almost instantly—in less than 2 seconds.
   —With an arterial disorder, it will take more than 2 seconds for the color to return.

ings with previous ones or correlate them with the patient's signs and symptoms.

A for **appearance:** Note whether the extremity is pale, mottled, cyanotic, or discolored red, black, or brown. Document areas of necrosis or bleeding and the size, depth, and location of ulcers. When assessing ulcers, note whether the edges are jagged or smooth and whether the area is painful to touch.

Shiny skin often marks the presence of edema; a dull appearance may signal inadequate arterial blood supply. Look for superficial veins, erythema, or inflammation anywhere on the affected extremity. Standing allows the saphenous veins to fill, so varicosities in the saphenous system are best evaluated with the patient standing. If a line of color change is present, mark it with a skin marker and monitor for changes in location.

T for **temperature:** If the patient has an arterial problem, the affected extremity will feel cool; if the problem is venous, the extremity will feel normal or abnormally warm. However, problems in arteries and veins are not the only reasons for temperature changes in an extremity; aortoiliac disease, HF, hypovolemia, pulmonary embolism, and other conditions can also affect skin temperature by interfering with peripheral blood flow.

C for **capillary refill:** Capillary refill is normally less than 2 seconds, but it may be extended when the patient has PVD. Press on a nail until the nailbed blanches, then release and count how many seconds it takes for normal color to return. Other sites to check capillary refill are the pads of the toes and fingers, the heel, and the thenar eminence on the palm of the hand proximal to the thumb. Although abnormal capillary refill is not diagnostic in itself, it adds valuable data to the assessment (see Box 8-7).

H for **hardness:** Palpate the extremity to determine whether the tissues are supple or hard and inelastic. Hardness may indicate longstanding PVD, chronic venous insufficiency, lymphedema, or chronic edema. Hardened subcutaneous skin also increases the risk of stasis ulcers.

E for **edema:** Pitting edema frequently indicates an acute process, and nonpitting edema may be seen with chronic conditions, such as venous insufficiency. Assess both extremities for edema and compare and document the findings.

To assess for pitting edema, gently press the skin on the affected extremity for at least 5 seconds. Release and grade pitting as follows: +1, 2-mm indentation; +2, 4-mm indentation; +3, 6-mm indentation; and +4, 8-mm indentation (see Figure 8-17). The most accurate way to determine the degree of nonpitting edema is to measure the circumference of the extremity and compare measurements with the other extremity and sub-

sequent measurements. Measure at the point of edema, and then mark the point with a skin marker so everyone will assess the same area. Accuracy is greatest if the measurements are taken at the same time every day, preferably in the morning before the patient ambulates.

S for **sensation:** Vascular discomfort can originate in arteries, in veins, or in the microcirculation if the patient has diabetes mellitus. In addition to asking the patient about pain, ask if he or she has other abnormal sensations, such as numbness or tingling. Tingling or tenderness can result from peripheral tissue ischemia, and the patient may say the extremity feels abnormally hot or cold (Willis, 2001).

Venous Assessment

Decreased venous circulation leads to edema. When the venous system does not return sufficient blood from the tissues to the heart and the lungs (venous insufficiency), excess fluid is left in the tissues of the affected extremity (edema). Assess for edema in the affected extremity and compare it with the unaffected extremity.

Venous insufficiency may lead to changes in skin pigmentation. Assess the skin for darker pigmentation, dryness, and scaling in the affected extremity. Chronic edema and stasis of blood from venous insufficiency may lead to ulceration of the tissues. These ulcers are referred to as **stasis ulcers.** Peripheral pulses are usually present with venous insufficiency. Pain, aching, and cramping associated with venous disorders are usually relieved by activity and/or elevating the extremity. Refer to Table 8-10 for a comparison of signs and symptoms associated with arterial and venous disorders.

Diagnostic Tests

Diagnostic tests for peripheral vascular disorders include noninvasive procedures and invasive procedures.

Noninvasive procedures include the following:

- **Treadmill test:** This exercise test is used to determine blood flow in the extremities after exercising. It identifies pain associated with exercise such as claudication.
- **Plethysmography:** Plethysmography is used to assess changes in blood volume in the veins of the calf or other body extremities.
- **Digital subtraction angiography:** Initially an IV contrast solution is administered. This allows blood vessels in the extremities to be visualized by radiography using an image intensifier video system and a television monitor.
- **Doppler ultrasound:** A Doppler ultrasound flowmeter measures blood flow in arteries or veins to assess intermittent claudication, obstruction of deep veins, and other disorders of peripheral veins and arteries.

Table 8-10   Comparison of Signs and Symptoms Associated with Arterial and Venous Disorders

SIGNS AND SYMPTOMS	ARTERIAL DISORDER	VENOUS DISORDER
Pain	Aching to sharp cramping; brought on by exercise; relieved by rest	Aching to cramping pain; relieved by activity or elevating extremity
Pulses	Diminished or absent	Usually present
Edema	Usually absent	Usually present; increases at the end of the day and when extremity is in a dependent position
Skin changes	Cool or cold Dry, shiny Hairless Pallor develops with elevation; becomes erythematous with dangling	Warm, thick, and toughened Darkened pigmentation Stasis ulcers

Invasive procedures include the following:

- **Venography:** A contrast medium is administered through a catheter placed in a foot vein. Films are taken to detect filling defects. Venography is the gold standard to assess the condition of the deep leg veins and to diagnose deep-vein thrombosis (DVT). Venography is invasive, is costly, can be unpleasant, and may cause phlebitis. Other diagnostic tests may be used to diagnose DVT.
- **Angiography:** This is done by injection of a contrast medium intravascularly and then visualizing the arteries using radiography.
- **D-dimer:** A serum test. D-dimer is a product of fibrin degradation (change to a less complex form). When a thrombus is present, plasma D-dimer concentrations are usually greater than 1591 ng/mL. The normal range for D-dimer is 68 to 494 ng/mL.
- **Duplex scanning:** This is a combination of ultrasound imaging techniques and Doppler capabilities to determine location and extent of thrombi within veins (most widely used test to diagnose DVT).

HYPERTENSION

Hypertension is considered with peripheral vascular disorders, since it is a risk factor in atherosclerosis, which leads to peripheral vascular disease.

Etiology and Pathophysiology

Normal blood pressure is a reading of less than 120 mm Hg systolic and 80 mm Hg diastolic. Hypertension (or high blood pressure) occurs when a sustained elevated systolic blood pressure is greater than 140 mm Hg and/or a sustained elevated diastolic blood pressure is greater than 90 mm Hg. Stage 1 hypertension is defined as a systolic blood pressure of 140 to 159 mm Hg or a diastolic blood pressure of 90 to 99 mm Hg. Stage 2 and Stage 3 hypertension have been combined into a single category, called stage 2, that is defined as a systolic blood pressure of 160 mm Hg or higher or a diastolic of 100 mm Hg or higher (Wright, 2006). A diagnosis is not based on a one-time elevated blood pressure reading, but on an average of two or more elevated blood pressure readings taken on separate occasions. The guidelines adapted from the Seventh Report of the Joint National Committee on Prevention, Detection, Evaluation, and Treatment of High Blood Pressure, National Institutes of Health, National Heart, Lung, and Blood Institute, May 2003, identify people with a blood pressure of 120 to 139 mm Hg systolic or 80 to 89 mm Hg diastolic as being prehypertensive. People whose blood pressure is in the prehypertensive range are at twice the risk for developing hypertension as people with normal values. The prehypertensive category was created to help patients understand the considerable health risks associated with small increases in blood pressure. Every 20/10 mm Hg increase in blood pressure doubles the risk for cardiovascular events for people ages 40 to 70 (Wright, 2006). Although there is no way of predicting who will develop high blood pressure, hypertension can be detected easily.

Approximately 60 million Americans have hypertension, and an additional 25 million have prehypertension. It has been estimated that up to 30% of the adult population in the United States have undiagnosed hypertension. It is difficult to determine exact numbers because most people are symptom free.

Arterial blood pressure is the pressure exerted by the blood on the walls of blood vessels. Systolic blood pressure is the greatest force caused by the contraction of the left ventricle of the heart. Diastolic blood pressure occurs during the relaxation phase between heartbeats. Blood flow is determined by the amount of blood the heart pumps with each contraction and how fast the heart beats. Peripheral vascular resistance is affected by the diameter of the blood vessel and the viscosity of the blood. Blood flow and peripheral vascular resistance play an important role in regulating blood pressure. Increased peripheral vascular resistance resulting from vasoconstriction, or narrowing of peripheral blood vessels, is a common factor in hypertension.

Vasoconstriction and vasodilation are controlled by the sympathetic nervous system and the renin-angiotensin system of the kidney. Stimulation of the sympathetic nervous system and the release of epinephrine and/or norepinephrine cause blood vessel constriction and increased peripheral vascular resistance. The activation of the renin-angiotensin system occurs with decreased blood flow to the kidney. Renin leads to the formation of angiotensin, which is a potent vasoconstrictor. Angiotensin stimulates the secretion of aldosterone, leading to the retention of sodium and water. The result is an increase in blood pressure.

The two main types of hypertension are **essential (primary)** hypertension and **secondary** hypertension. The incidence of hypertension increases with age and other risk factors.

Essential (Primary) Hypertension

Essential (primary) hypertension makes up 90% to 95% of all diagnosed cases. Although there is no general agreement on the cause of essential hypertension, theories to explain the mechanisms involved include arteriolar changes, sympathetic nervous system activation, hormonal influence (renin-angiotensin-aldosterone system stimulation), genetic factors, greater-than-ideal body weight, sedentary lifestyle, increased sodium intake, and excessive alcohol intake. For a long time many experts believed that an increase in systolic blood pressure was a normal part of aging. In fact, some believed that "100 mm Hg plus the patient's age" was a tolerable systolic blood pressure in the older adult. Treatment for hypertension was based primarily on the diastolic reading, and isolated systolic hypertension (ISH) was often not treated.

Clinical trials have re-emphasized that ISH is believed to raise the risk of cardiovascular disease and stroke (Gennari & Gennari, 2000). ISH is actually a better overall predictor of cardiovascular morbidity and mortality than diastolic pressure. (Diastolic pressure remains the better predictor of CAD in people younger than 45 years.) ISH is defined as an elevated systolic blood pressure of 140 mm Hg or more with a diastolic blood pressure below 90 mm Hg. The value of treating ISH in older patients has only recently been established, but now those findings are widely circulated.

Prognosis

With prolonged untreated essential hypertension, the elastic tissue in the arterioles is replaced by fibrous tissue. This process leads to decreased tissue perfusion and deterioration, especially in the target organs—the heart, the kidney, and the brain. CAD and cerebrovascular accident (stroke), the great causes of death and disability, are much more frequent in those who have elevated blood pressure than in those who are normotensive. With treatment, the prognosis is usually good. Risk factors that contribute to the development of essential hypertension are listed in Box 8-8.

Secondary Hypertension

Secondary hypertension is attributed to an identifiable medical diagnosis. Conditions associated with secondary hypertension are given in Table 8-11.

Box 8-8 **Risk Factors for Essential Hypertension**

NONMODIFIABLE RISK FACTORS
- **Age:** Risk increased as age advances past 30 years old
- **Gender:** Men more at risk than women
- **Race:** Risk twice as high in blacks as in whites
- **Family history:** Risk increased with a family history of hypertension

MODIFIABLE RISK FACTORS
- **Smoking:** Nicotine constricts blood vessels
- **Obesity:** Associated with increased blood volume
- **High-sodium diet:** Increases water retention, which increases blood volume
- **Elevated serum cholesterol:** Leads to atherosclerosis and narrowing of blood vessels
- **Oral contraceptives or estrogen therapy:** May contribute to elevated blood pressure
- **Alcohol:** Increases plasma catecholamines (biologically active amines, epinephrine, and norepinephrine), which leads to blood vessel constriction
- **Emotional stress:** Stimulates the sympathetic nervous system, which leads to blood vessel constriction
- **Sedentary lifestyle:** Regular exercise helps lower blood pressure over time

---

Table 8-11 **Causes of Secondary Hypertension**

CONDITION OR DISORDER	MECHANISM
Renal vascular disease	Kidney disease (glomerulonephritis, renal failure, renal artery stenosis, physiologic changes related to type of disease) affects renin and sodium and results in hypertension
Diseases of the adrenal cortex • Primary aldosteronism • Cushing's syndrome • Pheochromocytoma	Atherosclerotic changes in renal arteries cause increase in peripheral vascular resistance Increase in aldosterone causes sodium and water retention and increases blood volume Increase in blood volume Excess secretion of catecholamines increases peripheral vascular resistance
Coarctation of the aorta	Causes marked elevated blood pressure in upper extremities with decreased perfusion in lower extremities
Head trauma or cranial tumor	Increased intracranial pressure reduces cerebral blood flow and stimulates medulla oblongata to raise blood pressure
Pregnancy-induced hypertension	Cause unknown; generalized vasospasm may be a contributing factor

Prognosis

In most instances, secondary hypertension subsides when the primary disease process is treated or corrected.

Malignant Hypertension

Malignant hypertension is a severe, rapidly progressive elevation in blood pressure (diastolic pressure greater than 120 mm Hg) that causes damage to the small arterioles in major organs (heart, kidneys, brain, eyes). A primary distinguishing finding is inflammation of arterioles (arteriolitis) in the eyes. This type of hypertension is most common in black men under 40 years of age.

Prognosis

Unless medical treatment is successful, the course is rapidly fatal. The most common causes of death are MI, HF, stroke, and renal failure.

Clinical Manifestations

Hypertension is essentially a disease without symptoms until vascular changes occur in the heart, the brain, the eyes, or the kidneys. Longstanding, untreated hypertension can cause target organ damage. Advanced target organ damage may account for left ventricular hypertrophy, angina pectoris, MI, HF, stroke or transient ischemic attack, nephropathy, peripheral arterial disease, or retinopathy. Signs and symptoms usually occur as a result of advanced hypertension. These signs and symptoms may include awakening with a headache, blurred vision, and spontaneous epistaxis (nosebleed).

Assessment

Collection of **subjective data** includes assessing for morning headache in the occipital area and blurred vision. Assess the patient for risk factors (see Box 8-8). Determine the patient's understanding of hypertension, including the definition, meaning of systolic and diastolic readings, complications of hypertension, and possible concerns regarding treatment.

Collection of **objective data** includes measuring the blood pressure in both arms with the patient in supine and sitting positions. Compare the reading with previous blood pressure results. Take two or more blood pressure measurements on two separate occasions. Also measure and record height and weight. Assess and record heart sounds, and palpate and record peripheral pulses.

Diagnostic Tests

Diagnostic tests associated with hypertension evaluate the functions of the brain, the heart, and the kidneys. The results indicate the effects of hypertension on these organs and provide baseline information for future reference. These tests include CBC; serum levels of sodium, potassium, calcium, and magnesium; lipid profile; fasting blood glucose level; creatinine, BUN, urinalysis, and IV pyelography (effect on kidneys); re-

nal arteriography (the gold standard for confirming renal artery stenosis); and chest radiography, ECG, and possible echocardiography (effect on heart).

Medical Management

Medical management is directed at controlling hypertension and preventing complications. The goal in older adults is to keep the blood pressure at less than 140/90 mm Hg. The general goal for younger adults with mild hypertension is to achieve blood pressure of less than 130/80 mm Hg. Treatment is based on the severity of the hypertension, associated risk factors, and damage to major organs. Antihypertensive medications and nonpharmacologic measures are used to lower blood pressure.

Drug Therapy

For stage 1 or 2 hypertension, drug treatments may include the following (Lewis et al., 2007):

- Diuretics (thiazides, loop diuretics, potassium-sparing drugs)
- Beta-adrenergic blockers such as metoprolol, nadolol, propranolol, acebutolol (Sectral), atenolol, bisoprolol (Zebeta), timolol
- ACE inhibitors such as captopril, enalapril, lisinopril
- Angiotensin II receptor blockers such as valsartan, losartan, irbesartan, candesartan (Atacand), telmisartan (Micard)
- Calcium channel blockers such as diltiazem, amlodipine, nifedipine, felodipine (Plendil), verapamil
- Alpha-agonists such as clonidine
- Aliskiren hemifumarate (Tekturna), the first antihypertensive drug that is a direct renin inhibitor; decreases plasma renin activity and inhibits the conversion of angiotensinogen to angiotensin I (Hussar, 2008)

Special considerations include using ACE inhibitors for diabetes mellitus; using ACE inhibitors and diuretics for HF; using beta blockers and ACE inhibitors for MI; using calcium channel blockers and diuretics for blacks; and using diuretics and long-acting calcium channel blockers for older adults with ISH.

Nonpharmacologic Therapy

Nonpharmacologic therapy for hypertension includes the following:

- **Lose excess weight.** Being overweight is associated with increased blood pressure, abnormally high blood lipid levels, diabetes mellitus, and CAD. Limiting calorie intake and increasing physical exercise are the keys to losing weight.
- **Exercise regularly.** Thirty to 45 minutes of aerobic exercise three or four times a week—helps decrease the risk of hypertension and cardiovascular disease.
- **Reduce saturated fat.** A patient with high blood lipid levels may require dietary modification or drug therapy to normalize them. A cardinal

rule is to limit fat intake to less than 30% of total calories. According to the Dietary Approaches to Stop Hypertension (DASH) study, a low-fat diet rich in fruits and vegetables is recommended(www.webmd.com/hypertension-high-blood-pressure/dash-diet).

- **Consume enough potassium, calcium, and magnesium.** Plenty of potassium in the diet helps decrease blood pressure, so eating potassium-rich fruits and vegetables may improve blood pressure control. Administering potassium supplements to a patient who is hypokalemic as a result of diuretic therapy also combats hypertension. A word of caution: Anyone receiving ACE inhibitors or potassium-sparing diuretics should receive potassium supplements only with extreme caution and close monitoring for hyperkalemia. Low dietary calcium and magnesium may contribute to hypertension (http://www.dashdiet.org); the National Heart, Lung, and Blood Institute suggests consuming adequate amounts of calcium and magnesium but does not recommend supplementation to combat hypertension.
- **Limit alcohol intake.** Excessive alcohol consumption may contribute to hypertension. A man of normal weight should not drink more than 1 ounce of ethanol per day (the equivalent of 24 ounces of beer, 10 ounces of wine, or 2 ounces of 100-proof whiskey). Women and lightweight men should restrict their intake to half this amount.
- **Reduce sodium intake.** High sodium intake can increase blood pressure, especially in blacks, older adult patients with existing hypertension, and patients with diabetes mellitus. It is recommended limiting sodium intake to 2.4 g/day. Encourage your patient to eat unsalted, unprocessed foods and to read labels when shopping.
- **Stop smoking.** Cigarette smoking is one of the leading risk factors for hypertension and heart disease. Smoking also inhibits the effect of antihypertensive medication, so techniques for stopping are an integral part of patient education. Counseling, support groups, and aids to stop smoking are effective. Because many people who stop smoking gain weight, make certain a weight management and exercise program is part of the plan.
- **Use relaxation techniques and stress management.** Stress management and relaxation techniques have also been shown to offset hypertension and its symptoms.

Nursing Interventions and Patient Teaching

The main focus of nursing interventions is to maintain blood pressure management through patient teaching about hypertension, risk factors, and drug therapy. Patient compliance is improved with education about side effects of medications, dietary instruction, exercise, and stress-reduction techniques (Box 8-9).

Box 8-9	**Measures to Increase Compliance with Antihypertensive Therapy**

- Be certain that patient understands that absence of symptoms does not indicate control of blood pressure; remind patient that symptoms do not occur until advanced stages of the disease.
- Advise patient against abrupt withdrawal of medication; rebound hypertension can occur.
- Encourage patient to discuss unpleasant side effects of medication with a health care professional.
- If remembering to take medications is a problem, discuss alternate ways to remember, such as taking them with certain meals or placing medication in separate containers labeled with times of day.
- Suggest patient participate in an exercise program with a friend or pay for the program (more likely to participate "to get money's worth").
- Include family and significant others in the teaching process to provide support and promote adherence to regimen.
- Explain reason for regular health care follow-up (high blood pressure is a chronic disorder).
- Contact patients who consistently cancel follow-up appointments.

Nursing diagnoses and interventions for the patient with hypertension include but are not limited to the following:

Nursing Diagnoses	Nursing Interventions
Knowledge, deficient, related to: • disease process • therapeutic management	Assess level of understanding. Implement teaching plan for hypertension: • Disease process, risk factors • Prescribed medications and side effects; proper dosage and administration; necessity of taking medication, even when blood pressure readings are normal • Dietary restrictions • Exercise program • Relaxation techniques • Sexual dysfunction as a potential side effect of adrenergic inhibitors • Compliance with therapy and follow-up appointments Encourage the patient to promptly report any problems to health care professionals for counseling.

ARTERIAL DISORDERS

ARTERIOSCLEROSIS AND ATHEROSCLEROSIS

Arteriosclerosis (a common arterial disorder characterized by thickening, loss of elasticity, and calcification of arterial walls, resulting in a decreased blood supply) is the underlying problem associated with peripheral vascular disorders. **Arteriosclerosis** and **atherosclerosis** are frequently used interchangeably.

Atherosclerosis is characterized by yellowish plaques of cholesterol, lipids, and cellular debris in the inner layers of the walls of large and medium-sized arteries. The result is narrowing of the artery and reduced nutrients and oxygen reaching the tissue, resulting in ischemia to the tissue cells. The arterial wall also loses its elasticity and becomes less responsive to change in blood volume and pressure. Once plaque is formed in the arteries, it is thought to be irreversible. Lesions in the arteries formed from plaque may completely occlude an artery. Atherosclerosis can progress to obstruction, thrombosis, aneurysm, and rupture.

When the need for oxygen in the tissues exceeds the supply, ischemia occurs and may result in cell death and tissue necrosis. The degree of reduction in blood flow and oxygen determines the amount of ischemia and necrosis that occurs. Specific peripheral vascular disorders that stem from arteriosclerosis and atherosclerosis are discussed individually in this chapter.

PERIPHERAL ARTERIAL DISEASE OF THE LOWER EXTREMITIES

Etiology and Pathophysiology

PAD of the lower extremities is accompanied by narrowing or occlusion of the intima and the media of the blood vessel walls. Plaque, as a result of the arteriosclerotic process, forms on the internal wall of the blood vessel, causing partial or complete occlusion. The result is little or no blood flow to the affected extremity. The artery is unable to supply blood and oxygen to the tissues whether the patient is exercising or at rest. Thus signs and symptoms associated with tissue ischemia appear.

Patients with PAD have atherosclerosis of the coronary and carotid arteries. The most common arteries affected in PAD of the lower extremities are the iliac, common femoral arteries, and superficial femoral arteries. Patients with diabetes mellitus are especially prone to develop PAD below the knees. Arteries involved are the distal popliteal, anterior tibial, posterior tibial, and peroneal arteries (Figure 8-18) (Lewis et al., 2007).

Clinical Manifestations

The severity of the signs and symptoms of PAD depends on the location and the extent of the atherosclerosis and on the amount of collateral circulation.

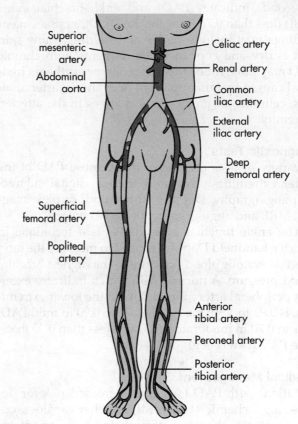

FIGURE 8-18 Common anatomic locations of atherosclerotic lesions (shown in yellow) of the abdominal aorta and lower extremities.

Pain is the first symptom that occurs from tissue ischemia. The pain generally occurs in the affected extremity in conjunction with sustained activity (see Table 8-6). This is because the demand of the tissue exceeds the available blood supply. The process of activity → ischemia → pain in an affected extremity is referred to as **claudication.** The pain of claudication subsides with rest; therefore it is frequently referred to as *intermittent claudication* (a weakness of the legs accompanied by cramping pains in the calves caused by poor circulation of the blood to the muscles). A burning pain at rest or at night occurs when the disease process is severe. Symptoms of coldness, numbness, and tingling may be associated with the pain. The signs and symptoms to watch for include the classic five P's of arterial occlusion: **pain, pulselessness, pallor, paresthesia,** and **paralysis.**

Assessment

Collection of **subjective data** focuses on pain associated with intermittent claudication. Does the pain occur with activity, and is it relieved by rest? Does pain occur at rest?

Collection of **objective data** includes assessment of pulses in the affected extremity, which may be weak or absent; comparison with pulses in the unaffected extremity; and assessment of capillary refill (more than

3 seconds indicates PAD) and ankle-brachial index (ABI) (less than 0.70 indicates PAD). Other assessment findings may include pallor and hairless, shiny skin that is dry and cool to touch. Patients with chronic PAD may have rubor (discoloration or erythema [redness] caused by inflammation) or cyanosis, arterial ulcers, cellulitis, or gangrenous changes in the affected extremity.

Diagnostic Tests

A variety of tests are useful to diagnose PAD of the lower extremities. Treadmill testing, digital subtraction angiography, Doppler ultrasound, duplex imaging, MRI, and angiography are likely choices.

The ankle brachial index (ABI) is a technique in which a handheld Doppler is used to measure the ratio of ankle systolic blood pressure to the highest brachial blood pressure. A normal ABI, which indicates excellent peripheral artery blood flow to the lower extremities, is 0.91 to 1.30; the ABI is 0.71 to 0.90 in mild PAD, 0.41 to 0.70 in moderate PAD, and less than 0.40 in severe PAD (Lewis et al., 2007).

Medical Management

A patient with PAD is also at increased risk for developing ischemic stroke, MI, or other cardiovascular problems; therefore the goals of treatment include decreasing the risk of cardiovascular disease and ischemic stroke (Belch, 2003; Treat-Jackson et al., 2003). Smoking cessation is an important aspect of treatment to decrease lower extremity ischemia in PAD and reduce the risk of MI (Belch, 2003; Willigendael et al., 2004).

The most effective oral antiplatelet treatment for patients with PAD is aspirin (160 to 325 mg/day) or clopidogrel (Tran et al., 2004).

ACE inhibitors (e.g., ramipril) are now being prescribed for the patient with PAD regardless of whether they have hypertension or left ventricular dysfunction (Hirsch, 2003). The use of ACE inhibitors decreases cardiovascular risks, improves arterial blood flow to the lower extremities, and improves walking distance (Lewis et al., 2007).

Two drugs approved for use in the United States to specifically treat intermittent claudication are pentoxifylline (Trental) and cilostazol (Pletal). These drugs improve the distance the patient can walk without pain (Lewis et al., 2007).

Fibrinolytics or thrombolytics are useful in dissolving existing thrombi. Urokinase (Abbokinase) is used in most patients with peripheral arterial occlusive disease. Unlike lytic therapy in MI or pulmonary embolism, in peripheral arterial occlusion the drug is administered directly into the thrombus through a central line that contains proximal and distal infusion wires (see Complementary & Alternative Therapies box).

 Complementary & Alternative Therapies

Cardiovascular and Peripheral Vascular Disorders

- A number of herbs have been studied for their circulatory effects. Ginkgo biloba has been found to be minimally effective for treating intermittent claudication and decreased cerebral circulation leading to reduced function. Manifestations of decreased cerebral circulation include decreased memory, vertigo, tinnitus, and mood swings with anxiety.

- In the treatment of chronic venous insufficiency, horse chestnut seed extract (HCSE, *Aesculus hippocastanum*) may be equivalent to compression stocking therapy. German health authorities have approved HCSE for the treatment of chronic venous insufficiency, pain and heaviness in the legs, and varicose veins. Gastrointestinal side effects may occur but are uncommon.

- Garlic has been studied for its effects on arteriosclerosis and lipids with varying results. The amount of fresh garlic a person would need to eat for a therapeutic dosage is high and likely to cause gastric upset. Garlic preparations vary widely in terms of their active constituents.

- Patients taking anticoagulants should be cautious regarding the use of herbs, including garlic, ginkgo, angelica, anise, bilberry, devil's claw, goldenseal, licorice root, parsley, and red clover. Although natural, these substances can have potent therapeutic activity. This may in part be due to anticoagulant effects, which may potentiate the action of anticoagulant medications. Be aware if patients are using such substances and monitor any interactions. Not enough controlled research is available to make definite predictions.

- Herbal remedies used to self-treat peripheral vascular disorders include those for hypertension, varicose veins, atherosclerosis, and vascular spasm. Herbs with antihypertensive action include garlic (*Allium sativum*), hawthorn (*Crataegus oxyacantha*), kudzu (*Pueraria lobata*), nettle (*Urtica dioica*), onion (*Allium cepa*), purslane (*Portulaca oleracea*), reishi mushroom (*Ganoderma lucidum*), and valerian (*Valeriana officinalis*). Ginkgo biloba has also been used for varicose veins and obliterative arterial disease of the lower extremities. HCSE is used for varicose veins and phlebitis, and valerian is used as an antispasmodic. Antihypertensive spices include basil, black pepper, fennel, and tarragon.

Data from Black, J.M., & Hawks, H.J. (2009). *Medical-surgical nursing.* Philadelphia: Saunders.

Surgical intervention for advanced disease includes embolectomy (removal of embolism) or endarterectomy (surgical removal of the lining of an artery, usually performed on any diseased or occluded major artery, such as the carotid, femoral, or popliteal), arterial bypass (Figure 8-19), PCTA, or amputation. If gangrene is extensive or all major arteries in the extremity are occluded, amputation, although the least desirable end-stage surgical option, may be required.

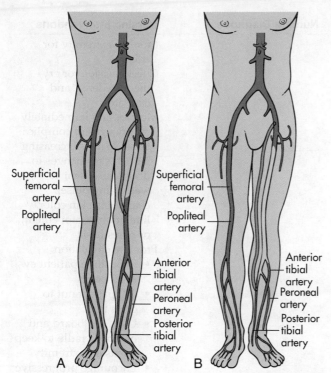

FIGURE 8-19 A, Femoral-popliteal bypass graft around an occluded superficial femoral artery. **B,** Femoral posterior tibial bypass graft around occluded superficial femoral, popliteal, and proximal tibial arteries.

Nursing Interventions and Patient Teaching

Nursing interventions are based on assessment findings and nursing diagnoses. Nursing diagnoses and nursing interventions for the patient with PAD of the lower extremities include but are not limited to the following:

Nursing Diagnoses	Nursing Interventions
Activity intolerance, related to: • ischemic pain • immobility	Prevent hazards of immobility by turning, positioning, deep breathing, and performing isometric and range-of-motion exercises. Encourage program of balanced exercise and rest to promote circulation. Instruct the patient to use pain or intermittent claudication as a guide to limiting activity during exercise.
Ineffective tissue perfusion, peripheral, related to decreased arterial blood flow	Place patient's legs in a dependent position relative to the heart to improve peripheral blood flow. Avoid raising feet above heart.

Nursing Diagnoses	Nursing Interventions
	Promote vasodilation by providing warmth to extremities and keeping room warm. Teach the patient to avoid vasoconstriction from nicotine, caffeine, stress, or chilling. Teach the patient to avoid constrictive clothing such as garters, tight stockings, or belts. Administer prescribed medications. Teach the patient to avoid crossing the legs.

Prognosis

In advanced disease, ischemia may lead to necrosis, ulceration, and gangrene (particularly of the toes and distal foot) because of the decreased circulation.

ARTERIAL EMBOLISM

Etiology and Pathophysiology

Arterial emboli are blood clots in the arterial bloodstream. They may originate in the heart from an atrial dysrhythmia, MI, valvular heart disease, or HF. Other foreign substances such as a detached arteriosclerotic plaque or tissue may result in arterial emboli. An embolus becomes dangerous when it lodges within and occludes a blood vessel. Blood flow to the area distal to the lodged embolus is impaired, and ischemia occurs. Signs and symptoms depend on the size of the embolus and the amount of circulation that is compromised.

Clinical Manifestations

Sudden loss of blood flow to tissues causes severe pain. Distal pulses are absent, and the affected extremity may become pale, cool, and numb. Necrotic changes may occur. Shock may result if the embolus occludes a large artery.

Assessment

Collection of **subjective data** includes determining the onset of pain and numbness and the location, quality, and duration of these symptoms.

Collection of **objective data** includes assessing pulses in the affected extremity. Compare both extremities to determine skin temperature and color, in addition to pulse volume.

Diagnostic Tests

Doppler ultrasonography and angiography are indicated to obtain a diagnosis.

Medical Management

Medications used to treat obstructed arteries include anticoagulants and fibrinolytics or thrombolytics. Anticoagulants prevent further clot formation and inhibit extension of a clot. Thrombolytics/fibrinolytics dissolve an existing clot. See Table 8-7 for more information on anticoagulants and fibrinolytics.

Endarterectomy (the surgical removal of the intimal lining of an artery) may be the treatment of choice. This involves stripping arteriosclerotic plaque from the intima or inner media of arteries affected by atherosclerosis. Balloon catheters and other instruments are used to accomplish this. Removal of plaque and thrombi increases blood flow and lessens the danger of complications from further emboli or occlusion of an artery.

Embolectomy is another treatment used when larger arteries are obstructed. It is the surgical removal of a blood clot. Surgery must be done within 6 to 10 hours of the event to prevent necrosis and loss of the extremity. Endarterectomy and embolectomy may be done together to deal with the existing emboli and prevent recurrence.

Nursing Interventions and Patient Teaching

Nursing interventions are similar to those for PAD in terms of preventing further arterial problems. During the acute phase monitor the patient for changes in skin color and temperature of the extremity distal to the embolus. Increasing pallor, cyanosis, and coolness of the skin indicate worsening or occlusion of arterial circulation to the extremity. Keep the extremity warm, but do not apply direct heat.

Nursing diagnoses and postoperative nursing interventions for the patient requiring an embolectomy and/or endarterectomy include but are not limited to the following:

Nursing Diagnoses	Nursing Interventions
Ineffective tissue perfusion, peripheral, related to decreased arterial blood flow	Monitor skin color and temperature of affected extremity every hour. Assess sensation and movement in the distal extremity. Assess peripheral pulses and capillary refill in the involved extremity: • Sudden absence of pulse may indicate thrombosis. • Mark location of peripheral pulse with a pen to facilitate frequent assessment. • Use Doppler to monitor whether pulses of involved extremity are nonpalpable and compare with pulses of noninvolved extremity.

Nursing Diagnoses	Nursing Interventions
	Monitor extremity for edema. Check incision for erythema, edema, and exudates. Monitor and immediately report signs of complications, such as increasing pain, fever, changes in drainage, absent or weakening pulse, changes in skin color, limitation of movement, or paresthesia. Promote circulation: • Reposition patient every 2 hours. • Tell patient not to cross legs. • Use a footboard and overbed cradle to keep linens off extremity. • Encourage progressive activity when permitted. Avoid sharp flexion in area of graft. Monitor for signs of bleeding secondary to anticoagulation therapy.
Deficient knowledge, related to anticoagulant therapy	Teach patient general action and side effects of prescribed drug; instruct patient to avoid taking anticoagulant medications with aspirin, which also has anticoagulant effect. Instruct patient to take anticoagulant at same time every day and to not stop taking it until advised by physician. Have patient check for signs of bleeding (gums, epistaxis [nosebleed], ecchymosis [bruising], cuts that do not stop bleeding with direct pressure, blood in urine or stool); report promptly to health care professional. Encourage patient to wear a medical-alert bracelet or carry an identification card containing the drug name, drug dosage, and physician's name in case of emergency.

Nursing Diagnoses	Nursing Interventions
Deficient knowledge, related to anticoagulant therapy—cont'd	Have patient report for prescribed blood tests (PTT, PT, INR) used to adjust drug dosage. Tell patient not to add dark green and yellow vegetables to diet (these contain vitamin K, which counteracts the anticoagulant drug effect). Instruct patient to restrict alcohol intake (increases anticoagulant effect).

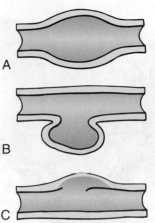

FIGURE 8-20 Types of aneurysms. **A,** Fusiform. **B,** Saccular. **C,** Dissecting.

Patient teaching is the same as for PAD with an emphasis on anticoagulant therapy.

Prognosis

Prognosis depends on the size of the embolus, the presence of collateral circulation, and the proximity to a major organ.

ARTERIAL ANEURYSM

Etiology and Pathophysiology

An **aneurysm** is an enlarged, dilated portion of an artery that is more than one and a half times the artery's circumference. To be a true aneurysm, the defect must involve all three layers, or tunics (Croce, 2007). Aneurysms may be the result of arteriosclerosis, trauma, or a congenital defect. Aneurysms of the lower extremities commonly affect the popliteal artery. Other areas predominantly affected are the thoracic and abdominal aorta and the coronary and cerebral arteries. The aorta is especially prone to aneurysm and rupture because it is continuously exposed to high pressures. Aortic aneurysms are most common in men in their 60s and 70s, especially if they have ever smoked. Other risk factors are hypertension, atherosclerosis, family history of aortic aneurysm, infarction, and trauma (Croce, 2007). Dissections and ruptures are more likely in the thoracic portion of the aorta than in the abdominal portion. An aneurysm starts with a weakened arterial wall that becomes dilated from blood flow and pressure in the area. The pathologic effect of this condition is differentiated according to shape and site of presentation (Figure 8-20).

Clinical Manifestations

A large pulsating mass may be the only identifiable factor. Clinical signs and symptoms of a thoracic aortic aneurysm depend on its location. If it compresses adjacent structures, it can cause chest pain, shortness of breath, cough, hoarseness, or dysphagia. If it compresses the superior vena cava, the patient may have edema of the face, the neck, and the arms. In the early stages an abdominal aneurysm is unlikely to cause symptoms. As it expands, however, it may cause pain in the chest, the

lower back, or the scrotum. A pulsatile, nontender upper abdominal mass may be palpated.

Assessment

Collection of **subjective data** may reveal no subjective symptoms unless the aneurysm is large and impinges on other structures, causing pain and inequality of pulses. A thoracic aortic aneurysm can result in chest pain, shortness of breath, or dysphagia.

Collection of **objective data** includes palpation of a large, nontender, pulsating mass at the site of the aneurysm.

Diagnostic Tests

Fluoroscopy, chest radiographic studies, CT scan, ultrasound, contrast aortography, arteriography, MRI, and TEE are used to diagnose an aneurysm. It is recommended that all men who have ever smoked have an abdominal aneurysm screening (Croce, 2007).

Medical Management

Aneurysms are monitored for complications such as dissection, rupture, formation of thrombi, and ischemia. Control of hypertension is the first priority of care. An oral beta blocker reduces blood pressure, heart rate, and myocardial contractility. Surgical intervention may be necessary. The blood vessel may be ligated or grafts used to replace the section of the artery that contains the aneurysm or to bypass the aneurysm.

A fusiform or circumferential aneurysm (in which all the walls of the blood vessel dilate more or less equally, creating a tubular swelling) can be removed and repaired with a graft of synthetic fiber, such as Dacron or Teflon, or with a vessel taken from another region of the patient's body. Saccular aneurysms (an aneurysm, usually caused by trauma, that consists of a weak area on only one side of the vessel, causing an outpouching of the vessel wall that is attached to the artery by a narrow neck) can be removed and the vessel then sutured, or a patch graft can be used to replace the deformity (Figures 8-21 and 8-22).

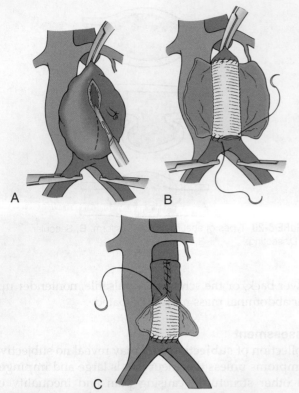

FIGURE 8-21 Surgical repair of an abdominal aortic aneurysm. **A,** Incising the aneurysmal sac. **B,** Insertion of synthetic graft. **C,** Suturing native aortic wall over synthetic graft.

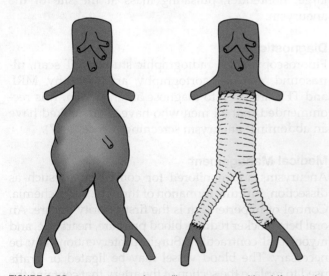

FIGURE 8-22 Replacement of aortoiliac aneurysm with a bifurcated synthetic graft.

In repair of a popliteal aneurysm, popliteal blood flow is enhanced when a homograft (or allograft, tissue transferred between two genetically dissimilar individuals of the same species, such as two humans who are not identical twins) is used.

Nursing Interventions and Patient Teaching
Initial nursing interventions include monitoring the status of an existing aneurysm. Monitor the patient for signs of rupture of the aneurysm, such as paleness, weakness, tachycardia, hypotension, sudden onset of abdominal or chest pain, back pain, or groin pain and a pulsating mass in the abdomen.

Postoperative nursing diagnoses and interventions for the patient with arterial aneurysm include but are not limited to the following:

Nursing Diagnoses	Nursing Interventions
Ineffective tissue perfusion, peripheral, related to decreased arterial blood flow	Assess circulation (especially in extremities) by pedal pulse checks and capillary refill assessments. Be alert for complications.
Anxiety, related to feelings of impending death	Examine coping ability Provide active listening and genuine interest. Maintain therapeutic environment. Administer antianxiety medications as ordered.

Because aneurysm formation is most commonly associated with atherosclerosis, patient teaching focuses on managing risk factors, including control of hypertension, promotion of tissue perfusion, maintenance of skin integrity, and prevention of infection and injury.

Prognosis
An aneurysm may rupture and cause hemorrhage, resulting in death unless emergency surgical intervention occurs. With surgical intervention, the prognosis is often good.

THROMBOANGIITIS OBLITERANS (BUERGER'S DISEASE)
Etiology and Pathophysiology
Thromboangiitis obliterans (Buerger's disease) is an occlusive vascular condition in which the small and medium-sized arteries become inflamed and thrombotic. The cause is not fully understood, but men between the ages of 25 and 40 years who smoke are most commonly affected by the disorder. Women, however, make up as much as 40% of patients with Buerger's disease. The disorder develops in the small arteries and veins of the feet and hands. Buerger's disease causes inflammation and damage to the arterial walls and is a type of arteritis (Lewis et al., 2007). The wrists and lower legs may also be involved. Occlusion of the arteries leads to ischemia; pain; and, in later stages, infection and ulceration. There is a strong relationship between Buerger's disease and tobacco use. It is thought that the disease occurs only in smokers, and when smoking is stopped, the disease improves.

Clinical Manifestations
The main characteristic is inflammation of vessel walls. The most common symptom is pain with exercise affecting the arch of the foot, also called **instep claudication.** When the hands are involved, the pain is usually

bilaterally symmetric (equal). Pain may occur at rest and be frequent and persistent, particularly when the patient also has atherosclerosis. The skin in the affected extremity may be cold and pale, and ulcers and gangrene may be present. Sensitivity to cold is an outstanding clinical manifestation. An early sign of Buerger's disease may be superficial thrombophlebitis.

Assessment

Subjective data include information about pain, claudication, and sensitivity to cold in affected extremities and risk factor assessment.

Objective data include presence of pulses, skin color, and temperature in the affected extremities.

Diagnostic Tests

No diagnostic tests are specific to Buerger's disease. Diagnosis is based on age of onset; history of tobacco use; clinical symptoms; involvement of distal vessels; presence of ischemic ulcerations; and exclusion of diabetes mellitus, autoimmune disease, and proximal source of emboli. Patients with Buerger's disease have a higher level of hematocrit blood viscosity and red blood cell rigidity than patients with PAD (Bozkurt et al., 2004).

Medical Management

Medical management is directed at preventing disease progression. Modifying risk factors and smoking cessation are a major focus. Smoking causes vasoconstriction and decreases blood supply to the extremities. Treatment includes complete cessation of tobacco use in any form (including secondhand smoke and nicotine-replacement products). Tell patients that they have a choice between cigarettes and their affected limbs; they cannot have both. The amputation rate in patients who continue tobacco use is 84%, compared with 30% in patients who discontinue tobacco use (Cooper, 2004). Trauma to the extremities must be avoided. Exercise to develop collateral circulation is encouraged. Surgical intervention, such as amputation of gangrenous fingers and toes, may be indicated. A sympathectomy (a surgical interruption of part of the sympathetic nerve pathways) to alleviate pain and vasospasm may also be performed.

Nursing Interventions and Patient Teaching

Nursing interventions focus on managing risk factors, promoting tissue perfusion, providing comfort measures, and patient teaching. Care of the extremities to prevent necrosis and gangrene includes hydration and cleanliness. Well-fitting shoes and socks alleviate pressure.

The hazards of cigarette smoking and its relationship to Buerger's disease are the primary focus of patient teaching. None of the palliative treatments are effective if the patient does not stop smoking. Nowhere are the cause and effect of smoking so dramatically seen as with Buerger's disease.

Prognosis

Buerger's disease is a chronic condition. Amputation may be necessary if the condition progresses to gangrene with chronic infection and extensive tissue destruction.

RAYNAUD'S DISEASE

Etiology and Pathophysiology

Raynaud's disease is caused by intermittent arterial spasms. Intermittent attacks of ischemia, especially of the fingers, the toes, the ears, and the nose, are caused by exposure to cold or by emotional stimuli. Raynaud's disease is either primary or secondary. The cause of primary Raynaud's is unknown, and the condition is usually mild. When symptoms occur in association with autoimmune diseases, a diagnosis of secondary Raynaud's disease is made. Primary Raynaud's disease usually occurs before 30 years of age, whereas secondary Raynaud's disease usually occurs after age 30. Secondary Raynaud's disease is associated with other conditions such as scleroderma (a relatively rare autoimmune disease affecting blood vessels and connective tissue), rheumatoid arthritis, systemic lupus erythematosus, drug intoxication, and occupational trauma. It usually affects women and is more prevalent during the winter months. The exact cause is unknown, but emotional stress, alterations in the nervous system and immunologic system, and hypersensitivity to cold may play a role in the development of signs and symptoms. Few arterial changes occur initially, but as the disease progresses, the intimal wall thickens and the medial wall hypertrophies.

Clinical Manifestations

The patient typically complains of chronically cold hands and feet. During arterial spasms, pallor, coldness, numbness, cutaneous cyanosis, and burning, throbbing pain occur. Chronic Raynaud's disease may result in ulcerations on the fingers and toes.

Assessment

Collection of **subjective data** includes determining underlying disease processes and evaluating risk factors. The patient may complain of cold hands or feet and a throbbing, aching pain with a tingling sensation (Lewis et al., 2007).

Collection of **objective data** includes assessment of pallor; edema; coldness; blanching; cyanosis; and reactive hyperemia (increased blood in part of the body, caused by increased blood flow), which instigates rubor, following an arterial spasm. Inspect the fingers and toes for ulceration because of circulatory inadequacy and residual waste products.

Diagnostic Tests

A cold stimulation test is used to diagnose Raynaud's disease. Skin temperature changes are recorded by a thermistor attached to each finger. Submerge the patient's hand in an ice water bath for 20 seconds, and record ongoing temperatures. A comparison is made for baseline data.

Medical Management

Medical therapy is aimed at prevention. Drug therapy may be prescribed to reduce pain and promote circulation. Currently the first-line drug therapy involves calcium channel blockers, such as nifedipine and diltiazem, to relax smooth muscles of the arterioles. Nifedipine is preferred over diltiazem because it has a stronger vasodilating effect and less effect on the calcium channels in the conduction system in the heart (Lewis et al., 2007). Biofeedback techniques have been used to increase skin temperature and thereby prevent spasms. Relaxation training and stress management are effective for some patients. Temperature extremes should be avoided. The patient should stop using all tobacco products and avoid caffeine and other drugs with vasoconstrictive effects such as amphetamines and cocaine. Possible surgical interventions include sympathectomy for symptomatic relief. If the disease is advanced, with ulcerations and gangrene, the involved area may have to be amputated.

Nursing Interventions and Patient Teaching

Nursing interventions are similar to those for other arterial disorders: promoting tissue perfusion, maintaining comfort, and preventing injury and infection. Risk factor management includes stress-reduction techniques and smoking cessation.

Nursing diagnoses and interventions stress patient teaching for the patient with Raynaud's disease, including but not limited to the following:

Nursing Diagnosis	Nursing Interventions
Deficient knowledge, related to: • effects of cigarette smoking • stress reduction • avoidance of exposure to cold	Develop teaching plan to include the following: • Effects of smoking on vasoconstriction and arterial blood flow • Techniques for smoking cessation: stop smoking programs, biofeedback, hypnosis • Techniques for stress reduction: massage, imagery, music, exercise, lifestyle changes • Ways of avoiding exposure to cold: layer clothing, wear mittens and warm socks during winter, use caution when cleaning the refrigerator and freezer, wear gloves when handling frozen food, and avoid occupations requiring constant exposure to cold

Prognosis

Raynaud's disease persists but may be controlled by protecting the body and extremities from the cold and using mild sedatives and vasodilators. No serious disability develops, but this condition is sometimes associated with rheumatoid arthritis or scleroderma.

VENOUS DISORDERS

Venous disorders occur when the blood flow is interrupted in returning from the tissues to the heart. Changes in smooth muscle and connective tissue make the veins less distensible. The valves in the veins may malfunction, causing backflow of blood. The major venous disorders are thrombophlebitis and varicose veins (Table 8-12).

THROMBOPHLEBITIS

Etiology and Pathophysiology

Thrombophlebitis is inflammation of a vein in conjunction with the formation of a thrombus. It occurs more frequently in women and affects people of all races. The incidence increases with aging. Other factors associated with thrombophlebitis include venous stasis, hypercoagulability (excessive clotting) of the blood, and trauma to the blood vessel wall. Immobilized patients who have had surgical procedures involving pelvic blood vessel manipulation, such as total hip replacement or pelvic surgery, or patients with MI are prone to thrombophlebitis. Thrombophlebitis develops in deep veins (DVT) or in superficial veins (superficial thrombosis) (Figure 8-23). Thrombophlebitis usually occurs in an extremity, most frequently a leg. Superficial thrombophlebitis is often minor and is treated with elevation, anti-inflammatory agents, and warm compresses. DVT is a condition involving a thrombus in a deep vein such as the iliac or femoral veins (Lewis at al., 2007). It is of greater significance and can become dislodged, carried to the lungs in the bloodstream, and cause a pulmonary embolus. Pulmonary embolism is a life-threatening complication.

Clinical Manifestations

Pain and edema occur when the vein is obstructed. The circumference of the calf or thigh may increase. Active dorsiflexion of the foot may result in calf pain. This is referred to as a positive Homans' sign and may indicate thrombophlebitis. Homans' sign is a classic but unreliable sign because it is not specific for DVT and appears in only 10% of DVT patients. Superficial thrombophlebitis may show signs of inflammation such as erythema, warmth, and tenderness along the course of the vein.

Assessment

Subjective data include characteristics of pain in the affected extremity, noting onset and duration and any history of venous disorders.

Table 8-12   Venous Disorders

SIGNS AND SYMPTOMS	MEDICAL MANAGEMENT AND NURSING INTERVENTIONS
THROMBOPHLEBITIS Entire extremity may be pale, cold, and edematous. Area along vein may be erythematous and warm to touch. Patient may have Homans' sign: pain in calf on dorsiflexion. Superficial veins feel indurated (hard) and thready or cordlike and are sensitive to pressure. Extremities have difference in circumference.	Maintain bed rest during acute phase. Apply warm, moist heat to reduce discomfort and pain per physician's orders. Elevate extremity, but do not use pillows under the knees, and never bend knees. Assess circulation of the affected extremity, and skin condition and pulses in all extremities. Measure calf circumference daily and record. Use antiembolism stocking on unaffected extremity. Administer heparin or enoxaparin (Lovenox) and warfarin (Coumadin) per physician's orders. Administer fibrinolytics (streptokinase) to resolve the thrombus per physician's orders. Begin exercise program after acute phase per physician's orders.
VARICOSE VEINS Veins appear as darkened, tortuous, raised blood vessels; more pronounced on prolonged standing. Legs feel heavy. Patient has fatigue. Patient has pain and muscle cramps. Legs are edematous. Ulcers are seen on skin.	Conservative treatment: • Elevate legs 10-15 minutes at least every 2-3 hours. • Wear elastic stockings. • Unna's paste boot is recommended for older or debilitated person with cutaneous ulcers (see Figure 8-25). • Avoid standing for long periods. • Avoid anything that impedes venous flow, such as garters, tight girdles, crossing the legs, and prolonged sitting. • Reduce weight if obese. • Inject sclerosing solutions for small varicosities. Surgery: • Venous ligation and stripping

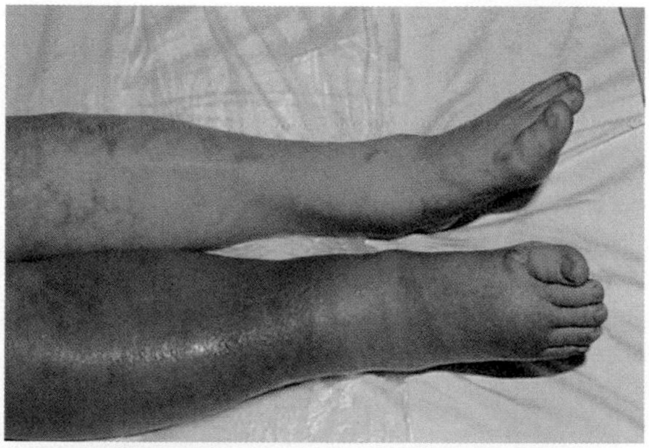

FIGURE 8-23 Deep-vein thrombophlebitis.

Collection of **objective data** includes inspecting the extremity and determining color and temperature (pale and cold if vein is occluded; erythematous and warm if superficial vein is inflamed). Measure both legs for circumference and comparison and to detect edema. If a thrombus involves the inferior vena cava, the lower extremities may become edematous and cyanotic. Involvement of the superior vena cava may result in cyanosis and edema of the arms, the neck, the face, and the back (Lewis et al., 2007).

Diagnostic Tests

Diagnostic tests for DVT include venous Doppler, duplex scanning (the most widely used test), and venogram (phlebogram). A serum D-dimer test will be elevated in DVT. D-dimer is a fibrin degradation fragment that is made from fibrolysis. When a thrombus is undergoing lysis (destruction), it results in increased D-dimer fragments.

Medical Management

Anticoagulant therapy is used for DVT prevention and treatment. For an existing DVT, anticoagulant therapy prevents extension of the clot, development of a new clot, or embolization (embolus traveling through the bloodstream). Anticoagulants do not dissolve a clot. Lysis (destruction) of the clot begins immediately by the body's own fibrinolytic system (Lewis et al., 2007).

Warm compresses may be applied intermittently to the affected extremity. Previously, treatment consisted of bed rest and elevation of the affected area above the level of the heart for 2 to 4 days until the thrombus was stable, therapeutic anticoagulation had occurred, and edema was decreased (Lewis et al., 2007). Current studies report no difference in the incidence of development of a pulmonary embolism in patients with a

---

⚠ **Safety Alert!**

Patient on Anticoagulant Therapy

1. Teach patient on oral warfarin requirements for frequent follow-up with blood tests (PT, INR) to assess blood clotting and whether change in drug dosage is required.
2. Teach patient side effects and adverse effects of anticoagulant therapy requiring medical attention.
   - Any bleeding that does not stop after a reasonable time (usually 10 to 15 minutes)
   - Blood in urine or stool or black, tarry stools
   - Unusual bleeding from gums, throat, skin, or nose, or heavy menstrual bleeding
   - Severe headaches or stomach pains
   - Weakness, dizziness, mental status changes
   - Vomiting blood
   - Cold, blue, or painful feet
3. Avoid any trauma or injury that might cause bleeding (e.g., vigorous brushing of teeth, contact sports, inline rollerskating).
4. Do not take aspirin-containing drugs or NSAIDs.
5. Limit alcohol intake to small amounts.
6. Wear a medical-alert bracelet or necklace indicating what anticoagulant is being taken.
7. Avoid marked changes in eating habits, such as dramatically increasing foods high in vitamin K (e.g., broccoli, spinach, kale, greens). Do not take supplemental vitamin K.
8. Inform all health care providers, including dentist, of anticoagulant therapy.
9. Correct dosing is essential and supervision may be required (e.g., for patients experiencing confusion).
10. Do not use herbal products that may alter coagulation (see Complementary & Alternative Therapies box).

DVT who were on anticoagulant therapy and who were on bed rest, compared with those allowed to ambulate (Trujillo et al., 2005). Drug therapy may include NSAIDs. DVT usually requires hospital treatment.

Low-molecular-weight heparin (LMWH) is effective for prevention of venous thrombosis and any extension or recurrence. Enoxaparin, and dalteparin are two types of LMWH. LMWH is administered subcutaneously in fixed doses, once or twice daily. LMWH has the practical advantage that it does not require anticoagulant monitoring and dose adjustment. LMWH has a greater bioavailability, more predictable dose response, and longer half-life than heparin with less risk of bleeding complications.

The affected extremity is elevated periodically above heart level to prevent venous stasis and to reduce edema. Specific orders depend on the physician's preference. When the patient ambulates, elastic stockings (antiembolism stockings) are used to compress the superficial veins, increase blood flow through the deep veins, and prevent venous stasis.

Surgery is indicated only when conservative measures have been unsuccessful. A thrombectomy or the **transvenous placement of a grid** or umbrella in the vena cava may be done to prevent the flow of emboli into the lungs. This inferior vena caval interruption device can be inserted percutaneously through superficial femoral or internal jugular veins. When the filter device is opened, the spokes penetrate the vessel walls. The device creates a "sieve-type" obstruction, filtrating clots without interrupting blood flow.

Nursing Interventions and Patient Teaching

Early mobilization is the easiest and most cost-effective method to decrease the risk of DVT. Patients on bed rest need to be instructed to change position, dorsiflex their feet, and rotate ankles every 2 to 4 hours. Ambulatory patients should ambulate at least three times per day. Elastic compression stockings (e.g., thromboembolic disease hose) and/or an intermittent compression device are used for hospitalized patients at risk for DVT. The major emphasis for the patient with thrombophlebitis is preventing complications, promoting comfort, and teaching about the disease and prevention of recurrence.

Nursing diagnoses and interventions for the patient with thrombophlebitis include but are not limited to the following:

Nursing Diagnoses	Nursing Interventions
Ineffective tissue perfusion, peripheral, related to decreased venous blood flow	Confine patient to bed in acute phase.
	Elevate affected extremity according to physician's orders.
	Check circulation frequently (monitor pedal pulses, capillary refill).
	Administer prescribed anticoagulants, and fibrinolytics.
	Measure calf or thigh circumference daily.
	Assess site for signs of inflammation and edema.
	Have patient wear elastic stockings when ambulatory.
	Implement graded exercise program as ordered.
Deficient knowledge, related to disease process and risk factors	Develop a teaching plan to prevent venous stasis, including the following:
	• Avoid prolonged sitting or standing; begin weight reduction if obese.
	• Avoid crossing the legs at the knee and wearing tight stockings or garters.
	• Elevate legs when sitting.
	• Do flexion-extension exercises of feet and legs when sitting or lying down to promote circulation and venous return.

Nursing Diagnoses	Nursing Interventions
Deficient knowledge, related to disease process and risk factors—cont'd	• Do not massage extremities because of danger of embolization of clots (thrombus breaking off and becoming an embolus). • Take prescribed medication.

Prognosis

A major risk during the acute phase of DVT is dislodgment of the thrombus, which can migrate to the lungs, causing a pulmonary embolus.

VARICOSE VEINS

Etiology and Pathophysiology

A varicose vein is a tortuous, dilated vein with incompetent valves. The highest incidence of varicose veins occurs in women ages 40 to 60 years. Approximately 15% of the adult population is affected. Causes of varicose veins include congenitally defective valves, an absent valve, or a valve that becomes incompetent. External pressure on the legs from pregnancy or obesity can place a strain on the vessels, and they become elongated and dilated. Poor posture, prolonged standing, and constrictive clothing may also contribute to this problem. The great and small saphenous veins of the legs are most often affected. The vessel wall weakens and dilates, stretching the valves and leaving the vessel unable to support a column of blood. Pooling of blood in the veins or varicosities is the result. Chronic blood pooling in the veins is referred to as **venous stasis**. Hemorrhage can occur if a varicose vein suffers trauma.

Clinical Manifestations

Varicose veins may be primary or secondary. Primary varicosities have a gradual onset and occur in superficial veins. Secondary varicosities affect the deep veins and result from chronic venous insufficiency or venous thrombosis. Often the only symptom is the appearance of darkened veins on the patient's legs. Symptoms include fatigue, dull aches, cramping of muscles, and a feeling of heaviness or pressure arising from decreased blood flow to the tissues. Signs and symptoms such as edema, pain, changes in skin color, and ulceration may occur from venous stasis.

Assessment

Collection of **subjective data** includes gathering information about predisposing factors: a family history of varicose veins, pregnancy, or other conditions that could cause pressure on the veins. Also include symptoms the patient is experiencing such as aches, fatigue, cramping, heaviness, and pain.

Collection of **objective data** includes inspecting the legs for varicosities, edema, color, and temperature of the skin and observing for ulceration.

Diagnostic Tests

Trendelenburg's test is done to diagnose the ability of the venous valves to support a column of blood by measuring venous filling time. The patient lies down with the affected leg raised to allow for venous emptying. A tourniquet is applied above the knee, and the patient stands. The direction and filling time of the veins are recorded both before and after the tourniquet is removed. When the veins fill rapidly from a backward blood flow, the veins are determined to be incompetent.

Medical Management

Mild signs and symptoms may be controlled with elastic stockings, rest periods, and leg elevation. Sclerotherapy consists of injection of a sclerosing solution at the sites of the varicosities. It is done as an outpatient procedure and produces permanent obliteration (complete occlusion of a part) of collapsed veins and good cosmetic results. Elastic bandages are applied for continuous pressure for 1 to 2 weeks. Surgical intervention is indicated for pain, progression of varicosities, edema, stasis ulcers, and cosmetic reasons. Surgery consists of vein ligation and stripping. The great saphenous vein is ligated (tied) close to the femoral junction. The great and small saphenous veins are stripped out through small incisions made in the inguinal area, above and below the knee and the ankle. The incisions are covered with sterile dressings, and an elastic bandage is applied and worn for at least 1 week.

Nursing Interventions and Patient Teaching

Nursing interventions focus on care of the patient after a surgical procedure, including maintaining comfort, maintaining peripheral circulation and venous return, and patient teaching regarding varicosity prevention and maintenance.

Nursing diagnoses and interventions for the patient with varicose veins include but are not limited to the following:

Nursing Diagnoses	Nursing Interventions
Ineffective tissue perfusion, peripheral, related to impaired venous blood return	Monitor for signs and symptoms of bleeding postoperatively. If bleeding occurs, apply pressure to the wound, elevate the leg, and notify the physician. Keep elastic bandage snug and wrinkle free; do not remove bandage for daily dressing change. Encourage deep breathing exercises and early ambulation to facilitate venous return. Encourage dorsiflexion exercises while in bed or sitting to facilitate venous return.

Continued

Nursing Diagnoses	Nursing Interventions
Deficient knowledge, related to disease process and measures to avoid venous stasis and promote venous return	Develop teaching plan to include the following: • Avoid anything that can increase pressure above the knees (crossing the legs, sitting in chairs that are too high, wearing garters and knee-high stockings). • Begin regular exercise to promote venous return by contraction of leg muscles. • Avoid prolonged sitting or standing. • Elevate legs when sitting. • Maintain ideal weight. • Wear elastic stockings for support for activities that require prolonged standing or when pregnant.

Prognosis

Varicosities are chronic conditions; the affected person must know how to prevent venous stasis and encourage venous return.

VENOUS STASIS ULCERS

Etiology and Pathophysiology

Venous stasis ulcers or leg ulcers occur from chronic deep vein insufficiency and stasis of blood in the venous system of the legs. Other causes include severe varicose veins, burns, trauma, sickle cell anemia, diabetes mellitus, neurogenic disorders, and hereditary factors. A leg ulcer is an open, necrotic lesion that results when an inadequate supply of oxygen-rich blood and nutrients reaches the tissue (Figure 8-24). The re-

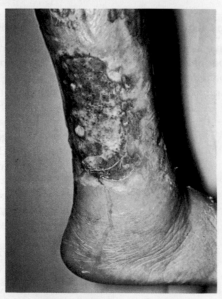

FIGURE 8-24 Venous leg ulcer.

sult is cell death, tissue sloughing, and skin impairment. Decreased circulation to the area contributes to the development of infection and prolonged healing.

Clinical Manifestations

Patients may report varying degrees of pain, from mild discomfort to a dull, aching pain relieved by elevation of the extremity. The skin is visibly ulcerated and has a leathery appearance and dark pigmentation. Edema may be present. Ulcerations often occur around the medial aspect of the ankle. Pedal pulses are present.

Assessment

Subjective data include onset and duration of pain and successful relief measures. Predisposing factors such as thrombophlebitis, venous insufficiency, and diabetes mellitus are noted.

Collection of **objective data** includes inspection of ulcerated areas: size, location, and condition of skin; color; and temperature. Palpate pedal pulses, and observe for edema.

Diagnostic Tests

Venography and Doppler ultrasonography are used to confirm venous insufficiency and stasis.

Medical Management

Management focuses on promoting wound healing and preventing infection. Diet is important to ensure adequate protein intake, since large amounts of protein in the form of albumin are lost through the ulcers. Also vitamin A and C and the mineral zinc are administered to promote tissue healing. Debridement of necrotic tissue, antibiotic therapy, and protection of the ulcerated area are usual treatments. Debridement can be mechanical, such as applying gauze moistened with saline dressing to the wound. When dry, the dressing is removed, pulling off the debris that has adhered to it. Debridement can also be chemical; enzyme ointments such as fibrinolysin deoxyribonuclease (Elase) are placed over the ulcer to break down necrotic tissue. Surgical debridement using a scalpel is done when other measures are not successful.

Applying compression to the affected area is essential to promote venous ulcer healing and prevent ulcer recurrence. Compression options include elastic wraps, custom-fitted compression stockings, intermittent compression devices, Velcro wraps, and a multilayer bandage system (e.g., Profore) (Wipke-Tevis et al., 2004). An Unna's paste boot can be used to protect the ulcer and provide constant and even support to the area (Figure 8-25). Moist, impregnated gauze is wrapped around the patient's foot and leg. It hardens into a "boot" that may be left on for 1 to 2 weeks, although it may be changed more often if there is copious drainage. It is essential that a patient with a venous leg ulcer has a balanced diet with adequate protein calories and nutrients to promote healing (Lewis et al., 2007).

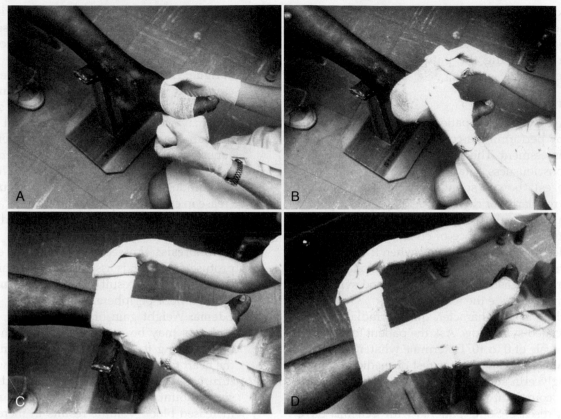

FIGURE 8-25   Nurse applying Unna's paste boot using specially impregnated gauze. Most ulcers are on inferior aspect of patient's foot.

Nursing Interventions and Patient Teaching

Nursing interventions focus on promoting wound healing, promoting comfort, maintaining peripheral tissue perfusion, preventing infection, and patient teaching.

Nursing diagnoses and interventions for the patient with venous stasis ulcers include but are not limited to the following:

Nursing Diagnoses	Nursing Interventions
Impaired skin integrity, related to open ulceration	Perform dressing changes per physician's order, using gauze, moistened with saline, topical drug treatments, and Unna's boot therapy. Assess wound for signs and symptoms of infection. Provide antibiotic therapy as prescribed. Encourage nutritional intake to promote wound healing.
Ineffective tissue perfusion, peripheral, related to insufficient venous circulation	Elevate extremities when sitting or lying to promote venous return and decrease risk of edema and venous stasis. Use overbed cradle to protect extremities from pressure of bed linens.

Nursing Diagnoses	Nursing Interventions
	Use cotton between toes to prevent pressure on a toe ulcer. Assess level of discomfort.

Patient teaching focuses on preventing infection, maintaining peripheral tissue circulation, avoiding venous stasis, and providing proper wound care and dressing changes. See previous nursing diagnoses and interventions.

Prognosis

Venous stasis ulcers are a chronic condition caused by chronic venous insufficiency and delayed healing. Most venous ulcers heal with therapy.

❖ NURSING PROCESS *for the Patient with a Cardiovascular Disorder*

The role of the licensed practical nurse/licensed vocational nurse (LPN/LVN) in the nursing process as stated is that the LPN/LVN will:

- Participate in planning care for patients based on patient needs
- Review patient's care plan and recommend revisions as needed
- Review and follow defined prioritization for patient care

- Use clinical pathways, care maps, or care plans to guide and review patient care

Systemic cardiac assessment provides baseline data useful for identifying the patient's physiologic and psychosocial needs.

▪ Assessment

Begin assessment of the patient with a cardiovascular disorder by performing a complete health history and physical assessment. The physical assessment includes level of consciousness, vital signs, lung sounds (crackles, wheezes), bowel sounds, apical heart sounds (strength, regularity of rhythm), pedal pulses, capillary refill, skin color (pallor, cyanosis), turgor, temperature and moisture, and presence of edema. The history includes a description of symptoms, when they occurred, their course and duration, location, precipitating factors, and relief measures. Specific signs and symptoms to be aware of include the following:

- **Pain:** Note the character, quality, radiation, and associated symptoms. Ask the patient to rate pain on a scale of 0 to 10. Determine what, if anything, relieved the pain, such as rest or medication (e.g., nitroglycerin sublingually). Chest pain is the primary complaint when patients have symptoms of heart disease. Some patients with ischemia have pain in the jaw and left shoulder. The patient may describe the pain as dull, sharp, pressure, squeezing, crushing, viselike, grinding, or radiating. Note any factors precipitating the onset. Pain originating from cardiac muscle ischemia (decreased blood supply to a body organ or part) produces anxiety. It may lead to other signs and symptoms such as nausea, vertigo, or diaphoresis. Chest pain is significant in indicating cardiac ischemia or damage.
- **Palpitations:** Characterized by rapid, irregular, or pounding heartbeat, palpitations may be associated with cardiac dysrhythmias (any disturbance or abnormality in a normal rhythmic pattern) or cardiac ischemia. Patients may begin to notice the heartbeat and describe it as "pounding" or "racing." This can be frightening for the patient.
- **Cyanosis:** A bluish discoloration of the skin and mucous membranes caused by an excess of deoxygenated hemoglobin in the blood, cyanosis results from decreased cardiac output and poor peripheral perfusion.
- **Dyspnea:** Dyspnea is characterized by difficulty breathing or shortness of breath. Observe for dyspnea with activity, referred to as **exertional dyspnea,** which is commonly associated with decreased cardiac function.
- **Orthopnea:** Orthopnea is an abnormal condition in which a person must sit or stand to breathe deeply or comfortably.
- **Cough:** The cough may be dry or productive and results from a fluid accumulation in the lungs. The patient may describe it as irritating or spasmodic. Dyspnea may be associated with it. The production of sputum should be observed for frothiness or hemoptysis (see discussion of pulmonary edema).
- **Fatigue:** Exhaustion and activity intolerance are associated with decreased cardiac output. The patient may be unable to perform ADLs. Depression may accompany this or be a result of it.
- **Syncope:** Syncope or fainting is a brief lapse of consciousness caused by transient cerebral hypoxia. It is usually preceded by a sensation of lightheadedness. It can result from a sudden decrease in cardiac output to the brain as a result of dysrhythmia (bradycardia or tachycardia) or decreased pumping action of the heart.
- **Diaphoresis:** The secretion of sweat, especially profuse sweating, is associated with clamminess. Diaphoresis is a result of decreased cardiac output and poor peripheral perfusion.
- **Edema:** Weight gain of more than 3 pounds in 24 hours may be indicative of HF. The mechanism leading to edema in HF is the inability of the heart to pump efficiently or accept venous return, causing retrograde blood flow and an excessive amount of circulating blood volume. This increased blood volume results in increased hydrostatic pressure and an increase of fluid in the interstitial spaces.

▪ Nursing Diagnosis

Assess the patient's cardiovascular system and identify characteristics that reveal a nursing diagnosis. Nursing diagnoses for cardiovascular problems may include the following:

- Activity intolerance
- Anxiety
- Decreased cardiac output
- Ineffective coronary tissue perfusion
- Excess fluid volume
- Impaired gas exchange
- Deficient knowledge (specify)
- Pain

▪ Expected Outcomes and Planning

Plan appropriate interventions to meet the needs of patients with cardiovascular problems. The nurse is in the unique position of ongoing patient monitoring and is able to participate in the development of nursing diagnoses, help select appropriate interventions, and document the care plan. Teaching throughout the hospital stay and when preparing for discharge is important. Reinforcement of good health habits improves the likelihood for compliance with the care plan.

▪ Implementation

Nursing interventions for the patient with a cardiovascular disorder include enhancing cardiac output, promoting tissue perfusion, promoting adequate gas exchange, improving activity tolerance, and promoting comfort. Patient teaching emphasizes adherence to diet and exercise and medication protocols and strategies for balancing activity, getting rest, and reducing stress.

▪ Evaluation

Evaluate the expected outcomes as the final step of the nursing process and determine their effectiveness. Participate in the revision of the plan and nursing interventions when necessary.

Get Ready for the NCLEX® Examination!

Key Points

- The cardiovascular system is composed of the heart, blood vessels, and lymphatic structures.
- The functions of the cardiovascular system are to deliver oxygen and nutrients to the cells and to remove carbon dioxide and waste products from the cells.
- The heart is a large pump (the size of a human fist) that propels blood through the circulatory system.
- The heart is composed of four chambers: two atria and two ventricles.
- There are two coronary arteries; they supply the heart with nutrition and oxygen.
- The electrical pattern of impulse starts with the SA node, which is the pacemaker of the heart; it initiates the heartbeat. This impulse travels to the AV node. From here the impulse travels to a bundle of fibers called the bundle of His and divides into right and left bundle branches and finally to the Purkinje fibers.
- Three kinds of blood vessels are organized for carrying blood to and from the heart: the arteries, the veins, and the capillaries.
- Risk factors for developing CAD are classified as nonmodifiable and modifiable.
- Nonmodifiable risk factors for CAD include advancing age, male gender, black race, and a positive family history of CAD.
- Major modifiable risk factors for CAD include cigarette smoking, hyperlipidemia, stress, obesity, sedentary lifestyle, and hypertension. A diet high in cholesterol and saturated fats contributes to risk.
- An important aspect of caring for the patient with a cardiovascular disorder is understanding the risk factors and incorporating them into patient teaching.
- Major diagnostic tests to evaluate cardiovascular function include chest radiograph, arteriography, cardiac catheterization, ECG, echocardiogram, telemetry, stress test, PET, and thallium scanning.
- Common laboratory examinations to evaluate cardiovascular function are blood cultures, CBC, PT, INR, PTT, ESR, serum electrolytes, lipids (VLDL, LDL, HDL), triglycerides, arterial blood gases, BNP, and serum cardiac markers. Troponin I is a myocardial muscle protein released into circulation after myocardial injury and is useful in diagnosing an MI.
- CAD is the term used to describe a variety of conditions that obstruct blood flow in the coronary arteries.
- When the myocardial oxygen demand exceeds the myocardial oxygen supply, ischemia of the heart muscle occurs, resulting in chest pain or angina.
- Patient teaching to minimize the pain of angina pectoris includes taking nitroglycerin before exertion, eating small

amounts rather than two or three larger meals, balancing exercise periods with rest, stopping activity at first sign of chest pain, avoiding exposure to extreme weather conditions, ceasing to smoke, and seeking a calm environment.
- Subjective data of a patient with MI may include heavy pressure or squeezing pressure in the chest, retrosternal pain radiating to left arm and jaw, anxiety, nausea, and dyspnea.
- Objective data for the patient with MI include pallor, hypertension, cardiac rhythm changes, vomiting, fever, and diaphoresis.
- Possible nursing diagnoses for the patient with MI include *pain (acute), tissue perfusion (ineffective), activity intolerance, decreased cardiac output, anxiety,* and *constipation.*
- Cardiac rehabilitation services are designed to help patients with heart disease recover faster and return to full and productive lives. Cardiac rehabilitation improves patient compliance.
- HF leads to the congested state of the heart, lungs, and systemic circulation as a result of the heart's inability to act as an effective pump. The most recent definition is that HF should be viewed as a neurohormonal problem that progresses as a result of chronic release in the body of substances such as catecholamines (epinephrine and norepinephrine). These substances may have toxic effects on the heart.
- It is important to realize that 1 L of fluid equals 1 kg (2.2 pounds); a weight gain of 2.2 pounds signifies a gain of 1 L of body fluid.
- Signs and symptoms of HF with left ventricular failure include dyspnea; cough; frothy, blood-tinged sputum; pulmonary crackles; and evidence of pulmonary vascular congestion with pleural effusion.
- Signs and symptoms of HF with right ventricular failure include edema in feet, ankles, and sacrum, which may progress into the thigh and external genitalia; liver congestion; ascites; and distended jugular veins.
- Medical management of HF includes increasing cardiac efficiency with digitalis, vasodilators, and ACE inhibitors; administering a beta blocker (carvedilol) for mild to moderate HF; lowering oxygen requirements through bed rest; providing oxygen to the tissues through oxygen therapy if the patient is hypoxic; treating edema and pulmonary congestion with a diuretic and a sodium-restricted diet; and weighing daily to monitor fluid retention.
- Nursing interventions for the patient with valvular heart disease include administering the prescribed medications (diuretics, digoxin, and antidysrhythmics); monitoring I&O and daily weight; auscultating breath sounds and heart sounds; taking blood pressure; and assessing capillary perfusion, pedal pulses, and presence of edema.

- Patient teaching for the patient with valvular heart disease includes dietary management, activity limitations, and the importance of antibiotic prophylaxis before invasive procedure.
- Most patients with cardiomyopathy have a severe, progressively deteriorating course, and the majority older than age 55 years die within 2 years of the onset of signs and symptoms.
- PVD is any abnormal condition that affects the blood vessels outside the heart and the lymphatic vessels.
- Arteriosclerosis is the underlying problem associated with PVD.
- Hypertension occurs when there is a sustained elevated systolic blood pressure greater than 140 mm Hg and/or sustained elevated diastolic blood pressure of greater than 90 mm Hg on two or more readings.
- Nursing interventions for hypertension primarily focus on blood pressure management through patient teaching, risk factor recognition, drug therapy, dietary management, exercise, and stress-reduction techniques.
- An aneurysm is an enlarged, dilated portion of an artery and may be the result of arteriosclerosis, trauma, or a congenital defect.
- The hazards of cigarette smoking and its relationship to thromboangiitis obliterans (Buerger's disease) are the primary focuses of patient teaching.
- The two major venous disorders are thrombophlebitis and varicose veins.
- Thrombophlebitis may result in calf pain on dorsiflexion of the foot, which is referred to as a positive Homans' sign. A positive Homans' sign appears in only 10% of DVT patients.
- Patient teaching to avoid thrombophlebitis includes avoid prolonged sitting or standing, avoid dehydration, reduce weight if obese, do dorsiflexion-extension exercises of feet and legs, do not cross legs at the knees, and elevate legs when sitting.

Additional Learning Resources

 Go to your Companion CD for an audio glossary, animations, video clips, and more.

evolve   Be sure to visit the Evolve site at http://evolve.elsevier.com/Christensen/adult/ for additional online resources.

Review Questions for the NCLEX® Examination

1. The blood that is pumped out of the left ventricle contains:
   1. a full supply of oxygen.
   2. impurities that must be removed by the liver.
   3. a high percentage of carbon dioxide.
   4. all the wastes to be delivered to the organs of excretion.

2. The heart contracts in the following patterns:
   1. right atrium, left atrium, then the ventricles.
   2. both atria, then both ventricles.
   3. right atrium, right ventricle, then the left atrium, left ventricle.
   4. ventricles, then atria.

3. The interior lining of the heart, the valves, and the large vessels of the heart are together called the:
   1. endocardium.
   2. myocardium.
   3. pericardium.
   4. epicardium.

4. Valve flaps prevent the backflow of blood from the pulmonary artery into the:
   1. lung.
   2. right atrium.
   3. right ventricle.
   4. left atrium.

5. The normal period in the heart cycle during which the muscle fibers lengthen, the heart dilates, and the cavities fill with blood, roughly the period of relaxation, is called:
   1. systole.
   2. pulse pressure.
   3. diastose.
   4. diastole.

6. The right atrium receives blood from the:
   1. superior and inferior venae cavae.
   2. pulmonary veins, pulmonary arteries.
   3. superior and inferior venae cavae and coronary sinus.
   4. membranous septum, coronary sinus.

7. When a patient is receiving heparin therapy, the nurse should:
   1. observe him for cyanosis.
   2. remember that a sedimentation rate is ordered for monitoring blood coagulation.
   3. give the injection intramuscularly.
   4. observe emesis, urine, and stools for blood.

8. A 72-year-old patient is admitted to the medical floor with a diagnosis of HF. In HF an increase in abdominal girth, increase in total body weight, and pitting edema are indications of:
   1. fluid retention.
   2. electrolyte imbalance.
   3. disorganized ventricle pulsation.
   4. AV node dysfunction.

9. A 10-year-old patient is diagnosed with rheumatic fever. Of all the manifestations seen in rheumatic fever, the one that can lead to permanent complications is:
   1. Sydenham's chorea.
   2. erythema marginatum.
   3. subcutaneous nodules.
   4. carditis.

10. A 67-year-old patient has a diagnosis of hypertension. She is being dismissed from the hospital. Her teaching should include:
    1. instruction in consuming a bland diet.
    2. instruction of sodium intake up to 4g/day.
    3. encouragement to begin a vigorous exercise program.
    4. education on continuing to take antihypertensive medications as prescribed.

11. An 86-year-old patient is receiving D5½ NS per IV at 83 mL/hr on the electronic infusion pump. It is vitally important that the IV lines of older adult patients be monitored carefully because:

   1. these patients do not get dehydrated very easily.
   2. they may get a fluid overload of the circulatory system.
   3. of the increased risk of infection in the veins.
   4. of the danger of thrombophlebitis developing in the peripheral system.

12. A 34-year-old patient with a history of IV drug use is diagnosed with acute infective endocarditis. Nursing interventions for this patient include:

   1. early ambulation and activity progression.
   2. restricted activity for several weeks.
   3. low-calorie diet.
   4. dilution of blood by increased fluid intake.

13. A 62-year-old patient has a history of angina pectoris. To decrease the pain from angina pectoris, the patient should:

   1. take a cardiac glycoside at first symptom of cardiac pain.
   2. avoid taking more than three or four nitroglycerin pills daily.
   3. take nitroglycerin sublingually qid.
   4. take nitroglycerin sublingually prophylactically before strenuous exercise.

14. A patient has peripheral arterial disorder (PAD) of the lower extremities. Patient teaching for PAD includes:

   1. encouraging the patient to ambulate frequently.
   2. the importance of avoiding exposure to cold and chilling.
   3. teaching self-massage of the legs with lotion.
   4. maintaining a reduced-calorie diet.

15. A 75-year-old patient is diagnosed with heart failure. The nursing diagnosis of *activity intolerance,* related to dyspnea and fatigue, would be appropriate. Choose the appropriate nursing intervention in keeping with this diagnosis.

   1. Plan frequent rest periods.
   2. Allow patient to shower.
   3. Encourage patient to perform all ADLs.
   4. Encourage fluid intake of 3000 L/day.

16. A patient recovering from an MI is being prepared for discharge and should be instructed to:

   1. remain inactive until healing is complete.
   2. remain at home and avoid exposure to cold temperatures.
   3. begin a cardiac rehabilitation program.
   4. perform isometric exercises in a relaxed environment.

17. Dependent edema of the extremities, enlargement of the liver, oliguria, jugular vein distention, and abdominal distention are signs and symptoms of:

   1. right-sided heart failure.
   2. left-sided heart failure.
   3. cardiac dysrhythmias.
   4. valvular heart disease.

18. The primary function of patient teaching after a myocardial infarction is:

   1. explaining the disease process.
   2. assisting the patient in developing a healthy lifestyle.
   3. describing the precipitating causes and onset of pain.
   4. educating the patient on causative factors that initiate cardiac vasoconstriction.

19. An important nursing intervention when caring for a patient with remote telemetry is to:

   1. encourage independence by permitting patient to shower.
   2. never remove telemetry and allow patient to shower unless physician has written an order to allow it.
   3. encourage use of stair climbing, aerobic exercise, and other forms of exertion to promote collateral circulation.
   4. be aware that special microphones, attached to the patient's chest, pick up cardiac sounds produced by pressure changes in the heart.

20. Signs and symptoms of cardiogenic shock include:

   1. warm, dry skin.
   2. decreasing blood pressure and weak, rapid pulse.
   3. flushed face, restlessness.
   4. polyuria and dysuria.

21. Modifiable risk factors for coronary artery disease (CAD) includes?

   1. Diabetes, family history
   2. Family history, smoking
   3. Smoking, heredity
   4. High cholesterol, obesity

22. The name of the neurohormone released from the left ventricle in response to volume expansion and pressure overload that has emerged as the blood marker for the identification of individuals with HF is:

   1. A-type natriuretic peptide (ANP).
   2. troponin I.
   3. B-type natriuretic peptide (BNP).
   4. CPK peptide.

23. The normal range for the above blood marker is:

   1. 0 to 100 pg/mL.
   2. 500 to 900 pg/mL.
   3. 0.003 to 1 pg/mL.
   4. 400 to 500 pg/mL.

24. _____ is a myocardial muscle protein released into circulation after myocardial injury and is useful in diagnosing a myocardial infarction.

25. In the United States, the two beta blocker medications specifically approved for heart failure are carvedilol (Coreg) and:

   1. benazepril (Lotensin).
   2. captopril (Capoten).
   3. long-acting metoprolol (Toprol X-L).
   4. verapamil (Calan).

26. The most useful noninvasive diagnostic tool for evaluating the patient with heart failure is:
    1. coronary angiography.
    2. echocardiogram.
    3. electrocardiogram.
    4. thallium scanning.

27. Electrocardiogram findings during an MI:
    1. are less likely to show ST-segment elevation in women than in men.
    2. always show ST-segment elevation in women, but not in men.
    3. always show ST-segment elevation in women and men.
    4. are easier to interpret in women than in men.

28. The nursing diagnosis of *decreased cardiac output,* related to loss of myocardial contractility, would be appropriate for the patient who has had an acute myocardial infarction. The correct nursing interventions for this nursing diagnoses would include: *(Select all that apply.)*
    1. Assess for and report decreased blood pressure and dysrhythmias.
    2. Assess for oliguria.
    3. Administer oxygen therapy as ordered.
    4. Give opioids sparingly.

29. Heart failure is usually treated with: *(Select all that apply.)*
    1. Cardiotonic drugs (digitalis)
    2. Diuretic agents
    3. Generous fluid intake
    4. ACE inhibitors, beta-adrenergic blockers (carvediol), nitrates

30. An invasive procedure in which a catheter from a femoral or brachial artery is placed in the coronary artery and a balloon is inflated against the narrowing wall, thus reducing the arterial constriction, is called:
    1. coronary artery bypass graft (CABG) surgery.
    2. pacemaker.
    3. vectorcardiogram.
    4. percutaneous transluminal coronary angioplasty (PTCA).

31. Thrombolytic agents such as streptokinase and tissue plasminogen activators such as alteplase and activase are agents used to dissolve blood clots. These agents are *most* effective in a patient with acute MI signs and symptoms:
    1. in the first 24 hours.
    2. in the first 30 minutes to 1 hour.
    3. in the first 72 hours.
    4. in the second 6 hours after an MI.

32. A 74-year-old patient with heart failure is admitted to the hospital because of a weight gain of 12 pounds in the past 2 weeks. After effective results from IV furosemide (Lasix), the patient has lost 8 pounds. This would reflect a loss of how much fluid?
    1. 1.6 L
    2. 6 L
    3. 3.6 or 4 L
    4. 2.2 L

33. A patient is admitted with a diagnosis of possible aortic abdominal aneurysm. In assessment for possible complications it is most important to monitor:
    1. body temperature.
    2. skin turgor.
    3. respiratory rate.
    4. blood pressure.

34. A 63-year-old patient has Buerger's disease. The most important aspect of patient compliance to decrease signs and symptoms of Buerger's disease is:
    1. low-fat diet.
    2. weight loss.
    3. cessation of tobacco use.
    4. keeping extremities warm.

35. An 83-year-old patient is diagnosed with venous stasis ulcers. The medical management includes the use of an Unna's paste boot. An Unna's boot: *(Select all that apply.)*
    1. hardens into a "boot" that may be left on for 1 to 2 weeks.
    2. is a moist, impregnated gauze wrapped around the patient's foot and leg.
    3. applies intermittent external pressure to the lower extremities; it pushes blood from the superficial veins into deep veins.
    4. protects the ulcer and provides constant and even support to the area.

36. A 58-year-old patient is admitted with Raynaud's disease. The correct patient teaching information includes: *(Select all that apply.)*
    1. avoid cold.
    2. warm hands and feet with heating pad.
    3. practice stress-reduction techniques.
    4. comply with smoking cessation.

37. A patient is admitted with HF and chronic arterial fibrillation. What medication is his physician likely to order to prevent thrombus formation?
    1. An ACE inhibitor
    2. Nitroglycerin
    3. An antihypertensive
    4. An anticoagulant

Care of the Patient with a Respiratory Disorder

Barbara Lauritsen Christensen

Objectives

Anatomy and Physiology

1. Differentiate between external and internal respiration.
2. Describe the purpose of the respiratory system.
3. List and define the parts of the upper and lower respiratory tracts.
4. List the ways in which oxygen and carbon dioxide are transported in the blood.
5. Discuss the mechanisms that regulate respirations.

Medical-Surgical

6. Identify those signs and symptoms that indicate a patient is experiencing hypoxia.
7. Differentiate among sonorous wheezes, sibilant wheezes, crackles, and pleural friction rub.
8. Describe the purpose, significance of results, and nursing interventions related to diagnostic examinations of the respiratory system.
9. Describe the significance of arterial blood gas values and differentiate between arterial oxygen tension (PaO_2) and arterial oxygen saturation (SaO_2).
10. Discuss the etiology and pathophysiology, clinical manifestations, assessment, diagnostic tests, medical management, nursing interventions, and prognosis of the patient with disorders of the upper airway.
11. Discuss nursing interventions for the patient with a laryngectomy.
12. Discuss the etiology and pathophysiology, clinical manifestations, assessment, diagnostic tests, medical management, nursing interventions, and prognosis of the patient with disorders of the lower airway.
13. List five nursing interventions to assist patients with retained pulmonary secretions.
14. Differentiate between tuberculosis infection and tuberculosis disease.
15. List four medications commonly prescribed for the patient with tuberculosis.
16. List five nursing assessments or interventions pertaining to the care of the patient with closed-chest drainage.
17. Discuss three risk factors associated with pulmonary emboli.
18. Compare and contrast the etiology and pathophysiology, clinical manifestations, assessment, diagnostic tests, medical management, nursing interventions, and prognosis for the patient with chronic obstructive pulmonary disease, including emphysema, chronic bronchitis, asthma, and bronchiectasis.
19. Differentiate between medical management of the patient with emphysema and the patient with asthma.
20. Discuss why low-flow oxygen is required for patients with emphysema.
21. State three possible nursing diagnoses for the patient with altered respiratory function.

Key Terms

adventitious (ăd-vĕnt-TĬ-shŭs, p. 379)

atelectasis (ă-tĕ-LĔK-tā-sĭs, p. 410)

bronchoscopy (brŏng-KŎS-kō-pē, p. 381)

cor pumonale (kŏr pŭl-mō-NĂ-lē, p. 421)

coryza (kō-RĪ-ză, p. 391)

crackles (KRĂK-ŭlz, p. 379)

cyanosis (sī-ă-NŌ-sĭs, p. 388)

dyspnea (DĬSP-nē-ă, p. 378)

embolism (ĔM-bō-lĭz-ŭm, p. 416)

empyema (ĕm-pī-Ē-mă, p. 408)

epistaxis (ĕp-ĭ-STĂK-sĭs, p. 384)

exacerbation (ĕg-zăs-ĕr-BĀ-shŭn, p. 424)

extrinsic (ĕk-STRĬN-zĭk, p. 426)

hypercapnia (hī-pĕr-KĂP-nē-ă, p. 424)

hypoventilation (hī-pō-vĕn-tĭ-LĀ-shŭn, p. 410)

hypoxia (hī-PŎK-sē-ă, p. 379)

intrinsic (ĭn-TRĬN-zĭk, p. 426)

orthopnea (ŏr-thŏp-NĒ-ă, p. 379)

pleural friction rubs (PLŪ-răl FRĬK-shŭn rŭbz, p. 379)

pneumothorax (nū-mō-THŌ-răks, p. 411)

sibilant wheezes (SĬB-ĭ-lănt wēz-ĕz, p. 379)

sonorous wheezes (sŏ-NŎR-ŭs wēz-ĕz, p. 379)

stertorous (STĔR-tĕr-ŭs, p. 385)

tachypnea (tăk-ĭp-NĒ-ă, p. 410)

thoracentesis (thŏ-ră-sĕn-TĒ-sĭs, p. 378)

virulent (VĬR-ū-lĕnt, p. 398)

ANATOMY AND PHYSIOLOGY OF THE RESPIRATORY SYSTEM

For the millions of cells throughout the body to carry out their specialized activities, they must have a continuous supply of oxygen. External respiration, or breathing, is the exchange of oxygen and carbon dioxide between the lung and the environment. As air is inhaled, it is warmed, moistened, and filtered to prepare it for use by the body. The respiratory system works with the cardiovascular system to deliver oxygen to the cells, where it provides energy to carry out metabolism. Internal respiration is the exchange of oxygen and carbon dioxide at the cellular level. Oxygen enters the cells while carbon dioxide leaves them. The gases diffuse across the cell membrane into the bloodstream, which plays the role of transporter. Failure of the respiratory system or cardiovascular system has the same result: rapid cell death from oxygen starvation. Figure 9-1 shows the structure of the respiratory organs.

UPPER RESPIRATORY TRACT

Nose

Air enters the respiratory tract through the nose. The air is filtered, moistened, and warmed as it enters the two nasal openings (nares) and travels to the nasal cavity. The nasal septum separates the nares. This entire area is lined with mucous membrane, which is vascular. The mucous membrane provides warmth and moisture and secretes 1 L of moisture every day.

Lateral to the nasal cavities are three scroll-like bones called **turbinates** or **conchae** (Figure 9-2), which cause

the air to move over a larger surface area. This increase in surface area provides more time for warming and moisturizing the air. Lining the nasal cavities are tiny hairs, which trap dust and other foreign particles and prevent them from entering the lower respiratory tract.

Communicating with the nasal structures are paranasal sinuses (Figure 9-3). They are called the **frontal, maxillary, sphenoid,** and **ethmoid cavities.** These are hollow areas that make the skull lighter and are believed to give resonance to the voice. They are lined with mucous membranes that are continuous with the nasal cavity. Because of this, nasal infections can cause sinusitis, which is uncomfortable and difficult to treat.

The receptors for the sense of smell are located in the mucosa of the nasal cavities. They are the nerve endings of the olfactory nerve, the first cranial nerve. The nasolacrimal ducts, or tear ducts, communicate with the upper nasal chamber. Hence, when an individual cries, there are copious nasal secretions.

Pharynx

The **pharynx,** or throat (a tubular structure about 5 inches [13 cm] long extending from the base of the skull to the esophagus and situated just in front of the vertebrae), is the passageway for both air and food. At the distal end of the pharynx are three subdivisions: (1) **nasopharynx** (superior portion), (2) **oropharynx** (posterior to mouth), and (3) **laryngopharynx** (directly superior to larynx) (see Figure 9-2).

The eustachian tubes enter either side of the nasopharynx, connecting it to the middle ear. Because the inner linings of the pharynx and the eustachian tube are continuous, an infection of the pharynx can spread easily to the ear. This is common in children. The adenoids (pharyngeal tonsils) are in the nasopharynx, whereas the palatine tonsils are in the oropharynx.

Larynx

The **larynx** (Figure 9-4, *A*), or organ of voice, is supported by nine areas of cartilage and connects the pharynx with the trachea. The largest area of cartilage is composed of two fused plates and is called the **thyroid cartilage,** or **Adam's apple.** It is the same size in girls and boys until puberty, when it enlarges in boys and produces a projection in the neck. The **epiglottis,** a large leaf-shaped area of cartilage, protects the larynx when swallowing. It covers the larynx tightly to prevent food from entering the trachea and directs the food to the esophagus (Figure 9-4, *B*).

The larynx contains the vocal cords. During expiration, air rushes over the vocal cords, causing them to vibrate. This enables speech to occur. The opening between the vocal cords is the glottis.

Trachea

The **trachea** (Figure 9-5), or windpipe, is a tubelike structure that extends approximately 4⅓ inches (11 cm) to the midchest, where it divides into the right and left

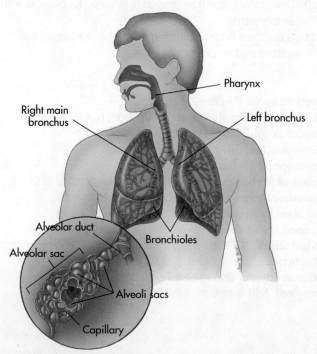

FIGURE 9-1 Structural plan of the respiratory organs showing pharynx, trachea, bronchi, and lungs. Inset shows the grapelike alveolar sacs where the interchange of oxygen and carbon dioxide takes place through the thin walls of the alveoli. Capillaries surround the alveoli.

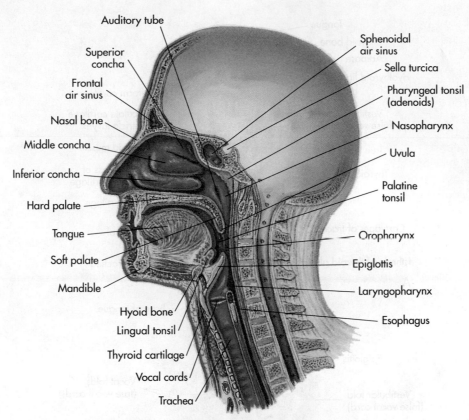

FIGURE 9-2 Sagittal section through the face and the neck.

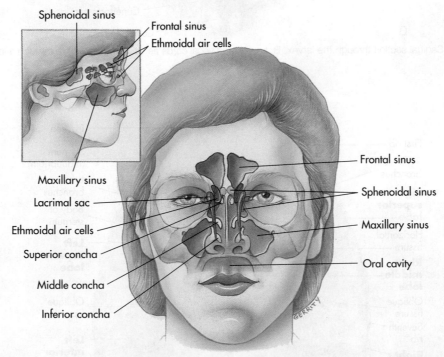

FIGURE 9-3 Projections of paranasal sinuses and oral nasal cavities on the skull and the face. Note the connection between the sinuses and the nasal cavity.

bronchi. It lies anterior to the esophagus and connects the larynx with the bronchi. The ventral (anterior) surface of the tube is covered in the neck by the isthmus (narrow connection) of the thyroid gland. It contains C-shaped cartilaginous rings that keep it from collapsing. The open part of the C-shaped rings lies posterior to the column anterior to the esophagus, which allows the esophagus to expand during swallowing while maintaining patency of the trachea. This is necessary for uninterrupted breathing.

The entire structure is lined with mucous membranes and tiny **cilia** (small, hairlike processes on the

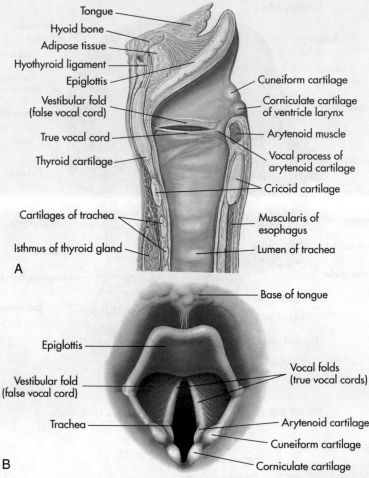

Tongue
Hyoid bone
Adipose tissue
Hyothyroid ligament
Epiglottis
Vestibular fold
(false vocal cord)
True vocal cord
Thyroid cartilage
Cartilages of trachea
Isthmus of thyroid gland

Cuneiform cartilage
Corniculate cartilage
of ventricle larynx
Arytenoid muscle
Vocal process of
arytenoid cartilage
Cricoid cartilage
Muscularis of
esophagus
Lumen of trachea

A

Base of tongue
Epiglottis
Vestibular fold
(false vocal cord)
Trachea

Vocal folds
(true vocal cords)
Arytenoid cartilage
Cuneiform cartilage
Corniculate cartilage

B

FIGURE 9-4 A, Sagittal section through the larynx. **B,** Larynx and vocal cords as viewed from above through a laryngeal mirror.

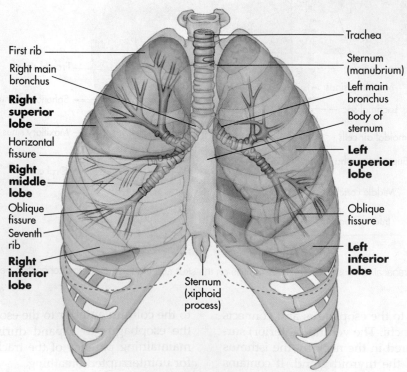

First rib
Right main
bronchus
**Right
superior
lobe**
Horizontal
fissure
**Right
middle
lobe**
Oblique
fissure
Seventh
rib
**Right
inferior
lobe**

Trachea
Sternum
(manubrium)
Left main
bronchus
Body of
sternum
**Left
superior
lobe**
Oblique
fissure
**Left
inferior
lobe**

Sternum
(xiphoid
process)

FIGURE 9-5 Projection of the lungs and trachea in relation to ribcage and clavicles. *Dotted line* shows location of dome-shaped diaphragm at the end of expiration and before inspiration. Note that apex of each lung projects above the clavicle. Ribs 11 and 12 are not visible in this view.

outer surfaces of small cells, which produce motion or current in a fluid) that sweep dust or debris upward toward the nasal cavity. Any large particles initiate the cough reflex, which aids in the evacuation of foreign material. Sometimes, because of an airway obstruction, a physician performs a tracheostomy (a surgical opening into the trachea through which an indwelling tube may be inserted). Once this procedure is completed, the individual breathes through the tracheal opening rather than the nose. The opening is below the larynx, so air cannot pass over the vocal cords. The vocal cords cannot vibrate, and speech becomes physiologically impossible.

LOWER RESPIRATORY TRACT
Bronchial Tree
As the trachea enters the lungs, it divides into the right and left bronchi. The right bronchus enters the right lung. It is larger in diameter and more vertical in descent. The left bronchus enters the left lung. It is smaller in diameter and slightly horizontal in position. Because of this design, foreign objects that are aspirated generally enter the right bronchus.

The large bronchi continue to divide into smaller structures called **bronchioles.** These structures divide into smaller, tubelike structures called **terminal bronchioles** or **alveolar ducts.** All these structures are lined with ciliated mucous membrane, as is the trachea. The end structures of the bronchial tree are called **alveoli.** These saclike structures resemble a bunch of grapes. A single grapelike structure is called an alveolus (Figures 9-1 and 9-6). In this terminal structure of the bronchial tree, gas exchange takes place. Each alveolus is surrounded by a blood capil-

lary, where diffusion of carbon dioxide and oxygen occurs. Alveoli are effective in gas exchange, mainly because they are extremely thin walled; each alveolus lies in contact with a blood capillary. In addition, each alveolus is coated with a thin covering of surfactant. Surfactant reduces the surface tension of the alveolus and prevents it from collapsing after each breath (see Figure 9-6).

The lungs contain millions of alveoli; they give shape and form to the lungs. They are filled with air, and lung tissue would float if it was put in water. This tiny, grapelike structure is the most important feature of the respiratory system. It is here that the oxygen diffuses into the cardiovascular system.

MECHANICS OF BREATHING
Thoracic Cavity
The lungs occupy almost all the thoracic cavity except the centermost area, the mediastinum, which contains the heart and the great vessels. This cavity, the interpleural space, is enclosed by the sternum, the ribs, and the thoracic vertebrae.

Lungs
The lungs are large, paired, spongy cone-shaped organs (see Figure 9-5). The right lung weighs approximately 625 g; the left lung weighs approximately 570 g. The right lung contains three lobes; the left lung contains only two lobes. Located approximately 1 inch (2.5 cm) above the first rib is the narrow part (the apex) of each lung. The broad, inferior part (the base) lies in the diaphragm.

The lungs receive their blood supply, which comes directly from the heart, through the pulmonary ar-

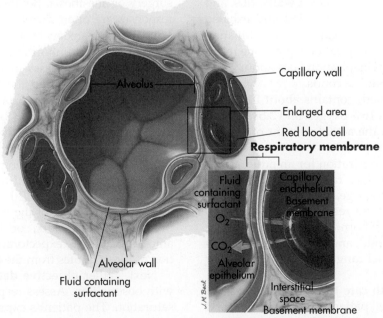

FIGURE 9-6 Each alveolus is continuously ventilated with fresh air. Inset shows a magnified view of the respiratory membrane composed of the alveolar wall (surfactant, epithelial cells, and basement membrane), interstitial fluid, and the wall of a pulmonary capillary (basement membrane and endothelial cells). Carbon dioxide and oxygen diffuse across the respiratory membrane.

teries. By the time the blood reaches the lung capillaries, it is low in oxygen content. Because alveolar air is rich in oxygen, diffusion causes movement of oxygen from the area of high concentration. Carbon dioxide also diffuses between blood and lung capillaries and alveolar air. Blood flowing through the lung capillaries is high in carbon dioxide. After carbon dioxide is diffused into the alveoli and oxygen is diffused into the blood, carbon dioxide leaves the body by expiration of air from the lungs. The blood, now rich in oxygen, returns to the heart for circulation to the body via the pulmonary veins to the left atrium.

The surface of each lung is covered with a thin, moist, serous membrane called the **visceral pleura.** The walls of the thoracic cavity are covered with the same type of membrane called the **parietal pleura.** The pleural cavity around the lungs is an airtight vacuum that contains negative pressure. The air in the lungs is at atmospheric pressure—higher than in the pleural cavity. The negative pressure assists in keeping the lungs inflated. The visceral and parietal pleura produce a serous secretion, which allows the lung to slide over the walls of the thorax while breathing. Usually the body produces the exact amount of serous secretion needed. If too much serous secretion is produced, fluid accumulates in the pleural space; this is called **pleural effusion.** The pleural space becomes distended and puts pressure on the lungs, making it difficult to breathe. The physician may decide to remove the fluid by performing a **thoracentesis**—inserting a needlelike instrument into the pleural space and removing the fluid.

Respiratory Movements and Ranges

The rhythmic movements of the chest walls, ribs, and associated muscles when air is inhaled and exhaled make up the respiratory movements. The combination of one inspiration and one expiration equals one respiration. At rest the normal inspiration lasts about 2 seconds and expiration about 3 seconds.

Room air, when inhaled, contains about 21% oxygen; exhaled air contains 16% oxygen and 3.5% carbon dioxide. This represents the actual amount of oxygen used in a single breath.

The normal range of respiration for an adult at rest is 14 to 20 breaths/min. This rate can be affected by many variables, including age, sex, activity, disease, and body temperature. The respiratory rate is 40 to 60 breaths/min for a newborn, 22 to 24 breaths/min for an early school-age child, and 20 to 22 breaths/min for a teenager. The normal range for women is higher than that for men.

Members of the health care team should assess all factors influencing the patient's respirations and should count the respirations without the patient's awareness to prevent alterations in the breathing pattern.

REGULATION OF RESPIRATION

Nervous Control

The medulla oblongata and pons of the brain are responsible for the basic rhythm and depth of respiration. The body's demands can modify the rhythm. Other parts of the nervous system help coordinate the transfer from inspiration to expiration. Chemoreceptors in the carotid and aortic bodies are specialized receptors. When stimulated by increasing levels of blood carbon dioxide, decreasing levels of blood oxygen, or increasing blood acidity, these receptors send nerve impulses to the respiratory centers, which in turn modify respiratory rates.

Carbon dioxide, which is present in the blood as carbonic acid, is considered the chemical stimulant for regulation of respiration. Therefore the more carbon dioxide in the blood, the more acidic the blood becomes. After exhalation the blood becomes more alkaline. The normal pH of the blood is 7.35 to 7.45—a narrow range. Deviation from this range causes the patient to develop either acidosis or alkalosis.

ASSESSMENT OF THE RESPIRATORY SYSTEM

The function of the respiratory system is gas exchange (oxygen and carbon dioxide) at the alveolar-capillary level. This function depends on the lungs' capability for contraction and expansion, which in turn is influenced by musculoskeletal and neurologic functions.

Physical assessment of the patient's general health always includes the respiratory system. More extensive assessments are required for patients with acute or chronic respiratory or cardiac conditions, those with a history of respiratory impairment related to trauma or allergic reactions, or those who have recently undergone surgery or anesthesia. Because physical and emotional responses are often correlated, also inquire about any accompanying anxiety or stress. This information should be obtained in an unhurried, matter-of-fact manner.

The respiratory assessment includes collection of **subjective data.** During the interview, encourage the patient to describe any symptoms, such as shortness of breath, dyspnea on exertion, or cough. **Dyspnea,** or difficulty breathing, is a subjective experience that only the patient can accurately describe. Data should include onset; duration; precipitating factors; and relief measures, such as position and use of over-the-counter or prescribed medications. If the patient reports a cough, ask for a description of the cough: productive or nonproductive; harsh, dry, or hacking; and color and amount of mucus expectorated. Record this information as direct quotes from the patient when possible.

Next, gather **objective data.** Begin the assessment with observation. Assess respiratory rate and oxygen saturation. The patient's expression, chest movement, and respirations all provide valuable visual clues. At times the patient cannot verbalize distress, but has a wide-eyed, anxious look that reflects the fear of suffocating. Flaring nostrils indicate the patient is struggling to breathe, which is usually a late sign of respiratory distress. Initial observation yields information on the patient's skin color and turgor. Note any obvious respiratory distress, wheezes, or **orthopnea** (an abnormal condition in which a person must sit or stand to breathe deeply or comfortably).

To continue the assessment, auscultate all lung fields, anteriorly and posteriorly, noting the presence of **adventitious** sounds (abnormal sounds superimposed on breath sounds, including sibilant wheezes [formerly called simply **wheezes**], sonorous wheezes [formerly called **rhonchi**], crackles [formerly called **rales**], and pleural friction rubs) (Table 9-1). **Sibilant wheezes** are musical, high-pitched, squeaking or whistling sounds, caused by the rapid movement of air through narrowed bronchioles. **Sonorous wheezes** are low-pitched, loud, coarse, snoring sounds. They are often heard on expiration. **Crackles** are short, discrete, interrupted crackling or bubbling sounds that are most commonly heard during inspiration. Crackles sound like hairs being rolled between the fingers close to the ear. They are thought to occur when air is forced through respiratory passages narrowed by fluid, mucus, or pus. They are associated with inflammation or infection of the small bronchi, bronchioles, and alveoli. **Pleural friction rubs** are low-pitched, grating or creaking lung sounds that occur when inflamed pleural surfaces rub together during respiration.

Also assess chest movement. Note whether the chest expands equally on both sides; chest expansion on one side only may indicate serious pulmonary complications. Look for retraction of the chest wall between the ribs and under the clavicle during inspiration. This can signal late-stage respiratory distress. Be alert for signs and symptoms of **hypoxia** (oxygen deficiency) (Box 9-1).

LABORATORY AND DIAGNOSTIC EXAMINATIONS

A variety of tests are used to evaluate respiratory status and identify respiratory conditions. Other tests include diagnostic imaging, laboratory work, and more invasive measures. Nurses should be familiar with these tests so they can adequately prepare the patient.

CHEST ROENTGENOGRAM

Usually referred to as chest radiographs, chest roentgenograms are an essential diagnostic tool for evaluating disorders of the chest. A chest radiograph provides

Table 9-1 Adventitious Breath Sounds

TYPE	CHARACTERISTICS	COMMENTS
Crackles (rales)	Brief, not continuous; more common in inspiration; interrupted crackling or bubbling sounds, similar to those produced by hairs being rolled between the fingers close to the ear	Caused by fluid, mucus, or pus in the small airways and alveoli.
Fine crackles	As described above; high-pitched, sibilant crackling at end of inspiration	Found in diseases affecting bronchioles and alveoli.
Medium crackles	As described above; medium pitch, more sonorous, moisture sound during midinspiration	Associated with diseases of small bronchi.
Coarse crackles	As described above; loud, bubbly sound in early inspiration	Associated with diseases of small bronchi.
Sonorous wheezes (rhonchi)	Deep, running sound that may be continuous; loud, low, coarse sound (like a snore) heard at any point of inspiration or expiration	Caused by air moving through narrowed tracheobronchial passages (caused by secretions, tumor, spasm); cough may alter sound if caused by mucus in trachea or large bronchi.
Sibilant wheezes (wheezes)	High-pitched, musical, whistlelike sound during inspiration or expiration; sound may be several notes or one, and may vary from one minute to the next	Caused by narrowed bronchioles; bilateral wheeze often result of bronchospasm; unilateral, sharply localized wheeze may result from foreign matter or tumor compression.
Pleural friction rub	Dry, creaking, grating, low-pitched sound with a machinelike quality during both inspiration and expiration; loudest over anterior chest	Sound originates outside respiratory tree, usually caused by inflammation; over the lung fields it suggests pleurisy; over the pericardium it suggests pericarditis with a pericardial friction rub. To distinguish the two, ask the patient to hold the breath briefly. If the rubbing sound persists, it is a pericardial friction rub because the inflamed pericardial layers continue rubbing together with each heartbeat; a pleural rub would stop when breathing stops.

Box 9-1 **Signs and Symptoms of Hypoxia**

- Apprehension, anxiety, restlessness
- Decreased ability to concentrate
- Disorientation
- Decreased level of consciousness
- Increased fatigue
- Vertigo
- Behavioral changes
- Increased pulse rate; bradycardia as hypoxia advances
- Increased rate and depth of respiration; shallow, slow respirations as hypoxia progresses
- Elevated blood pressure; with continuing oxygen deficiency, decreased blood pressure
- Cardiac dysrhythmias
- Pallor
- Cyanosis (may not be present until hypoxia is severe)
- Clubbing
- Dyspnea

visualization of the lungs, ribs, clavicles, humeri, scapulae, vertebrae, heart, and major thoracic vessels. This test gives information on alterations in size and location of the pulmonary structures and blood flow, and it identifies lesions, infiltrates, foreign bodies, or fluid. A chest radiograph also shows whether a disorder involves the lung parenchyma (the tissue of an organ, as distinguished from supporting or connective tissue) or the interstitial spaces. Chest radiographs can confirm pneumothorax, pneumonia, pleural effusion, and pulmonary edema.

The chest radiographic examination can be performed at different angles for greater clarification. Have the patient wear a hospital gown tied in back. Do not use pins. Any article of clothing containing metal (e.g., a bra with metal hooks) or jewelry must be removed, since the metal produces a shadow on the film.

COMPUTED TOMOGRAPHY

Chest CT Scan

Computed tomography (CT) **scans** of the lungs take pictures of small layers of pulmonary tissue, usually to identify a pulmonary lesion. These views can be diagonal or cross-sectional, with a scanner rotating at various angles. Although this test is painless and noninvasive and results in little radiation exposure, patient teaching is necessary before the procedure to offer explanations and allay anxiety.

Helical or Spiral CT Chest Scan

Helical (also called spiral or volume-averaging) **CT scanning** represents a marked improvement over standard CT scanning. The helical CT scan continuously obtains images. This produces faster and more accurate images. Because the helical CT can scan the abdomen and chest in less than 30 seconds, the entire study can be performed with one breath-hold. Furthermore, when contrast material is used, the entire region can be

imaged in just a few seconds after the contrast injection (Pagana & Pagana, 2007).

Pulmonary Angiography (Pulmonary Arteriography)

Pulmonary angiography (pulmonary arteriography) uses a radiographic contrast material injected into the pulmonary arteries to permit visualization of the pulmonary vasculature. Angiography is used to detect pulmonary embolism (PE) and a variety of congenital and acquired lesions of the pulmonary vessels.

When PE is suspected, lung scanning is performed first. If the lung scan is normal, PE is ruled out. If the scan is uncertain however, the diagnosis of PE is questionable because pathologic processes (e.g., emphysema, pneumonia) also may cause abnormalities on the lung scan. Definitive diagnosis for PE may require pulmonary angiography (Pagana & Pagana, 2007).

Ventilation-Perfusion Scan (V/Q Scan)

Ventilation-perfusion (V/Q) scanning is used primarily to check for a PE. An intravenous (IV) radioisotope is given for the perfusion portion of the test, and the pulmonary vasculature is outlined and photographed. For the ventilation portion of the test, the patient inhales a radioactive gas that outlines the alveoli, and another photograph is taken. Normal scans show homogeneous radioactivity. Diminished or absent radioactivity suggests lack of perfusion or airflow (Lewis et al., 2007).

PULMONARY FUNCTION TESTING

Pulmonary function tests (PFTs) are performed to assess the presence and severity of disease in the large and small airways. PFTs include various procedures to obtain information on lung volume, ventilation, pulmonary spirometry, and gas exchange. Lung volume tests refer to the volume of air that can be completely and slowly exhaled after a maximum inhalation (**vital capacity**). **Inspiratory capacity** is the largest amount of air that can be inhaled in one breath from the resting expiratory level. **Total lung capacity** is calculated to determine the volume of air in the lung after a maximal inhalation. Ventilation tests evaluate the volume of air inhaled or exhaled in each respiratory cycle. Pulmonary spirometry tests evaluate the amount of air that can be forcefully exhaled after maximum inhalation. These tests require the use of a spirometer.

One of the most important tools for diagnosing respiratory diseases is gas exchange, which identifies the capacity for diffusion of carbon dioxide. This component of PFT determines the degree of function in the pulmonary capillary beds in contact with functioning alveoli.

MEDIASTINOSCOPY

Mediastinoscopy is a surgical endoscopic procedure in which an incision is created in the suprasternal notch, allowing the endoscope to be passed into the upper mediastinum. This is performed to gather a sample of lymph nodes for biopsy for tumor diagnosis. Because these lymph nodes receive lymphatic drainage from the lungs, they help diagnose malignant tumors. Tumors in the mediastinum (e.g., thymoma or lymphoma) can also be biopsied through the mediastinoscope (Pagana & Pagana, 2007). This procedure is performed in the operating room, with the patient under general anesthesia.

LARYNGOSCOPY

Laryngoscopy can be performed for either direct or indirect visualization of the larynx. Indirect laryngoscopy is probably the most common procedure for assessing respiratory difficulties; this entails using a laryngeal mirror in the awake patient's mouth for visualization. This procedure can be used for biopsy or polyp excision. Direct laryngoscopy requires local or general anesthesia and exposes the vocal cords with a laryngoscope passed down over the tongue.

BRONCHOSCOPY

Bronchoscopy is performed by passing a bronchoscope into the trachea and bronchi. Using either a rigid bronchoscope or a flexible fiberoptic bronchoscope (the instrument of choice in most cases) allows visualization of the larynx, the trachea, and the bronchi (Figure 9-7). Diagnostic bronchoscopic examination includes observation of the tracheobronchial tree for (1) abnormalities, (2) tissue biopsy, and (3) secretions collected for cytologic (cell) or bacteriologic examination. A local anesthetic agent may be used, but an IV general anesthetic agent is usually given. The patient is treated as a surgical patient.

Nursing interventions for patients after bronchoscopy include (1) keeping the patient on NPO (nothing by mouth) status until gag reflex returns, usually about 2 hours after the procedure; (2) keeping the patient in a semi-Fowler's position and turning on either side to facilitate removal of secretions (unless the phy-

sician specifies another position); (3) monitoring the patient for signs of laryngeal edema or laryngospasms, such as stridor or increasing dyspnea; and (4) if lung tissue biopsy is taken, monitoring sputum for signs of hemorrhage (blood-streaked sputum is expected for a few days after biopsy).

SPUTUM SPECIMEN

Sputum samples frequently are obtained for microscopic evaluation, such as Gram stain and culture and sensitivity (Box 9-2). For the range of sputum characteristics, see Box 9-3.

| Box 9-2 | Guidelines for Sputum Specimen Collection |

1. Explain to the patient that the sputum must be brought up from the lungs. Patients who have difficulty producing sputum or who have tenacious sputum may be dehydrated. Encourage fluid intake.
2. Collect the sputum specimen before prescribed antibiotics are started.
3. Collect specimens before meals to avoid possible emesis from coughing.
4. Instruct patient to inhale and exhale deeply three times, then inhale swiftly, cough forcefully, and expectorate into the sterile sputum container. Usually early morning samples are collected on 3 consecutive days.
5. If the patient cannot raise sputum spontaneously, a hypertonic saline aerosol mist may help produce a good specimen. Instruct the patient to take several normal breaths of the mist, inhale deeply, cough, and expectorate.
6. Instruct patient to rinse mouth with water before expectorating into sterile specimen bottle to decrease sputum contamination.
7. Properly label and send to the laboratory without delay.
8. Sputum samples can also be obtained indirectly, such as with nasotracheal suctioning with a catheter or transtracheal aspiration. Take care to ensure that the suction catheters remain sterile. A physician's order must be obtained for endotracheal suctioning.

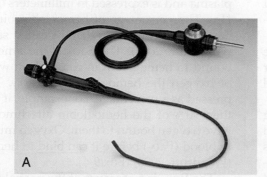
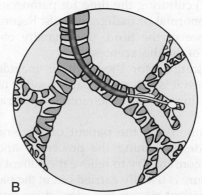

FIGURE 9-7 Fiberoptic bronchoscope. **A,** The transbronchoscopic balloon-tipped catheter and the flexible fiberoptic bronchoscope. **B,** The catheter is introduced into a small airway and the balloon is inflated with 1.5 to 2 mL of air to occlude the airway. Bronchial alveolar lavage is performed by injecting and withdrawing 30-mL aliquots of sterile saline solution, gently aspirating after each instillation. Specimens are sent to the laboratory for analysis.

Box 9-3	Range of Sputum Characteristics

COLOR
- Clear
- White
- Yellow
- Green
- Brown
- Red
- Pink tinged
- Streaked with blood

ODOR
- None
- Malodorous

CONSISTENCY
- Frothy
- Watery
- Tenacious

BLOOD
- All the time
- Occasionally
- Early morning

CYTOLOGIC STUDIES

Cytologic tests can be performed on any body secretion, such as sputum or pleural fluid, to detect abnormal or malignant cells.

LUNG BIOPSY

Lung biopsy may be done transbronchially or as an open-lung biopsy. The purpose is to obtain tissue, cells, or secretions for evaluation. Transbronchial lung biopsy involves passing a forceps or needle through the bronchoscope to obtain a specimen. Specimens can be cultured or examined for malignant cells. Nursing interventions are the same as for fiberoptic bronchoscopy. Open-lung biopsy is used when pulmonary disease cannot be diagnosed by other procedures. The patient is anesthetized, the chest is opened with a thoracotomy incision, and a biopsy specimen is obtained.

THORACENTESIS

Thoracentesis is the surgical perforation of the chest wall and pleural space with a needle for the aspiration of fluid for diagnostic or therapeutic purposes or for the removal of a specimen for biopsy (Figure 9-8). Indications for fluid removal for diagnostic purposes include (1) examining the pleural fluid for specific gravity, white blood cell count, red blood cell count, protein, and glucose; and (2) culturing the fluid for pathogens and checking for abnormal or malignant cells. Record the gross appearance of the fluid, the quantity obtained, and the site of the thoracentesis.

Therapeutic indications for thoracentesis include removal of fluid when it is a threat to patient safety or comfort and instillation of medication into the pleural space.

Nursing interventions for the patient undergoing thoracentesis include explaining the procedure and obtaining a written consent. Try to relieve the patient's anxiety. The procedure is usually carried out in the patient's room. The patient sits on the edge of the bed with the head and arms resting on a pillow placed on an overbed table. If the patient cannot sit up, turn him or her to the unaffected side with the head of the bed elevated 30 degrees.

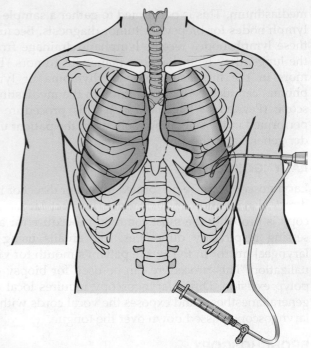

FIGURE 9-8 Thoracentesis. The needle has penetrated the fluid-filled pleural space to remove fluid.

Monitor vital signs, general appearance, and respiratory status throughout the procedure. Usually no more than 1300 mL of pleural fluid should be removed within a 30-minute period because of the risk of intravascular fluid shift with resultant pulmonary edema. After thoracentesis, position the patient on the unaffected side. Label the specimen and send it immediately to the laboratory per physician's orders.

ARTERIAL BLOOD GASES

Blood gas analysis is an essential test in diagnosing and monitoring patients with respiratory disorders. The lungs' ability to oxygenate arterial blood adequately is determined by examination of the arterial oxygen tension (Pao_2) and arterial oxygen saturation (Sao_2). Oxygen is carried in the blood in two forms: dissolved oxygen and oxygen in combination with hemoglobin. The Pao_2 represents the amount of oxygen dissolved in the plasma and is expressed in millimeters of mercury (mm Hg). The percentage of hemoglobin binding sites that have oxygen bound to them is called saturation (Sao_2) (Woodruff, 2006). The Sao_2 is the amount of oxygen bound to hemoglobin in comparison with the amount of oxygen the hemoglobin can carry. The Sao_2 is expressed as a percentage. For example, if the Sao_2 is 90%, then 90% of the hemoglobin attachments for oxygen have oxygen bound to them. Oxygen must first dissolve in blood (Pao_2) before it can bind to hemoglobin (Sao_2) (Woodruff, 2006) (Box 9-4).

The Pco_2 is a measure of the partial pressure of carbon dioxide in the blood. Pco_2 is referred to as the respiratory component in acid-base determination because this value is primarily controlled by the lungs. As the carbon dioxide level increases, the pH de-

Box 9-4   **Guidelines for Interpreting Arterial Blood Gas Values**

1. Examine each value by itself.
   Normal arterial blood gas values (ABGs)
   - pH: 7.35-7.45
   - $Paco_2$: 35-45 mm Hg
   - Pao_2: 80-100 mm Hg
   - HCO_3^- : 21-28 mEq/L
   - Sao_2: 95%
2. Determine whether the pH reflects acidity or alkalinity.
   - pH ≤7.35 = acidity
   - pH ≥7.45 = alkalinity
3. Which other value corresponds with that condition?
   NOTE: $Paco_2$ reflects respiratory factors; HCO_3^- reflects metabolic factors.
   - Carbon dioxide is a potential acid, so carbon dioxide greater than 45 = more acidity.
   - HCO_3^- is a basic (alkaline) substance, so HCO_3^- greater than 45 = more alkalinity.
   EXAMPLE: A patient with acute exacerbation of chronic obstructive pulmonary disease has the following ABGs:
   - pH: 7.42
   - $Paco_2$: 49 mm Hg
   - Pao_2: 50 mm Hg

   - HCO_3^-: 31 mEq/L
   - Sao_2: 84%
   Because the pH is within a normal range, this is a compensated respiratory problem. The kidneys have increased the amount of bicarbonate they put into the blood to bring the pH to a normal level. The Pao_2 and the Sao_2 are low, indicating hypoxemia.
   EXAMPLE:
   - pH: 7.21
   - $Paco_2$: 58 mm Hg
   - Pao_2: 70 mm Hg
   - HCO_3^-: 24 mEq/L
   - Sao_2: 84%
   The pH is less than 7.35, indicating acidosis. The $Paco_2$ is higher than 45 mm Hg, indicating acidosis. The $Paco_2$ matches the pH, making it a respiratory acidosis. The HCO_3^- is normal, indicating there is no compensation. The $Paco_2$ and the Sao_2 are low, indicating hypoxemia. The full diagnosis for a patient with these ABG results is uncompensated respiratory acidosis with hypoxemia.

Woodruff, D. (2006). Take these 6 easy steps to ABG analysis. *Nursing Made Incredibly Easy!* 4(1):4–7.

creases. Therefore the carbon dioxide level and pH are inversely proportional. The Pco_2 level is elevated in primary respiratory acidosis and decreased in primary respiratory alkalosis. Because the lungs compensate for primary metabolic acid-based derangements, Pco_2 levels are affected by metabolic disturbances as well. In metabolic acidosis the lungs attempt to compensate by "blowing off" carbon dioxide to raise pH. In metabolic alkalosis the lungs attempt to compensate by retaining carbon dioxide to lower pH.

The bicarbonate ion (HCO_3^-) is a measure of the metabolic (renal) component of the acid-base equilibrium. This ion can be measured directly by the bicarbonate value or indirectly by the carbon dioxide content. As the HCO_3^- level increases, the pH also increases; therefore the relationship of bicarbonate to pH is directly proportional. HCO_3^- is elevated in metabolic alkalosis and decreased in metabolic acidosis. The kidneys also compensate for primary respiratory acid-base derangements. For example, in respiratory acidosis, the kidneys attempt to compensate by reabsorbing increased amounts of HCO_3^-. In respiratory alkalosis the kidneys excrete HCO_3^- in increased amounts in an attempt to lower pH through compensation (Table 9-2).

Arterial blood gas (ABG) testing yields definitive information on the patient's respiratory status and metabolic balance. The procedure is performed at the bedside. A heparinized syringe and needle are used to withdraw 3 to 5 mL of arterial blood, usually from the radial artery. Other possible sites include femoral or brachial arteries. After the sample is obtained, place direct pressure on the puncture site for a minimum of 5 minutes to prevent hematoma formation and blood loss. If the patient is taking

Table 9-2   **Acid-Base Disturbances and Compensatory Mechanisms**

ACID-BASE DISTURBANCE	MODE OF COMPENSATION
Respiratory acidosis	Kidneys retain increased amounts of HCO_3^- to increase pH.
Respiratory alkalosis	Kidneys excrete increased amounts of HCO_3^- to lower pH.
Metabolic acidosis	Lungs "blow off" carbon dioxide to raise pH.
Metabolic alkalosis	Lungs retain carbon dioxide to lower pH.

anticoagulants, maintain pressure for 20 minutes or longer until bleeding stops. Place the capped syringe in a basin of crushed ice and water to preserve the gas and pH levels of the specimen. Send the properly labeled specimen to the laboratory immediately.

The blood gas values (see Box 9-4) assess the patient's metabolic (acid-base) status by measuring the pH. Carbon dioxide tension is measured by $Paco_2$ and indicates the patient's ventilation. Oxygen saturation (Pao_2 and Sao_2) is also measured.

PULSE OXIMETRY

Pulse oximetry is a noninvasive method of providing continuous monitoring of Sao_2 (saturation of oxygen) for assessment of gas exchange. The system consists of a probe that looks like a large clothespin and is applied to a finger, a toe, an earlobe, or the bridge of the nose. The noninvasive probe has a light-emitting sensor that shoots narrow beams of red and infrared light through the tissue and a light-receiving sensor that measures the amount of light being absorbed by oxygenated and deoxygenated hemoglobin in pulsating arterial blood. The probe is connected to a computer with a monitor that displays hemoglobin oxygen saturation and pulse rates (Figure 9-9). A pulse oximeter beeps if the patient's SaO_2 registers outside of the limits set according to the physician's order.

For decades, physicians have relied on ABG analysis to evaluate gas exchange and oxygen transport. As valuable as this test is, ABG results reflect a patient's oxygenation status at only one moment in time. Today, pulse oximetry permits continuous, noninvasive monitoring of SaO_2. Oximetry technology allows the nurse to assess minute-to-minute changes in arterial saturations, intervene before hypoxemia produces obvious and serious signs and symptoms, and evaluate the patient's response to treatment. Pulse oximetry alone does not provide data about PaO_2 and acid-base balance. Therefore, ABGs are also needed periodically (Woodruff, 2006).

An SaO_2 of 90% to 100% is needed to adequately replenish oxygen in plasma. The ability of hemoglobin to feed oxygen to the plasma weakens significantly when the SaO_2 drops below 85%. An SaO_2 of less than 70% is considered life threatening.

Arterial oxygen saturation can be quickly and noninvasively determined through pulse oximetry. Severe circulatory problems may diminish the accuracy of the reading. If oximetry results seem questionable, the physician usually orders ABG tests. A pulse oximeter can detect a change within 6 seconds. To get optimal results, remember these points:

- Do not attach the transducer to an extremity that has a blood pressure cuff or arterial catheter in place; these devices reduce blood flow.
- Place the probe over a pulsating vascular bed.
- While the probe is on the patient, protect it from strong light (such as direct sunlight), which can affect the reading.

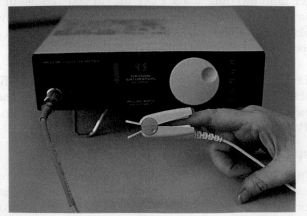

FIGURE 9-9 Portable pulse oximeter with spring-tension digit probe displays oxygen saturation and pulse rate.

- Avoid excess patient movement to ensure accuracy.
- Remember that hypothermia, hypotension, and vasoconstriction can affect readings.

DISORDERS OF THE UPPER AIRWAY

EPISTAXIS

Etiology and Pathophysiology

The underlying cause of epistaxis (bleeding from the nose) is congestion of the nasal membranes, leading to capillary rupture. This condition is frequently caused by injury and occurs more frequently in men.

Epistaxis can be either a primary disorder or secondary to other conditions. It can be related to menstrual flow in women or hypertension. Other causes include local irritation of nasal mucosa, such as dryness, chronic infection, trauma (e.g., injury, vigorous nose blowing, or nose picking), topical corticosteroid use, nasal spray abuse, or street drug use. If the patient has a disorder that results in a prolonged bleeding time or reduction in platelet counts, this could predispose the patient to epistaxis (Kucik, 2005). Bleeding may also be prolonged if the patient takes aspirin or nonsteroidal antiinflammatory drugs (NSAIDs). A major factor in epistaxis is the many capillaries in the nasal passages.

Clinical Manifestations

The primary observation is bright red blood draining from one or both nostrils. With a severe nasal hemorrhage, adults can lose as much as 1 L of blood per hour, but this loss is not prolonged. Exsanguination (loss of blood to the point at which life can no longer be sustained) from epistaxis is rare.

Assessment

Collection of **subjective data** includes asking the patient to relate the duration and severity of bleeding and identifying precipitating factors, if possible.

Collection of **objective data** involves assessing the presence of bleeding from one or both nostrils. Determine whether the bleeding is occurring in the anterior or posterior portion of the nasal passageway. Assess the patient's blood pressure, temperature, pulse, respirations, and any evidence of hypovolemic shock. Severe bleeding results in a drop in blood pressure, which may cause the bleeding to stop. Hypotension is a late sign of shock.

Diagnostic Tests

A hemoglobin and hematocrit determination will aid in establishing an estimate of the blood loss. Prothrombin time (PT), International Normalized Ratio (INR), and partial thromboplastin time (PTT) assist in identifying contributing factors, such as a bleeding tendency and clotting abnormalities. A rhinoscopy may be performed to locate the bleeding site and possible causes and treatment. This procedure involves inserting a lighted nasal speculum into the nasal cavity.

Medical Management

Epistaxis has many possible treatments, including nasal packing with cotton saturated with 1:1000 epinephrine to promote local vasoconstriction. Cautery can be either electrical (burning [cauterizing] the bleeding vessel) or chemical (applying a silver nitrate stick to the site of the bleeding). Posterior packing of the nasal cavity may be needed. A balloon tamponade may be done by inserting a Foley-like catheter into the nose and inflating the balloon after it is placed posteriorly. Traction is then placed on the catheter to compress the vessel in the area. Also, some physicians prescribe antibiotics (penicillin) after the bleeding is controlled to minimize risk of infection.

Nursing Interventions and Patient Teaching

Nursing interventions include keeping the patient quiet. Place the patient in a sitting position, leaning forward, or in a reclining position with head and shoulders elevated. Apply direct pressure by pinching the entire soft lower portion of the nose for 10 to 15 minutes. Apply ice compresses to the nose and have the patient suck on ice. Partially insert a small gauze pad into the bleeding nostril, and apply digital pressure if bleeding continues. Monitor for signs and symptoms of hypovolemic shock.

Nursing diagnoses and interventions for the patient with epistaxis include but are not limited to the following:

Nursing Diagnoses	Nursing Interventions
Ineffective tissue perfusion, cerebral and/or cardiopulmonary, related to blood loss	Assess vital signs and level of consciousness every 15 minutes and report any changes. Document estimated blood loss.
Risk for aspiration, related to bleeding	Elevate head of bed; place patient in Fowler's position with the head forward; encourage patient to let the blood drain from the nose. Pinch nostrils; have the patient breathe through the mouth; apply ice compresses over the nose (however, the primary benefit of the application of ice is that it requires the patient to remain still); assist patient in clearing secretions. Maintain airway patency. Instruct patient to expectorate any blood or clots rather than swallow them, which could cause nausea and vomiting.

Instruct the patient (and the family, if possible) not to pick, scratch, or otherwise irritate the nares. To prevent recurrent hemorrhage, warn the patient not to blow the nose vigorously and to avoid dryness of the nose. Instruct the patient and the family regarding the risks of foreign objects inserted in the nose (this is especially important in pediatric patients). Encourage the patient to use a vaporizer and saline or nasal lubricants to keep nasal mucous membranes moist. Advise the patient to avoid using aspirin-containing products or NSAIDs, and teach him or her to sneeze with the mouth open.

Prognosis

With treatment, prognosis is good.

DEVIATED SEPTUM AND NASAL POLYPS

Etiology and Pathophysiology

Common conditions that cause nasal obstruction include nasal polyps or a deviated septum caused by congenital abnormality or, more likely, injury. The septum deviates from the midline and can partially obstruct the nasal passageway. Nasal polyps are tissue growths on the nasal tissues that are frequently caused by prolonged sinus inflammation; allergies are often the underlying cause.

Clinical Manifestations

The major manifestations of nasal septal deviations and polyps are **stertorous** (characterized by a harsh snoring sound) respirations, dyspnea, and sometimes postnasal drip.

Assessment

Collection of **subjective data** includes establishing the presence of previous injuries or infections, allergies, and sinus congestion. The patient complains of dyspnea.

Collection of **objective data** involves identifying the condition and its location. Note the rate and character of the patient's respirations.

Diagnostic Tests

Sinus radiographic studies depict the presence of shadowy sinuses when nasal polyps are present. A shift of the nasal septum is evident with a septal defect. A deviated septum may also be seen on visual examination.

Medical Management

These conditions frequently require surgical correction. Nasoseptoplasty is the operation of choice to reconstruct, align, and straighten the deviated nasal septum. A nasal polypectomy is performed to remove the polyps. Actions include nasal packing to control bleeding for 24 hours, and then maintaining nasal mucosa hydration with nasal irrigation of saline or application of a light layer of petroleum jelly to the external nares to prevent drying. Medications include (1) corticosteroids (prednisone), which cause polyps to decrease or disappear; and (2) antihistamines for allergy signs and symptoms, to decrease congestion in both septal deviations and polyps. Antibiotic agents (penicillin) may be used in both conditions to prevent infection. Analgesics (acetaminophen [Tylenol]) may be given to relieve the headache that occurs with septal deviation.

Nursing Interventions and Patient Teaching
Nursing interventions are generally aimed at maintaining airway patency and preventing infection. Postoperative interventions for nasal surgery include monitoring closely for infection or hemorrhage and maintaining patient comfort.

Nursing diagnoses and interventions for the patient with deviated septum or nasal polyps include but are not limited to the following:

Nursing Diagnoses	Nursing Interventions
Ineffective airway clearance, related to nasal exudates	Document patient's ability to clear secretions, and note respiratory status. Elevate head of bed, and apply ice compresses to the nose to decrease edema, discoloration, discomfort, and bleeding. Change nasal drip pad as needed, documenting color, consistency, and amount of exudates.
Risk for injury, related to trauma to bleeding site associated with vigorous nose blowing	Assess and report exudates (as stated above). Instruct patient against blowing nose in immediate postoperative period, since this could increase bleeding, edema, and ecchymosis.

Instruct the patient to contact the physician if bleeding or infection develops. The patient should use nasal sprays and drops judiciously because of the possible rebound effect on nasal mucous membranes. Remind the patient to avoid nose blowing, vigorous coughing, or Valsalva's maneuver (holding the breath and bearing down as if straining during a bowel movement) for 2 days postoperatively. Remind the patient that facial ecchymosis and edema may persist for several days after surgery.

Prognosis
With surgical correction, the prognosis is excellent.

ANTIGEN-ANTIBODY ALLERGIC RHINITIS AND ALLERGIC CONJUNCTIVITIS (HAY FEVER)
Etiology and Pathophysiology
Allergic rhinitis and allergic conjunctivitis (hay fever) are atopic allergic conditions that result from antigen-antibody reactions in the nasal membranes, nasophar-

ynx, and conjunctiva from inhaled or contact allergens. Many infants, children, and adults have these seasonal or perennial conditions, which often result in absences from school and work.

During the antigen-antibody reaction of rhinitis and conjunctivitis, ciliary action slows; mucosal gland secretion increases; leukocyte (eosinophil) infiltration occurs; and, because of increased capillary permeability and vasodilation, local tissue edema results. Common allergens are tree, grass, and weed pollens; mold spores; fungi; house dusts; mites; and animal dander. Some foods, drugs, and insect stings can also cause these reactions.

Clinical Manifestations
Acute ocular manifestations include edema, photophobia, excessive tearing, blurring of vision, and pruritus. Individuals with rhinitis complain of excessive secretions or inability to breathe through the nose because of congestion and/or edema. Otitis media symptoms can occur if the eustachian tubes are occluded. These symptoms occur more in childhood, with the individual complaining of ear fullness, ear popping, or decreased hearing.

Assessment
The initial complaints of seasonal rhinitis and conjunctivitis include severe sneezing, congestion, pruritus, and lacrimation (watery eyes). Cough, epistaxis, and headache may also occur. More chronic signs and symptoms include headache, severe nasal congestion, postnasal drip, and cough. If these are not treated, chronic sufferers eventually develop secondary infections, such as otitis media, bronchitis, sinusitis, and pneumonia.

Diagnostic Tests
In allergic rhinitis, on physical examination the mucosa of the turbines is usually pale because of venous engorgement, which is in contrast to the erythema of viral rhinitis. When symptoms are extremely bothersome, a search for offending allergens may be helpful. This can be done by skin testing or serum radioallergosorbent test.

Medical Management
Treatment goals are to relieve signs and symptoms and prevent infections and other complaints, such as malaise, extreme fatigue, and severe headaches. Avoiding the allergen is effective. Perennial use of antihistamines, intranasal corticosteroids, and leukotriene receptor antagonists such as zafirlukast (Accolate) or montelukast (Singulair) is recommended. Changing from one antihistamine to another seasonally may help impede tolerance to any one medication.

Decongestants may be added and used intermittently for 3 to 5 days if congestion occurs. Common over-the-counter decongestants—such as phenylephrine, pseudoephedrine, chlorpheniramine, and phenyl-propanolamine—are contained in familiar products such as Actifed, Triaminic, and Robitussin.

Lodoxamide (Alomide) four times a day is the recommended treatment for mild to moderately severe allergic conjunctivitis.

Long-term, consistent use of topical or nasal corticosteroids is highly recommended. Included are beclomethasone (Vancenase, Beconase), dexamethasone (Decadron, Turbinaire), flunisolide (Nasalide), fluticasone (Flonase), and budesonide (Rhinocort). Corticosteroids require a prescription.

Pressure headaches may require opioid analgesics until signs and symptoms are relieved. Hot packs over facial sinuses offer relief if headache is related to sinus congestion.

Nursing Interventions and Patient Teaching

These illnesses are self-limiting, so focus on health promotion and maintenance teaching to provide for self-care management. Include ways to avoid allergens, self-care management through symptom control, and medication action and usage.

OBSTRUCTIVE SLEEP APNEA
Etiology and Pathophysiology

Obstructive sleep apnea (OSA) is characterized by partial or complete upper airway obstruction during sleep, causing apnea and hypopnea. **Apnea** is the cessation of spontaneous respirations; **hypopnea** is abnormally shallow and slow respirations. Airflow obstruction occurs when the tongue and the soft palate fall backward and partially or completely obstruct the pharynx. The obstruction may last from 15 to 90 seconds. During the apneic period, the patient experiences severe hypoxemia (decreased Pao_2) and hypercapnia (increased $Paco_2$). These changes are ventilatory stimulants and cause the patient to partially awaken. The patient has a generalized startle response, snorts, and gasps, which causes the tongue and soft palate to move forward and the airway to open. Apnea and arousal cycles occur repeatedly, as many as 200 to 400 times during 6 to 8 hours of sleep.

Sleep apnea occurs in 2% to 10% of the population, but is considered underreported. Sleep apnea affects 18 million adults in the United States, but as many as 90% of them are undiagnosed (Dugan, 2007).

Clinical Manifestations and Assessment

Clinical manifestations of sleep apnea include frequent awakening at night, insomnia, excessive daytime sleepiness, and witnessed apneic episodes. The patient's bed partner may complain about loud snoring, sometimes so loud that both people cannot sleep in the same room. Other symptoms include morning headaches (from hypercapnia, which causes vasodilation of cerebral blood vessels), personality changes, and irritability. Systemic hypertension, cardiac dysrhythmias,

right-sided heart failure from pulmonary hypertension caused by nocturnal hypoxemia, and stroke are serious complications that may occur.

Symptoms of sleep apnea alter many aspects of a patient's lifestyle. With chronic sleep loss, the patient may have diminished ability to concentrate, impaired memory, failure to accomplish daily tasks, and interpersonal difficulties. Men may experience impotence. Driving accidents are more common in habitually sleepy people. Family life and the patient's ability to maintain employment are also often compromised. As a result, the patient may experience severe depression. Risk factors for OSA include the following (Tate & Tasota, 2002):

- Male gender: About twice as many men as women have OSA.
- Older age: Although younger patients can develop OSA, the incidence increases with age over 65 years, probably because of weight gain and loss of pharyngeal muscle strength.
- Obesity: An obese person's pharynx may be infiltrated with fat, and the tongue and soft palate may be enlarged, crowding the air passages. An obese individual may also have a short, thick neck (more than 17 inches), which increases the susceptibility to obstruction.
- Nasal conditions: Nasal allergies, polyps, or septal deviation decrease the diameter of the pharynx.
- Receding chin: A person with a receding chin may not have enough room in the pharynx for the tongue, thus contributing to obstruction.
- Pharyngeal structural abnormalities: A person with OSA may have enlarged tonsils, an elongated uvula, an especially long tongue, or a soft palate that rests on the base of the tongue. Any of these structural abnormalities can impinge on the airway.

Appropriate referral should be made if problems are identified. Cessation of breathing reported by the bed partner is usually a source of great anxiety because of fear that breathing may not resume.

Diagnostic Tests

Diagnosis of sleep apnea is made during sleep with the use of polysomnography. Electrodes are placed on the patient's scalp, mandibular area, and lateral area of the eyelids. A nasal cannula measures airflow, and pulse oximetry measures Sao_2 (Holcomb, 2006). The patient's chest and abdominal movement, oral airflow, nasal airflow, Spo_2, ocular movement, muscle activity, brain activity, and heart rate and rhythm are monitored, and time in each sleep stage is determined. A diagnosis of sleep apnea requires documentation of multiple episodes of apnea (no airflow with respiratory effort) or hypopnea (airflow diminished 30% to 50% with respiratory effort). Polysomnography may be carried out in a sleep laboratory, or the patient may be taught to attach monitoring leads for a home sleep study.

Medical Management and Nursing Interventions

Mild sleep apnea may respond to simple measures. Instruct the patient to avoid sedatives and alcoholic beverages for 3 to 4 hours before sleep. Referral to a weight loss program may help, since excessive weight exacerbates symptoms. Symptoms resolve in half of the patients with OSA who use an oral appliance during sleep that brings the mandible and tongue forward to enlarge the airway space, thereby preventing airway occlusion. Some individuals find a support group beneficial so they can express concerns and feelings and discuss strategies for resolving problems.

In patients with more severe symptoms, nasal continuous positive airway pressure (nCPAP) may be used. With nCPAP the patient applies a nasal mask that is attached to a high-flow blower (Figure 9-10). The blower is adjusted to maintain sufficient positive pressure (5 to 15 cm H_2O) in the airway during inspiration and expiration to prevent airway collapse. Some patients cannot adjust to exhaling against the high pressure. A technologically more sophisticated therapy, bilevel positive airway pressure (BiPAP), capable of delivering higher pressure during inspiration (when the airway is most likely to be occluded) and lower pressure during expiration, may be helpful and is better tolerated. Although nCPAP is highly effective, compliance is poor even if symptoms of sleep apnea are relieved.

If other measures fail, sleep apnea may be managed surgically. The most common procedures are uvulopalatoplasty, pharyngoplasty (UPP, UPPP, or UP^3) and genioglossal advancement and hyoid myotomy (GAHM). UPPP involves excision of the tonsillar pillars, uvula, and posterior soft palate with the goal of removing the obstructing tissue. GAHM involves advancing the attachment of the muscular part of the tongue on the mandible. When GAHM is performed, UPPP is generally done as well. Symptoms are relieved in up to 60% of patients. Laser-assisted uvulopalatoplasty is a new surgical procedure that has been used to treat OSA (Lewis et al., 2007).

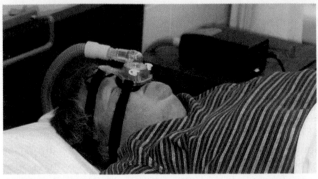

FIGURE 9-10 Nasal continuous positive airway pressure (nCPAP). The patient applies a nasal mask attached to a blower to maintain positive pressure.

UPPER AIRWAY OBSTRUCTION

Etiology and Pathophysiology

Upper airway obstruction is precipitated by a recent respiratory event, such as traumatic injury to the airway or surrounding tissues. Common airway obstructions include choking on food; dentures; aspiration of vomitus or secretions; and, the most common airway obstruction in an unconscious person, the tongue.

Altered physiology includes any condition that could produce airway obstruction, such as laryngeal spasm caused by tetany resulting from hypocalcemia. Another cause may be laryngeal edema caused by injury.

Clinical Manifestations

The main signs are stertorous respirations, altered respiratory rate and character, and apneic periods.

Assessment

Subjective data are limited because a patient is unable to talk when the airway is obstructed. The nurse therefore must make a prompt and accurate assessment of objective data.

Collection of **objective data** includes prompt assessment for the classic sign of choking in which the patient places a hand over throat. Also monitor for signs of hypoxia (an inadequate, reduced tension of cellular oxygen; see Box 9-1), **cyanosis** (slightly bluish, grayish, slatelike, or dark purple discoloration of the skin resulting from excessive amounts of deoxygenated hemoglobin in the blood), stertorous respirations, and wheezing or stridor (harsh, high-pitched sounds during respiration, caused by obstruction). As hypoxia progresses, the respiratory centers in the brain (medulla oblongata and pons) are depressed, resulting in bradycardia and shallow, slow respirations.

Diagnostic Tests

Because this is a medical emergency, no diagnostic tests are needed. This condition is diagnosed by a prompt and accurate assessment.

Medical Management

The patient may require abdominal thrusts (Heimlich maneuver) or an emergency tracheostomy to remove the obstruction. Depending on the cause of the obstruction, an artificial airway may be inserted to maintain patency. Pharyngeal, endotracheal, or tracheal artificial airways may be used.

Nursing Interventions and Patient Teaching

The most immediate nursing intervention is opening the airway and restoring patency. This may be accomplished by properly repositioning the patient's head and neck, or it may require further maneuvers. The head-tilt/chin-lift technique recommended by the American Heart Association minimizes further damage in the presence of a suspected cervical neck fracture. With a foreign body airway obstruction, the Heimlich maneuver is used.

Nursing diagnoses and interventions for the patient with an airway obstruction include but are not limited to the following:

Nursing Diagnoses	Nursing Interventions
Ineffective airway clearance, related to obstruction in airway	Reestablish and maintain secure airway.
	Administer oxygen as ordered.
	Suction as needed and assess patient's ability to mobilize secretions.
	Monitor vital signs and breath sounds closely.
Risk for aspiration, related to partial airway obstruction	Monitor respiratory rate, rhythm, and effort.
	Assess patient's ability to swallow secretions by elevating the head of the bed.
	Assess and document breath sounds.
	Facilitate optimal airway and functional swallowing by elevating head of bed.
	Note amount, color, and characteristics of secretions
	Suction as needed.

The goal of education is prevention. Teach the patient and the family how to assess for airway patency. Describe appropriate use of the Heimlich maneuver. Explain the rationale for all treatments and procedures.

Prognosis

With immediate medical and nursing intervention, the prognosis is good; without emergency intervention, the condition is life threatening.

CANCER OF THE LARYNX

Etiology and Pathophysiology

The American Cancer Society (2009) estimated that about 12,290 new cases of laryngeal cancer and about 3,660 deaths due to this disease would occur in 2009.

Squamous cell carcinoma of the larynx is increasing in frequency. Laryngeal cancers occur most often in people older than age 60; 90% of laryngeal cancers occur in men. The incidence appears to be correlated to prolonged tobacco use (cigarettes, pipes, cigars, chewing tobacco, smokeless tobacco) and heavy alcohol use, chronic laryngitis, vocal abuse, and family history. Because of the increase in the number of women who are heavy smokers, their incidence of carcinoma of the larynx is increasing.

Laryngeal cancer limited to the true vocal cords is slow growing because of decreased lymphatic supply; however, elsewhere in the larynx there is an abundance of lymph tissue, and cancer in these tissues spreads rapidly and metastasizes early to the deep lymph nodes of the neck.

Clinical Manifestations

Progressive or persistent hoarseness is an early sign. Any person who is hoarse longer than 2 weeks should seek medical treatment. Signs of metastasis to other areas include pain in the larynx radiating to the ear, difficulty swallowing (dysphagia), a feeling of a lump in the throat, and enlarged cervical lymph nodes.

Assessment

Collection of **subjective data** includes assessing the onset and duration of symptoms. Complaints of referred pain to the ear (otalgia) and difficulty breathing (dyspnea) or swallowing should be noted.

Collection of **objective data** includes examining sputum for blood (**hemoptysis,** or blood expectorated from the respiratory tract).

Diagnostic Tests

Visual examination of the larynx with direct laryngoscopy, with a fiberoptic scope, is done to determine the presence of laryngeal cancer. Other diagnostic tests to detect local and regional spread of laryngeal cancer are CT scan, magnetic resonance imaging (MRI), or positron emission tomography (PET). The patient may also have a chest x-ray study and a CT scan to determine whether there is lung or liver metastasis (Scheich, 2007). A health history helps in making the diagnosis, and a biopsy and microscopic study of the lesion are definitive.

Medical Management

Treatment is determined by the extent of tumor growth. If the tumor is confined to the true cord without limitation of cord movement, then radiation therapy is the best course of treatment. Surgical intervention is considered when extension of the tumor becomes affixed to one of the cords or extends upward or downward from the larynx; surgical options include a total or partial laryngectomy or a radical neck dissection. A partial laryngectomy is done to remove the diseased vocal cord and possibly a portion of thyroid cartilage. This requires placement of a temporary tracheostomy, which is closed when the edema has decreased. A total laryngectomy is performed when the cancer of the larynx is advanced; this requires placement of a permanent tracheostomy. Because the patient can no longer breathe through the nose, the sense of smell is lost. The voice is also absent once the larynx is removed. There is no connection between the patient's mouth and trachea.

A radical neck dissection to remove cervical lymph nodes is often done in conjunction with a total laryngectomy in patients who have a high risk of metastasis to the neck from carcinoma of the larynx. This surgery entails removal of the submandibular salivary gland, the sternocleidomastoid muscle, the spinal accessory nerve, and the internal jugular vein, which results in one-sided shoulder droop.

Chemotherapy using cisplatin and 5-fluorouracil (5-FU) before and after surgery or radiation has achieved a positive response in many cases (Scheich, 2007).

Nursing Interventions and Patient Teaching

Airway maintenance through proper suctioning techniques is important. Assess skin integrity surrounding the tracheal opening; be alert for signs of infection.

Monitor intake and output (I&O) balance and assist with tube feedings as ordered. Explain to the patient that the tube feedings are temporary and that normal eating may begin again when healing occurs in a few weeks. Weigh the patient daily and assess hydration status for the need for additional fluids; note skin turgor and observe for diarrhea.

Because of neck and facial disfigurement and loss of voice, a thorough psychosocial assessment and resultant interventions are beneficial. Encourage communication through writing and facial and hand gestures. Often no one can reassure a patient that speech can be regained as well as a fellow patient who has undergone the same surgical intervention. Many cities have a Lost Chord Club or a New Voice Club, whose members are willing to visit hospitalized patients. A speech therapist should meet with the patient after a total laryngectomy to discuss voice restoration options, including a voice prosthesis, esophageal speech, and an electrolarynx.

Nursing diagnoses and interventions for the patient with a tracheostomy include but are not limited to the following:

Nursing Diagnoses	Nursing Interventions
Ineffective airway clearance, related to secretions or obstruction	Suction secretions as needed.
	Provide tracheostomy care according to protocol; ensure the availability of emergency equipment (oxygen and tracheostomy tray).
	Offer small, frequent feedings, and give liquid or pureed food as tolerated to avoid choking.
	Teach patient stoma protection.
	Assess respiratory rate and characteristics every 1 to 2 hours.

Nursing Diagnoses	Nursing Interventions
	Auscultate lung sounds, monitor SaO_2 every 4 hours.
	Elevate head of bed 30 degrees or higher.
	Turn patient and encourage coughing and deep breathing every 2 to 4 hours.
	Auscultate lung sounds.
	Provide constant humidity.
	Suction tracheostomy tube as needed, using aseptic technique; instruct patient to inhale as catheter is advanced.
	Clean inner cannula of tracheostomy tube every 2 to 4 hours and as needed, using a solution of normal saline and hydrogen peroxide.
	Suction trachea as needed.
Impaired communication, verbal, related to removal of larynx	Provide patient with implements for communication, including pencil, paper, Magic slate; picture books, or electronic voice device.
	Keep call signal by patient's hand at all times.
	If possible, ask patient questions that require only a yes or no response to avoid fatigue and frustration.
	Refer patient to local support groups and the local chapter of the American Cancer Society.
	Assist with speech rehabilitation.
	Review instructions about esophageal and electroesophageal speech. Reinforce need for regular follow-up with speech pathologist and surgeon after discharge.

Explain techniques of airway maintenance, such as oxygen usage, deep breathing, and coughing. Discuss the importance of dietary management in relationship to airway maintenance. Encourage optimal communication through speech rehabilitation and community support groups.

Prognosis

If tumor is limited to the true cord, the cure rate is 80% to 90%. The prognosis in primary supraglottic and subglottic cancer is poorer. The 5-year survival rate is 65%.

RESPIRATORY INFECTIONS
ACUTE RHINITIS
Etiology and Pathophysiology
Acute rhinitis (or acute **coryza**), known as the **common cold,** is an inflammatory condition of the mucous membranes of the nose and accessory sinuses. It is typically characterized by edema of the nasal mucous membrane. The common cold is usually caused by one or more viruses; however, it may become complicated by a bacterial infection. Signs and symptoms usually are evident within 24 to 48 hours after exposure. Sinus congestion causes increased sinus drainage, leading to postnasal drip. The postnasal drip causes throat irritation, headache, and earache. Most people with colds contaminate their hands when coughing or sneezing, thus contaminating everything they touch. Others become infected when touching the telephone, computer, or anything else that has been touched by the person with a cold. Also, many colds are believed to be spread by shaking hands with a person who has a cold.

Clinical Manifestations
An increased amount of thin, serous nasal exudate and a productive cough are two of the most common signs. Sore throat and fever are often present. If the infection remains uncomplicated, it generally subsides in a week.

Assessment
Subjective data include the patient's complaints of sore throat, dyspnea, and congestion of varying duration.

Collection of **objective data** includes noting the color and consistency of the nasal exudate. A visual examination of the throat may reveal erythema, edema, and local irritation. Also document the presence and duration of fever.

Diagnostic Tests
Throat and sputum cultures indicate the presence and nature of microorganisms.

Medical Management
Medical management is aimed at accurate diagnosis and prevention of complications. No specific treatment is available for the common cold. Among the medications used are (1) aspirin or acetaminophen for analgesia and reduction of temperature (aspirin is not used in infants, children, and adolescents because of the danger of developing Reye's syndrome); and either (2) a cough suppressant for a dry, nonproductive cough; or (3) an expectorant for a productive cough. If a secondary bacterial infection is confirmed, an antibiotic agent (e.g., erythromycin) is prescribed (see Complementary & Alternative Therapies box).

Nursing Interventions and Patient Teaching
Nursing interventions are aimed at promoting comfort. Such measures include encouraging fluids and applying warm, moist packs to sinuses.

Complementary & Alternative Therapies
Respiratory Disorders

- Herbal medicines for respiratory problems include remedies for nasal discharge and congestion, cough, sore throat, fever and headache, and immunostimulant effects. Ephedra (*Ephedra sinica, Ephedra vulgaris*) is a stimulant and is illegal in some areas. Expectorants include anise (*Pimpinella anisum*), coltsfoot (*Tussilago farfara*), and horehound (*Marrubium vulgare*). Coltsfoot and horehound are also believed to have antitussive action.
- Sore throat remedies include mint (*Mentha piperita* [peppermint], *Mentha spicata*, [spearmint]) and slippery elm (*Ulmus rubra*). Remedies for the fever and the headache that may accompany colds and influenza include boneset (*Eupatorium perfoliatum*), feverfew (*Tanacetum parthenium*), and willow (*Salix purpurea, S. fragilis, S. daphnoides*).
- Stimulants of the immune system, believed to help ward off colds and flu, include echinacea (*Echinacea angustifolia, E. pallida, E. purpurea*) and goldenseal (*Hydrastis canadensis*).
- Some interventions that contribute to comfort in patients experiencing dyspnea include the following:
  - —Breathing exercises
  - —Relaxation therapy
  - —Massage
  - —Acupuncture
  - —Hypnosis
  - —Visualization
- Some people believe that reflexology helps relieve congestion.
- Facial massage with diluted aromatic oils is believed by some to open occluded sinuses and relieve congestion. These essential oils include lavender, eucalyptus, peppermint, and tea tree oil.

Nursing diagnoses and interventions for the patient with acute rhinitis include but are not limited to the following:

Nursing Diagnoses	Nursing Interventions
Ineffective airway clearance, related to nasal exudates	Encourage fluids to liquefy secretions and aid in their expectoration. Use vaporizer to moisten mucous membranes and prevent further irritation.
Health-seeking behaviors: illness prevention, related to preventing exacerbation or spread of infection	Remind patient and family of health maintenance behaviors to decrease risk of illness, such as adequate fluid and nutritional management and sufficient rest. Teach importance of hygiene measures to decrease spread of infection.

Teach the patient the correct handwashing technique and proper disposal of tissues used for nasal secretions. Instruct the patient to limit exposure to others during the first 48 hours and to check the temperature every 4 hours.

Prognosis

Signs and symptoms resolve in 2 to 10 days. Even though the common cold does not cause death, its economic importance is vast because it is the greatest cause of absenteeism in industry and schools.

ACUTE FOLLICULAR TONSILLITIS
Etiology and Pathophysiology

Acute follicular tonsillitis can be an acute inflammation of the tonsils. It is the result of an airborne or foodborne bacterial infection, often streptococci. Less frequently, it can also be viral. If it is caused by group A β-hemolytic streptococci, sequelae such as rheumatic fever, carditis, and nephritis must be considered. It appears to be most common in school-age children. Signs and symptoms of tonsillitis include sore throat, fever, chills, and anorexia. The tonsils become enlarged and often contain purulent exudate.

Clinical Manifestations

Acute follicular tonsillitis manifests itself clinically with enlarged, tender cervical lymph nodes. Fever may be present with chills, general muscle aching, and malaise. Laboratory data reveal an elevated white blood cell count.

Assessment

Collection of **subjective data** includes monitoring the severity of throat pain and the possibility of referred pain to the ears. Note headache or joint pain.

Collection of **objective data** includes a visual examination that shows increased throat secretions and enlarged, erythematous tonsils.

Diagnostic Tests

Throat cultures identify the causative microorganism, most commonly β-hemolytic streptococci. A complete blood count (CBC) is done to determine whether the white blood cell count is elevated. Commonly the white blood cell count is 10,000 to 20,000/mm³.

Medical Management

If antibiotics to which the offending organism is sensitive are administered early, infection subsides. An elective tonsillectomy and adenoidectomy (T&A), where the tonsils and adenoids are surgically excised, is performed in people who have recurrent attacks of tonsillitis. The procedure is usually performed from 4 to 6 weeks after an acute attack has subsided. Either general or local anesthesia is used. Hemostasis is of utmost importance, since the patient can lose a large amount of blood through hemorrhage without demonstrating any signs of bleeding. The physician may be able to control minor postoperative bleeding by applying a sponge soaked in a solution of epinephrine to the site. The patient who is bleeding excessively often is returned to the operating room for surgical treatment to stop the hemorrhage.

Medications used in tonsillitis include analgesics and antipyretics (e.g., acetaminophen) and antibiotic agents (e.g., penicillin). Warm saline gargles are also beneficial.

Nursing Interventions and Patient Teaching

One of the primary nursing goals for acute tonsillitis is to provide meticulous oral care, which promotes comfort and assists in combating infection. Observe and report if the patient swallows frequently, since this is often a subtle but reliable indication of excessive bleeding.

Postoperative care for tonsillectomy includes maintaining IV fluids until the nausea subsides, at which time the patient may begin drinking ice cold clear liquids. The diet is advanced to custard and ice cream and then to a normal diet as soon as possible. Apply an ice collar to the neck for comfort and to reduce bleeding by vasoconstriction. Monitor vital signs to assess for hemorrhage, postoperative fever, or other complications. Comfort measures are important, and emotional support is essential.

Nursing diagnoses and interventions for the patient with acute follicular tonsillitis include but are not limited to the following:

Nursing Diagnoses	Nursing Interventions
Pain, related to inflammation and irritation of the pharynx	Assess degree of pain and need for analgesics. Document effectiveness of medication, and offer analgesic as ordered. Maintain bed rest, and promote rest. Offer warm saline gargles, ice chips, and ice collar as needed.
Risk for deficient fluid volume, related to inability to maintain usual oral intake because of painful swallowing	Assess hydration status by noting mucous membranes, skin turgor, and urinary output. Encourage Popsicles, ice chips, and increased oral intake; cold liquids, sherbet, and ice cream are best tolerated; carbonated drinks may be taken if patient tolerates; avoid offering citrus juices because they may burn the throat.

Nursing Diagnoses	Nursing Interventions
Risk for aspiration, related to postoperative bleeding	Maintain patent airway; keep patient lying on side as much as possible to prevent aspiration. Observe for vomiting of dark brown fluid; patient may have "swallowed" blood during surgery. Watch for frequent swallowing, which may indicate bleeding; check frequently with flashlight to see if blood is trickling down posterior pharynx.

Instruct the patient (or the family for a child) that the patient should complete the entire course of the prescribed antibiotic. If patient had surgery (T&A), offer dietary instruction regarding appropriate foods and liquids. Tell the patient to avoid attempting to clear the throat immediately after surgery (may initiate bleeding) and to avoid coughing, sneezing, or vigorous nose blowing for 1 to 2 weeks. Most surgeons no longer prescribe aspirin for pain after tonsillectomy, since it increases the tendency to bleed; acetaminophen or another aspirin substitute is usually ordered. Analgesics are usually given orally in liquid form. Remind the patient to avoid overexertion, and make certain that the patient and the family know how to reach the physician in case of increased pain, fever, or bleeding.

Prognosis
Tonsillitis is usually self-limiting, but may have serious complications, such as sinusitis, otitis media, mastoiditis, rheumatic fever, nephritis, or peritonsillar abscess.

LARYNGITIS
Etiology and Pathophysiology
Laryngitis often occurs secondary to other respiratory infections. Laryngeal inflammation is a common disorder that can be either chronic or acute. Acute laryngitis may cause severe respiratory distress in children younger than 5 years of age because the relatively small larynx is subject to spasm when irritated or infected and readily becomes partially or totally obstructed.

Acute laryngitis often accompanies viral or bacterial infections. Other causes include excessive use of the voice or inhalation of irritating fumes. Chronic laryngitis is usually associated with inflammation of laryngeal mucosa or edematous vocal cords.

Clinical Manifestations
Clinical manifestation includes hoarseness of varying degrees or even complete voice loss. The throat feels scratchy and irritated, and the patient may have a persistent cough.

Assessment
Subjective data include the patient reporting progressive hoarseness and a cough that may be productive or may be dry and nonproductive. Attempt to identify any precipitating factors such as excessive voice use or exposure to inhaled irritants.

Collection of objective data includes evaluating the patient's voice quality and the characteristics (color, consistency, and amount) of sputum produced.

Diagnostic Tests
Laryngoscopy reveals abnormalities (edema, drainage) of vocal cords and erythematous laryngeal mucosa.

Medical Management
If the laryngitis is due to a virus, there is no specific therapy; if it is bacterial, medications include antibiotics (such as erythromycin or levofloxacin [Levaquin]). Analgesics or antipyretics for comfort, antitussives to relieve cough (such as promethazine [Phenergan] with codeine), and throat lozenges to promote comfort and decrease irritation are useful.

Nursing Interventions and Patient Teaching
General interventions include use of warm or cool mist inhalation via vaporizer. Encourage the patient to rest the voice by limiting verbal communication.

Nursing diagnoses and interventions for the patient with laryngitis include but are not limited to the following:

Nursing Diagnoses	Nursing Interventions
Pain, related to pharyngeal irritation	Assess level of pain, and offer medications to promote comfort. Use steam inhalation as ordered. Instruct patient on the importance of resting the voice.
Impaired communication, verbal, related to edematous vocal cord	Instruct patient on the importance of resting the voice. Provide other means for communication (written word, gestures). Anticipate patient's needs whenever possible.

If the patient receives antibiotic agents, instruct him or her to finish the entire prescribed course. Remind the patient of the need to limit use of the voice. Encourage patients who smoke to quit and to limit exposure to irritating fumes.

Prognosis
The prognosis is good in adults. In the infant and young child, respiratory edema can result in respiratory distress.

PHARYNGITIS

Etiology and Pathophysiology

Pharyngitis may be either chronic or acute. It is the most common throat inflammation and frequently accompanies the common cold. Pharyngitis is usually viral but can be caused by β-hemolytic streptococci, staphylococci, or other bacteria. There is increased evidence of gonococcal pharyngitis caused by the gram-negative diplococcus *Neisseria gonorrhoeae*. A severe form of acute pharyngitis often is referred to as **strep throat** because the streptococcus organism is commonly the cause. This disorder is contagious for 2 or 3 days after the onset of signs and symptoms.

Clinical Manifestations

Pharyngitis manifests itself clinically by a dry cough, tender tonsils, and enlarged cervical lymph glands. The throat appears erythematous, and soreness may range from slight scratchiness to severe pain with difficulty swallowing.

Assessment

Subjective data include any reported pharyngeal discomfort, fever, or difficulty swallowing.

Collection of **objective data** includes palpating for enlarged, edematous glands and associated tenderness and noting elevated temperature.

Diagnostic Tests

A rapid step screen is performed to determine the presence of β-hemolytic streptococci. Two throat swabs are obtained so a culture can be performed if the rapid strep screen test is negative (Kamienski, 2007).

Medical Management

Commonly ordered medications include antibiotics, such as penicillin or erythromycin, to (1) treat severe infections; or (2) prevent superimposed infections, particularly in people who have a history of rheumatic fever or bacterial endocarditis. Analgesics and antipyretics, such as acetaminophen, are used to promote comfort.

Nursing Interventions and Patient Teaching

Offer throat rinses or gargles and encourage oral intake. Emphasize the importance of adequate rest and use of a vaporizer to increase humidity.

Nursing diagnoses and interventions for the patient with pharyngitis include but are not limited to the following:

Nursing Diagnoses	Nursing Interventions
Impaired oral mucous membrane, related to edema	Provide warm saline gargles to promote comfort. Assess level of pain and provide medications as ordered. Encourage oral intake of fluids. Offer frequent oral care.

Nursing Diagnoses	Nursing Interventions
Deficient fluid volume, risk for, related to decreased oral intake as a result of painful swallowing	Observe and record patient's hydration status. Monitor I&O and patient's temperature. Maintain IV therapy if indicated.

Perform and document medication teaching, including the importance of completing the entire prescribed course of antibiotics and any side effects of medications. Instruct the patient to avoid exposure to inhaled irritants and to use preventive measures, such as using a vaporizer and maintaining adequate fluid intake.

Prognosis

Signs and symptoms usually resolve in 4 to 6 days unless secondary complications develop.

SINUSITIS

Etiology and Pathophysiology

Sinusitis can be chronic or acute, involving any sinus area, such as maxillary or frontal. This infection can be either viral or bacterial in origin and often is a complication of pneumonia or nasal polyps. The underlying pathophysiology begins with an upper respiratory tract infection that leads to a sinus infection.

Clinical Manifestations

The patient with sinusitis often complains of a constant, severe headache with pain and tenderness in the particular sinus region, and often has purulent exudate.

Assessment

Subjective data include patient reporting decreased appetite or nausea. The patient may also complain of generalized malaise, headache, diminished sense of smell, and pain in the sinus region when bending forward.

Collection of **objective data** involves assessing vital signs, particularly temperature, and also assessing the character and amount of drainage. Purulent nasal secretions, elevated temperature, facial congestion, and eyelid edema are often noted (Lewis et al., 2007).

Diagnostic Tests

Sinus radiographic studies are frequently done to depict cloudy or fluid-filled sinus cavities. A simple way to diagnose sinusitis is with transillumination. This procedure involves shining a light in the mouth with the lips closed around it; infected sinuses will look dark, whereas normal sinuses will transilluminate. To confirm the diagnosis, a sinus CT scan may be performed.

Medical Management

Nasal windows or other surgical incisions can be created to allow better drainage and removal of diseased mucosal tissue. A common surgical procedure to relieve chronic maxillary sinusitis, the Caldwell-Luc operation, is a radical antrum operation involving the creation of an incision under the lip to remove diseased mucosal and bone tissue.

Medications used to treat sinusitis include antibiotic agents (amoxicillin), analgesics to relieve headache (acetaminophen, possibly with codeine), antihistamines (azatadine [Optimine]) to reduce congestion and secretions, and vasoconstrictors in the form of nasal sprays (oxymetazoline hydrochloride [Afrin]) to reduce local vascular congestion. If symptoms do not resolve in 10 to 14 days, the antibiotic—amoxicillin—should be changed to a broader-spectrum agent such as sulfamethoxazole-trimethoprim (Bactrim) or erythromycin (Lewis et al., 2007).

Nursing Interventions and Patient Teaching

Steam inhalation and warm, moist packs facilitate drainage and promote comfort.

Nursing diagnoses and interventions for the patient with sinusitis include but are not limited to the following:

Nursing Diagnoses	Nursing Interventions
Ineffective breathing pattern, related to nasal congestion	Assess respiratory status frequently, noting any changes; mouth breathing may be necessary because of nasal airway and sinus discomfort.
Pain, related to sinus congestion	Document comfort level. Assess need for analgesics, and document patient response. Elevate head of bed to promote drainage of secretions. Apply warm, moist packs four times a day to promote secretion drainage and provide relief.

The aim of patient education is to prevent recurrence or complications of sinus infection. Instruct the patient to be alert to signs and symptoms of sinusitis so early treatment can be obtained.

Prognosis

Prognosis for uncomplicated sinusitis is good; complications include cavernous sinus thrombosis and spread of infection to bone, brain, or meninges, which can result in meningitis, osteomyelitis, or septicemia.

DISORDERS OF THE LOWER AIRWAY

ACUTE BRONCHITIS

Etiology and Pathophysiology

Usually acute bronchitis is secondary to an upper respiratory tract infection, but it can be related to exposure to inhaled irritants. Inflammation of the trachea and bronchial tree causes congestion of the mucous membranes, which results in retention of tenacious secretions. These secretions can become a culture medium for bacterial growth.

Clinical Manifestations

Acute bronchitis manifests itself with symptoms such as a productive cough, diffuse rhonchi and wheezes, dyspnea, chest pain, and low-grade temperature. Generalized malaise and headache are also common symptoms.

Assessment

Subjective data include the patient's complaints of feeling poorly and experiencing headache and aching tightness in the chest.

Collection of **objective data** includes monitoring vital signs frequently, checking breath sounds, and noting the presence of wheezes or basilar crackles.

Diagnostic Tests

The usual diagnostic aids include a chest radiographic examination to ensure clear lung fields and a sputum specimen to determine the presence of associated bacterial infections.

Medical Management

A quick recovery is promoted by preventing further infectious complications. The physician may order sputum cultures periodically to ascertain that there is no secondary infection.

Medications that are frequently prescribed are cough suppressants (codeine), antitussives (dextromethorphan [Pertussin]), antipyretics (acetaminophen), and bronchodilators (albuterol [Ventolin, Proventil]). Antibiotics such as ampicillin may be ordered to combat or prevent an infectious process.

Nursing Interventions and Patient Teaching

The goal of nursing interventions is to facilitate recovery and prevent secondary infections. Such actions include placing the patient on bed rest to conserve energy, using a vaporizer to add humidity to inhaled air, and increasing fluid intake.

Nursing diagnoses and interventions for the patient with acute bronchitis include but are not limited to the following:

Nursing Diagnoses	Nursing Interventions
Risk for infection, related to retained pulmonary secretions	Assess for signs and symptoms of infection: fever, dyspnea, color and characteristics of sputum production. Administer antipyretics and antibiotics as ordered.

Continued

Nursing Diagnoses	Nursing Interventions
Ineffective airway clearance, related to tenacious pulmonary secretions	Assess patient's ability to move secretions; also note any increase in retained pulmonary secretions. Facilitate airway clearance by elevating head of bed and liquefying secretions by use of humidifier and adequate fluid intake (3000 to 4000 mL/day). Suction as needed. When offering fluids, avoid dairy products, which tend to produce more tenacious secretions.

Instruct the patient on measures that will prevent exacerbation or recurrence of infection. Such measures include increasing oral fluid intake, incorporating rest periods between activities, and recognizing the signs that may indicate worsening infection (purulent sputum and increased dyspnea). Also emphasize the importance of adhering to prescribed medication regimen and using analgesics and antipyretics to reduce fever and malaise. Advise the patient to limit exposure to others, who may spread infection, and to avoid smoking or other irritating fumes.

Prognosis
Prognosis for acute bronchitis is good.

LEGIONNAIRES' DISEASE

Etiology and Pathophysiology
The causative microorganism of legionnaires' disease is *Legionella pneumophila*, first identified in 1976 when it caused a pneumonia outbreak at a convention of the American Legion in Philadelphia. *L. pneumophila* is a gram-negative bacillus not previously recognized as an agent of human disease. This organism thrives in water reservoirs, such as in air conditioners, humidifiers, and whirlpool spas. It is transmitted through airborne routes. The *Legionella* microbe can progress in two different forms: influenza or legionnaires' disease. The latter characteristically results in life-threatening pneumonia that causes lung consolidation and alveolar necrosis. The disease progresses rapidly (less than 1 week) and can result in respiratory failure, renal failure, bacteremic shock, and ultimately death.

Clinical Manifestations
Clinical manifestations include significantly elevated temperature, headache, nonproductive cough, diarrhea, and general malaise.

Assessment
Collection of **subjective data** includes noting the patient's complaints of dyspnea, headache, and chest pain on inspiration.

Objective data include many significant signs associated with this infectious process. A significantly elevated temperature (102° to 105° F [38.8° to 40.5° C]) bears close watching and may require immediate interventions. The patient also has a nonproductive cough with difficult and rapid breathing. Auscultation of lungs reveals crackles or wheezes. Because of the high fever and extreme respiratory effort, tachycardia and signs of shock may be present. Hematuria may develop, indicative of renal impairment.

Diagnostic Tests
Diagnostic tests to confirm *L. pneumophila* infection are cultures of blood, sputum, and pulmonary tissue or fluid. Chest radiographic studies show patchy infiltrates and small pleural effusions.

Medical Management
The physician may need to place the patient on assisted ventilation, which requires intubation through an oral or nasal airway or directly via the trachea. Close observation for disease progression is required. The patient may also require temporary renal dialysis because of acute kidney failure.

To control and compensate for impaired and ineffective respiratory function, the patient requires oxygen therapy, possibly even mechanical ventilation. The patient needs adequate IV fluid therapy to maintain hydration and electrolyte status.

Antibiotic agents (erythromycin) are given intravenously early in the course of the disease and then orally for a prolonged period to treat the infection. Rifampin is also beneficial. Antipyretics are administered to reduce the patient's temperature. The patient may also require vasopressors (dopamine or dobutamine) and analgesics to treat shock signs and promote comfort.

Nursing Interventions and Patient Teaching
Maintain the patient on bed rest, and monitor I&O.

Nursing diagnoses and interventions for the patient with legionnaires' disease include but are not limited to the following:

Nursing Diagnoses	Nursing Interventions
Ineffective tissue perfusion, cardiopulmonary or renal, related to lack of oxygen	Monitor and report signs and symptoms of impending shock (decreased blood pressure and increased pulse). Administer vasopressor drugs as ordered. Maintain hydration status and urinary output. Assess changes in level of consciousness. Assist with acute hemodialysis if indicated.

Nursing Diagnoses	Nursing Interventions
Ineffective breathing pattern, related to respiratory failure	Assess signs and symptoms of respiratory failure. Note respiratory rate, rhythm, and effort. Be alert for cyanosis and dyspnea. Assist with oxygen therapy or mechanical ventilation as ordered. Facilitate optimal ventilation; place patient in semi-Fowler's position if tolerated; suction as needed. Have patient cough and deep breathe every 2 hours if able. Identify associated factors, such as ineffective airway clearance, pain, and altered level of consciousness.

Because of the many alarming actions necessary to treat this disease and its complications, patient and family education is important. Instruct the patient and the family on the purpose of respiratory support (oxygen therapy or ventilator assistance) and how to use these procedures for the greatest benefit. Before their implementation, explain all procedures, including the purpose of hemodialysis and why it is required. Stress the importance of controlling the patient's temperature and fluid and electrolyte status. Offer emotional support to the patient and the family as needed.

Prognosis
Usually the disease is self-limiting, but legionnaires' disease can be severe and fatal. The mortality rate has been 15% to 20% in a few localized epidemics.

SEVERE ACUTE RESPIRATORY SYNDROME
Etiology and Pathophysiology
Severe acute respiratory syndrome (SARS) is an infection caused by a coronavirus. The virus spreads by close contact between people, most likely via droplets in the air. It is possible that SARS may also spread by touching contaminated objects.

Clinical Manifestations
In general, SARS begins with a fever greater than 100.4° F (38° C). Other manifestations may include headache, an overall feeling of discomfort, and muscle aches. Some people also experience mild respiratory symptoms. After 2 to 7 days, SARS patients may develop a dry cough and shortness of breath, difficulty breathing, or hypoxia. About 20% of patients with SARS need intubation and mechanical ventilation (Lewis et al., 2007).

Diagnostic Tests
A chest radiograph is ordered. In the early stages of SARS, the chest radiograph may be normal. In some patients a chest radiograph may later reveal some interstitial infiltrates that progress to a patchy appearance.

A SARS diagnosis can later be made from detection of serum antibodies or positive tissue cultures. Blood specimens for laboratory tests, nasopharyngeal and oropharyngeal swabs, and nasopharyngeal aspirate are obtained. Bronchoalveolar lavage may be used to obtain secretions from the lower respiratory tract. Reverse transcription polymerase chain reaction tests may be done on serum, stool, and nasal secretions.

Initially, the patient's white blood cell count will be normal or low. In about 50% of cases, platelet counts are 50,000 to 150,000/mm^3 (normal range, 150,000 to 400,000/mm^3). Early in the respiratory phase, creatine phosphokinase levels may be as high as 3000 units/L (normal, 5 to 200 units/L) (Parini, 2003).

Additional criteria to establish a diagnosis of SARS include travel within 10 days of symptom onset to an area with current community transmission of SARS—in the recent past, these areas included mainland China (particularly Beijing), Hong Kong, Vietnam, Singapore, Taiwan, and Toronto—or close contact within 10 days of symptom onset with a person suspected of having SARS (Katz & Hirsch, 2003).

Medical Management
Because the disease is severe, treatment is started based on the symptoms before the cause of the illness is confirmed. First, people who are suspected of having SARS are placed in respiratory isolation, including use of an appropriate disposable particulate respirator mask to protect other patients and health care workers. Although no definitive treatment exists, antiviral medications (such as ribavirin) and corticosteroids may be given. Antibiotics will not help with SARS (because it is believed to be caused by a *virus*), but they may be used when the patient also has a bacterial infection.

Nursing Interventions and Patient Teaching
The infection control nurse must notify the local public health department. Respiratory isolation with meticulous hand hygiene is carried out to prevent the spread of SARS. When the patient's respiratory status returns to baseline, he or she is discharged home. The patient can go out in public and return to work 10 days after the fever has resolved and respiratory symptoms are improving or absent (Parini, 2003).

Prognosis
About 80% to 90% of infected people start to recover after 6 to 7 days. However, 10% to 20% go on to develop severe breathing problems and may need mechanical ventilation. The risk of death is higher for this group and appears to be linked to preexisting health conditions. People older than age 40 are more likely to develop severe breathing problems (Lewis et al., 2007).

ANTHRAX

Etiology and Pathophysiology

Anthrax infection is caused by the spore-forming bacterium *Bacillus anthracis*. Found in nature, anthrax most commonly infects wild and domestic hoofed animals. It is spread through direct contact with the bacteria and its spores—dormant, encapsulated bacteria that become active when they enter a living host.

In humans, anthrax gains a foothold when spores enter the body via the skin, intestines, or lungs. It is not contagious by person-to-person contact, so treating family members and others in contact with an infected person is not recommended unless they were exposed to the same source of infection.

Three Types of Anthrax

Anthrax symptoms depend on the initial site of infection. The three types of anthrax are as follows:

1. **Cutaneous anthrax,** the most common type, occurs after bacteria or spores enter the skin through a cut or abrasion. Within several days of exposure, a pruritic reddened macule or papule develops, followed by vesicle formation. The lesion resembles an insect bite at first, until black eschar appears at the center of the lesion and the site becomes edematous. Although a patient may develop bacteremia if the organism enters his or her bloodstream, cutaneous anthrax is rarely fatal if it is treated with antibiotics.
2. **Gastrointestinal anthrax,** the least common type, occurs after ingestion of the organism in contaminated, undercooked food. Spores can germinate in the mouth, the esophagus, the stomach, or the small and large intestines, causing ulcers. Inflammation of the gastrointestinal tract can cause nausea, vomiting, fever, abdominal pain, and diarrhea. Unless treated early, a patient may die from sepsis.
3. **Inhalational anthrax,** seen in global germ warfare, is the most deadly type. It develops when spores are inhaled deeply into the lungs. Immune cells sent to fight the lung infection carry some bacteria back to the lymph system, which spreads the infection to other organs.

Initial symptoms of inhalational anthrax resemble those of the common cold or influenza, except that the patient usually does not develop an increased amount of thin, clear nasal exudate. Subsequent breathing problems may be mistaken for pneumonia, delaying diagnosis. Other severe symptoms, including hemorrhage, tissue necrosis, and lymphedema, are caused by bacterial toxins. Death usually results from blood loss and shock.

Diagnostic Tests

A chest x-ray helps differentiate inhalational anthrax from pneumonia. A widening mediastinum from lymphadenopathy is characteristic of inhalational anthrax infection; infiltrates characterize pneumonia.

No single reliable screening test for anthrax is currently available, although the Mayo Clinic recently announced development of a rapid deoxyribonucleic acid test to identify anthrax in people and the environment. Using standard precautions, obtain specimens for a blood smear and culture and a chest x-ray for anyone with symptoms of inhalational anthrax. A nasal swab is not recommended to diagnose anthrax infection. For a patient suspected of cutaneous anthrax, obtain a culture specimen from the lesion's vesicular fluid. Obtain a stool specimen for culture if intestinal anthrax is suspected.

Medical Management

Antibiotic treatment is indicated for anyone diagnosed with anthrax or exposed to anthrax spores. For both children and adults, ciprofloxacin (Cipro) has been considered the treatment of choice for all three forms of anthrax because of concerns that genetically engineered anthrax strains might resist older antibiotics. Most anthrax strains are susceptible to many other antibiotics, including penicillin and doxycycline (Vibramycin). Concerned about drug resistance, in 2002, health experts in the United States urged health care providers to avoid prescribing antibiotics indiscriminately because of the danger of antimicrobial resistance (www.excellenthealth.com/news011102a.htm).

The Centers for Disease Control and Prevention (CDC) recommend a 60-day course of therapy to ensure eradication of inactive spores and bacteria. An alternative treatment for postexposure prophylaxis is 30 days of antibiotics and three doses of the anthrax vaccine if it is available. (The anthrax vaccine is not currently recommended for the general public in the absence of anthrax exposure.) Consult the U.S. Food and Drug Administration (FDA) and CDC websites for the prescribing information for children and other treatment updates.

TUBERCULOSIS

Etiology and Pathophysiology

In 1882 Robert Koch identified the tubercle bacillus (*Mycobacterium tuberculosis*) as the causative agent for tuberculosis (TB). TB is a chronic pulmonary and extrapulmonary (outside of the lung) infectious disease acquired by inhalation of a dried droplet nucleus containing a tubercle bacillus, coughed or sneezed into the air by a person whose sputum contains virulent (capable of producing disease) tubercle bacilli, and inhaled into the alveolar structure of the lung. It is characterized by stages of early infection (frequently asymptomatic), latency, and a potential for recurrent postprimary disease. It most commonly affects the respiratory system, but other parts of the body such as gastrointestinal and genitourinary tracts, bones, joints, nervous system, lymph nodes, and skin may become infected (see Cultural Considerations box).

It is important to differentiate **infection** with TB from **active disease.** Although infection always pre-

Cultural Considerations

Tuberculosis

- Tuberculosis in the United States tends to be a disease of the older population, urban poor, minority groups, and patients with acquired immunodeficiency syndrome.
- At all ages the incidence of tuberculosis among nonwhites is at least twice that of whites.
- Ethnic groups that have a high incidence of tuberculosis include foreign-born people from Asia, Africa, and Latin America.
- Southeastern Asian, Haitian, and Hispanic immigrants have incidence rates of tuberculosis similar to those of the countries from which they came.

cedes the development of active disease, only about 10% of infections progress to active disease. TB infection is characterized by mycobacteria in the tissue of a host who is free of clinical signs and symptoms and who demonstrates the presence of antibodies against the mycobacteria. TB disease is manifested as pathologic and functional signs and symptoms indicating destructive activity of mycobacteria in host tissue.

A common misconception about TB is that it is easily transmitted. In fact, most people exposed to TB do not become infected. The body's first line of defense, the upper airway, prevents most inhaled TB organisms from ever reaching the lungs. If the inhaled particles are small enough, the organisms can survive in the upper respiratory tract, reach the alveoli, and establish infection. Less commonly, transmission may occur by ingestion or by invasion of the skin or mucous membranes.

TB had been epidemic in the Western world. With the introduction of pharmacologic management in the late 1940s and early 1950s, the prevalence of TB decreased dramatically. TB had been responsible for one third of the deaths of young adults in Europe. After Koch's discovery, improvement in living conditions, sanitation, and the development of effective drug therapy and treatment brought about a steady decline in mortality attributable to TB. Shortly after the centennial of Koch's work, eradication of the disease in the United States by the year 2010 was considered a realistic goal.

Although the overall rate of TB in the United States has declined substantially since 1992, the rates of decrease among foreign-born persons have remained virtually level, with approximately 7000 to 8000 cases per year. In contrast, the number in U.S.-born persons decreased from more than 6000 in 2006. The total number of TB cases reported in the United States in 2006 was 13,779 (CDC, 2007). TB still presents a serious health problem. Most alarming, a growing percentage of new cases of TB are resistant to the drugs that are traditionally used to fight the disease.

TB has been particularly prevalent among people infected with the human immunodeficiency virus (HIV). The status of the host's immune system is the major determinant for the development of active TB. The disease occurs most often in individuals with incompetent immune systems, such as HIV-infected people, older adults, people receiving immunosuppressive therapy, and the malnourished.

Hospitals are a high-risk setting for TB transmission, and health care workers are at high occupational risk for TB infection. Until recently the vulnerability of hospital workers to TB infection had not been emphasized. This complacency is changing with the wide publicity accompanying the increase in TB (Box 9-5).

In the lung, pulmonary macrophages ingest TB bacteria. Macrophages engulf the organisms, but do not kill them. Instead they surround them and wall them off in tiny, hard capsules called **tubercles.** Macrophages activate lymphocytes, and within 2 to 10 weeks, activated lymphocytes usually control the initial infection in the lung and nonpulmonary sites. Nonmultiplying tubercle bacilli can survive more than 50 years in human tissue.

Most people who become infected with the TB organism do not progress to the active disease stage. They remain asymptomatic and noninfectious. They will have a positive tuberculin skin test, and chest radiographs will be negative. These people still retain a lifelong risk of developing reactivation of TB if the immune system is compromised.

Clinical Manifestations

The clinical manifestations are insidious. Generally patients have fever, weight loss, weakness, and a productive cough. Later in the disease, daily recurring fever with chills, night sweats, and hemoptysis is seen.

Assessment

Subjective data include the patient reporting loss of muscle strength and weight loss.

| Box 9-5 | High-Risk Groups to Screen for Tuberculosis |

- People infected with the human immunodeficiency virus
- Close contacts (especially children and adolescents) of people with active infectious tuberculosis (TB)
- People with conditions that increase the risk of active TB after infection, such as silicosis, diabetes, chronic renal failure, history of gastrectomy, weight 10% below ideal body weight, prolonged corticosteroid or other immunosuppressive therapy, some hematologic disorders (e.g., leukemia and lymphomas), and other malignancies
- People born in countries with a high prevalence of TB
- Substance abusers, such as alcoholics, intravenous drug users, and cocaine or crack users
- Residents of long-term care facilities, nursing homes, prisons, mental institutions, homeless shelters, and other congregate housing settings
- Medically underserved low-income populations, including racial and ethnic minorities, homeless people, and migrant workers
- Health care workers and others who provide services to any high-risk group

Collection of **objective data** includes evaluating and recording the amount, color, and characteristics of sputum produced.

Diagnostic Tests

Diagnostic evaluation includes the tuberculin skin test (Mantoux), using purified protein derivative (PPD), to identify people infected with the TB organism. A positive reaction indicates infection 2 to 10 weeks after exposure to the tubercle bacillus. To read the test 48 to 72 hours later, measure and record the subsequent induration (an area of hardened tissue); do not measure the erythema (redness). A negative reaction is less than 5 mm. If the patient is infected with TB (whether active or dormant), lymphocytes recognize the PPD antigen in the skin test and cause a local indurated reaction. Generally, the larger the reaction is, the greater the likelihood that the person is infected with the TB organism. However, a negative reaction does not rule out infection. An infected person whose immune system has been weakened by disease, drugs, or old age may have a limited or negative reaction. If the test is negative and the physician strongly suspects TB, a "second-strength" tuberculin test can be used. If this test is negative, the patient does not have TB.

Other diagnostic tests used to confirm the diagnosis of pulmonary TB are chest radiograph and evaluation of sputum specimens for mycobacterial organisms. Sputum specimens can be rapidly smeared, stained, and screened for the presence of acid-fast organisms. Mycobacteria are one of the few organisms that are characteristically acid fast. Three positive acid-fast smears constitute a presumptive diagnosis of TB and indicate the need for treatment. The diagnosis of TB is confirmed if tubercle bacilli grow in culture, a process that may take 6 to 8 weeks.

QuantiFERON-TB Gold Test

In May 2005 the FDA approved a blood test to aid in the diagnosis of latent TB. This blood test, the QuantiFERON-TB Gold (QFT-G), is more specific for *Mycobacterium* tubercle bacillus than the PPD skin test (Todd, 2006). The advantages of QFT-G are greater specificity and results 24 hours after blood is collected. The PPD skin test requires a 2- to 3-day wait and a return visit to the health care provider (Todd, 2006). Sputum smears and cultures are still done, but the QFT-G offers a quick and reliable diagnosis for the patient and health care provider.

All patients diagnosed with TB must be reported to the public health personnel for appropriate investigation and follow-up care (Todd, 2006).

Medical Management

Drug therapy is the mainstay of TB treatment. Infectiousness declines rapidly once drug therapy is initiated, even before sputum smears become negative. Cough frequently also declines with drug therapy.

TB isolation (acid-fast bacillus [AFB]) is isolation for patients with pulmonary TB who have a positive sputum smear or a chest radiograph that strongly suggests current (active) TB. Laryngeal TB is also included in this isolation category. In general, infants and young children with pulmonary TB do not require isolation precautions because they rarely cough and their bronchial secretions contain few AFB, compared with adults with pulmonary TB. If there is question of infectiousness in the adult TB patient, hospitalized patients usually remain in respiratory isolation during their hospital stay.

Compared with most other infectious diseases, treatment for TB is lengthy, typically 6 to 9 months, and sometimes longer for extrapulmonary disease. If treatment is not continued for a long time, some of the TB organisms survive and the patient is at risk for a relapse.

Treatment therapy now involves multiple drugs to which the organisms are susceptible. If only one drug is given, the patient may become resistant to it. Treatment usually consists of a combination of at least four drugs, each of which helps prevent the emergence of organisms resistant to the others, thus increasing the therapeutic effectiveness. The drugs that are used to treat TB are categorized as first-line drugs and second-line drugs. First-line drugs are isoniazid (INH); rifampin (rifampicin); rifampin and isoniazid (Rifamate), with a fixed combination of 300 mg rifampin and 150 mg isoniazid per capsule; pyrazinamide; ethambutol; and streptomycin. In 1998 the FDA approved rifapentine (Priftin), the first new TB drug to become available in the United States in 10 years. Although it is similar to rifampin, rifapentine has a longer half-life and can be taken less frequently. Second-line drugs are ethionamide, para-aminosalicylate sodium (PAS), cycloserine, capreomycin, kanamycin, amikacin, levofloxacin, ofloxacin, and ciprofloxacin (Table 9-3).

Monitoring patients with TB is critically important; failure to complete prescribed medication treatment is a major factor in the emergence of multi-drug resistance and treatment failures (Todd, 2006). To ensure compliance and to help prevent the development of drug-resistant strains of the tubercle bacillus, in some cases the health care worker may need to watch the patient take the medications; this is referred to as directly observed therapy.

Nursing Interventions and Patient Teaching

If TB is suspected, immediately ask permission to place the patient in AFB isolation precautions. These precautions include the use of isolation rooms with a negative air pressure so that air flows into, rather than out of, the room. Keep doors and windows closed to maintain airflow control. Room air should be exhausted directly to the outside and not recirculated to other rooms. Also included in AFB isolation precautions is the use of high-efficiency particulate respiration masks (because AFB particles pass through standard masks). Although TB is not easily transmitted, it

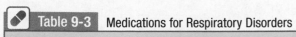

Table 9-3 **Medications for Respiratory Disorders**

Generic (Trade)	Action	Side Effects	Nursing Implications
Acetylcysteine (Mucomyst)	Mucolytic agent; also used as antidote in acetaminophen overdose	Nausea, vomiting, rhinorrhea, mucorrhea, bronchospasm	Store product in refrigerator; bad taste may be masked by mixing with soft drink when using as antidote.
Aminophylline	See theophylline	See theophylline	See theophylline
Azatadine (Optimine); also available in numerous combination allergy and cold preparations	Antihistamine; blocks allergic response through histamine receptor blockade	Drowsiness, confusion, dry mouth, constipation, urinary retention, blurred vision, increased viscosity of respiratory secretions	Avoid use with alcohol or other CNS depressants; avoid driving and other hazardous activities.
Short-acting beta$_2$-receptor agonists; albuterol (Proventil, Ventolin), others	Beta$_2$-receptor agonists; cause bronchodilation, cardiac palpitations, angina or chest pain, cardiac dysrhythmias	Anxiety, headache, insomnia, dizziness, restlessness, tachycardia	Use with caution in cardiac disease. Teach patient that paradoxic bronchospasm may occur and to stop drug immediately and call physician. Teach proper use of metered dose inhaler to achieve an excellent therapeutic response.
Long-acting beta$_2$-receptor agonists: salmeterol (Serevent)	Causes bronchodilation; used in prevention of exercise-induced asthma	Tremors, anxiety, insomnia, headache, stimulation, tachycardia, dry mouth, bronchospasm	Avoid use of OTC medications; overstimulation may occur. Use with caution in cardiac disorders, hyperthyroidism, hypertension, and narrow-angle glaucoma.
Corticosteroids: Prednisone (Deltasone), methylprednisolone (Medrol), hydrocortisone (Cortef)	Antiinflammatory agent	Short-term: Sodium and water retention, hypokalemia, hyperglycemia, euphoria	Do not discontinue medication abruptly; dosage must be tapered slowly. Have patient carry identification signaling steroid use. Take with food or milk to minimize upset.
Fluticasone (Flovent) (inhaled corticosteroid)		Long-term: Osteoporosis, increased susceptibility to infection, poor wound healing, bruising, thinning of skin, Cushingoid weight distribution, cataracts, glaucoma, peptic ulcer disease, myopathy, muscle weakness, suppression of endogenous glucocorticoid production	
Epinephrine (Adrenalin, others)	Beta$_1$- and beta$_2$-receptor agonist; causes bronchodilation and cardiac stimulation; alpha$_1$-agonist activity may cause vasoconstriction	Tachycardia, palpitations, angina, chest pain, myocardial infarction, cardiac dysrhythmias, hypertension, restlessness, agitation, anxiety	Use with extreme caution in cardiac disease; do not use OTC cough or cold preparations; do not use discolored preparations.
Ethambutol (Myambutol)	Antitubercular agent	Optic neuritis, blurred vision or decreased visual acuity, hyperuricemia, exacerbation of gout, drowsiness, confusion, GI effects, hepatoxicity, thrombocytopenia	Patient should have baseline visual examination at start of therapy. Emphasize that long-term therapy is required for cure.

GI, Gastrointestinal; *OTC,* over-the-counter.

Continued

Table 9-3 Medications for Respiratory Disorders—cont'd

Generic (Trade)	Action	Side Effects	Nursing Implications
Isoniazid (INH) (Nydrazid, others)	Antitubercular agent	Peripheral neuropathy, hepatotoxicity, SLE-like syndrome, hyperglycemia, bone marrow suppression	Monitor liver function. Emphasize that long-term therapy is required. Instruct patient to report numbness or tingling of extremities.
Leukotriene modifiers; leukotriene receptor antagonists (zafirlukast [Accolate] montelukast [Singulair]); leukotriene synthesis inhibitors (zileuton [Zyflo])	Interferes with the synthesis or blocks the action of leukotrienes, causing both bronchodilator and antiinflammatory effects; for long-term treatment of asthma	Zafirlukast: Hepatic dysfunction, systemic eosinophilia, headache, infection, nausea, asthenia, abdominal pain Montelukast: Tiredness, fever, abdominal pain, dizziness Zileuton: Headache, abdominal pain, asthenia, dyspepsia	Monitor for eosinophilia, worsening pulmonary symptoms, cardiac complications, and neuropathy. Administer after meals for GI symptoms.
Oxymetazoline (Afrin, others)	Vasoconstrictor, used for nasal congestion	Local nasal irritation, dryness, rebound congestion	Do not use for more than 4 consecutive days to minimize rebound congestion.
Para-aminosalicylate sodium (PAS)	Antitubercular agent	Nausea, vomiting, diarrhea, abdominal pain, hypersensitivity reactions, hepatotoxicity, leukopenia, thrombocytopenia	Take with food. Discard if discolored. Use with caution in peptic ulcer disease or congestive heart failure. Emphasize that long-term therapy is required.
Potassium iodide (many; also available in numerous combination preparations)	Expectorant, mucokinetic agent	Hypersensitivity, rash, metallic taste, burning in mouth or throat, GI irritation, headache, parotitis, hyperkalemia	Do not use in pregnant women. Mix with fruit juice to mask taste.
Pyrazinamide (PMS-Pyrazinamide Tebrazid)	Antitubercular agent	Hyperuricemia, exacerbation of gout, hepatotoxicity	Monitor liver function tests and serum uric acid levels; instruct patient not to use alcohol; emphasize that long-term therapy is required.
Rifampin (Rifadin, Rimactane)	Antitubercular agent	Flulike syndrome, hematopoietic reactions, hepatotoxicity, rash, red-orange coloration of body fluids, shortness of breath, heartburn, sore mouth and tongue, dizziness, confusion	Give on empty stomach; emphasize that long-term therapy is required. May accelerate metabolism of other drugs, including theophylline, oral contraceptives, and warfarin. Instruct patient that body fluids may be discolored; may cause permanent staining of soft contact lenses.
Rifapentine (Priftin)	Antitubercular agent	Hepatotoxicity, hyperuricemia, neutropenia, pyuria, proteinuria, rash, anemia, leukopenia, arthralgias, nausea, vomiting, dyspepsia, pseudomembranous colitis	Monitor liver function tests and serum uric acid. Monitor WBC count. Tell the patient that rifapentine may produce red-orange discoloration of body tissues or fluids (e.g., skin, teeth, tongue, urine, feces, saliva, sputum, tears, cerebrospinal fluid). Emphasize importance of not missing any doses.

SLE, Systemic lupus erythematosus; *WBC,* white blood cell.

Table 9-3	Medications for Respiratory Disorders—cont'd		
Generic (Trade)	**Action**	**Side Effects**	**Nursing Implications**
Theophylline (Accurbron, Bronkodyl, Theo-Dur) (Aminophylline is a salt of theophylline.)	Bronchodilator	Anxiety, restlessness, insomnia, headache, seizures, tachycardia, cardiac dysrhythmias, nausea, epigastric pain, hematemesis, gastroesophageal reflux, tachypnea	Do not crush sustained-release preparations; contents of pellet-containing capsules may be sprinkled over food. Avoid caffeine; use with caution in peptic ulcer disease or cardiac dysrhythmias. Metabolism is affected by other medications (erythromycin, ciprofloxacin, cimetidine, rifampin); monitor serum concentrations.

is more easily transmitted in closed spaces and in areas with poor ventilation and no environmental controls.

Perhaps the simplest, most effective technique for stopping TB at the source is kindly insisting that patients cover their noses and mouths when coughing or sneezing.

To help the patient comply with the prescribed medication regimen, develop a supportive relationship. Nursing interventions focus on preventing complications and illness transmission.

Nursing diagnoses and interventions for the patient with TB include but are not limited to the following:

Nursing Diagnoses	Nursing Interventions
Ineffective breathing pattern, related to pulmonary infection process	Monitor breathing for evidence of dyspnea or signs and symptoms of pneumothorax. Evaluate degree of respiratory effort and assist as needed. Assess expectorated sputum for hemoptysis. Help immobile patient to turn, cough, and deep breathe every 2 to 4 hours to prevent pooling of secretions.
Risk for infection, (patient contacts), related to viable *M. tuberculosis* in respiratory secretions	Obtain specimen for culture (incorrect collection and handling may destroy or contaminate specimen, thus interfering with diagnostic results). Employ AFB isolation until antimicrobial therapy is successfully initiated for sputum-positive patients to prevent transmission of organisms. Employ drainage and secretion precautions until wounds from patient with extrapulmonary TB stop draining to prevent transmission of organism.

Nursing Diagnoses	Nursing Interventions
	Instruct the patient to cough and sneeze into tissue and properly dispose of it to prevent organism transmission.

Teach the patient techniques of proper disposal and handwashing related to coughing and sneezing. These measures will decrease the spread of infection. Explain the vital importance of adhering to the medication regimen as ordered and the need for prolonged treatment. Instruct the patient on medication, dosage, frequency, and possible side effects. Emphasize the need to report hemoptysis, dyspnea, vertigo, or chest pain. Remind the patient to maintain adequate fluid and nutritional intake.

Prognosis

Active TB requires a long course of drug ingestion—6 to 9 months minimum, and often longer—to stop the disease. As many as 50% of patients fail to complete therapy as prescribed. Numerous drug-resistant TB cases have been reported in HIV-infected people. These infections are characterized by rapid disease progression, with 4 to 16 weeks from diagnosis to death and mortality rates of 72% to 89%.

Nonmultiplying tubercle bacilli can survive more than 50 years in human tissue and can be reactivated when the patient has a compromised immune system.

PNEUMONIA

Etiology and Pathophysiology

Pneumonia is an inflammatory process of the respiratory bronchioles and the alveolar spaces that is caused by an infection. It can also be caused by oversedation, inadequate ventilation, or aspiration.

Pneumonia can occur in any season but is most common during winter and early spring. People of all ages are susceptible, but pneumonia is more common among infants and older adults. Pneumonia is often caused by aspiration of infected materials into the distal bronchioles and alveoli. High-risk people include those whose normal respiratory defense mechanisms are damaged or altered (those with chronic obstructive pulmonary disease [COPD], influenza, or tracheostomy and those who have recently had anesthesia); people who have a disease affecting antibody response; people with alcoholism, in whom there is increased danger of aspiration; and people with delayed white blood cell response to infection. Increasingly, nosocomial pneumonia (acquired in the hospital) is a cause of morbidity and mortality (see Health Promotion box).

Pneumonia is a communicable disease; the mode of transmission depends on the infecting organism. Pneumonia is classified according to the offending organism rather than the anatomical location (lobar or bronchial), as was the practice in the past. Pneumonia can be caused by bacteria, viruses, mycoplasma, fungi, and chemicals. Currently, about half of pneumonia cases are caused by bacteria and half by virus. Up to 96% of bacterial pneumonia is caused

---

Health Promotion

Pneumonia

- A number of nursing interventions can help prevent the occurrence of, as well as the morbidity associated with, pneumonia.
- Teach the patient to practice good health habits, such as proper diet and hygiene, adequate rest, and regular exercise, to maintain the natural resistance to infecting organisms.
- Encourage the individual at risk for pneumonia (e.g., the chronically ill, older adult) to obtain both influenza and pneumococcal vaccines.
- In the hospital, identify the patient at risk and take measures to prevent the development of pneumonia.
- Place the patient with altered consciousness in positions that will prevent or minimize the risk of aspiration (e.g., side lying, upright). Turn and reposition the patient at least every 2 hours to facilitate adequate lung expansion and to discourage pooling of secretions.
- The patient who has difficulty swallowing (e.g., stroke patient) needs assistance in eating, drinking, and taking medication to prevent aspiration.
- The patient who has recently had surgery and others who are immobile need assistance with turning and deep breathing measures at frequent intervals and use of incentive spirometer.
- Aspiration pneumonia can occur as a result of nasogastric tube feedings. Always check for correct placement and keep the head of bed elevated to 30 degrees.
- Be careful to avoid overmedication with opioids or sedatives, which can cause a depressed cough reflex and accumulation of fluid in the lungs.
- Before providing food or fluids, ensure the gag reflex has returned to the patient who had local anesthesia to the throat.
- Practice strict medical asepsis and adherence to infection control guidelines to reduce the incidence of nosocomial infections. Health care providers should wash their hands each time before they provide care to a patient. Comply with current Centers for Disease Control and Prevention hand hygiene guidelines.

---

by four organisms: *Streptococcus pneumoniae* (pneumococcal), hemolytic streptococcus type A, *Staphylococcus aureus*, and *Haemophilus influenzae* type B. Nonbacterial or atypical pneumonia is caused by *Mycoplasma pneumoniae*, *L. pneumophila* (legionnaires' disease), and *Pneumocystis jiroveci* (formerly *carinii*) pneumonia.

Aspiration pneumonia is frequently called necrotizing pneumonia because of the pathologic changes in the lungs. Aspiration pneumonia occurs most commonly as a result of aspiration of vomitus when the patient is in an altered state of consciousness due to a seizure, drugs, alcohol, anesthesia, acute infection, or shock. Aspiration pneumonia may be acquired through foreign body aspiration or may follow aspiration of toxic materials, such as gasoline or kerosene.

The causative agents of bacterial aspiration pneumonia include *S. aureus*, *Escherichia coli*, *Klebsiella pneumoniae*, *Pseudomonas aeruginosa*, and *Proteus* species.

The pathophysiology of pneumonia depends on the causative agent. Bacterial pneumonia is marked by an alveolar suppurative (process of pus formation) exudate with consolidation of infection. Mycoplasmal and viral pneumonia produce interstitial inflammation with no consolidation or exudate. Fungal and mycobacterial pneumonias are marked by patchy distribution that may undergo necrosis with the development of cavities. Aspiration pneumonia manifests with various physiologic responses depending on the pH of the aspirated substance.

An overview of the pathophysiology is as follows: (1) pulmonary cilia cannot remove accumulating secretions from the respiratory tract; (2) these retained secretions then become infected; (3) inflammation of some part of the respiratory tract develops, leading to a localized edema; and (4) this causes decreased oxygen–carbon dioxide exchange. This process can begin in the bronchi or in the lobe of one lung, and it can become more extensive.

Clinical Manifestations

Many significant signs and symptoms are seen in pneumonia. A productive cough is common; color and consistency of sputum vary depending on the type of pneumonia present. Severe chills, elevated temperature, and increased heart and respiratory rates may accompany the painful, productive cough (see Life Span Considerations box).

Clinical manifestations depend on the type of pneumonia:

- **Streptococcal, pneumococcal:** Sudden onset; chest pain; chills; fever; headache; cough; rust-colored sputum; crackles and possibly friction rub; hypoxemia as blood is shunted away from area of consolidation; cyanosis; area of consolidation visible on chest radiograph; sputum culture needed to determine causative agent

Life Span Considerations

Older Adults

Respiratory Disorder

- Signs and symptoms of pneumonia are often atypical in older adults. Fever, cough, and purulent sputum may be absent. Generalized signs and symptoms such as lethargy, disorientation, dyspnea, tachypnea, chills, chest pain, and vomiting, as well as an unexpected exacerbation of coexisting conditions, should be viewed with suspicion because they may indicate pneumonia in the older adult.
- Adequate hydration is important for the older person with pneumonia. It helps liquefy secretions and promotes expectoration.
- Many older adults have difficulty expectorating. This slows resolution of congestion and increases the difficulty of obtaining sputum specimens. Because deep breathing and coughing are difficult, the older person may require suctioning to remove respiratory secretions. Perform this with caution, since too-frequent suctioning can stimulate increased production of secretions.
- Older adults, particularly those living in an institution, should have routine skin tests for tuberculosis. Many older adults were exposed to tuberculosis during their childhood and have positive results on skin tests. These individuals should receive routine chest radiographic studies. Older adults who have histories of inactive tuberculosis should be watched for recurrence of active tuberculosis. Signs and symptoms are often vague and include loss of appetite and weight loss.
- Closely watch older immigrants and immunosuppressed older adults for drug-resistant strains of tuberculosis.
- Provided that there is no serious disease of the respiratory tract, the older person is generally able to maintain adequate ventilation and oxygenation. However, changes of aging do have an effect on respiratory function:
  - Drier mucous membranes and decreased number of cilia affect the older individual's ability to humidify inhaled air and trap debris. This increases the risk for inflammation and irritation of the upper respiratory tract.
  - Kyphosis and calcification of costal cartilage are common changes. These restrict expansion of the thoracic cavity and lead to a barrel-chested appearance.
  - Intercostal muscles and the diaphragm lose elasticity, resulting in a decreased ability to breathe deeply and cough.
  - The elasticity of airways and alveoli decreases, alveoli thicken, and pulmonary blood flow decreases, resulting in an increased risk for impaired gas exchange.
- Years of exposure to air pollution, smoke, and mechanical irritants increase the risk for respiratory disease in older adults, particularly those who have emphysema or chronic bronchitis.
- Inactivity and immobility increase the risk of stasis pooling of respiratory secretions. This increases the risk of pneumonia.
- Neurologic damage as a result of strokes, Parkinson's disease, and other conditions is increasingly common in the older adult. Any neurologic disorder that decreases the gag or swallow reflexes increases the risk of aspiration of fluids and food, with resultant trauma to the respiratory tract.
- Cor pulmonale with right-sided heart failure, as well as left-sided heart failure with pulmonary congestion, are common complications of chronic obstructive pulmonary disease in the older adult.

- **Staphylococcal:** Many of the same signs as streptococcal; sputum copious and salmon colored
- **Klebsiella:** Many of the same signs and symptoms as streptococcal; onset more gradual; more bronchopneumonia (inflammation of the terminal bronchioles and alveoli) visible on chest radiograph; if treatment delayed beyond second day after onset, patient becomes critically ill and mortality rate is high
- **Haemophilus:** Commonly follows upper respiratory tract infection; low-grade fever; croupy cough; malaise; arthralgias; yellow or green sputum
- **Mycoplasmal:** Gradual onset; headache; fever; malaise; chills; cough severe and nonproductive; decreased breath sounds and crackles; chest radiograph clear; white blood cell count normal
- **Viral:** Signs and symptoms generally mild; cold symptoms; headache; anorexia; myalgia (tenderness or pain in muscles); irritating cough that produces mucopurulent or bloody sputum; bronchopneumonic type of infiltration on chest radiograph; white blood cell count usually normal; rise in antibody titers

Assessment

Subjective data include the patient's description of the onset and duration of cough. The patient may complain of fever and night sweats.

Collection of **objective data** includes checking the level of consciousness and vital signs, especially temperature and respirations, every 2 hours or as ordered. Note the color, consistency, and amount of sputum produced. Inspect the thorax to determine the patient's use of accessory muscles (abdominal or intercostal) in respiratory effort, and note any cyanosis or dyspnea. Perform auscultation; the patient will have crackles on inspiration and possibly a pleural effusion.

Diagnostic Tests

Blood and sputum cultures help identify organisms. Collect sputum for culture and sensitivity before starting antibiotic therapy. Chest radiographic studies reveal changes in density, primarily in the lower lobes. White blood cell count is normal or even low in viral or mycoplasmal pneumonia, whereas it is elevated in bacterial pneumonia. Leukocytosis is found in the majority of patients with bacterial pneumonia, usually with a white blood cell count greater than 15,000/mm^3 with a shift to the left. PFTs may be done to determine whether lung volume is decreased, and ABG values are determined to identify altered gas exchange. Pulse oximetry is ordered to monitor oxygen saturation of arterial blood levels. Oximetry is invaluable for rapid and continuous assessment of oxygen needs.

Medical Management

If pus accumulates in the pleural space (empyema), the physician inserts a chest tube for drainage. The physician also prescribes oxygen therapy and physiotherapy (chest percussion and postural drainage). Encourage patients to cough and breathe deeply to maximize ventilatory capabilities.

Commonly prescribed medications include antibiotics (penicillin, erythromycin, cephalosporin, and tetracycline), depending on causative organism and sensitivity. With prompt treatment and appropriate antibiotics, bacterial and mycoplasmal pneumonia patients usually respond to therapy in 48 to 72 hours (Lewis et al., 2007). Currently viral pneumonia has no definitive treatment. Analgesics and antipyretics (acetaminophen or aspirin), expectorants, and bronchodilators are often prescribed. Humidification with a humidifier or a nebulizer if secretions are tenacious and copious is useful. Oxygenation is prescribed if the patient has an oxygen saturation of less than 91%. Venturi mask or nasal cannula is commonly used.

A vaccine is now available for the most common and important bacterial pneumonia, streptococcal (or pneumococcal) pneumonia. Pneumococcal vaccine is indicated primarily for the individual considered at risk who (1) has chronic illnesses such as lung and heart disease and diabetes mellitus, (2) is recovering from a severe illness, (3) is 65 years of age or older, or (4) is in a nursing home or other long-term care facility. This is particularly important because the rate of drug-resistant streptococcal pneumonia is increasing. The vaccine is 50% to 80% effective in preventing pneumococcal disease. The current recommendation is that pneumococcal vaccine is good for the person's lifetime. However, in the immunosuppressed individual or the older adult at risk for development of fatal pneumococcal infection, revaccination should be considered every 5 years. When given in different arms, the influenza vaccine and the pneumococcal vaccine may be administered at the same time.

Nursing Interventions and Patient Teaching

Nursing strategies are aimed at helping the patient conserve energy. Allow rest periods and facilitate optimal air exchange by placing the patient in a high Fowler's position. Place the patient on the side with the "good lung down." This position benefits those with unilateral pulmonary disease, including unilateral pneumonia. In pneumonia and many other pulmonary problems, Pao$_2$ rises when the healthy lung is dependent (or "good lung down"). When the unimpaired lung is down, this better ventilated lung also is vastly better perfused. Studies have revealed that hypoxia worsened when patients were placed on their back or side with the affected (sick) lung down.

Assess the patient's ability to move secretions. If the patient is unable to expectorate secretions, assist with appropriate measures (such as coughing, positioning, suctioning, and liquefying secretions). Promptly administer bronchodilators, mucolytics, and expectorants as prescribed to dilate bronchioles and remove secretions. Carefully and frequently auscultate the chest for quality of breath sounds and adventitious sounds. Note cough and sputum characteristics and document. Provide hydration to liquefy secretions and replace fluids. Fluid intake of at least 3 L/day is important in the supportive treatment of pneumonia. If oral intake cannot be maintained, IV administration of fluids and electrolytes may be necessary for the acutely ill patient. Fluid intake must be individualized for patients with heart failure.

An intake of at least 1500 calories per day should be maintained to provide energy for the patient's increased metabolic processes. Small, frequent meals are better tolerated by the dyspneic patient.

Nursing diagnoses and interventions for the patient with pneumonia include but are not limited to the following:

Nursing Diagnoses	Nursing Interventions
Ineffective breathing pattern, related to inflammatory process and pleuritic pain	Assess ventilation, including breathing rate, rhythm, and depth; chest expansion; and presence of respiratory distress such as dyspnea, shortness of breath, nasal flaring, pursed-lip breathing, or prolonged expiratory phase and use of accessory muscles. Auscultate lungs for crackles, wheezes, and pleural friction rub. Identify contributing factors such as airway clearance or obstruction problem or weakness. Encourage increased fluid intake to 3 L/day, unless contraindicated, to liquefy secretions for easier expectoration. Maintain patient in position that facilitates ventilation (head of bed in semi-Fowler's position or sitting and leaning forward on overbed table).

Nursing Diagnoses	Nursing Interventions
Impaired gas exchange, related to alveolar-capillary membrane changes secondary to inflammation	Assess patient to identify signs (e.g., restlessness, disorientation, and irritability) that may indicate the body's response to altered blood gas states (hypoxia). If necessary and with physician consultation, administer oxygen by nasal cannula or Venturi mask to maintain oxygen saturations above 90%. Carefully monitor body temperature, which may fluctuate due to alterations in metabolism or infection.

Teach the patient and the family about (1) deep breathing and coughing techniques and the use of an incentive spirometer; (2) the importance of hand-washing to prevent the spread of the disease; (3) prescribed medications such as antibiotics, including the purpose, action, dosage, frequency of administration, and side effects; (4) the specific type of pneumonia the patient has, treatment, anticipated response, possible complications, and probable disease duration; (5) the importance of consuming large quantities of fluid; (6) adaptive exercise and rest techniques; and (7) the availability of pneumococcal vaccine. Also inform the patient about changes in health status that must be reported to the health care provider. These include a change in sputum characteristics or color, decreased activity tolerance, fever despite the antibiotics, increasing chest pain, or a feeling that things are not getting better.

Prognosis

Improvement occurs in 48 to 72 hours with appropriate antibiotics in uncomplicated cases (Lewis et al., 2007). The disease usually resolves within 2 to 3 weeks with proper treatment. However, pneumonia is the most common cause of death from infectious disease in North America. It is also the major cause of disease and death in critically ill or older adult patients. Even with treatment with new antimicrobial agents, pneumonia and influenza still remain the seventh leading cause of death in the United States (Lewis et al., 2007).

PLEURISY

Etiology and Pathophysiology

Pleurisy is an inflammation of the visceral and parietal pleura. Pleurisy can be caused by either a bacterial or viral infection. The underlying physiologic change is an inflammation of any portion of the pleura. It may occur spontaneously but more frequently is a compli-

cation of pneumonia, pulmonary infarctions, viral infections of the intercostal muscles, pleural trauma, or early stages of TB or lung tumor.

Clinical Manifestations

One of the first symptoms of pleurisy may be a sharp inspiratory pain, often radiating to the shoulder or abdomen of the affected side. The pain is caused by stretching of the inflamed pleura. If pleural effusion develops, pain subsides and fever and dry cough occur. Other signs and symptoms include dyspnea, cough, and elevated temperature.

Assessment

Subjective data include the patient's complaint of chest pain on inspiration. The patient may also report an elevated temperature.

Collection of **objective data** includes assessment of the inspiratory pain, noting its radiation points. Monitor vital signs, especially temperature, every 2 or 4 hours. Monitor and document respiratory rate and rhythm, including dyspnea. On auscultation of the lungs, a pleural friction rub is heard.

Diagnostic Tests

The presence of a pleural friction rub may be considered diagnostic. Chest radiographic examination is of limited value in diagnosing pleurisy unless pleural effusion is present if fluid accumulates.

Medical Management

The physician may inject an anesthetic block around the vertebrae to block the intercostal nerves, thus relieving pain. Prescribed medications may include antibiotics (penicillin) to combat the infection and analgesics (meperidine [Demerol] or morphine) to decrease pain when the patient takes deep breaths and coughs. Antipyretics (acetaminophen) are used for fever. Oxygen may be administered.

Nursing Interventions and Patient Teaching

Position the patient comfortably on the affected side to splint the chest, and apply heat to the area.

Nursing diagnoses and interventions for the patient with pleurisy include but are not limited to the following:

Nursing Diagnoses	Nursing Interventions
Pain, related to stretching of the pulmonary pleura as a result of fluid accumulation	Assess patient's pain level and need for analgesics; administer as needed, documenting effectiveness. Assist with splinting affected side when patient coughs and deep breathes.

Continued

Nursing Diagnoses	Nursing Interventions
Impaired gas exchange, related to pain on inspiration and expiration	Assess patient's level of consciousness, noting any increase in restlessness or disorientation, which may indicate ineffective breathing. Auscultate lungs for wheezes, crackles, and pleural friction rub. Reposition patient every 2 hours to prevent pooling of secretions and to promote optimal lung expansion. Elevate head of bed to facilitate optimal ventilation.

Instruct the patient to be alert to signs and symptoms of exacerbation: purulent sputum production, further increase in temperature, and increased pain. Teach the patient to effectively cough every 2 hours and to splint the affected side.

Prognosis
Prognosis is usually excellent. Complications of atelectasis or secondary infection such as pneumonia may develop.

PLEURAL EFFUSION/EMPYEMA
Etiology and Pathophysiology
Once the pleural lining is inflamed (as in pleurisy), fluid can accumulate in the pleural space. This accumulation of fluid is known as **pleural effusion.** Pleural effusion is rarely a disease by itself but occurs as a secondary problem when the physiologic pressure in the lungs and pleurae is disturbed. If the fluid becomes infected, it is called **empyema,** which is the accumulation of pus in a body cavity, especially the pleural space.

The pathophysiology of pleural effusion lies in the alteration of pressure gradients or surface characteristics of capillaries. Empyema may be acute or chronic. In acute empyema the affected area is inflamed with a thin layer of fluid. If this goes untreated, the fluid thickens and the pleura becomes scarred and fibrosed, losing its elasticity.

Clinical Manifestations
Pleural effusion is generally associated with other disease processes, such as pancreatitis, cirrhosis of the liver, pulmonary edema, congestive heart failure, kidney disease, or carcinoma involving altered capillary permeability. Empyema is usually seen as a result of bacterial infection, as in pneumonia, TB, or blunt chest trauma. The patient may have a persistent fever in spite of receiving antibiotics.

Assessment
Subjective data include patient complaints of dyspnea and air hunger. The patient may also report fear and anxiety related to decreased levels of oxygen.

Collection of **objective data** in both pleural effusion and empyema includes assessment of signs and symptoms of respiratory distress, such as nasal flaring, tachypnea, and decreased breath sounds. Assess breath sounds and vital signs, especially temperature, frequently.

Diagnostic Tests
Effusions or pleural fluid will be evident on chest radiographic examination. Often a thoracentesis (needle inserted into pleural space to aspirate excess fluid) will be done to obtain a specimen for culture to identify the causative agent, and also to relieve dyspnea and discomfort.

Medical Management
Usually this condition requires a thoracentesis to remove fluid from the pleural space. A possible danger from this procedure is removing fluid too rapidly; less than 1300 to 1500 mL at one time is recommended.

A chest tube or tubes may be inserted for continuous drainage of fluid, blood, or air from the pleural cavity and for medication instillation. The tubes are sutured in place and covered with a sterile dressing. To prevent the lung from collapsing, a closed drainage system is used, which maintains the lung cavity's normal negative pressure. Under normal conditions, intrapleural pressure is below atmospheric pressure (approximately 4 to 5 cm H_2O below atmospheric pressure during expiration and approximately 8 to 10 cm H_2O below atmospheric pressure during inspiration). If intrapleural pressure becomes equal to atmospheric pressure, the lungs will collapse. The chest tubes and attached closed drainage system restore normal intrapleural pressure and facilitate expansion of the lung.

With this procedure one or, more commonly, two thoracotomy tubes are inserted into the pleural space and are attached to a closed-system, water-seal drainage. One catheter is inserted through a stab wound in the anterior chest wall; this is referred to as the **anterior tube.** It removes air from the pleural space. The second tube, the **posterior tube,** is inserted through a stab wound in the posterior chest. It is primarily for the drainage of serosanguineous fluid or purulent exudate. The posterior (lower) tube may be larger in diameter than the anterior (upper) tube to prevent it from becoming occluded with exudate or clots (Figure 9-11). The chest tubes are connected to a pleural drainage system with collection, water-seal, and suction control chambers to drain secretions and reestablish negative pressure in the pleural space (Coughlin, 2006) (Figure 9-12).

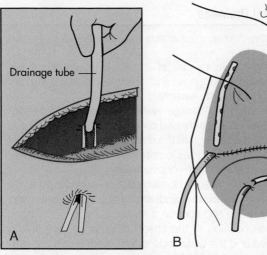

FIGURE 9-11 **A,** Drainage tube inserted into pleural space. **B,** Note that anterior and posterior tubes are placed well into pleural space.

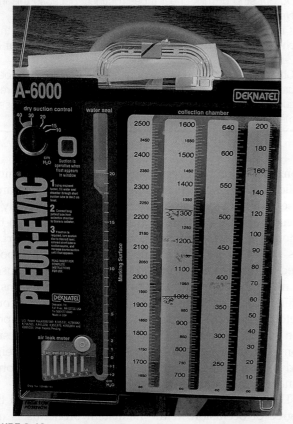

FIGURE 9-12 Pleur-Evac, a disposable, commercial chest drainage system.

Nursing Interventions and Patient Teaching

General nursing measures include placing the patient on bed rest. If the patient is receiving oxygen therapy, provide frequent oral care to keep mucous membranes moist. Also encourage effective coughing and deep-breathing techniques and respiratory treatments. If the patient has had a thoracentesis, apply a large sterile dressing and assess it for drainage, noting the color and amount.

Ensure that patency of the chest tube system is maintained so that it can drain fluid adequately. Areas of concern are the following:

- **Proper system function:** Ensuring that the water in the water-seal chamber fluctuates when suction is applied. There should not be any bubbling in the water seal, since this indicates an air leak.
- **Potential atelectasis resulting from hypoventilation:** Assessing for increased dyspnea; checking chest radiographic studies frequently to compare degree of lung consolidation.
- **Increased air in the pleural space:** Noting any air leaks in the system; ensuring tubing is secure and remains patent.
- **Infection:** Noting an increase in white blood cells, elevated temperature, and presence of purulent drainage.

A patient with a chest tube in place is usually positioned on the unaffected side to keep the tube from becoming kinked; however, the patient may assume any position of comfort in bed. There is no contraindication to ambulation with a chest tube in place, as long as the water-seal bottle remains below the level of the chest. Never elevate the drainage system to the level of the patient's chest, since this would cause fluid to drain back into the pleural cavity. Facilitate coughing and deep-breathing procedures at least every 2 hours and auscultate breath sounds frequently. Document the amount and characteristics of pleural fluid drainage by marking the drainage level on the container at the end of each shift, along with the date and the hour (Box 9-6). Prevent a chest tube from being accidentally removed by paying careful attention to securing connections and positioning drainage tubes. Be careful to keep tubing as straight as possible and coiled loosely. Do not let the patient lie on it. Tubing should never be placed over the side rails.

Administer antibiotic agents as ordered.

Nursing diagnoses and interventions for the patient with pleural effusion or empyema include but are not limited to the following:

Nursing Diagnoses	Nursing Interventions
Impaired gas exchange, related to ineffective breathing pattern	Assess for changes in level of consciousness, such as disorientation, restlessness, or irritability, since these may indicate increasing hypoxia as a result of ineffective breathing. Monitor ABGs and pulse oximetry. Encourage coughing and deep breathing to remove secretions and facilitate lung expansion.

Continued

Box 9-6 **Guidelines for Care of Patient with Chest Tubes and Water-Seal Drainage**

- Keep all tubing as straight as possible and coiled loosely below chest level. Do not let patient lie on it.
- Keep all connections between chest tubes, drainage tubing, and the drainage collector tight, and tape at connections.
- Keep the water-seal and suction control chamber at the appropriate water levels by adding sterile water as needed because water loss by evaporation may occur.
- Mark the time measurement and the fluid level with a black marker pen on the drainage chamber according to the prescribed orders. Marking intervals may range from every hour to every 8 hours. Any change in the quantity or characteristics of drainage (e.g., clear yellow to serosanguineous) should be reported to the physician and recorded. Record output on chart.
- Observe for air bubbling in the water-seal chamber and fluctuations (tidaling). If no tidaling is observed (rising with inspiration and falling with expiration in the spontaneously breathing patient; the opposite occurs during positive-pressure mechanical ventilation), the drainage system is occluded or the lungs are reexpanded. If bubbling increases, there may be an air leak.
- Bubbling in the water seal may occur intermittently. When bubbling is continuous and constant, the source of the air leak may be determined by momentarily clamping the tubing at successively distal points away from the patient until the bubbling ceases. Retaping tubing connections or re-

placing the drainage apparatus may be necessary to correct the air leak.
- Monitor the patient's clinical status. Take vital signs frequently, auscultate lungs, and observe the chest wall for any abnormal chest movements.
- Never elevate the drainage system to the level of the patient's chest because this will cause fluid to drain back into the pleural space. Secure the drainage system to the metal drainage stand or racks. Do not empty the drainage chamber unless it is in danger of overflowing.
- Encourage the patient to breathe deeply periodically to facilitate lung expansion, and encourage range-of-motion exercises to the shoulder on the affected side.
- Check the position of the chest drainage system. If it is overturned and the water seal is disrupted, return the system to an upright position and encourage the patient to take a few deep breaths, followed by forced exhalations and cough maneuvers.
- Do not strip or milk chest tubes routinely because this increases pleural pressures.
- If the drainage system breaks, place the distal end of the chest tubing connection in a sterile water container at a 2-cm level as an emergency water seal.
- Chest tubes are not clamped routinely. Clamps with rubber protection are kept at the bedside for special procedures such as changing the chest drainage system and assessment before removal of chest tubes.

Nursing Diagnoses	Nursing Interventions
Impaired gas exchange, related to ineffective breathing pattern— cont'd	Reposition patient every 2 hours to prevent pooling of secretions. Assess for atelectasis.
Self-care deficit, related to mobility restriction	Assess patient's ability to care for self, and assist when needed. Encourage increasing activity level when fever is reduced.

Explain all procedures before their implementation. Prepare the patient emotionally for chest tube insertion. Teach the patient and the family about this condition and the healing process. Instruct the patient on effective coughing and deep-breathing techniques.

Prognosis
The prognosis is variable, depending on the patient's overall health status.

ATELECTASIS

Etiology and Pathophysiology
Atelectasis (the collapse of alveoli, preventing the respiratory exchange of carbon dioxide and oxygen) occurs from occlusion of air (blockage) to a portion of the lung. Atelectasis is a common postoperative complication

from a mucous plug resulting from shallow breathing, which interferes with coughing and effective clearance of secretions. All or part of the lung collapses, usually as a result of hypoventilation (the condition in which the amount of air that enters the alveoli and takes part in gas exchange is not adequate for the body's metabolic needs), which then leads to bronchial obstruction caused by mucus accumulation. Accumulation of secretions, a foreign body, or a tenacious plug of mucus may completely occlude a bronchus, closing off all air to a portion of the patient's lung. Atelectasis can also result from obstruction of the airway by aspiration of a foreign body or compression of lung tissue caused by emphysema, pneumothorax, or tumor.

The altered physiology depends on the site and the degree of occlusion. If the mainstem bronchus is obstructed, severe ventilatory compromise occurs. When a small bronchiole becomes obstructed, as with secretion accumulation, fewer signs and symptoms are seen because the respiratory system tries to compensate. However, in either case, atelectasis can lead to stasis pneumonia (because the retained secretions are rich in nutrients for the growth of bacteria) and lung damage.

Clinical Manifestations
The patient displays dyspnea, tachypnea (an abnormally rapid rate of breathing), pleural friction rub, restlessness, hypertension, and elevated temperature.

Assessment

Subjective data include patient complaints of severe shortness of breath (dyspnea) requiring much effort, which results in fatigue. The patient may also verbalize a feeling of air hunger and resulting anxiety.

Objective data include decreased breath sounds and crackles on auscultation. Assess vital signs frequently because tachycardia and hypertension are present at first, followed by hypotension and bradycardia. Note respiration rate and amount of effort required for breathing. The patient may exhibit altered levels of consciousness caused by hypoxia.

Diagnostic Tests

Serial chest radiographic studies (repeated radiographic examinations of same area done for comparison) demonstrate atelectatic changes. A chest CT scan can detect compression in the airway and may also reveal the underlying pathologic condition contributing to the problem. ABGs reveal a Pao_2 of less than 80 mm Hg initially; this generally improves within the first 24 hours. Pulse oximetry reveals oxygen saturation levels below 90%. $Paco_2$ is normal or low because of hypoventilation. A flexible fiberoptic bronchoscopy may reveal a bronchial obstruction; this procedure can also remove a mucous plug or retained secretions.

Medical Management

Ventilation maintenance with intubation is often required. Incentive spirometry 10 times every hour while awake helps provide visual feedback of respiratory effort. Respiratory therapy with oxygen is ordered. Chest physiotherapy with postural drainage is administered. The patient may require suctioning, coughing, and vigorous respiratory and physical therapy if a mechanical obstruction is present. Prescribed medications may include bronchodilators (albuterol) to facilitate secretion removal, antibiotics to prevent infection, and mucolytic agents (acetylcysteine [Mucomyst]) to reduce viscosity of secretions. A bronchoscope can be used to remove a thick, tenacious secretion or a mucous plug.

Nursing Interventions and Patient Teaching

Postoperatively, remind patients to cough, breathe deeply, use their incentive spirometer, and change positions every 1 to 2 hours. Effective coughing is essential in mobilizing secretions. If secretions are present in the respiratory passages, deep breathing and use of the incentive spirometer often will move them up to stimulate the cough reflex, and then they can be expectorated. Administer analgesics to relieve pain and increase the patient's ability to carry out respiratory exercises and to clear airway passages. Provide emotional support. Encourage early ambulation.

Nursing diagnoses and interventions for the patient with atelectasis include but are not limited to the following:

Nursing Diagnoses	Nursing Interventions
Ineffective airway clearance, related to inability to clear secretions	Assess patient's ability to move secretions, and assist if needed. Encourage use of incentive spirometer 10 times every hour while awake. Encourage coughing and deep breathing every 1 to 2 hours while awake. Encourage adequate hydration to liquefy secretions. Auscultate breath sounds frequently, documenting and reporting any changes. Assess color, consistency, and amount of secretions removed via either coughing or suction.
Ineffective coping, related to invasive medical regimen	Assess the patient's ability to comply with the prescribed regimen and to cooperate with caregivers. Identify patient's emotional support systems.

Instruct the patient on proper techniques for effective coughing and deep breathing and other measures to facilitate optimal air exchange, such as increasing movement and changing position. Medication teaching should address the rationale and side effects of prescribed medications.

Prognosis

Prognosis depends on the patient's age and preexisting illness.

PNEUMOTHORAX

Etiology and Pathophysiology

Pneumothorax is a collection of air or gas in the pleural space, causing the lung to collapse. It can be secondary to a ruptured bleb on the lung surface (as in emphysema) or a severe coughing episode. It can be caused by a penetrating chest injury that punctures the pleural lining, fractured ribs, or injury to the pleura from insertion of a subclavian catheter. A spontaneous pneumothorax can also occur suddenly without an apparent cause (Figure 9-13).

When the pleural space is penetrated, air enters, thus interrupting the normal negative pressure. Consequently the lung cannot remain fully inflated.

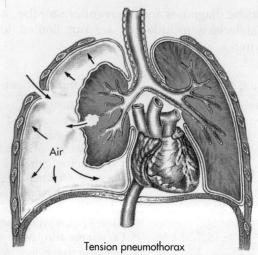

Tension pneumothorax

FIGURE 9-13 Pneumothorax (complete collapse of the right lung).

Clinical Manifestations

The patient may be seen with a recent chest injury. He or she will have decreased breath sounds on the affected side and a sudden, sharp, pleuritic chest pain with dyspnea. The patient may be diaphoretic and exhibit an increased heart rate, tachypnea, and dyspnea. Normal chest movements on the affected side cease. With a pneumothorax resulting from penetrating injury, a sucking sound is heard on inspiration.

As intrathoracic pressure increases in the pleural space, the lung collapses. Because lung tissue no longer expands, the mediastinum may shift to the unaffected side (mediastinal shift), which is subsequently compressed. As the intrathoracic pressure increases, cardiac output is altered because of decreased venous return and compression of the great vessels.

Assessment

Collection of **subjective data** includes reporting a precipitating respiratory condition such as COPD, a recent penetrating chest injury, or severe coughing episode. The patient may complain of chest pain, shortness of breath of sudden onset, and feelings of anxiety associated with air hunger.

Collection of **objective data** involves taking frequent vital signs, noting any change in respiratory and cardiac rate and rhythm. A small pneumothorax usually manifests with mild tachycardia and dyspnea. A larger pneumothorax causes reparatory distress, including rapid shallow respirations, air hunger, dyspnea, and oxygen desaturation. Hemoptysis and cough may be present (Lewis et al., 2007). Findings on auscultation are bilaterally unequal breath sounds, with no breath sounds over the affected area. Note color, characteristics, and amount of sputum.

Diagnostic Tests

Chest radiographic examination shows the presence of pneumothorax. ABGs show a decrease in pH and Pao_2, with an increased $Paco_2$.

Medical Management

Surgery may be done to insert a chest tube (thoracotomy). The chest tube is inserted in the fifth and sixth intercostal spaces at the midaxillary line. The chest tube is attached to a water-seal drainage system (see Figures 9-11 and 9-12).

Another approach to correcting a pneumothorax is the use of a Heimlich valve, which is typically used as a stopgap measure until chest tube therapy can be started. The valve attaches to a chest tube and is inserted into the chest. As the patient exhales, air and fluid drain through the valve into a plastic bag. When the patient inhales, however, the flexible tubing in the valve collapses, preventing secretions and air from reentering the pleura.

Nursing Interventions and Patient Teaching

General measures include maintaining airway patency and providing adequate oxygenation. Assess and document patency of the chest tube system, keeping it free from kinks. Note the color and amount of drainage and assess integrity of the drainage system. Monitor blood pressure and place the patient in a high Fowler's position to promote airway clearance and lung expansion. Control pain by administering appropriate analgesics, but avoid the use of respiratory depressants.

Nursing diagnoses and interventions for the patient with pneumothorax include but are not limited to the following:

Nursing Diagnoses	Nursing Interventions
Ineffective breathing pattern, related to nonfunctioning lung	Assess respiratory rate and rhythm, and note any signs of respiratory distress, such as dyspnea, use of accessory muscles, nasal flaring, and anxiety.
	Provide chest tube care, maintaining secure placement.
	Facilitate ventilation by elevating head of bed, and administer oxygen as ordered.
	Suction as needed to remove secretions.
	Encourage adaptive breathing techniques to decrease respiratory effort.
	Encourage rest periods interspersed with activities.
Fear, related to feeling of air hunger	Assess patient's feelings of fear related to health concerns and feeling of air hunger.
	Identify positive coping methods, and support their use.
	Determine support systems available to patient.

Explain the rationale for treatments (oxygen therapy and chest tube drainage) before their implementation. Reinforce effective breathing techniques and the need for ongoing medical care. Instruct the patient to limit exposure to people who may have infections, such as upper respiratory tract infection or influenza. Advise the patient to not smoke but to drink a lot of fluids, to avoid fatigue and strenuous activity, and to report any signs and symptoms of recurrence (e.g., chest pain, difficulty breathing, or fever) to the physician.

Prognosis

The lung usually reexpands within several days. The physician removes the chest tube when a chest radiograph shows that the lungs are completely expanded.

LUNG CANCER

Etiology and Pathophysiology

The incidence of lung cancer has been steadily increasing during the past 50 years in both men and women. In 1987, cancer of the lung surpassed breast cancer to become the number one cancer killer of women. Thus lung cancer is now the leading cause of death from cancer in both men and women. Lung cancer causes 34% of cancer deaths in men. The American Cancer Society estimated that in 2009 about 219,440 Americans would be diagnosed with lung cancer and 159,390 would die of this devastating disease. Seventy-two percent of people have regional or distant metastases at diagnosis. Tumors may result from metastasis anywhere in the body or may appear as primary tumors. Metastasis from the colon and kidney is common. Metastasis to the lung may be discovered before the primary lesion is known, and sometimes the location of the primary lesion is not determined during the person's life.

Approximately 87% of lung tumors are linked to cigarette smoking. A history of smoking, especially for 20 years or more, is considered to be a prime risk factor. The more cigarettes someone smokes each day, the higher the risk. "Passive smoking" (breathing in sidestream smoke) is qualitatively similar to mainstream smoking; involuntary (secondhand) smoking poses a risk for the development of lung cancer in nonsmokers. Occupational exposures, such as asbestos, radon, and uranium, are also risk factors. It is suspected that air pollutants may increase risk. Most people who develop the disease are older than 50 years of age.

Many studies suggest the importance of certain antioxidant vitamins, especially vitamins A and E, to reduce the risk of developing lung cancer. Studies report that an increased intake of fruits; green and yellow vegetables; and perhaps micronutrients such as total carotenoids, beta-carotene, and vitamins can significantly lower the risk of lung cancer in cigarette smokers as well as nonsmokers (Edmondson, 2007).

The mortality of people with lung cancer depends primarily on the specific type of cancer and the size of the tumor when detected. Lung cancer is classified by microscopic study of the tumor. Treatment is based on the type and extent of the disease, using two major classifications. Small cell lung cancer (SCLC) (oat cell cancer), mixed small cell–large cell carcinoma, and combined small cell carcinoma are the three types of small cell lung cancers (Edmondson, 2007). SCLC is very aggressive and occurs in approximately 20% of patients with lung cancer; non–small cell lung cancer (NSCLC), including adenocarcinoma, accounts for 30% to 32% of lung cancer; squamous cell carcinoma accounts for 30% of lung cancers; and large cell undifferentiated carcinoma occurs in about 9% of cases.

Clinical Manifestations

Lung cancer is insidious because it is usually asymptomatic in the early stages. If the lesion is located peripherally, it produces few symptoms and may not be discovered until visualized on a routine chest radiographic examination. If the peripheral lesion perforates the pleural space, pleural effusion and severe pain will occur. Central lesions originate from a larger branch of the bronchial tree. These lesions cause obstruction and erosion of the bronchus. Signs and symptoms are cough, hemoptysis, dyspnea, fever, and chills. Auscultation may reveal wheezing on the affected side. Phrenic nerve involvement causes paralysis of the diaphragm.

As the disease progresses, metastasis may occur, along with weight loss, fatigue, decreased stamina, and changes in functional status. Pain is unlikely unless the tumor is pressing on a nerve or the cancer has spread to the bones. Primary lung tumors usually metastasize to the liver or to nearby structures, such as the esophagus, the pericardium, skeletal bone, and the brain.

Assessment

Subjective data include the patient's complaints of a chronic cough and of hoarseness. The patient may also report weight loss and extreme fatigue. Interview the patient regarding a family history, especially a history of cigarette smoking and of exposure to occupational irritants.

Collection of **objective data** includes assessing the cough, noting color (especially blood streaked) and consistency of sputum, as well as frequency, duration, and precipitating factors. Also assess the characteristics of the cough (moist, dry, hacking) and effect of body position and identify with the patient what, if anything, helps to relieve the cough. Auscultate the lungs to determine if unilateral wheezing or crackles are present. Invasion of the superior vena cava causes edema of the neck and face and is called **superior vena cava syndrome.**

Diagnostic Tests

Chest radiographic studies and spiral CT scan of the chest are used to identify the location and size of the tumor. MRI may be used along with or instead of spiral CT scans and endobronchial ultrasound. PET may become the standard imaging study to detect lung cancer once enough data are accumulated to confirm its efficacy. When the lesion is on the lung periphery, the physician can obtain specimens via percutaneous fine needle aspiration guided by fluoroscopy or CT. Bronchoscopy with biopsy or brushings for cytologic findings indicates the presence of malignant cells. Sputum cytologic study can identify malignant cells, but results are positive in only 20% to 30% of lung cancer cases. A mediastinoscopy may be done to determine whether the tumor has spread to the lymph nodes. Scalene lymph node biopsy is also done to identify metastasis. This biopsy is performed in the supraclavicular area.

Medical Management

The treatment of lung cancer depends on the type and stage. Unfortunately, most patients are not diagnosed early enough for curative surgical intervention. It is estimated that one third of the patients are inoperable when first seen, and one third are found to be inoperable on exploratory thoracotomy. Of the third who are operable, the surgical mortality is 10% for pneumonectomy and 2% to 3% for lobectomy. A pneumonectomy is the most common surgical treatment. This consists of removing the entire lung. Because there is no lung left to require reexpansion, drainage tubes are usually not necessary. The fluid remaining in that area consolidates eventually, which helps prevent a mediastinal shift. A lobectomy is performed when one lobe is involved rather than the entire lung. If only a portion of a lobe of a lung is involved, a segmental resection is done. Both a lobectomy and a segmental resection require chest tube insertion with water-seal drainage to facilitate lung reexpansion (see Figures 9-11 and 9-12). Video-assisted thoracoscopic surgery allows surgeons to remove tumors through a small keyhole incision in the chest cavity.

Radiation therapy and chemotherapy are often done in conjunction with surgery to enhance recovery for NSCLC. An oral drug called gefitinib (Iressa) has been approved as monotherapy in patients with locally advanced or metastatic NSCLC after failure of first-line treatment with both platinum-based and docetaxel chemotherapies (see Home Care Considerations box). In SCLC, chemotherapy alone or combined with radiation has largely replaced surgery as a treatment of choice because, regardless of staging, SCLC is considered to be metastatic at diagnosis. A large percentage of these patients experience remission; in a few cases the remission has been long lasting. At present about one third of the patients who have surgery experience tumor spread.

Among the promising biologic response modifiers are interferon-α, interleukin-2, interleukin-4, tumor necrosis factor, and monoclonal antibodies. The last

---

⌂ Home Care Considerations

Lung Cancer

- If the patient with lung cancer smokes, teach her or him that stopping smoking can improve pulmonary function, minimize postoperative complications, decrease the risk of pneumonia, and improve appetite during treatment.
- The patient who has had a surgical resection of the lung with intent to cure should be followed up carefully after discharge for manifestations of metastasis.
- Instruct the patient and the family to contact the physician if symptoms such as hemoptysis, dysphagia, chest pain, and hoarseness develop.
- For many individuals who have lung cancer, little can be done to significantly prolong their lives.
- Many people with lung cancer require palliative and hospice care. Encourage the patient and his or her family to adjust their expectations and adapt their goals from controlling disease to improving symptom relief.
- Radiation therapy and chemotherapy can provide palliative relief from distressing symptoms.
- Constant pain becomes a major problem, requiring measures to relieve pain.

---

are being investigated alone and in combination with radioisotopes, toxins, and standard chemotherapeutic drugs to see if they can identify and destroy cancer cells with specific antigens (Dest, 2000).

Nursing Interventions and Patient Teaching

Whether treatment offers comfort or cure, the patient needs comprehensive nursing interventions. From patient education to symptom management to emotional support, nursing care can improve the quality of life and help the patient and the family cope with a frightening diagnosis. Nursing interventions are often directed at postsurgical interventions, including facilitating recovery and preventing complications by promoting effective airway clearance through frequent repositioning, coughing, and deep breathing.

Encourage the use of incentive spirometry. Explain the importance of changing position (to prevent atelectasis) and exercising the legs and feet (to prevent deep-vein thrombosis [DVT]). Administer supplemental oxygen and monitor oxygen saturation levels. If a patient has chest tubes to water-seal drainage, assess for patency, and record the amount, color, and consistency of drainage. Carefully assess lung sounds and record findings. Assess vital signs frequently. After checking routine postoperative vital signs, check the patient every 2 hours until he or she is stable, and then every 4 hours.

Prescribed medications are primarily antineoplastic agents to prevent or reduce tumor growth. Medications are also given for symptomatic relief: opioid analgesics for pain control, antipyretics for fever, and antiemetics for nausea.

Nursing diagnoses and interventions for the patient with lung cancer include but are not limited to the following:

Nursing Diagnoses	Nursing Interventions
Ineffective airway clearance, related to lung surgery	Facilitate optimal breathing by placing patient in a sitting position. Assist with position changes frequently. Promote coughing and deep breathing, providing necessary splinting. Encourage early ambulation to mobilize secretions. Encourage use of an incentive spirometer.
Fear, related to cancer, treatment, and prognosis	Monitor changes in communication patterns with others. Monitor expression of feelings, such as worthlessness, anxiety, powerlessness, abandonment, or exhaustion. Listen and accept expressions of anger without taking it personally. Encourage patient to identify problem, redefine the situation, obtain needed information, generate alternatives, and focus on solutions.

Teach the patient effective coughing techniques. Instruct the patient and the family regarding nutritional needs and importance of maintaining physical mobility. If the patient smokes, encourage him or her to quit; encourage family members to stop also. Encourage the patient to eat a diet high in protein and calories. Instruct the patient and the family regarding signs and symptoms that could indicate recurrence of metastasis, such as fatigue, weight loss, increased coughing or hemoptysis, central nervous system changes, and arm or shoulder pain. Identify resources in the community, such as the American Cancer Society and the American Lung Association, that can assist the patient and the family with information, support groups, and equipment needed.

Prognosis
Only 10% to 15% of lung cancer patients live 5 years or longer after diagnosis. The survival rate is 40% for cases detected in a localized stage; only 20% of lung cancers are discovered that early.

PULMONARY EDEMA
Etiology and Pathophysiology
Pulmonary edema is an accumulation of serous fluid in interstitial lung tissue and alveoli resulting from the following (Lewis et al., 2007):
- Severe left ventricular failure resulting from a weakened myocardium due to a myocardial infarction. The most common cause of pulmonary edema is left-sided heart failure.
- Hypoalbuminemia, hepatic disease, and nutritional disorders.
- Rapid administration of IV fluids (packed red blood cells, plasma, or fluids).
- Altered capillary permeability of lungs: inhaled toxins, inflammation (e.g., pneumonia), severe hypoxia, near drowning.
- Opioid overdose.

Cardiogenic pulmonary edema usually accompanies underlying cardiac disease in which the failure of the left ventricle causes pooling of fluid to back up into the left atrium and into pulmonary veins and capillaries. The most common cause of pulmonary edema is increased capillary pressure from left ventricular failure. As the pulmonary capillary pressure exceeds the intravascular pressure, serous fluid is rapidly forced into the alveoli. Fluid rapidly reaches the bronchioles and bronchi, and patients literally begin to drown in their own secretions. As oxygen decreases, the person shows signs of severe respiratory distress. Pulmonary edema is acute and extensive and may lead to death unless treated immediately.

Clinical Manifestations
The primary signs and symptoms of pulmonary edema are dyspnea and related breathing disturbances. Labored respirations; tachypnea; tachycardia; cyanosis; and, especially, pink (or blood-tinged), frothy sputum are the most obvious signs. The patient may also exhibit restlessness or agitation because of the altered tissue perfusion and resulting hypoxia and respiratory failure.

Assessment
Subjective data include the patient's complaints of severe dyspnea and a feeling of impending death.

Collection of objective data involves assessing for signs of respiratory distress, including nasal flaring and sternal retractions with inspiration; rapid, stertorous respirations; hypertension; tachycardia; restlessness; and disorientation. On auscultation the nurse will most likely hear wheezing and crackles. The patient may have a sudden gain weight because of fluid retention; decreased urinary output as a result of retained fluid in the pulmonary vasculature; and a productive cough of frothy, pink sputum.

Diagnostic Tests

Chest radiographic examination reveals fluid infiltrates, indicating alveolar edema, increased pleural space fluid (pleural effusion), and enlarged heart (cardiomegaly). ABGs are altered, with varying Pao_2 and $Paco_2$ levels. The patient may have respiratory alkalosis or acidosis. Sputum cultures are done periodically to rule out a bronchopulmonary infection.

Medical Management

The physician orders oxygen therapy and may intubate the patient for adequate ventilation support. Medications include diuretics to reduce alveolar and systemic edema by increasing urinary output (furosemide [Lasix]). Patients are also given an opioid analgesic, usually morphine sulfate, to decrease respiratory rate; lower the anxiety level; reduce venous return; and dilate both the pulmonary and systemic blood vessels, thus improving the exchange of gases. IV nitroprusside (Nipride) is a potent vasodilator that improves myocardial contraction and reduces pulmonary congestion. Because of its effects on the vascular system, it is the drug of choice for the patient with pulmonary edema. Medications for treatment of heart failure are used to treat underlying cardiac conditions.

Nursing Interventions and Patient Teaching

An important nursing measure is accurate assessment and documentation to identify changes in the patient's condition. This includes assessment of respiratory status and frequent monitoring of cardiac status, I&O, vital signs, ABGs, pulse oximetry, and electrolyte values. Maintain oxygenation therapy as ordered—commonly delivered by Venturi mask at 40% to 70% concentration. Mechanical ventilation may be required; in this case provide the intubated patient with oral and tracheostomy care according to protocol. Facilitate optimal air exchange by placing the patient in a high Fowler's position. Maintain a patent IV line (saline block) for administering prescribed IV medications. IV fluids are usually withheld to prevent adding even more fluid to the overloaded patient.

Nursing diagnoses and interventions for the patient with pulmonary edema include but are not limited to the following:

Nursing Diagnoses	Nursing Interventions
Impaired gas exchange, related to excess fluid in pulmonary vessels interfering with oxygen diffusion	Be alert to any signs indicating altered ventilation, such as restlessness, irritability, disorientation, or apprehension. Monitor ABGs and notify physician of any change. Frequently monitor vital signs, including cardiac rhythm.
Excess fluid volume, related to altered tissue permeability	Administer oxygen therapy as ordered and document patient response. Administer diuretics, bronchodilators, morphine sulfate, cardiotonic glycosides, and other medications as ordered. Assess indicators of patient's fluid volume status, such as breath sounds and skin turgor. Monitor I&O accurately. Monitor electrolyte values closely, and notify physician of alterations. Administer diuretics as ordered, and note patient response. Weigh patient daily on same scale at same time of day with same amount of bed linen and patient clothing. Provide low-sodium diet to prevent excess fluid retention.

Teach the patient effective breathing techniques. Inform the patient and the family about actions, side effects, and dosage of prescribed medications. Instruct the patient and the family about a low-sodium diet and refer them to a dietitian for follow-up. Emphasize the signs and symptoms to observe that would indicate alteration in health, such as productive cough (noting the color and characteristics of sputum), activity intolerance, or dyspnea.

Prognosis

The prognosis for acute pulmonary edema is guarded; it may lead to death unless treated rapidly.

PULMONARY EMBOLISM

Etiology and Pathophysiology

The most common pulmonary perfusion abnormality, pulmonary embolism (PE), is caused by the passage of a foreign substance (blood clot, fat, air, tumor tissue, or amniotic fluid) into the pulmonary artery or its branches, with resulting obstruction of the blood supply to lung tissue and subsequent collapse. PE usually occurs in patients identified to be at risk, such as those with prior thrombophlebitis; those who have recently had surgery, been pregnant, or given birth; women who are taking contraceptives on a long-term basis; and those with a history of congestive heart failure, obesity, or immobilization from fracture. Immobilization appears to be a key consideration.

Venous stasis, venous wall injury, and increased coagulability of blood cause the formation of a venous thrombus. The thrombus (usually in the deep veins of the lower extremities) dislodges and travels through the venous circulation; it passes through the right side of the heart and enters the pulmonary artery, where it becomes lodged.

Once an embolus obstructs pulmonary blood flow, a V/Q mismatch develops: an area of lung is ventilated but not perfused. The obstruction hinders oxygenation of the blood. Atelectasis develops, and pulmonary vascular resistance increases. Arterial hypoxia is the result.

Clinical Manifestations

The classic signs and symptoms of dyspnea, hemoptysis, and chest pain occur in less than 20% of patients with a PE, making diagnosis difficult (Lewis et al., 2007). A PE may manifest itself by a sudden, sharp, constant, nonradiating, pleuritic chest pain that worsens with inspiration. Because PE impairs gas exchange, the patient may have acute, unexplained dyspnea. The respiratory rate is rapid. In small areas of infarction, presenting signs and symptoms are a small amount of hemoptysis, pleuritic chest pain, elevated temperature, and increased white blood cell count. In large areas of infarction, symptoms include hypoxia, hemoptysis, hypotension, tachycardia, diaphoresis, and tachypnea. Regional bronchoconstriction, atelectasis, and pulmonary edema develop, along with decreased surfactant production. Lung sounds are diminished, and wheezes may be present.

Assessment

Subjective data include the patient's report of presence and degree of dyspnea and pleuritic chest pain. The patient may complain of a sense of impending doom. Nursing assessment also includes identifying associated risk factors.

Collection of **objective data** involves assessing for pleuritic pain and noting the nature of the patient's cough. Also assess breath sounds and vital signs, and be alert for tachycardia, hypotension, and tachypnea. Auscultation reveals crackles, decreased breath sounds over the affected area, and a pleural friction rub. In assessing the patient's psychological response, document the presence and degree of anxiety, which is often associated with air hunger. Other objective data may include hemoptysis, elevated temperature, increased white blood cell count, and diaphoresis.

Diagnostic Tests

ABGs are significantly altered, indicating hypoxia. The pH remains normal unless respiratory alkalosis develops early from hyperventilation as respiratory drive diminishes. Respiratory acidosis with hypoxemia often follows.

Initially, the chest radiograph is normal. After 24 hours the radiograph may reveal small infiltrates secondary to atelectasis. Chest radiographic examination also shows an enlarged main pulmonary artery. In most cases of PE, the chest radiograph is normal and is useful only to rule out pulmonary edema or pneumothorax.

A helical (or spiral) CT scan of the lung to visualize the pulmonary vasculature is ordered. This new type of noninvasive scan can be performed in a few seconds and is replacing the V/Q scan, although the V/Q scan is still used in smaller facilities where spiral CT is not available. If the V/Q scan result is intermediate or low probability but the physician still suspects a PE based on the patient's signs, symptoms, and risk factors, he or she may order a pulmonary angiogram.

Pulmonary angiogram is the gold standard for detecting PE because it provides a direct anatomical view of the pulmonary vessels to assess perfusion defects. Pulmonary angiography is an invasive procedure that is performed as follows: (1) insert a catheter through the antecubital or femoral vein, (2) advance the catheter to the pulmonary artery, and (3) inject contrast medium. This procedure allows visualization of the pulmonary vascular system and location of the embolus. ABG analysis is important. A D-dimer serum test is drawn. D-dimer is a product of fibrin degradation (a change to a less complex form). When a thrombus or embolus is present, plasma D-dimer concentrations are usually greater than 1591 ng/mL. The normal range for D-dimer is 68 to 494 ng/L. If the D-dimer levels are elevated, a venous ultrasound is indicated to look for a DVT. Positive results from venous ultrasound are helpful in diagnosing DVT.

Medical Management

When multiple PEs are present, an umbrella filter may be placed in the inferior vena cava to retain the emboli, preventing their migration to other parts of the body.

The physician prescribes anticoagulant therapy, for example, oral warfarin (Coumadin) or subcutaneous low-molecular-weight heparin (enoxaparin sodium [Lovenox]) or dalteparin (Fragmin), to prevent clot formation. Initially heparin may be administered intravenously, by way of a continuous infusion on a pump.

Heparin does not dissolve an existing thrombus; its role is to keep it from enlarging and to prevent more thrombi from forming while the body's natural fibrinolytic mechanism lyses (destroys red blood cells) the existing clot. The effectiveness of heparin is determined by monitoring PTT values, which should be maintained at 1½ to 2 times the control (or normal) values. In the event of overheparinization resulting in profound bleeding, the treatment is IV administration of protamine sulfate. Heparin therapy is gradually tapered (it may take several days). Oral anticoagulation (warfarin) is initiated. The patient takes warfarin for up to 1 year. Effectiveness of warfarin therapy is determined by monitoring PT and INR values, with the goal being 1¼ to 1½ times the control (or normal) values. Vitamin

K reverses the effects of warfarin. Fresh frozen plasma may be required in cases of severe bleeding.

A massive PE must be dissolved using thrombolytics such as the tissue plasminogen activator alteplase (Activase).

Nursing Interventions and Patient Teaching

General nursing interventions include applying thromboembolic disease (TED) stockings and elevating the lower extremities. Check peripheral pulses and frequently measure bilateral calf circumference to monitor for occlusion caused by a clot. Slightly elevate the head of the bed, and administer oxygen by mask or nasal cannula to facilitate optimal gas exchange. Promote lung expansion by encouraging the patient to cough and breathe deeply.

Related nursing interventions include assessing for signs of bleeding: epistaxis, hemoptysis, bleeding from gums or rectum, and ecchymosis. Keep the patient adequately hydrated; place the patient on bed rest for the first few days, and gradually increase activity.

Nursing diagnoses and interventions for the patient with PE include but are not limited to the following:

Nursing Diagnoses	Nursing Interventions
Impaired gas exchange, related to alteration in pulmonary vasculature	Assess sensorium and vital signs every 2 hours or as needed, noting any changes indicative of altered oxygenation or ventilation. Elevate head of bed 30 degrees to improve ventilation. Administer oxygen as ordered. Monitor ABGs frequently, reporting any increase or decrease of $Paco_2$ and Pao_2 of more than 10 mm Hg.
Ineffective protection, related to risk of prolonged bleeding or hemorrhage secondary to anticoagulation therapy	Monitor vital signs for indicators of profuse bleeding or hemorrhage resulting from anticoagulant therapy: hypotension, tachycardia, and tachypnea. At least once a shift, check stool, urine, sputum, and vomitus for occult blood using agency-approved method for testing. At least once a shift, inspect wounds, oral mucous membranes, any entry site of an invasive procedure, and nares for evidence of bleeding.

Nursing Diagnoses	Nursing Interventions
	To prevent hematoma formation, avoid giving intramuscular injection unless it is unavoidable. Teach patient the necessity of using sponge-tipped applicators and mouthwash for oral care to minimize the risk of gum bleeding. Instruct patient to shave with an electric rather than a bladed razor.

Medication teaching regarding long-term anticoagulant therapy is a major nursing concern. Patients with recurrent emboli are treated indefinitely; typical anticoagulant therapy continues for at least 3 to 6 months. Oral anticoagulation often becomes a lifelong regimen that bears close monitoring. Assess the patient's present knowledge base and expand on it. Preventive measures are also important, especially in the postoperative period. Teach the patient techniques to reduce venous pooling (which could precipitate thrombophlebitis), such as changing positions and wearing nonrestrictive clothing. Tell the patient to avoid crossing the legs while sitting or lying down and also to avoid standing in one place for a prolonged period, since these activities increase venous pooling. Teach the rationale and application procedure for TED hose. Explain that the patient should put them on in the morning before getting out of bed. Instruct the patient and the family on signs and symptoms of PE to report to the physician, such as chest pain; dyspnea; and blood-tinged sputum or blood in the urine, which could result from anticoagulant therapy.

Prognosis

Early diagnosis and appropriate treatment reduce mortality to 2% to 8%. Untreated PE carries a 30% mortality rate (Thompson et al., 2006). It is one of the most common causes of preventable death in hospitalized patients (Valentine et al., 2006). Although most PEs resolve completely and leave no residual deficits, some patients may be left with chronic pulmonary hypertension.

ACUTE RESPIRATORY DISTRESS SYNDROME

Etiology and Pathophysiology

Acute respiratory distress syndrome (ARDS) is not a disease but a complication that occurs as a result of other disease processes. ARDS has many causes, which result from either a direct or an indirect pulmonary injury. Possible causes include viral or bacterial pneumonia, chest trauma, pulmonary contusion, aspiration, inhalation injury, near drowning, fat emboli, sepsis, or any type of shock. Drug overdoses, renal failure, and pancreatitis are also known causative factors, as are COPD, neuromuscular defects with Guillain-Barré syndrome, and myasthenia gravis. Among these, sepsis is the most common precursor of ARDS.

Regardless of the cause of ARDS, the body's response follows a similar sequence. The surface of the alveolar capillary membrane is altered, causing increased permeability, which then allows fluid to leak into the interstitial spaces and alveoli. This creates pulmonary edema and hypoxia. The alveoli lose their elasticity and collapse, which causes the blood to be shunted through the impaired alveoli, interfering with oxygen transport. The damaged capillaries allow plasma and red blood cells to leak out, resulting in hemorrhage. ARDS is characterized by pulmonary artery hypertension, which results from vasoconstriction.

Clinical Manifestations

ARDS manifests 12 to 24 hours after injury, resulting in lung tissue damage or hypovolemic shock; 5 to 10 days after sepsis development, the patient experiences respiratory distress with altered breath sounds. There may be altered sensorium as a result of an elevated $Paco_2$ and decreased Pao_2. Additional signs are cardiovascular: tachycardia, hypotension, and decreased urinary output.

Assessment

Subjective data include background information and a history of the present illness (obtained from family members, since the patient is usually too ill to give details).

Collection of **objective data** involves being an astute observer of any change in the patient's condition, no matter how small or gradual. Make an accurate and thorough initial assessment so such changes will be quickly recognized. Initial assessment includes identifying and documenting respiratory rate, rhythm, and effort. Note signs of dyspnea, such as nasal flaring, sternal and subclavicular retractions, or cyanosis. Auscultate the lungs and document the presence of crackles or wheezing. Closely observe vital signs. Frequent assessment of the level of consciousness, with particular attention to increased restlessness or lethargy, is necessary.

Diagnostic Tests

PFTs are done to determine the ease or difficulty of oxygen crossing the alveolar capillary membrane. ABGs show definitive changes: Pao_2 is decreased (less than 70 mm Hg), $Paco_2$ is increased (greater than 35 mm Hg), and HCO_3^- is decreased (less than 22 mEq/L). Initially, HCO_3^- increases in an attempt to buffer the elevated $Paco_2$ level, thereby maintaining pH in the normal range. The pH is elevated initially but steadily decreases as the patient's condition deteriorates. A chest radiographic examination depicts thickened bronchial margins and possibly diffuse infiltrates.

Medical Management

The medical plan focuses on supportive treatment by maintaining adequate oxygenation and treating the cause: drug overdose, infections, or inhaled toxins. Medications commonly used to treat associated conditions include corticosteroids, antibiotics, vasodilators like nitroprusside, bronchodilators, mucolytics, and diuretics to treat pulmonary edema, aiding in restoring lung tissues to their normal structure and function. Morphine sulfate is commonly given to sedate restless patients and decrease respiratory rate. When the patient is intubated and ventilator dependent, a neurologic blocking agent, such as pancuronium (Pavulon), may be administered to suppress the patient's own respiratory effort, relying on the controlled ventilator assistance. Positive endexpiratory pressure is the most important ventilator treatment component for the patient with ARDS (Jacobs, 2005). Other medications may include cardiotonic glycosides (digoxin) to enhance cardiac function.

An experimental treatment is being used in which nitric oxide gas is inhaled, causing local vasodilation and maximizing perfusion in ventilated areas of the lungs and often significantly improving oxygenation. Nitric oxide is usually administered via a face mask; if the patient is ventilator dependent, however, the ventilator is the mode of delivery.

Nursing Interventions and Patient Teaching

The goal of nursing interventions is to provide adequate oxygenation and ventilation and to treat the multisystem responses caused by ARDS. Nurses must be knowledgeable about mechanical ventilator settings and effects. Care for intubated patients includes suctioning, providing oral care, and assessing for signs of inadequate ventilation. Closely monitor ABGs and pulse oximetry and report any changes.

To improve gas exchange, frequently reposition the patient from side to side, thus preventing one region of the lung from being in a dependent position for prolonged periods (Jacobs, 2005). Studies suggest some people with ARDS demonstrate a marked improvement in Pao_2 when turned from the supine to prone position. Not all patients respond to prone positioning (Balas, 2000). Also, an accurate, ongoing assessment of cardiac function is important. Be alert for and document any rate or rhythm changes. The registered nurse will notify the physician of any changes.

Assess vital signs and identify elevated temperatures so that cultures can be obtained to treat infections.

Nursing diagnoses and interventions for the patient with ARDS include but are not limited to the following:

Nursing Diagnoses	Nursing Interventions
Impaired gas exchange, related to tachypnea	Monitor ABGs and report any changes. Address any factors that would contribute to restlessness and anxiety, since they increase the body's oxygen demand and exacerbate the patient's already serious condition. Administer oxygen as ordered, assessing and recording patient response. Monitor electrocardiogram (ECG) changes. Report any changes in vital signs and any change in patient's response, no matter how small or gradual.
Ineffective breathing pattern, related to respiratory distress	Assess respiratory rate, rhythm, and effort, being alert to signs of dyspnea. Facilitate optimal ventilation by proper positioning. Maintain airway patency by encouraging frequent coughing and deep breathing, if able, or suctioning as needed.

Teach the patient effective breathing techniques, emphasizing the importance of frequent position changes, coughing, and deep breathing. If the patient is intubated, explain all procedures before their implementation and explain the importance of working with the ventilator and not trying to breathe independently. Reassure the patient that the ventilator will breathe for him or her and that those breaths will be more effective than his or her own. Explain to the patient and the family the importance of using rest and activity appropriately. Also explain the purpose and side effects of all medications.

Prognosis
ARDS affects an estimated 150,000 to 200,000 people each year, with mortality rates of 40% with severe ARDS when trauma is the cause and 55% to 70% when the condition is associated with sepsis.

CHRONIC OBSTRUCTIVE PULMONARY DISEASE
COPD is a progressive and irreversible condition characterized by diminished inspiratory and expiratory capacity of the lungs. It is a chronic respiratory condition that obstructs the flow of air to or from the patient's bronchioles (Figure 9-14). COPD includes emphysema, chronic bronchitis, asthma, and bronchiectasis. All these diseases are characterized by **chronic airflow limitation.** The mantra of the American Lung Association is, "When you can't breathe, nothing else matters." Still, more than 35 million Americans live with chronic lung disease.

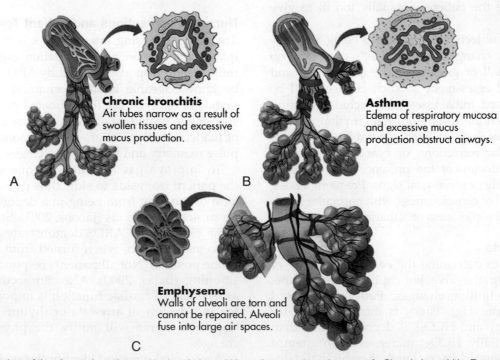

Chronic bronchitis
Air tubes narrow as a result of swollen tissues and excessive mucus production.

Asthma
Edema of respiratory mucosa and excessive mucus production obstruct airways.

Emphysema
Walls of alveoli are torn and cannot be repaired. Alveoli fuse into large air spaces.

FIGURE 9-14 Disorders of the airways in patients with chronic bronchitis, asthma, and emphysema. **A,** Chronic bronchitis: Excessive amounts of mucus accumulate in the airways, obstructing airflow and impairing ciliary function. **B,** Asthma: Bronchial smooth muscle constricts in response to irritants, resulting in airflow obstruction and wheezing. **C,** Emphysema: Alveoli become overinflated and destructive changes occur in alveolar walls.

EMPHYSEMA

Etiology and Pathophysiology

Emphysema symptoms usually develop when the patient is in his or her 40s, with disability increasing by age 50 to 60. This condition is characterized by changes in the alveolar walls and capillaries: thus emphysema is primarily an **alveolar disease** (see Figure 9-14, C).

Emphysema is an abnormal permanent enlargement of the alveoli distal to the terminal bronchioles, accompanied by destruction of their walls. There is usually an overlap between chronic bronchitis and emphysema. The bronchi, bronchioles, and alveoli become inflamed as a result of chronic irritation. Because of bronchiole lumen narrowing, air becomes trapped in the alveoli during expiration, causing alveolar distention (Figure 9-15). The alveoli then rupture and scar, losing their elasticity. Oxygen in the arterial blood decreases and carbon dioxide increases.

This process is worsened by cigarette smoking and other inhaled irritants. There is a lag of 30 to 35 years, on average, between taking up smoking and onset of signs and symptoms. Cigarette smoking is by far the most common cause of emphysema and chronic bronchitis; 90% of COPD cases are caused by smoking, whereas as few as 25% of smokers develop the disorder. This suggests that genetic susceptibility plays a role in the risk for COPD (Sharma, 2006). Risk factors for emphysema are the same as for chronic bronchitis, with one addition: heredity. An inherited form of emphysema is caused by a deficiency of alpha$_1$-antitrypsin (ATT), a lung protective protein produced by the liver, which acts predominantly by inhibiting neutrophil elastase in the lungs. ATT deficiency accounts for less than 1% of emphysema in the United States.

The patient with emphysema is disabled because all available energy must be used for breathing. COPD can lead to **cor pulmonale,** an abnormal cardiac condition characterized by hypertrophy of the right ventricle of the heart as a result of hypertension of the pulmonary circulation. Cor pulmonale results in edema in the lower extremities and in the sacral and perineal area, distended neck veins, and enlargement of the liver with ascites. Cor pulmonale is a late complication of emphysema.

Clinical Manifestations

The primary symptom of emphysema is dyspnea on exertion, which becomes progressively more severe. Eventually dyspnea occurs at rest. Initially there is little sputum production, but later it becomes copious. The patient eventually appears barrel chested (an increased anteroposterior diameter caused by overinflation) and begins using accessory muscles for breathing (Figure 9-16). Spontaneous pursed-lip breathing and chronic weight loss with emaciation ensue.

Assessment

Subjective data include a history of onset of symptoms. Note the duration and intensity of dyspnea, cough, and sputum production (documenting color and amount). Also determine the patient's reported history of smoking and exposure to inhalants and the family history of respiratory disorders.

Collection of **objective data** includes assessment of presenting signs, such as tachycardia, tachypnea, orthopnea, peripheral cyanosis, and clubbing of fingers. The most outstanding feature of clubbing is a lateral and longitudinal curvature of the nails accompanied by soft tissue enlargement, presenting a bulbous (bulb-

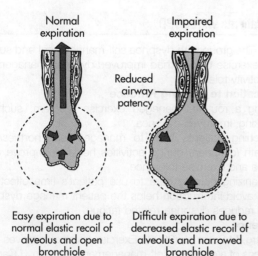

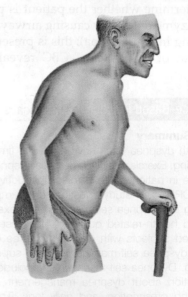

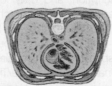

FIGURE 9-15 Mechanisms of air trapping in emphysema. Damaged or destroyed alveolar walls no longer support and hold airways open. Alveoli lose their property of passive elastic recoil. Both these factors contribute to collapse during expiration.

Normal expiration — Impaired expiration
Reduced airway patency
Easy expiration due to normal elastic recoil of alveolus and open bronchiole — Difficult expiration due to decreased elastic recoil of alveolus and narrowed bronchiole

FIGURE 9-16 Barrel chest. Note increase in anteroposterior diameter.

shaped), shiny appearance. This occurs late in the disease. Hypoxemia (especially during exercise) may be present, but hypercapnia does not develop until late in the disease. The person is characteristically underweight, but the exact cause for this is not well understood. One possibility is that the patient is in a hypermetabolic state with increased energy requirements that are partly due to the increased work of breathing. A therapeutic position for the patient with COPD is to lean forward with the head tilted and the arms resting on the patient's legs or a table. Expiration is prolonged as the patient forces his or her breath out through obstructed airways (Crawford, 2008).

Diagnostic Tests

An important goal of the diagnostic workup is to determine the major disease component of COPD, the severity of the disease, and the impact of the disease on the patient's quality of life. A history and physical examination are extremely important.

PFTs are done to measure total lung capacity, which is decreased with COPD. Residual volume is increased, as are compliance and airway resistance. Ventilatory response is decreased. Pulse oximetry is useful in assessing oxygen saturation in arterial blood.

ABGs are usually assessed in the severe stages and are monitored in hospitalized patients with acute exacerbations. ABGs reveal a decreased Pao_2 and $Paco_2$; increased HCO_3^-; and low-normal, elevated, or decreased pH. A chest radiographic examination shows hyperinflation of the lungs, widened intercostal spaces, and flattened diaphragm with increased anteroposterior diameter (barrel chest). Hematological studies are done to determine whether the patient is positive for AAT (an enzyme deficiency causing airway abnormalities resulting in emphysema); this is present in an inherited form of emphysema. CBC reveals elevated erythrocytes and hemoglobin and hematocrit levels (secondary polycythemia, as a compensatory response to chronic hypoxia). This is also a late manifestation of emphysema.

Medical Management

The medical plan includes long-term management with home oxygen therapy and chest physiotherapy as needed. In an acute exacerbation the patient may require mechanical ventilation.

Prescribed medications include bronchodilators such as beta-adrenergic agonists (e.g., short-acting albuterol and long-acting inhaled salmeterol [Serevent]) or theophyllines. Anticholinergics such as ipratropium (Atrovent) are also effective bronchodilators. Bronchodilators enlarge the bronchioles for greater oxygenation and ease of secretion clearance, and corticosteroids decrease pulmonary inflammation and obstruction. Corticosteroids are usually prescribed only during an acute exacerbation because of the many side effects seen in long-term steroid therapy. Antibiotics are frequently ordered to reduce the risk of infection related to retained pulmonary secretions. Diuretics assist with fluid removal. Pulmonary therapy can help mobilize secretions and improve oxygenation.

Many physicians prescribe pulmonary rehabilitation therapy that includes aerobic exercise such as walking. This increases the body's capacity to take up and use oxygen through the sustained rhythmic contraction of large muscle groups. Prescribed exercise training improves aerobic capacity, endurance, and strength; improves and maintains functional performance in day-to-day life; and reduces breathlessness and fatigue during exertion (see Evidence-Based Practice box).

During an acute exacerbation, severe dyspnea can produce considerable anxiety, restlessness, or irritabil-

---

🔍 Evidence-Based Practice | The Efficacy of Exercise Training in Patients with COPD

Evidence Summary

Patients with dyspnea often have a difficult time controlling their breathing. Exercise training improves dyspnea and activity tolerance in patients with chronic obstructive pulmonary disease (COPD). This study investigated the impact of exercise training on dyspnea self-management, exercise performance, and health-related quality of life. Researchers randomly placed subjects with COPD into three groups. One group had dyspnea self-management and supervised exercise training. Dyspnea self-management included individualized education about dyspnea management strategies, a home-walking prescription, and daily logs. The other two groups received standard care. Researchers measured outcomes (symptoms) at baseline and every 2 months for a year. Patients measured their symptoms through three questionnaires: Chronic Respiratory Questionnaire (CRQ), Shortness of Breath Questionnaire, and Baseline/Transitional Dyspnea Index. The group with dyspnea self-management and supervised exercise training had improved dyspnea management and activity tolerance.

Application to Nursing Practice

• Using a routine, managed exercise program, such as walking, improves dyspnea.
• Teaching patients how to manage their shortness of breath (dyspnea) during activities helps to improve dyspnea and exercise tolerance.
• Organizing nursing care to use patient's time effectively and avoid interruption helps the patient manage dyspnea and reduces dyspnea-related fatigue.

Reference

Stulbarg, M.S., et al. (2002). Exercise training improves outcomes of a dyspnea self-management program. *J Cardiopulm Rehabil 22*(2), 109.

From Potter, P.A., & Perry, A.G. (2009). *Fundamentals of nursing: concepts, process, and practice.* (7th ed.). St. Louis: Mosby.

ity. Carefully monitor the patient with COPD because of the increased risk for respiratory failure from central nervous system depressants. Careful evaluation for hypoxemia is necessary before a central nervous system depressant is prescribed (see Clinical Pathway 9-1 on Evolve).

Nursing Interventions and Patient Teaching

Nursing interventions are directed toward decreasing the patient's anxiety and promoting optimal air exchange. **Such measures include elevating the head of the bed and administering low-flow (1 to 2 L by nasal cannula) oxygen as ordered.** This is extremely important for COPD patients because a higher flow of oxygen delivery can be dangerous, since it diminishes the brain's respiratory (regulatory) center and can cause respiratory failure. Avoid use of respiratory depressants to ensure adequate alveolar ventilation. Assist with chest physiotherapy, which includes percussion, vibration, and postural drainage. All three techniques help loosen secretions to be expectorated; sometimes it takes several hours after chest physiotherapy before the patient can expectorate loosened secretions. Increasing oral intake of fluids liquefies secretions, thus aiding in their removal. Additionally, the use of a humidifier enhances this process. Allow sufficient rest periods and assist the patient in activities of daily living to prevent a decrease in oxygen saturation levels.

Assist the patient in maintaining nutritional intake by advising rest for 30 minutes before eating. This conserves energy and decreases dyspnea. The patient with emphysema has a markedly increased need for protein and calories to maintain an adequate nutritional status. A high-protein, high-calorie diet should be divided into five or six small meals a day. Oral fluid intake should be 2 to 3 L/day unless contraindicated (e.g., because of congestive heart failure). Instruct the patient to drink fluids between meals, rather than with meals, to reduce gastric distention and pressure on the diaphragm. Perform frequent oral hygiene to freshen the patient's mouth after coughing exercises and before meals.

Cessation of cigarette smoking in the early stages is probably the most significant factor in slowing the progression of the disease and improving pulmonary function. The use of nicotine replacement therapy and the newer, nonnicotine medication bupropion (Zyban) may minimize the effects of nicotine withdrawal. These adjunctive therapies should be combined with other modalities such as support groups, education materials, and behavior modification programs. Regardless of the method used to stop smoking, the most important factor is the patient's commitment.

The patient with COPD should have a vaccination with influenza virus vaccine yearly and a pneumococcal revaccination every 5 years.

Nursing diagnoses and interventions for the patient with emphysema include but are not limited to the following:

Nursing Diagnoses	Nursing Interventions
Ineffective airway clearance, related to narrowed bronchioles	Assess patient's ability to mobilize secretions, intervening as needed. Encourage coughing and deep breathing, frequent position changes, and increased oral intake (up to 2 to 3 L/day). Elevate head of bed; suction as needed. Assist with respiratory treatments. Auscultate lungs, and report any changes in lung sounds.
Activity intolerance, related to imbalance between oxygen supply and demand, secondary to inefficient work of breathing	Organize care so that periods of activity are interspersed with at least 90 minutes of undisturbed rest. Assist patient with active range-of-motion exercises to build stamina and prevent complications of decreased mobility. Monitor patient's respiratory response to activity. Activity intolerance is indicated by excessively increased respiratory rate (e.g., increased more than 10 breaths/min above patient's baseline) and depth, dyspnea, and use of accessory muscles of respiration.

Instruct the patient and the family on (1) the importance of not smoking and of reducing exposure to other inhaled irritants, (2) effective breathing techniques (such as pursed-lip breathing), and (3) relaxation exercises for anxiety control. Teach the patient about the dangers of increased oxygen intake for a patient dependent on hypoxic drive (stimulation of respiration by low Pao$_2$) for ventilation. Also teach the patient and the family how to prevent infection and symptoms that should be reported to the physician (see Home Care Considerations box, Communication box, and Nursing Care Plan 9-1).

Prognosis

Emphysema is usually irreversible. COPD is the fourth leading cause of death in the United States. COPD affects about 16 million Americans with about 120,000 deaths each year.

Home Care Considerations

Chronic Oxygen Therapy at Home

- Improved prognosis has been noted in patients with chronic obstructive pulmonary disease who receive nocturnal or continuous oxygen to treat hypoxemia.
- The longer the continuous daily use of oxygen is maintained, the greater the improvement.
- Periodic reevaluations are necessary for the patient who is using chronic supplemental oxygen in the home.
- Home oxygen systems are usually rented from a company that sends a respiratory therapist or pulmonary nurse specialist to the patient's home.
- The therapist teaches the patient how to use the oxygen system, how to care for it, and how to recognize when the supply is running low and needs to be reordered.
- Post "No smoking" warning signs where they can be seen in the home.
- Do not use electric razors, portable radios, open flames, wool blankets, or mineral oils in the area where oxygen is in use.
- Do not allow smoking in the home.

Communication

Mr. Oden, a 91-year-old, lives at home with his wife of 38 years. He was admitted to the hospital with acute **exacerbation** (an increase in the seriousness of a disease or disorder as marked by greater intensity in the signs or symptoms) of emphysema. Mr. Oden has a 24-year history of emphysema, with progression of signs and symptoms, including exertional dyspnea, expectoration of copious amounts of tenacious mucus, fatigue, and fear of suffocation.

Mr. Oden: Will it always be like this? I'm so short of air.

Ms. Lessing: Are you frightened?

Mr. Oden: I'm not afraid of dying, but I worry about having to fight for my air.

Ms. Lessing: (gently touches Mr. Oden's arm) Try taking slow, deep breaths, and concentrate on remaining calm.

Mr. Oden: Sometimes I can't even get to the bathroom and do my business—much less help my wife with the dishes or even fill the bird feeder.

Ms. Lessing: Do you feel you are becoming a burden?

Mr. Oden: I have to be good to my wife. I want to have something left to give her.

Ms. Lessing: I notice you are breathing more easily. I will be back to check on you, and perhaps we can continue this conversation.

CHRONIC BRONCHITIS

Etiology and Pathophysiology

Chronic bronchitis is characterized by a recurrent or chronic productive cough for a minimum of 3 months a year for at least 2 years. It is caused by physical or chemical irritants and recurrent lung infections. Cigarette smoking is by far the most common cause of chronic bronchitis. Workers exposed to dust, such as coal miners and grain handlers, also are at higher risk. The underlying process is an impairment of cilia, so they can no longer move secretions. Mucous gland hypertrophy causes hypersecretion, altering cilia function (see Figure 9-14, *A*). Excessive mucus is trapped in edematous airways, obstructing airflow. The lining of the bronchial tubes becomes inflamed and eventually scarred. The patient cannot clear tenacious mucus and it becomes a medium for bacteria and infection. This increased airway resistance leads to bronchospasm. The condition results in an altered oxygen–carbon dioxide exchange, hypoxia (an inadequate, reduced tension of cellular oxygen), and **hypercapnia** (greater than normal amounts of carbon dioxide in the blood).

Clinical Manifestations

Primary signs include a productive cough, most pronounced in the mornings (this is often overlooked by cigarette smokers). The patient also has increased dyspnea and use of accessory muscles. A complication of chronic bronchitis is cor pulmonale, which is hypertrophy of the right side of the heart resulting from pulmonary hypertension. Cyanosis develops, often accompanied by right ventricular failure. The patient with chronic bronchitis often has a characteristic reddish blue skin (resulting from chronic hypoxia, which stimulates erythropoiesis, thus resulting in polycythemia, cyanosis, and dependent edema).

Assessment

Subjective data include a detailed history of smoking or exposure to irritants and family history of respiratory disorders. Also determine the patient's current medication and treatment regimen.

Collection of **objective data** includes assessing the patient's productive cough, noting characteristics and amount of sputum. Assess the severity of dyspnea and presence of wheezing, and note the patient's level of restlessness. Also, when checking vital signs, pay special attention to tachycardia, tachypnea, and elevated temperature.

Diagnostic Tests

Chest radiographs taken early in the disease may not show abnormalities; later in the disease they will. An ECG may be normal or show signs indicative of right ventricular failure. An echocardiogram can be used to evaluate right and left ventricular function.

A CBC shows increased erythrocytes, hemoglobin, hematocrit, and white blood cell count. Polycythemia develops as a result of increased production of red blood cells as the body attempts to compensate for chronic hypoxemia. Hemoglobin concentrations may reach 20 g/dL or more. ABG values reveal respiratory acidosis, hypoxia, and hypercapnia. Pulse oximetry is valuable to assess oxygen saturation levels in arterial blood. PFTs will have an alteration that reveals airflow limitation on expiration, increased airway resistance and residual volume, and often electrolyte abnormalities. Monitor oximetry levels on all patients with hypoxia.

Nursing Care Plan 9-1   **The Patient with Emphysema**

Mr. Oden is a 91-year-old patient admitted with an exacerbation of chronic obstructive pulmonary disease (COPD). His respirations are 32 breaths/min and labored. He has nasal flaring, and his nailbeds are cyanotic. He has a barrel chest and digital clubbing. He states he has a productive cough and "can't get my air." It is noted he expectorates tenacious yellow mucus. He appears anxious during the assessment.

NURSING DIAGNOSIS *Ineffective airway clearance, related to tenacious secretions and expiratory airflow obstruction*

Patient Goals and Expected Outcomes	Nursing Interventions	Evaluation
Patient will maintain patent airway as evidenced by decreased wheezes, tachypnea, dyspnea, and arterial blood gas (ABG) values within limits (for this patient)	Assess lung sounds every 2 to 4 hours. Encourage turning, coughing, and deep breathing every 2 to 4 hours. Suction as needed. Explain all medications used in inhalation therapy and assist with treatment. Monitor effectiveness. Ensure hydration: oral intake of 2 to 3 L/day to liquefy secretions for easier expectoration.	Patient's respiratory status remains within baseline for this patient. Patient has normal breath sounds on auscultation. Patient is able to expectorate sputum without difficulty.

NURSING DIAGNOSIS *Ineffective breathing pattern, related to decreased lung expansion secondary to chronic airflow limitations*

Patient Goals and Expected Outcomes	Nursing Interventions	Evaluation
After treatment intervention, patient's breathing pattern will improve as evidenced by patient maintaining respiratory rate within 5 breaths/min of baseline Patient will demonstrate relaxed appearance	Assess for indicators of respiratory distress (agitation, restlessness, decreased level of consciousness, and use of accessory muscles of respiration). Auscultate breath sounds; report a decrease in breath sounds or an increase in adventitious breath sounds. Instruct patient in the use of pursed-lip breathing, which provides internal stability to the airways and may prevent airway collapse during expiration. Administer bronchodilator therapy as prescribed. Monitor patient's response to prescribed oxygen therapy. Be aware that high concentrations of oxygen can depress the respiratory drive in individuals with chronic carbon dioxide retention. Avoid use of respiratory depressants to ensure adequate alveolar ventilation.	Patient's arterial blood gases are within normal values. Patient has absence of adventitious breath sounds. Patient is sleeping for 5 to 6 hours without respiratory distress.

Critical Thinking Questions

1. Mr. Oden turns on his call light and states that he is "unable to get my air." The nurse notes subclavicular retractions and a respiratory rate of 36 breaths/min. His oxygen is flowing at 1 L/min via nasal cannula. What nursing interventions would decrease his dyspnea?
2. While the nurse is performing an assessment on Mr. Oden, he states, "I'm so tired of fighting to breathe that I wish I could just go to sleep and never wake up." What is an appropriate response?
3. During vital signs assessment, the nurse notes that Mr. Oden's temperature is 102° F (38.8° C), the pulse rate is 110 bpm, and the respiratory rate is 44 breaths/min. The nurse knows that Mr. Oden's COPD places him at a high risk for:

Medical Management

The medical plan is aimed at slowing the disease progression and facilitating optimal air exchange by reducing spasms and secretions.

Three main classes of bronchodilators are typically used to treat COPD. To reverse bronchospasm, the health care provider may order beta-adrenergic agonists such as short-acting albuterol and long-acting salmeterol. The theophyllines as well as anticholinergics such as ipratropium are also effective as bronchodilators. Corticosteroids are helpful in reducing airway inflammation. Long-term use of systemic steroids can lead to many adverse reactions, including osteoporosis. Inhaled steroids have fewer systemic effects and are preferred. Mucolytics such as guaifenesin to break up tenacious mucus may be helpful (Wisniewski, 2004). Antibiotic agents (erythromycin) are commonly ordered.

Nursing Interventions and Patient Teaching

Provide adequate hydration to liquefy secretions and aid in their removal. Suction the patient as needed, and provide low-flow oxygen to maintain SaO_2 above 90%. Offer frequent oral hygiene and provide rest periods. The nutritional needs are similar to those of the patient with emphysema.

Nursing diagnoses and interventions for the patient with chronic bronchitis include but are not limited to the following:

Nursing Diagnoses	Nursing Interventions
Ineffective breathing pattern, related to retained pulmonary secretions	Assess degree of dyspnea, noting nasal flaring, sternal retractions, and pursed-lip breathing. Instruct on effective breathing techniques. Suction as needed.
Fatigue, related to increased respiratory effort	Assess degree of fatigue, and use problem-solving techniques with patient to explore ways to decrease fatigue. Provide treatments in calm, unhurried manner. Identify support systems and provide referrals if needed. Encourage adequate periods of rest.

Teach the patient effective breathing techniques, and instruct the patient and the family on avoidance of infection exposure. Instruct the patient to notify the physician at the first sign of a respiratory infection. Usually the best indication of such an infection is a change in the color, consistency, or amount of sputum. Provide medication teaching, including action, rationale, and side effects. Stress the importance of increasing fluid intake, unless contraindicated. Encourage the patient and the family not to smoke. Encourage a patient who smokes to join a smoking cessation program, and teach about prescription and over-the-counter medications to assist with quitting smoking.

Prognosis

Chronic bronchitis is usually irreversible. COPD is the fourth leading cause of death in the United States, after heart disease, cancer, and traumatic injuries.

ASTHMA

Etiology and Pathophysiology

Asthma is a broad clinical syndrome and an airway pathologic condition. It involves episodic increased tracheal and bronchial responsiveness to various stimuli, resulting in widespread narrowing of the airways. Asthma usually improves either spontaneously or with treatment. It is classified as extrinsic or intrinsic. **Extrinsic** means it is caused by external factors, such as environmental allergens (pollen, dust, feathers, animal dander, foods, etc.); **intrinsic** asthma is from internal causes, not fully understood but often triggered by respiratory tract infection. Recurrence of attacks is greatly influenced by secondary factors, by mental or physical fatigue, and by emotional factors.

Asthma can result from an altered immune response or increased airway resistance and altered air exchange. Gastroesophageal reflux disease (GERD) can trigger an asthma attack (Lewis et al., 2007). The actual course of GERD resulting in an asthma attack is unknown, but it is assumed that the gastric acid reflux in the esophagus is aspirated into the lungs, resulting in vagal stimulation and bronchoconstriction (Lewis et al., 2007). An acute asthma attack may be caused by an antigen-antibody reaction in which histamine is released. There are three mechanisms involved (see Figure 9-14, *B*):

- Recurrent, reversible obstruction of airflow in the bronchioles and smaller bronchi secondary to bronchospasm. The muscles around the bronchioles tighten and narrow the air passages.
- Increased capillary permeability resulting in edema of mucous membranes with increased narrowing of airways and increased mucus secretion.
- An acute inflammatory response in the mast cells of the lungs, caused by exposure to an asthma trigger. These cells release histamine and other inflammatory agents. Systemic immune system cells release substances that cause circulating inflammatory cells to migrate to the lungs.

Clinical Manifestations

Mild asthma is manifested by dyspnea on exertion and wheezing. Symptoms are usually controlled by medications. An acute asthma attack usually occurs at night and includes tachypnea, tachycardia, diaphoresis, chest tightness, cough, expiratory wheezing, use of accessory muscles, and nasal flaring. The wheezing sound characteristic of asthma is caused by air forcing its way through the narrowed bronchioles and by vibrating mucus. The patients also has increased anxiety; diaphoresis; and a productive cough of copious, thick mucus. Asthma can be triggered by external factors (e.g., dust, mold, or lint) or precipitated intrinsically by a respiratory tract infection or exercise.

Status asthmaticus is a severe, unrelenting, life-threatening attack that fails to respond to usual treatment and places the patient at risk for respiratory failure. Symptoms of an acute attack are present, and the trapped air leads to exhaustion and respiratory failure. An axiom describes status asthmaticus: "The longer it lasts, the worse it gets, and the worse it gets, the longer it lasts" (Lewis et al., 2007).

Assessment
Subjective data include complaints of anxiety, fear of suffocation, breathlessness, chest tightness, and cough, particularly at night and in the early morning (Lewis et al., 2007).

Collection of **objective data** includes assessing for signs of hypoxia, which may include restlessness, inappropriate behavior, increased pulse and blood pressure, and tachypnea. The patient may assume a "hunched forward" position in an attempt to get more air. Auscultate the lungs for inspiratory and expiratory wheezing. Coughing produces thick, stringy mucus (Lewis et al., 2007).

Diagnostic Tests
To diagnose asthma, the physician orders ABGs and PFTs. The chest radiographic examination reveals lung hyperinflation related to air trapping, and a flat diaphragm related to increased intrathoracic volume. PFTs establish the diagnosis of asthma by determining the reversibility of bronchoconstriction. Normal values for these tests vary, depending on the patient's age, weight, and sex. In an acute asthma episode the patient will not be able to perform a complete pulmonary function study, but the nurse can check the peak expiratory flow rate. ABGs may be ordered during an acute exacerbation of asthma. Pulse oximetry is used to monitor the patient's Sao_2.

Obtain a sputum culture from the patient to rule out any secondary infection. A CBC and differential reveal an increased eosinophil count, which is indicative of an allergic response. If the patient has been taking theophylline, draw a blood sample to determine whether the prescribed dosage is maintained at a therapeutic level; the acceptable therapeutic range is 10 to 20 mcg/mL. This also reduces the risk of complications as a result of toxicity.

Medical Management
Medication management of asthma can be placed in two categories: maintenance therapy and acute (or rescue) therapy. **Maintenance therapy** prevents and minimizes symptoms; the medications are taken on a regular basis. These include the long acting beta$_2$-agonist salmeterol and formoterol (Foradil), which are used prophylactically only; inhaled corticosteroids, such as fluticasone; cromolyn; and theophylline. A combination of fluticasone and salmeterol (Advair Diskus) is also sometimes prescribed.

A recent group of drugs called leukotriene modifiers is now available for the prophylaxis and chronic treatment of asthma. Leukotrienes are chemicals present in the body that are powerful bronchoconstrictors and vasodilators; some also cause airway edema and inflammation, thus contributing to the symptoms of asthma. The two types of leukotriene modifiers are leukotriene receptor antagonists (zafirlukast, montelukast) and leukotriene synthesis inhibitors (zileuton [Zyflo]). These drugs interfere with the synthesis or block the action of leukotrienes. A major advantage is that they have both bronchodilator and antiinflammatory effects. These drugs are not recommended as the only treatment for persistent asthma. A broad range of patients, with mild to severe asthma, can benefit from leukotriene modifiers. Leukotriene modifiers are not indicated for use in the reversal of bronchospasms in acute asthma attacks. They are indicated for the chronic treatment of asthma (see Table 9-1).

Acute (or **rescue**) **therapy** works immediately to relieve symptoms of an asthma attack. The drugs involved include short-acting inhaled beta$_2$-agonist albuterol, metaproterenol (Alupent, Metaprel), and pirbuterol (Maxair) taken by a metered dose inhaler using spacer devices or by a nebulizer; oral or IV corticosteroids; and epinephrine. A study showed that inhaled corticosteroids, given with short-acting beta$_2$-agonists, may be better and faster than IV corticosteroids at treating an acute exacerbation (Miracle & Winston, 2000). Short-acting beta$_2$-agonists quickly relax the muscles around the airway and are the most effective drugs for relieving acute bronchospasms (see Table 9-3). Epinephrine, given subcutaneously or intramuscularly, may be considered in an emergency when symptoms have not been relieved by the use of a beta$_2$-agonist. Epinephrine acts as a bronchodilator. Although the value of administering aminophylline in the treatment of acute asthma has been questioned, IV aminophylline may be considered if the asthma is severe or there is minimal or no response to short-acting inhaled beta$_2$-agonists.

In acute asthma, oxygen therapy should be started immediately and its administration monitored by pulse oximetry and, in severe cases, by measurement of ABGs.

Using a peak flowmeter can help the patient manage asthma. This device measures peak expiratory flow rate—the flow of air in a forced exhalation in liters per minute, which is a good indicator of lung function. Peak flow monitoring measures how well air moves out of the lungs when blown out as hard and fast as possible. Peak flow measurement can help the patient detect early signs of asthma episodes before symptoms occur. Normal peak flow is 80% to 100% of the value predicted for the patient based on height, weight, age, and sex. Severe, persistent asthma is characterized by a peak flow of less than 60% of the value predicted. A severe, life-threatening exacerbation of asthma is characterized by a peak flow of less than 50% of the patient's predicted value.

Once the acute event is over, the medical plan includes identifying precipitating factors and promoting optimal health. Elimination of allergen or countermeasures, such as desensitization or hyposensitization, are desirable.

Nursing Interventions and Patient Teaching

Nursing interventions include administering prescribed medications and ensuring adequate fluid intake and optimal ventilation. To accomplish these goals, incorporate rest periods into activities and interventions; elevate the head of the bed; teach effective breathing techniques, such as pursed-lip breathing and correct use of the peak flowmeter; and provide oxygen therapy as ordered. Monitor vital signs and electrolytes. Kind and empathic emotional support is vital.

Nursing diagnoses and interventions for the patient with asthma include but are not limited to the following:

Nursing Diagnoses	Nursing Interventions
Ineffective breathing pattern, related to narrowed airway	Assess ventilation, and be alert for signs of increasing dyspnea, such as using accessory muscles, nasal flaring, dyspnea, pursed-lip breathing, or prolonged expiration. Maintain position to facilitate ventilation. Administer prescribed medications. Assist with administration of respiratory treatments. Provide care in calm, unhurried manner. Attempt to minimize exposure to dust and other irritants by maintaining clean environment and use of humidifier. Maintain adequate hydration.
Ineffective health maintenance, related to possible allergens in the home	Implement mutual problem solving to explore with patient and family what stimulants may be in home environment, such as allergens. Facilitate allergy testing if needed. Teach the patient and the family importance of avoiding exposure to known irritants.

Educate the patient and the family to identify signs and symptoms and recognize asthma "triggers" and avoid them or lessen their effects to prevent recurrent attacks. Instruct the patient on relaxation techniques to manage anxiety. Stress the importance of health maintenance measures, such as adequate fluid intake and effective breathing techniques. Teach the patient to take prescribed medications correctly and on time, to monitor the peak flowmeter to recognize the early signs of an asthma attack and begin treatment immediately, and to follow the program treatment steps during an attack. The goal is to provide a good control of symptoms with the least possible medication.

Prognosis

Although the incidence of asthma has steadily increased, the mortality and morbidity rates are currently decreasing. There are still more than 4,000 deaths per year from asthma (Lewis et al., 2007), which is disheartening, since treatment and education can reduce or eliminate asthma attacks. If status asthmaticus is not reversed, death will ensue.

BRONCHIECTASIS

Etiology and Pathophysiology

Bronchiectasis is a disease characterized by abnormal permanent dilation of one or more large bronchi. This dilation eventually destroys muscular elements and bronchial elastic that support the bronchial wall. Pulmonary muscle tone is gradually lost after one or, more often, repeated pulmonary infections in children and adults. Because of the disease, it is much more difficult to clear mucus from the lungs, and the lungs experience decreased expiratory airflow.

This condition is usually secondary to failure of normal lung tissue defenses (as caused by cystic fibrosis, foreign body, or tumor). It occurs as a complication of recurrent inflammation and infection process that gradually alters the pulmonary structures.

Clinical Manifestations

Signs and symptoms occur after a respiratory tract infection. The late signs and symptoms usually seen are dyspnea, cyanosis, and clubbing of fingers. The patient has paroxysms of coughing on arising in the morning and when lying down. This severe coughing produces copious amounts of foul-smelling sputum. Fatigue, weakness, and a loss of appetite are also noted.

Assessment

Subjective data include the patient's report of difficulty breathing, weight loss, and fever.

Objective data include fine crackles and wheezes in the lower lobes on auscultation. The patient exhibits a prolonged expiratory phase and increased dyspnea. Hemoptysis is seen in 50% of the patients.

Diagnostic Tests

Chest radiographic examination is essentially normal, but inflammation and mediastinal shift may result from overinflation of specific lobes. High-resolution CT scan of the chest is the gold standard for diagnosing bronchiectasis. Sputum cultures can rule out a bacterial infection. PFTs show a decreased forced expiratory volume.

Medical Management

Medical management of bronchiectasis involves treatment of exacerbations with antibiotics. A sputum culture is preferable before treatment with antibiotics, but if a culture is not obtainable, an antibiotic is still prescribed (Lewis et al., 2007).

Oxygen may be ordered at low-flow volume. The patient may require surgery if he or she does not respond to more conservative measures, such as medications, chest physiotherapy, and adequate hydration. If surgery is needed, the affected area is removed (lobectomy).

Medications also include mucolytic agents (acetylcysteine) and bronchodilators.

Nursing Interventions and Patient Teaching

General nursing interventions include using a cool mist vaporizer to provide humidity and increasing oral intake of fluids to aid in secretion removal. Assess vital signs and lung sounds every 2 to 4 hours. Suction the patient as needed and provide assistance in turning, coughing, and deep breathing every 2 hours. Assist with chest physiotherapy.

Nursing diagnoses and interventions for the patient with bronchiectasis include but are not limited to the following:

Nursing Diagnoses	Nursing Interventions
Ineffective airway clearance, related to retained pulmonary secretions	Assess patient's ability to mobilize secretions, assisting as needed. Encourage postural drainage and coughing; suction if needed. Encourage frequent position changes to facilitate secretion mobility and removal. Maintain adequate hydration. Administer mucolytic agents as ordered, and note patient response.
Impaired physical mobility, related to decreased exercise tolerance	Assess patient's activity tolerance, and promote adaptive techniques, such as incorporating rest periods into activities. Promote a gradual increase of activity, noting patient tolerance.

Nursing Diagnoses	Nursing Interventions
	Problem solve with patient and family to identify methods of energy conservation and ways to integrate them into lifestyle.

Teach the patient and the family environmental awareness (avoidance of smoke, fumes, and irritating inhalants). Discourage smoking, and advise the patient on appropriate rest and exercise practices. Perform medication teaching, including dosage, rationale, and side effects. Instruct the patient and the family on signs and symptoms of a secondary infection, and ensure the patient knows how to reach the physician after discharge.

Prognosis

Bronchiectasis is a chronic disease. Surgical removal of a portion of the patient's lung is the only cure.

❖ NURSING PROCESS *for the Patient with a Respiratory Disorder*

The role of the licensed practical nurse/licensed vocational nurse (LPN/LVN) in the nursing process as stated is that the LPN/LVN will:

- Participate in planning care for patients based on patient needs
- Review patient's care plan and recommend revisions as needed
- Review and follow defined prioritization for patient care
- Use clinical pathways, care maps, or care plans to guide and review patient care

▪ Assessment

When a patient is admitted with a respiratory disorder, a thorough, immediate, and accurate nursing assessment is an essential first step. The assessment should include the patient's level of consciousness, vital signs, lung sounds (crackles, wheezes, pleural friction rub), and oximetry level. Ask the patient if he or she has shortness of breath, dyspnea on exertion, or cough. If the patient has a cough, ask whether it is productive or nonproductive and the amount and the color of the sputum expectorated. Observe the patient's facial expressions and for signs of respiratory distress such as flaring nostrils, substernal or clavicular retractions, asymmetrical chest wall expansion, and abdominal breathing.

▪ Nursing Diagnosis

Assist in the development of nursing diagnoses. Nursing diagnoses specific to the patient with a respiratory disorder include but are not limited to the following:

- Ineffective airway clearance
- Ineffective breathing pattern
- Impaired gas exchange

- Anxiety
- Activity intolerance
- Imbalanced nutrition: less than body requirements

■ **Expected Outcomes and Planning**

The overall goals are that the patient with a respiratory disorder will have (1) effective breathing patterns, (2) adequate airway clearance, (3) adequate oxygenation of tissues, and (4) a realistic attitude toward compliance to treatment. The care plan may include the following goals:

Goal 1: Patient will achieve improved activity tolerance.

Outcome: Patient reports less discomfort with exercise.

Goal 2: Patient will maintain a patent airway.

Outcome: Patient clears airway by coughing.

■ **Implementation**

Maintaining the patient's optimal health is important in reducing respiratory symptoms. Nursing interventions may include improving the patient's activity tolerance. This enables the patient to perform activities of daily living while not increasing dyspnea.

■ **Evaluation**

Evaluate the expected outcomes and determine their effectiveness. Notify the physician if the patient's respiratory status does not improve immediately.

Goal 1: Patient will achieve improved activity tolerance.

Evaluative measure: Assess patient's exercise tolerance.

Goal 2: Patient will maintain a patent airway.

Evaluative measure: Auscultate lungs after hearing patient cough.

Get Ready for the NCLEX® Examination!

Key Points

- When air is inhaled, it is warmed, moistened, and filtered to prepare it for use by the body.
- The most important structure of the respiratory system is the alveolus, where actual air exchange occurs.
- For breathing to occur, pressure changes must take place within the thoracic cavity.
- The combination of one inspiration plus one expiration equals one respiration, or one respiratory movement.
- The primary function of the respiratory system is to exchange oxygen and carbon dioxide at the alveolar-capillary level.
- The lungs' ability to expand and contract depends on musculoskeletal and neurologic functions, as well as physiologic conditions affecting the respiratory system.
- Activity tolerance is frequently altered as a result of decreased oxygenation-ventilation.
- Anxiety can exacerbate pulmonary disorders, increasing the body's need for oxygen.
- Breathing exercises can improve ventilation.
- Effective breathing techniques include elevating the head and chest to maintain airway patency; deep breathing and coughing exercises to facilitate lung expansion; and pursed-lip breathing to decrease the effort of breathing.
- Adequate fluid intake and humidity help moisten secretions, thus aiding in their clearance.
- A thorough psychosocial assessment and resultant interventions are necessary for the patient with a laryngectomy because of loss of voice and neck and facial disfigurement.
- In May 2005 the FDA approved a new version of a blood test to aid in diagnosing latent TB infection and active TB. It is called QFT-G, and it can be used in place of the traditional PPD skin test. The QFT-G may detect TB with greater specificity than the PPD test.

- SARS is a serious acute respiratory infection caused by a coronavirus.
- People who are suspected of having SARS should be placed in respiratory isolation, including use of an appropriate disposable particulate respirator to protect other patients and health care workers.
- Clinical manifestations of sleep apnea include frequent awakening at night, insomnia, excessive daytime sleepiness, witnessed apneic episodes, morning headaches, personality changes, and irritability.
- Chest drainage serves a twofold purpose: it (1) drains air, blood, or fluid from the pleural space; and (2) restores negative pressure. It requires a water seal to prevent air from reentering the pleural space.
- Techniques used in chest physiotherapy include percussion, vibration, and postural drainage.
- Nursing interventions after thoracic surgery that assist in preventing complications by promoting effective airway clearance are (1) frequent repositioning, (2) coughing, and (3) deep breathing.
- Studies have revealed that hypoxia worsens when patients are placed on their backs or sides with the affected (sick) lung down.
- Low-flow oxygen therapy is required for patients with COPD because higher oxygen concentrations depress the body's own respiratory regulatory centers.
- Hospitals are a high-risk setting for TB transmission, and health care workers are at high occupational risk for TB infection.
- Because PE impairs gas exchange, its hallmark is acute, unexplained dyspnea with abrupt, constant, nonradiating pain that worsens with inspiration.
- Patients with respiratory disorders must reduce exposure to infection, which increases the body's oxygen demands.
- COPD includes emphysema, chronic bronchitis, asthma, and bronchiectasis.

- Transmission of TB is primarily by inhalation of minute droplet nuclei (each containing a single tubercle bacillus) coughed or sneezed by a person whose sputum contains tubercle bacilli.
- Pulse oximetry is a noninvasive method providing continuing monitoring of SaO_2 (saturation of oxygen).

Additional Learning Resources

 Go to your Companion CD for an audio glossary, animations, video clips, and more.

evolve Be sure to visit the Evolve site at http://evolve.elsevier.com/ Christensen/adult/ for additional online resources.

Review Questions for the NCLEX® Examination

1. Rapid and deeper respirations are stimulated by the respiratory center of the brain when:
   1. oxygen saturation levels are greater than 90%.
   2. carbon dioxide levels increase.
   3. the alveoli contract.
   4. the diaphragm contracts and lowers its dome.

2. The tendency of molecules of a substance (gaseous, liquid, or solid) to move from a region of high concentration to one of lower concentration is the passive process at work in the exchange of gases between the blood capillary and alveolar area. This process is called:
   1. osmosis.
   2. filtration.
   3. diffusion.
   4. transport.

3. Each alveolus is coated with a thin lipoprotein covering that prevents it from collapsing after each breath; this covering is:
   1. LDH.
   2. isoenzyme.
   3. surfactant.
   4. sebum.

4. The walls of the thoracic cavity are lined with a serous membrane composed of tough endothelial cells called:
   1. visceral pleura.
   2. apneustic serosa.
   3. pneumotaxic serosa.
   4. parietal pleura.

5. The exchange of oxygen and carbon dioxide in external respiration takes place in the:
   1. lungs.
   2. bronchioles.
   3. capillaries and body cells.
   4. alveoli and pulmonary capillaries.

6. A 73-year-old patient is diagnosed with chronic bronchitis. He is very dyspneic and must sit up to breathe. An abnormal condition in which there is discomfort in breathing in any but an erect sitting position is:
   1. orthopnea.
   2. dyspnea.

3. orthopsia.
4. Cheyne-Stokes.

7. A 45-year-old patient is being evaluated to rule out pulmonary tuberculosis (TB). Which finding is most closely associated with TB?
   1. Leg cramps
   2. Night sweats
   3. Skin discoloration
   4. Green-colored sputum

8. The health care workers caring for a patient with active TB, are instructed in methods of protecting themselves from contracting TB. The Centers for Disease Control and Prevention currently recommend that health care workers who care for TB-infected patients:
   1. ask the patient to wear a mask while in isolation.
   2. wear a surgical mask.
   3. wear a small-micron, fitted filtration mask.
   4. receive the BCG vaccine.

9. The physician ordered a blood culture and sputum specimen for a patient who has pneumonia. These diagnostic tests should be collected:
   1. after initiation of antibiotic therapy.
   2. the morning after admission.
   3. before initiation of antibiotic therapy.
   4. at the first elevated temperature.

10. A 62-year-old patient has just returned to her room after a bronchoscopy. No food or fluids should be given after the examination until:
   1. total absence of blood-streaked sputum.
   2. the head nurse gives the order.
   3. her gag reflex returns.
   4. she is up and about and steady on her feet.

11. A patient who was in a motor vehicle accident and has a lacerated pleura secondary to fractured ribs. To promote reexpansion of his lung, what type of thoracic drainage system was used?
   1. Open system to promote negative pressure
   2. Closed system to maintain the lungs' normal negative pressure
   3. Closed system to maintain the lungs' positive pressure
   4. Closed system to allow air to enter the pleural cavity for reexpansion

12. A 45-year-old, second-day postoperative patient is recovering from thoracic surgery. A therapeutic nursing intervention would include:
   1. helping the patient cough and deep breathe by splinting the anterior and posterior chest.
   2. splinting the anterior chest for coughing.
   3. placing the patient in a supine position.
   4. allowing the patient to sleep uninterrupted for 8 hours.

13. A 71-year-old patient is admitted with an exacerbation of COPD. He has dependent edema, ascites, and dyspnea. A complication that may occur in COPD, in which some of the capillaries surrounding the alveoli are destroyed, resulting in pulmonary hypertension,

blood returning to the right side of the heart, and signs and symptoms of right-sided HF, is:

1. pulmonary edema.
2. cor pulmonale.
3. tetralogy of Fallot.
4. acyanotic heart disease.

14. A 52-year-old patient had a laryngectomy due to cancer of the larynx. Discharge instructions are given to the patient and his family. Which response, by written communication from the patient or verbal response by the family, indicates that the instructions need to be clarified?

1. Report swelling, pain, or excessive drainage.
2. The suctioning at home must be a clean procedure, not sterile.
3. Cleanse skin around stoma bid, use hydrogen peroxide and rinse with water, pat dry.
4. It is acceptable to take over-the-counter medications now that condition is stable.

15. Most pulmonary embolisms (PEs) originate from:

1. deep-vein thrombosis (DVT).
2. ventilation/perfusion (V/Q) mismatch.
3. increased pulmonary vascular resistance.
4. right-sided heart failure.

16. Chest pain from pulmonary embolism (PE) typically:

1. radiates to the neck and jaw.
2. is unchanged by deep breathing.
3. is pleuritic and worsens on inspiration.
4. radiates to the abdomen and back.

17. In the treatment of asthma, peak flow monitoring is important to help the patient manage the asthma. Peak flow monitoring measures:

1. the inspiratory capacity of the lungs.
2. the residual volume of the lungs.
3. the vital capacity of the lungs.
4. how well air moves out of the lungs during forceful exhalation.

18. The primary goal for the patient with bronchiectasis is that the patient will:

1. have no recurrence of disease.
2. have normal pulmonary function.
3. maintain removal of bronchial secretions.
4. avoid environmental agents that precipitate inflammation.

19. A patient was seen in clinic for an episode of epistaxis, which was controlled by placement of anterior nasal packing. During discharge teaching, the nurse instructs the patient to:

1. avoid vigorous nose blowing and strenuous activity.
2. use aspirin or aspirin-containing compounds for pain relief.
3. apply ice compresses to the nose every 4 hours for the first 48 hours.
4. leave the packing in place for 7 to 10 days until it is removed by the physician.

20. TB is spread by:

1. contact with clothing, bedding, or food.
2. eating from utensils used by an infected person.
3. inhaling the TB bacteria after a person coughs, speaks, or sneezes.
4. talking with an individual with TB.

21. Which type of medication is used as rescue medication in an acute asthma exacerbation?

1. Methylxanthines
2. Leukotriene modifiers
3. Long-acting beta$_2$-agonists
4. Short-acting beta$_1$-agonists

22. Asthma is best characterized as:

1. an inflammatory disease.
2. a steady progression of bronchoconstriction.
3. an obstructive disease with loss of alveolar walls.
4. a chronic obstructive disorder characterized by mucus production.

23. A patient with COPD asks why the heart is affected by the respiratory disease. The nurse's response to the patient is based on the knowledge that cor pulmonale is characterized by:

1. pulmonary congestion secondary to left ventricular failure.
2. excess serous fluid collection in the alveoli caused by retained respiratory secretions.
3. right ventricular hypertrophy secondary to increased pulmonary vascular resistance.
4. right ventricular failure secondary to compression of the heart by hyperinflated lungs.

24. A patient with TB has a nursing diagnosis of noncompliance. The nurse recognizes that the most common etiologic factor for this diagnosis in patients with TB is:

1. fatigue and lack of energy to manage self-care.
2. lack of knowledge about how the disease is transmitted.
3. little or no motivation to adhere to a long-term drug regimen.
4. feelings of shame and the response to the social stigma associated with TB.

25. Three types of anthrax are:

1. cutaneous, gastrointestinal, inhalational.
2. renal, gastrointestinal, CNS.
3. musculoskeletal, inhalational, adrenal.
4. cutaneous, endocrine, gastrointestinal.

26. To get optimal results from pulse oximetry, which statements are correct? *(Select all that apply.)*

1. Do not attach the transducer to an extremity that has a blood pressure cuff in place.
2. While the probe is in place, protect it from decreased light, which can affect the reading.
3. Place the probe over a pulsating vascular bed.
4. Remember that hypothermia, hypotension, and vasoconstriction can affect readings.

27. *Ineffective airway clearance,* related to tracheobronchial obstruction or secretions, is a nursing diagnosis for a patient with COPD. Which of the following nursing interventions are correct? *(Select all that apply.)*
    1. Offer small, frequent, high-calorie, high-protein feedings.
    2. Encourage generous fluid intake.
    3. Restrict fluid intake to decrease congestion.
    4. Have patient turn and cough every 2 hours; teach effective coughing technique.

28. *Ineffective breathing pattern,* related to decreased lung expansion during an acute attack of asthma, is an appropriate nursing diagnosis. Which nursing interventions are correct? *(Select all that apply.)*
    1. Place patient in a supine position.
    2. Administer oxygen therapy as ordered.
    3. Remain with patient during acute attack to decrease fear and anxiety.
    4. Incorporate rest periods into activities and interventions.
    5. Maintain semi-Fowler's position to facilitate ventilation.

29. The patient with respiratory acidosis demonstrates: *(Select all that apply.)*
    1. disorientation.
    2. pH of less than 7.35.
    3. pH of more than 7.44.
    4. rapid respirations.

30. The appropriate nursing intervention for a 40-year-old patient with active TB, would be to:
    1. place the patient in drainage and secretion precautions.
    2. place the patient in acid-fast bacilli (AFB) isolation precautions.
    3. maintain the patient in enteric isolation.
    4. not use any isolation precautions.

31. Patient teaching after a tonsillectomy and adenoidectomy would include which instruction(s)? *(Select all that apply.)*
    1. Avoid attempting to clear the throat, coughing, and sneezing.
    2. Avoid vigorous nose blowing for 1 to 2 weeks.
    3. Resume foods and fluids as tolerated.
    4. Take aspirin, gr 10, every 4 hours.
    5. Notify the physician in case of increased pain, fever, or bleeding.

32. If the patient has an epistaxis, the correct nursing intervention(s) would be to: *(Select all that apply.)*
    1. place the patient in Fowler's position with the head forward.
    2. place the patient in Fowler's position with the head extended.

3. compress the nostrils tightly below the bone and hold for 10 minutes or longer.
    4. place ice compresses over the nose.

33. In pulmonary edema, the medical management often include(s): *(Select all that apply.)*
    1. IV infusion at 150 mL/hr.
    2. furosemide (Lasix) IV.
    3. oxygen therapy.
    4. orthopneic position.
    5. morphine sulfate to decrease respiratory rate.

34. An appropriate nursing diagnosis for a patient with pulmonary edema is *excess fluid volume,* related to altered tissue permeability. Which nursing intervention(s) for this diagnosis are correct? *(Select all that apply.)*
    1. Assess indicators of patient's fluid volume status, such as breath sounds; skin turgor; and pedal, sacral, and periorbital edema.
    2. Monitor intake and output accurately.
    3. Administer diuretics as ordered.
    4. Weigh daily.
    5. Provide regular diet with normal sodium intake.

35. The nurse should educate the patient in the proper techniques to use for the collection of a sputum specimen. Which guideline(s) are correct? *(Select all that apply.)*
    1. Explain to the patient the need to bring the sputum up from the lungs.
    2. Encourage fluid intake.
    3. Collect specimens after meals when patient feels stronger.
    4. Notify staff as soon as specimen is collected so it can be sent to the laboratory without delay.
    5. Place sputum specimen in sterile container.

36. Medical management and nursing interventions of the patient with pulmonary embolism usually include: *(Select all that apply.)*
    1. bed rest
    2. administration of intravenous heparin per protocol
    3. semi-Fowler's position
    4. administration of vitamin K subcutaneously
    5. oxygen per mask or nasal cannula

37. A new blood assay test that offers a promising alternative in TB testing is:
    1. QuantiFERON-TB Gold Test.
    2. Relenza Test.
    3. HPV DNA Test.
    4. BNP Test.

Objectives

Anatomy and Physiology

1. Describe the structures of the urinary system, including functions.
2. List the three processes involved in urine formation.
3. Name three hormones and their influence on nephron function.
4. Compare the normal components of urine with the abnormal components.

Medical-Surgical

5. Identify the effects of aging on urinary system function.
6. Appraise the changes in body image created when the patient experiences an alteration in urinary function.
7. Incorporate pharmacotherapeutic and nutritional considerations into the nursing care plan of the patient with a urinary disorder.

8. Prioritize the special needs of the patient with urinary dysfunction.
9. Describe the alterations in kidney function associated with disorders of the urinary tract.
10. Discuss the effect of renal disease on family function.
11. Address patient concerns in teaching about altered sexuality secondary to urinary disorders and treatments.
12. Investigate community resources for support for the patient and significant others as they face lifestyle changes from chronic urinary disorders and treatments.
13. Select nursing diagnoses related to alterations in urinary function.
14. Design culturally sensitive care of the patient with a urinary disorder.

Key Terms

anasarca (ăn-ă-SĂR-kă, p. 467)
anuria (ă-NŪ-rē-ă, p. 471)
asthenia (ăs-THĒ-nē-ă, p. 451)
azotemia (ă-zō-TĒ-mē-ă, p. 455)
bacteriuria (băk-tēr-ē-Ū-rē-ŭh, p. 451)
costovertebral angle (CVA) (kŏs-tō-VĔR-tě-brăl ĂNG-gŭl, p. 455)
cytologic evaluation (sī-tŏ-LŎJ-ĭk ě-văl-ū-Ā-shŭn, p. 461)
dialysis (dī-ĂL-ĭ-sĭs, p. 474)
dysuria (dĭs-Ū-rē-ă , p. 441)
hematuria (hěm-ă-TŪ-rē-ă, p. 451)

hydronephrosis (hī-drō-ně-FRŌ-sĭs, p. 457)
ileal conduit (ĭl-ē-ăl KŎN-dū-ĭt, p. 478)
micturition (mĭk-tū-RĬSH-ŭn, p. 457)
nephrotoxins (něf-rō-TŎK-sĭnz, p. 480)
nocturia (nŏk-TŪ-rē-ă, p. 451)
oliguria (ŏl-ĭ-GŪ-rē-ă, p. 467)
prostatodynia (prŏs-tě-tō-DĬN-ē-ă, p. 454)
pyuria (pĭ-Ū-rē-ă, p. 451)
residual urine (rě-ZĬ-dū-ăl Ū-rĭn, p. 448)
retention (rē-TĔN-shŭn, p. 448)
urolithiasis (ū-rō-lĭ-THĬ-ă-sĭs, p. 457)

ANATOMY AND PHYSIOLOGY OF THE URINARY SYSTEM

Each day, the cells throughout the body metabolize ingested nutrients. This process provides energy for the body and produces waste products. As proteins break down, nitrogenous waste—urea, ammonia, and **creatinine** (a nitrogenous compound produced by metabolic processes in the body)—is produced. The primary function of the kidneys is excretion of these waste products. The kidneys also assist in regulating the body's water, electrolytes, and acid-base balance. The urinary system is probably the most important system in maintaining homeostasis.

The urinary system consists of two kidneys, which produce urine by removing waste, excess water, and

electrolytes from the blood; two ureters, which transport urine from the kidneys to the bladder; one bladder, which collects and stores urine; and one urethra, which transports urine from the bladder to the outside of the body for elimination (Figure 10-1). This chapter explores the filtering process, the composition of urine, and the pathway of urine removal from the body.

KIDNEYS

The kidneys lie behind the parietal peritoneum (retroperitoneal), just below the diaphragm on each side of the vertebral column. Kidneys are dark red, bean-shaped organs that are 4 to 5 inches (10 to 12 cm) long, 2 to 3 inches (5 to 7.5 cm) wide, and about 1 inch (2.5 cm) thick. Because of the liver, the right kidney

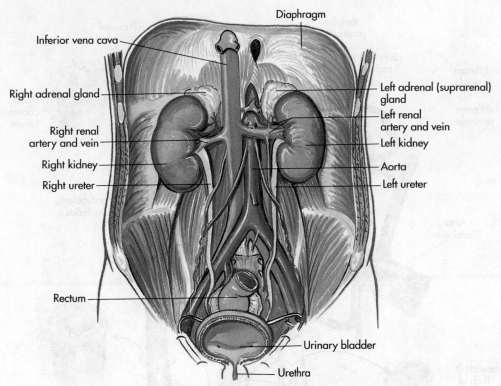

FIGURE 10-1 Locations of urinary system organs.

lies slightly lower than the left. The kidneys are surrounded and anchored in place by a layer of adipose tissue. Near the center of the kidney's medial border is a notch or indentation called the **hilus** where the renal artery enters and the renal vein and the ureter exit the kidney.

The adrenal glands, a part of the endocrine system, sit near the top of each kidney. The adrenal glands secrete hormones that help control blood pressure and heart rate, among other functions. The primary mineralocorticoid secreted by the adrenal cortex is aldosterone. Plasma potassium concentration is the primary regulator of aldosterone. Changes evoked through the adrenal glands create changes in kidney function (see Chapter 11).

Gross Anatomical Structure

The outer covering of the kidney is a strong layer of connective tissue called the **renal capsule.** Directly beneath the renal capsule is the renal **cortex.** It contains 1.25 million renal tubules, which are part of the microscopic filtration system. Immediately beneath the cortex is the **medulla,** which is a darker color. The medulla contains the triangular **pyramids.** Continuing inward, the narrow points of the pyramids **(papillae)** empty urine into the calyces. The **calyces** are cuplike extensions of the renal pelvis that guide urine into the renal pelvis. The **renal pelvis** is an expansion of the upper end of the ureter; the ureter in turn drains the finished product, urine, into the bladder (Figure 10-2).

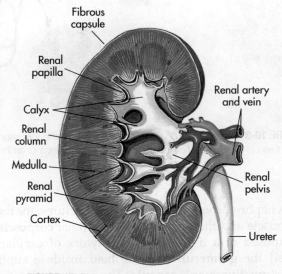

FIGURE 10-2 Coronal section through right kidney.

Microscopic Structure

Nephron

Each kidney contains more than 1 million nephrons. The **nephron** is the functional unit of the kidney, resembling a microscopic funnel with a long stem and two convoluted sections (Figure 10-3). It is responsible for filtering the blood and processing the urine. The nephron has three major functions: (1) controlling body fluid levels by selectively removing or retaining water, (2) assisting with the regulation of the pH of the blood, and (3) removing toxic waste from the blood. Approximately 60 times a day, the body's entire volume of blood is filtered through the kidneys.

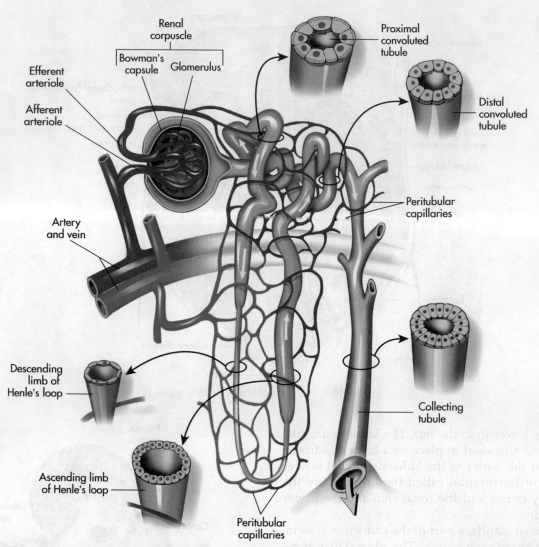

FIGURE 10-3 The nephron unit. Cross-sections from the four segments of the renal tubule are shown. The differences in appearance in tubular cells seen in a cross-section reflect the differing functions of each nephron segment.

A nephron consists of two main structures: the renal corpuscle and the renal tubule. The renal corpuscle is composed of a tightly bound network of capillaries called the **glomeruli** that are held inside a cuplike structure, **Bowman's capsule.** The renal arteries (right and left) branch off the abdominal aorta and enter the kidney at the hilus. The renal arteries continue branching until blood is delivered to the glomerulus by the afferent arteriole. The blood leaves the glomerulus through the efferent arteriole to the peritubular capillary. Blood finally reaches the renal veins and flows into the inferior vena cava.

The renal tubule becomes tightly coiled (at the proximal convoluted tubule), makes a sudden straight drop, and curves back upward like a hairpin (at Henle's loop, or nephron loop) and becomes tightly coiled again (at the distal convoluted tubule). The convoluted tubule terminates at the collecting tubule or duct. Several collecting ducts unite in a pyramid and open at the papilla to empty urine into the associated calyx.

The juxtaglomerular apparatus is the microscopic structure in the kidney, which regulates the function of each nephron. The juxtaglomerular apparatus is named for its proximity to the glomerulus; it is found between the vascular pole of the renal corpuscle and the returning distal convoluted tubule of the same nephron. This location is critical to its function in regulating renal blood flow and glomerular filtration rate. The juxtaglomerular apparatus is where the afferent arterioles come into direct contact with the distal convoluted tubule. The juxtaglomerular apparatus works to regulate systemic blood pressure and filtrate formation.

The specialized cells of the afferent arteriole at this region are called juxtaglomerular cells. These cells contain the enzyme renin and function as mechanoreceptors to sense blood pressure.

The specialized cells of the distal convoluted tubule at the point of contact with the afferent arteriole are the macula densa cells. These cells function as chemoreceptors to sense changes in the solute concentration and flow rate of the filtrate.

When systemic blood pressure decreases, the juxtaglomerular cells have a decreased stretch, which leads to their release of renin (Figure 10-4). Renin release causes the activation of the renin-angiotensin mechanism, which ultimately leads to an increased blood pressure.

Reabsorption begins as soon as the filtrate reaches the tubule system. The filtrate contains important products needed by the body: water, glucose, and ions may be absorbed. In fact, 99% of the filtrate is returned to the body (see Figure 10-4).

In summary, the three phases of urine formation (Table 10-1) and location of the processes are as follows:

1. **Filtration** of water and blood products occurs in the glomerulus of Bowman's capsule.

2. **Reabsorption** of water, glucose, and necessary ions back into the blood occurs primarily in the proximal convoluted tubules, Henle's loop, and the distal convoluted tubules. This process reclaims important substances needed by the body.

3. **Secretion** of certain ions, nitrogenous waste products, and drugs occurs primarily in the distal convoluted tubule. This process is the reverse of reabsorption; the substances move from the blood to the filtrate.

Hormonal Influence on Nephron Function. When the body has suffered increased fluid loss through hemorrhage, diaphoresis, vomiting, diarrhea, or other means, the blood pressure drops. These events decrease the amount of filtrate produced by the kidneys. The posterior pituitary gland releases antidiuretic hormone

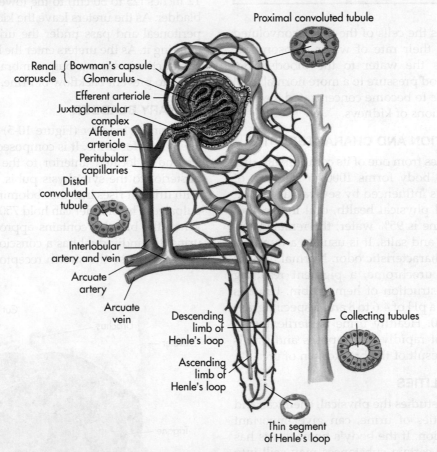

FIGURE 10-4 Cross-section from the four segments of the renal tubule.

PART OF NEPHRON	PROCESS IN URINE FORMATION	SUBSTANCES MOVED AND DIRECTION OF MOVEMENT
Glomerulus	Filtration	Water and solutes (sodium and other ions, nitrogen wastes, urea, uric acid, creatinine, glucose, and other nutrients) filter through the glomeruli into Bowman's capsule
Proximal convoluted tubule	Reabsorption	Water and solutes
Henle's loop	Reabsorption	Sodium and chloride ions
Distal convoluted and collecting tubules	Reabsorption	Water, sodium, and other chloride ions
	Secretion	Ammonia, potassium ions, urea, uric acid, creatinine, hydrogen ions, and some drugs

Table 10-1   Functions of Parts of the Nephron in Urine Formation

---

Box 10-1 Major Functions of the Kidneys

Urine formation: Glomerular filtration, tubular reabsorption, and secretion; 1000 to 2000 mL of urine formed each day

Fluid and electrolyte control: Maintain correct balance of fluid and electrolytes within a normal range by excretion, secretion, and reabsorption

Acid-base balance: Maintain pH of blood (7.35 to 7.45) at normal range by directly excreting hydrogen ions and forming bicarbonate for buffering

Excretion of waste products: Direct removal of metabolic waste products contained in the glomerular filtrate

Blood pressure regulation: Regulation of blood pressure by controlling the circulating volume and renin secretion

Red blood cell (RBC) production: Secretion of erythropoietin, which stimulates bone marrow to produce RBCs

Regulation of calcium-phosphate metabolism: Regulation of vitamin D activation

---

(ADH). ADH causes the cells of the distal convoluted tubules to increase their rate of water reabsorption. This action returns the water to the bloodstream, which raises the blood pressure to a more normal level and causes the urine to become concentrated. See Box 10-1 for major functions of kidneys.

URINE COMPOSITION AND CHARACTERISTICS

The word *urine* comes from one of its components, uric acid. Each day, the body forms 1000 to 2000 mL of urine; this amount is influenced by several factors, including mental and physical health, oral intake, and blood pressure. Urine is 95% water; the remainder is nitrogenous wastes and salts. It is usually a transparent yellow with a characteristic odor. Normal urine is yellow because of urochrome, a pigment resulting from the body's destruction of hemoglobin. Urine is slightly acidic, with a pH of 4.6 to 8 and a specific gravity of 1.003 to 1.030. Healthy urine is sterile, but at room temperature it rapidly decomposes and smells like ammonia as a result of the breakdown of urea.

URINE ABNORMALITIES

A urinalysis, which studies the physical, chemical, and microscopic properties of urine, can give important diagnostic information. If the body's homeostasis has been compromised, certain substances may spill into the urine. Some of the more common substances include the following:

- **Albumin** in the urine (albuminuria) indicates possible renal disease, increased blood pressure, or toxicity of the kidney cells from heavy metals.
- **Glucose** (sugar) in the urine (glycosuria) most often indicates a high blood glucose level. The blood glucose level rises above the renal threshold (the point at which the renal tubules can no longer reabsorb), and the glucose spills into the urine.

- **Erythrocytes** in the urine (hematuria) may indicate infection, tumors, or renal disease. Occasionally an individual may have a renal calculus (kidney stone), and irritation produces hematuria.
- **Ketone bodies** in the urine is called ketoaciduria (or ketonuria). It occurs when too many fatty acids are oxidized. This condition is seen with diabetes mellitus, starvation, or any other metabolic condition in which fats are rapidly catabolized.
- **Leukocytes** (white blood cells [WBCs]) are found in urine when there is an infection in the urinary tract.

URETERS

Once the urine has been formed in the nephrons, it passes to the paired ureters. Ureters are actually extensions of the renal pelvis and extend downward 10 to 12 inches (25 to 30 cm) to the lower part of the urinary bladder. As the ureters leave the kidneys, they are retroperitoneal and pass under the urinary bladder before entering it. As the ureters enter the bladder (ureterovesical junction), the mucous membrane folds, acting as a valve to prevent backflow of urine.

URINARY BLADDER

The urinary bladder (Figure 10-5) is a temporary storage pouch for urine. It is composed of collapsible muscle and is located anterior to the small intestine and posterior to the symphysis pubis. As the bladder fills with urine, it rises into the abdominal cavity and can be palpated. The bladder can hold 750 to 1000 mL of urine. When the bladder contains approximately 250 mL of urine, the individual has a conscious desire to urinate. This is because the stretch receptors become activated

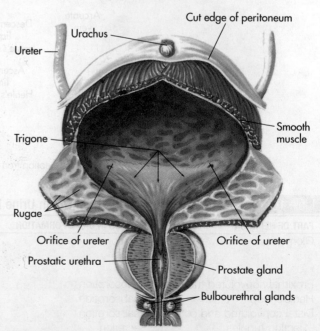

FIGURE 10-5 The male urinary bladder, cut to show the interior. Note how the prostate gland surrounds the urethra as it exits the bladder.

and a message is sent to the spinal cord. A moderately full bladder holds 450 mL (1 pint) of urine.

Two sphincters, the internal and external, control the release of the urine. The internal sphincter located at the bladder neck is composed of involuntary muscle. As the bladder becomes full, the stretch receptors cause contractions, pushing the urine past the internal sphincter. The urine then presses on the external sphincter, which is composed of skeletal or voluntary muscle at the terminus of the urethra.

URETHRA

The **urethra** is the terminal portion of the urinary system. It is a small tube that carries urine by peristalsis from the bladder out of its external opening, the **urinary meatus.** In females it is embedded in the anterior wall of the vagina vestibule and exits between the clitoris and the vaginal opening. The female urethra is approximately ¼ inch in diameter and 1½ inches long. In males the urethra is approximately 8 inches long, passing through the prostate gland and extending the length of the glans penis. In the male the urethra serves two functions: as a passageway for urine and a passageway for semen.

NORMAL AGING OF THE URINARY SYSTEM

With aging the kidneys lose part of their normal functioning capacity; in fact, by 70 years of age, the filtering mechanism is only 50% as efficient as at 40 years. This occurs because of decreased blood supply and loss of nephrons.

In the aging woman the bladder loses tone and the perineal muscles may relax, resulting in stress incontinence. In the aging man the prostate gland may become enlarged, leading to constriction of the urethra. Incomplete emptying of the bladder in both men and women increases the possibility of urinary tract infection (UTI) (see Life Span Considerations box).

LABORATORY AND DIAGNOSTIC EXAMINATIONS

Diagnostic tests for urinary tract conditions include laboratory tests, diagnostic imaging, and endoscopic procedures. Nursing responsibilities vary according to the studies performed. Be aware of specific patient variables that may influence test results: state of hydration, nutritional status, or trauma (see Cultural Considerations box). Prepare patients for diagnostic testing by briefly describing the purpose of the procedure and what the patient can expect to happen.

URINALYSIS

The most common urinary diagnostic study is the urinalysis. Table 10-2 describes normal and abnormal constituents in the urine and possible factors that influence test results. A urinalysis may be done during assessments of other body systems because of the role of the kidneys in maintaining homeostasis. Urine cul-

 Life Span Considerations

Older Adults

Urinary Disorder

- Urinary frequency, urgency, nocturia, retention, and incontinence are common with aging. These occur because of weakened musculature in the bladder and urethra, diminished neurologic sensation combined with decreased bladder capacity, and the effects of medications such as diuretics.
- Urinary incontinence is a leading reason for institutional placement of older adults.
- Urinary incontinence can lead to a loss of self-esteem and result in decreased participation in social activities.
- Older women are at risk for stress incontinence because of hormonal changes and weakened pelvic musculature.
- Older men are at risk for urinary retention because of prostatic hypertrophy.
- Urinary tract infections in older adults are often associated with invasive procedures such as catheterization, diabetes mellitus, and neurologic disorders.
- Inadequate fluid intake, immobility, and conditions that lead to urinary stasis increase the risk of infection in the older adult.
- Frequent toileting and meticulous skin care can reduce the risk of skin impairment secondary to urinary incontinence.

 Cultural Considerations

Urinary Disorder

A cultural assessment reflects a dynamic process in which the health care team seeks to understand the patient and gain insights to the meaning of care, health, and well-being. Integral components of a cultural assessment include communication, time orientation, personal space, pain, religious beliefs, taboos, customs, dietary practices, health practices, family roles, and views of death.

Professional discussion of urinary problems requires sensitivity because of the association of the urinary system with the reproductive system and the associated cultural taboos surrounding sexuality. Often the patient's self-image and sexual performance are affected by altered urinary function. Be sensitive to the patient's feelings, guiding the interview to ensure accurate assessment while maintaining the patient's dignity.

ture and sensitivity may be done to confirm suspected infections, to identify causative organisms, and to determine appropriate antimicrobial therapy. Cultures are also obtained for periodic screening of urine when the threat of a UTI persists. Various reagent strips are available to test urine for abnormal substances. The strips are a quick reference that can be used in a clinical setting or at home. Common substances measured to monitor kidney function include total urine protein, creatinine, urea, uric acid levels, and catecholamines.

Urinalysis is completed on a clean-catch or catheterized specimen. A sterile urine specimen is obtained either by inserting a straight catheter into the urinary bladder and removing urine or by obtaining a specimen from the port of an indwelling catheter via cathe-

Table 10-2	Urinalysis	
CONSTITUENT	**NORMAL RANGE**	**INFLUENCING FACTORS**
Color	Pale yellow to amber	Diabetes insipidus, biliary obstruction, medications, diet
Turbidity	Clear to slightly cloudy	Phosphates, white blood cells, bacteria
Odor	Mildly aromatic	Medication, bacteria, diet
pH	4.6-8	Stale specimen, food intake, infection, homeostatic imbalance
Specific gravity	1.003-1.030	State of hydration, medications
Glucose	Negative	Diabetes mellitus, medications, diet
Protein	Negative	Renal disease, muscle exertion, dehydration
Bilirubin	Negative	Liver disease with obstruction or damage, medications
Hemoglobin	Negative	Trauma, renal disease
Ketones	Negative	Diabetes mellitus, diet, medications
Red blood cells	Up to 2 LPF	Renal or bladder disease, trauma, medications
White blood cells	0-4 LPF	Renal disease, urinary tract infection
Casts	Rare	Renal disease
Bacteria	Negative	Urinary tract infection

ter port using sterile technique. Because the kidneys excrete substances in varying amounts and rates during a 24-hour period, the nurse may be responsible for collecting a 24-hour urine sample. Discard the first voiding and note the time at the beginning of the 24-hour urine collection. For the next 24 hours collect all urine and place it in a special laboratory container.

SPECIFIC GRAVITY

Specific gravity measures the patient's hydration status and gives information about the kidneys' ability to concentrate urine. Specific gravity is decreased by high fluid intake, reduced renal concentrating ability, diabetes insipidus, and diuretic use. It is increased in dehydration due to fever, diaphoresis, vomiting, diarrhea, and medical conditions such as diabetes mellitus (diabetic ketoacidosis or hyperglycemic hyperosmolar nonketotic coma) and inappropriate secretion of ADH. The value ranges between 1.003 and 1.030, with the lower values suggesting more dilute urine (Pagana & Pagana, 2008).

BLOOD (SERUM) UREA NITROGEN

Blood urea nitrogen (BUN) is a laboratory test used to determine the kidney's ability to rid the blood of nonprotein nitrogen (NPN) waste and urea, which result from protein breakdown (catabolism). The acceptable serum range for BUN is 10 to 20 mg/dL. For a more accurate test result, the patient should receive nothing by mouth (NPO) for 8 hours before blood sampling. If the BUN is elevated, institute preventive nursing measures to protect the patient from possible disorientation or seizures.

BLOOD (SERUM) CREATININE

Creatinine is a catabolic product of creatine, which is used in skeletal muscle contraction. The daily production of creatine, and subsequently creatinine, depends on muscle mass, which fluctuates little. Creatinine, as with BUN, is excreted entirely by the kidneys and is therefore directly proportional to renal excretory func-

tion. Thus, with normal renal excretory function, the serum creatinine level should remain constant and normal. Only renal disorders (such as glomerulonephritis, pyelonephritis, acute tubular necrosis, and urinary obstruction) cause an abnormal elevation in creatinine.

The serum creatinine test, as with BUN, is used to diagnose impaired kidney function. However, unlike BUN, the creatinine level is affected little by dehydration, malnutrition, or hepatic function. The creatinine level is interpreted in conjunction with the BUN. The acceptable serum creatinine range is 0.5 to 1.1 mg/dL (female) and 0.6 to 1.2 mg/dL (male) (Pagana & Pagana, 2008).

CREATININE CLEARANCE

Creatinine, an NPN substance, is present in blood and urine. Creatinine is generated during muscle contraction and then excreted by glomerular filtration. Levels are directly related to muscle mass and are usually measured for a 24-hour period. During the testing period, the patient avoids excessive physical activity. Draw a fasting blood sample at the onset of testing and another at the conclusion. Discard the initial specimen and start the 24-hour timing at that point. Collect all urine in the 24-hour period because any deviation will alter test results. An elevation in serum levels with a decline in urine levels indicates renal disease. Normal ranges are **serum,** 0.5 to 1.1 mg/dL (female), 0.6 to 1.2 mg/dL (male); **urine,** 87 to 107 mL/min (female), 107 to 139 mL/min (male) (Pagana & Pagana, 2008).

PROSTATE-SPECIFIC ANTIGEN

Prostate-specific antigen (PSA) is an organ-specific glycoprotein produced by normal prostatic tissue. Measurement of PSA has largely replaced that of prostatic acid phosphatase because it is a more accurate test. Test results rise with tissue manipulation; therefore obtain a blood sample before physical examination. Normal range is less than 4 ng/mL. Elevated PSA levels result from prostate cancer, benign prostatic hypertrophy (BPH), and prostatitis.

OSMOLALITY

Assessment of urine **osmolality** (the weight of the solute compared with its own weight) may be preferred over specific gravity. Plasma osmolality may be done in conjunction with the urine sampling when pituitary disorders are suspected. Results provide information on the concentrating ability of the kidney.

KIDNEY-URETER-BLADDER RADIOGRAPHY

A kidney-ureter-bladder (KUB) radiograph assesses the general status of the abdomen and the size, structure, and position of the urinary tract structures. No special preparation is necessary. Explain that the procedure involves changing position on the radiography table, which may be uncomfortably firm. Abnormal findings related to the urinary system may indicate tumors, calculi, glomerulonephritis, cysts, and other conditions.

INTRAVENOUS PYELOGRAM
OR INTRAVENOUS UROGRAPHY

Intravenous pyelogram (IVP) or intravenous urography (IVU) evaluates structures of the urinary tract, filling of the renal pelvis with urine, and transport of urine via the ureters to the bladder. It is vital to determine whether the patient has an allergy to iodine (or iodine-containing foods such as iodized salt, saltwater fish, seaweed products, vegetables grown in iodine-rich soils) because it is the base of the radiopaque dye that is injected into a vein for this and other radiologic examinations. If the patient has had an allergic reaction, the physician may order administration of a corticosteroid or an antihistamine before testing or, alternatively, may order ultrasonography.

Because kidneys and ureters are positioned in the retroperitoneal space, gas and stool in the intestines interfere with radiographic visualization. Preparation usually includes eating a light supper, taking a non–gas-forming laxative, and remaining NPO 8 hours before testing. In planning the testing regimen, schedule urography before barium-based studies. When the dye is injected, the patient experiences a warm, flushing sensation and a metallic taste. During the procedure, monitor vital signs frequently. Radiographs are taken at various intervals to monitor movement of the dye. Abnormal findings may indicate structural deviations, hydronephrosis, calculi within the urinary tract, polycystic renal (kidney) disease (PKD), tumors, and other conditions.

RETROGRADE PYELOGRAPHY

Retrograde pyelography involves examination of the lower urinary tract with a cystoscope under aseptic conditions. The urologist injects radiopaque dye directly into the ureters to visualize the upper urinary tract. Urine samples can be obtained directly from the renal pelvis. Additional retrograde studies include the following:

- **Retrograde cystography:** Radiopaque dye is injected through an indwelling catheter into the urinary bladder to evaluate its structure or to determine the cause of recurrent infections.
- **Retrograde urethrography:** A catheter is inserted and dye injected as with the cystography to assess the status of the urethral structure.

VOIDING CYSTOURETHROGRAPHY

Voiding cystourethrography is used in conjunction with other diagnostic studies to detect abnormalities of the urinary bladder and the urethra. Preparation includes an enema before testing. An indwelling catheter is inserted into the urinary bladder, and dye is injected to outline the lower urinary tract. Radiographs are taken, and the catheter is then removed. The patient is asked to void while radiographs are being taken. Some patients experience embarrassment or anxiety related to the procedure and should be given the opportunity to express their feelings. Structural abnormalities, diverticula, and reflux into the ureter may be detected.

ENDOSCOPIC PROCEDURES

Endoscopic procedures are visual examinations of hollow organs using an instrument with a scope and light source. Because of the invasive nature of the procedure, informed consent is necessary, and because the procedure is most often performed in the surgical suite, preoperative preparation is indicated (see Chapter 2). The urologist performs the procedure.

Cystoscopy is a visual examination to inspect, treat, or diagnose disorders of the urinary bladder and proximal structures. Patient preparation includes a description of the procedure. Usually the procedure is carried out using a local anesthetic after the patient has been sedated. Patient safety is paramount when the patient is sedated. The patient is placed in a lithotomy position for the procedure, which may produce embarrassment and anxiety. The thought of a scope being passed while the patient is awake may intensify these feelings. Provide an opportunity for the patient to verbalize feelings.

The scope is passed under aseptic conditions after a local anesthetic is instilled into the urethra. The patient experiences a feeling of pressure as the scope is passed. Continuous fluid irrigation of the bladder is necessary to facilitate visualization. Care after the procedure includes hydration to dilute the urine. Monitor the first voiding after the procedure, assessing time, amount, color, and any *dysuria* (painful or difficult urination). The first voiding is occasionally blood tinged due to the trauma of the procedure.

The urologist can perform a brush biopsy via a ureteral catheter during a cystoscopy. A nylon brush is inserted through the catheter to obtain specimens from the renal pelvis or calyces. Nephroscopy (renal endoscopy) is done using the percutaneous (through the skin) route and provides direct visualization of the upper urinary structures. The urologist can obtain biopsy or urine specimens or remove calculi.

RENAL ANGIOGRAPHY

Renal angiography aids in evaluating blood supply to the kidneys, evaluates masses, and detects possible complications after kidney transplantation. Withhold oral intake the night before the procedure. The procedure requires the passing of a small radiopaque catheter into an artery (usually the femoral artery) to provide a port for the injection of radiopaque dye. Therefore, when the procedure is completed, have the patient lie flat in bed for several hours to minimize the risk of bleeding. Assess the puncture site for bleeding or hematoma, and maintain the pressure dressing at the site. Assess circulatory status of the involved extremity every 15 minutes for 1 hour, then every 2 hours for 24 hours.

RENAL VENOGRAM

A renal venogram provides information about the kidney's venous drainage. Access for the radiopaque catheter is the femoral vein. Monitor the patient afterward for bleeding at the puncture site.

COMPUTED TOMOGRAPHY

A computed tomography (CT) scan differentiates masses of the kidney. Images are obtained by a computer-controlled scanner. A radiopaque dye may be injected to enhance the image. A serum urea and creatinine level are obtained before use of radiopaque dye. The dye is not used if inadequate kidney function is noted. Inform the patient that the table on which he or she is placed and the machine "taking pictures" will move at intervals and that it is important to lie still. The CT body-scanning unit takes multiple cross-sectional pictures at several different sites, creating a three-dimensional map of the renal structure. The adrenals, the bladder, and the prostate may also be visualized.

MAGNETIC RESONANCE IMAGING

Magnetic resonance imaging (MRI) uses nuclear magnetic resonance as its source of energy to obtain a visual assessment of body tissues. The patient requires no special preparation other than removal of all metal objects that might be attracted by the magnet. Patients with metal prostheses (such as heart valves, orthopedic screws, or cardiac pacemakers) cannot undergo MRI.

Emphasize that the examination area will be confining and that a repetitive "pounding" sound will be heard (somewhat like the sound of a muffled jackhammer). MRI can be used for diagnoses of pathologic conditions of the renal system.

RENAL SCAN

A radionuclide tracer substance that will be taken up by renal tubular cells or excreted by the glomerular filtrate is injected intravenously. A series of computer-generated images is then made. The scan provides data related to functional parenchyma (the essential parts of an organ that are concerned with its function). No special preparation is needed. Check facility policy concerning the disposal of the patient's urine for the first 24 hours. Pregnant nurses should refrain from caring for this patient during this time.

ULTRASONOGRAPHY

Ultrasonography is a diagnostic tool that uses the reflection of sound waves to produce images of deep body structures. Inform the patient that a conducting jelly will be applied on the skin over the area to be studied; this improves the transmission of sound waves. The sound waves are high frequency and inaudible to the human ear; the waves are converted into electrical impulses that are photographed for study.

Ultrasonography can visualize size, shape, and position of the kidney and delineate any irregularities in structure. Deviations from normal findings may indicate tumor, congenital anomalies, cysts, or obstructions. No special preparations are necessary.

TRANSRECTAL ULTRASOUND

Transrectal ultrasound instrumentation of the prostate gland provides clear images of prostatic tumors that otherwise might go undiagnosed. Transrectal ultrasound–guided biopsy is performed to obtain samples of prostatic tissue from various areas with minimal discomfort to the patient.

RENAL BIOPSY

The kidney can be biopsied by an open procedure similar to other surgical procedures on the kidney or by the less invasive method of needle biopsy, also called a **percutaneous biopsy**. Tell the patient that he or she may experience pain during the procedure and should follow instructions, such as holding the breath. Bed rest is instituted for 24 hours after the procedure. Mobility is restricted to bathroom privileges for the next 24 hours, and gradual resumption of activities is allowed after 48 to 72 hours.

URODYNAMIC STUDIES

Urodynamic studies are indicated when neurologic disease is suspected of being an underlying cause of incontinence. The studies evaluate detrusor reflex. The patient may experience embarrassment and slight discomfort. During cystometrogram a catheter is inserted into the bladder, then connected to a cystometer, which measures bladder capacity and pressure. The examiner asks the patient about sensations of heat, cold, and urge to void and instructs the patient at times to void and change position.

Cholinergic and anticholinergic medications may be administered during urodynamic studies to determine their effects on bladder function. (A cholinergic drug, such as bethanechol [Urecholine], stimulates the atonic bladder; an anticholinergic drug, such as atropine, brings an overactive bladder to a more normal level or function.)

Associated testing includes rectal electromyography, which involves placement of an electrode; and urethral pressure profile, in which a special catheter connected to a transducer evaluates urethral pressures.

MEDICATION CONSIDERATIONS

The kidneys filter a wide range of water-soluble products from the blood, including medications. The kidneys' effectiveness in removing certain medications from the blood may be affected by various conditions, such as renal disease, changes in the pH of urine, and age. Patients with renal disease are given reduced dosages of medications to minimize further damage or drug toxicity. Alteration in urinary pH affects the absorption rate of certain medications. Older patients may have decreased physiologic functioning, diminishing the kidneys' capacity to excrete drugs. Diminished kidney function interferes with the filtration of water-soluble medications.

The medications included in this discussion are representative of those that directly affect the function of the kidney or are used to treat urinary disorders (Table 10-3).

DIURETICS TO ENHANCE URINARY OUTPUT

Diuretics are administered to enhance urinary output. They achieve this by increasing the kidney's filtration of sodium, chloride, and water at different sites in the kidney. Diuretics are used in the management of a variety of disorders, such as heart failure and hyperten-sion. Diuretics are classified by chemical structure and by the site and type of action on the kidney.

Thiazide Diuretics

Thiazide diuretics act at the distal convoluted tubule to impair sodium and chloride reabsorption, leading to excretion of electrolytes and water. The thiazide diuretic chlorothiazide (Diuril) affects electrolytes to cause hypokalemia (extreme potassium depletion in blood), hyponatremia (decreased sodium concentration in blood), and/or hypercalcemia (excessive amounts of calcium in blood). Hypochloremic alkalosis occurs from a deficiency of chloride. The main uses are management of systemic edema and control of mild to moderate hypertension, although it may take a month to achieve the full antihypertensive effect. Chlorothiazide is contraindicated in anuria.

Loop (or High-Ceiling) Diuretics

Loop, or **high-ceiling, diuretics** act primarily in the ascending Henle's loop to inhibit tubular reabsorption of sodium and chloride. This group is the most potent of all diuretics and may lead to significant electrolyte depletion. These diuretics are effective for use in patients with impaired kidney function.

The loop diuretic furosemide (Lasix) affects electrolytes to cause hypokalemia, hypochloremia, hyponatremia, hypocalcemia (abnormally low blood calcium), and/or hypomagnesemia (decreased magnesium in the blood). The effect on acid-base balance is the development of hypochloremic alkalosis. Furosemide is used in nephrotic syndrome, heart failure, and pul-

Table 10-3   Medications that Affect the Urinary System

Generic (Trade)	Functional Class	Use	Special Considerations
Oxybutynin chloride (Ditropan)	Spasmolytic	Reduces bladder spasms (neurogenic bladder)	Assess voiding pattern.
Bethanechol chloride (Urecholine)	Cholinergic stimulant	Urinary bladder stimulant (urinary retention, neurogenic atony)	Assess for hypotension.
Phenazopyridine (Pyridium, Urogesic)	Nonnarcotic analgesic	Anesthetic on mucosa of urinary tract	Assess decrease in urinary symptoms. Urine may turn red-orange. Report yellowing of sclera.
Flavoxate (Urispas)	Spasmolytic	Relieves nocturia, incontinence, dysuria	Assess decrease of urinary symptoms.
Finasteride (Proscar)	Androgen hormone inhibitor	Prevents benign prostatic hyperplasia	Monitor urinary output. May cause impotence. Pregnant women should avoid handling crushed pills.
Terazosin hydrochloride (Hytrin)	Antihypertensive and benign prostatic hyperplasia agent	In benign prostatic hyperplasia, causes relaxation of smooth muscle and improves urine flow	Assess for hypotension. Assess voiding pattern.

monary edema. Side effects are those associated with rapid fluid loss: vertigo, hypotension, and possible circulatory collapse.

Potassium-Sparing Diuretics

Potassium-sparing diuretics act on the distal convoluted tubule to inhibit sodium reabsorption and potassium secretion. Potassium-sparing diuretics decrease the sodium-potassium exchange. Although the actions of these medications vary, they all conserve potassium that is usually lost with sodium in diuresis. But, because they are weak, they are usually used in combination with other diuretics. Potassium-sparing diuretics are contraindicated in patients who experience hyperkalemia, since further retention of potassium could cause a fatal cardiac dysrhythmia. There are two types of potassium-sparing diuretics: aldosterone antagonists and nonaldosterone antagonists.

The aldosterone antagonist spironolactone (Aldactone) blocks aldosterone in the distal tubule to promote potassium uptake in exchange for sodium secretion. Although it can be used in combination with other diuretics, primarily in the treatment of hypertension and edema, spironolactone is most frequently used for its potassium-sparing quality.

The nonaldosterone antagonist triamterene (Dyrenium) directly reduces ion transportation in the tubule, though it has little diuretic effect. Triamterene is instead used to help limit the potassium-wasting effect of other diuretics.

Osmotic Diuretics

Osmotic diuretics act at the proximal convoluted tubule to increase plasma osmotic pressure, causing redistribution of fluid toward the circulatory vessels. Osmotic diuretics are used to manage edema, promote systemic diuresis in cerebral edema, decrease intraocular pressure, and improve kidney function in acute renal failure (ARF). In ARF, osmotics are used to prevent irreversible failure, but they are contraindicated in advanced states of renal failure.

The osmotic diuretic mannitol (Osmitrol) increases osmolarity of glomerular filtrate; decreases reabsorption of water electrolytes; and increases urinary output, sodium, and chloride, which actually has minimal effect on acid-base balance. Mannitol is used to prevent or treat the oliguric phase of ARF, promote systemic diuresis in cerebral edema, and decrease intraocular pressure. Careful assessment of the cardiovascular system before administering mannitol is essential because of the high risk of inducing heart failure. Avoid extravasation (escape of the medication from the blood vessel into the tissues), which may lead to tissue irritation or necrosis.

Carbonic Anhydrase Inhibitor Diuretics

The **carbonic anhydrase inhibitor diuretic** acetazolamide (Diamox) interferes with the bonding of water and carbon dioxide by the enzyme carbonic anhydrase (present in red blood cells) at the proximal convoluted tubule. Although it has limited usefulness as a diuretic, acetazolamide is used to lower intraocular pressure.

Nursing Interventions

Because patients receiving diuretics often have complicated disease conditions such as heart failure and pulmonary edema, monitor for signs and symptoms of fluid overload: changes in pulse rate, respirations, cardiac sounds, and lung fields. Record daily morning weights for the patient receiving diuretics. Keep accurate intake and output (I&O) records, and document blood pressure, pulse, and respirations four times a day until the medication is regulated and the vital signs stabilize. Assess BUN, serum electrolytes, and urine as ordered. Diet instruction to the patient and the family should include a warning to avoid overuse of salt in cooking or as a table additive. A number of salt substitutes are currently on the market; however, the long-term effects of those potassium preparations are not known and could further complicate the renal patient's condition. The use of most diuretics, with the exception of the potassium-sparing diuretics, requires adding daily potassium sources (e.g., baked potatoes, raw bananas, apricots, or navel oranges). In some cases the physician orders potassium supplements to be taken with the diuretic.

When a diuretic is effective, the serum concentration of other medications may increase as a result. Carefully monitor this potentiating effect to prevent toxicity from other medications. For example, as diuretics effectively decrease the volume of extracellular fluid, the serum level of digoxin may increase proportionately, resulting in digitoxicity. Special care is required in the selection and management of diuretics in the treatment of children, adolescents, and older adults.

MEDICATIONS FOR URINARY TRACT INFECTIONS

Certain antimicrobial agents are administered primarily to treat infections within the urinary tract. The appropriate medication is selected according to Gramstain sensitivity of the organism. Urinary antiseptics inhibit bacteria growth and are used to prevent and treat urethritis and cystitis. Caution should be used to determine if the patient is pregnant, since all of these agents have not been sufficiently tested for use during pregnancy.

Urinary antiseptics are divided into four groups: quinolones, nitrofurantoins, methenamines, and fluoroquinolones. Examples of each group follow.

Quinolone

Nalidixic acid (NegGram) is used to treat UTIs caused by gram-negative microbes (e.g., *Escherichia coli* and *Proteus mirabilis*). The common side effects are drowsiness, vertigo, weakness, nausea, and vomiting. The use of nalidixic acid is contraindicated in renal impairment.

Nitrofurantoin

Nitrofurantoin compound (Macrodantin) is effective against both gram-positive and gram-negative microbes (e.g., *Streptococcus faecalis*, *E. coli*, and *P. mirabilis*) in the urinary tract. Common side effects are loss of appetite, nausea, and vomiting.

Methenamine

Methenamine mandelate (Mandelamine) suppresses fungi and gram-negative and gram-positive organisms (e.g., *E. coli*, staphylococci, and enterococci). Acidification of the urine with an acid-ash diet or other acidifiers to a pH of less than 5.5 is necessary for effective action. Methenamine mandelate is used for patients with chronic, recurrent UTIs as a preventive measure after antibiotics have cleared the infection. Although side effects are rare, they include nausea, vomiting, skin rash, and urticaria (hives).

Fluoroquinolone

Norfloxacin (Noroxin) is a broad-spectrum antibiotic effective against gram-positive and gram-negative organisms (e.g., *E. coli*, *P. mirabilis*, *Pseudomonas* organisms, *Staphylococcus aureus*, and *Staphylococcus epidermidis*). It is used in the treatment of UTIs, gonorrhea, and gonococcal urethritis. It is administered with a full glass of water 1 hour before or 2 hours after meals or with antacids.

Nursing Interventions

Before administering antibiotics for UTIs, be certain to check all medications the patient is using for potential negative drug interactions. Instruct the patient to take all the medication, even though the symptoms may subside quickly. Hydrate the patient to produce daily urinary output of 2000 mL, unless contraindicated. When indicated, teach the patient to use the acid-ash diet to help maintain a urine pH of 5.5. Soothe skin irritations with cornstarch or a bath of bicarbonate of soda or dilute vinegar. Report continuing signs of infection.

Observe the patient receiving nalidixic acid for visual disturbances and offer appropriate assistance for ambulation or transfer. Monitor the patient receiving nitrofurantoin for signs of allergic response (such as erythema, chills, fever, and dyspnea). If these signs or symptoms develop, discontinue the medication and notify the physician (trial doses of this medication may be used to detect possible allergic reaction before administering full dosage).

NUTRITIONAL CONSIDERATIONS

The nutritional needs of the patient with a urinary tract disorder vary with each disease process. Some general guidelines include provision of food choices

---

> **Box 10-2**   **Acid-Ash and Alkaline-Ash Foods**
>
> **ACID-ASH FOODS***
> Meat, whole grains, eggs, cheese, cranberries, prunes, and plums
>
> **ALKALINE-ASH FOODS**
> Milk, vegetables, fruits (except cranberries, prunes, and plums)

*Acid-ash diets should be supplemented with vitamins C and A and folic acid.

and number of servings as recommended by the U.S. Department of Agriculture's MyPyramid nutrition planning tool (www.mypyramid.gov) and daily intake of 2000 mL of water, unless contraindicated. Unique nutritional requirements are discussed with each disorder. Box 10-2 gives an example of dietary modifications for urinary lithiasis. Patients with other systemic diseases, such as diabetes mellitus, require strict adherence to those restrictions as well.

MAINTAINING ADEQUATE URINARY DRAINAGE

Urine clears the body of waste materials and helps balance electrolytes. Conditions that interfere with urinary drainage may create a health crisis. Therefore it is important to reestablish urine flow as soon as possible to prevent the buildup of toxins in the bloodstream. Patients at risk for difficulty with urine elimination include those who have undergone surgical procedures of the bladder, the prostate, or the vagina; patients with primary urologic problems, such as urethral stricture; and those who are critically ill with multisystem problems.

Urinary catheters are used to maintain urine flow, to divert urine flow to facilitate healing postoperatively, to introduce medications by irrigation, and to dilate or prevent narrowing of some portions of the urinary tract. Catheters may be used for intermittent or continuous urinary drainage. Urinary catheters may be introduced into the bladder, the ureter, or the kidney. The type and size of urinary catheter are determined by the location and cause of the urinary tract problem. Catheters are measured by the French (F) system. Urethral catheters range from 14 to 24 F for adult patients. Ureteral catheters are usually 4 to 6 F. The physician always inserts ureteral catheters, whereas the nurse usually inserts indwelling urethral catheters.

TYPES OF CATHETERS

Different types of catheters are used for different purposes (Figure 10-6). The **coudé catheter** has a tapered tip and is selected for ease of insertion when enlargement of the prostate gland is suspected. The coudé catheter is less traumatic during insertion because it is stiffer and more easily controlled than the straight-tip catheter (Potter & Perry, 2009). The **Foley catheter** has

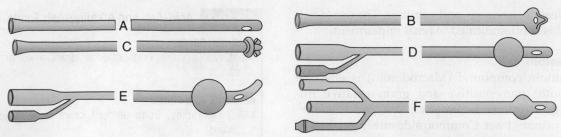

FIGURE 10-6 Commonly used catheters. **A,** Simple urethral catheter. **B,** Mushroom or de Pezzer (can be used for suprapubic catheterization). **C,** Winged-tip or Malecot. **D,** Indwelling with inflated balloon. **E,** Indwelling with coudé tip. **F,** Three-way indwelling (the third lumen is used for irrigation of the bladder).

a balloon near its tip that may be inflated after insertion, holding the catheter in the urinary bladder for continuous drainage. **Malecot** and **de Pezzer,** or **mushroom, catheters** are used to drain urine from the renal pelvis of the kidney. The **Robinson catheter** has multiple openings in its tip to facilitate intermittent drainage. **Ureteral catheters** are long and slender to pass into the ureters. The **whistle-tip catheter** has a slanted, larger orifice at its tip to be used if there is blood in the urine. The **cystostomy, vesicostomy,** or **suprapubic catheter** is introduced by the physician through the abdominal wall above the symphysis pubis. This catheter diverts urine flow from the urethra as needed to treat injury to the bony pelvis, the urinary tract, or surrounding organs; strictures; or obstruction. The catheter is inserted via surgical incision or puncture of the abdominal and bladder walls with a trocar cannula. The catheter is connected to a sterile closed drainage system and secured to avoid accidental removal; the wound is covered with a sterile dressing. When the lower urinary tract has healed, the patient's ability to void is tested by clamping the catheter so the patient can try to void naturally. When the measured residual urine is consistently less than 50 mL, the catheter is usually removed and a sterile dressing is placed over the wound.

An **external (Texas** or **condom)** catheter is not actually a catheter but rather a drainage system connected to the external male genitalia. This noninvasive appliance is used for the incontinent male to minimize skin irritation from urine and to reduce risk of infection from an indwelling catheter. The appliance is removed daily for cleansing and inspecting the skin. Use of the external catheter allows the patient to have a more normal lifestyle.

NURSING INTERVENTIONS AND PATIENT TEACHING

Problems of the urinary tract may be indicative of a primary disorder or may be one of multiple symptoms of complex, chronic disease. Therefore it is important to assess urinary elimination at the time of admission. Because of embarrassment and sociocultural taboos, some patients may be reluctant to share information with the nurse. Often the medical system intensifies this discomfort by repeatedly asking the patient to describe the

problem to staff in the laboratory, radiology, and other departments. Discretion during the admission interview and health assessment with strict adherence to Health Insurance Portability and Accountability Act standards enhance patient privacy and comfort.

Nursing interventions for the patient with a urinary drainage system involve a number of principles to prevent and detect infection and trauma:

1. Follow aseptic technique to avoid introducing microorganisms from the environment. Never rest the collecting bag on the floor.
2. Record I&O. For precision monitoring, such as hourly urinary output, add a urometer to the drainage system. If urinary output falls below 50 mL/hr, check the drainage system for proper placement and function before contacting the physician.
3. Adequately hydrate the patient to flush the urinary tract.
4. Do not open the drainage system after it is in place except to irrigate the catheter, and then only with physician orders. It is important to maintain a closed system to prevent UTIs.
5. Perform catheter care twice daily and as needed, using standard precautions. Each institution has a specific protocol for catheter care. Cleanse the perineum with mild soap and warm water, rinse well, and pat dry. At times an antiseptic solution or ointment may be ordered to use at the catheter incision site.
6. Check the drainage system daily for leaks.
7. Avoid placement of the urinary drainage bag above the level of the catheter insertion, which would cause urine to reenter the drainage system and contaminate the urinary tract.
8. Prevent tension on the system or backflow of urine while transferring the patient.
9. Ambulate the patient if possible to facilitate urine flow. If the patient's activity must be restricted, turn and reposition every 1½ hours.
10. Avoid kinks or compression of the drainage tube that may cause pooling of the urine within the urinary tract. Gently coil excess tubing, secure with a clamp or pin to avoid dislodging the catheter, and release the tubing before transferring or repositioning the patient.

11. Gently inspect the catheter entry site for blood or exudate that may indicate trauma or infection. Observe the color and composition of the urine for blood or sediment. During drainage of the collection bag, note the presence of malodor.

12. Collect specimens from the catheter by cleansing the drainage port with alcohol, then withdrawing the urine using a sterile adapter and a sterile 10-mL syringe, using standard precautions. Send the urine specimen immediately to the laboratory.

13. Report and record assessment findings and interventions initiated.

After the urinary catheter is removed, the patient may experience difficulty voiding until bladder tone and sensation return. If the patient complains of urinary retention, stimulate urination by running water, placing the patient's hands in water, or pouring water over the perineum. With the last method, subtract the amount of water used in calculating the correct amount voided. If the patient's condition permits, a woman can sit on a bathroom stool or commode, and a male can stand, to void.

The patient may experience some dribbling of urine after voiding as a result of dilation of the sphincter from the catheter. Record the time, amount, and color of the urinary output.

Nursing diagnoses and interventions for the patient with a urinary catheter include but are not limited to the following:

Nursing Diagnoses	Nursing Interventions
Risk for trauma, related to insertion and maintenance of the catheter	Maintain sterile technique during insertion. Use smallest size catheter possible. Lubricate catheter. Secure catheter to leg, as appropriate. Provide adequate fluids. Administer urinary analgesic as ordered. Allow enough slack in tubing for patient to move about freely while in bed. Inspect insertion site to determine if area is clean and without signs of possible infection or bleeding.
Risk for infection, related to invasive use of catheter	Use aseptic technique and meticulous catheter care. Maintain closed urinary drainage system. Avoid placement of drainage bag above level of catheter insertion (meatus). Avoid reflux of urine.

Nursing Diagnoses	Nursing Interventions
	Encourage adequate fluid intake. Administer antimicrobials as ordered. Monitor patient's temperature and the color, odor, and clarity of urine.

Instruct the patient about proper transfer from bed, chair, or stretcher and the principles of catheter care. Encourage fluid intake to flush the urinary system.

Self-Catheterization

Self-catheterization may be the intervention of choice for the patient who experiences spinal cord injury or other neurologic disorders that interfere with urinary elimination. Intermittent self-catheterization promotes independent function. At home there is less risk of cross-contamination than in the hospital, so the catheterization procedure can be safely modified as a clean technique. Still, instruct the patient using strict surgical asepsis in the hospital because of the risk of infection there. Emphasize the need for the patient to be alert for signs and symptoms of infection and to have periodic evaluations by the physician. Follow institutional guidelines for catheter insertion.

Bladder Training

Bladder training involves developing the muscles of the perineum to improve voluntary control over voiding; bladder training may be modified for different problems. In preparation for removal of a urethral catheter, the physician may order a clamp-unclamp routine to improve bladder tone. A patient with stress incontinence can learn to control leakage by performing **Kegel,** or **pubococcygeal, exercises** that tighten the muscles of the perineal floor. The patient can develop awareness of the appropriate muscle group by trying to stop the flow of urine during voiding. Once the patient has identified the correct muscles and the feeling of their contraction, direct her to tighten the muscles of the perineum, hold that tension for 10 seconds, then relax for 10 seconds. The exercises should be done initially in groups of 10, building to groups of 20, four times a day. Because muscle control develops gradually, it may take 4 to 6 weeks to learn to control leakage.

For habit training, establish a voiding schedule. Monitor the patient's voiding for a few days to identify patterns, or schedule voiding times to correlate with the patient's activities. Typical voiding times are on arising, before each meal, and at bedtime. Help the patient void as scheduled. After a few days, evaluate whether the scheduled voiding pattern keeps the patient continent. Modify the schedule until continence is established. Fluid intake and medications may influence voiding patterns (e.g., the patient may need to void 30 minutes after ingesting coffee or furosemide in response to the diuretic effect). Reduction of fluid intake before bedtime may help keep the patient dry during sleep.

PROGNOSIS

The outcome for patients with urinary disorders depends on many variables: age, preexisting health conditions, general health status, complications, compliance, and available family and community support.

DISORDERS OF THE URINARY SYSTEM

ALTERATIONS IN VOIDING PATTERNS

URINARY RETENTION

Etiology and Pathophysiology

Urinary retention is the inability to void even with an urge to void. It may be acute or chronic. The patient may not be able to empty the bladder, creating urinary stasis and increasing the possibility of infection.

Urinary retention has a variety of causes: a response to stress; interference with the sphincter muscles during surgery to the perineum; occlusion of the urethra by calculi, infection, or tumor; medication side effects; or perineal trauma secondary to vaginal delivery. With chronic urinary retention the bladder capacity may be exceeded and the urine may overflow the bladder, causing incontinence.

Clinical Manifestations

The signs and symptoms of urinary retention are sometimes vague and easily overlooked. The bladder becomes increasingly distended and may be palpated above the symphysis pubis. Urinary retention may cause the patient considerable discomfort and anxiety.

Assessment

Subjective data include patient complaints of frequency with or without symptoms of burning, urgency, nocturia, and occasionally acute discomfort. Initial symptoms may not seem to be directly associated with urinary retention.

Collection of **objective data** includes assessing urinary bladder distention (palpable ovoid [egg-shaped] bladder arising suprapubically). The patient may void frequently, void small amounts, and have episodes of incontinence. Patients with diminished sensorium, as from spinal cord injury or organic brain disorder, may be restless and irritable without direct complaints about difficulty voiding.

Medical Management

Mechanical methods, such as the use of urinary catheters or the surgical release of obstructions, may be needed to treat urinary retention. Administer urinary analgesics and antispasmodics as prescribed to enhance patient relaxation and comfort.

Nursing Interventions

The primary goal of nursing interventions is the reinstitution of normal voiding patterns. Regardless of the pathologic findings and medical intervention, the nurse can help the patient achieve adequate voiding by providing a private, relaxed environment. Bladder training approaches may assist the patient in emptying the bladder. Warm showers or sitz baths may promote relaxation of the abdominal, gluteal, and sphincter muscles. Provide warm beverages to help the patient relax. If possible, permit the patient whatever position is preferred for voiding: for women, sitting on a commode or bathroom stool is best; for men, standing may be more natural.

When continence is established, the patient may be catheterized intermittently to determine whether the bladder is emptying. Have the patient void and measure the amount. Catheterize the patient immediately after the voiding and measure the amount. The amount retained in the bladder is residual urine and should be less than 50 mL. If the underlying pathologic condition remains unchanged, this patient may be at risk for again developing retention. Teach the patient or primary caretaker to observe for signs and symptoms of urinary retention and to notify the physician immediately if they return.

A nursing diagnosis and interventions for the patient with urinary retention include but are not limited to the following:

Nursing Diagnosis	Nursing Interventions
Impaired urinary elimination, related to: • sensory or motor impairment • neuromuscular impairment • mechanical trauma	Establish urinary drainage. Develop a voiding schedule. Teach the patient Kegel exercises. Assist with skin care. Suggest use of protective clothing. Engage patient in social activities. Teach importance of adequate fluid intake. Ensure that patient verbalizes an understanding of factors that alter urinary pattern.

URINARY INCONTINENCE

Urinary incontinence (UI) may be the most common health problem in women. Although stress incontinence is not the only cause of UI, it is the one most frequently mentioned. Stress incontinence is the involuntary loss of urine during physical exertion or when coughing, sneezing, or laughing. Because of embarrassment, stress UI may be underreported, and thus its sociologic and economic influence is impossible to assess. However, UI is a major reason older adults are admitted to long-term care facilities.

Etiology and Pathophysiology

UI is the involuntary loss of urine from the bladder. The patient may be totally incontinent, have dribbling, or experience leakage while lifting or sneezing (stress incontinence). Incontinence may arise as a complication of many disorders, such as UTI, loss of sphincter control, or sudden change of pressure within the abdomen. Incontinence may be permanent, as with spinal cord trauma, or temporary, as with pregnancy. Women with weakened structures of the pelvic floor are prone to stress incontinence. Although incontinence may occur at any age, loss of control of urination is a particular problem for older adults (see Evidence-Based Practice box).

Physical exertion such as heavy lifting, jobs that require long periods of standing, and high-impact sports may increase an individual's risk for UI. UI may also result from physiologic conditions such as obesity, chronic lung disease, smoking, pelvic floor injury, and surgery. Lack of estrogen in postmenopausal women contributes to atrophy of the vaginal and urethral walls with subsequent loss of muscle tone that may result in postvoiding urine retention and possible prolapse of the bladder.

Clinical Manifestations

The cardinal sign of UI is the involuntary loss of urine, which may or may not be the primary reason the patient seeks treatment.

Assessment

Subjective data include information concerning the patient's inability to control the urine. A woman may complain of urine leaking when she coughs, sneezes, lifts heavy objects, or has intercourse.

Collection of **objective data** requires alertness for clues that the patient is experiencing difficulty controlling the flow of urine. Follow the assessment guidelines to clarify the patient's complaints. Although more common in women, UI is a common symptom for men who have BPH and should be included in the assessment.

Medical Management

The management of incontinence depends on the underlying cause. If the problem arises from a disorder within the neck of the bladder, surgical repair may be necessary. Stress incontinence related to sphincter weakness may be treated with collagen implant injections. The patient may require temporary or permanent urinary diversion or management with an indwelling catheter. New appliances and drugs on the market are being used for the control of UI.

The incontinence pessary, which is inserted into the vagina to support the bladder, may help manage episodes of stress incontinence in some women. Close-fitting absorbent pads may be effective in managing mild leakage.

Management of stress incontinence should include behavior modification, pelvic floor muscle therapies, medications, and mechanical devices before resorting to surgical procedures. If these strategies are not effective, surgical interventions offer other treatment options. One procedure is the transvaginal tape sling procedure. The surgeon passes a permanent polypropylene mesh tape, covered by a protective plastic sheath with stainless steel needles attached at each end, through a small incision in the anterior vaginal wall. The U-shaped sling supports the urethra during stress and increased intraabdominal pressure during routine activities. This procedure is not without difficulties. Careful patient teaching is important before any surgical treatment.

 Evidence-Based Practice

The majority of older adults have bladder control, but changes due to aging, chronic diseases, and related conditions place them at risk for bladder control problems, especially urinary incontinence and/or frequency. Many persons do not seek treatment because of embarrassment or the mistaken belief that there is no treatment available. In this research study nurses wanted to determine the educational needs of older adults. Focus groups were held in senior centers, churches, and in senior apartment buildings. Questions that guided the discussion included items related to general health and specific questions related to bladder control issues. After the discussion session, the nurses showed the groups a self-help video that included causes of urinary incontinence, treatment, and prevention strategies. The results of the study demonstrated that given the opportunity, older adults will discuss their concerns about bladder control and are willing to learn methods of control.

Although the participants in the focus groups were mainly active older adults in an urban setting, the information gathered was helpful as a starting point for designing educational programs for that population. The participant groups included both men and women and were diverse in ethnicity and race.

Application to Nursing Practice
- Incontinence and/or frequency are experienced by adults of all ages, ethnicities, educational levels, economic status, and health status.
- Many adults wrongly believe that urinary incontinence and/or frequency are an expected part of the aging process and that there are no treatments available.
- Older adults of culturally diverse backgrounds are willing to discuss bladder control issues with nurses.
- Older adults are receptive to different forms of education and are interested in learning.

Reference
Palmer, M.H., & Newman, D.K. (2006). Bladder control: educational needs of older adults, *J Gerontol Nurs*, 32(1), 28.

Estrogen replacement for the treatment of UI is controversial and its reported effectiveness varies. Topical administration of prednisone and estrogen may help restore turgor and elasticity of the vaginal submucosa. Transdermal oxybutynin (Oxytrol) is effective in reducing the symptoms of an overactive bladder with few side effects. A new self-catheterization system, the Self-Cath Closed System, is available for patients who must maintain intermittent self-catheterization. It is designed for patient convenience and minimization of bacterial contamination. An artificial urinary sphincter is a surgical option to reestablish continence, though there is controversy over its use.

Nursing Interventions

The incontinent patient may reduce fluid intake to decrease voiding, but without adequate fluids, urine may become more concentrated, irritating the bladder mucosa and increasing the urge to urinate. Teach the patient bladder training exercises to improve the tone of the perineal muscles. For the female patient, Kegel exercises are helpful; 10 repetitions, 5 to 10 times a day is suggested to improve muscle tone. Establish a 2-hour schedule for the patient to go to the bathroom. Once continence has been achieved, the goal may be raised to 3 hours.

Incontinence pads of different absorbancy are available in most grocery stores and pharmacies. They can increase the patient's confidence to participate in social activities. Use of protective undergarments may help keep the patient and the patient's clothing dry.

Alcoholic and caffeinated drinks stimulate urgency and urination; advise the patient not to drink too much liquid just before bedtime.

Many patients who are incontinent have low self-esteem. Be supportive by listening, encouraging the patient to express feelings, and providing kind reassurances. Never scold.

NEUROGENIC BLADDER

Etiology and Pathophysiology

Neurogenic bladder means the loss of voluntary voiding control, resulting in urinary retention or incontinence. Neurogenic bladder is caused by a lesion of the nervous system that interferes with normal nerve conduction to the urinary bladder. The lesion may be caused by a congenital anomaly (e.g., spina bifida), a neurologic disease (e.g., multiple sclerosis), or trauma (as in spinal cord injury). The two types of neurogenic bladder are **spastic** and **flaccid.**

Spastic (reflex or automatic) bladder is caused by a lesion above the voiding reflex arc (upper motor neuron) that results in a loss of the urge to void and a loss of motor control. The bladder wall atrophies, decreasing bladder capacity. Urine is released on reflex, with little or no conscious control.

A flaccid (atonic, nonreflex) bladder, caused by a lesion of a lower motor neuron, continues to fill and distend, with pooling of urine and incomplete emptying. Because of the accompanying loss of sensation, the patient may not experience discomfort that would indicate retention.

Clinical Manifestations

Identification of the disease process is the first step in assessing the potential problem of neurogenic bladder. Prevention of complications is a major concern; infection occurs from urinary stasis and repeated catheterization. Retention of urine may lead to backup of urine (reflux) into the upper urinary tract and to the distention of the structures of the urinary tract.

Assessment

Subjective data include patient complaints of diaphoresis, flushing and nausea before reflex incontinence, or infrequent voiding.

Collection of **objective data** involves investigating the urinary status of the patient at risk for neurogenic bladder; this includes patients with a congenital anomaly, a neurologic disease, or a spinal cord injury. The patient with a spastic bladder experiences UI, whereas the patient with a flaccid bladder describes infrequent voiding.

Diagnostic Tests

To assess the type and extent of damage to the urinary tract, chemistry studies monitor change in BUN and creatinine levels. Radiographic studies outline structural changes that occur.

Medical Management

Closely monitor patients identified as at risk for neurogenic bladder. Assess urinary function early in the course of treatment, and give antibiotics to treat signs of infection. The patient is aided by the use of parasympathomimetic medication (e.g., bethanechol) to increase the bladder's contractility. The patient may need to use intermittent self-catheterization or a urinary collection system if continence is not achieved.

Sacral Nerve Modulation (Sacral Neuromodulation) and Stimulation

A number of electronic devices to modulate nerve impulses are being used experimentally and in clinical practice for treating various bladder problems: urinary frequency, urgency, incontinence, chronic pain, and interstitial cystitis (IC).

Sacral nerve stimulation for urinary urge incontinence is the use of a permanently implantable electrical stimulation device to change neuronal activity in the sacral efferent and afferent nerves to reduce urinary urge incontinence. The Interstim device, marketed by Medtronic Inc., delivers continuous low-level electrical impulses to the bladder and urethral sphincters via the sacral nerve. It corrects UI by modulating the neural reflexes, reducing stimulation to an overactive bladder, or boosting stimulation to an underactive one. The action of the impulses is unknown.

Four electrodes are connected to a battery-operated generator. The wire is inserted into the sacral foramen through a 2-cm incision. The end of the wire is tunneled across subcutaneous tissue, exits on the patient's back, and is connected to a temporary generator attached to the outside of the body. The patient tests this temporary implant for 1 to 2 weeks. If the patient achieves 50% continence, a permanent implant is put in place.

Nursing Interventions and Patient Teaching

The management goal for the patient with neurogenic bladder is to establish urinary elimination and prevent complications. Because neurologic function is disturbed, it may not be possible to reinstate normal voiding. The patient with a spastic bladder may be placed on a bladder training program, with self-stimulation used every 2 hours to empty the bladder: The patient tries to initiate voiding using bladder compressions by applying pressure to the abdomen suprapubically or by digital stimulation of the anal sphincter. Residual urine is then measured by catheterization. As the patient becomes more proficient in emptying the bladder, the time between catheterizations is increased until voiding is independent. It is important to educate the patient to be alert for signs of the bladder becoming distended.

Management of the patient with a flaccid bladder is similar. Place the patient on a 2-hour voiding schedule for bladder training. Issues of self-esteem are crucial for this patient to remain in social settings. Provide a supportive, sensitive environment for the patient to discuss ways to adapt to an altered self-image.

INFLAMMATORY AND INFECTIOUS DISORDERS OF THE URINARY SYSTEM
URINARY TRACT INFECTIONS

A UTI is the presence of microorganisms in any urinary system structure. Bacteriuria (bacteria in the urine) is the most common of all nosocomial infections; most are associated with the use of urinary catheters. UTIs are common in older patients, related to bladder obstruction, insufficient bladder emptying, decreased bactericidal secretions of the prostate, and increased perineal soiling in women. Immobility, sensory impairment, and multiple organ impairment may increase the chances of infection in older adults. Women are more susceptible to UTIs than men because the urethra is short and proximal to the vagina and rectum.

Etiology and Pathophysiology

UTIs are caused by pathogens that enter the urinary tract, with or without symptoms. Normally the flushing of the urinary tract with urine is sufficient to wash away pathogens. However, some conditions interfere with this process; urinary obstruction, neurogenic bladder, ureterovesical or urethrovesical reflux, sexual intercourse, and catheterization may introduce bacteria into the urinary system. Many chronic health problems predispose the patient to a UTI: diabetes mellitus, multiple sclerosis, spinal cord injuries, hypertension, and renal diseases.

Changes in urinary tract homeostasis allow the concentration of bacteria and increase the risk of infection. The patient with a compromised immune system does not seem to be predisposed to UTI infections, but once the infection is established, that patient has difficulty recovering. Infections of the lower urinary tract increase the risk of infection of the upper urinary tract, especially if untreated.

Gram-negative microorganisms that commonly infect the urinary tract (e.g., E. coli and Klebsiella, Proteus, or Pseudomonas organisms) are usually from the gastrointestinal tract and ascend through the urinary meatus. Normally the body's defenses keep infections in check and clear them from the system before signs and symptoms appear. If there is incomplete emptying of the bladder or reflux of urine, the retained urine supports growth of bacteria.

Clinical Manifestations

The common signs and symptoms associated with UTI are urgency, frequency, burning on urination, and microscopic to gross (visible without aid of microscope) hematuria. UTIs are identified by the location of the infection: urethritis (urethra), cystitis (urinary bladder), pyelonephritis (kidney), and prostatitis (prostate gland). Infections of the bladder are said to be *lower* UTIs, whereas infections of the kidneys are *upper* UTIs.

Assessment

Subjective data include patient complaints of pain or burning on urination, urgency, frequency, and nocturia (excessive urination at night). The patient may also have related asthenia (a general feeling of tiredness and listlessness). Abdominal discomfort, perineal pain, or back pain may be present, depending on the extent of the disease process and site of infection.

Collection of **objective data** involves palpation of the lower abdomen, which may produce discomfort over the urinary bladder. Urine may be cloudy or blood tinged.

Diagnostic Tests

Urine culture and bacteriologic tests confirm the diagnosis. For patients with recurrent UTIs or systemic disease, more detailed urologic studies, such as an IVP and a voiding cystogram, are completed to assess the extent of involvement and damage to the structures of the urinary tract. Microscopic inspection of the urine often reveals bacteria, hematuria (blood in the urine), and pyuria (pus in the urine). Prostatitis is confirmed by patient history and culture of prostatic fluid or tissue.

Medical Management

The goal of medical management is to eliminate bacteria from the urinary tract, thereby relieving symptoms, preventing damage to renal structures, and preventing spread of infection to other body systems. The physician prescribes antiinfective medications in either oral or parenteral single or multiple doses, depending on the severity of the infection, microbial sensitivity, cost, and patient tolerance. Urinary antiseptics, such as methenamine mandelate, may be used prophylactically in recurrent infections. Some of these medications are instilled directly into the bladder. If the infection is complicated by obstruction, that obstruction should be removed. For neurogenic bladder or other retention, intermittent catheterization permits urinary drainage (see Complementary & Alternative Therapies box).

Nursing Interventions

Nursing interventions should be supportive, with patient education for adequate hydration and hygiene. Because these infections tend to recur or persist, patient education must include early detection. Comfort measures include a regimen of antiinfective agents, urinary analgesics (e.g., phenazopyridine [Pyridium]), adequate fluid intake, and perineal care. If treatment is effective, the patient should receive relief quickly. Infection may spread from the urinary system to other parts of the body. **Urosepsis** is septic poisoning due to retention and absorption of urinary products in the tissues.

Complementary & Alternative Therapies

Urinary Disorders

- Cranberry (Cranberry Plus, Ultra Cranberry) has been used to prevent urinary tract infections (UTIs), particularly in women prone to recurrent infection. It has also been used to treat acute UTI. Monitor patients for lack of therapeutic effect.
- Echinacea stimulates the immune system and treats UTI. Patients with human immunodeficiency virus infections, including acquired immunodeficiency syndrome, tuberculosis, collagen disease, multiple sclerosis, or other autoimmune disease, should avoid use. Echinacea should not be used in place of antibiotic therapy.
- Sea holly (Eryngium campestre) aboveground plant parts have a mild diuretic effect. Roots have an antispasmodic effect. Aboveground parts are used in UTI and prostatitis; roots are used to treat kidney and bladder calculi, renal colic, kidney and urinary tract inflammation, and urinary retention.
- Nettle (Urtica dioica) is currently being investigated as an irrigation for the urinary tract and also to treat benign prostatic hypertrophy. Patients with fluid retention caused by reduced cardiac or renal activity should not use this herb.
- Caffeine increases urine production.
- Some believe that acupuncture applied to the abdominal meridian may help relieve cystitis.
- Some advocate massage with diluted rosemary, juniper, or lavender to aid in relieving pain associated with cystitis.

Because of the high incidence of nosocomial UTIs, regular staff in service review of basic procedures for catheter insertion and maintenance is important. Patient education for those who practice self-catheterization should include return demonstration to evaluate the success of maintaining clean technique.

URETHRITIS

Etiology and Pathophysiology

Urethritis, inflammation of the urethra, is classified by the presence or absence of gonorrhea. Nongonorrheal urethritis is called **nonspecific urethritis (NSU).** NSU may be caused by candidal or trichomonal infections in women. Bacteria are present normally in the urethra but do not cause problems unless the integrity of the mucous membrane or tissues is interrupted, as when a catheter is in place or trauma has occurred.

Clinical Manifestations

The clinical manifestations include inflammation of the urethra with pus formation in the mucus-forming glands within the urethral lining. With gonorrheal urethritis, acute infection of the mucous membrane of the urethra causes a purulent exudate from the meatus; the patient feels discomfort, frequency, and burning on urination.

Assessment

Subjective data vary, since the patient may be asymptomatic or may complain of dysuria, urethral pruritus, and urethral discharge. Women may complain of vaginal discharge or vulvar irritation.

Collection of **objective data** includes light palpation of the lower abdomen, which may produce discomfort over the urinary bladder. Inspection of the urethra may reveal purulent exudates or inflammation. Culture and sensitivity may be ordered; follow the institution's procedure.

Diagnostic Tests

Diagnostic tests are usually limited to a Gram stain of the exudate to identify the pathogen.

Medical Management

The first step in medical management is prevention of injury to the urethra during catheterization or sexual intercourse. Treatment is based on identifying and treating the cause and providing symptomatic relief. Drugs that may be prescribed are sulfamethoxazole-trimethoprim (Bactrim, Septra), metronidazole (Flagyl), clotrimazole (Mycelex), and nystatin (Mycostatin). Comfort measures include antibiotics, adequate fluid intake to flush the system, warm sitz baths, and special care of the perineum using clean technique.

Patients with continuous catheter drainage use either a bedside bag or a leg bag for urine collection. Studies are under way to test a drainage system designed with the bag worn around the waist. This experimental drainage system can be maintained closed for 24 hours and offers improvements in ambulation, activities of daily living (ADLs), and social and mental well-being.

Nursing Interventions

Nursing interventions focus on patient education: Avoid sexual activity until the infection clears; take all medications, especially antibiotics, to ensure the infection is resolved; and use condoms for protection from reinfection. Instruct patients with sexually transmitted urethritis to refer their sexual partners for evaluation and testing if they had sexual contact in the 60 days preceding onset of the patient's symptoms or diagnosis.

CYSTITIS

Etiology and Pathophysiology

Cystitis is an inflammation of the wall of the urinary bladder, usually caused by urethrovesical reflux, introduction of a catheter or similar instrument, or contamination from feces. The most common microorganism causing acute cystitis is *E. coli*. Cystitis is most common in women because of the ease of entrance of pathogens through the short urethra, even during voiding. Conflicting data exist about the role of bubble baths, clothing, and hygiene in increasing the risk of cystitis in women. Cystitis in men usually occurs secondary to another infection, such as prostatitis or epididymitis (see Safety Alert box).

Clinical Manifestations

The common signs and symptoms associated with cystitis are dysuria, urinary frequency, and pyuria.

Assessment

Collection of **subjective data** includes assessment of the lower abdomen, which may produce discomfort over the urinary bladder. Patient complaints include burning on urination, dysuria, frequency, urgency, and nocturia.

Collection of **objective data** includes a clean-catch or catheterized urinalysis with culture and sensitivity to aid in confirming the diagnosis and in determining the appropriate treatment.

! **Safety Alert!**

Cystitis

- Teach the woman to cleanse the perineal area anteriorly to posteriorly to prevent contamination of pathogens (especially *E. coli*) from the rectum to the short urethra.
- Encourage drinking 2000 mL of liquids per day unless contraindicated.
- Instruct the patient to take all the prescribed medications even though symptoms may subside quickly.
- Instruct the patient about early detection and testing with Chemstrip LN.

Diagnostic Tests

Microscopic inspection of the urine often reveals bacteria and hematuria. A voiding cystogram may be used to identify reflux of urine into the bladder. Diagnosis is confirmed by a clean-catch, midstream urinalysis that reveals a bacterial count greater than 100,000 organisms/mL.

Medical Management

For cystitis without the complications of obstruction or other underlying pathologic conditions, medical management consists of short-term therapy with an antiinfective agent. If the treatment is effective, the patient should receive relief quickly. A repeat urinalysis 1 to 3 days after initiation of the medication confirms the effectiveness of the intervention.

Nursing Interventions and Patient Teaching

Nursing interventions focus on teaching that these infections tend to recur by either reinfection or persistent infection. Encourage the patient to drink 2000 mL of fluid per day. Record accurate I&O. Include early detection in the teaching. Long-term prophylaxis with low doses of medication may be necessary. A simple urine test, Chemstrip LN, allows the patient to test the urine at the first sign of infection and to call the physician for a prescription.

Prognosis

Successful treatment depends on the patient's ability to adequately flush the urinary tract and completion of the antibiotics prescribed.

INTERSTITIAL CYSTITIS

Etiology and Pathophysiology

IC is a chronic pelvic pain disorder with recurring discomfort or pain in the urinary bladder and surrounding region. It mostly affects middle-age white women. The pathophysiology is unknown, but bacteria do not trigger it. Instead, it seems to be caused by a breech in the bladder's protective mucosal lining that allows urine to seep through to the bladder wall, resulting in pain, inflammation, and small vessel bleeding. The bladder wall is infiltrated by inflammatory cells, resulting in ulceration and scarring of the mucosa, spasm of the detrusor muscle, hematuria, urgency, frequency, and pain on urination.

If a patient has signs and symptoms of a UTI but no bacteriuria, pyuria, or positive urine culture, IC is suspected. Other disorders that produce signs and symptoms similar to those of IC (such as UTI or endometriosis) must be excluded (Lewis et al., 2007). Small bleeding sites may be visualized via endoscopy.

ADLs and personal relationships may be disrupted by voiding patterns; some patients report voiding 60 times a day. IC can affect people of any age or gender, but most patients are women with a median age of 40 years.

Clinical Manifestations

The common signs and symptoms associated with IC are similar to those of cystitis: dysuria, urinary frequency, and microscopic bleeding. IC is characterized by urinary frequency, urgency, suprapubic pain, and dyspareunia (an abnormal pain during sexual intercourse); it is often associated with fibromyalgia and irritable bowel syndrome. Autoimmune, allergic, and infectious etiologies are being studied (Janos & Higgins, 2007).

Assessment

Subjective data include complaints of discomfort over the urinary bladder, dysuria, frequency, urgency, and nocturia.

Collection of **objective data** includes assessment of the lower abdomen, which may produce discomfort over the urinary bladder and the lower quadrants of the abdomen. A clean-catch midstream sample for urinalysis is used to rule out infection. Cystoscopy and tissue biopsy are used to establish a differential diagnosis.

Medical Management

IC is difficult to treat. Medications are prescribed for pain relief and inflammation, including low-dose cyclosporine (Neoral, Sandimmune), doxycycline (Vibramycin), and pentosan polysulfate sodium (Elmiron) (Page et al., 2005).

Amitriptyline (Elavil) and nortriptyline (Aventyl) are two antidepressants that reduce the burning pain and frequency of urination. The only oral medication approved by the FDA to treat the pain or discomfort of IC is pentosan. It improves the bladder's protective mucosal layer and relieves pain from IC by decreasing the irritative effects of urine on the bladder wall. It takes between 4 weeks to 3 months for significant improvement to occur (Page et al., 2005). For immediate relief, a brief course of opioid analgesics may be prescribed (Lewis et al., 2007).

Surgical interventions include studies of the effect of sacral nerve root stimulation via implantation of electrodes; cystectomy, with the creation of a urostomy; and urinary diversion. Some patients continue to experience pain even after surgery.

Nursing Interventions and Patient Teaching

Nursing interventions focus on pain control and comfort measures. Because all medications have side effects, patients must consult their physician before taking any prescription or over-the-counter medication. Pelvic floor exercise may help decrease urgency and nocturia. Patients may be asked to keep a daily bladder diary; this information can be used to make treatment decisions.

Potential dietary irritants include spicy and acidic floods, such as tomatoes, alcohol, citrus fruits, dark chocolate, and coffee. An elimination diet may help identify foods that trigger pain. A complete IC diet,

self-management strategies, and other nonmedical management tools are available from the Interstitial Cystitis Association (www.ichelp.com).

IC is often associated with a reduced quality of life. Embarrassment, pain, and inability to manage elimination may lead to withdrawal from business, social, and intimate relationships. The patient and significant others need psychosocial support to face an uncertain outcome.

Prognosis

Only about half of patients with IC recover fully. Until researchers find a cause and an effective treatment, symptoms will continue.

PROSTATITIS

Etiology and Pathophysiology

Prostatitis, defined as inflammation and/or infection of the prostate gland, is actually a group of diseases. Bacterial prostatitis is caused by infectious organisms such as *Pseudomonas* organisms and *S. faecalis* traveling up the urethra. Nonbacterial prostatitis may result from a variety of conditions related to occlusion of the urethra (e.g., enlargement of the prostate gland).

Prostatodynia (pain in the prostate gland) manifests with neither inflammation nor infection but demonstrates the other symptoms typical of prostatitis.

Clinical Manifestations

The signs and symptoms vary in number and intensity. The patient may experience fever; chills; malaise; arthralgia; myalgia; perineal prostatic pain; dysuria; obstructive urinary tract symptoms, including frequency, urgency, dysuria, nocturia, hesitancy, weak stream, and incomplete voiding; low back pain; low abdominal pain; spontaneous urethral discharge; ejaculatory pain; and erectile dysfunction. Chronic bacterial prostatitis may be asymptomatic. Edema of the prostate gland may serve as an obstruction, causing urinary retention as a complication to the prostatitis. Pooling of urine may also foster stone formation. Other complications are epididymitis, pyelonephritis, and bacteremia (the presence of bacteria in the blood). The patient may be asymptomatic, but the symptoms of acute bacterial prostatitis are often the same as those of UTI, with pain in the low back, perineum, or rectum. The condition may become chronic.

Diagnostic Tests

Diagnosis is confirmed by patient history and culture of prostatic fluid or tissue. The expressed prostate secretion (EPS) is considered useful in the diagnosis of prostatitis. EPS is obtained using a premassage and postmassage test. The patient is asked to void into a specimen cup just before and just after a vigorous prostate massage. Prostatic massage (for EPS) should be avoided if acute bacterial prostatitis is suspected, since compression is extremely painful and increases the risk of bacterial spread. Transabdominal ultrasound or MRI may be done to rule out an abscess on the prostate. A urinalysis and urine culture, WBC count, and blood cultures may also be performed.

Assessment
Subjective data include complaints of chills and low back and perineal pain. Chronic bacterial prostatitis causes dysuria; urgency; frequency; nocturia; and pain in the lower abdomen or back, perineum, or genitalia.

Collection of **objective data** involves assessing for elevated temperature and rectal palpation of the prostate gland by the physician, which may reveal it to be firm, edematous, and tender.

Medical Management
If the condition is infectious, management focuses on control of the infection and prevention of the complications of abscess formation or bacteremia. Antibiotics commonly used for acute and chronic bacterial prostatitis include trimethoprim-sulfamethoxazole, ciprofloxin (Cipro), and ofloxacin (Floxin). Doxycycline or tetracycline may be prescribed for patients with multiple sex partners. Antibiotics are usually given orally for up to 4 weeks for acute bacterial prostatitis. However, if the patient has high fever or other signs of impending sepsis, hospitalization and intravenous antibiotics are prescribed. Patients with chronic bacterial prostatitis are given oral antibiotic therapy for 4 to 16 weeks.

Antiinflammatories are the most common agents used for pain control in prostatitis, but these provide only moderate pain relief. Opioid analgesics can be given, but cautiously, since this pain can be chronic. The pain resolves as the infection is treated.

Nursing Interventions and Patient Teaching
Regardless of the pathologic basis, comfort measures used are analgesics, sitz baths, and stool softeners to reduce pain, edema, spasm, and straining pressure in the pelvis.

Teaching includes the medication regimen. Warn the patient with acute prostatitis to avoid sexual arousal and intercourse so the prostate can rest; however, intercourse may be beneficial in the treatment of chronic prostatitis. Follow-up with the physician is crucial because of the likelihood that the disorder will become chronic.

Prognosis
Prostatitis is difficult to cure and requires long periods of antibiotic treatment. Stress the importance of taking all the antibiotics prescribed, even after the initial symptoms have subsided.

PYELONEPHRITIS
Etiology and Pathophysiology
Pyelonephritis is an inflammation of the structures of the kidney—renal pelvis, renal tubules, and interstitial tissue. Pyelonephritis is almost always caused by *E. coli*. The kidney becomes edematous and inflamed, and the blood vessels are congested. The urine may be cloudy and contain pus (pyuria), mucus, and blood. Small abscesses may form in the kidney.

Pyelonephritis is usually seen in association with pregnancy; chronic health problems, such as diabetes mellitus or polycystic or hypertensive renal disease; insult to the urinary tract from catheterization; or infection, obstruction, or trauma. Careful management of these disorders is important to prevent pyelonephritis.

Clinical Manifestations
Acute pyelonephritis may be unilateral or bilateral, causing chills, fever, prostration, and flank pain. Repeated episodes of pyelonephritis lead to a chronic disease pattern, with atrophy of the kidney as the nephrons are destroyed. Azotemia (the retention of excessive amounts of nitrogenous compounds in the blood) develops if enough nephrons are nonfunctional.

Assessment
Subjective data in acute pyelonephritis includes a patient who is acutely ill, with malaise and pain in the costovertebral angle (CVA) (one of two angles that outline a space over the kidneys). CVA tenderness to percussion is a common finding in pyelonephritis. In the chronic phase the patient may show unremarkable symptoms, such as nausea and general malaise.

Collection of **objective data** includes assessing the patient for signs of infection: elevated temperature, vomiting, and chills. The chronic disease results in systemic signs: elevated blood pressure and gastrointestinal irritation such as vomiting and diarrhea.

Diagnostic Tests
Diagnosis is confirmed by bacteria and pus in the urine, varying degrees of hematuria, WBCs and WBC casts in the urine (indicating involvement of the renal parenchyma), and leukocytosis. A clean-catch or catheterized urinalysis with culture and sensitivity identifies the pathogen and determines appropriate antimicrobial therapy. To prevent spread of infection in the early stages of acute pyelonephritis, imaging examinations such as an IUP or CT scan requiring intrauterine injection of contrast materials are usually not performed. Ultrasound of the urinary system is often done to identify anatomical abnormalities such as renal abscesses, obstructing calculus, or hydronephrosis (Lewis et al., 2007). BUN and creatinine levels of the blood and urine may be assessed to monitor kidney function.

Medical Management
The patient with mild signs and symptoms may be treated on an outpatient basis with antibiotics for 14 to 21 days. Parenteral antibiotics are often given initially in the hospital to establish high serum and urinary medication levels. When initial treatment resolves the acute symptoms and the patient is able to tolerate oral fluids and medications, he or she may be discharged on a regi-

men of oral antibiotics for an additional 14 to 21 days. Antibiotics are selected according to results of urinalysis culture and sensitivity and may include broad-spectrum medications such as ampicillin or vancomycin combined with an aminoglycoside (e.g., tobramycin [Nebcin], gentamicin [Garamycin]); other treatment options include trimethoprim-sulfamethoxazole and fluoroquinolones such as ciprofloxin and ofloxacin.

Adequate fluids (at least eight 8-ounce glasses per day) are encouraged. Urinary analgesics such as phenazopyridine are helpful. Follow-up urine culture is indicated.

Nursing Interventions and Patient Teaching

Nursing diagnoses and interventions for the patient with pyelonephritis include but are not limited to the following:

Nursing Diagnoses	Nursing Interventions
Risk for infection, related to bacteria in the urinary tract	Monitor urine character and odor. Encourage oral fluids. Instruct patient to void when he or she feels the urge. Encourage perineal hygiene.
Health-seeking behaviors, related to desire for prevention of further renal disease	Assess knowledge level concerning measures to prevent recurrence of symptoms. Discuss personal health habits: diet, exercise. Discuss treatment plan with patient and family.

Teach the patient to identify the signs and symptoms of infection: elevated temperature, flank pain, chills, fever, nausea and vomiting, urgency, fatigue, and general malaise. Also teach the patient indications, dose, length of course, and side effects of the medications. Emphasize the importance of follow-up care with the physician on a routine basis and when signs of infection arise.

Prognosis

Prognosis depends on early detection and successful treatment. Baseline assessment for every patient must include urinary assessment because pyelonephritis can occur as a primary or secondary disorder.

OBSTRUCTIVE DISORDERS OF THE URINARY TRACT

URINARY OBSTRUCTION

Etiology and Pathophysiology

Obstruction at any point within the urinary tract can adversely affect function and alter structure. Causes of obstruction include strictures, kinks, cysts, tumors, calculi, and prostatic hypertrophy. Obstruction may lead to alterations in blood chemistry, infection that thrives as a result of urine stasis, ischemia due to compression, or atrophy of renal tissue.

Clinical Manifestations

The patient may be unaware of any problems at first if the obstruction is partial, allowing urine to drain and kidney function to remain within normal limits. With prostatic hypertrophy the obstructive process may be so gradual that the patient ignores the vague symptom of dull flank pain and seeks medical attention only when urination becomes acutely difficult. Acute pain occurs as the musculature is stretched by increasing pressure from urine accumulation and as muscular contractions increase in an attempt to move urine past the obstruction. This acute pain is called renal colic and is a classic symptom of renal calculi.

Assessment

Subjective data include the patient's cardinal complaint of a sensation of needing to void but only being able to void small amounts. Pain may range from dull flank pain to acute, incapacitating pain. Nausea often accompanies acute pain.

Collection of **objective data** includes noting on physical assessment if the bladder is palpable suprapubically because of urine retention. The affected kidney may also be palpable. Retention with overflow occurs when the patient is unable to completely empty the urinary bladder and it quickly refills, causing the urge to void again. Assess time and amount of voidings.

Diagnostic Tests

As a quick evaluation, the physician may order a KUB radiograph. Renal ultrasonography or IVP provides definitive information about structural changes. Other diagnostic tests may include visual examinations with the aid of endoscopy and a blood chemistry profile.

Medical Management

Initial intervention is aimed at establishing urine drainage and relieving discomfort. Conservative measures include inserting an indwelling catheter and administering an analgesic (usually opioid) and an anticholinergic agent (atropine) to decrease smooth muscle motility. It may be necessary to establish urine drainage surgically by inserting a catheter directly into the bladder through the abdominal wall (suprapubic cystostomy), into a ureter (ureterostomy), or into the kidney (nephrostomy).

Surgical correction of an obstruction in the urinary system may involve a tube, called a stent. Stent insertion is used for patients who are poor operative risks. A meshlike tube or coil-shaped device is inserted through an endoscope into the ureter. The stent holds the tubular structure open to facilitate drainage. Stents may be permanent or temporary. Closely monitor the patient for signs of infection, obstruction, and pain.

Nursing Interventions

After surgery, observe the patient for hemorrhage, provide aseptic care of the surgical site, and provide a safe environment to prevent injury and infection.

Prognosis

The prognosis varies, depending on the cause of the obstruction. If surgical correction is successful, the prognosis is excellent.

HYDRONEPHROSIS

Etiology and Pathophysiology

Hydronephrosis (the dilation of the renal pelvis and calyces) may be congenital or may develop at any time. It can occur unilaterally or bilaterally. Hydronephrosis is caused by obstructions in the lower urinary tract, the ureters, or the kidneys. The location of the obstruction determines whether one or both kidneys are affected.

An obstruction generates pressure from accumulated urine that cannot flow past it. This pressure may cause functional and anatomical damage to the renal system. The renal pelvis and ureters dilate and hypertrophy. This pressure, if prolonged, causes fibrosis and loss of function in affected nephrons. If the condition is left untreated, the kidney may be destroyed.

Clinical Manifestations

Hydronephrosis can occur without any symptoms as long as kidney function is adequate and urine can drain. The amount of pain is proportional to the rate of stretching of urinary tract structures. Slowly developing hydronephrosis may cause only a dull flank pain, whereas a sudden occlusion of the ureter, such as from a calculus, causes a severe stabbing (colicky) pain in the flank. Nausea and vomiting, which often accompany hydronephrosis, are a reflex reaction to the pain and usually subside when the pain is controlled.

Assessment

Subjective data include patient reports of pain, including location, intensity, and character, and nausea. Discuss the patient's voiding pattern: frequency, difficulty starting a stream of urine, dribbling at the end of micturition (voiding), nocturia, and burning on urination. Note any history of obstructive disorders.

Collection of **objective data** includes assessing patients suspected of having hydronephrosis for vomiting, hematuria, urinary output, edema, a palpable mass in the abdomen, bladder distention (detected on palpation), and tenderness over the kidneys or bladder.

Diagnostic Tests

A urinalysis and serum kidney function studies that include measurement of urea and creatinine are obtained. Cystoscopy may be performed with or without retrograde pyelogram. Radiographic examinations may include IVP or IVU, KUB radiograph, CT scan, or ultrasound evaluation. Sometimes a renal biopsy is performed.

Medical Management

Management is usually conservative if the condition is not severe. Surgery relieves the obstruction and preserves kidney function. If the kidney is severely damaged, a nephrectomy may be necessary. If infection is present, antiinfective medications are administered: penicillin in combination with sulfasoxazole (Gantrisin) or sulfamethoxazole-trimethoprim (Bactrim). Opioids, such as morphine and meperidine, in combination with antispasmodic drugs, such as propantheline (Pro-Banthine) and belladonna preparations, are usually necessary to relieve severe, colicky pain.

Nursing Interventions and Patient Teaching

Nursing interventions for the patient with hydronephrosis include administering medications as ordered, monitoring I&O, observing for signs and symptoms of infection, and monitoring vital signs. Encourage the patient to take fluids, and assess the patient for pain. Keep any drainage tubes open and anchored to avoid inadvertent displacement. If a catheter is present, provide catheter care. If surgery has been performed, observe the dressing because drainage of urine may continue for some time. Keep the area clean and dry to avoid excoriation of the skin. Explain all procedures to the patient and the family.

Patient teaching includes explaining the abnormality and the signs and symptoms of infection or obstruction. Describe measures to prevent infection, such as adequate fluid intake, perineal hygiene daily with mild soap and water (drying thoroughly), and regular emptying of the bladder.

Prognosis

Prognosis depends on the degree of urinary system destruction and the need for surgical intervention.

UROLITHIASIS

Urolithiasis (formation of urinary calculi) can develop in any area of the urinary tract. *Urolithiasis* is a general term that encompasses all urinary calculi, but specific names are also used to indicate where they are located or formed: nephrolithiasis (stones in the kidney), ureterolithiasis (stones in the ureter), and cystolithiasis (stones in the bladder). Other descriptive terms are **lithiasis** and **calculi** (the formation of stones).

Etiology and Pathophysiology

Urolithiasis develops from minerals that have precipitated out of solution and adhere, forming stones that vary in size and shape. The event that initiates stone formation remains unknown. However, some individuals are predisposed to urolithiasis: people who are immobile, are hyperparathyroid (calcium leaves the bones and accumulates in the bloodstream), or have recurrent UTIs. Individual history and some foods, nutrients, and medications contribute to development of stones. Thorough assessment and analysis of the composition of the stones guides medical and nursing management.

Clinical Manifestations

Symptoms depend on the stones' size and degree of mobility. The patient with renal colic seeks care immediately, whereas a person with a less mobile stone may not seek assistance until signs of infection or hydronephrosis occur.

Assessment

Subjective data include the patient with mobile calculi complaining of intractable pain (pain that is unrelieved by ordinary medical measures and is usually accompanied by nausea and vomiting). The patient describes the pain as starting in the flank and radiating into the groin, the genitalia, and the inner thigh. The patient with a less mobile stone may develop signs and symptoms associated with UTI secondary to hydronephrosis.

Collection of **objective data** includes assessing for hematuria and vomiting.

Diagnostic Tests

Diagnostic tests include KUB and IVP or IVU radiography, ultrasound, cystoscopy, and urinalysis. Other tests may be ordered to determine stone content, presence of infection, and alterations in blood chemistry that influence stone formation. Twenty-four-hour urine examination may be done to detect abnormal excretion of calcium oxalate, phosphorus, or uric acid.

Medical Management

Antiinfective agents may be administered to treat infection or prophylactically. If stones are not passed, invasive techniques may be indicated (Figure 10-7). Stones in the lower tract can be removed by cystoscopy with stone manipulation or by surgical incision.

Terminology describes the location: ureterolithotomy, pyelolithotomy, and nephrolithotomy. Chemolytic agents, either alkylating or acidifying agents, may be instilled to dissolve stones.

Extracorporeal shock wave lithotripsy is an alternative to surgery. The patient is submerged in a special tank of water, and ultrasonic shock waves are used to pulverize the stone. Urine must still be strained, even if a catheter is in place. Renal colic may occur as the patient passes the stone fragments.

Long-term management may include dietary adjustments to alter urine pH or to decrease availability of certain substances that cause stone formation. Moderate reduction of foods containing calcium phosphorus and purine may help when stones are caused by metabolic abnormalities. Foods to avoid include cheese, greens, whole grains, carbonated beverages, nuts, chocolate, shellfish, and organ meat. Daily fluid intake of 2000 mL (unless clinically contraindicated) helps cleanse the urinary tract.

Drug therapy depends on stone composition. In calcium stone formation, sodium cellulose phosphate binds with ingested calcium and prevents its absorption; aluminum hydroxide gel binds with excess phosphorus, allowing intestinal excretion rather than urinary excretion; and allopurinol (Zyloprim) reduces serum urate levels, thereby facilitating reabsorption of urate crystals.

Nursing Interventions and Patient Teaching

Stones are more likely to be passed if the patient remains active and increases fluid intake. If pain is so severe that it requires opioid medication, be cautious when allowing the patient out of bed. If nausea inhibits oral intake, the physician may order supplemental intravenous fluids. All urine is strained. Because stones may be any size, save even the smallest speck for assessment. Encourage fluids and administer analgesics as ordered. Assess urine for possible hematuria. Monitor BUN and creatinine for indications of continuing urinary tract obstruction.

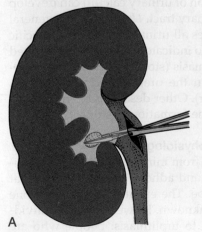 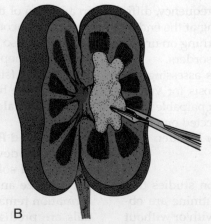 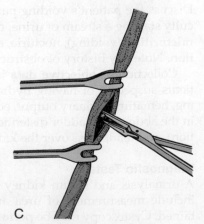

A   B   C

FIGURE 10-7 Location and methods of removing renal calculi from upper urinary tract. **A,** Pyelolithotomy, removal of stone through renal pelvis. **B,** Nephrolithotomy, removal of staghorn calculus from renal parenchyma (kidney split). **C,** Ureterolithotomy, removal of stone from ureter.

Nursing diagnoses and interventions for the patient with urolithiasis include but are not limited to the following:

Nursing Diagnoses	Nursing Interventions
Risk for infection, related to bacteria in the urinary tract	Monitor urine character and odor. Encourage oral fluids. Instruct the patient to void when urge is felt. Encourage perineal hygiene.
Health-seeking behaviors, related to desire for prevention of further renal disease	Assess knowledge level concerning measures to prevent recurrence of symptoms. Discuss personal health habits (diet, exercise). Discuss treatment plan with patient and family.

Discuss the prescribed diet, including fluid intake, and home medications (their purpose, dosage, refills, and side effects). The patient should avoid inactivity by walking frequently. Emphasize the need for follow-up with the physician, including keeping scheduled appointments and reporting difficulty with urination.

Although opinions vary greatly as to benefits of dietary restrictions, the nurse may be responsible for clarifying diet instructions. Encourage a fluid intake of at least 2000 mL in 24 hours, unless contraindicated. People who are calcium stone formers may need to curtail their intake of dietary calcium (dairy products, antacids) to within minimum recommended dietary allowance guidelines. New research on the impact of diet on the development of calcium oxalate kidney stones concludes that restricting consumption of animal protein and salt in combination with normal calcium intake reduces the risk of kidney stones better than the traditional low-calcium diet (Moyad, 2003).

Prognosis

Prognosis is related to the location of the stone and the extent of invasive procedures necessary to remove the stone. A certain population, categorized as "stone formers," is at risk for recurrence.

TUMORS OF THE URINARY SYSTEM

RENAL TUMORS

Etiology and Pathophysiology

The majority of renal tumors are malignant adenocarcinomas, also known as renal cell carcinoma, that develop unilaterally and are often large when first detected. Renal cell carcinoma as a primary malignant tumor appears to arise from cells of the proximal convoluted tubules. This is the tenth most common cancer, accounting for 3% of all cancers in adults, with a median age at diagnosis of 65 years. Twice as many men as women are diagnosed with renal cancer.

No strong risk factors have been identified, although some studies have suggested a relationship to obesity and smoking (American Institute of Cancer Research, 2007). The strongest risk factors appear to be genetic; multifocal renal adenocarcinomas have a hereditary basis, which is being studied intensively. Several multiorgan syndromes are associated with a high risk of renal malignancies; the most prominent is von Hippel–Lindau disease, an autosomally dominant hereditary disease originating from chromosome 3p. von Hippel–Lindau disease is characterized by central nervous system hemangioblastomas, renal adenocarcinomas, and other anomalies.

Because of the isolated anatomical location of the kidney, renal adenocarcinomas can grow large while remaining clinically silent. Most demonstrate a characteristic hypervascularity. Renal adenocarcinomas tend to grow intravascularly within the renal vein and into the inferior vena cava. These tumor thrombi may extend as far as the right atrium, presenting a unique surgical challenge. Although essentially every organ site can be affected, the most common sites of metastases are the lungs, the adrenal glands, the liver, and bones.

Clinical Manifestations

The historic sign and symptom triad of renal adenocarcinoma is hematuria, flank pain, and a flank mass. Most cases with these symptoms are advanced and incurable. Other common signs and symptoms are hypercalcemia, fever, anemia, weakness, and erythrocytosis. Gross hematuria is rarely a sign of renal adenocarcinoma until the malignancy is advanced. Check the patient's home medications for anticoagulant therapy, since this may be the cause of hematuria.

Assessment

Subjective data include a patient history of blood in the urine, which "comes and goes." When the bleeding occurs, there is usually no associated pain. In advanced stages of the illness, the patient experiences weight loss, fatigue, and dull flank pain.

Collection of **objective data** involves a physical assessment that reveals a mass in the patient's flank in the advanced stages of the illness. Hematuria and signs related to systemic metastasis may be obvious.

Diagnostic Tests

Localized adenocarcinoma is being diagnosed in patients who have no signs and symptoms specifically related to the tumor; these tumors are often discovered incidentally during evaluation of other complaints. Patients with gross hematuria should be assessed by a urologist. A cystoscopy followed by an IVP with tomography should be performed.

The vast majority of solid masses are malignant and require definitive evaluation and treatment. Percutaneous biopsy on a solid renal mass is rarely done because it is unlikely to change the future treatment unless there is evidence of advanced disease. A CT (with or without contrast), a chest x-ray, and, in some cases, a bone scan are used to stage renal adenocarcinoma.

Medical Management

Because renal adenocarcinoma is relatively radioresistant, radiation therapy has little or no role in its treatment. Surgery is the sole intervention capable of cure. The standard procedure is radical nephrectomy along with removal of adjacent lymph nodes and tissue. In the patient with renal insufficiency or a solitary kidney, partial nephrectomy (a far more complex procedure) may be indicated.

Nursing Interventions and Patient Teaching

Care of the patient with surgery of the urinary tract is addressed later in this chapter.

Nursing diagnoses and interventions for the patient with renal tumors include but are not limited to the following:

Nursing Diagnoses	Nursing Interventions
Ineffective coping, related to powerlessness	Encourage patient to express feelings.
	Assist patient in identifying personal strengths and coping skills.
	Actively listen.
	Support realistic hope; answer questions honestly.
Decisional conflict, with verbalized uncertainty about choice to have renal surgery	Assess patient's capacity to make decisions.
	Assess knowledge of procedure.
	Review outline of surgical procedure and what nursing interventions the patient and significant others can expect postoperatively.
Impaired physical mobility, related to pain and discomfort	Plan activities when pain control is greatest.
	Encourage active or passive range-of-motion exercises.
	Assess need for assistive devices.

Instruct the patient about community resources, support groups, and home health care. Emphasize the importance of follow-up care, including following discharge instructions and keeping return appointment.

Prognosis

In most cases of localized renal adenocarcinoma, the 5-year survival rate is more than 60%. The natural history of renal adenocarcinoma is far more unpredict-

able than that of most solid tumors. Disease may recur more than 15 years after removal of the original primary lesion. Metastatic disease has a poor prognosis and is rarely curable. Metastatic recurrence at a remotely distant time is not uncommon.

RENAL CYSTS

Etiology and Pathophysiology

Acquired renal cysts are simple cysts that must be distinguished from more serious causes of cystic disease. Acquired cysts are usually simple: round and sharply demarcated with smooth walls. They may be single or multiple. Single cysts are isolated and are most often detected incidentally. They are clinically insignificant, but must be distinguished from other more significant cystic renal disorders and renal masses such as renal cell carcinoma. Renal cell carcinoma is typically irregular or multiloculated with irregular walls and areas of unclear demarcation.

Acquired cysts are significant only because patients have a higher incidence of renal carcinoma; whether the cysts become malignant is unknown. For this reason, some physicians periodically screen patients with acquired cysts for renal carcinoma using ultrasonography or CT.

Multiple cysts are most common in patients with chronic renal failure, especially those undergoing hemodialysis. The cause is unknown, but the cysts may be due to compensatory hyperplasia of residually functioning nephrons. A criterion for diagnosis is more than four cysts in each kidney on ultrasonography or CT.

The most significant problems arise with **PKD.** PKD is a genetic disorder characterized by the growth of numerous fluid-filled cysts, which can slowly replace much of the kidney. A patient with longstanding renal insufficiency or a dialysis patient may develop polycystic disease. Kidney function is compromised by the pressure of the cysts on renal structures, secondary infections, and tissue scarring caused by rupture of the cysts. The patient may progress to end-stage renal disease (ESRD).

Clinical Manifestations

Signs and symptoms are influenced by the degree of renal structure involvement. The most common site is the collecting ducts, which fill with urine and/or blood. As the disease progresses, fewer nephrons are available to maintain normal kidney function.

The Bosniak Classification of Renal Cysts classifies lesions according to their character. Class I lesions are simple, benign cysts and do not warrant further workup. Class II lesions are minimally complicated with some features that cause concern. They have smooth, sharp margins; are thicker; and require follow-up scanning. Class III lesions have irregular and thickened walls and multiloculated cysts; they require surgical exploration. Class IV lesions show nonuniform wall thickening and irregular margins; they contain solid components visible on CT. These lesions are clearly malignant, and a total nephrectomy is warranted.

Assessment

Subjective data include the most common symptoms of abdominal and flank pain, followed by headache, gastrointestinal complaints, voiding disturbances, and a history of recurrent UTIs.

Collection of **objective data** involves observation for systemic changes. Closely monitor blood pressure, which is usually elevated, and hematuria. Document patient complaints and response to intervention.

Diagnostic Tests

Diagnosis is established by family history, physical examination, excretory urography, and imaging of cysts on radiographic examination or sonography. Blood chemistry results, such as urea and creatinine levels, are used to monitor the level of kidney function.

Medical Management

PKD has no specific treatment. Medical treatment is aimed at relief of pain and other symptoms. Heat and analgesics may relieve some of the discomfort caused by the enlarging kidneys. If the patient bleeds, discontinue heat and place the patient on bed rest. Hypertension is treated vigorously with antihypertensive agents, diuretics, and fluid and dietary modifications. Because infections are common, antibiotics are often prescribed. As the disease progresses, dialysis or kidney transplantation may be required.

Nursing Interventions

Individual complaints and the severity of the disease process influence nursing interventions. Provide information to patients and family members about the availability of genetic counseling. Emphasize the need to report any changes in health status to the physician.

Prognosis

Prognosis is favorable with a single cyst but guarded with polycystic disease because of its chronic nature.

TUMORS OF THE URINARY BLADDER

Etiology and Pathophysiology

The bladder is the most common site of cancer in the urinary tract. A bladder tumor is an excess growth of cells that line the inside of the bladder, in many cases because the cells were exposed to certain chemicals. Tumors of the urinary bladder range from benign papillomas to invasive carcinomas. Papillomas have the potential to become cancerous and are removed when detected. A noncancerous bladder tumor is usually a small, wartlike growth that does not spread (National Cancer Institute, 2008).

The overall incidence and mortality for bladder cancer have changed little for most racial and ethnic groups over the past 20 years. Recent research has shown black patients were 35% more likely to die of bladder cancer than white patients. Men are more likely to develop bladder cancer than women; cigarette smoking is a major factor (National Cancer Institute, 2008).

Several types of carcinoma arise on the bladder surface. The most common type diagnosed in North America is transitional cell carcinoma (TCC), which can occur anywhere in the urinary tract, but is usually found in the urinary bladder. TCC involves development of a papillary tumor that projects into the bladder lumen and, if untreated, continues into the bladder muscle, where it can metastasize.

Clinical Manifestations

The patient may delay seeking medical attention because the primary sign of bladder cancer is painless, intermittent hematuria.

Assessment

Subjective data include symptoms such as changes in voiding patterns, signs of urinary obstruction, or renal failure, depending on the extent of the disease process.

Collection of **objective data** includes assessing the patient's understanding of current health status, which will aid in planning teaching interventions. Accurately document the time and amount of voiding, including the urine description.

Diagnostic Tests

Diagnostic tests include a urine cytologic evaluation (study of cells) and/or one of several available bladder cancer markers. Bladder biopsies are needed to confirm a diagnosis.

Bladder cancer tumors are most commonly staged using the system developed by the American Joint Committee on Cancer. The stage of the tumor is the most important indicator of prognosis and overall survival for invasive tumors. Staging is an assessment of how far the tumor has spread.

Medical Management

Local disease may be treated by removing the tissue by burning with an electric spark (fulguration), laser, instillation of chemotherapy agents, or radiation therapy. Closely monitor these patients with cytologic studies and cystoscopy, since the recurrence rate is as high as 60%. A partial or total cystectomy may be performed to remove invasive lesions. With complete removal of the urinary bladder, urinary diversion is necessary. (See the discussion of the ileal conduit or sigmoid conduit, pp. 478-479, and Figure 10-13.)

Nursing Interventions and Patient Teaching

Care of the patient with bladder cancer is influenced by the extent of the disease process, medical treatment, coincidental illness, and the patient's response to treatment. Observe voiding patterns and urine characteristics to monitor response to these therapies. Provide teaching and support so that the patient can return to optimum performance of ADLs. Emphasize the importance of follow-up care for the patient with papillomas.

Prognosis

The prognosis is directly related to the extent of the disease process when diagnosed. Another important aspect in recovery is the patient's adaptability to any changes in urinary elimination as a result of treatment.

CONDITIONS AFFECTING THE PROSTATE GLAND

BENIGN PROSTATIC HYPERTROPHY

Etiology and Pathophysiology

The prostate gland encircles the male urethra at the base of the urinary bladder. It secretes an alkaline fluid that helps neutralize seminal fluid and increases sperm motility. BPH, enlargement of the prostate gland, is common in men older than 50 years of age. The cause is unclear but may be influenced by hormonal changes. The prostate enlarges, exerting pressure on the urethra and vesicle neck of the urinary bladder, which prevents complete emptying.

Clinical Manifestations

The patient has symptoms associated with urinary obstruction. Other clinical manifestations include complications of urinary obstruction, such as UTI, hematuria, oliguria, and signs of renal insufficiency.

Assessment

Subjective data include the patient describing the urine stream as difficult to start, slow, and painful, with complaints of frequency and nocturia. Collectively these symptoms may be referred to as **prostatism** (any condition of the prostate gland that causes retention of urine in the bladder).

Collection of **objective data** involves eliciting information about voiding patterns to aid in determining the severity of the obstruction.

Diagnostic Tests

On rectal examination the physician may palpate the enlarged prostate gland, which has an elastic consistency. The hypertrophied prostate is symmetrically enlarged with a uniform, boggy presentation. Severity of the process can be determined by detecting alterations in blood chemistry, by measuring residual urine, or by cystoscopy or IVP. Cytologic evaluation determines whether the process is benign or malignant.

Medical Management

Treatment is based on the degree of occlusion and on signs and symptoms. Pharmacologic agents such as dutasteride (Avodart) convert testosterone to dihydrotestosterone, a key enzyme in the development and growth rate of prostatic hyperplasia. This medication may take 3 to 6 months to shrink the prostate gland, decreasing its size as much as 25%. Terazosin (Hytrin) is an antihypertensive that dilates arteries and veins and decreases contractions in smooth muscle of the prostatic capsule. This decreases symptoms of prostatic hyperplasia (urinary urgency, hesitancy, nocturia).

Deciding which treatment intervention to choose is difficult. Transurethral resection of the prostate (TURP) is still considered the standard for surgical intervention. The newer, less-invasive treatments are still being evaluated. In general, these treatments are considered to cause less morbidity, but the results are not considered as effective or long lasting as those of TURP.

Transurethral Microwave Thermotherapy

Transurethral microwave thermotherapy (TUMT) is one of various procedures used for the treatment of lower urinary tract symptoms due to BPH. TUMT involves the insertion of a specially designed urinary catheter into the bladder, allowing a microwave antenna to be positioned within the prostate; there, it heats and destroys hyperplastic prostate tissue. The goal of TUMT is to provide a one-time treatment. Candidates for TUMT include persons with moderate-to-severe voiding symptoms due to BPH, those with side effects to medical therapy, those in whom medical therapy has failed, and those who choose to not be treated medically. There are a number of exclusions to the use of TUMT, so all patients require a thorough history and physical examination.

Patients should return to the clinic for follow-up. If a catheter is placed, it can be removed at home or in the clinic. Instruct patients to watch for an inability to void, painful voiding, high fevers, abdominal pain, or other problems. Posttreatment convalescence is relatively rapid, with most patients able to void and recover in less than 5 days at home. Thus some patients return to full activity relatively early (Rubenstein & McVary, 2008).

Transurethral Needle Ablation (TUNA)

Transurethral needle ablation (TUNA) of the prostate is another procedure used to treat BPH. It is performed by placing interstitial radiofrequency needles through the urethra and into the lateral lobes of the prostate, causing heat-induced coagulation necrosis. The tissue is heated to 230° F (110° C) for approximately 3 minutes per lesion. A coagulation defect is created. A comprehensive history and physical examination must be done to determine the benefits of using this procedure. Urethrocystoscopy may be indicated to help select the optimal form of therapy.

Photoselective Vaporization of the Prostate

Photoselective vaporization of the prostate (PVP) using the GreenLight laser is another option for the treatment of BPH. PVP is a safe alternative for patients who are seriously ill, are taking anticoagulants, or have unfavorable anatomy (i.e., a large prostate). The technique employs a laser beam, which emits a visible green light at a wavelength that has shallow tissue penetration and is selectively absorbed by blood. A urologist delivers the laser's energy by way of a thin fiber inserted into the urethra through a 23-F continuous-flow cystoscopy. The GreenLight laser vaporizes the prostate tissue.

Nursing Interventions

Initial management is aimed at relieving the obstruction, usually by insertion of a Foley catheter. Take care to avoid rapid decompression of the bladder to prevent rupture of mucosal blood vessels. Usually no more than 1000 mL of urine should be removed from a distended bladder initially. Follow physician's orders for the individual patient.

Prostatectomy (removal of the prostate gland) is indicated to relieve or prevent further obstruction of the urethra. The physician chooses the surgical approach for the prostatectomy after thorough appraisal of the patient. Preoperatively the physician may order an enema to reduce the possibility of the patient's straining to

defecate after surgery, which could cause bleeding. Other preoperative preparations are standard, as noted in Chapter 2. A prostatectomy may be done using any of four surgical techniques (Box 10-3 and Figure 10-8).

With BPH, TURP is the resection most often chosen because it is less invasive and less stressful for the pa-

Box 10-3 Four Prostatectomy Techniques

1. **Transurethral prostatectomy** is done by approaching the gland through the penis and bladder using a resectoscope, a surgical instrument with an electric cutting wire for resection and cautery to resect the lobes away from the capsule (see Figure 10-8, A).
2. **Suprapubic prostatectomy** is accomplished by an incision through the abdomen; the bladder is opened, and the gland is removed from above with the finger (see Figure 10-8, B).
3. **Radical perineal prostatectomy** requires an incision through the perineum between the scrotum and the rectum (see Figure 10-8, C).
4. **Retropubic prostatectomy** requires a low abdominal incision, but the bladder is not opened. The gland is removed by making an incision into the capsule encasing the prostate gland (see Figure 10-8, D).

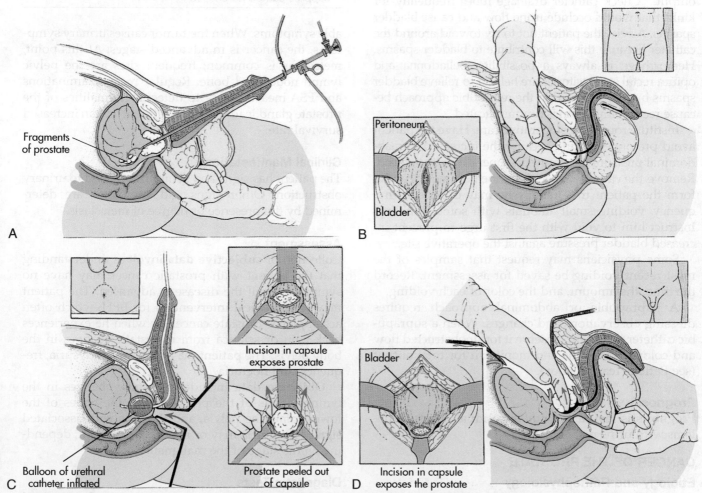

FIGURE 10-8 Four types of prostatectomies. **A,** Transurethral resection of prostate gland by means of resectoscope. Note enlarged prostate gland surrounding urethra and tiny pieces of prostatic tissue that have been cut away. **B,** Suprapubic. **C,** Radical perineal. **D,** Retropubic prostatectomy.

tient, especially the older patient or the patient with coincidental illness. The tissue is removed through the urethra. With this procedure the outer capsule of the prostate gland is left in place, maintaining the continuity between the bladder and the lower urethra (see Figure 10-8, A). Care of this patient centers on observing urine characteristics and maintaining patency of the Foley catheter.

The patient who has a TURP may have continuous closed bladder irrigation or intermittent irrigation to prevent occlusion of the catheter with blood clots, which would cause bladder spasms. Inform the patient and the family that hematuria is expected after prostatic surgery. Monitor vital signs and urine color every 2 hours for the first 24 hours to detect early signs of complications. With continuous bladder irrigation the urine will be light red to pink, and with intermittent irrigation the urine will be a clear, cherry red. Continuous irrigation is achieved with a three-way catheter (one lumen for irrigation fluid, one for urine drainage, and one to the retention balloon) or by using two catheters (Foley and suprapubic—one for irrigation fluid and one for urine drainage). The irrigant is an isotonic solution. To determine urinary output, subtract the amount of irrigation fluid used from the Foley catheter output. This is reported as "actual urinary output." Check catheter drainage tubes frequently for kinks that would occlude urine flow and cause bladder spasms. Advise the patient not to try to void around the catheter because this will contribute to bladder spasms. Hemorrhage is always a possibility. Belladonna and opium rectal suppositories are helpful to relieve bladder spasms but are not used in the retropubic approach because rectal stimulation is contraindicated.

Institute routine postoperative care. Have the patient avoid prolonged sitting because the increased intraabdominal pressure may cause the operative site to bleed. Remove the catheter when the urine becomes clear. Inform the patient that initially he may experience frequency, voiding small amounts with some dribbling. Instruct him to void with the first urge to prevent increased bladder pressure against the operative site.

Some physicians may request that samples of the most recent voiding be saved for assessment. Record the time, the amount, and the color of each voiding.

A suprapubic or abdominal approach requires dressing observations and changes. When a suprapubic catheter is present, observe it for unobstructed flow and color of the urine and monitor it for total output (see Patient Teaching box).

Prognosis

Prognosis is favorable without residual effects. Problems with urine dribbling vary.

CANCER OF THE PROSTATE

Etiology and Pathophysiology

Prostatic cancer is common in men older than 50 years of age. This insidious cancer usually starts as a nodule on the posterior portion of the prostate without notice-

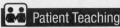

Patient Teaching

Postprostatectomy

Written Instructions with Frequently Asked Questions
- Rest for 48 hours to help prevent postoperative bleeding.
- Do not take aspirin or anticoagulant medications.
- Do not drive for 48 hours.
- Avoid sexual activity for 2 weeks, or as directed by physician.
- If prescribed antibiotics, take medication as prescribed until all are gone.
- Prevent constipation.
- Observe for signs and symptoms of urinary tract infection.
- A list of contact numbers.
- An appointment card for follow-up visit.

Managing Urinary Incontinence
- It usually takes several weeks to achieve urinary continence. Continence may improve for up to 12 months.
- Maintain oral fluids between 2000 and 3000 mL/day (unless contraindicated).

Erectile Dysfunction
- Sexual counseling and treatment options may be necessary if erectile dysfunction becomes a chronic or permanent problem.

Indwelling Catheter
- If the patient goes home with an indwelling catheter, send instructions for the catheter care and local stores where the supplies can be purchased.

able symptoms. When the tumor causes urinary symptoms, the cancer is in advanced stages. At this point, metastasis is common; frequent sites are the pelvic lymph nodes and bone. Regular rectal examinations and PSA measurement to detect abnormalities of the prostate gland lead to early treatment and an increased survival rate.

Clinical Manifestations

The patient has signs and symptoms related to urinary obstruction. Other signs and symptoms are determined by the presence or degree of metastasis.

Assessment

Collection of **subjective data** involves understanding that the patient with prostatic cancer may have no symptoms until the disease is advanced. The patient may seek medical intervention for BPH, which often accompanies prostate cancer, or when he experiences back pain or sciatica from metastatic changes in the bony pelvis. The patient may complain of dysuria, frequency, and nocturia.

Objective data include metastatic changes in the lymph glands of the pelvis and in the bones of the lower spine, the pelvis, and the hips with associated signs. Hematuria may or may not be present, depending on the stage of the malignancy.

Diagnostic Tests

On rectal examination by the physician, the involved area of the prostate gland feels firm and fixed with hardened nodules typically in the posterior lobe of the gland.

Definitive diagnosis is made by cytologic examination. Prostate cells can be obtained by needle aspiration.

Men should consider a yearly PSA and digital rectal examination starting at age 50 or at age 45 if at high risk (blacks or men with a father or brother diagnosed with prostate cancer at an early age). PSA is greatly increasing the odds of early diagnosis. PSA, normally secreted and disposed of by the prostate, increases in the bloodstream in cancer of the prostate as well as in the harmless condition of BPH. The normal PSA is 0 to 4 ng/mL. It is important to monitor even a slight increase in PSA levels. Elevated PSA levels mean further diagnostic evaluation is needed. When PSA levels are high but a digital examination is normal, transrectal ultrasound is proving increasingly helpful in detecting cancer of the prostate gland too small to be palpated rectally. Other tests, such as a bone scan and serum alkaline phosphatase, are performed to assess the degree of metastasis.

The Gleason Grading System is the most widely used system for grading prostate cancer. Based on microscopic identification of glandular differentiation in tumor cells, tumors are graded from 1 to 5. Grade 1 represents the most well differentiated (most like the original cells), and grade 5 represents the most poorly differentiated (undifferentiated). Gleason grades are given to the two most commonly occurring patterns of cells and added together. The Gleason score, a number from 2 to 10, is used to predict how quickly the cancer will progress. A score of 2 to 4 indicates a slowly growing tumor. Grades 5 to 7 are associated with a more aggressive tumor with a 40% chance of metastasis. Grades 8 to 10 indicate an aggressive tumor with a 75% chance of metastasis (Lewis et al., 2007).

Medical Management

Treatment is based on the stage of the cancer—whether it has spread beyond the wall of the prostate, and to what extent—and the patient's age. In an older man with an estimated remaining life span of 5 to 10 years, controlling the disease with radiation or hormone therapy may be enough. In many cases, particularly in men older than 70 years of age, prostate cancer grows slowly, and hormone therapy can hold the disease at bay for several years.

Localized prostate cancer can be cured by radiation therapy or surgery. A treatment in which radioactive seed implants are placed directly in the prostate gland while sparing the surrounding tissue (rectum and bladder) is called brachytherapy. The seeds are accurately placed with a needle through a grid template guided by a transrectal ultrasound. Brachytherapy is a convenient, one-time outpatient procedure, whereas external radiation can take 5 to 6 weeks (Lewis et al., 2007). The seeds remain in the body, but their radioactivity declines over a period of months. Patients are advised to refrain from having children (or adults) sit in their lap and to avoid intercourse during the first 2 months after therapy. Radiation therapy also is used when the cancer has spread to just outside the gland, in an attempt to destroy cancer cells and shrink the prostate.

The operation to remove the prostate is a radical prostatectomy. Radical prostatectomy by the perineal approach is used in patients with early-stage clinical disease and is considered one of the most effective ways of eradicating the tumor. This procedure involves removing the entire prostate, including the true prostatic capsule, seminal vesicles, and a portion of the bladder neck. The remaining portion of the bladder neck is reanastomosed to the urethra. The retropubic approach is often the first choice because it provides access to the pelvic lymph nodes (pelvic lymphadenectomy) and affords more urinary control and less stricture formation. A third, nerve-sparing prostatectomy procedure uses a retropubic and perineal approach in an attempt to prevent impotence and reduce the likelihood of UI.

The three goals of a radical prostatectomy are removing all the tumor, preserving urine control, and preserving sexual function. Extent of sexual function may not be known for 6 to 12 months postoperatively. The patient needs emotional support related to the cancer and the possibility of impotence after surgery. Preoperative teaching should include an opportunity for the patient and his partner to discuss treatment options and mortality rate.

When the capsule of the prostate gland is removed, as with the perineal approach, the bladder and the lower urethra are no longer connected. The area where these two structures are reconnected is usually supported by placement of a Foley catheter. Extreme care must be taken to avoid placing tension on the catheter, which would disturb the surgical area. The catheter remains indwelling for several postoperative days.

In cases of advanced prostatic cancer, hormonal deprivation therapy may be used in an attempt to alter the tumor growth by blocking androgen (testosterone) production. Hormone deprivation therapy includes estrogens, gonadotropin-releasing hormone analogs, and antiandrogens. Luteinizing hormone–releasing hormone (LHRH) drugs act by causing an initial surge in luteinizing hormone and testosterone, rapidly followed by a decline in testosterone level similar to that achieved by castration. The primary forms of LHRH agonists are leuprolide (Lupron) and goserelin (Zoladex). Alternatives to LHRH agonists include oral nonsteroidal antiandrogens, including bicalutamide (Casodex), flutamide (Eulexin), and nilutamide (Nilandron) (Black & Hawks, 2009). Palliative therapy for patients with metastatic disease also may include orchiectomy (removal of the testes). Bilateral orchiectomy eliminates 95% of testosterone production, a step that is useful in managing metastatic disease. The patient may receive relief from such symptoms as pain or obstruction, but may experience feminization, increased incidence of cardiac disease, thrombophlebitis, pulmonary embolus, and stroke. Additional therapies are instituted to treat these side effects.

Radiation therapy may be used in advanced stages of the illness as primary or palliative treatment. Management of disseminated disease with cytotoxic drugs has been marginally successful.

Because cure for cancer of the prostate is possible only when the tumor is discovered early, it is important to teach all male patients older than the age of 40 to have annual or biannual rectal examinations and yearly PSA serum levels.

Nursing Interventions and Patient Teaching

Postoperative nursing management is similar to that for perineal surgery, with special attention to maintenance of bowel and bladder function while keeping the surgical wound clean and avoiding pressure on the perineum and wound. Adequate fluid intake, modification of dietary selections, and perineal exercises may be used to promote regulation of bowel and bladder function. Take extreme care to prevent trauma to the perineum, which could lead to fistula formation. Rectal temperature-taking, enemas, and use of rectal tubes are therefore forbidden. Also take care not to place tension on the Foley catheter, which would disturb the surgical area. Observe the color of the urine for signs of bleeding. The patient will also have a tissue drain inserted during surgery to promote drainage from the wound in the perineum. Initially there may be a small amount of urine from the drain, but this should cease in 1 or 2 days. Follow surgical asepsis during dressing changes. Irrigation of the perineum may be ordered to cleanse the wound and soothe the patient. Administer comfort measures and analgesics as ordered for pain control in the lower back, pelvis, upper thighs, and operative site.

Nursing diagnoses and interventions for the patient undergoing prostate surgery include but are not limited to the following:

Nursing Diagnoses	Nursing Interventions
Risk for fluid volume, deficient, related to hemorrhage or decreased fluid intake	Monitor signs and symptoms of fluid deficit: decreasing or increasing blood pressure, dyspnea. Observe catheter for urine color and amount. Avoid manipulation of rectum by thermometer or rectal tube.
Ineffective sexuality patterns, related to surgical trauma and altered body function	Encourage verbalization of sexual concerns. Provide privacy with significant other to discuss concerns. Inform physician of patient concerns. Explore professional resources: clergy, sexual counselors.

Because UI may occur postoperatively, teach the patient how to keep himself clean. He may need to discuss feelings of depression about his altered body function. Modifying lifestyle and maintaining confidence are important for his return to preillness function. Discuss alternate expressions of sexuality, the value of sexual counseling, and the possibility of recovering some or all of sexual function after treatment is completed.

Emphasize the need for adequate fluid intake, exercise, and rest. Instruct the patient in pain-relieving measures (e.g., exercise, warmth, and medication). Discuss new pharmacologic agents that act as adjuvants in the treatment of cancer and for pain relief during the postoperative recovery period.

Prognosis

Prognosis is directly correlated to the extent of the disease process when diagnosed. Grading of the tumors (well, moderately, or poorly differentiated) correlates with the prognosis; the more poorly differentiated the tumor, the poorer the prognosis is. Under the Gleason system discussed previously, a low score of 2 through 4 is good; a high score of 7 through 10 is not. The treatment goal for the localized disease process is a cure; palliation is used for the extended disease process.

URETHRAL STRICTURES

Etiology and Pathophysiology

A urethral stricture is a narrowing of the lumen of the urethra that interferes with urine flow. Narrowing may be congenital or acquired. Acquired strictures may be caused by chronic infection, trauma, or tumor or occur as a complication of radiation treatment of the pelvis.

Clinical Manifestations

Signs and symptoms include dysuria, weak stream, splaying (spreading out) of the urine stream, nocturia, and increasing pain with bladder distention. In the presence of infection, fever and malaise may be apparent.

Assessment

Subjective data include patient complaints of difficulty initiating the urine stream and the stream seeming to splay more than usual or even seeming to "fork."

Collection of **objective data** includes assessing for signs that may indicate an infectious process and for information indicating the extent of the stricture and possible presence of an obstruction.

Diagnostic Tests

Diagnosis can be confirmed by a voiding cystourethrogram, which demonstrates stricture. Additional diagnostic studies help evaluate damage caused by the obstruction.

Medical Management

Correction of the stricture may be achieved by dilation with metal sounds or surgical release (internal urethrotomy).

Nursing Interventions

Care includes adequate hydration to decrease discomfort when voiding and monitoring urinary output. Mild analgesics should relieve discomfort. Sitz baths may encourage voiding. Reconstruction of the urethra (urethroplasty) may require temporary urinary diversion. After the procedure a splinting catheter supports the suture line. Take care not to place tension on the catheter.

Prognosis

Prognosis after surgical correction or dilation is favorable.

URINARY TRACT TRAUMA

Etiology and Pathophysiology

Assess any patient with a history of traumatic injury for involvement of the urinary tract. Such injuries may include contusions or rupture of the urinary structures. Also observe a patient who has undergone abdominal surgery for incidental injury sustained during the operation. Traumatic invasion of the urinary tract may be evident in open wounds to the lower abdomen, such as gunshot or stab wounds. Trauma to the bladder can occur from a fractured pelvis. Contusion or laceration of the urethra may lead to urethral stricture and possible impotence in men secondary to soft tissue, blood vessel, and nerve damage.

Clinical Manifestations

Monitor urinary output hourly for amount and color. Report any evidence of hematuria. Assess the patient for abdominal pain and tenderness, which may indicate internal hemorrhage, peritonitis, or seepage of urine into the tissues.

Assessment

Collection of **subjective data** involves understanding that the trauma patient may be unable to relate any symptoms that would aid in the assessment of urinary tract involvement. If the patient is able to respond, asking about signs of hematuria is extremely important.

Collection of **objective data** includes a comprehensive assessment of the trauma patient, reviewing all body systems. Assessment related to the urinary tract includes hourly measurement of I&O; observation of urine character or difficulty voiding; evaluation of complaints of abdominal, flank, or referred shoulder pain; and evaluation of abdominal distention and girth.

Diagnostic Tests

Diagnosis of traumatic involvement of the urinary tract may be aided by KUB radiograph, IVP, urinalysis, excretory urogram, and cystoscopy.

Medical Management

Surgical intervention is necessary for correction of tears or rupture of the urinary tract to reinstate urine flow. If damage is severe, removal of the kidney or the bladder may be necessary with the creation of urinary diversion, as discussed later in this chapter. Management of possible hemorrhage and prevention of infection are necessary both before and after surgery.

Nursing Interventions

Nursing responsibility centers on identifying individuals at risk and detecting variations in assessment findings that indicate trauma to the urinary tract. Document and report all findings.

Prognosis

Prognosis depends on the extent and location of the trauma.

IMMUNOLOGIC DISORDERS OF THE KIDNEY

NEPHROTIC SYNDROME

Etiology and Pathophysiology

Nephrotic syndrome (nephrosis) is characterized by marked proteinuria, hypoalbuminemia, and edema. Several events may precipitate nephrotic syndrome; the primary form of nephrosis occurs in the absence of glomerulonephritis or systemic disease, with the inciting event being an upper respiratory tract infection or allergic reaction.

Nephrotic syndrome is characterized by proteinuria, hypoalbuminemia, hyperlipidemia, and edema. The most common sign is excess fluid in the body. This may take several forms: edema around the eyes, characteristically in the morning; pitting edema over the legs; fluid in the pleural cavity (pleural effusion); or fluid in the peritoneal cavity (ascites).

In nephrotic syndrome, the glomeruli become damaged due to inflammation, so that small proteins, such as albumins, immunoglobulins, and antithrombin, can pass through the kidneys into urine. Physiologic changes in the glomeruli interfere with selective permeability. Blood protein is allowed to pass into the urine (proteinuria), causing a loss of serum protein (hypoalbuminemia). This decreases serum osmotic pressure, thus allowing fluid to seep into interstitial spaces, and edema occurs.

Immune responses, both humoral and cellular, are altered in nephrotic syndrome; as a result, infection is an important cause of morbidity and mortality.

Clinical Manifestations

The patient has severe generalized edema (anasarca), anorexia, fatigue, and altered kidney function.

Assessment

Subjective data include patient complaints of loss of interest in eating, constant fatigue, foamy urine from the presence of protein, and decreased urinary output (oliguria), less than 500 mL in 24 hours.

Collection of **objective data** includes assessing the degree of fluid retention by monitoring daily weight, I&O, respiratory effort, and level of consciousness. The patient may relate problems with "swelling" of the face, hands, and feet. Assess skin integrity to determine special needs.

Diagnostic Tests

Blood chemistry findings include hypoalbuminemia and hyperlipidemia. Renal biopsy provides identification of the type and extent of tissue change. Other diagnostic testing is performed to identify the specific underlying cause.

Medical Management

Medical management depends on the extent of tissue involvement and may include the use of corticosteroids (prednisone); antineoplastic agents for immunosuppressive effect; loop diuretics; and a low-sodium, high-protein diet for therapeutic management of edema. Hypoproteinemia may be treated with normal serum albumin and protein-rich nutrition replacement therapy.

Nursing Interventions and Patient Teaching

Nursing interventions include monitoring fluid balance (weight, measurement of abdominal girth, I&O), maintaining bed rest in the presence of extreme edema (recumbent position may initiate diuresis), and assessing for electrolyte imbalance. Skin care is important, as is a gradual increase in activity as the edema is resolved.

Diet includes protein replacement using foods that provide high biologic value (meat, fish, poultry, cheese, eggs) and restriction of sodium to decrease edema. Blood pressure is often elevated and should be monitored closely for changes.

As the patient begins to convalesce, the teaching plan includes the medication regimen (type, dosage, side effects, and need to finish all prescriptions), nutrition (high protein, low sodium), self-assessment of fluid status (monitor weight, presence of edema), signs and symptoms indicating need for medical attention (increase in edema, fatigue, headache, infection), and the need for follow-up care.

Prognosis

In approximately 25% of children and 50% to 75% of adults who develop nephrosis, the disease progresses to renal failure within 5 years. Other patients (particularly children) may have remissions or chronic nephrotic syndrome. Aside from treating the underlying illness, little can be done to prevent a recurrence of nephrosis.

NEPHRITIS

Nephritis encompasses a number of renal disorders characterized by inflammation of the kidney—involving the glomeruli, tubules, or interstitial tissue—and abnormal function. Included in this group of disorders is acute and chronic glomerulonephritis.

Acute Glomerulonephritis
Etiology and Pathophysiology

The health history commonly reveals that the onset of acute glomerulonephritis was preceded by an infection, such as a sore throat or skin infection (most commonly β-hemolytic streptococci) 2 to 3 weeks earlier, or other preexisting multisystem diseases, such as systemic lupus erythematosus. The infectious disease process triggers an immune response that results in inflammation of glomeruli that allows excretion of red blood cells and protein in the urine. This condition is common in children and young adults.

Clinical Manifestations

Often family members first note that the individual has "swelling" of the face, especially around the eyes. Some patients may be acutely ill with a multitude of symptoms, whereas others may be diagnosed on routine examination with only vague symptoms.

Assessment

Subjective data include symptoms indicative of anorexia, nocturia, malaise, and exertional dyspnea.

Collection of **objective data** includes assessment of skin integrity and general condition of skin; the presence and degree of edema with associated difficulty in breathing on exertion, when recumbent, or as evidenced by changes in lung and heart sounds (unusual heart sounds, crackles over lung fields, distention of neck veins); hematuria with changes in urine color from "cola" to frank sanguineous; or changes in voiding, decrease in amount of urinary output, or dysuria.

Diagnostic Tests

Diagnostic tests reveal elevation of BUN, serum creatinine, potassium, erythrocyte sedimentation rate, and antistreptolysin-O titer. Urinalysis shows red blood cells, casts, and/or protein.

Medical Management

Medical management includes treatment of primary symptoms while preventing complications to cerebral and cardiac function. Serum electrolyte levels (sodium and potassium) may indicate a need to adjust dietary intake of sodium and potassium. Level of consciousness should be monitored when the BUN is elevated. Bed rest and fluid intake adjustments are guided by urinary output until diuresis is adequate.

A prophylactic antimicrobial agent, such as penicillin, may be administered for several months after the acute phase of the illness to protect against recurrence of infection. Diuretics may be prescribed to control fluid retention and antihypertensives to reduce blood pressure.

Nursing Interventions and Patient Teaching

Nursing interventions are guided by individual patient needs, focusing on control of symptoms and prevention of complications. Dietary intake includes pro-

Health Promotion

The Patient with Nephritis

Activity
- Keep patient on bed rest until edema and blood pressure are reduced.
- Encourage quiet diversional activities.
- Ambulate gradually with assistance.
- Space activity to lessen fatigue.

Fluid Balance Maintenance
- Implement dietary restrictions.
- Monitor intake and output.
- Document reactions to medication.

Diet Therapy
- Restrict protein to decrease nitrogenous wastes.
- Restrict sodium to prevent further fluid retention.
- Increase calories for energy source.

Drug Therapy
- Prophylactic antibiotics
- Antihypertensives
- Diuretics
- Drug interactions, side effects to expect and report

Health Maintenance
- Recovery may be extended.
- Physician will monitor urine for albumin and red blood cells (RBCs).
- Teach early signs of fluid retention.
- Signs and symptoms may resolve and then become worse.
- Normal activities may be resumed after urine is free of albumin and RBCs for 1 month, although the patient is not considered cured until the urine is free of albumin and RBCs for 6 months.
- Report hematuria, headache, edema.

tein restrictions (to decrease blood urea levels), with carbohydrates providing a source of energy.

Monitor I&O and vital signs. Determine the level of activity based on the degree of edema, hypertension, proteinuria, and hematuria, since excessive activity may increase these signs (see Health Promotion box).

Because of the long-term nature of glomerulonephritis, patient teaching is important. Proteinuria and hematuria may exist microscopically even when other symptoms subside. Although fatigue may be present, these patients usually feel well; therefore they often must be convinced of the need to continue prescribed treatment and to return for follow-up care. Explain the nature of the illness and the effect of diet and fluids on fluid balance and sodium retention. Teach about prescribed sodium and fluid restrictions (provide written information regarding sodium content of foods, as necessary). Include information about protein restrictions and carbohydrate sources. Also discuss the medication regimen (dose, frequency, side effects, need to continue per physician instructions). Stress the need to pace activities with rest if fatigue is present; to avoid trauma and infection (which may exacerbate the illness); and to obtain follow-up health care. Teach the patient about the signs and symptoms indicating the need for medical attention (hematuria, headache, edema, hypertension).

Prognosis
The prognosis of acute poststreptococcal glomerulonephritis is generally good; however, some patients develop chronic glomerulonephritis and ESRD, requiring dialysis or kidney transplantation.

Chronic Glomerulonephritis
Etiology and Pathophysiology
With chronic glomerulonephritis there is usually no indication of an inciting event. Occasionally the patient with acute glomerulonephritis progresses to a chronic phase. Because other chronic illnesses (e.g., diabetes mellitus or systemic lupus erythematosus) may mask the symptoms of renal degeneration, many patients do not seek medical attention until kidney function is compromised. Chronic glomerulonephritis is characterized by slow, progressive destruction of glomeruli with related loss of function. The kidneys atrophy (actually decrease in size).

Clinical Manifestations
Signs and symptoms may include malaise, morning headaches, dyspnea with exertion, visual and digestive disturbances, edema, and fatigue. Physical findings include hypertension, anemia, proteinuria, anasarca, and cardiac and cerebral manifestations.

Assessment
Subjective data include patient complaints of fatigue and a decreased ability to perform ADLs as a result of dyspnea and decreasing ability to concentrate. Investigate complaints of morning headaches (their location, pattern, and character), and note the presence of any visual disturbance.

Collection of **objective data** includes clarifying outward manifestations of the headache and respiratory effort that may interfere with daily task performance. Assess mental functioning, irritability, slurred speech, ataxia, or tremors. Carefully assess and document the degree of edema, noting specific location and response to pressure by pressing the fingers into the edematous area and observing for pitting (see Figure 8-17). Note skin color, ecchymoses (irregularly formed hemorrhagic areas of the skin) or rash, dry skin, and scratching. Observe urine color and amount. Monitor vital signs, including a chest assessment for cardiac and pulmonary signs of fluid retention: unusual heart sounds, crackles over lung fields, and distention of neck veins.

Diagnostic Tests
Early disease shows albumin and red blood cells in the urine, although kidney function test results are within normal limits. With advanced destruction of nephrons, the specific gravity becomes fixed and blood levels of

NPN wastes (creatinine and urea) increase. Creatinine clearance may be as low as 5 to 10 mL/min, compared with the normal range of 107 to 139 mL/min in men and 87 to 107 mL/min in women.

Medical Management

Medical management includes control of secondary side effects as discussed with acute glomerulonephritis, with the use of renal dialysis and possible kidney transplantation to provide elimination of wastes from the body.

Nursing Interventions and Patient Teaching

Nursing interventions for the patient with chronic glomerulonephritis represent a special challenge. This patient has already suffered major damage to the kidney filtration system. It is crucial that the patient's condition not be further compromised by infection or other complications. Monitor changes in vital signs and diagnostic tests to aid in choosing proper nursing interventions. Interventions parallel those noted with nephrotic syndrome and acute glomerulonephritis. Chronic glomerulonephritis may progress to ESRD, necessitating related nursing interventions (see Health Promotion box, p. 472).

Nursing diagnoses and interventions for the patient with chronic glomerulonephritis include but are not limited to the following:

Nursing Diagnoses	Nursing Interventions
Excess fluid volume, related to decreased urinary output	Assess the patient's understanding of therapeutic interventions.
	Note I&O every hour (or more often).
	Monitor signs and symptoms of fluid excess: weight gain, hypertension, edema, dyspnea.
	Provide ice chips for thirst with prescribed diet.
	Monitor and report abnormal laboratory results.
Activity intolerance, related to kidney dysfunction	Assess level of activity tolerance.
	Encourage patient to report activities that increase his or her fatigue.
	Plan activities to minimize fatigue.

Patient teaching focuses on preventive health maintenance, emphasizing a health-promoting lifestyle, with prevention and early treatment of infections.

Prognosis

Some people with minimal impairment in kidney function continue to feel well and show little progression of disease. With other patients the progression of renal de-

terioration may be slow but steady and end in renal failure. In still others the disease progresses rapidly.

RENAL FAILURE

Renal failure is characterized by the kidneys' inability to remove wastes, concentrate urine, and conserve or eliminate electrolytes. Diabetes mellitus is the most common cause of renal failure, accounting for more than 40% of new cases. Other predisposing concurrent illnesses include burns, trauma, heart failure, volume depletion, and renal disease. Nursing interventions to prevent the development of renal failure include providing adequate hydration, preventing infections, monitoring for signs and symptoms of shock, and teaching drug side effects to report immediately.

ACUTE RENAL FAILURE

Etiology and Pathophysiology

Kidney function may be altered by interference with the kidney's ability to be selective in filtering blood or by an actual decrease in blood flow to the kidneys. ARF can be caused by a number of medical conditions, such as hemorrhage, trauma, infection, and decreased cardiac output.

The course of ARF is divided into phases. In the **oliguric phase,** BUN and serum creatinine levels rise while urinary output decreases to less than 20 mL/hr (less than 400 mL/24 hr). The oliguric phase may last from several days to 4 weeks to several months. Some patients may experience the nonoliguric form, usually caused by nephrotoxic antibiotics, in which urinary output may exceed 2 L/24 hr. In the **diuretic phase,** blood chemistry levels begin to return to normal and urinary output increases to 1 to 2 L/24 hr. The diuretic phase usually lasts 1 to 3 weeks. Return to normal or near-normal function occurs in the **recovery phase.** Recovery begins as the glomerular filtration rate rises. Recovery can take up to 1 year.

Clinical Manifestations

The patient may experience anorexia, nausea, vomiting, edema, and associated signs and symptoms of diminished kidney function.

Assessment

Subjective data include patient reports of lethargy, loss of appetite, nausea, and headache.

Objective data involve physical findings of progression of the disease process. Assess for dry mucous membranes, poor skin turgor, urinary output of less than 400 mL/24 hr, vomiting, diarrhea, and anasarca. Assessment findings may include central nervous system manifestations of drowsiness, muscle twitching, and seizures.

Diagnostic Tests

Physical assessment, history, and elevated blood chemistry tests such as BUN and creatinine (azotemia) confirm the diagnosis. After the patient is stabilized, further studies may be done to assess for residual damage.

Medical Management

Measures include administration of fluids and osmotic preparations to prevent decreased renal perfusion, manage fluid volume, and treat electrolyte imbalances. Renal dialysis may be necessary to manage systemic fluid shifts, especially cardiac and respiratory, and may be effective in removing some nephrotoxins.

Diet should be protein sparing, high in carbohydrates, and low in potassium and sodium. Drug therapy may include diuretics to increase urinary output (e.g., furosemide, hydrochlorothiazide [HydroDIURIL]). Potassium-lowering agents are used to remove potassium through the gastrointestinal tract; sodium polystyrene sulfonate (Kayexalate) is administered orally, per nasogastric tube, or as a retention enema. Antibiotics that are not dependent on kidney excretion are used to eradicate or prevent infection. Whatever combination of drug therapy is used, dosage and administration times require adjustment according to the level of kidney function.

Nursing Interventions and Patient Teaching

Accurately document urinary output to identify the level of kidney function. Azotemia may be revealed by blood chemistry studies. Observe the patient with azotemia for changes in level of consciousness. Closely monitor fluid status, vital signs, and response to therapies. Frequent skin care with tepid water to remove urea crystals will be comforting. Dialysis presents special nursing challenges, discussed later in this chapter.

Teaching includes identifying preventable environmental or health factors contributing to the illness (such as hypertension, nephrotoxic drugs). Teach the patient about activity restrictions, dietary restrictions, and the medication regimen. Provide nutritional support with specialized enteral formulas, which may contain essential amino acids and minerals, in addition to replacement of electrolytes (especially sodium to match insensible loss) and provision of caloric needs. Make a nutritional assessment with appropriate modifications daily.

Stress the need to report signs and symptoms of infection and of returning renal failure to the physician. Emphasize the need for ongoing follow-up care.

Prognosis

Recovery from an episode of ARF depends on the underlying illness, the patient's condition, and careful supportive management given during the period of kidney shutdown. The leading cause of death is infection, such as that of the urinary tract, lungs, and peritoneum. Mortality from fluid overload and acidosis has been reduced as a result of dialysis and other forms of therapy. Patients who survive the acute episode of tubular insufficiency have a chance of recovering kidney function. Although renal tissue may regenerate more completely after toxic injury than ischemia, both forms usually show return to normal or near-normal kidney function.

For those in whom ARF has been caused by glomerular disease or severe infection of renal tissue, the prognosis may not be as favorable. Return of kidney function is determined by the extent of scarring and destruction of functional renal tissue that has occurred during the acute episode of renal failure.

CHRONIC RENAL FAILURE (END-STAGE RENAL DISEASE)

Etiology and Pathophysiology

Chronic renal failure, or ESRD, exists when the kidneys are unable to regain normal function. ESRD develops slowly over an extended period as a result of renal disease or other disease processes that compromise renal blood perfusion. As much as 80% of nephrons may be severely impaired before loss of kidney function is detected. The most common causes of ESRD are pyelonephritis, chronic glomerulonephritis, glomerulosclerosis, chronic urinary obstruction, severe hypertension, diabetes mellitus, gout, and PKD. Whatever the cause, dialysis or kidney transplantation is needed to maintain life.

ESRD represents a significant health problem worldwide, resulting in the death of thousands and financial crisis for patients and their families. The government actively helps defray costs through the Medicare program.

Clinical Manifestations

The onset of signs and symptoms may be so gradual and the signs and symptoms so vague that the patient is unable to identify when the problems started. When questioned, the patient may be able to relate occurrences that seemed insignificant at the time. The clinical picture is usually unique to the individual. Common symptoms are headache; lethargy; asthenia (decreased strength or energy); anorexia; pruritus; elimination changes; anuria (urinary output of less than 100 mL/day); muscle cramps or twitching; impotence; characteristic dusky yellow-tan or gray skin color from retained urochrome pigments; and signs and symptoms characteristic of central nervous system involvement, such as disorientation and mental lapses.

Other associated conditions are responsible for many of the symptoms. Azotemia develops as excessive amounts of nitrogenous compounds build in the blood. Anemia occurs when the production of renal erythropoietin is decreased as a result of loss of kidney function. Acidosis, hypertension, and glucose intolerance may be present as a result of the insult to homeostasis.

Assessment

Subjective data include patient complaints of joint pain and edema; severe headaches; nausea; anorexia; intermittent chest pain; weakness; and in particular, fatigue, intractable singultus (hiccups), decreased libido, menstrual irregularities, and impaired concentration. The clinical consequences of renal failure are far reaching, affecting nearly every body system.

Collection of **objective data** involves a nursing assessment that may yield unremarkable results, except for signs and symptoms that support the patient complaints. Uremic encephalopathy affects the central nervous system. Usually the first sign is a reduction in alertness and awareness. The patient exhibits Kussmaul's respirations (abnormally deep, very rapid sighing respirations), and coma develops. The accumulation of urates results in halitosis with a urine odor and "uremic frost" on the skin in the form of a white powder.

Diagnostic Tests

Diagnosis of ESRD is confirmed by elevated BUN of at least 50 mg/dL and serum creatinine levels greater than 5 mg/dL, electrolyte imbalance (including a decreased number of bicarbonate and magnesium and an increased number of potassium, sodium, and phosphatase ions), and other indicators related to the underlying cause. Kidney function studies assess the degree of damage or level of kidney function.

Medical Management

Medical management is instituted to conserve kidney function as long as possible. Renal dialysis is initiated when necessary, and the patient may be prepared for kidney transplantation. Drug therapy may include anticonvulsants to control seizure activity (phenytoin [Dilantin], diazepam [Valium]), antianemics, vitamin supplements to counteract nutritional deficiencies, antiemetics (prochlorperazine [Compazine]), antipruritics (cyproheptadine [Periactin]), and biologic response modifiers to stimulate red cell production (epoetin alfa [Epogen, EPO]) to treat anemia caused by a reduced production of erythropoietin. Iron deficiency anemia must be treated with ferrous sulfate orally or iron dextran (DexFerrum per Z-track intramuscular method) before epoetin alfa will be effective.

Nursing Interventions and Patient Teaching

Nursing interventions focus on restoring homeostasis. Measures to control fluid and electrolyte balance vary greatly, according to individual patient needs. Nutritional therapy is aimed at preserving protein stores and preventing production of additional protein waste products that the kidney would have to clear. High biologic proteins are used to provide the essential amino acids.

The diet is high in calories from carbohydrates and fats from polyunsaturated sources (to maintain weight and spare protein), at least 2500 to 3000 calories daily. Other dietary restrictions are related to the patient's degree of acidosis. Potassium is retained, so foods high in potassium are restricted. Sodium is controlled at a level sufficient to replace sodium loss without causing fluid retention.

Nursing interventions for ARF are also instituted for ESRD. Provide emotional support for the patient who faces role changes and invasive treatments such as dialysis or kidney transplantation. As discussed in the Health Promotion box, fluid balance is of prime importance. The patient may have fluid equal to the amount excreted in the urine plus about 300 to 600 mL to compensate for **insensible** (imperceptible) **fluid loss** (fluid lost through the lungs, perspiration, and feces). Salt substitutes are not advised because most contain potassium. If seizure activity occurs, institute safety measures to protect the patient (Nursing Care Plan 10-1) (see also Chapter 14).

Patient teaching should emphasize food exchanges and fluid intake within restrictions prescribed for that patient. Encourage the patient to increase activity as tolerated; maintain impeccable skin care; prevent infection and injury; and develop coping behaviors to adapt to lifestyle changes for patient, family, and caregiver.

 Health Promotion

The Patient with Renal Failure

Fluid and Electrolyte Balance
- Assess intake and output (hourly may be indicated).
- Weigh daily (same time, same clothing, same scale).
- Assess overt (open to view) signs of hydration status: edema, turgor.
- Assess covert (hidden) signs of hydration status: breath sounds, laboratory studies, and so on.

Nutrition
- Provide prescribed diet.
- Guide patient food selection.
- Plan fluid intake per shift within prescribed limits and according to patient preference.
- Reinforce diet instructions as indicated.

Comfort and Safety
- Provide quiet environment (sound and lighting).
- Space nursing interventions to conserve patient energy.
- Medicate as needed for comfort.
- Provide skin care to alleviate discomfort from pruritus.
- Provide mouth care as needed.
- Maintain asepsis during procedures.
- Prevent exposure to pathogens.

Coping Behaviors
- Listen (to patient and significant others).
- Refer to pastoral care or religious support group.
- Provide private times with significant others.
- Offer interview with social services.

Documentation and Reporting
- Document all relevant findings.
- Maintain open communications with supervisory staff.
- Adjust nursing care plan as indicated to meet changing patient needs.
- Maintain dietary restrictions: food exchange, measuring fluids, food diary.
- Take health promotion–illness prevention measures.

Nursing Care Plan 10-1   The Patient with End-Stage Renal Disease

Mr. Jerrod, a 37-year-old high school basketball coach, visited his family physician with complaints of weight gain, decreasing strength, increasing inability to concentrate, and morning headaches. Physical examination revealed severe hypertension, yellow-gray skin color, and pale mucous membranes. After diagnostic studies reveal chronic glomerulonephritis with end-state renal disease (ESRD), Mr. Jerrod is admitted to the hospital to stabilize his condition.

NURSING DIAGNOSIS *Excess fluid volume, related to compromised renal regulatory mechanism, as evidenced by systemic edema*

Patient Goals and Expected Outcomes	Nursing Interventions	Evaluation
The patient will be able to reduce fluid to precrisis level	Record baseline assessment data. Create chart for patient to monitor: • Daily weight • Intake and output • Edema	Patient is able to complete daily self-monitoring with 1 pound weight loss daily × 3.
The patient will modify diet to exclude foods and fluids that foster sodium, potassium, and water retention	Teach nutritional guidelines for dietary and fluid parameters with scheduling. Evaluate daily or as needed for systemic edema: girth, skin turgor, respiratory rate and quality. Monitor for manifestations of electrolyte imbalance. Teach patient and significant other about the type, cause, and treatment for fluid and electrolyte imbalance, as appropriate.	Patient is able to order daily diet and fluids within prescribed parameters.

NURSING DIAGNOSIS *Powerlessness, related to sudden onset of life-altering illness as evidenced by patient statements: "I've always tried to take care of myself—look where it got me. Nowhere! Now I have to face my own death!"*

Patient Goals and Expected Outcomes	Nursing Interventions	Evaluation
The patient will be empowered to assist in planning own care and in goal achievement	Provide support for the patient. Explain plans and procedures before scheduled times, according to patient's ability to understand. Negotiate with patient when changes are necessary. Accept patient's expression of self and values. Include significant other in planning for the patient's maximum role in self-management. Communicate unique patient planning arrangements for continuity with all treatment team members.	Patient voices a sense that the staff is sensitive to his needs. Patient seems able to plan modifications in work and home schedules to accommodate health needs.

NURSING DIAGNOSIS *Deficient knowledge, related to health education and home maintenance for ESRD*

Patient Goals and Expected Outcomes	Nursing Interventions	Evaluation
The patient will describe the fundamental characteristics of ESRD and treatment options	Assess the amount and depth of the patient's information about ESRD. Collaborate with physician and treatment team in individualizing established institutional protocol for care of the patient with ESRD: 1. What happens when kidneys fail? 2. Treatment options • Hemodialysis • Peritoneal dialysis • Kidney transplantation	Patient is able to correctly answer basic questions about treatment options. Patient is able to correctly answer questions from teaching and is open to pose new questions.

Continued

⭐ **Nursing Care Plan 10-1** | **The Patient with End-Stage Renal Disease—cont'd**

Patient Goals and Expected Outcomes	Nursing Interventions	Evaluation
The patient will describe the fundamental characteristics of ESRD and treatment options—cont'd	3. Inpatient versus outpatient care 4. Financing treatment 5. Teaching aids 6. Organizations that can help Plan time to listen to the patient's and family's concerns and fears. Allow time for questions and answers and teaching reinforcement each day. Arrange (with patient's permission) opportunity for patient and family to meet with a patient or family who is positively adapting to ESRD. Be consistent in scheduling treatments with primary health care providers. Participate in end-of-life planning, when and if appropriate.	

Critical Thinking Questions

1. Mr. Jerrod complains of loss of appetite and limited food choices. What would be some helpful suggestions to improve his nutritional status?
2. Mr. Jerrod established a therapeutic nurse-patient relationship with the nurse and confided that he is having marital problems partly due to his inability to have a satisfactory sexual relationship with his wife. What would be an appropriate response?
3. The nurse notes Mr. Jerrod's lack of interest in his therapeutic regimen of diet, medications, and fluid restrictions. He states, "What's the use? I will never be well again." What would be some therapeutic interventions?

CARE OF THE PATIENT REQUIRING DIALYSIS

Dialysis is a medical procedure for the removal of certain elements from the blood; the process is based on the difference in their rates of diffusion through an external semipermeable membrane or, in the case of peritoneal dialysis, through the peritoneum. Dialysis mimics kidney function, helping to restore balance when normal kidney function is interrupted temporarily or permanently. Dialysis involves either diffusion of wastes, drugs, and/or excess electrolytes and/or osmosis of water across a semipermeable membrane into a dialysate fluid that is prescribed to meet individual needs. Dialysis is achieved by the process of hemodialysis or peritoneal dialysis.

HEMODIALYSIS

Hemodialysis is used for patients with acute or irreversible renal failure and fluid and electrolyte imbalances. Hemodialysis requires access to the patient's circulatory system to route blood through the artificial kidney (dialyzer) for removal of wastes, fluids, and electrolytes; the blood is then returned to the patient's body. Box 10-4 lists nursing intervention guidelines. Temporary methods include subclavian or femoral catheters or an external shunt placed in the nondominant forearm (Figure 10-9). In ESRD, access can be achieved by constructing a direct or a graft arteriovenous (AV) fistula (Figure 10-10). The AV fistula is preferred for permanent access. Hemodialysis is usually scheduled three times a week for 3 to 6 hours. Patients can be maintained on dialysis therapy indefinitely or while waiting for kidney transplantation.

In a comparative study of the use of daily versus traditional hemodialysis on alternative days, researchers found that more frequent hemodialysis decreased the risk of fatal nonrenal complications of ARF (Schiffl et al., 2002).

Medical Management

Medical management includes continuation of previously instituted therapies. Closely monitor blood levels of drugs excreted by the kidney to maintain therapeutic levels and prevent toxic accumulations. Dose adjustments are affected by glomerular filtration rate, dialysis, vomiting, and doses missed during hospital treatments. Medication may include antihypertensives, cardiac glycosides, antibiotics, and antidysrhythmics. Instruct the patient not to take over-the-counter medications without consulting the physician.

Box 10-4 Nursing Intervention Guidelines for the Patient Undergoing Hemodialysis

PATIENT TEACHING
- Reinforce explanation of dialysis procedure.
- Inform of community resources.
- Explain dietary restrictions.
- Teach about self-care, general information.

MONITORING DURING DIALYSIS
- Maintain asepsis and universal precautions.
- Weigh before and after treatment.
- Obtain vital signs every 30 to 60 minutes (take blood pressure in arm without fistula).
- Maintain orientation (thought processes may be altered).
- Assess for hemorrhage resulting from heparin use during dialysis.
- Monitor equipment (interruption of procedure).

ACTIVITY
- Provide diversions (reading, television, sleep).
- Ensure patient comfort (reclining, sitting, lying).
- Monitor dietary intake (may be hungry or nauseated).

CARE AFTER DIALYSIS OR BETWEEN TREATMENTS
- Schedule fluid intake within restrictions.
- Monitor for signs of fluid and electrolyte imbalance.
- Assess the access site for signs of infection, adequate circulation.
- Post signs regarding location of access site; do not take blood pressure or perform a venipuncture on arm with access site.
- Auscultate arteriovenous fistula for bruit (adventitious sound of venous or arterial origin heard on auscultation); palpate arteriovenous fistula for thrill (abnormal tremor).
- Assess, document, and report changes in general status.
- Provide skin care: bathe with tepid water to remove urea deposit.

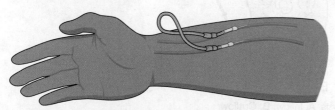

FIGURE 10-9 External arteriovenous shunt.

Nursing Interventions

Nursing interventions are dictated by individual patient conditions, including other acute or chronic problems. Most patients are dialyzed on an outpatient basis. (General nursing intervention guidelines are noted in Box 10-4 and in Nursing Care Plan 10-1.) Psychosocial aspects of care for patients receiving dialysis are illustrated in the Communication box on p. 476.

Nurses have a key responsibility for maintaining access sites and preventing or managing infection. Use a structured teaching program, with individualized patient teaching strategies to accommodate culture and knowledge level.

PERITONEAL DIALYSIS

Peritoneal dialysis can be performed with a minimum of equipment and by an ambulatory patient. Unlike hemodialysis, peritoneal dialysis is performed four times a day, 7 days a week. One exchange cycle usually requires 30 to 40 minutes. The principle of osmosis and diffusion through a semipermeable membrane is the same as in hemodialysis, but the peritoneum is used as the semipermeable membrane instead of the artificial kidney. Peritoneal dialysis is contraindicated for patients with systemic inflammatory disease, previous abdominal surgery, and chronic back pain, among other conditions.

To facilitate peritoneal dialysis, the physician places a catheter into the peritoneal space under aseptic conditions (Figure 10-11). The dialyzing fluid is instilled for a predetermined period, then drained. The patient with ESRD may be maintained on peritoneal dialysis, continuous ambulatory peritoneal dialysis (CAPD), or continuous cycle peritoneal dialysis (CCPD). Nocturnal intermittent peritoneal dialysis can be done three to five times per week for 10 to 12 hours. The patient is taught how to do the dialysis, which allows for more freedom. Although hemodialysis can also be done at home using strict aseptic technique, it is much more expensive and confining than CAPD.

Nursing Interventions

Common complications associated with peritoneal dialysis guide nursing interventions. Hypotension may occur with excessive sodium and fluid removal. Perito-

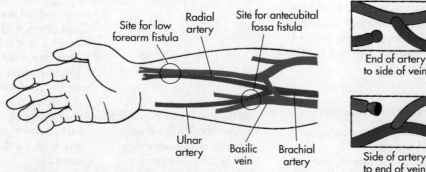
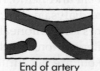
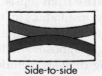
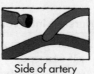

FIGURE 10-10 Internal arteriovenous fistula. Types of fistula construction.

Communication

Psychosocial Aspects of Care for Patients Receiving Dialysis

Mr. Jonas, a student nurse, enters Mr. Klauss's room to complete the initial morning assessment and finds him crying while struggling to get out of bed.

Nurse: Mr. Klauss, what's wrong? (general lead, allows patient to describe)

Patient: Oh, nothing!

Nurse: (therapeutic silence, remains attentive, gives time)

Patient: Nothing is going right. I might as well be dead!

Nurse: What's wrong? (general lead, patient did not answer, encourages description)

Patient: I was trying to get up to take a shower, but I'm so weak I can't get myself out of bed.

Nurse: That must be frustrating. (voicing the implied)

Patient: That's an understatement! Look at me! I'm 37 years old; I should be in my prime but instead I'm gaining weight; can't do my job because I can't concentrate. How am I supposed to feel?

Nurse: It must be frightening to experience all these changes. It would be understandable for you to be scared. (validating feelings)

Patient: I am scared! What if I never get better? I read this article about someone younger than I am who had the same thing and he died when he had to go on dialysis.

Nurse: What do you think will happen to you? (general lead, encourages description without prescribing response)

Patient: Well, I don't know. The doctor keeps avoiding my questions and I see myself being less able to do anything. Maybe I am afraid—afraid of dying.

Nurse: (therapeutic silence, allows time for reflection)

Patient: Well, I never thought I'd say that—being afraid to die. It doesn't seem so frightening to say. I guess I didn't trust myself to be honest with myself or anyone else.

Nurse: Being honest with yourself is an important step to understanding. (pause) It seems, too, that you may not have accurate information about your illness. Let's plan to talk with your doctor about what you can reasonably expect—things you will be able to do, limitations, and things that you can do to enhance your physical and emotional health. (summarizing and goal setting for individualized patient teaching and discharge planning)

Patient: That sounds great, Mr. Jonas. I really do want to do whatever I can to improve my chances of a better life. Would you help me get up to shower?

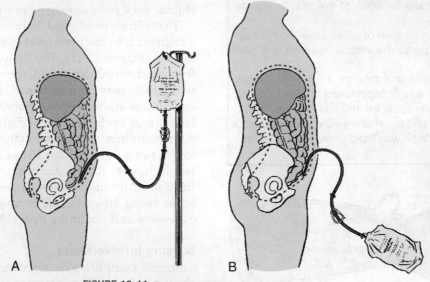

FIGURE 10-11 Peritoneal dialysis. **A,** Inflow. **B,** Outflow.

nitis may arise from sepsis. Pain and hemorrhage may accompany instillation of the dialysate. Box 10-5 lists nursing intervention guidelines for peritoneal dialysis.

Nursing diagnoses and interventions for the patient undergoing dialysis include but are not limited to the following:

Nursing Diagnoses	Nursing Interventions
Ineffective role performance, related to: • chronic illness • treatment side effects	Encourage verbalization of self-concept. Assist in identifying personal strengths.

Nursing Diagnoses	Nursing Interventions
	Assist patient and significant others with clarifying expected roles and those that must be relinquished or altered. Support grief work if loss of role has occurred.
Ineffective tissue perfusion, peripheral, related to: • risk of disconnection • clotting of vascular access	Avoid taking blood pressure and venipuncture in arm with fistula or cannula. Auscultate for bruits.

Box 10-5	Nursing Intervention Guidelines for the Patient Undergoing Peritoneal Dialysis

PATIENT TEACHING
- Explanation of procedure
- Signs of complications
- Diet or fluid restrictions
- Medication (schedule in relation to dialysis time)
- Dialysate kept at body temperature to lessen discomfort

MONITORING DURING DIALYSIS
- Weight before and after procedure
- Hemorrhage (smoky, pink, or red-tinged dialysate)
- Type of dialysate (tailored to patient needs)
- Amount and timing of dialysate instillation
- Vital signs

CARE BETWEEN DIALYSES
- Signs of peritonitis (pain, fever, cloudy fluid)
- Strict aseptic care of catheter site
- Weigh daily

Nursing Diagnoses	Nursing Interventions
Ineffective tissue perfusion, peripheral, related to: • risk of disconnection • clotting of vascular access	Observe access site for skin color and condition. After dialysis, inspect needle puncture sites for bleeding.

Prognosis

The patient with effective medical management can be maintained indefinitely on dialysis.

SURGICAL PROCEDURES FOR URINARY DYSFUNCTION

If damage to the urinary system cannot be corrected by medical management, surgical intervention may be necessary for temporary or permanent resection of the affected organ, such as when kidney function is lost. Dialysis is a viable management alternative, but a kidney transplant is preferable. The patient may require a kidney from a live or cadaver donor to replace the damaged kidney. Common surgical interventions and nursing intervention priorities are listed in Table 10-4. Pre-

operative and intraoperative management measures are the same as for major abdominal surgery with general anesthesia (see Chapter 2). Suggested nursing diagnoses include those for abdominal surgery.

NEPHRECTOMY

Nephrectomy is the surgical removal of the kidney, either a small portion or the entire organ and surrounding tissues. In partial nephrectomy, only the diseased or infected portion of the kidney is removed. Radical nephrectomy involves removing the entire kidney, a section of the ureter, the adrenal gland, and the fatty tissue surrounding the kidney.

Postoperative management for surgical removal of the kidney is based on the prevention and detection of hemorrhage by monitoring vital signs, especially pulse and blood pressure; observation for restlessness and for gastrointestinal complications of nausea, vomiting, and abdominal distention; and establishment of adequate urinary drainage. Record I&O. If the thoracic cavity is opened during surgery, the patient will have chest tubes (see Chapter 9). Pain may compromise respiratory efficiency. Administer analgesics as ordered to facilitate lung expansion and the patient's activity level. Reposition the patient every 2 hours and ambulate as ordered. Change dressings according to the physician's order, and record the amount and color of any drainage. Maintain close surveillance on the function of the remaining kidney.

Patient Teaching

Instruct the patient to avoid heavy lifting, drink 2000 mL of fluid each day (unless contraindicated), monitor output, avoid use of alcohol, and avoid respiratory tract infections and hazardous activities that could damage the remaining kidney.

Prognosis

Complete recovery from nephrectomy is expected in the absence of any complication.

NEPHROSTOMY

A nephrostomy is an incision created between the kidney and the skin to drain urine directly from the renal pelvis. A nephrostomy is performed when an occlu-

Table 10-4	Surgical Procedures for Urinary Dysfunction	
SURGICAL INTERVENTION		**NURSING INTERVENTION PRIORITIES**
Nephrostomy: Surgical procedure in which an incision is made on the patient's flank, so that a catheter can be inserted into the renal pelvis for drainage		Meticulous skin care, assessment for hemorrhage, accurate intake and output (I&O)
Nephrectomy: Surgical removal of the kidney		Assessment for hemorrhage, promotion of respiratory effort, accurate I&O
Cystectomy: Surgical removal of the bladder		Promotion of urinary drainage via ileal conduit, I&O
Ureterosigmoidostomy: Surgical procedure in which a ureter is implanted in the sigmoid colon of the intestinal tract		Meticulous skin care, monitoring of electrolyte imbalance, assessment of signs and symptoms of infection
Cutaneous ureterostomy: Surgical implantation of the terminal ends of the ureter under the skin		Meticulous skin care, assessment of urinary obstruction, accurate I&O

sion keeps urine from passing from the kidney, through the ureter, and into the urinary bladder. Without a way for urine to drain, pressure would rise within the urinary system and damage the kidneys. The most common cause of obstruction is cancer. This procedure can also be used to remove kidney stones.

Catheters are used to drain the wound. Take care to prevent obstruction of the catheters with blood clots postoperatively. Measure and record the amount and nature of drainage from the catheters, and change dressings frequently, keeping the skin clean using surgical sepsis. Turn the patient and position on the affected side as ordered to facilitate drainage and assist in respiratory ventilation. Never clamp a nephrostomy catheter (tube); acute pyelonephritis may result. If ordered by the physician, irrigate a nephrostomy catheter using strict aseptic technique. Gentle instillation of no more than 5 mL of sterile saline solution at one time prevents renal damage.

KIDNEY TRANSPLANTATION

Kidney transplantation is performed as an intervention in irreversible renal failure. The kidney is surgically placed retroperitoneally in the iliac fossa. The renal artery is anastomosed to the recipient's internal or external iliac artery and the renal vein to the recipient's iliac vein. Usually, the kidney begins to function immediately.

Selection of a transplant recipient is based on careful evaluation of the patient's medical, immunologic, and psychosocial status. Usually a recipient is younger than age 70, has an estimated life expectancy of 2 years or more, and is expected to have an improved quality of life after transplantation. Through conservative management and dialysis, the patient's state is as nontoxic as possible. Preoperative nursing intervention is complicated by the patient's fear and anxiety about transplantation and about possible rejection of the implanted organ. The patient is dialyzed until surgery can be satisfactorily completed. In surgery the nonfunctioning kidney remains in place and the donor kidney is positioned in the iliac fossa anterior to the crest of the ileum. The ureter is anastomosed into either the patient's ureter or bladder (Figure 10-12). However, bilateral nephrectomy may be performed before the transplantation procedure for persistent or active bacterial pyleonephritis, uncontrolled reninmediated hypertension, polycystic kidneys, or rapidly progressive glomerulonephritis.

Postoperatively, assess the patient for signs of rejection and infection: apprehension, generalized edema, fever, increased blood pressure, oliguria, edema, and tenderness over the graft site. An immunosuppressive agent, such as cyclosporine, is used alone or in conjunction with steroids. Cyclosporine is considered an effective drug in suppressing the immune system's efforts to reject tissue while leaving the recipient sufficient immune activity to combat infection. Mycopheno-

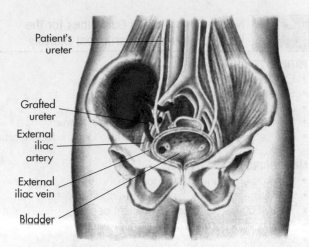

FIGURE 10-12 Kidney transplantation.

late (CellCept) and tacrolimus (Prograf) are drugs used to prevent rejection of kidney transplants; they are used in combination with corticosteroids. Immunosuppressive therapy increases the risk for infection and possible steroid-induced bleeding.

Patient Teaching

Postoperative care includes special assessment of kidney function and electrolyte balance. The function of the transplanted kidney is the primary concern after surgery. Home follow-up becomes a life pattern for the transplantation patient. Patient education is extensive: diet, fluids, daily weights, strict I&O measurements, prevention of infection, and avoidance of activities that may compromise the integrity of the urinary tract. Community support groups, sponsored by the American Association of Kidney Patients, help the patient and the family adapt to living with dialysis and transplantation. The National Kidney Foundation has a written protocol for the procurement of organs for donation.

Prognosis

Success of kidney transplantation parallels the individual patient's general health status and compliance with the treatment plan. Transplantation offers the only possibility of return to a normal lifestyle for the ESRD patient. Successful kidney transplantation prolongs and markedly improves quality of life, freeing the patient from the restrictions of dialysis.

URINARY DIVERSION

Several types of procedures are used to divert the flow of urine when required for treatment of bladder cancer, invasive cervical cancer, neurogenic bladder, and congenital anomalies. Often a cystectomy (the surgical removal of the bladder) is performed.

The cystectomy patient presents a unique challenge because of the need to create an artificial port for urine elimination. The most common urinary diversion procedure is the **ileal conduit** (Bricker's procedure or ileal loop), the ureters are implanted into a loop of the il-

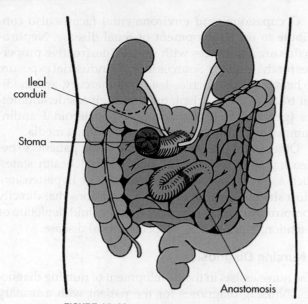

FIGURE 10-13 Ileal conduit or ileal loop.

eum that is isolated and brought to the surface of the abdominal wall (Figure 10-13). Occasionally a segment of the sigmoid colon is isolated and used instead of the ileum to form a sigmoid conduit. Bowel function is maintained with anastomosis of the remaining intestine. A drainage bag (urostomy bag or appliance) is fitted over the stoma to contain the constant drainage of urine. Continuous urine drainage prevents increased pressure within the conduit that would cause backflow to the kidneys, compromise the circulatory integrity of the conduit, or rupture the surgical anastomosis. Decreased urinary output and low abdominal pain may signal the onset of such problems. Complications of this procedure are wound infection, dehiscence, urinary leakage, ureteral obstruction, small bowel obstruction, stomal gangrene or atrophy, pyelonephritis, renal calculi, and compromised respiratory status secondary to incisional pain.

Postoperatively, measure urine flow hourly. Report output less than 30 mL/hr to the physician immediately. A healthy stoma appears moist and pink and may even bleed slightly. Inspect the skin around the stoma daily for signs of bleeding, excoriation, and infection. Mucus is present in the urine from the intestinal secretions. The patient should ingest large quantities of water to flush the ileal conduit. Any odor of urine about the patient may indicate an infection or leak of urine from the drainage bag. Early signs of urinary leakage (indicating a leak in an anastomosis) include increased abdominal girth; fever; and drainage through the incision, tubes, or drains. Ureteral separation from the conduit may cause urine to seep into the peritoneal cavity; observe the patient for signs and symptoms of peritonitis such as fever, abdominal pain and rigidity, and absence of bowel sounds.

Care of the patient with an ileal conduit is a nursing challenge because of the continuous drainage of urine through the stoma.

To change the urostomy bag, remove and drain it. Cleanse the skin with water, and apply the new appliance as outlined in the institution's standards of care. When the peristomal skin is healed, the bag is emptied at 2- to 3-hour intervals. At night a straight drainage tube is connected to a drainage bag. A permanent urostomy bag can be left in place 4 to 7 days if it remains sealed. Recommend that the patient have two bags, so one can be worn while the other is washed. Some patients prefer to use disposable bags. Odor is controlled by using deodorant drops or tablets in the urostomy bag; avoiding odor-producing foods, such as beans, onions, cabbage, asparagus, high-fiber wheat, simple sugars, and milk in the lactose-intolerant patient; and cleansing the urostomy bag with a vinegar and water rinse and thoroughly drying.

The **continent ileal urinary reservoir,** or **Kock pouch,** is created by implantation of the ureters into a segment of the small intestine that has been surgically removed from the rest of the bowel and anastomosed to the abdominal wall. Urine flow is controlled by a nipplelike valve that prevents leakage. To drain urine from the reservoir, the patient inserts a catheter through the valve at regular intervals, thus minimizing the reabsorption of waste materials from the urine and reflux into the ureters (Figure 10-14).

Patient Teaching
Patient teaching centers on the tasks of lifestyle adaptation: care of the stoma, nutrition, fluid intake, maintenance of self-esteem in light of altered body image, modification of sexual activities, and early detection of complications. Patient teaching begins with selecting an appliance, sizing the stoma, and changing the appliances. The home health nurse can assist the patient in modifying care in the home environment and by providing support during this stressful adjustment period (see Home Care Considerations box).

Prognosis
Although the patient may fully recover without recurrence, the day-to-day challenges of managing a urinary diversion are permanent.

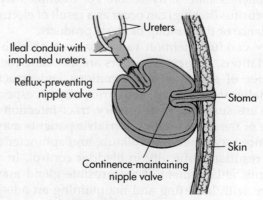

FIGURE 10-14 Kock pouch.

Home Care Considerations

Urinary Diversion Warning Signs

- Provide the patient and significant other with a list of warning signs and symptoms to report to the physician when home. Be certain to compose the list in clear, concise language.
- Keep this list handy and call the physician (phone number _____-_____) if you notice any of the following signs or symptoms:
  —Decrease in urinary output
  —Change in urine color: bloody, cloudy
  —Fever greater than 101° F
  —Change in appearance of stoma: pale color, swelling, "drawing-in" of stoma
  —Skin changes around stoma: redness, burning, breakdown
  —General feeling of weakness
  —Nausea and vomiting
  —Abdominal distention or pain
  —Any other health changes that are new or worse

❖ NURSING PROCESS for the Patient with a Urinary Disorder

The role of the licensed practical nurse/licensed vocational nurse (LPN/LVN) in the nursing process as stated is that the LPN/LVN will:

- Participate in planning care for patients based on patient needs
- Review patient's care plan and recommend revisions as needed
- Review and follow defined prioritization for patient care
- Use clinical pathways, care maps, or care plans to guide and review patient care

■ Assessment

Assessment of the urinary tract is included in baseline data for all patients. The assessment includes **subjective data:** the patient's description of urination patterns and associated sensations, such as complaints of burning or pain on urination or difficulty maintaining the urine stream. Supplement subjective data with **objective data** by assessing for signs of fluid overload or depletion. The skin provides easily assessed clues about the patient's state of hydration. For example, dryness and pruritus (itching) can occur as a result of electrolyte imbalance or the buildup of waste products.

Pay careful attention to assessment of high-risk populations. Urinary disorders are associated with a number of systemic malformations and structural anomalies in newborns. Pediatric patients, especially girls, are susceptible to urinary tract infections because of the short urethra. Geriatric patients may experience weakened musculature and sphincter tone, with resultant difficulty in bladder control. In male patients, enlargement of the prostate gland may interfere with initiating and maintaining an adequate urine stream.

Occupational and environmental factors also contribute to the development of renal disease. Nephrotoxins are substances with specific destructive properties for the kidneys. Sources include industrial exposure to heavy metals, such as lead and mercury, and medical treatment with cisplatin, aminoglycoside antibiotics (gentamicin or kanamycin), nonsteroidal antiinflammatory drugs, or radiopaque contrast media.

Other vulnerable populations include patients experiencing systemic changes from altered health states, such as pregnancy, diabetes mellitus, or hypertension. Most susceptible are those with conditions that directly compromise kidney function: trauma, fluid depletion or retention, and active or suspected renal disease.

■ Nursing Diagnosis

The nurse assists in the development of nursing diagnoses. Nursing diagnoses for the patient with a urinary disorder include but are not limited to the following:

- Impaired urinary elimination
- Ineffective tissue perfusion: renal
- Acute pain; chronic pain
- Risk for infection
- Risk for deficient fluid volume
- Excess fluid volume
- Ineffective sexuality patterns
- Deficient knowledge

■ Expected Outcomes and Planning

For the patient with a urinary disorder, the nursing care priority is the short-term goal of reestablishing urinary flow and kidney function. Long-term planning for the patient and the family or significant other focuses on prevention of complications and quick response to recurrent problems. Goals are individualized for each patient and are modified to adapt to the patient's changing health status and urinary elimination management. The care plan may include the following goals:

Goal 1: The patient will achieve control of the elimination of urine.

Outcome: Patient reports effective management of normal patterns of urination.

Goal 2: The patient will practice proper protocol such as drinking adequate fluids and correct methods of perineal cleansing for the female to prevent UTI.

Outcome: Patient reports no signs or symptoms of recurrent urinary difficulty.

■ Implementation

The nurse will assist patient in bladder training to promote normal patterns of urination. The patient will be educated in importance of drinking 2 to 3 L of water daily (unless contraindicated). Teach the female patient the importance of cleansing from anterior to posterior in the perineal area after a bowel movement to prevent contamination of the urethra with *Escherichia coli.*

■ Evaluation

Evaluation of urinary status is determined by success in attaining expected outcomes. Monitoring of urinary output and character is continual. Because some urinary disorders become chronic, patient involvement in the prevention of complications is vitally important. Avoidance of risk factors and early detection of symptoms are essential to limit damage to the urinary tract.

Goal 1: The patient will experience normal patterns of urinary elimination.
Evaluative measure: Patient reports return to own normal voiding.
Goal 2: The patient will monitor self for early signs and symptoms of recurrent UTI.
Evaluative measure: Patient is able to correctly answer questions about signs and symptoms and appropriate measures to take for treatment.

Get Ready for the NCLEX® Examination!

Key Points

- The kidneys lie retroperitoneally, just below the diaphragm.
- The functioning unit of the kidney is the nephron.
- The kidneys rid the body of wastes and excess electrolytes, maintain water and electrolyte balance, and maintain acid-base balance.
- Kidney function is achieved by the processes of filtration, secretion, and reabsorption.
- Assessment of the urinary tract is included in baseline data for all patients.
- The subject of urinary problems is an embarrassing topic for many patients. Be sensitive to the patient's feelings and be supportive.
- Aging may have a negative influence on urinary function, but many problems can be corrected.
- Hydration status is monitored by daily weights, I&O, laboratory studies, inspection of the skin and mucous membranes, and assessment of the level of consciousness.
- A large percentage of nosocomial infections involve the urinary tract.
- Proper care of urinary catheters decreases the chance of UTIs.
- Surgical intervention may be indicated for urinary dysfunction that cannot be corrected by medical management.
- Dialysis, which mimics kidney function, may be used temporarily or as a long-term therapy.
- Dietary, fluid, and medication modifications may be necessary for the patient with urinary dysfunction.
- Sacral nerve stimulation for urinary urge incontinence is conducted with a permanently implanted electrical stimulation device that changes neuronal activity in the sacral efferent and afferent nerves.

Additional Learning Resources

Go to your Companion CD for an audio glossary, animations, video clips, and more.

evolve   Be sure to visit the Evolve site at http://evolve.elsevier.com/ Christensen/adult/ for additional online resources.

Review Questions for the NCLEX® Examination

1. When reading the urinalysis report, the nurse recognizes this result as abnormal:
   1. turbidity clear.
   2. pH 6.0.
   3. glucose negative.
   4. red blood cells, 15 to 20.

2. After renal angiography, the patient assessment priority is the:
   1. blood pressure.
   2. respiratory effort.
   3. puncture site.
   4. urinary output.

3. The nursing care plan includes teaching the patient Kegel exercises. The nurse teaches the patient to alternately tighten and relax which group of muscles?
   1. Perineal floor
   2. Pubococcygeal
   3. Abdominis rectus
   4. Detrusor

4. The physician has talked to the patient and his wife about the treatment plan for his bladder cancer. Later, the patient tells the nurse he does not understand what the doctor is going to do. The most appropriate response by the nurse would be:
   1. "Okay. I'll explain it to you again."
   2. "Make a list of questions for the doctor."
   3. "Try not to think about the treatment."
   4. "Tell me what you know about the treatment."

5. Which activity would be harmful for the incontinent patient?
   1. Restricting fluid intake
   2. Drinking only water
   3. Fluid intake of 2000 mL/day
   4. Restricting acidic fruit juice intake

6. The nurse recognizes that the most common causative organism in pyelonephritis is:
   1. *Candida albicans.*
   2. *Klebsiella.*
   3. *Escherichia coli.*
   4. *Pseudomonas.*

7. The most important factor to foster patient compliance with the treatment plan is to provide the patient with:

   1. a set time schedule to follow.
   2. data on success rates.
   3. written information of the plan.
   4. an active role in the planning.

8. When scheduling the administration of furosemide (Lasix), it would be in the patient's best interest to schedule the medication to be given at:

   1. 9 AM.
   2. 12 PM (noon).
   3. 2100.
   4. 12 AM (midnight).

9. In discussion with the patient with ESRD about dietary needs, the nurse recognizes that foods highest in potassium include:

   1. apples, applesauce, grapes, and raisins.
   2. bananas, nuts, and chocolate.
   3. grapefruit, tomatoes, oranges, and bananas.
   4. milk, grapefruit, orange juice, and sugar.

10. Which patient report indicates that phenazopyridine hydrochloride (Pyridium) is being effective?

    1. Decreased bladder spasms
    2. Decrease in burning
    3. Increased urinary output
    4. Increased pain tolerance

11. When calculating actual urinary output during continuous bladder irrigations, the nurse would:

    1. measure and record all fluid output in the drainage bag.
    2. measure the total output and deduct the amount of irrigation solution used.
    3. add the total of all intravenous and irrigation solutions and deduct output.
    4. measure total output and deduct the total intravenous solutions.

12. What statement by the patient indicates the need for further teaching before renal angiography?

    1. "I will miss having breakfast."
    2. "I know the nurse will be checking my pulse after the test."
    3. "I'm glad I don't have to stay in bed after the test."
    4. "I had a test similar to this 3 years ago."

13. The nurse performs a catheterization immediately after the patient voids and obtains 30 mL residual urine. The next step would be to:

    1. document the procedure with outcome data.
    2. continue the catheterization routine after each voiding.
    3. restrict fluid intake after dinner.
    4. immediately notify the physician of the results.

14. Which goal would have priority in planning care of the aging patient with urinary incontinence?

    1. Recognizes the urge to void
    2. Mobility necessary for toileting independently

3. Episodes of incontinency decrease
4. Drinks a minimum of 2000 mL of fluid per day

15. The goal for peritoneal dialysis is to:

    1. remove toxins and metabolic waste.
    2. produce rapid fluid shifts.
    3. increase clearance of dialysate flow.
    4. restore normal kidney function.

16. In postoperative care of the patient with an arteriovenous shunt, the nurse should:

    1. secure the shunt with an elastic bandage.
    2. notify the physician if a bruit or thrill is present.
    3. change the shunt if clotting occurs.
    4. use strict surgical asepsis for dressing changes.

17. The teaching priority for the patient with acute renal failure is:

    1. treatment of hyponatremia.
    2. prevention of infection.
    3. maintenance urinary output at 50 mL/hr.
    4. control of caloric intake.

18. The patient with ESRD receiving hemodialysis is at risk for:

    1. sepsis.
    2. renal insufficiency.
    3. anemia.
    4. *Klebsiella* infection.

19. The primary function of the kidney is:

    1. regulation of enzymes.
    2. filtration of water and blood products.
    3. collection of urine from the body.
    4. control of the adrenal glands.

20. The priority short-term goal for disorders of the urinary system is:

    1. patient confidentiality.
    2. privacy.
    3. education for patient and family.
    4. normal patterns of urinary elimination.

21. Assessment of the patient with a urinary disorder may be complicated by:

    1. European practices to withhold personal information.
    2. marital status.
    3. coexisting pathologic condition.
    4. social taboos surrounding sexuality.

22. The nurse making rounds discovers that there is no urine drainage from a postoperative patient's Foley catheter. The first nursing action is to:

    1. ensure patency.
    2. irrigate until clear.
    3. call the physician.
    4. insert larger lumen catheter.

23. Which problem constitutes a medical emergency?

    1. Anuria
    2. Polyuria
    3. Dysuria
    4. Dyspnea

24. The most common cause of renal failure is:
    1. trauma.
    2. diabetes mellitus.
    3. cancer.
    4. heart failure.

25. The clinical findings in the oliguric phase of acute renal failure include:
    1. BUN and creatinine levels rise.
    2. urinary output increases.
    3. signs of impending shock.
    4. increased blood flow to the kidneys.

26. During postoperative care of the patient with an ileoconduit, which finding represents an emergency?
    1. Abdominal pain
    2. Presence of mucus in the urine
    3. Nausea and vomiting
    4. Absence of bowel sounds

27. Choose all of the correct patient teachings for the patient with cystitis.
    1. Teach the patient to drink cranberry juice to treat and prevent UTIs.
    2. Teach the female patient to cleanse the perineal area from anterior to posterior to prevent rectal *E. coli* contamination of the urethra.
    3. Encourage the patient to drink 2000 mL of fluid per day, unless contraindicated.
    4. Instruct the patient that it is acceptable to stop taking prescribed medications when symptoms subside.

28. Renal calculi may result from: *(Select all that apply.)*
    1. Stasis of urine caused by obstruction or quadriplegia
    2. Infections of urinary tract
    3. Hyperparathyroidism, which causes increase in calcium metabolism
    4. Diabetes mellitus

29. The collection of subjective and objective data for the patient with acute glomerulonephritis could include: *(Select all that apply.)*
    1. Periorbital edema
    2. Anorexia
    3. Hypotension
    4. Frankly sanguineous urine

30. Careful preparation of the patient for an IVP is necessary. Nursing interventions would include: *(Select all that apply)*
    1. NPO for about 12 hours before examination
    2. Ascertaining whether patient has allergy to magnesium
    3. Giving prescribed bowel prep
    4. Instructing patient concerning IVP

31. A patient with diabetes is admitted for evaluation of kidney function because of recent fatigue, weakness, and elevated BUN and serum creatinine levels. While obtaining a nursing history, the nurse identifies an early symptom of renal insufficiency when the patient states:
    1. "I get up several times every night to urinate."
    2. "I wake up in the night feeling short of breath."
    3. "My memory is not as good as it used to be."
    4. "My mouth and throat are always dry and sore."

32. A patient diagnosed with ESRD is treated with conservative management, including erythropoietin injections. After teaching the patient about management of ESRD, the nurse determines teaching has been effective when the patient states:
    1. "I will measure my urinary output each day to help calculate the amount I can drink."
    2. "I need to take the erythropoietin to boost my immune system and help prevent infection."
    3. "I need to try to get more protein from dairy products."
    4. "I will try to increase my intake of fruits and vegetables."

33. As the nurse reviews a diet plan with a patient with diabetes mellitus and renal insufficiency, the patient states that with diabetes and renal failure there is nothing that is good to eat. The patient says, "I am going to eat what I want; I'm going to die anyway!" The best nursing diagnosis for this patient is:
    1. imbalanced nutrition: more than body requirements, related to knowledge deficit about appropriate diet.
    2. risk for noncompliance, related to feelings of anger.
    3. grieving, related to actual and perceived losses.
    4. risk for ineffective health maintenance, related to complexity of therapeutic regimen.

34. The nurse has instructed a patient who is receiving hemodialysis about dietary management. Which diet choices by the patient indicate that the teaching has been successful?
    1. Scrambled eggs, English muffin, and apple juice
    2. Cheese sandwich, tomato soup, and cranberry juice
    3. Split-pea soup, whole-wheat toast, and nonfat milk
    4. Oatmeal with cream, half a banana, and herbal tea

35. To determine glomerular filtration rate for a patient with chronic renal disease, the nurse plans to:
    1. schedule frequent blood urea nitrogen (BUN) tests.
    2. initiate a 24-hour collection of the patient's urine.
    3. check the specific gravity on serial urine specimens.
    4. use a bladder scanner to check for residual urine.

Care of the Patient with an Endocrine Disorder

evolve

http://evolve.elsevier.com/Christensen/adult/

Barbara Lauritsen Christensen

Objectives

Anatomy and Physiology

1. List and describe the endocrine glands and their hormones.
2. Define the negative feedback system.
3. Explain the action of the hormones on their target organs.
4. Describe how the hypothalamus controls the anterior and posterior pituitary glands.

Medical-Surgical

5. Discuss the etiology and pathophysiology, clinical manifestations, assessment, diagnostic tests, medical management, nursing interventions, patient teaching, and prognosis for patients with acromegaly, gigantism, dwarfism, diabetes insipidus, syndrome of inappropriate antidiuretic hormone, hyperthyroidism, hypothyroidism, goiter, thyroid cancer, hyperparathyroidism, hypoparathyroidism, Cushing's syndrome, and Addison's disease.
6. List four tests used in the diagnosis of hyperthyroidism.
7. Explain how to test for Chvostek's sign, Trousseau's sign, and carpopedal spasms.
8. List two significant complications that may occur after thyroidectomy.
9. Discuss the medications commonly used to treat hyperthyroidism and hypothyroidism.
10. Differentiate between the clinical manifestations of Cushing's syndrome and Addison's disease.
11. Describe the etiology and pathophysiology, clinical manifestations, assessment, diagnostic tests, medical management, nursing interventions, patient teaching, and prognosis for the patient with diabetes mellitus.
12. Differentiate between the signs and symptoms of hyperglycemia and hypoglycemia.
13. Differentiate among the signs and symptoms of diabetic ketoacidosis, hyperglycemic hyperosmolar nonketotic coma, and hypoglycemic reaction.
14. Explain the roles of nutrition, exercise, and medication in the control of diabetes mellitus.
15. Discuss how oral agents work to improve the mechanisms by which insulin and glucose are produced and used by the body.
16. Discuss the two new subcutaneous insulin-enhancing drugs exenatide (Byetta) and pramlintide (Symlin) and their mechanisms of action.
17. Discuss the various insulin types and their characteristics.
18. Describe the correct way to draw up and administer insulin.
19. Discuss the various classes of oral hypoglycemic medications to treat type 2 diabetes mellitus.
20. Discuss the acute and long-term complications of diabetes mellitus.
21. List five nursing interventions that foster self-care in the activities of daily living of the patient with diabetes mellitus.

Key Terms

Chvostek's sign (KHVŎS-tĕks sīn, p. 498)
dysphagia (dĭs-FĀ-jē-ă, p. 497)
endocrinologist (ĕn-dō-krĭ-NŎL-ŏ-jĭst, p. 491)
glycosuria (glī-kōs-Ū-rē-ă, p. 511)
hirsutism (HĔR-sōōt-ĭszm, p. 505)
hyperglycemia (hī-pĕr-glī-SĒ-mē-ă, p. 511)
hypocalcemia (hī-pō-kăl-SĒ-mē-ă, p. 503)
hypoglycemia (hī-pō-glī-SĒ-mē-ă, p. 518)
hypokalemia (hī-pō-kă-LĒ-mē-ă, p. 504)
idiopathic hyperplasia (ĭd-ē-ō-PĂTH-ĭk hī-pĕr-PLĀ-zhă, p. 489)

ketoacidosis (kē-tō-ă-sĭ-DŌ-sĭs, p. 511)
ketone bodies (KĒ-tōn bŏd-ēz, p. 510)
lipodystrophy (lĭp-ō-DĬS-trŏ-fē, p. 517)
neuropathy (nū-RŎP-ĕ-thē, p. 522)
polydipsia (pŏl-ē-DĬP-sē-ă, p. 511)
polyphagia (pŏl-ē-FĀ-jă, p. 511)
polyuria (pŏl-ē-Ū-rē-ă, p. 511)
Trousseau's sign (trū-SŌZ sīn, p. 498)
turgor (TŬR-gŏr, p. 493)
type 1 diabetes mellitus (tīp 1 dī-ă-BĒ-tēz MĔL-ĭ-tŭs, p. 509)
type 2 diabetes mellitus (tīp 2 dī-ă-BĒ-tēz MĔL-ĭ-tŭs, p. 510)

ANATOMY AND PHYSIOLOGY OF THE ENDOCRINE SYSTEM

ENDOCRINE GLANDS AND HORMONES

Glands can be divided into two broad categories: exocrine and endocrine. **Exocrine glands** secrete through a series of ducts (sebaceous and sudoriferous glands of the skin). Their secretions are protective and functional. **Endocrine glands** are ductless; they release their secretions directly into the bloodstream. Their secretions have a regulatory function.

The endocrine system is composed of a series of ductless glands whose work is closely related to the nervous system. Both systems control homeostasis through communication within the systems. The endocrine system communicates more slowly through the use of **hormones,** which are chemical messengers that travel through the bloodstream to their target organ. When the hormone reaches its target, a metabolic change occurs.

The total weight of all the endocrine glands is less than half a pound, yet they have a powerful influence. The slightest change in hormonal levels can upset the metabolic balance of the entire body. Hormones can increase or decrease a normal body process by affecting a target organ. Too much or too little of a given hormone can affect other hormones, and for this reason they are somewhat interrelated. The endocrine glands (Figure 11-1) have a generalized effect on the patient's metabolism, growth, development, reproduction, and many other bodily activities.

The amount of hormonal release is controlled by a **negative feedback** (a decrease in function in response to stimuli) system. Information is constantly being exchanged between the target organ and the pituitary gland via the bloodstream regarding the effect of the hormone on the target organ.

Pituitary Gland

The pea-sized **pituitary gland** (hypophysis) is one of the most powerful glands in the body. It has been called the "master gland" because, through the negative feedback system, it controls the other endocrine glands. It works closely with the hypothalamus of the brain and is located in the cranial cavity in a small saddlelike depression in the sphenoid bone. It is divided into two segments, the **anterior pituitary** (adenohypophysis) and the **posterior pituitary** (neurohypophysis). Each segment has specialized hormones. The hypothalamus actually produces the hormones of the posterior pituitary and releases them for storage in the posterior pituitary gland; they are released from here as a result of nerve impulses received from the hypothalamus.

Anterior Pituitary Gland

Six major hormones are secreted by the anterior pituitary gland; the hormones make up about 75% of the gland's total weight. Five hormones are called **tropic** hormones, because they are responsible for the stimulation of other endocrine glands. Prolactin, the remaining hormone, causes the mammary glands to produce milk. These hormones and their functions are shown in Figures 11-2 and 11-3.

Posterior Pituitary Gland

Two hormones are released by the posterior pituitary when the hypothalamus stimulates their release. They are **oxytocin** and **antidiuretic hormone** (ADH) (see Figure 11-2). Oxytocin promotes the release of milk and stimulates uterine contractions during labor. ADH, also called vasopressin, causes the kidneys to conserve water by decreasing the amount of urine produced. ADH/vasopressin also causes constriction of the arterioles in the body and a pressor effect, which results in increased blood pressure.

Thyroid Gland

The **thyroid gland** is butterfly shaped, with one lobe lying on either side of the trachea just below the larynx (Figure 11-4). The lobes are connected by the **isthmus.** The gland is very vascular and receives approximately 80 to 120 mL of blood per minute.

The thyroid gland secretes the hormones **thyroxine** (T_4) and **triiodothyronine** (T_3). Adequate oral intake of iodine is necessary for the formation of thyroid hormones. These hormones regulate three main functions: (1) growth and development, (2) metabolism, and (3) activity of the nervous system. Their function

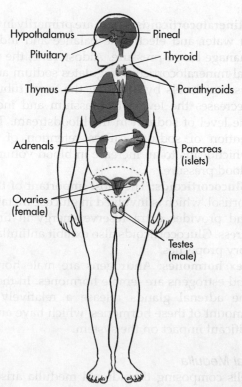

FIGURE 11-1 Location of the endocrine glands in the female and male bodies. Thymus gland is shown at maximal size at puberty.

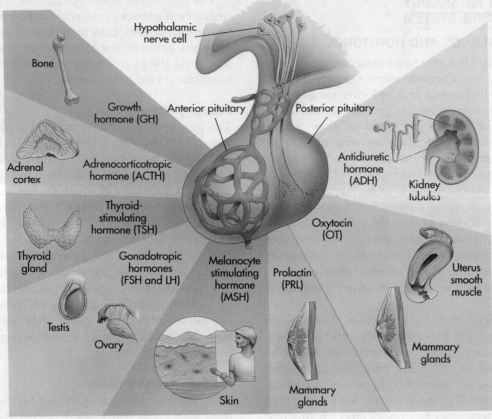

FIGURE 11-2 Pituitary hormones. Principal anterior and posterior pituitary hormones and their target organs.

is controlled by the release of thyroid-stimulating hormone (TSH) from the pituitary gland.

Calcitonin is a hormone also released by the thyroid gland. It decreases blood calcium levels by causing calcium to be stored in the bones.

Parathyroid Glands

The four parathyroid glands are located on the posterior surface of the thyroid gland (see Figure 11-4) and secrete **parathyroid hormone** (PTH, parathormone). As an antagonist to calcitonin from the thyroid, PTH tends to increase the concentration of calcium in the blood. It also regulates the amount of phosphorus in the blood.

The delicate balance of calcium in the blood is extremely important for normal body function. When calcium blood levels are low, the nerve cells become excited and stimulate the muscles with too many impulses, resulting in spasms **(tetany).** When blood calcium levels are abnormally high, heart function becomes impaired; this can result in death. Under the influence of PTH, two changes occur in the kidneys: It increases the reabsorption of calcium and magnesium from the kidney tubules and accelerates the elimination of phosphorus in the urine.

Adrenal Glands

The adrenal glands (suprarenal glands) are small, yellow masses that lie atop the kidneys. Both glands contain an outer section, the adrenal cortex, and a smaller inner section, the adrenal medulla (Figure 11-5).

Adrenal Cortex

The adrenal cortex is divided into three separate layers. Each layer secretes a particular hormone, called a **steroid:**

- **Mineralocorticoids:** These are primarily involved in water and electrolyte balance and indirectly manage blood pressure. Aldosterone, the principal mineralocorticoid, regulates sodium and potassium levels by affecting the renal tubules. It decreases the level of potassium and increases the level of sodium in the bloodstream. The retention of sodium causes retention of water, which leads to an increase in blood volume and blood pressure.

- **Glucocorticoids:** The most important of these is cortisol, which is involved in glucose metabolism and provides extra reserve energy in times of stress. Glucocorticoids also exhibit antiinflammatory properties.

- **Sex hormones:** Androgens are male hormones and estrogens are female hormones. In the adult the adrenal glands release a relatively small amount of these hormones, which have an insignificant impact on the system.

Adrenal Medulla

The cells composing the adrenal medulla arise from the same type of cells as the sympathetic nervous system. Two hormones are released during times of stress: (1) epinephrine (adrenaline), and (2) norepinephrine.

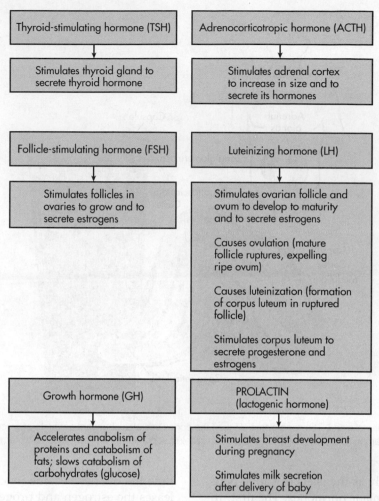

Thyroid-stimulating hormone (TSH)	Adrenocorticotropic hormone (ACTH)
Stimulates thyroid gland to secrete thyroid hormone	Stimulates adrenal cortex to increase in size and to secrete its hormones

Follicle-stimulating hormone (FSH)	Luteinizing hormone (LH)
Stimulates follicles in ovaries to grow and to secrete estrogens	Stimulates ovarian follicle and ovum to develop to maturity and to secrete estrogens Causes ovulation (mature follicle ruptures, expelling ripe ovum) Causes luteinization (formation of corpus luteum in ruptured follicle) Stimulates corpus luteum to secrete progesterone and estrogens

Growth hormone (GH)	PROLACTIN (lactogenic hormone)
Accelerates anabolism of proteins and catabolism of fats; slows catabolism of carbohydrates (glucose)	Stimulates breast development during pregnancy Stimulates milk secretion after delivery of baby

FIGURE 11-3 Names and functions of anterior pituitary hormones.

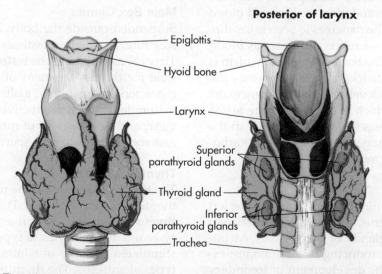

FIGURE 11-4 Thyroid and parathyroid glands. Note their relations to each other and to the larynx and trachea.

They cause the heart rate and blood pressure to increase, the blood vessels to constrict, and the liver to release glucose reserves for immediate energy. This is a systemic preparation of the body for a "fight-or-flight" response needed in times of crisis.

Pancreas

The pancreas is an elongated gland that lies posterior to the stomach. It is an active organ, composed of both exocrine and endocrine tissue. The endocrine tissue of the pancreas contains more than a million tiny clusters

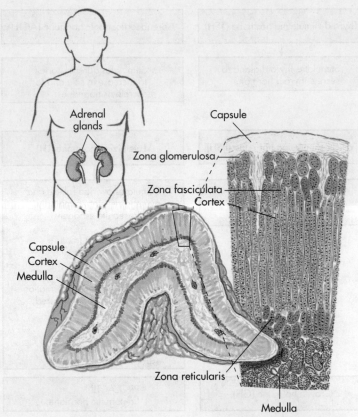

FIGURE 11-5 Structure of the adrenal gland. The zona glomerulosa of the cortex secretes abundant amounts of glucocorticoids, chiefly cortisol. The zona reticularis secretes minute amounts of sex hormones and glucocorticoids. A portion of the medulla is visible at the bottom of the illustration.

of cells known collectively as the islets of Langerhans. These cells secrete two major hormones. The first, **insulin,** is secreted by the **beta cells** in response to increased levels of glucose in the blood. Insulin's secretion pattern is a physiologic example of negative feedback between insulin and glucose. Elevated blood glucose levels stimulate the pancreas to secrete insulin. The stimulus for insulin secretion decreases as blood glucose levels decrease. The homeostatic mechanism is considered negative feedback because it reverses the change in blood glucose level. The second pancreatic hormone is **glucagon,** which is secreted by the **alpha cells** in response to decreased levels of glucose in the blood. Insulin and glucagon play a major role in carbohydrate, fat, and protein metabolism.

Female Sex Glands

Deep in the lower abdominal region, lying to the left and the right of the uterus, are two almond-shaped **ovaries,** the major sex glands of the woman. At puberty the ovaries begin producing two hormones: **estrogen** (responsible for the development of secondary sex characteristics, such as axillary hair and pubic hair, and for maturation of the reproductive organs) and **progesterone** (continues the preparation of the reproductive organs that was initiated by the estrogen). (See Chapter 12 for more information.)

The **placenta** is a temporary endocrine gland that forms and functions during pregnancy. During this time the ovaries become inactive and the placenta releases the estrogen and progesterone needed to maintain the pregnancy. (For a more in-depth discussion, refer to Chapter 12.)

Male Sex Glands

Suspended outside the body in the **scrotum,** a saclike structure, are the two oval sex glands called the **testes.** They release the hormone **testosterone,** which is responsible for the development of the male secondary sex characteristics, including axillary, pubic, and facial hair; maturation of the reproductive organs; deepening of the voice; and development of muscle and bone mass. Testosterone is necessary for sperm formation.

Thymus Gland

The thymus gland lies in the upper thorax, posterior to the sternum (see Figure 11-1). It produces the hormone **thymosin,** which plays an active role in the immune system. T lymphocytes (a type of white blood cell) are stimulated to carry out immune reactions to certain types of antigens. The thymus gland programs this information into the T lymphocytes in utero and during the first few months of life.

Pineal Gland

The pineal gland is a small, cone-shaped gland located in the roof of the third ventricle of the brain (see Figure 11-1). It secretes the hormone **melatonin,** which seems to inhibit reproductive activities by inhibiting the gonadotropic hormones. This is particularly important in preventing the sexual maturation of the child's body until adulthood. It is thought to induce sleep, may affect mood, and has an impact on menstrual cycles.

DISORDERS OF THE PITUITARY GLAND (HYPOPHYSIS)

ACROMEGALY

Etiology and Pathophysiology

An overproduction of somatotropin (growth hormone [GH]) in the adult causes acromegaly, a condition that affects an estimated 250 people in the United States each year. The cause may be either (1) idiopathic hyperplasia (an increase in number of cells without a known cause) of the anterior lobe of the pituitary gland or (2) tumor growth. Unfortunately, growth changes that occur in acromegaly are irreversible, even with adequate medical or surgical intervention.

Clinical Manifestations

Manifestations of acromegaly begin gradually, usually in the third or fourth decade of life. Typically an average of 7 to 9 years passes between the initial onset of signs and symptoms and final diagnosis. The subsequent overabundance of GH produces many changes throughout the patient's body, including enlarged cranium and lower jaw, separated and maloccluded teeth, bulging forehead, bulbous nose, thick lips, enlarged tongue, and generalized coarsening of the facial features (Figure 11-6). Enlargement of the tongue results in speech difficulties, and the voice deepens as a result of hypertrophy of the vocal cords. The hands and feet grow larger; the fingertips develop a tufted or clubbed appearance (Lewis et al., 2007). There is enlargement of the heart, the liver, and the spleen. Muscle weakness usually develops. Joints may hypertrophy and become painful and stiff. Male patients may become impotent, and female patients may develop a deepened voice, increased facial hair,

and amenorrhea. If a tumor is present, pressure on the optic nerve may cause partial or complete blindness. Severe headaches are common.

Assessment

Subjective data include headaches or visual disturbances and painful, stiff joints. Evaluate muscle weakness and its effect on the patient's ability to perform activities. Encourage patients to share their emotional responses to sexual problems (such as impotence in men and masculinization in women).

Collection of **objective data** includes ongoing assessment of bone enlargement and joint involvement, evidenced by gait changes and decreasing ability to perform activities. Changes in vital signs that may herald the onset of early heart failure include dyspnea, tachycardia, weak pulse, and hypotension.

Diagnostic Tests

Diagnosis of acromegaly is based on the history and the clinical manifestations, computed tomography (CT) scan, magnetic resonance imaging (MRI), and cranial radiographic evaluation. A complete ophthalmologic examination, including visual fields, is usually performed because a large tumor of the pituitary gland potentially causes pressure on the optic chiasm or optic nerves. Laboratory tests confirm the elevated levels of serum GH and plasma insulin-like growth factor–1. The definitive test for acromegaly is the oral glucose challenge test. Normally GH concentration falls during an oral glucose challenge test, but in acromegaly these levels do not fall (Lewis et al., 2007). Restrict the patient's oral intake for 8 hours before this test.

Medical Management

Medical treatments include dopamine agonists such as cabergoline (Dostinex) and somatostatin analogs (which inhibit GH), such as octreotide (Sandostatin, Sandostatin Depot) (Table 11-1), especially in patients who are not candidates for surgery or radiation therapy. These drugs are used in an attempt to suppress GH secretion. Surgical treatment to remove pituitary tumors associated with acromegaly is accomplished with the transsphenoidal removal of tumor tissue. The goal of transsphenoidal surgery is to remove only the tumor that is causing GH secretion. Irradiation procedures using proton beam therapy have been used to destroy GH-secreting tumors. Proton beam treatment uses very low doses of radiation and therefore is much less destructive to adjacent tissues, such as the hypothalamus and temporal lobes, than conventional radiation therapy.

Nursing Interventions and Patient Teaching

Nursing interventions are mainly supportive. Muscle weakness, joint pain, or stiffness warrant assessment of the ability to perform activities of daily living (ADLs). Headache may impair the patient's ability to socialize and may also impede education. Worsening headaches

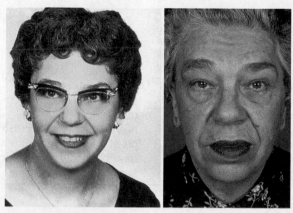

FIGURE 11-6 *Right:* This patient has coarse facial features typical of acromegaly. *Left:* Compare the patient's face many years before she developed the pituitary tumor.

Table 11-1   Medications for Endocrine Disorders

Generic/Trade	Action	Side Effects	Nursing Implications
Bromocriptine (Parlodel)	Inhibits prolactin secretion, lowers serum levels of growth hormone, dopamine receptor agonist	Nausea, headache, dizziness, abdominal cramping, orthostatic hypotension	Give with meals to prevent GI effects; change positions carefully to prevent orthostatic hypotension; contraindicated with hypersensitivity to ergot derivatives.
Calcium salts (gluconate, lactate, chloride gluceptate)	Calcium electrolyte replacement	Hypercalcemia, phlebitis, necrosis, and burning at IV site; bradycardia, hypotension, and dysrhythmias with rapid IV administration	Monitor cardiac status and blood pressure and for extravasation when giving intravenously.
Fludrocortisone (Florinef)	Adrenal corticosteroid with mineralocorticoid activity; promotes sodium and water retention	Hypertension, edema, sweating, rash, hypokalemia	Monitor for hypokalemia and fluid retention or depletion; do not discontinue abruptly; patient should carry identification signaling use.
Levothyroxine (Eltroxin, Synthroid, Levothroid) Liothyronine (Cytomel) Liotrix (Thyrolar) Thyroid (Thyrar, Armour Thyroid)	Thyroid hormone replacement	Most side effects due to therapeutic overdose; include anxiety, insomnia, headache, hypertension, tremors, angina, dysrhythmias, tachycardia, menstrual irregularities	Give in morning to minimize insomnia; use caution in older adults or patients with coronary artery disease; monitor for signs of overdose; do not switch brands unless instructed.
Mitotane (Lysodren)	Adrenal cytotoxic agent; reduces production of adrenal steroids	Anorexia, nausea, vomiting, diarrhea, lethargy, somnolence, vertigo, rash	Tell patient to use contraception; instruct patient to use caution when driving or performing tasks requiring alertness; monitor for dehydration.
Potassium iodide (SSKI)	Blocks release of thyroid hormone in thyroid storm and hyperthyroidism; also used as an expectorant	Hypersensitivity reactions, rash, metallic taste, burning in mouth or throat, GI irritation, headache, parotitis, hyperkalemia	Do not use in pregnant women; mix with fruit juice to mask taste.
Somatostatin analogs: octreotide (Sandostatin)	A secretory inhibitory growth hormone suppressant that suppresses secretion of serotonin, gastroenteropancreatic peptides; enhances fluid and electrolyte absorption from the GI tract; used for carcinoid tumors, VIPomas, and high-output fistulas	Nausea, diarrhea, abdominal pain, headache, injection site discomfort, hyperglycemia, hypoglycemia	SubQ route of administration is preferred, but may also be given IV.
Antidiuretic hormone: vasopressin (Pitressin)	Synthetic pituitary hormone with antidiuretic effects on the kidney (used to treat diabetes insipidus); also a potent vasoconstrictor (used to treat bleeding esophageal varices)	Nasal irritation and congestion with nasal preparations; hypertension; ischemia to heart, mesenteric organs, and kidneys; angina; myocardial infarction; water retention; hyponatremia	Use with caution in older adults or patients with coronary artery disease or heart failure; discontinue if chest pain develops; monitor urinary output and serum sodium.

GI, Gastrointestinal; *IV*, intravenous; *subQ*, subcutaneous.

may indicate tumor progression. The diet should be soft and easy to chew, since jaw muscles and the temporomandibular joint may be involved. Encourage the patient to chew thoroughly, and allow adequate time during meals, assisting when necessary. Encourage frequent fluid intake. Nonopioid analgesics may be given for pain relief. Visual impairment may increase the risk of injury for these patients, so take care to prevent them from stumbling into furniture or dropping objects.

As the body changes, the patient may develop problems with self-esteem and may feel physically unattractive. He or she may have difficulty communicating with significant others, which can disrupt individual or family coping methods. Other complications of acromegaly are related to enlargement of the liver, the spleen, and the heart. Cardiac dysrhythmias may develop, and the patient may experience heart failure. Abdominal girth may increase as a result of weight gain and inactivity, and respiratory difficulty may occur.

Nursing diagnoses and interventions for the patient with acromegaly include but are not limited to the following:

Nursing Diagnoses	Nursing Interventions
Disturbed body image, related to enlargement of hands, feet, tongue, jaw, and soft tissue	Convey respect and nonjudgmental acceptance of patient as a person. Help the patient set achievable short-term goals.
Activity intolerance, related to physical weakness	Assess patient's current activity level and priorities for activity performance. Discuss with patient alternate ways of performing activities.

The patient should remain under the supervision of a physician so that any complications can be promptly diagnosed and adequately treated. Teach the patient exercises that can be performed at home, such as active range-of-motion of joints of the extremities and of the neck, to help prevent muscle atrophy and loss of movement.

Prognosis
Even with adequate medical or surgical treatment, the physical changes are irreversible, and the patient is prone to developing complications.

GIGANTISM
Etiology and Pathophysiology
Gigantism usually results from an oversecretion of GH as a result of hyperplasia of the anterior pituitary; this hyperplastic tissue may develop into a tumor. Another possible cause is a defect in the hypothalamus, which directs the anterior pituitary to release excess amounts of GH.

Clinical Manifestations
When overproduction of GH occurs in a child before closure of the epiphyses, there is an overgrowth of the long bones. This results in the attainment of great height, accompanied by increased muscle and visceral development. Weight increases, but body proportions are usually normal. Despite their size, these patients are usually weak. Other kinds of gigantism may be caused by certain genetic disorders or by disturbances in sex hormone production. Once identified, these children should be referred for further medical evaluation and follow-up.

Assessment
Collection of **subjective data** includes assessment of the patient's understanding of the disease process and his or her ability to verbalize emotional responses.

Collection of **objective data** requires frequent measurement of height. Assess the patient's use of adaptive coping measures and family interactions.

Diagnostic Tests
The GH-suppression test (also called the **glucose-loading test**) may be done to evaluate GH levels. In the patient with gigantism, baseline levels of GH are high.

Medical Management
Medical management of children with gigantism may include surgical removal of tumor tissue or irradiation of the anterior pituitary gland, with subsequent replacement of pituitary hormones as indicated. The physician then observes the child for the development of related complications, such as hypertension, heart failure, osteoporosis, thickened bones, and delayed sexual development.

Nursing Interventions and Patient Teaching
Nursing interventions primarily include early identification of children who are experiencing increased growth rates compared with other children their age. The condition causes potential problems with self-image, especially if the child is a preteen who is a great deal taller than peers. Girls usually suffer more emotional trauma in this situation than boys do. Be understanding and compassionate and accentuate the positive aspects of being tall.

Early diagnosis of these patients is essential, since proper medical management can retard the height a child will reach. Stress to the parents the importance of regular visits to the pediatrician or pediatric endocrinologist (a physician who specializes in endocrinology).

Prognosis
With new medical and surgical advances, the expected life span of these patients is longer than it was previously. However, their life expectancy is still shorter than that of the average individual.

DWARFISM

Etiology and Pathophysiology

Hypopituitary dwarfism is a condition caused by deficiency in GH. Most cases are idiopathic, but a small number can be attributed to an autosomal recessive trait. In some cases the patients also lack adrenocorticotropic hormone (ACTH), TSH, and the gonadotropins.

Clinical Manifestations

The most common clinical manifestation of dwarfism is that the child is a great deal shorter than his or her peers. These patients usually appear well proportioned and well nourished but appear younger than their chronologic age. They may have problems with dentition as the permanent teeth erupt, since the jaws are underdeveloped. Sexual development is usually normal but delayed. Many people with hypopituitary dwarfism are able to reproduce normal offspring, unless there is an accompanying deficiency in gonadotropins. Because only a small number of children who experience short stature or delayed growth suffer from dwarfism, a thorough diagnostic workup is crucial.

Assessment

Subjective data include the patient's understanding of the disease process and emotional responses to it. A family history of dwarfism may reveal previously successful coping strategies. Encourage the patient to verbalize feelings. Most of these children display normal intelligence. The child's history usually reveals a normal birth weight. It is important to determine when the child's growth retardation was first noted.

Collection of **objective data** includes regular measurement of height and weight to determine responses to GH and other hormones that may be administered. Compare current height and weight with standard growth charts, and compare the child's growth pattern with that of siblings and other relatives at comparable age periods.

Diagnostic Tests

Diagnostic tests include radiographic evaluation of the wrist for bone age and an MRI or a CT scan to rule out a pituitary tumor. Definitive diagnosis is based on decreased plasma levels of GH. Restrict the patient's oral intake after midnight for this test.

Medical Management

Medical treatment involves replacement of GH by injection and the addition of other hormones as needed to correct deficiencies. If a tumor is the cause of dwarfism, surgery is usually indicated.

Nursing Interventions and Patient Teaching

Exercise particular care to identify children with growth problems. The physician correlates the onset of growth retardation with symptoms of headache, visual disturbances, or behavior changes that might indicate tumor, so be alert for these symptoms. Be careful not to make the parents feel guilty about any delay in seeking medical attention for their child.

Encourage the child to wear age-appropriate clothing and engage in activities with peers, since major problems with self-esteem can occur in dwarfism. Emphasize the child's abilities and strengths instead of his or her physical size.

Prognosis

Most of these patients lead fairly normal lives, and many become parents of normal children. Complications experienced are often of the musculoskeletal and cardiovascular systems.

DIABETES INSIPIDUS

Etiology and Pathophysiology

Diabetes insipidus (*diabetes*, "like a sieve or siphon"; and *insipidus*, "tasteless") is a transient or permanent metabolic disorder of the posterior pituitary in which ADH is deficient. The condition may be either primary or secondary to other conditions, such as head injury, intracranial tumor, intracranial aneurysm, or infarct. Infections such as encephalitis or meningitis have been known to cause diabetes insipidus. Diabetes insipidus occurs when either the secretion or action of ADH goes awry. A decrease in ADH results in electrolyte and fluid imbalances. The imbalances are caused by increased plasma osmolality and increased urinary output.

Clinical Manifestations

Diabetes insipidus is characterized by marked polyuria and intense polydipsia. The urine is very dilute, looking much like water, with a low specific gravity (1.001 to 1.005; the normal range is 1.003 to 1.030). Urinary output may exceed 5 to 20 L/24 hr, whereas the average is 1.5 L/24 hr. Patients typically lose as much as 200 mL of urine an hour for more than 2 consecutive hours. The patient craves cold or iced water and may drink 4 to 20 L of fluid daily, yet may become severely dehydrated and have increased levels of sodium in the blood (hypernatremia). Even when unconscious after surgery or head trauma, these patients continue to produce copious quantities of urine. If untreated, diabetes insipidus can lead to signs and symptoms of hypovolemic shock, including changes in level of consciousness, tachycardia, tachypnea, and hypotension. However, unlike hypovolemic shock, diabetes insipidus causes an increase in urinary output rather than a decrease.

Assessment

Subjective data include the patient's understanding of the relationship of symptoms (such as thirst and polyuria) to the underlying cause. The patient should be able to state the importance of not restricting oral fluids. Assess the severity of thirst. The patient may be embarrassed about the constant need to drink and then empty the bladder and may voluntarily restrict social contacts and work activities. The patient is weak, tired, and lethargic.

Collection of **objective data** includes assessment of skin turgor (the normal resiliency of the skin) and color and specific gravity of the urine. Carefully monitor intake and output (I&O). The skin is dry, turgor is poor, and body weight is lost. Constipation may occur. Weigh the patient daily in the early morning, before breakfast. Determine whether the patient has nocturia.

Diagnostic Tests
Diagnosis is based on clinical manifestations, urine specific gravity, and urine ADH measurement. The urine specific gravity often drops below 1.003, and the serum sodium level increases to more than 145 mEq/L (normal serum sodium level is 135 to 145 mEq/L). The serum osmolality may be greater than 300 mOsm/kg (normal is 280 to 300 mOsm/kg). The fluid deprivation (water deprivation) test may be ordered to determine how well the pituitary is producing ADH and to help rule out other causes. A CT scan and radiographic evaluation of the sella turcica (the "Turkish saddle"–shaped depression in the sphenoid bone that houses the pituitary gland) may be done.

Medical Management
Medical treatment involves intravenous (IV), subcutaneous, intranasal, or oral administration of ADH preparations in the form of desmopressin acetate (DDAVP). Several other drugs are available for ADH replacement, including aqueous vasopressin (Pitressin intramuscular [IM] or intranasal), vasopressin tannate IM, and lypressin (Diapid intranasal). Coffee, tea, and other beverages containing caffeine are usually eliminated from the diet because of their possible diuretic effect. If the patient cannot match the urinary losses through oral intake, he or she is at risk for dehydration and severe hypernatremia. IV fluids of hypotonic saline or dextrose 5% in water are needed.

Nursing Interventions and Patient Teaching
Because of the potential for fluid volume deficiency, carefully monitor the urinary output of pediatric and unconscious patients. Assess skin turgor frequently, along with the condition of oral mucous membranes. Weigh the patient and record I&O daily. Do not limit oral fluids in an effort to reduce urinary output.

Nursing diagnoses and interventions for the patient with diabetes insipidus include but are not limited to the following:

Nursing Diagnoses	Nursing Interventions
Deficient fluid volume, risk for, related to excessive urine production	Assess for signs and symptoms of dehydration (dry oral mucous membranes, poor skin turgor, soft eyeballs, lowered blood pressure, rapid pulse). Monitor electrolyte status carefully. Measure I&O.

Nursing Diagnoses	Nursing Interventions
Impaired skin integrity, risk for, related to altered state of hydration	Inspect skin for erythema, cyanosis, vesicles, and lesions. Prevent pressure on skin and skeletal prominences by turning and ambulating patient and using sheepskin, eggcrate mattress, or other measures. Increase fluid intake up to 2600 mL/day if possible. Encourage patient to eat food adequate in calories, protein, and vitamin C to promote healthy skin.

Instruct the patient to wear medical-alert jewelry, such as a necklace or bracelet, stating the diagnosis of diabetes insipidus. Stress that the patient must remain under medical supervision for monitoring of the metabolic state, since the condition may worsen with time.

Prognosis
The prognosis depends on the etiology. Patients who survive usually are dependent on medication for the rest of their lives. With proper treatment, most patients can expect to live a relatively normal life.

SYNDROME OF INAPPROPRIATE ANTIDIURETIC HORMONE
Syndrome of inappropriate ADH (SIADH) occurs when the pituitary gland releases too much ADH. In response to ADH, the kidneys reabsorb more water, decreasing urinary output and expanding the body's fluid volume. The patient experiences hyponatremia, hemodilution, and fluid overload without peripheral edema.

Etiology and Pathophysiology
ADH regulates the body's water balance. Synthesized in the hypothalamus, ADH is stored in the posterior pituitary gland. When released into the circulation, it acts on the kidney's distal tubules and collecting ducts, increasing their permeability to water. This decreases urine volume, since more water is reabsorbed and returned to the circulation, which increases blood volume. This syndrome occurs more commonly in older adults.

When the body's system of checks and balances malfunctions—whether from a tumor, medication, unrelated disease process, or some other cause—ADH may be released continuously, causing SIADH.

ADH is released in response to stress. Be alert to patients who have the following risk factors and who are also in pain or undergoing stressful procedures:
- Medications
  —General anesthetics
  —Opiates
  —Barbiturates

—Thiazide diuretics
—Oral hypoglycemics
—Oxytocin
- Malignancies (the most common cause of SIADH; cancerous cells are capable of producing, storing, and releasing ADH):
  —Small cell cancer of the lung
  —Hodgkin's lymphoma, non-Hodgkin's lymphoma, lymphocytic leukemia
  —Prostate cancer
  —Colorectal cancer
  —Duodenal cancer
  —Pancreatic cancer
- Nonmalignant pulmonary diseases
  —Chronic obstructive pulmonary disease
  —Tuberculosis
  —Lung abscess
  —Pneumonia
- Nervous system disorders
  —Head trauma
  —Cerebrovascular thrombosis
  —Cerebral atrophy
  —Acute encephalitis
  —Meningitis
  —Guillain-Barré syndrome
- Miscellaneous
  —Hypothyroidism
  —Lupus erythematosus
  —Adrenal insufficiency

Clinical Manifestations

Clinically, SIADH is characterized by hyponatremia and water retention that progresses to water intoxication. The severity of the patient's condition depends on how hyponatremic he or she becomes and how rapidly fluid accumulates. Most signs and symptoms appear when serum sodium levels fall below 125 mEq/L.

Assessment

Subjective data include vague complaints. Hyponatremia triggers the earliest symptoms, which are nonspecific and could indicate other disorders. These symptoms include weakness, muscle cramps, anorexia, nausea, and headache.

Collection of **objective data** includes assessment for hyponatremia. Hyponatremia may trigger diarrhea. The patient may also be disoriented and irritable and may gain weight. Fluid intake exceeds urinary output. The patient does not develop peripheral edema because excess fluid is accumulating in the vascular system, not in the interstitial spaces.

As water intoxication progresses and serum becomes more hypotonic, brain cells expand (become edematous), so later signs of SIADH are neurologic. The patient becomes progressively lethargic, with marked personality changes. The patient has seizures, and the deep tendon reflexes diminish or disappear altogether.

Diagnostic Tests

The diagnosis of SIADH is made by simultaneous measurements of urine and serum osmolality. Laboratory tests show hyponatremia (sodium less than 134 mEq/L). Serum osmolality is less than 280 mmol/kg (normal is 285 to 295 mmol/kg). The serum is diluted and the urine is concentrated (Lewis et al., 2007). Urine specific gravity is greater than 1.032, and urine sodium is elevated.

Medical Management

The physician orders fluid restriction, initially 800 to 1000 mL/day. However, with severe hyponatremia fluids may be restricted to 500 mL/day. Daily fluid intake should equal fluid output. If fluid restriction is adequate, tests show a gradual increase in serum sodium along with a decrease in body weight.

A hypertonic saline solution (3% to 5%) may be ordered via IV infusion pump at a very slow rate to avoid too rapid a rise in sodium. This is necessary to correct sodium imbalance and to pull water out of edematous brain cells.

The physician may order medications such as demeclocycline (Declomycin), a tetracycline derivative, in a dosage of 300 mg orally four times daily. The physician may also prescribe lithium carbonate. Both drugs interfere with the antidiuretic action of ADH and cause polyuria. Diuretics such as furosemide (Lasix)—40 to 80 mg/day orally in divided dosages or 20 to 40 mg IV daily—may be prescribed, but only if the serum sodium is at least 125 mEq/L, or the drug may promote more loss of sodium. Taking furosemide increases losses of potassium, magnesium, and calcium; supplements may be needed.

Treatment must also be directed at eliminating the underlying problem. Surgical resection, radiation, or chemotherapy may be indicated for malignant neoplasms. If the causative factor is a medication, it is discontinued.

Monitor the loss of potassium and other electrolytes from diuresis, as well as I&O, to prevent hypovolemia.

Nursing Interventions and Patient Teaching

Nursing interventions for SIADH focus on a continual assessment of the patient's condition to determine whether it is improving or deteriorating. Every 3 to 4 hours perform a neurologic examination and assess the patient's hydration status. Auscultate lung sounds every 2 to 4 hours to check for crackles that would indicate overhydration. Document any changes and report them immediately. Carefully observe serum electrolytes, urine sodium, and urine specific gravity because overcorrection can cause hypernatremia. Take a daily weight at the same time and on the same scales. Closely monitor I&O; output is the guide to regulating intake.

The nursing goal is to control the patient's intake and to minimize discomfort. Explain why fluids are being restricted; allow the patient to divide allotted fluids and to choose the fluids, if possible. Supplement the diet with sodium and potassium, especially if diuretics are prescribed. Advise the patient to avoid salty foods (e.g., potato chips or bacon) because they will make the patient more thirsty.

Frequent mouth care is essential to maintain the integrity of oral mucous membranes. Take steps to prevent skin impairment. Inform the patient and family members with simple explanations, such as that pain and anxiety can aggravate SIADH. If nausea is present (because of water intoxication), obtain an order for an antiemetic to be administered 30 minutes before meals.

Nursing diagnoses and interventions for the patient with SIADH include but are not limited to the following:

Nursing Diagnoses	Nursing Interventions
Excess fluid volume, related to decreased urinary output	Obtain daily weight, same scales, same time. Assess and record I&O. Monitor laboratory results. Administer medications as ordered. Maintain dietary and fluid restrictions (fluids should be high in sodium; avoid salty foods). Monitor IV infusions (such as 3% to 5% sodium chloride over several hours).
Risk for impaired oral mucous membrane, related to fluid restrictions of 500 mL/day	Provide frequent oral care; avoid alcohol-based mouthwashes and lemon glycerin swabs. Allow patient to choose fluids and to divide the allotted amount (such as half in morning, one third in evening, and the remainder at night). Offer simple explanation for fluid restrictions. If ordered, administer antiemetics 30 minutes before meals.

Patient teaching should be an ongoing part of nursing care. Be certain the patient understands the treatment plan, the rationale behind it, and the expected outcome. Provide information about signs and symptoms of SIADH, and tell the patient to alert the physician if any changes are noted. SIADH can recur after discharge.

Prognosis
SIADH resulting from an adverse reaction to medication or secondary to a head trauma, is self-limiting. If it occurs as a result of metabolic conditions or tu-mors, however, it tends to become chronic (Lewis, et al., 2007).

SIADH is potentially dangerous but treatable. If signs and symptoms are recognized early and intervention is appropriate, the prognosis is good; without treatment, coma and death occur.

DISORDERS OF THE THYROID AND PARATHYROID GLANDS

HYPERTHYROIDISM

Etiology and Pathophysiology
Hyperthyroidism—also called **Graves' disease,** exophthalmic goiter, and thyrotoxicosis—is a condition in which there is increased activity of the thyroid gland, with overproduction of the thyroid hormones T_4 and T_3. As a result, all of the patient's metabolic processes are exaggerated. It may occur during pregnancy or in adolescence. Graves' disease occurs most frequently in women in the 20- to 40-year-old age-group. Two percent of the female population is affected by Graves' disease, compared with 0.2% of the male population. Graves' disease is an autoimmune disorder of unknown etiology. It may be caused by genetic factors interacting with precipitating factors such as inadequate iodine, infection, and extreme physical or emotional stress (Lewis et al., 2007).

Clinical Manifestations
Clinical manifestations are numerous and varied, from mild to severe. The patient usually has visible edema of the anterior portion of the neck as a result of enlargement of the thyroid. In severe cases, exophthalmos (bulging of the eyeballs) may occur, usually attributable to periorbital edema (Figure 11-7). Twenty percent to 40% of patients with Graves' disease manifest the classic finding of exophthalmos. The eyeballs are forced outward, resulting in incomplete closure of the eyelids; the exposed corneas become dry with subsequent development of corneal ulcers and loss of vision (Lewis et al., 2007).

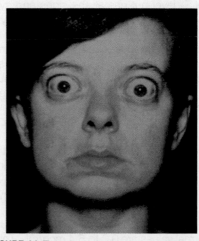

FIGURE 11-7 Exophthalmos of Graves' disease.

Assessment

Subjective data include an inability to concentrate and memory loss. The patient may complain of dysphagia or may be hoarse. There is usually weight loss, even with a voracious appetite. The patient reports feeling nervous, jittery, and excitable and may experience insomnia. These patients are emotionally labile and may overreact to stressful situations.

Objective data include changes in vital signs. The pulse is usually rapid, blood pressure is elevated, and a bruit may be auscultated over the thyroid. The skin is warm and flushed, and the hair is fine and soft. Female patients may cease to menstruate. Elevated body temperature may be accompanied by intolerance to heat, with profuse diaphoresis. Note tremors of the hands. Behavior changes may include hyperactivity and clumsiness. Daily weighing usually shows weight loss.

Diagnostic Tests

Hyperthyroidism is confirmed by a decrease in TSH levels and an elevation of free T_4 (FT_4) levels. Total T_3 and T_4 levels may be evaluated but are not as helpful in the diagnosis. With the radioactive iodine uptake (RAIU) test, the patient demonstrates an uptake of 35% to 95% of the drug (Lewis et al., 2007) (Box 11-1).

Medical Management

Medical management for hyperthyroidism may include administration of drugs that block the production of thyroid hormones, such as propylthiouracil (PTU) or methimazole (Tapazole). PTU must be taken three times per day, but it lowers hormone levels more quickly. Methimazole is usually preferred because only one dose daily is required (Lewis et al., 2007) (Table 11-2). The patient usually begins to notice a decrease in symptoms within 6 to 8 weeks after the dose of the drug. This may be followed after the acute stage by ablation therapy using a therapeutic dose of radioactive iodine ($^{131}INaI$ or $^{125}INaI$), based on the patient's age, clinical manifestations, and estimated weight of the thyroid. Ablation therapy using radioactive iodine is the gold standard for treating hyperthyroidism. The goal is to destroy some of the hypertrophied thyroid tissue. Because the therapeutic dose of radioactive iodine is low, no radiation safety precautions are necessary.

An unfortunate outcome of this treatment in most patients is the development of hypothyroidism. Thus the patient must have adequate follow-up medical supervision. If a patient develops hypothyroidism after treatment, levothyroxine therapy will be needed. **^{131}I is not a radiation hazard to the nonpregnant patient but is absolutely contraindicated during pregnancy. Pregnant nurses should not care for this patient for several days after treatment.**

Surgery has fallen out of favor because of possible serious complications, such as hemorrhage, hypoparathyroidism, and vocal cord paralysis. However, surgery may still be indicated for patients who cannot tolerate antithyroid drugs, are not good candidates for radioactive iodine therapy, have a possible malignancy, or have large goiters causing tracheal compression.

Surgical treatment for hyperthyroidism is subtotal thyroidectomy, a procedure in which approximately five sixths of the thyroid is removed. If too much tissue is taken, the gland will not regenerate after surgery and hypothyroidism will result. Surgery is usually delayed, if possible, until the patient is in a normal thyroid (euthyroid) state because of the risk

---

| Box 11-1 | Diagnostic Tests for Hyperthyroidism |

- **T_3 (serum triiodothyronine):** Measures the T_3 level in the blood. Normal is 65 to 195 ng/dL. As with the thyroxine (T_4 test), the serum T_3 is an accurate measurement of thyroid function. T_3 is less stable than T_4. An elevated T_3 determination is clinically important in the patient who has a normal T_4 level but has all the signs and symptoms of hyperthyroidism. In this patient the test may identify T_3 thyrotoxicosis.
- **T_4 (serum thyroxine):** Measures the T_4 level in the blood. Normal is 5 to 12 mcg/dL. Some medications such as oral contraceptives, steroids, estrogens, and sulfonamides may be withheld for several hours before the T_3 and T_4 tests, but food and fluids are not withheld. Elevated levels of these tests usually indicate hyperthyroidism.
- **Free T_4 (FT_4):** Measures active component of total T_4. Normal values are 1 to 3.5 ng/dL. Because this level remains constant, this is considered a better indication of function than T_4 and is useful in diagnosing hyperthyroidism and hypothyroidism. High FT_4 suggests hyperthyroidism; low FT_4 suggests hypothyroidism.
- **Thyroid-stimulating hormone (TSH):** Measures level of TSH. Normal values are 0.3 to 5.4 mcg/mL. This is considered the most sensitive method for evaluating thyroid disease. It is generally recommended as the first diagnostic test for thyroid dysfunction. TSH is suppressed in hyperthyroidism and elevated in hypothyroidism.
- **Radioactive iodine uptake (RAIU) test:** Radioactive iodine, ^{131}I, is given by mouth to the fasting patient. After 2, 6, and 24 hours, a scintillation camera is held over the thyroid to measure how much of the isotope has been removed from the bloodstream. A hyperactive thyroid may remove 35% to 95% of the drug. This test may be affected by prior ingestion of iodine-containing substances or foods. Obtain a signed consent form for this test. Also note any allergy to iodine on the request form, along with medications currently being taken. No radiation precautions are necessary.
- **Thyroid scan:** ^{131}I is given to the patient either orally or intravenously. If an IV dose is given, the scan may be done in 30 to 60 minutes. A scintillation camera positioned over the patient's thyroid sends images that are received on an oscilloscope and may be printed out on special paper. Obtain a signed consent form for this test. No radiation precautions are necessary.

Table 11-2	Medications Commonly Used to Treat Hyperthyroidism and Hypothyroidism
MEDICATIONS	**COMMON SIDE EFFECTS**
HYPERTHYROIDISM	
Iodine or iodine products (potassium or sodium iodide with strong iodine solution, potassium iodide, Lugol's solution)	Nausea, vomiting, diarrhea, abdominal pain
Radioactive iodine (^{131}I or ^{125}I)	Sore throat, edema or pain in neck, temporary loss of taste, nausea, vomiting, painful salivary glands
Methimazole (Tapazole), propylthiouracil (PTU)	Rash or pruritus, vertigo, nausea, vomiting, loss of taste, paresthesias, abdominal pain
HYPOTHYROIDISM	
Levothyroxine (Levothroid, Synthroid, Eltroxin, Levo-T, Unithroid) Liothyronine (Cytomel) Liotrix (Thyrolar) Thyroid (Armour Thyroid, Thyrar)	Nervousness, irritability, tremors, insomnia, tachycardia, hypertension, palpitations, cardiac dysrhythmias, vomiting, diarrhea, nausea, appetite changes, weight loss, menstrual irregularities, leg cramps, fever

of excess bleeding during thyroidectomy and postoperative thyroid crisis.

Patients who have only mild hyperthyroidism are rarely admitted to the acute care hospital. They are treated by the physician in an office or clinic setting. However, the hospital nurse may come in contact with the patient because of admission for a different condition and also cares for these patients before and after thyroidectomy.

Nursing Interventions and Patient Teaching

The hyperthyroid patient needs more nutrients because of increased metabolism, so diet therapy usually consists of food high in calories, vitamins (especially the B vitamins), minerals, and carbohydrates. Offer between-meal snacks. Food should be soft and easily swallowed if the patient has dysphagia (difficulty swallowing). Coffee, tea, and colas should be avoided because of their stimulant effect.

Preoperative teaching is extremely important for the patient who is scheduled for a thyroidectomy. Keep the environment as stable as possible to prevent emotional strain. Include instructions on how to properly support the head while turning in bed or rising to a sitting or standing position. The nurse (or patient) places both hands behind the head and maintains anatomical position while the rest of the body is being moved. Also teach the patient to deep breathe, but the physician will determine whether coughing is to be done postoperatively, since it strains the suture line. Inform the patient that a period of "voice rest" may be enforced for 48 hours postoperatively and that pencil and paper will be provided for writing notes instead of talking. Do voice checks every 2 to 4 hours, as ordered by the physician. Ask the patient to say "ah" and check for excessive hoarseness or voice change. Slight hoarseness is expected and should not cause alarm. Approximately 12.4% of patients suffer some damage to the laryngeal nerve during surgery, but this is not always permanent.

Postoperative management includes keeping the bed in semi-Fowler's position, with pillows supporting the head and shoulders. Caution the patient to avoid hyperextending the head to prevent excess tension on the incision, which is usually made in a horizontal crease in the anterior neck. Have a suction apparatus and tracheotomy tray available for emergency use. A cool-mist humidifier at the bedside may help soothe the throat and prevent coughing. Check vital signs frequently, with special attention paid to the rate and depth of respirations and observations for any dyspnea (shortness of breath or difficulty breathing) related to edema in the operative site. Before giving any liquid orally, be sure the swallowing and cough reflexes have returned. Be alert for signs of internal or external bleeding; early signs of internal bleeding include restlessness, apprehension, increased pulse rate, decreased blood pressure, and a feeling of fullness in the neck. Later, cyanosis may develop, signaling an obstructed airway; notify the surgeon immediately. Inspect the dressing on the neck frequently for obvious external bleeding. Also check for bleeding at the sides and back of the neck and on top of the patient's shoulders, since oozing blood may pool there as a result of gravity. Most surgeons allow a dressing to be reinforced as needed and loosened slightly if the patient complains that it is too tight.

Postoperatively, the diet initially consists of clear, cool liquids, progressing to soft food as tolerated. This is followed by a regular diet as soon as possible to help the patient regain lost weight and correct any nutritional deficiencies.

Another significant postoperative complication after thyroidectomy is tetany. One possible cause of tetany is the inadvertent removal of one or more of the parathyroid glands during surgery. Another is edema in the operative area, which occludes release of PTH into the bloodstream, resulting in a low serum calcium level (normal serum calcium is 9.0 to 10.5 mg/dL). The symptoms include numbness and tingling in the fingertips and toes and around the mouth. The patient may also have **carpopedal spasms** (muscle spasms in the wrists and feet) and increased pulse, respirations, and blood pressure, accompanied by anxiety and agitation. Laryngeal spasm and stridor may occur. Chvostek's sign is positive (an abnormal spasm of the facial muscles elicited by light taps on the facial nerve in patients who are hypocalcemic), and Trousseau's sign may also be positive (assesses for latent tetany; carpal spasm is induced by inflating a sphygmomanometer cuff on the upper arm to a pressure exceeding systolic blood pressure for 3 minutes; a positive result may be seen in hypocalcemia and hypomagnesemia). If untreated, the condition may progress to convulsions or lethal cardiac dysrhythmias. Emergency treatment of tetany is the IV administration of calcium gluconate, which should always be available postoperatively.

The other serious complication after thyroidectomy is thyroid crisis, or thyroid storm. Fortunately, it occurs rarely and can usually be attributed to manipulation of the thyroid during surgery, which causes the release of large amounts of thyroid hormones into the bloodstream. If thyroid crisis occurs, it usually does so within the first 12 hours postoperatively. In thyroid crisis, all the signs and symptoms of hyperthyroidism are exaggerated. Additionally, the patient may develop nausea, vomiting, severe tachycardia, severe hypertension, and occasionally hyperthermia up to 106° F (41° C). Extreme restlessness, cardiac dysrhythmia, and delirium may also occur. The patient may develop heart failure and die. Diagnostic tests indicate increased FT_4 and decreased TSH.

The three goals of thyroid storm management are (1) to induce a normal thyroid state, (2) prevent cardiovascular collapse, and (3) prevent excessive hyperthermia. Emergency treatment of thyroid crisis includes administration of IV fluids, sodium iodide, corticosteroids, antipyretics, an antithyroid drug (such as PTU or methimazole), and oxygen as needed. Prompt, adequate treatment usually results in dramatic improvement within 12 to 24 hours.

Nursing diagnoses and interventions for the patient having a thyroidectomy include but are not limited to the following:

Nursing Diagnoses	Nursing Interventions
Preoperative	
Risk for hyperthermia, related to increased metabolism	Assess body temperature at regular intervals.
	Regulate environment (room temperature, linens, clothing) to help keep patient comfortable.
	Administer acetaminophen as prescribed.
Imbalanced nutrition: less than body requirements, related to increased metabolism	Encourage patient to eat prescribed diet and avoid caffeine.
	Assess daily weight and food intake.

Nursing Diagnoses	Nursing Interventions
Postoperative	
Impaired swallowing, related to postoperative edema	Ensure swallowing and cough reflexes are present before oral intake.
	Encourage patient to drink slowly and chew food thoroughly.
Ineffective breathing pattern, risk for, related to: • postoperative edema • pain	Monitor rate and depth of respirations.
	Assess breath sounds and skin color.
	Encourage slow, deep breaths at least once an hour.
	Position patient to maximize respiratory effort.

Patient education after thyroidectomy includes stressing the importance of follow-up medical supervision. Thyroid function tests are done periodically to check for both hyperthyroidism and hypothyroidism, which occurs in approximately 43% of surgical cases. Before discharge, teach the patient proper care of the incision site and symptoms that might indicate development of an infection, in which case he or she should notify the surgeon immediately. Discuss with the patient the need for a high-calorie, high-protein, high-carbohydrate diet until weight is stable.

Prognosis

With adequate, appropriate medical or surgical treatment, these patients usually have a normal life expectancy. However, exophthalmos, if present, may remain to a lesser degree in some patients.

HYPOTHYROIDISM

Etiology and Pathophysiology

Hypothyroidism is one of the most common medical disorders in the United States, affecting 10% of women and 3% of men older than 65 years of age. It occurs most often in women 30 to 60 years of age and is more common in older adults than previously thought. Hypothyroidism is the clinical state that occurs when the thyroid fails to secrete sufficient hormones, slowing all of the body's metabolic processes. It may be caused by a condition of the thyroid itself or by a failure of the pituitary gland to furnish sufficient TSH for proper stimulation of thyroid secretion. It is sometimes an unfortunate outcome of the medical or surgical treatment of hyperthyroidism. Severe hypothyroidism in adults is called **myxedema** (Figure 11-8). It is characterized by edema of the hands, the face, the feet, and periorbital tissues. Congenital hypothyroidism is called **cretinism** (Figure 11-9) and is estimated to occur in 1 of every 4000 to 5000 newborns. All infants in the United States are screened for decreased thyroid function at birth.

Clinical Manifestations

Clinical manifestations range from mild to severe and depend on the degree of thyroid hormone deficiency present. All the body's metabolic processes slow, resulting in decreased production of body heat, intolerance to cold, and weight gain. Atherosclerotic changes may result in coronary artery disease. Hypothyroidism may have adverse effects on the heart with decreased cardiac output and contractility; the patient experiences decreased exercise tolerance and dyspnea on exertion (Lewis et al., 2007).

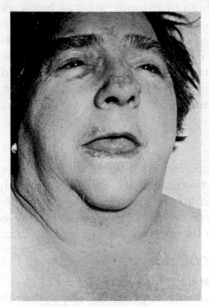

FIGURE 11-8 Person with myxedema.

Assessment

Subjective data include the patient's mental and emotional status, which may include depression, paranoia, impaired memory, and general slowing of thought processes. Speech and hearing may be deficient. The patient is lethargic, forgetful, and irritable. Because of the body's slowed metabolism, cold intolerance, anorexia, and constipation may develop. Both sexes may experience decreased libido and reproductive difficulty. Assess the patient's adaptive coping methods.

Collection of **objective data** includes assessment of the skin and hair. The hair thins and may fall out; the skin becomes thickened and dry. Facial features may enlarge to give the patient an edematous appearance with a masklike facial expression. The voice is characteristically low and hoarse. Decreased metabolism usually causes bradycardia, decreased blood pressure and respirations, and exercise intolerance. The patient has decreased ability to perform activities because of weakness, clumsiness, and ataxia. Assess the respiratory rate after administration of any central nervous system depressant. Evaluate the abdomen for distention, since **myxedema ileus** may occur. Menorrhagia (excessive menstrual flow) is a frequent complaint of women with hypothyroidism. Also inhibition of ovulation with subsequent infertility may occur (Lewis et al., 2007).

Diagnostic Tests

Diagnosis of hypothyroidism is based on the physical examination and history and on appropriate laboratory tests, such as TSH, T_3, T_4, and FT_4 levels. Low levels of T_3, T_4, and FT_4 are the underlying stimuli for TSH.

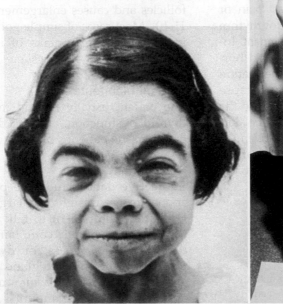

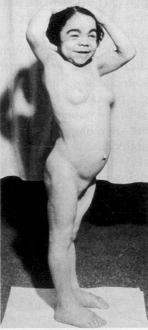

FIGURE 11-9 Adult cretin (33 years old, untreated). Note characteristic cretinoid features: dwarfism (44 inches in height), absent axillary and scant pubic hair, poorly developed breasts, protruding abdomen, and small umbilical hernia.

Therefore a compensatory elevation of TSH occurs in patients with primary hypothyroid states, and low levels of T_3, T_4, and FT_4 are present. Subclinical cases may go undiagnosed for years, so be aware of subtle clues while interviewing and caring for the patient.

Medical Management

The treatment for hypothyroidism is replacement therapy, with desiccated animal thyroid (Armour Thyroid); T_4; or synthetic products, such as levothyroxine (Levothroid, Synthroid, Levo-T, Eltroxin) (see Table 11-2). These drugs are usually given in the morning to enhance utilization of nutrients ingested during the daily meals. The patient initially is given a low dose, with increases as necessary until the desired effect is achieved. A maintenance dose is then established. Early in treatment, monitor hormone levels about every 6 to 8 weeks until the patient's TSH level is normal and at least yearly after that. Watch the patient for adverse effects of drug therapy, which mimic the signs and symptoms of hyperthyroidism. There is usually a dramatic change in the patient within a short time after replacement therapy begins. Lifelong thyroid replacement therapy is usually required.

Nursing Interventions and Patient Teaching

Nursing interventions for the hospitalized severely hypothyroid patient center mainly on symptomatic relief. Keep the room at least 70° to 74° F (21° to 23° C), and be certain the patient is not chilled during the bath or other procedures. Allow extra time for physical care, so the patient does not feel rushed. Keep accurate records of bowel elimination, since constipation may be severe. Stool softeners and bulk laxatives may be ordered. Provide a high-protein, high-fiber, low-calorie diet, and encourage increased fluid intake. The patient should avoid concentrated carbohydrates, such as sweets, to help prevent excess weight gain. Watch for chest pain or dyspnea, accompanied by changes in the rate or rhythm of the heart; this may indicate cardiac involvement. Instruct the patient not to stop taking the thyroid hormone without consulting a physician. This medication must be taken for the rest of the patient's life. Because most hypothyroid patients are more susceptible to the effects of sedatives, hypnotics, and anesthetics, be alert for possible adverse effects if these agents are given.

Nursing diagnoses and interventions for the patient with hypothyroidism include but are not limited to the following:

Nursing Diagnoses	Nursing Interventions
Decreased cardiac output, related to decreased metabolism	Assess pulse, blood pressure, skin color, and temperature. Schedule nursing activities around patient's activity cycle, with rest periods as needed to conserve energy.

Nursing Diagnoses	Nursing Interventions
Constipation, related to decreased peristaltic action	Assess frequency and character of stools. Encourage increased intake of oral fluids and high-fiber foods.

Regular checkups are essential because drug dosage may have to be adjusted from time to time. The patient and significant other should understand the desired effects and major adverse effects of the medication. Instruct the patient to eat well-balanced meals of high-fiber foods, such as fruits, vegetables, and whole-grain cereals and breads; the patient also needs adequate intake of iodine, in foods such as saltwater fish, milk, and eggs, and increased fluids to prevent constipation. Tell the patient and the family that mental and physical slowness may still be present but should improve with thyroid replacement therapy.

Prognosis

Most hypothyroid patients do well with proper medical supervision, although they will probably have to take medication for the rest of their lives. In children, when T_4 replacement begins before epiphyseal fusion, the chance for normal growth is greatly improved.

SIMPLE (COLLOID) GOITER

Etiology and Pathophysiology

A simple, or colloid, goiter develops when the thyroid gland enlarges in response to low iodine levels in the bloodstream or when it is unable to utilize iodine properly. When the blood level of T_3 is too low to signal the pituitary to decrease TSH secretion, the thyroid gland responds by increasing the formation of thyroglobulin (colloid), which accumulates in the thyroid follicles and causes enlargement of the gland (Figure 11-10). Most cases of simple goiter can be attributed to insufficient dietary intake of iodine, leading to this overgrowth of thyroid tissue.

Clinical Manifestations

The patient usually has no manifestations of overt thyroid dysfunction, and the diagnosis is essentially based on the patient's physical manifestations.

Assessment

Subjective data include the patient's emotional response to the unsightly enlargement of the thyroid. Encourage the patient to talk about his or her feelings. The patient may complain only of symptoms of dysphagia, hoarseness, or dyspnea related to the pressure of the enlarged gland against the esophagus and trachea. Dysphagia may make it difficult to eat and drink adequate amounts. Assess the patient for increasing dyspnea. Determine the patient's understanding of the need for medication, diet therapy, and medical follow-up.

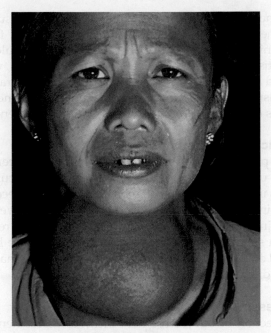

FIGURE 11-10 Simple goiter.

Collection of **objective data** includes assessment of increased goiter size, voice changes, and adequacy of food and fluid intake.

Medical Management

The thyroid may be only slightly enlarged, or it may be so enlarged that surgery must be done to improve respiration or swallowing. Surgery also is sometimes performed for cosmetic effect, since this type of goiter can be unsightly and damage the patient's self-image and self-esteem. If thyroidectomy is done, most of the gland is removed. Medical treatment consists of oral administration of potassium iodide and foods high in iodine.

Nursing Interventions and Patient Teaching

Nursing interventions after thyroidectomy (previously discussed) are aimed at prevention of complications such as bleeding, tetany, and thyroid crisis.

Nursing diagnoses and interventions for the patient with simple (colloid) goiter include but are not limited to the following:

Nursing Diagnoses	Nursing Interventions
Risk for noncompliance, related to therapeutic regimen	Provide opportunities for patient to express feelings about treatment plan. Correct misconceptions and reinforce previous medical instruction. Stress importance of taking prescribed medications, having regular checkups, and avoiding any identified goitrogenic foods.

Nursing Diagnoses	Nursing Interventions
Risk for disturbed body image, related to altered physical appearance	Develop open and trusting relationship so that the patient will express his or her feelings. Discuss ways to disguise thyroid enlargement (scarves, high collars, makeup).

Stress the importance of adequate dietary intake of iodine by the patient. Medical supervision is recommended at regular intervals.

Prognosis

Most patients can expect to live a normal life after adequate treatment of goiter.

CANCER OF THE THYROID

Etiology and Pathophysiology

Cancer of the thyroid is a relatively rare malignancy, affecting approximately 25 of each 1 million people in the United States each year. However, more cases are expected, since between 1949 and 1960, many infants and children through adolescence were irradiated to shrink enlarged thymus tissue, tonsils, or adenoids and to treat severe cases of acne vulgaris. Cancer of the thyroid occurs more frequently in females and in whites. The incidence rises as age increases. About 75% of malignancies of the thyroid are papillary, well-differentiated adenocarcinomas, a type of cancer that grows slowly, is usually contained, and does not spread beyond the adjacent lymph nodes. Cure rates after thyroidectomy in these cases are excellent. Other cancers, follicular and anaplastic, are more rare and have extremely low cure rates.

Clinical Manifestations

The principal clinical manifestation of thyroid cancer is a firm, fixed, small, rounded, painless mass or **nodule** that is felt during palpation of the gland. Only in rare instances are the symptoms of hyperthyroidism seen.

Assessment

Subjective data include the patient's use of adaptive coping methods to deal with the diagnosis. Also observe the support system provided by the patient's significant others. Assess the patient's understanding of the importance of medical follow-up.

Objective data include progressive enlargement of the tumor area preoperatively, response to ^{131}I therapy, and skin involvement in the neck and torso after radiation therapy.

Diagnostic Tests

Papillary thyroid cancer is suspected when a thyroid scan shows a "cold" nodule, indicating decreased uptake of [131]I. Benign adenomas and follicular cancers are usually visualized as "hot" nodules because of their increased uptake of the isotope. Thyroid function tests usually yield normal results. To confirm the diagnosis, a thyroid needle biopsy may be done, but only by a skilled practitioner to avoid seeding of adjacent tissues. Metastasis could result, with the prognosis becoming much more grave.

Medical Management

Treatment of thyroid cancer is a total thyroidectomy, with subsequent lifelong thyroid hormone replacement therapy. If metastasis is present at the time of the initial surgery, a radical neck dissection may be performed. In addition, radiation therapy, chemotherapy, and administration of ^{131}I may be done.

Nursing Interventions and Patient Teaching

Nursing interventions are like those for the patient who has undergone thyroidectomy (see pp. 497 to 498). As with a thyroidectomy for noncancerous lesions, the major postoperative complications are respiratory distress, recurrent laryngeal damage, hemorrhage, and hypoparathyroidism.

Nursing diagnoses and interventions for the patient with cancer of the thyroid include but are not limited to the following:

Nursing Diagnoses	Nursing Interventions
Anxiety, related to situational crisis	Encourage patient to discuss feelings about upcoming surgery. Monitor level of anxiety. Maintain a calm environment; try to decrease stressors.
Ineffective coping, related to personal vulnerability in crisis	Help patient identify previously successful coping methods. Teach new coping methods as needed.

Stress the importance of proper medical follow-up to monitor thyroid hormone replacement therapy and to help ensure prompt diagnosis of any metastatic lesions. Before discharge from the hospital, teach the patient proper care of the surgical incision.

Prognosis

The prognosis after treatment for thyroid cancer depends on the type of tumor. For papillary carcinoma the prognosis is excellent; for follicular and anaplastic carcinomas, the prognosis is much less favorable.

HYPERPARATHYROIDISM

Etiology and Pathophysiology

Hyperparathyroidism involves overactivity of the parathyroid glands, with increased production of PTH. The cause of this condition may be a primary hypertrophy

of one or more of the tiny parathyroid glands, usually in the form of an adenoma. It may also result from chronic renal failure, pyelonephritis, or glomerulonephritis. Parathyroid carcinoma is a rare condition, with rapid progress and a grave prognosis. Hyperparathyroidism usually occurs in adults between 30 and 70 years of age, and it occurs twice as often in women.

Clinical Manifestations

The primary clinical manifestation is hypercalcemia. This occurs as calcium leaves the bones and accumulates in the bloodstream. As a result, the bones become demineralized, causing skeletal pain, pain on weight bearing, and pathologic fractures (fractures that result from slight or no trauma to diseased bone). The high level of calcium in the blood may lead to the formation of kidney stones.

Assessment

Collection of **subjective data** includes assessment of the severity of skeletal pain, the degree of muscle weakness, and the effectiveness of analgesics. It is important to determine nursing measures that contribute to the patient's comfort and mobility. As neuromuscular function decreases, the patient has generalized fatigue, drowsiness, apathy, nausea, and anorexia; assess the degree of anorexia and nausea. There may be constipation, personality changes, disorientation, and even paranoia. Renal colic and dull back pain may indicate calculus formation.

Collection of **objective data** includes careful observation for any skeletal deformity or abnormal movement of bone that might indicate a pathologic fracture. Observe the urine for quantity and the presence of hematuria and stones. There may be vomiting and weight loss. Hypertension and cardiac dysrhythmias may present significant problems. Changes in the serum calcium level may cause bradycardia and other cardiac irregularities. The level of consciousness may decrease to the level of stupor or coma.

Diagnostic Tests

Radiographic examination may reveal skeletal decalcification. Blood PTH levels are increased, as are alkaline phosphate levels. The patient should receive nothing by mouth for 8 to 12 hours before these tests. The serum calcium level is elevated, whereas the serum phosphorus level is decreased. Bone density measurements may also be used to detect bone loss. Imaging, such as MRI, CT, and ultrasound, may be used to localize the adenoma. A differential diagnosis should be made to rule out multiple myeloma, Cushing's syndrome, vitamin D excess, and other causes of hypercalcemia.

Medical Management

The treatment for hyperparathyroidism is surgical removal of an existing tumor or of one or more parathyroid glands. Normal parathyroid tissue taken from the patient is transplanted in the forearm or near the sternocleidomastoid muscle. This autotransplantation allows the parathyroid tissue to continue to secrete PTH to regulate the concentration of calcium and phosphorus in the blood. If autotransplantation is not possible, or it fails, the patient needs to take calcium replacement for life (Lewis et al., 2007).

Nursing Interventions and Patient Teaching

Preoperative nursing interventions include helping restore fluid and electrolyte balance by encouraging increased oral fluid intake and by carefully monitoring the IV fluid therapy. Monitor the patient's I&O because diuretics may be used. Furosemide is the diuretic of choice. Thiazide diuretics are not used because they decrease renal excretion of calcium and thus increase the hypercalcemic state. Urine may be strained because development of kidney calculi is not uncommon. Daily serum calcium levels may be ordered. The diet should be low in calcium, eliminating milk and other dairy products. Cranberry juice may help promote acidic urine, thereby lessening the possibility of calculus formation. Some antacids are high in calcium and should not be used. Accurately assess the patient's pain and administer prescribed analgesics as needed. Postoperatively, care for the patient in the same manner as after a thyroidectomy, with careful monitoring of I&O. These patients commonly retain fluid in the tissues after surgery and often have decreased urinary output. It is important to avoid overhydration at this point. Assess the patient frequently for signs of hypocalcemia (a deficiency of calcium in the blood serum), such as tetany, cardiac dysrhythmias, and carpopedal spasms. If tetany does occur, administer calcium gluconate intravenously.

Nursing diagnoses and interventions for the patient with hyperparathyroidism include but are not limited to the following:

Nursing Diagnoses	Nursing Interventions
Activity intolerance, related to neuromuscular dysfunction	Help patient to identify factors that increase or decrease activity tolerance and to eliminate or reduce painful, fatiguing activities. Encourage patient to follow prescribed individualized activity or exercise program.
Acute pain: skeletal, joint; renal colic, related to physiologic variables	Assess factors that cause or worsen pain, and help patient adjust body mechanics or activity. Encourage adequate fluid intake while assessing cardiac and urinary output.

Teach the patient the principles of good body mechanics to prevent pathologic fractures during ambulation. Reassure the patient that bone pain should gradually decrease as electrolyte balance is restored and the condition is alleviated. Encourage the patient to participate in mild exercise as prescribed by the physician to regain muscle strength and a feeling of well-being. Teach the patient how to check the urine for stones or blood and how to monitor the pulse for any changes. Evaluate the home environment and develop a plan of changes necessary to prevent accidents.

Prognosis

With proper medical or surgical treatment, the patient can lead a fairly normal life. In patients with parathyroid carcinoma, the prognosis is grave.

HYPOPARATHYROIDISM

Etiology and Pathophysiology

Hypoparathyroidism occurs when there is decreased PTH, resulting in decreased levels of serum calcium. Idiopathic hypoparathyroidism is a rare condition, thought to be either autoimmune or familial in origin. The most common cause is the inadvertent removal or destruction of one or more of the tiny parathyroid glands during thyroidectomy.

Clinical Manifestations

Decreased PTH levels in the bloodstream cause an increased serum phosphorus level and a decreased serum calcium level, resulting in neuromuscular hyperexcitability, involuntary and uncontrollable muscle spasms, and hypocalcemic tetany. Severe hypocalcemia may result in laryngeal spasm, stridor, cyanosis, and an increased possibility of asphyxia. Some patients have calcification of the basal ganglia in the brain, causing a parkinsonian syndrome with bizarre posturing and spastic movements.

Assessment

Collection of **subjective data** includes assessment of neuromuscular activity for symptoms such as dysphagia and numbness or tingling of the lips, fingertips, and occasionally feet and increased muscle tension leading to paresthesias and stiffness. The patient may feel anxious, irritable, or depressed. The patient may experience headaches and nausea. Abdominal or flank pain may occur if a renal calculus attempts to pass down the ureter into the bladder. Assess the effectiveness of narcotics used to relieve renal colic.

Objective data include a positive Chvostek's sign or Trousseau's sign. If laryngeal spasm and stridor occur, cyanosis may appear. Cardiac output may decrease as a result of hypocalcemia, and the patient may develop dysrhythmias. Tetanic spasms of the extremities may be observed.

Diagnostic Tests

Diagnostic laboratory studies confirm the decreased serum calcium and PTH with increased urinary calcium, and increased serum phosphorus with decreased urinary phosphorus. Rule out other possible causes of hypocalcemia, such as vitamin D deficiency, kidney failure, and acute pancreatitis.

Medical Management

The immediate treatment of hypoparathyroid tetany is IV administration of calcium gluconate or calcium chloride (10%). This drug irritates the vessel wall and should always be given slowly, at a rate not to exceed 1 mL/min. The patient may complain of a hot feeling of the skin or tongue. If given too rapidly, IV calcium can precipitate hypotension, serious cardiac dysrhythmias, or cardiac arrest. Thus electrocardiographic monitoring is indicated when administering calcium. Take care that none of the drug escapes the vein and extravasates into the tissues, since sloughing may occur. After the initial IV dose, calcium may be continued in a slow IV infusion until tetany is controlled; then it is given orally. Vitamin D is usually also given orally to increase the absorption and blood level of calcium.

Nursing Interventions and Patient Teaching

Monitor any patient receiving calcium, especially intravenously, for signs of hypercalcemia. The most common clinical manifestations of this are vomiting, disorientation, anorexia, abdominal pain, and weakness. Assess the patient for respiratory distress; renal involvement; and adverse reactions to calcium therapy, such as bradycardia, syncope, and hypotension. Use calcium cautiously in digitalized patients, since it may cause digitalis toxicity. Cimetidine (Tagamet) interferes with normal parathyroid functioning and should be used carefully in these patients. Vitamin D supplements are prescribed to improve the absorption of calcium in the intestinal tract and improve bone resorption in patients with chronic and resistant hypocalcemia. Dihydrotachysterol (Hytakerol) and calcitriol (Rocaltrol) are the preferred medications (Lewis et al., 2007). The diet should contain foods high in calcium, such as dairy products, dark green vegetables, soybeans, tofu, and canned fish with the bones included. Offer high-calcium snacks.

Nursing diagnoses and interventions for the patient with hypoparathyroidism include but are not limited to the following:

Nursing Diagnoses	Nursing Interventions
Risk for injury, related to postoperative hypocalcemia	Assess for signs and symptoms of hypocalcemia (muscle spasms, laryngeal stridor, convulsion). Institute prescribed calcium therapy if needed.

Nursing Diagnoses	Nursing Interventions
Imbalanced nutrition: less than body requirements, related to calcium intake	Give calcium replacement agents as scheduled. Monitor for Chvostek's and Trousseau's signs. Arrange for dietitian to discuss dietary sources of calcium. Assess patient's intake of high-calcium foods.

Teach the patient the early symptoms of hypocalcemia, with instructions to notify the nurse or physician if they occur. Draw blood levels of calcium and phosphorus periodically while the patient is hospitalized. Teach the patient to monitor the pulse for changes, maintain fluid balance, and use calcium supplements at home. Stress the need for life long treatment and follow-up care, including monitoring calcium levels three or four times a year (Lewis et al., 2007).

Prognosis

For most patients, a fairly normal lifestyle and life expectancy are possible.

DISORDERS OF THE ADRENAL GLANDS

ADRENAL HYPERFUNCTION (CUSHING'S SYNDROME)

Etiology and Pathophysiology

Cushing's syndrome is a spectrum of clinical abnormalities caused by excess corticosteroids, particularly glucocorticoids. This syndrome may be caused by hyperplasia of adrenal tissue resulting from overstimulation by the pituitary hormone ACTH, by a tumor of the adrenal cortex, by ACTH-secreting neoplasms outside the pituitary (such as small cell carcinoma of the lung), and by prolonged administration of high doses of corticosteroids. The body's protective feedback mechanism fails, resulting in excess secretion of the adrenal hormones: glucocorticoids, mineralocorticoids, and sex hormones.

Clinical Manifestations

This overabundance of corticosteroids produces the signs and symptoms commonly associated with Cushing's syndrome, including moon face and buffalo hump. Weight gain, the most common feature, results from accumulation of adipose tissue in the trunk, face, and cervical spine area (Figure 11-11). The arms and legs become thin as a result of muscle wasting. Hypokalemia (a condition in which an inadequate amount of potassium, the major intracellular cation, is found in the circulating bloodstream) is usually present. Hyperglycemia occurs because of glucose intolerance (associated with cortisol-induced insulin resistance) and increased glucose release by the liver. The patient usually has protein in the urine and increased urinary calcium

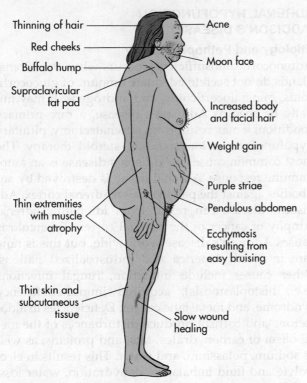

Thinning of hair

Red cheeks

Buffalo hump

Supraclavicular fat pad

Acne

Moon face

Increased body and facial hair

Weight gain

Purple striae

Pendulous abdomen

Thin extremities with muscle atrophy

Ecchymosis resulting from easy bruising

Thin skin and subcutaneous tissue

Slow wound healing

FIGURE 11-11 Common characteristics of Cushing syndrome.

excretion, which may lead to the development of renal calculi. Osteoporosis results from abnormal calcium absorption, and kyphosis may develop. The patient is susceptible to infections, but the symptoms may be masked and the infection not detected until it is life threatening.

Assessment

Collection of **subjective data** includes assessment of the patient's ability to concentrate. Patients may have mood disturbances such as irritability, anxiety, euphoria, insomnia, irrationality, and occasionally psychosis. Depression is common, and the possibility of suicide is an ever-present concern. Be alert to subtle changes in the patient's affect, and keep the environment free from objects with which the patient can inflict self-harm. Patients of both sexes may experience loss of libido and alterations in self-esteem with concerns about sexual dysfunction. Encourage the patient to verbalize concerns about altered body image. Severe backache is often present and may signal a compression fracture of a vertebral body. Assess the severity of back pain and nursing measures that contribute to the patient's comfort. Appetite usually increases. Ensure that the patient understands dietary restrictions and the importance of medical follow-up.

Collection of **objective data** includes observation of the skin for ecchymoses and petechiae. The skin becomes thin and fragile, and wound healing is delayed. The patient may have weight gain and abdominal enlargement, with development of **striae** (a streak or linear scar that often results from stretching of the skin); this increased girth may contribute to difficulty with mobility. Monitor weight, since peripheral edema and associated hypertension are common. Impaired carbohydrate metabolism results in hyperglycemia. Women may experience hirsutism (excessive body hair in a masculine distribution), menstrual irregularities, and deepening of the voice. Elevated body temperature may indicate an undetected infection.

Diagnostic Tests

Diagnosis is usually based on the patient's clinical appearance and laboratory test results. Plasma cortisol levels are usually elevated. Plasma ACTH levels may be increased or decreased, depending on the location of a tumor. Skull radiographic evaluation may detect erosion of the sella turcica in the presence of a pituitary tumor. Adrenal angiography aids in diagnosing an adrenal tumor. A 24-hour urine test for 17-ketosteroids and 17-hydroxysteroids shows increased levels. Blood glucose for hyperglycemia and urinalysis for glycosuria are other diagnostic tests associated with but not diagnostic of Cushing's syndrome. Abdominal CT scan and ultrasound may help localize an abdominal tumor.

Medical Management

Treatment is directed toward the causative factor. If an adrenal tumor is present, adrenalectomy is usually indicated for its removal. Pituitary tumors may be irradiated or removed surgically by transsphenoidal microsurgery. If the patient is unable to undergo surgery because of inoperable cancer elsewhere in the body or another preexisting condition, mitotane (Lysodren) therapy may be used. Mitotane alters peripheral metabolism of cortisol, decreases plasma and corticosteroid level, and suppresses cortisol production—essentially providing a "medical adrenalectomy." This cytotoxic agent is toxic to the adrenal glands and is given for at least 3 months, during which time the patient must be monitored for symptoms of hepatotoxicity, such as jaundice, gastrointestinal upset, and pruritus. The diet should be low in sodium to help decrease edema. Reduced calories and carbohydrates help control hyperglycemia, and foods high in potassium help correct hypokalemia. If Cushing's syndrome has developed during the course of prolonged administration of corticosteroids (e.g., prednisone), one or more of the following alternatives may be tried: (1) gradually discontinuing corticosteroid therapy, (2) reducing the corticosteroid dose, and (3) converting to an alternate-day regimen. Gradually tapering the corticosteroids is necessary to avoid potentially life-threatening adrenal insufficiency.

Nursing Interventions and Patient Teaching

Important nursing interventions include gentle handling to prevent skin impairment or excessive ecchymosis and frequent assessment for erythema, edema, or early signs of infection. Encourage the patient to turn frequently and ambulate as tolerated to eliminate undue pressure on bony prominences. Elbow and heel protectors and an eggcrate mattress pad may help prevent decubitus ulcers in the bedridden patient. Encourage the patient to participate as fully as possible in normal ADLs, interspersing personal hygiene tasks with rest periods to prevent overtiring.

Nursing diagnoses and interventions for the patient with Cushing's syndrome include but are not limited to the following:

Nursing Diagnoses	Nursing Interventions
Deficient knowledge, related to therapeutic regimen	Assess patient's understanding of prescribed medication and diet. Encourage patient to wear medical-alert jewelry and carry wallet identification card.
Activity intolerance, related to weakness and immobility	Assess patient's current activity tolerance, and identify priorities for energy expenditures. Plan activity and rest periods with patient.
Risk for infection, related to: • suppression of immune system • lowered resistance to stress	Monitor patient for complaints of pain, purulent exudates, or decrease of function because the usual signs and symptoms of inflammation, such as fever and erythema, may not be present (Lewis et al., 2007). Practice meticulous handwashing before caring for patient.

The patient's mental attitude is extremely important. Encourage verbalization of concerns and watch for the development of depression and suicidal thoughts. Help the patient understand prescribed medications, such as mitotane, as well as possible side effects. It is important for the patient to wear a medical-alert bracelet or necklace and to carry a wallet card stating the diagnosis of Cushing's syndrome. The patient may need to adjust to a major lifestyle change, and the aid of a social worker may be enlisted. Before adrenalectomy, teach the patient the importance of avoiding stress and infections. Postoperative teaching includes proper wound care and the symptoms of Addison's disease, which is sometimes an unavoidable sequela after this type of surgery.

Prognosis

Depending on whether the cause of the disease was benign or malignant and whether the treatment was successful or unsuccessful, the patient with Cushing's syndrome can expect to have major lifestyle changes, possibly with many complications and a shortened life expectancy.

ADRENAL HYPOFUNCTION (ADDISON'S DISEASE)

Etiology and Pathophysiology

Adrenocortical insufficiency occurs when the adrenal glands do not secrete adequate amount of glucocorticoids, mineralocorticoids, and androgens. It may initially be seen as Addison's disease, a rare primary condition; it may result from adrenalectomy, pituitary hypofunction, or longstanding steroid therapy. The most common cause of Addison's disease is an autoimmune response. Adrenal tissue is destroyed by antibodies against the patient's own adrenal cortex. Addison's disease can result from idiopathic adrenal atrophy or cancer of the adrenal cortex. Tuberculosis causes Addison's disease worldwide, but this is now rare in North America and industrialized nations. Other causes include infarction, fungal infections (e.g., histoplasmosis), acquired immunodeficiency syndrome, and metastatic cancer. Deficiencies in aldosterone and cortisol produce disturbances of the metabolism of carbohydrates, fats, and proteins, as well as sodium, potassium, and water. This results in electrolyte and fluid imbalance, dehydration, water loss, and hypovolemia. Adrenal insufficiency most often occurs in adults less than 60 years of age and affects both genders equally.

Clinical Manifestations

Because manifestations are usually not evident until 90% of the adrenal cortex is destroyed, the disease is often advanced before it is diagnosed. Clinical manifestations are directly related to imbalances in adrenal hormones, nutrients, and electrolytes.

Assessment

Subjective data include progressive weakness, fatigue, nausea, anorexia, and craving for salt. Postural hypotension may be associated with vertigo, weakness, and syncope, resulting in reluctance to attempt normal activities. The patient may complain of severe headache, disorientation, abdominal pain, or lower back pain, which could represent early symptoms of adrenal crisis. This patient tolerates stress poorly and feels anxious and apprehensive. It is important to assess emotional status and allow the patient to share feelings about altered self-image. Also assess the patient's overall understanding of the disease process and the importance of medical treatment and follow-up.

Collection of **objective data** includes observation of changes in the color of the mucous membranes and the skin. Skin hyperpigmentation, a common feature, is seen primarily in sun-exposed areas of the body; at pressure points; over joints; and in creases, especially in palmar creases. The patient usually loses weight, often with vomiting and diarrhea. Hypoglycemia may contribute to fatigue; assess the patient's ability to perform ADLs. An abnormally low or abnormally high body temperature, orthostatic hypotension, hyponatremia, and hyperkalemia are signs of impending **adrenal crisis,** a life-threatening emergency caused by insufficient adrenocortical hormones or a sudden sharp decrease in these hormones. Precipitating factors that can trigger an addisonian crisis are stress-producing situations such as infections, surgery, trauma, hemorrhage, psychological stress, sudden withdrawal of corticosteroid hormone replacement therapy, postadrenal surgery, or sudden pituitary gland destruction (Lewis et al., 2007). See Table 11-3 for a comparison of Cushing's syndrome and Addison's disease.

Diagnostic Tests

Laboratory studies show decreased serum sodium, increased serum potassium, and decreased serum glucose. A 24-hour urine specimen shows decreased levels of 17-ketosteroids and 17-hydroxysteroids. Fasting plasma cortisol levels and aldosterone levels are low with an ACTH stimulation test. A glucose tolerance test may yield abnormal results.

Medical Management

Medical treatment involves the prompt restoration of fluid and electrolyte balance and replacement of the deficient adrenal hormones. The most common form of replacement therapy is hydrocortisone, which has both mineralocorticoid and glucocorticoid properties. Glucocorticoid dosage must be increased during times of physiologic stress to prevent addisonian crisis. Fludrocortisone (Florinef) (a mineralocorticoid) is also administered. The diet should be high in sodium and low in potassium.

Treatment for the life-threatening emergency of an addisonian crisis includes shock management, high-dose hydrocortisone replacement therapy, and large volumes of 0.9% saline and 5% dextrose solutions to improve electrolyte imbalances and reverse hypotension (Lewis et al., 2007).

Nursing Interventions and Patient Teaching

Carefully assess the patient's circulatory status, keep accurate I&O records, and record daily weight. Check skin turgor and offer fluids frequently. Monitor vital signs at regular intervals, paying particular attention to temperature and blood pressure. Also monitor the patient for response to prescribed steroid drugs, and promptly report any adverse effects to the physician. Keep the environment as free from stress as possible. Visitors and hospital personnel should be screened for infectious disease and excluded from the patient's room. Continually assess the patient for signs of developing adrenal (addisonian) crisis, manifested by a sudden, severe drop in blood pressure; nausea and vomiting; an extremely high temperature; and cyanosis, progressing to vasomotor collapse and possibly death. The patient should carry an emergency kit at all times with 100 mg of IM hydrocortisone, syringes, and instructions for use. Teach the patient and significant others to give an IM injection in case replacement therapy cannot be taken orally. Also advise the patient that he or she will need extra medications to tolerate periods of physical or emotional stress (Lewis et al., 2007). Patient education is imperative for long-term compliance in the management of Addison's disease.

Nursing diagnoses and interventions for the patient with Addison's disease include but are not limited to the following:

Nursing Diagnoses	Nursing Interventions
Risk for infection, related to altered metabolic processes	Assess environment for stressors. Screen visitors and personnel for contagious disease. Monitor temperature routinely. Stress the importance of taking prescribed medications.

Continued

Table **11-3** **Nursing Assessment of Patients with Cushing's Syndrome or Addison's Disease**

AREA OF ASSESSMENT	CLINICAL MANIFESTATIONS IN CUSHING'S SYNDROME	CLINICAL MANIFESTATIONS IN ADDISON'S DISEASE
Cardiovascular	Mild to moderate hypertension	Postural hypotension, vertigo, syncope
Neurologic	Impaired memory and concentration, insomnia, irritability	Lethargy, headache
Musculoskeletal	Muscle weakness, muscle wasting in extremities, back and rib pain, kyphosis	Muscle weakness, fatigue, muscle aches, muscle wasting
Integumentary	Thin skin, red cheeks, acne, frequent petechiae and ecchymoses, increased body and facial hair, poor wound healing	Hyperpigmentation, decreased body hair
Self-care and self-concept	Tires easily; insomnia, malaise, negative feelings regarding changes in body	Tires easily; profound weakness, lack of interest in usual activities and relationships
Nutrition and fluid balance	Increased appetite, moderate weight gain, edema, buffalo hump, moon face, obesity of trunk, hyperglycemia; need for decreased salt intake, reduced calories and carbohydrate intake, increased potassium intake	Nausea and vomiting, fluid and electrolyte imbalance, dehydration, weight loss, hypoglycemia; need for increased salt and decreased potassium intake

Nursing Diagnoses	Nursing Interventions
Ineffective tissue perfusion, peripheral, related to electrolyte imbalance	Monitor vital signs and I&O. Have patient make position changes slowly; monitor for vertigo, visual changes.

Before discharge from the hospital, teach the patient the importance of adhering to the prescribed drug therapy; having regular medical checkups; and immediately reporting all illnesses, even a cold, to the physician. Emphasize that stress is one of the major precipitating factors in adrenal crisis, and encourage the patient to minimize stress through cognitive behavior therapy, relaxation therapy, biofeedback, and mental imagery. Other conditions to avoid include overexertion, diarrhea, infection, decreased intake of salt, exposure to cold, and surgery. It is critical that the patient wear a medical-alert bracelet and carry a wallet card stating that the patient has Addison's disease so that appropriate therapy be initiated in case of trauma, accident, or crisis.

Prognosis

With long-term steroid therapy, adequate medical care, and follow-up, this patient has a fair prognosis.

PHEOCHROMOCYTOMA

Etiology and Pathophysiology

A pheochromocytoma is a rare tumor of the adrenal medulla that causes excessive secretion of catecholamines (epinephrine and norepinephrine). These tumors occur most often in adults between 20 and 60 years of age and are almost always benign; only about 10% are malignant. The secretion of excessive catecholamines results in severe hypertension.

Clinical Manifestations

Pheochromocytoma results in severe hypertension because of sympathetic nervous system stimulation. Other classic clinical signs and symptoms include anxiety, severe headache, diaphoresis, tachycardia, and unexplained abdominal or chest pain (Lewis et al., 2007). Hypertensive crisis may occur, during which the blood pressure may fluctuate widely, sometimes as high as 300/175 mm Hg. Signs and symptoms may be triggered by an identifiable factor, such as overexertion or emotional trauma, or they may occur for no apparent reason. Extreme hypertension may result in stroke, kidney damage, and retinopathy. Cardiac damage may occur, resulting in heart failure.

Assessment

Subjective data during a hypertensive crisis include severe headache and palpitations. The patient may feel nervous, dizzy, and dyspneic and may experience paresthesias, nausea, and intolerance to heat. Anxiety is common, and the patient may have trouble sleeping. Question the patient about the occurrence of symptoms in relation to identifiable factors, such as excess stress or overexertion, and identify the coping methods used.

Collection of **objective data** includes frequent measurement of blood pressure and respiratory rate for increases and of pulse for tachycardia. The patient may have tremors, diaphoresis, dilated pupils, glycosuria, and hyperglycemia. Assess responses to prescribed medications.

Diagnostic Tests

The measurement of urinary metanephrines (catecholamine metabolites), usually performed as a 24-hour urine collection, is the simplest and most reliable test. Values are elevated in at least 90% of those with pheochromocytoma. Vanillylmandelic acid (VMA) may also be measured in a 24-hour urine sample. However, this test has more false negatives than that for urine metanephrines. Plasma catecholamines are also elevated. It is preferable to measure serum catecholamines during an "attack." CT scan and MRI of the adrenal glands may help in locating the tumor.

Medical Management

Treatment is usually the surgical removal of the tumor. Surgery is more commonly done via laparoscopic adrenalectomy than via open abdominal incision. Preoperatively, the patient may be given calcium channel blockers such as nicardipine (Cardene) or alpha-adrenergic blocking agents such as phentolamine mesylate (Regitine) or phenoxybenzamine hydrochloride (Dibenzyline) in an effort to control hypertension. Beta blockers (e.g., propranolol [Inderal]) to decrease tachycardia and other dysrhythmias are also used. Metyrosine (Demser) may be given to help inhibit catecholamine production, and the drug must be continued on a long-term basis if the tumor is inoperable.

Nursing Interventions and Patient Teaching

Postoperative care is carried out in the same manner as for any major abdominal surgery, with the following special concerns. If the patient has undergone adrenalectomy, large amounts of hydrocortisone will be given. Watch carefully for fluctuations in blood pressure caused by adrenal manipulation during surgery, with subsequent release of epinephrine and norepinephrine. These fluctuations may be severe and life threatening if cardiovascular collapse occurs. The patient should avoid excess stress and must be allowed adequate time to rest; give sedatives to ensure this. Keep a careful I&O record and administer IV solutions exactly as ordered. Vasopressors and corticosteroids may be given. The diet should be free from stimulants, such as coffee, tea, and soft drinks containing caffeine.

Nursing diagnoses and interventions for the patient with pheochromocytoma include but are not limited to the following:

Nursing Diagnoses	Nursing Interventions
Ineffective tissue perfusion, cardiopulmonary, renal, related to hypertension	Monitor blood pressure and pulse and record I&O.
	Eliminate smoking and caffeine-containing beverages.
Activity intolerance, related to hypertension	Assist with gradual position changes from lying to sitting or standing.
	Limit activity, as needed, to prevent increased hypertension.

Follow-up 24-hour urine tests (catecholamine metabolites or VMA) may determine when the levels have returned to normal. The patient is then pronounced cured and may resume normal activities. If the tumor is inoperable, the patient remains under lifelong medical supervision. Stress the importance of compliance with prescribed treatment. The patient should wear medical-alert jewelry and carry a wallet card. Teach the patient self-monitoring of blood pressure and when to call the physician if elevation occurs.

Prognosis

If undiagnosed and untreated, pheochromocytoma may lead to diabetes mellitus, cardiomyopathy, and death. The prognosis after successful removal of the causative tumor is good; for an inoperable tumor, the prognosis depends on adequate medical management of hypertension.

DISORDERS OF THE PANCREAS

DIABETES MELLITUS

Etiology

Diabetes mellitus (DM) (*diabetes,* "like a sieve or siphon"; *mellitus,* "sweet or related to honey") is a systemic metabolic disorder that involves improper metabolism of carbohydrates, fats, and proteins. This is a chronic multisystem disease related to a decrease or absolute lack of insulin production by the beta cells of the islets of Langerhans in the pancreas or by impaired insulin utilization, or both. In nondiabetic people the beta cells are stimulated by increased blood glucose levels; insulin secretion reaches peak levels about 30 minutes after meals and returns to normal in 2 to 3 hours. Between meals or during a period of fasting, insulin levels remain low, and the body uses its supply of stored glucose and amino acids to provide energy for the tissues. The beta cells of the pancreas continuously release insulin into the bloodstream in small amounts. A bolus of insulin is released after the intake of food. The average

amount of insulin secreted by the beta cells of the pancreas in an adult is 40 to 50 units every 24 hours. The release of insulin in this systematic manner results in the body maintaining a normal blood sugar between 70 to 120 mg/dL (Lewis et al., 2007). In people with diabetes, the body's insulin supply is either absent or deficient, or target cells resist the action of insulin. There are several types of DM, but in each type, hyperglycemia is the principal clinical manifestation.

Although the exact cause of DM is unknown, a number of factors contribute to its development: genetic predisposition, viruses (such as coxsackievirus B, rubella, and mumps), the aging process, diet and lifestyle, and ethnicity. Obesity is believed to be a major factor. The T lymphocytes may play a role in the autoimmune destruction of the pancreatic insulin-producing cells.

Complications of diabetes are: blindness; nephropathy; amputation of a lower extremity; cardiovascular complications including heart disease, hypertension, and stroke (Lewis et al., 2007).

Types of Diabetes Mellitus

There are two main types of DM: **type 1** and **type 2.** Type 1 was formerly called juvenile diabetes, juvenile-onset diabetes, or insulin-dependent DM. Type 2 was formerly called adult-onset diabetes, maturity-onset diabetes, or non–insulin-dependent DM. Because this disease is becoming more common in children, and because some people with type 2 diabetes use insulin, these terms are no longer appropriate. About 80% to 90% of type 2 diabetes patients are overweight at the time of diagnosis. Other DM patients have conditions such as pancreatitis, genetic syndromes, malnutrition, chemical- or drug-induced disease, and pregnancy. Type 1 and type 2 diabetes have some distinct differences (Table 11-4). In type 1 an autoimmune disease (probably stimulated by a virus) eventually results in destruction of beta cells in the pancreatic islets and results in deficient insulin **production;** the patient retains normal sensitivity to insulin action. Within 5 years of diagnosis, all of the patient's beta cells have been destroyed and no insulin is produced. In type 2 the main problem seems to be an abnormal resistance to insulin **action.**

Regardless of the type of DM, all of these patients have impaired glucose tolerance. Only 5% to 10% of all people with diabetes have type 1. About 90% of people with DM in the United States have type 2, with a high incidence among blacks; Hispanic Americans; and Native Americans, especially members of the Pima tribe. The American Diabetes Association (ADA) estimates that as many as 20.8 million Americans (7% of the population) have DM, and 41 million more people have prediabetes.

Type 1 Diabetes Mellitus

Type 1 diabetes mellitus results from progressive destruction of beta-cell function in the pancreas as a result of an autoimmune process in a susceptible in-

Table 11-4 Comparison of Type 1 and Type 2 Diabetes Mellitus

FACTOR	TYPE 1	TYPE 2
Age at onset	Usually 30 years or younger, but can occur at any age	Usually age 35 years or older, but can occur at any age. Incidence is increasing in children
Body weight	Normal or underweight	80% are overweight
Symptoms at onset	Sudden; polyphagia, polydipsia, polyuria, weight loss, weakness, fatigue; glycosuria, hyperglycemia; acidosis, progressing to DKA	Gradual; may be asymptomatic at onset; later, may develop signs and symptoms of type 1; others include slow wound healing, blurred vision, pruritus, boils or other skin infections; vaginal infections in women
Treatment	Diet, exercise, and insulin; may add subcutaneous insulin-enhancing drug (pramlintide [Symlin])	Diet and exercise; or diet, exercise, and oral hypoglycemic agents; or diet, exercise, oral hypoglycemic agents, and insulin during times of illness or stress; may add a subcutaneous insulin-enhancing agent such as exenatide (Byetta) or pramlintide
Incidence of complications	Frequent	Frequent
Psychosocial and sexual concerns	Irritability; disturbed body image; mood swings, depression; menstrual irregularities; decreased libido	Disturbed body image; amenorrhea; decreased libido; poor tolerance to stress

DKA, Diabetic ketoacidosis.

dividual. The pancreatic islets of Langerhans cell antibodies and insulin autoantibodies cause an 80% to 90% reduction in beta cells before hyperglycemia and symptoms occur. Type 1 DM is characterized by autoimmune beta-cell destruction, which is attributed to a genetic predisposition. Genetics plus infection of one or more viral agents and possibly chemical agents are believed to cause type 1 DM. It is not known whether these are the only factors involved. The onset and progression of hyperglycemic signs and symptoms are usually more rapid and acute in type 1 DM than in type 2. Type 1 diabetes may occur at any age, but signs and symptoms usually appear before 30 years of age. The patient is usually thin. The patient often has strongly positive urine ketone tests with hyperglycemia and depends on insulin therapy to prevent ketoacidosis and to sustain life (Lewis et al., 2007). Because they do not produce adequate amounts of endogenous (produced by the body) insulin, patients with type 1 DM must take regular injections of exogenous (from outside the body) insulin or they will die.

Type 2 Diabetes Mellitus

The pathophysiologic factors that have been identified in **type 2 diabetes mellitus** include (1) decreased tissue (e.g., fat, muscle) responsiveness to insulin as a result of a receptor or postreceptor defects; (2) overproduction of insulin early in the disease, but eventual decreased secretion of insulin from beta-cell exhaustion; and (3) abnormal hepatic glucose regulation. These factors result in what is often referred to as peripheral insulin resistance. This resistance stimulates increased insulin production as a compensatory response, which may also predispose the patient to weight gain. Weight loss for the obese patient with type 2 diabetes tends to reverse

this problem. The patient with type 2 diabetes may benefit from oral antidiabetic agents, which increase insulin production, improve cell receptor binding, regulate hepatic glucose production, and delay carbohydrate absorption from the small intestine. Type 2 usually occurs in people who are older than 35 years of age, with about half of the people diagnosed being older than 55 at diagnosis. Eighty percent to 90% of these patients are overweight, with a familial history of diabetes. Patients have few classic symptoms. The patient is usually not prone to ketoacidosis except during periods of stress. Individuals with type 2 diabetes are not dependent on exogenous insulin for survival, but may require it for adequate control of hyperglycemia.

These patients can usually achieve good control of their disease by diet, exercise, and oral hypoglycemics, using insulin only when first diagnosed and during times of illness, surgery, or other periods when the body's insulin level is out of control (Lewis et al., 2007). Most newly diagnosed type 2 diabetic patients have had the disease for as long as 10 years without treatment and have therefore been at risk for serious complications before diagnosis.

Pathophysiology

In normal metabolism the end products of digestion (glucose, fatty acids and glycerol, and amino acids) are absorbed into the venous circulation and carried to the liver, where they may be either used immediately or stored for later use. The liver can change glycerol and fatty acids into glucose, and glucose into triglycerides, as needed. Fatty acids may also be changed into **ketone bodies** (normal metabolic products, such as β-hydroxybutyric acid and aminoacetic acid, from which acetone may arise spontaneously), which serve as fuel for the muscles and as an energy source for the brain. Glucose is stored in the form of glycogen in the liver. Free glucose in the bloodstream can always be used by the brain and kidney because insulin is not needed for glucose molecules to enter the brain cells or the glomeruli. But insulin must be present for muscle cells and other body cells to utilize glucose. Glycogen can be changed back into glucose as needed by the body for energy. In the patient with diabetes, lack of proper amounts of insulin, or its inadequate utilization, impairs the use of glucose by the body. Thus the excess glucose accumulates in the bloodstream, and hyperglycemia (greater than normal amounts of glucose in the blood) exists.

To rid the body of this abnormal amount of glucose, the kidneys excrete it in the urine. This is called glycosuria (abnormal presence of a sugar, especially glucose, in the urine), a condition that necessitates an extra amount of water for proper dilution of the urine. The patient thus develops polyuria (excretion of an abnormally large quantity of urine) and also polydipsia (excessive thirst). Often the patient is unable to drink enough fluid to compensate for polyuria and may become dehydrated. Even though excess glucose is available in the bloodstream, the body tissues cannot utilize it without the help of insulin. Thus the cells are not properly nourished, and polyphagia (eating to the point of gluttony) develops. In spite of increased food intake, metabolism remains faulty, and the patient loses weight. Because carbohydrates cannot be utilized properly, proteins and fats are broken down and ketone bodies are used excessively for heat and energy. Because ketone bodies are acid substances, the patient may develop acidosis. Diabetic ketoacidosis (DKA) (acidosis accompanied by an accumulation of ketones in the blood), formerly called diabetic coma, may develop, and the patient could die. DKA is a severe metabolic disturbance caused by an acute insulin deficiency, decreased peripheral glucose utilization, and increased fat mobilization and ketogenesis.

Clinical Manifestations

The hallmark symptoms of type 1 DM include the three classic "polys": polyuria, polydipsia, and polyphagia. As ketone bodies accumulate in the bloodstream, imbalances of sodium, potassium, and bicarbonate result. People with type 2 DM, most of whom are more than 35 years of age, experience different signs and symptoms. The patient may be asymptomatic in the early stages of the disease, but later may complain of symptoms associated with type 1, plus a number of others. These patients may not seek medical care until a severe complication such as kidney involvement, retinopathy, impotence, neuropathy, or gangrene occurs.

Assessment

Subjective data include hunger, thirst, and nausea. In addition to frequent urination of large amounts, the patient may complain of nocturia, weakness, and fatigue.

The patient may have blurred vision, the appearance of halos around lights, and headache. Symptoms such as cold extremities, cramping pain in the calves and feet during exercise or walking, decreased sensation to pain and temperature in the feet, and numbness and tingling of the lower extremities may occur. Symptoms of delayed stomach emptying such as nausea, vomiting, and early satiety (feeling of being full after eating) may develop. Male patients may become impotent. The patient may verbalize negative feelings about his or her body and the ability to cope with the illness. Assess coping methods and knowledge about the disease process. Misunderstandings and lack of interest may result in inadequate skills—such as diet planning, injections, and exercise programs—to manage the necessary diabetic lifestyle. Assess the patient's understanding of the importance of adhering to prescribed medical treatment and obtaining adequate follow-up.

Collection of objective data includes assessment of the skin, since slow wound healing, furuncles, carbuncles, and ulcerations are common. Women with DM may experience frequent urinary tract and vaginal infections, and vaginal discharge is often bothersome. In type 1 patients, weight loss and muscle wasting may be seen, but many type 2 patients remain obese. The skin on the lower extremities may appear shiny and thin, with less hair present. The legs and feet may feel cold to the touch, and there may be ulcerated areas. Gangrene of the toes is a dreaded sign. Assess the patient's ability to perform blood glucose testing and proper injection of insulin.

Diagnostic Tests

Diagnosis of DM is made on the basis of clinical manifestations, plus the patient's history and laboratory findings. The patient with random blood glucose greater than 200 mg/dL, a fasting plasma glucose level greater than 126 mg/dL, or a glucose 2-hour postload (75 g anhydrous) level greater than 200 mg/dL should be further evaluated. Blood tests commonly performed include those in Box 11-2.

The ADA recommends self-monitoring of blood glucose (SMBG) instead of urine testing in any patient with DM. This is accomplished in a number of ways. Blood from a fingerstick may be placed on a reagent strip and compared with a color chart, or it may be placed into a reflectance meter. Another type of meter uses a glucose sensor, and test strips are not used; instead, a drop of blood is placed directly into the machine. SMBG is the monitoring tool of choice because it provides an accurate picture of current blood glucose levels (Figure 11-12).

The frequency of monitoring depends on the glycemic goals the patient and health care provider set and the intensity of the treatment regimen. The patient receiving two or more injections of insulin per day may want to test before meals and at bedtime every day. If

Box 11-2	Diagnostic Tests for Diabetes Mellitus

- **Fasting blood glucose (FBG):** After an 8-hour fast, blood is drawn. Normal is 60 to 110 mg/dL of venous blood; 126 mg/dL or greater is considered abnormal.
- **Oral glucose tolerance test (OGTT):** When patient shows overt signs and symptoms of hyperglycemia, polyuria, polydipsia, and polyphagia, together with FBG levels of 126 mg/dL or greater, further OGTTs are usually not warranted. However, whenever OGTTs are used, the accuracy depends on adequate patient preparation and attention to the many factors that may influence the outcome of such tests.
- **Serum insulin:** Absent in type 1 diabetes mellitus (DM); normal to high in type 2 DM.
- **Postprandial (after a meal) blood glucose (PPBG):** Give a fasting patient a measured amount of carbohydrate solution orally, or have the patient eat a measured amount of foods containing carbohydrates, fats, and proteins. Draw a blood sample 2 hours after completion of the meal. Elevated plasma glucose over 160 mg/dL may indicate the presence of DM.
- **Patient self-monitoring of blood glucose (SMBG):** A blood sample is obtained by the fingerstick method, by either the patient or the nurse, and tested using a blood glucose-monitoring device.
- **Glycosylated hemoglobin (HbA$_{lc}$):** This blood test measures the amount of glucose that has become incorporated into the hemoglobin within an erythrocyte; these levels are reported as a percentage of the total hemoglobin. Because glycosylation occurs constantly during the 120-

day life span of the erythrocyte, this test reveals the effectiveness of diabetes therapy for the preceding 8 to 12 weeks. Glycosylated hemoglobin levels remain more stable than plasma glucose levels and are evaluated by a venipuncture every 6 to 8 weeks. Normal HbA$_{lc}$ is approximately 4% to 6% of the total. There is an urgent need to reduce HbA$_{lc}$ values to below 7% to reduce complications. A result greater than 8% represents an average blood glucose level of approximately 200 mg/dL and signals a need for changes in treatment.
- **C-peptide test:** The production of insulin by the beta cells of the pancreas begins with proinsulin with an A chain of amino acids and a B chain of amino acids with a connecting peptide or C-peptide. The C-peptide allows the A and B proinsulin to fold and cleave together, creating the structure of insulin. After the connection has been made, the fusion occurs, creating insulin and a C-peptide by-product. C-peptide then gets secreted into the bloodstream by the pancreas along with insulin. The C-peptide level may be measured in a patient with type 2 DM to see if any insulin is being produced by the body. A newly diagnosed diabetic patient will often use this test to determine whether he or she has type 1 or type 2 DM. Normal values are 0.5 to 2 ng/mL. The patient with type 1 diabetes is unable to produce insulin and therefore has decreased levels of C-peptide; C-peptide levels in type 2 diabetic patients are normal or higher than normal. In type 2 diabetics, the problem seems to be an abnormal resistance to insulin action.

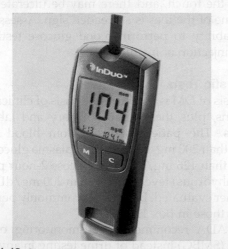

FIGURE 11-12 Glucose sensor for self-monitoring of blood glucose.

glycemic control is relatively stable, the patient may elect to test two or more times a day on certain days of the week. Testing is usually done before meals, but it can be done any time the patient needs to know the way a factor, such as stress, is affecting the blood glucose levels. The frequency of recording SMBG results to guide therapy decision should be jointly determined by the health care provider and the patient.

The technology used for SMBG changes rapidly, with newer and more convenient systems being introduced every year. Blood glucose monitoring technology using a noninvasive spectroscopy—or a laser light on a skin surface such as the forearm or space

between finger and thumb—is being researched for possible use in the future. Implantable sensors for continuous glucose monitoring are also being considered in research trials.

Urine testing for ketonuria is a valuable aid in determining the advent of DKA and is recommended for every patient with type 1 diabetes when the patient is experiencing hyperglycemia or acute illness. The amount of acetone is represented by a color change in shades of pink to purple. Acetone testing products include Ketostix and Acetest tablets.

Medical Management

Medical treatment for DM, no matter what type, consists mainly of education, monitoring, meal planning, medication, and exercise. The overall goal is to assist people with diabetes in making changes in nutrition and exercise habits leading to improved metabolic control. Additional goals include the following:

- Maintenance of as near-normal blood glucose levels as possible by balancing food intake with insulin or oral glucose-lowering medications and activity levels.
- Achievement of optimal serum lipid levels.
- Provision of adequate calories for maintaining or attaining reasonable weight for adults and normal growth and development rates for children and adolescents; and for meeting increased metabolic needs during pregnancy, lactation, and recovery from illnesses. Reasonable weight is de-

fined as the weight the patient and health care provider decide is achievable and maintainable in both the short term and the long term. This may not be the same as the usually defined desirable or ideal body weight.

- Prevention and treatment of acute complications such as hypoglycemia and long-term complications such as renal disease, neuropathy, hypertension, and cardiovascular disease.
- Improvement of overall health through optimal nutrition. The U.S. Department of Agriculture's MyPyramid food planning tool (www.mypyramid. gov) summarizes nutritional guidelines and nutrient needs for all healthy Americans and can be used by the patient with diabetes.

It is hoped that the patient will assume a large part of the responsibility for self-care, with emphasis on optimal wellness instead of illness. Since 1921, when Charles Best and Frederick Banting first isolated insulin, medical science has made many dramatic strides in the care of the patient with diabetes, but physicians depend on the help obtained from other members of the health care team, especially nurses. Every newly diagnosed patient must undergo an intensive and extensive education program to learn proper diet, medication routines, SMBG, and the role of exercise. The importance of the nurse as a teacher cannot be overemphasized (see Evidence-Based Practice box).

Diet

Nutritional therapy for the patient with diabetes is aimed at helping to achieve a normal blood glucose level of less than 126 mg/dL and at attaining or maintaining a reasonable body weight, while ensuring proper growth and body maintenance. Nutritional therapy is the cornerstone of care for the person with diabetes. A nutritionally adequate meal plan with a reduction of total fat, especially saturated fat, is important. Monitoring of blood glucose levels, glycosylated hemoglobin, and lipids is essential. Enlist the services of a dietitian for

each newly diagnosed diabetic. The menu must be individualized, taking into consideration the patient's age, weight, activity level, lifestyle, ethnic background, and food preferences. Assess the ability to choose and pay for groceries, prepare food, and properly store leftovers to ensure the patient can follow dietary instructions after discharge. If the patient is living with family, educate the person who plans and prepares the meals along with the patient, and teach this person how to accommodate the patient's dietary needs in the family menus. The physician and dietitian decide the proper amounts of each nutrient in the dietary prescription. Dietary treatment, also called **medical nutrition therapy for diabetes,** involves individualized meal plans. Diets are based on ADA recommendations, and patients may obtain additional information and menus from that organization at no cost.

Quantitative diabetic diets, following the food choices and number of servings recommended by the MyPyramid food planning tool, include 45% to 50% of total kilocalories from carbohydrates, 10% to 20% of total kilocalories from proteins, and no more than 30% of total kilocalories from fats. Rigid rules on carbohydrates have softened. Now the emphasis is on the total amount of carbohydrates consumed, rather than on the type. Once it was believed that a simple carbohydrate (sugar) would drive up blood glucose levels, so patients were advised to consume only complex carbohydrates. This has proven inaccurate, however, as: (1) some complex carbohydrates (rice, potatoes, and bread) produce a glycemic response similar to that caused by sucrose (table sugar), and (2) milk and fruit have less effect on blood glucose than most starches. As a result, sugars and complex carbohydrates are counted together as total carbohydrates.

Different carbohydrate foods affect the blood glucose level in different ways; this varying effect is termed the **glycemic index.** So emphasis may be placed not only on the amount of carbohydrate eaten but also on the glycemic index of those foods.

 Evidence-Based Practice   Changes in Diabetes Self-Care Behaviors

Evidence Summary

Diabetes self-management is critical, complex, and demanding. In a comparison between diabetes Treatment as Usual (TAU) with the Pathways to Change (PTC) intervention, the PTC group received stage-matched personalized assessment reports, self-help manuals, and newsletters. In addition, individual phone counseling helped determine readiness for self-monitoring of blood glucose (SMBG), healthy eating, and/or smoking cessation. Those in the PTC group were more likely to move into the action stages of those self-care behaviors, such as performing SMBG as instructed, eating more fruits and vegetables, and quitting smoking in order to manage their diabetes.

Application to Nursing Practice

As health care professionals, we need to help patients move through the stages of behavior change. It is important to as-

sess and determine the patient's readiness for change and target messages appropriately. When a patient is not even beginning to think about eating more fruits and vegetables in his or her diet, it is unrealistic to tell the patient to eat at least five fruits and vegetables every day. It would be more appropriate to inform the patient why this is important, have the patient identify a favorite fruit or vegetable, and give one or two simple suggestions as to how to incorporate the fruits or vegetables into his or her diet. By helping patients through the change process, we can reduce long-term complications of diabetes.

Reference

Jones, H., Edwards, L., Vallis, T.M., et al. (2003). Changes in diabetes self-care behaviors make a difference in glycemic control: the Diabetes Stages of Change (DiSC) study, *Diabetes Care,* 26(3):732.

From Potter, P.A., & Perry, A.G. (2009). *Fundamentals of nursing: concepts, process, and practice.* (7th ed.). St. Louis: Mosby.

The **qualitative** diet is unmeasured and more unrestricted, stressing moderation when selecting foods from the MyPyramid food planning tool and reducing the use of simple carbohydrates, saturated fats, and alcohol. This diet may be used for the patient whose blood glucose levels are not extremely high, for the pediatric patient, or for the patient who does not adhere to the ADA diet.

Insulin-dependent patients are usually given midafternoon and bedtime snacks in addition to their regular three meals a day. It is important to evenly distribute food intake throughout the day, taking insulin dosage and exercise into consideration. The patient who plans to engage in strenuous exercise should eat more food, since exercise increases the absorption rate of insulin, thereby enabling muscles to use glucose more effectively.

Exercise

The patient with diabetes should exercise regularly. The physician helps determine the best type of exercise for each patient. Exercise is beneficial not only because it aids in promoting proper utilization of glucose, but also because it is important to the overall functioning of the cardiovascular system and increases the patient's feeling of well-being. Of all the therapies available for treating type 2 diabetes, exercise is probably the least expensive and most cost effective. Exercise can reduce insulin resistance and increase glucose uptake for as long as 72 hours; it also reduces blood pressure and lipid levels. However, it can carry some risks, including hypoglycemia. Patients older than age 40 should have a complete physical examination before beginning a rigorous exercise program. Like medications, exercise can be adjusted to improve blood glucose control. With exercise, motivation is more important than facts and information.

Stress of Acute Illness and Surgery

Both emotional and physical stress can increase the blood glucose level and result in hyperglycemia. However, it is impossible to avoid stress in life situations such as death in the family, job, interviews, and final examinations. These situations may require extra insulin to avoid hyperglycemia.

Common stress-evoking situations include acute illness, pregnancy, and the controlled stress of surgery. The patient with diabetes who has a minor illness such as a cold or the flu should continue drug therapy and food intake. A carbohydrate liquid substitution such as regular soft drinks, gelatin dessert, or beverages such as Gatorade may be necessary. The patient should understand that food intake is important during this time because the body requires extra energy to deal with the stress of the illness.

Blood glucose monitoring should be done every 1 to 2 hours by either the patient or a person who can assume responsibility for care during the illness. Urinary output and the presence and degree of ketonuria should be monitored, particularly when fever is present. Increase fluid intake to prevent dehydration, with a minimum of 4 ounces per hour for an adult.

Instruct the patient to contact the health care provider when the blood glucose level exceeds 250 mg/dL; in such cases, fever, ketonuria, and nausea and vomiting may occur. The health care provider should supervise the necessary adjustments in the treatment regimen during times of stress. Eventually the well-informed patient will be able to make most adjustments independently on the basis of experience.

Surgery is controlled stress, and adjustments in the diabetes regimen can be planned to ensure glycemic control. The patient is given IV fluids and insulin immediately before, during, and after surgery when there is no oral intake. The type 2 diabetic patient receiving oral antidiabetic medications usually has the drugs discontinued 48 hours before surgery and is treated with insulin during the surgical period. Explain to the patient that this is a temporary measure, not a worsening of diabetes.

Medications

Insulin and oral hypoglycemic drugs are the drugs of choice for patients with diabetes. Insulin administration is necessary for all patients with type 1 and patients with type 2 whose condition cannot be controlled by diet, exercise, or hypoglycemic medications alone.

Insulin

Today only biosynthetic insulin is used. In the past, insulin was obtained from the pancreas of cows and pigs. Biosynthetic insulin is produced by genetically altering common bacteria or yeast using deoxyribonucleic acid (DNA) technology. This insulin exhibits chemical and biologic properties identical to those of human insulin produced by human B cells in the pancreas (Figure 11-13). Insulin is a hormone and is most commonly absorbed into the patient's bloodstream. Insulin is given subcutaneously, although IV administration of regular insulin can be done when immediate onset of action is desired. IV regular insulin is mixed in normal saline solution. The amount of solution depends on the institution's protocol.

Insulins differ in regard to onset, peak, action, and duration (Table 11-5). The specific preparation of each

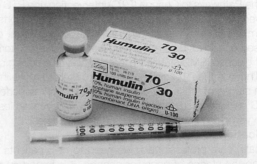

FIGURE 11-13 U/100 insulin and disposable U/100 insulin syringe.

Table 11-5   Types of Insulin

TYPE OF INSULIN	SOURCE AND COLOR	INJECTION TIME (BEFORE MEAL)	RISK TIME FOR HYPOGLYCEMIC REACTION	ACTION	START OF ACTION	PEAK ACTION	DURATION
RAPID OR SHORT ACTING							
Lispro (Humalog)	Human Clear	5-15 min	No meal within 30 min	Rapid	15-30 min	1-2 hr	3-4 hr
Aspart (NovoLog)	Human Clear	5-15 min	No meal within 30 min	Rapid	15-30 min	1-3 hr	3-5 hr
Glulisine (Apidra)	Human Clear	5-15 min	No meal within 30 min	Rapid	15-30 min	1-3 hr	3-5 hr
Regular Humulin R Novolin R ReliOn R	Human Clear	30 min	Delayed meal or 3-4 hr after injection	Short	30-60 min	2-4 hr	6-8 hr
MIXED							
Novolog Mix 70/30 (neutral protamine aspart and aspart)	Human Cloudy	15 min	No meal within 30 min	Rapid and intermediate	15-30 min	2-10 hr	12-16 hr
Humalog Mix 75/25 (neutral protamine lispro and lispro)	Human Cloudy	15 min	No meal within 30 min	Rapid and intermediate	15-30 min	2-10 hr	12-16 hr
NPH/regular Mix 70/30 Humulin Mix 70/30	Human Cloudy	30-60 min	Delayed meal or 3-4 hr after injection	Short and intermediate	30-60 min	6-12 hr	18-24 hr
Novolin Mix 70/30	Human Cloudy	30-60 min	Delayed meal or 3-4 hr after injection	Short and intermediate	30-60 min	6-12 hr	18-24 hr
ReliOn N Mix 70/30	Human Cloudy	30-60 min	Delayed meal or 3-4 hr after injection	Short and intermediate	30-60 min	6-12 hr	18-24 hr
NPH/Regular Mix 50/50	Human Cloudy	30-60 min	Delayed meal or 3-4 hr after injection	Short and intermediate	30-60 min	6-12 hr	18-24 hr
Humulin Mix 50/50	Human Cloudy	30-60 min	Delayed meal or 3-4 hr after injection	Short and intermediate	30-60 min	6-12 hr	18-24 hr
INTERMEDIATE ACTING							
NPH (Humulin N, Novolin N, ReliOn N)	Human Milky when mixed	30 min	4-6 hr after injection	Intermediate acting	2-4 hr	6-10 hr	12-16 hr
Lente	Human Milky when mixed	30 min	3-6 hr after injection	Intermediate acting	1-3 hr	6-12 hr	18-26 hr

From Lewis, S.M., et al. (2007). *Medical-surgical nursing: assessment and management of clinical problems.* (7th ed.). St. Louis: Mosby.   *Continued*

| Table 11-5 | Types of Insulin—cont'd | | | | | | |

TYPE OF INSULIN	SOURCE AND COLOR	INJECTION TIME (BEFORE MEAL)	RISK TIME FOR HYPOGLYCEMIC REACTION	ACTION	START OF ACTION	PEAK ACTION	DURATION
LONG ACTING							
Glargine (Lantus) Detemir (Levemir)	Synthetic Clear; do not mix with others	Usually take at 9 PM, once daily*	Starting dose should be 20% less than total daily dose of NPH	Long lasting	1-2 hr	No pronounced peak	24 hr†
Ultralente	Human Milky when mixed	30 min	6 hr after injection	Long lasting	4-6 hr	18 hr	24 hr

Proper timing of insulin and eating if on regular or 70/30 in relationship with blood glucose	Glucose	Primarily Covers
<50 mg/dL = when mealtime is complete 50-70 mg/dL = at mealtime 70-120 mg/dL = 15 min before mealtime 120-180 mg/dL = 30 min before meal >180 mg/dL = 45 min before meal	AM: Rapid and short acting AM: NPH or Lente Noon: Rapid and short PM: Rapid and short acting PM: NPH and Lente Bedtime: NPH or Lente Bedtime: glargine or detemir or Ultralente	Breakfast to lunch Lunch to evening meal Lunch to midafternoon Evening meal to bedtime Late evening to early morning Midnight to following morning Provides continuous coverage

*May take at other times.
†Type 1, once or twice daily; type 2, once daily.

type of insulin is matched with the patient's diet and activity. By adding zinc, acetate buffers, and protamine to insulin in various ways, the onset of activity, peak, and duration times can be manipulated. Different combinations of these insulins can be used to tailor treatment to the patient's specific pattern of blood glucose levels.

Formulas are classified as rapid acting (insulin lispro [Humalog], insulin aspart [NovoLog], insulin glulisine [Apidra]), short acting (regular insulin [Humulin R, Novolin R, ReliOn R]), intermediate acting (NPH insulin [Humulin N, Novolin N, and ReliOn N]), and long acting (glargine [Lantus], detemir [Levemir]). Glargine is used once a day at bedtime and works around the clock for 24 hours. It is a "peakless" insulin that provides a continuous insulin level similar to the slow, steady (basal) secretions of insulin from a normal pancreas. Glargine must not be mixed in the same syringe with other insulins because it will interfere with their action (Figure 11-14).

If hyperglycemia occurs, elevated blood glucose is covered with sliding-scale regular insulin. Premixed combinations are 70/30 (70% NPH and 30% regular) (see Figure 11-13) and 50/50 (50% NPH and 50% regular). Two recent combinations are available: 75/25 (75% lispro protamine [NPH] and 25% lispro [Humalog] [rapid acting], called Humalog mix 75/25) and 70/30 aspart protamine (70% protamine [NPH] and 30% aspart [rapid acting], called Novolog mix 70/30). The premixed insulins are most helpful for those who have stable insulin needs. Timing of insulin action to match food intake can be a challenge, and it tends to

be more difficult for people with type 1 diabetes because their only source of insulin is by injection. Regular insulin is prescribed when a rapid onset of glucose-lowering action is needed, such as before meals and during periods of acute illness, surgery, or stress. Only regular insulin can be administered intravenously; thus it is used in emergencies.

A human insulin formula called insulin lispro was approved in June 1996 by the U.S. Food and Drug Administration. Insulin lispro begins to take effect in less than half the time of regular, fast-acting insulin. The products previously on the market must be taken subcutaneously 30 to 60 minutes before a meal; the new formula can be injected 15 minutes before a meal. This timing more closely mimics the body's own hormone activity. Lispro brings the most benefit to people with type 1 diabetes who take short-acting insulin before meals combined with a longer-acting insulin once or twice a day. Two additional rapid-acting insulins, aspart (Novolog) and glulisine (Apidra) with similar onset of action as lispro (Humulog) are also now available. Insulins are commonly used in combination to mimic the normal pancreatic insulin secretion.

When giving insulin, be careful to inject into the **subcutaneous tissue** (space between the fat and muscle layers) only, avoiding depositing the medication directly into the fat or muscle. Insulin administration requires the appropriate syringe. Most commercial insulin is available as U/100, indicating that each milliliter contains 100 units of insulin. U/100 insulin must be used with a U/100-marked syringe. For a user tak-

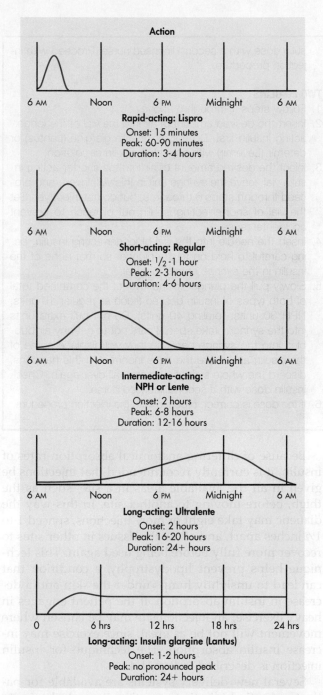

Action

Rapid-acting: Lispro
Onset: 15 minutes
Peak: 60-90 minutes
Duration: 3-4 hours

Short-acting: Regular
Onset: ½-1 hour
Peak: 2-3 hours
Duration: 4-6 hours

**Intermediate-acting:
NPH or Lente**
Onset: 2 hours
Peak: 6-8 hours
Duration: 12-16 hours

Long-acting: Ultralente
Onset: 2 hours
Peak: 16-20 hours
Duration: 24+ hours

Long-acting: Insulin glargine (Lantus)
Onset: 1-2 hours
Peak: no pronounced peak
Duration: 24+ hours

FIGURE 11-14 Commercially available insulin preparations, including onset, peak, and duration of action.

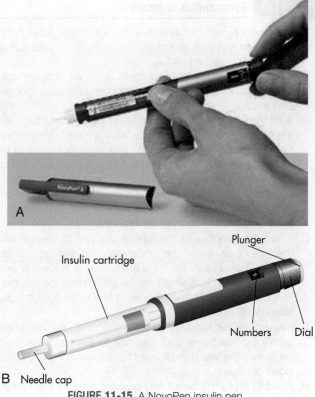

FIGURE 11-15 A NovoPen insulin pen.

ing smaller doses of insulin, insulin syringes marked for 25, 30, or 50 units are available for use with U/100 syringes. One important distinction is that the 100-unit syringe is marked in 2-unit increments, whereas the 50- and 30-unit syringes are marked in 1-unit increments. Be certain that the patient gets the correct size of syringe and does not switch syringes, thus avoiding serious dosing errors. The Joint Commission now recommends using **units** instead of the abbreviation U on medication orders and medication administration records to decrease errors in dosing.

Insulin pens are another popular method of administering insulin. The pen serves the same function as a needle and syringe but is compact and portable, thus

making it more convenient. Insulin pens are handy in that they contain all the necessary parts in one piece, but the user must also attach a needle and discard it after each use (Figure 11-15).

Needles are very fine, usually 25 to 32 gauge, to be as atraumatic to the tissue as possible. Disposable needles and syringes are now used in the hospital and the home. An open bottle of insulin currently being used does not have to be refrigerated. In fact, it is now believed that insulin should be administered at room temperature, not straight from the refrigerator, to help prevent insulin **lipodystrophy** (abnormality in the metabolism or deposition of fats; insulin lipodystrophy is the loss of local fat deposits). Extra bottles are stored in the refrigerator. Box 11-3 offers guidelines for preparation of a dose of insulin, one or two types at a time.

Patients who self-inject insulin at home may want to have a family member oversee the procedure. Nurses administering insulin injections must always have another licensed person check and document the dose drawn up in the syringe to prevent medication errors. The patient with diabetes should ideally be taught self-injection technique before discharge from the hospital. However, some patients are unable to perform this because of physical problems, intellectual incapacity, visual disturbances, or age. In these cases, family members or others have to administer the injections. Before discharge, either the patient or the significant other, or both, must display the ability to correctly draw up and inject insulin.

In a newly diagnosed patient, regular or rapid-acting insulin may be injected before each meal. After

Box 11-3 Preparation of Insulin

1. Thoroughly wash hands with warm water and soap. Bring the insulin to room temperature because an injection of cold insulin can be painful.
2. Assemble all equipment needed, such as properly calibrated insulin syringe with a prefitted needle, prep sponge, and insulin.
3. Turn the insulin vial onto its side and gently rotate between the hands several times to be certain it is mixed. The precipitate should be evenly blended. This does not need to be done with regular insulin because it has no precipitate. Never shake insulin vigorously because this creates air bubbles.
4. Clean the rubber stopper on the vial with a prep sponge.
5. Remove the needle cover and draw in the same amount of air as units of insulin to be injected.
6. Insert the needle into the rubber stopper of the vial and then inject air. Invert the bottle with the syringe unit attached, making sure the tip of the needle is below the level of the insulin so that air will not be drawn into the syringe.
7. Pull back slowly on the plunger, a few units past the desired dose of insulin.
8. Inspect for air bubbles in the syringe; if any are seen, gently tap the barrel until they rise to the top, then push back into the vial with plunger to the level of the desired dose of insulin.
9. Holding on to the barrel and plunger, remove the syringe unit and put the needle cover back on. **Always** check in-sulin dose with a second licensed nurse. Proceed with injection procedure.

TWO INSULINS
1. Follow steps 1 through 5 above.
2. Insert the desired amount of air into the vial of the longer-acting insulin first. Do not mix insulin glargine (Lantus) or detemir (Levemir) with any other insulin or solution.
3. Inject the desired amount of air into the shorter-acting insulin vial; leave the syringe unit in this vial; invert, and proceed through steps 6 through 9, but do not inject yet. Set the vial of shorter-acting insulin out of reach to prevent accidental reuse.
4. Insert the needle into the vial of longer-acting insulin, being careful to hold on to the plunger so that none of the insulin in the syringe enters that vial.
5. Slowly pull the plunger to the level of the combined total of both types of insulin desired (such as regular 10 units, NPH 30 units, totaling 40 units). Do not pull extra units into the syringe. Take special care not to get any air bubbles into the syringe because they will displace some of the insulin and make the dose incorrect. If this happens, discard the whole syringe and start all over again. Check insulin dose with a second licensed nurse.
6. If the dose is correct, proceed with the injection procedure.

---

reasonable control of hyperglycemia is achieved, the dosage schedule may be changed to once a day, in the morning before breakfast, with the type of insulin being intermediate or long acting (see Figure 11-14 and Table 11-5 for types of insulin). Sometimes patients with DM take two divided doses of insulin, one before breakfast and one before the evening meal. Be alert for signs of hypoglycemia (a less than normal amount of glucose in the blood, usually caused by administration of too much insulin, excessive secretion of insulin by the islet cells of the pancreas, or dietary deficiency) at the peak of action of whatever type of insulin the patient is taking. Instruct the patient to notify a member of the nursing staff if any of the following signs of hypoglycemic (insulin) reaction occur: faintness, sudden weakness, excessive perspiration, irritability, hunger, palpitations, trembling, or drowsiness.

After appropriate blood glucose testing, the patient chooses an injection site. The subcutaneous pocket is the desired layer into which insulin should be injected. Insulin should not be injected into the muscle, because it enters the bloodstream too quickly and could cause hypoglycemia. Site selection is crucial, as is site rotation. The patient may choose sites at the abdomen (except for 2 inches [5 cm] around the navel), the upper arms, the anterior or lateral aspects of the thighs, and the hips or buttocks. The abdomen provides the fastest, least variable absorption, followed by the arms, thighs, and buttocks. Patients may find it easier to keep track of their injection sites by recording each injection on a numbered chart (Figure 11-16).

Because of differing anatomical absorption rates of insulin, it is currently recommended that injections be given in all the available areas in a site, such as the thigh, before moving to another site. In this way the diabetic may take eight or more injections, spaced 1 to 1½ inches apart, and allow the tissues in other sites to recover more fully before being used again. This technique helps prevent lipodystrophy, a condition that can lead to unsightly lumps under the skin and a decrease in insulin absorption. If the patient engages in heavy exercise, an injection site may be chosen where movement will not be as great, since exercise may increase insulin absorption. The technique for insulin injection is described in Box 11-4.

Several new delivery systems are available for patients who find injections emotionally and physically uncomfortable. These include automatic injectors, the jet stream (needleless) injector, the Insuflon indwelling insulin delivery service, and the button infuser.

Another method of insulin administration is continuous subcutaneous insulin infusion using the external infusion pump (Figure 11-17). This small, battery-powered computerized device is worn on the user's body, usually in a pocket or on a belt. It is attached to a thin tube with a needle on the end, which is inserted into the subcutaneous tissue. A continuous, or basal, rate of rapid- or short-acting regular insulin delivery can be programmed, with bolus doses administered as needed. The insulin pump is as close a substitute as available to a healthy, working pancreas. It mimics the pancreas by releasing small amounts of rapid-acting

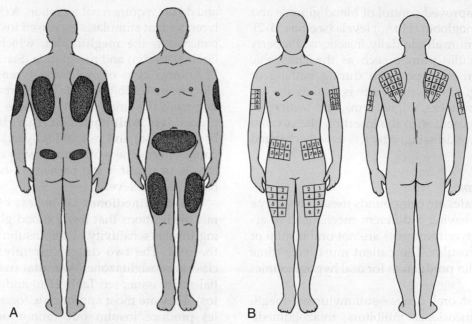

FIGURE 11-16 A, Rotation of sites for insulin injections. **B,** Injection diagram to track rotation of injection sites.

Box 11-4 Technique for Insulin Injection

1. Follow the steps in Box 11-3 to prepare the insulin dose.
2. Don disposable gloves.
3. Clean the injection site with a prep swab, using a circular motion. Allow the alcohol to dry. Place the swab between the last two fingers of the hand not used to inject the insulin.
4. Pick up the syringe and remove the needle cover and lay it aside. Hold the syringe like a dart.
5. Using the other hand, gently pinch up at least a 2-inch fold of tissue (not just the skin).
6. Quickly insert the needle into the top (apex) of the fold, entering the subcutaneous tissue. The "soft spot" technique is to insert the needle about 1 inch to the side of the apex of the fold, into softer tissue, entering the pocket. The needle should be inserted at a 90-degree angle unless the patient is very thin and has little subcutaneous tissue. In that case the angle may be reduced by up to 45 degrees to avoid intramuscular injection.
7. Release the skinfold and use that hand to steady the barrel of the syringe.
8. Inject the insulin over a period of 3 to 5 seconds.
9. Place the alcohol swab against the needle hub, at the injection site, and pull the syringe unit straight out in one swift motion. Gently press on the injection site for a few seconds, but do not massage the site.
10. Carefully place the entire unit, uncapped, into the sharps container provided.
11. Record the injection site and insulin dose on a chart, computer, or other documentation sheet. Include the second licensed nurse who witnessed the insulin dose during preparation. Have the nurse witness the dose given. Store insulin and other supplies properly.
12. When instructing patient to self-inject insulin, use the following guidelines (if appropriate):
    —Aspiration does not need to be done before injection.
    —The injection site does not need to be cleansed with alcohol. The use of an alcohol swab by the patient on the site before self-injection is no longer recommended. Routine hygiene such as washing with soap and rinsing with water is adequate (Lewis et al., 2007).

---

insulin every few minutes. Buffered regular insulin may be substituted in patients unable to use rapid-acting insulin to improve postprandial blood glucose levels and long-term glucose control (Bode et al., 2002). The basal rate is designed to keep the blood glucose level steady between meals and during sleep. When food is eaten, the pump is programmed (at the touch of a button) to deliver a larger quantity of insulin right away to cover the carbohydrate in the meal. This is called a bolus of insulin. The bolus can also be adjusted based on the blood glucose level and planned physical activity. For carefully selected and properly educated patients, the pump offers improved flexibil-

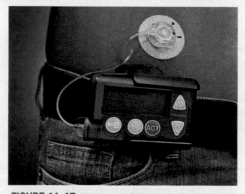

FIGURE 11-17 Medtronic MiniMed insulin pump.

ity in lifestyle, improved control of blood glucose and glycosylated hemoglobin (HbA$_{1c}$) levels (see Box 11-2), and freedom from multiple daily injections. Properly disassembled insulin pumps such as the Disetronic H-Tron V100 can even be worn during bathing or while swimming. The insertion site is usually the abdomen, but the buttocks, thighs, arms, and sections of the back may be used, with the insertion site covered by a clear occlusive dressing, which is usually changed every other day.

Oral Hypoglycemics

Oral hypoglycemics are compounds used to treat type 2 diabetes, each having a different mechanism of action. Oral hypoglycemic agents are not oral insulin or a substitute for insulin. The patient must have some functioning insulin production for oral hypoglycemics to be effective.

Five classes of oral drugs—sulfonylureas, meglitinides, alpha-glucosidase inhibitors, thiazolidinediones, and biguanide—are available for patients whose insulin production or utilization is inadequate due to type 2 diabetes mellitus (Table 11-6).

Sulfonylureas have blood glucose–lowering effects. They stimulate the pancreas to release insulin. A second generation of sulfonylureas, approved for use in the United States, includes glipizide (Glucotrol XL), glyBURIDE (Micronase, DiaBeta, Glynase), and glimepiride (Amaryl). They are more potent than previous drugs

and do not require renal excretion. A class of oral hypoglycemics that stimulates increased insulin release in the pancreas is the **meglitinides,** which includes repaglinide (Prandin) and nateglinide (Starlix).

Another class of oral hypoglycemics lowers blood glucose by inhibiting delay of carbohydrate absorption from the small intestine; these are called **alpha-glucosidase inhibitors.** This drug class includes acarbose (Precose) and miglitol (Glycet). The best way to gauge effectiveness of therapy with acarbose and miglitol is to monitor the patient's 2-hour postprandial blood glucose level.

Thiazolidinediones are a class of oral hypoglycemic medications that lower blood glucose by increasing insulin sensitivity at the insulin receptor sites on the cells. The two drugs currently available in this class are rosiglitazone (Avandia) (which has a potential safety issue; see Table 11-6) and pioglitazone (Actos). They are most appropriate for adults whose bodies produce insulin but cannot use it because of inadequate or ineffective insulin receptor sites.

Metformin (Glucophage) is a **biguanide** glucose-lowering agent. It works primarily by reducing hepatic glucose production and lowers fasting blood glucose levels. It also enhances tissue response to insulin and improves glucose transport into cells. Metformin usually does not promote weight gain and may help improve lipid levels. Metformin is widely used by itself and in combination with a sulfonylurea. Com-

Table 11-6 Five Classes of Oral Hypoglycemics

GENERIC AND BRAND NAME	MECHANICS OF ACTION
SULFONYLUREAS Glipizide (Glucotrol, Glucotrol XL) GlyBURIDE (DiaBeta, Micronase, Glynase) Glimepiride (Amaryl)	Insulin secretagogues primarily stimulate the beta cells of the pancreas to release insulin, particularly in the early course of type 2 diabetes mellitus. Sulfonylureas increase the sensitivity to insulin at receptor sites.
MEGLITINIDES Repaglinide (Prandin) Nateglinide (Starlix)	Insulin secretagogues, like the sulfonylureas, stimulate the beta cells in the pancreas to increase insulin release. Their effects, which are glucose dependent, decrease when the patient's blood glucose level decreases. Requires functioning pancreatic beta cells.
BIGUANIDE Metformin (Glucophage, Glucophage XR, Fotamet, Riomet)	It works primarily by reducing hepatic glucose production and lowers fasting blood glucose levels. It also enhances tissue response to insulin and improves glucose transport into the cells.
ALPHA-GLUCOSIDASE INHIBITORS Acarbose (Precose) Miglitol (Glyset)	Metabolized by intestinal bacteria and digestive enzymes; delay carbohydrate absorption from the small intestine.
THIAZOLIDINEDIONES Rosiglitazone (Avandia) (use with caution*) Pioglitazone (Actos)	Increases insulin sensitivity at insulin receptor sites on the cell. Thiazolidinediones are most appropriate for adults whose bodies produce insulin but cannot use it because of inadequate or ineffective insulin receptor sites.

Data from Funnel, M., & Barlage, D. (2002). Managing diabetes with "agent oral." *Nursing, 34*(3):36.
*The U.S. Food and Drug Administration announced a potential safety issue related to the use of rosiglitazone. Patients who are taking rosiglitazone, especially those with underlying cardiac disease or a high risk of myocardial infarction, should consult their diabetic care provider about whether to continue therapy with this medication (Scemons, 2007).

bined glyBURIDE-metformin (Glucovance) is another oral hypoglycemic agent that may be prescribed.

Once an oral drug becomes ineffective, simply substituting rarely works. But combination therapy can be highly effective. For example, oral drugs from two or more classes may be combined, or an oral drug may be combined with a bedtime dose of NPH or glargine insulin or detemir. Metformin and insulin are commonly chosen for combination therapy with sulfonylureas (Funnel & Barlage, 2004).

Other Treatments

Two subcutaneous agents act as adjuncts to insulin therapy, not a replacement for it. Pramlintide (Symlin) is used in type 1 and type 2 DM. It decreases gastric emptying, glucagon secretion, and glucose output from the liver and increases satiety. Exenatide (Byetta) is used only in type 2 DM. It stimulates release of insulin from the pancreatic B cells, decreases glucagon secretion, increases satiety, and decreases gastric emptying (Table 11-7). However, the FDA (2009) warns that it may increase the risk for kidney problems; labeling changes include dosing cautions and contraindications in patients with renal impairment.

Another drug that may be used to treat hypoglycemic reactions in DM is glucagon, a hormone normally secreted by the alpha cells of the pancreas. It stimulates the liver to change stored glycogen into glucose, which is then released into the bloodstream. Glucagon is available in a purified, crystallized form for reconstruction and subcutaneous, IM, or IV administration in the event of loss of consciousness as a result of hypoglycemic reaction. The usual dose is 0.5 to 1 mg for adults, with smaller doses for children. Some form of oral protein and carbohydrate, such as milk and crackers, should be

Table 11-7   Insulin-Enhancing Drugs

CLASSIFICATION	MECHANISM OF ACTION
Pramlintide (Symlin) Subcutaneous	A synthetic form of amylin, a pancreatic hormone that slows gastric emptying and suppresses the release of glucagon and the formation of glycogen in the liver. Used as an adjunct to insulin therapy. Used in type 1 and type 2 diabetics. It carries a black box warning because of potential to cause severe hypoglycemia within 3 hours of administration (Bass, 2007).
Exenatide (Byetta) Subcutaneous	Incretin mimetics. Designed for use in type 2 diabetics. Incretins are gut hormones that promote insulin secretion during a meal, suppress glucagon release, and delay gastric emptying, which effectively reduces postprandial blood sugars. It is not indicated for use with insulin (Bass, 2007).

Complementary & Alternative Therapies

Endocrine Disorders

- Herbal medicines used in the treatment of type 2 diabetes mellitus include aloe vera juice, beans (*Phaseolus* species), bitter gourd, karela (*Momordica charantia*), black tea (*Camellia sinensis*), fenugreek (*Trigonella foenum-graecum*), gurmar (*Gymnema sylvestre*), macadamia nut, and Madagascar periwinkle (*Catharanthus roseus*). Effects of these herbs include lowering of blood pressure (fenugreek), boosting of insulin production (gurmar), and increased use of available insulin (black tea).
- Kelp (*Fucus vesiculosus*) may help with weight loss in hypothyroid disorders. Milk thistle (*Silybum marianum*) is used for treatment and prophylaxis of chronic hepatotoxicity, inflammatory liver disorders, and certain types of cirrhosis.
- Yoga may help the patient with diabetes mellitus with diet control and may improve pancreatic function.

---

given after the patient regains consciousness. Many people with diabetes carry a commercially prepared kit containing glucagon and concentrated carbohydrate such as candy or glucose gel (see Complementary & Alternative Therapies box).

Selected patients with type 1 DM now have the option of a pancreas transplant. Usually a pancreas transplant is performed on a DM patient who has end-stage renal disease and has already had a kidney transplant or will have one in the near future. A kidney and pancreas transplant are usually done at the same time. Patients who undergo kidney and pancreas transplantation must have lifelong immunosuppression therapy to prevent rejection of the transplants (Lewis et al., 2007).

Nursing Interventions and Patient Teaching

People with diabetes may be hospitalized as a direct result of their disease process, or they may have a different primary diagnosis. The main focus of nursing interventions must always be on the primary diagnosis, but remember that the patient is also diabetic and is susceptible to a number of complications in addition to all those experienced by nondiabetic patients.

Daily routine for the patient with diabetes includes accurate monitoring of blood glucose levels, either by fingerstick specimens or by laboratory testing. Careful attention to diet is important; note the amount of food eaten at each meal and record it accurately.

If the patient with type 1 DM is ill, is nauseated, or cannot eat for any reason, consult with the physician or primary care provider. Physiologic and psychological stress raises the patient's blood glucose level. Do not withhold insulin in a patient with type 1 DM. Without insulin to promote glucose to enter the cells, the body must seek an alternative source for energy. Fats and protein are used. When these cells break down, ketones are formed. Accumulation of ketones results in ketosis and acidosis. If this situation is not corrected, the patient may develop DKA.

Often the primary care provider recommends providing Popsicles or apple juice, which can compensate for a decrease in calories when a regular diet cannot be consumed. If the patient does not like the types of food on the meal tray, arrange for a dietitian to consult.

Good skin care is essential for the person with diabetes, since poor circulation can lead to the development of skin problems. Compromised skin integrity makes a patient with DM more susceptible to infection. In diabetes, elevated glycosylated hemoglobin in the red blood cells impedes the release of oxygen to the tissues. Elevated blood glucose levels also make some pathogens thrive and proliferate. Vascular changes decrease blood, oxygen, and nutrient supply to the tissues and affect the supply of white blood cells in the area, because if white blood cells do not function properly, phagocytosis is defective (Brozenec, 1998).

Report to the physician any abnormalities such as cuts, scratches, or lesions anywhere on the body, and treat them before infection develops. Special foot care is crucial for this patient, since poor circulation and decreased nerve sensation or neuropathy (any abnormal condition characterized by inflammation and degeneration of the peripheral nerves) increase the danger of ulcers or other abnormal lesions developing into gangrene. Many patients seek the services of a podiatrist for their foot care. The patient should thoroughly wash the feet with soap and water every day; dry them thoroughly; and inspect them carefully for cracks, blisters, or foreign objects, paying special attention to the area between the toes. Foot soaks or powders are not recommended. The patient should wear clean socks daily and avoid tight garters. The toenails should be clipped straight across so that the edges do not become ingrown. The nurse should never trim the toenails of a patient with diabetes without a physician's written order. Do not put hot water bottles or heating pads on the feet, since burns may occur and not be felt. The patient should wear sturdy, properly fitting shoes, preferably with wide toe boxes or molded shoes that are less constrictive. Medicare now reimburses patients with DM who have certain conditions for the cost of specially molded shoes. The patient should not go barefoot at any time. Notify the physician immediately of any injury to the toes or feet (see Health Promotion box). Patients with DM are also advised to have an eye examination each year.

Carefully watch the patient who is receiving insulin for development of hypoglycemia, especially when the particular kind of insulin being injected is at its peak of action. Hypoglycemia is seen less frequently in patients receiving oral hypoglycemics, but it can occur.

The emotional aspects of diabetes are numerous, and many patients experience a period of denial after the initial diagnosis. Some patients become depressed. Because this disease affects all age-groups, nursing interventions are tailored to fit the needs of each patient (see Life Span Considerations box). Patients with diabetes must have help in working through their feelings, so be a good listener and supportive at all times. The patient who does not satisfactorily resolve any major problems in accepting the diagnosis of DM may be noncompliant with the treatment plan.

The nurse who supervises the patient in a home setting must encourage the patient to take the prescribed medication faithfully, eat the right kinds of food, test blood or urine correctly, and exercise regularly. If a family member is responsible for the patient's care, ensure that the caregiver is functioning adequately in this role. Some patients live alone and do well caring for themselves, with occasional visits from a home health or public health nurse. Others who have visual disturbances, circulatory problems, or other conditions may need daily visits and more actual nursing intervention, such as help with hygiene, meals, and insulin injections (Nursing Care Plan 11-1).

 Health Promotion

Foot Care for the Patient with Diabetes Mellitus

- Wash feet daily with a mild soap and **warm** water. Test water temperature with hands first.
- Pat feet dry gently, especially between toes.
- Examine feet daily for cuts, blisters, edema, erythema, and tender areas. If patient's eyesight is poor, have others inspect feet.
- Use lanolin on feet to prevent skin from drying and cracking. Do not apply between toes.
- Use mild foot powder on feet if perspiring.
- Do not use commercial remedies to remove calluses or corns.
- Cleanse cuts with **warm** water and mild soap, covering with clean dressing. Do not use iodine, rubbing alcohol, or strong adhesives.
- Report skin infections or nonhealing lesions to health care provider immediately.
- Cut toenails even with rounded contour of toes. Do not cut down corners. The best time to trim nails is after a shower or bath.

- Separate overlapping toes with cotton or lamb's wool.
- Avoid open-toe, open-heel, and high-heel shoes. Leather shoes are preferred to plastic ones. Wear slippers with soles. Do not go barefoot. Shake out shoes before putting on.
- Wear clean, absorbent (cotton or wool) socks or stockings that have not been mended. Colored socks must be colorfast.
- Do not wear clothing that leaves impressions or constricts circulation.
- Do not use hot water bottles or heating pads to warm feet. Wear socks for warmth.
- Guard against frostbite.
- Exercise feet daily either by walking or by flexing and extending feet in suspended position. Avoid prolonged sitting, standing, and crossing of legs.

Acute Complications

One of the acute complications of DM is coma, which may be attributed to three different causes. The first type of coma can occur during DKA, which results from inadequate amounts of insulin or from inadequate insulin utilization. The second type, hyperglycemic hyperosmolar nonketotic coma (HHNC), involves no acidosis or ketonemia, but results from excess glucose, diuresis, and dehydration without adequate fluid replacement. The third type may occur during hypoglycemic reaction, which results from an excess amount of insulin with an inadequate amount of glucose present. These three complications are compared and contrasted in Table 11-8. (See also Safety Alert boxes: Emergency Care for Hypoglycemic Reaction and Emergency Care for Hyperglycemic Reaction.)

Another acute complication faced by the patient with diabetes is the development of infections of any kind. Hyperglycemia and ketonemia hinder the phagocytic action of leukocytes. An infection can therefore

---

Life Span Considerations

Older Adults

Endocrine Disorder

- Diabetes mellitus is more prevalent in older adults. A major reason for this is that the process of aging involves insulin resistance and glucose intolerance, which are believed to be precursors to type 2 diabetes.
- The classic signs and symptoms of diabetes may not be obvious in older adults.
- Dietary management may be complicated by a variety of functional, social, economic, and financial factors.
- Hormone supplements must be administered with caution.
- Older adult diabetic patients are at increased risk for infection and should be counseled to receive proper immunizations and seek regular medical attention for even minor symptoms. The older adult often has considerable difficulty in managing diabetes.

- Some symptoms of hypothyroidism in the older adult are similar to those in a younger person but are more likely to be overlooked because the symptoms—fatigue, mental impairment, sluggishness, and constipation—are often attributed solely to aging. The older person with hypothyroidism has symptoms unique to the age set, including more disturbances of the central nervous system, such as syncope, convulsions, dementia, and coma. There is often pitting edema and deafness.
- The older patient with hyperthyroidism frequently has manifestations related only to the cardiovascular system, such as palpitations, angina, atrial fibrillation, and breathlessness. Signs and symptoms often attributed to "aging" may actually indicate an endocrine problem.

 Nursing Care Plan 11-1 | The Patient with Diabetes Mellitus

Ms. Thompson is an obese, 52-year-old married patient with type 2 diabetes mellitus (DM) diagnosed 3 years ago. She was referred to a short-term ambulatory diabetes education program by her physician for instruction on insulin administration because she has not achieved blood glucose control with dietary measures.

Objective data included blood glucose 220 mg/dL, weight 200 pounds, and blood pressure 134/84 mm Hg. Collaborative nursing actions include teaching Ms. Thompson measures that will help her control blood glucose (insulin, diet, and exercise) and how to detect, prevent, and treat hypoglycemic reactions. The nurse reported Ms. Thompson's work schedule to the physician and asked for insulin dosage alterations on weekends. The physician was unaware of her work schedule and stated that blood glucose control could not be optimum with this schedule.

NURSING DIAGNOSIS *Deficient knowledge: self-injections, SMBG, related to lack of exposure*

Patient Goals and Expected Outcomes	Nursing Interventions	Evaluation
Patient will independently self-administer insulin	Support patient as necessary to self-inject insulin.	Patient demonstrates safety in drawing up and self-administering insulin.
Patient will perform SMBG accurately	Observe patient's skill in SMBG; correct as necessary.	Patient demonstrates accuracy in SMBG.
Patient will use measurements obtained by SMBG to achieve blood glucose less than 126 mg/dL	Review with patient the effect of activity, dietary intake, and insulin on blood glucose.	Patient can verbalize the effect of activity, diet, and insulin on blood glucose.
Patient will be able to detect and treat hypoglycemia	Instruct patient on frequency and timing of SMBG.	Patient can recite signs and symptoms of hypoglycemia and the correct immediate treatment to pursue.
	Review with patient signs and symptoms and treatment measures.	
	Refer to dietitian for modification of diet necessary with insulin and for verification of diet knowledge.	

Continued

⬟ Nursing Care Plan 11-1   **The Patient with Diabetes Mellitus—cont'd**

NURSING DIAGNOSIS *Ineffective health maintenance, related to ineffective coping skills*

Patient Goals and Expected Outcomes	Nursing Interventions	Evaluation
Patient will state at least one change that will improve blood glucose control	Teach patient effects of stress, lack of exercise, and activity pattern on blood glucose. Explore with patient willingness and ability to change behaviors: sleep-activity, coping, and exercise. Engage patient in mutual problem solving; refrain from prescribing. Explore sources for long-term support in learning more effective coping skills; suggest support groups: • For patients with DM • For weight loss and maintaining weight loss • Available at work in health service program Suggest to patient that she seek a trial period on day shift on weekends.	Patient has enrolled in an exercise and weight-reduction program to assist in achieving a reasonable weight and beneficial exercise.

Critical Thinking Questions

1. Ms. Thompson received Humalog 75/25, 25 units subQ at 7:30 AM. She ate her American Diabetes Association diet at breakfast and lunch. At 3:00 PM she complains of being hungry, nervous, and tremulous. What are the immediate nursing interventions?
2. Ms. Thompson states, "I need to lose about 40 pounds, and I'm considering joining a weight-reduction club." What would be some helpful suggestions by the nurse?
3. In discharge planning, the nurse notes that Ms. Thompson has poorly fitting shoes. What would be some important discharge patient teaching for foot care?

❗ Safety Alert!

Emergency Care for Hypoglycemic Reaction

IMMEDIATE TREATMENT: IF CONSCIOUS

• Give patient 10 to 20 g of quick-acting carbohydrate in some form, such as 4 to 6 oz of orange juice or a regular soft drink (not a diet drink); half of a candy bar; commercially prepared concentrated dextrose tablets or glucose paste; one tube Cake Mate icing gel (small); 2 tsp sugar or honey; six jelly beans or gumdrops; five or six LifeSavers or other roll candy; four animal crackers; or one granola bar. Offer another 5 to 20 g of quick-acting carbohydrate in 15 minutes if no relief is obtained.

• Give patient additional food, a longer-acting carbohydrate (e.g., slice of bread, crackers with peanut butter), after symptoms subside.

IMMEDIATE TREATMENT: IF UNCONSCIOUS

• Squeeze one tube of glucagon gel between teeth and gums, in buccal space, or give glucagon 0.5 to 1 mg subQ or IM; get patient to hospital. Hospitalized patients may receive IV bolus of 20 mL of 50% glucose or 50 mL of 20% glucose; glucagon may be given intravenously. Patient may need IV 10% or 20% glucose at 100 mL/hr to follow.

NURSING INTERVENTIONS DURING AND AFTER HYPOGLYCEMIC EPISODE

• Stay with the patient; check vital signs and do fingerstick blood glucose levels.

• Monitor for worsening of condition or relief of symptoms.

• If patient becomes unconscious, administer glucagon buccally, subcutaneously, intramuscularly, or intravenously.

• Be certain patient ingests food such as milk, six crackers with peanut butter, or one slice cheese and six crackers after symptoms end.

• Observe closely for 1 to 2 hours after cessation of symptoms.

• Notify physician about the hypoglycemic reaction.

• Assess reason the reaction may have occurred.

Table 11-8   Comparison of Types of Diabetic Coma

ASSESSMENT	HYPERGLYCEMIC REACTION, DIABETIC KETOACIDOSIS	HYPOGLYCEMIC REACTION	HYPERGLYCEMIC HYPEROSMOLAR NONKETOTIC COMA
Type of diabetes	Type 1	Type 1 or type 2	Type 2
Cause	Inadequate insulin	Too much insulin or oral hypoglycemic agent	Inadequate insulin or oral hypoglycemic agent
Patient history	Omitted or insufficient dose of insulin, physical or emotional stress, gastrointestinal upsets, dietary noncompliance	Reduced food intake, delayed meal, too much exercise	Reduced fluid or food intake with increased urinary output, resulting in severe dehydration
Onset of symptoms	Hours to days	Minutes to hours	Days
Previous diagnosis of having diabetes	Almost always	Yes; on medication	Usually type 2, on hypoglycemic agent
Age of patient	Usually younger patient	Usually younger patient	Usually older adult patient
Appearance of skin	Hot, dry, flushed	Cool, moist	Hot, dry; body temperature elevated
Breath	Fruity (from ketones)	Normal	Normal
Mucous membranes	Dry	Moist	Very dry
Respirations	Deep; may have Kussmaul's respirations (air hunger) as a result of metabolic acidosis	Rapid, shallow	Normal
Neurosensory	Drowsiness to coma	Irritability, tremors, impaired consciousness, personality changes; may lose consciousness	Lethargy, decreased consciousness; may lose consciousness
Blood pressure	Low	Normal	Decreased
Glycosuria and ketonuria	Present	Absent	Glycosuria present; no ketonuria
Polyuria and polydipsia	Present	Absent	Present
Hunger	Absent; may have nausea and vomiting	Present; may be nauseated	Absent
Blood glucose level	Usually 300-800 mg/dL	Usually <50 mg/dL	600-2000 mg/dL; serum osmolality greatly increased
Emergency treatment	Insulin, usually regular	Glucose (oral or IV) or glucagon (subQ, IM, or IV)	Large amounts of intravenous fluids; regular insulin

GI, Gastrointestinal; *IM,* intramuscular; *IV,* intravenous; *subQ,* subcutaneous.

⚠ Safety Alert!

Emergency Care for Hyperglycemic Reaction (Diabetic Ketoacidosis)

USUAL TREATMENT DURING ACUTE STAGE
- Start an IV, using an 18-gauge needle, and begin fluid replacement, usually with 0.9% normal saline 1L/hr, until blood pressure is stabilized and urinary output is 30 to 60 mL/hr. When blood glucose levels approach 250 mg/dL, add 5% dextrose to the fluid regimen to prevent hypoglycemia.
- Give regular insulin (the only kind that can be given intravenously) as a piggyback infusion, using 100 units regular insulin in 500 mL normal saline. Administer the infusion with a pump controller. Adjust the infusion rate to obtain and maintain desired blood glucose levels.
- Determine blood glucose level hourly (SMBG method or venous sample).
- Provide IV replacement of potassium to help move insulin into cells; monitor serum potassium.
- Administer oxygen via nasal cannula or nonrebreather mask.
- Monitor cardiac status, with central venous pressure and Swan-Ganz monitoring if available.

- Insert Foley catheter and monitor I&O hourly.
- Assess vital signs and neurologic status.

NURSING INTERVENTIONS DURING AND AFTER DIABETIC KETOACIDOSIS
- Keep airway patent.
- Maintain patent IV infusion at prescribed rate.
- Keep accurate I&O record.
- Do accurate blood testing for glucose and urine testing for acetone.
- Monitor vital signs frequently, and assess cardiac status on monitor.
- Assess breath sounds for fluid overload.
- Assess level of consciousness frequently, and perform neurologic checks as ordered.
- Assess the cause of DKA.

become more severe and last longer, with poor wound healing taking place. Infection increases the possibility of DKA and makes it harder to control the disease. Patients with diabetes are often hospitalized for treatment of infections that might be handled on an outpatient basis for the nondiabetic patient.

Chronic Complications

Primary chronic complications associated with diabetes are those of end-organ disease, which results from damage to blood vessels (angiopathy) secondary to chronic hyperglycemia (Figure 11-18). Chronic complications of diabetes include blindness, cardiovascular problems, and renal failure.

Diabetes causes more cases of blindness in the United States than any other disease. Diabetic retinopathy involves progressive changes in the microcirculation of the retina, resulting in hemorrhages, scar tissue formation, and various degrees of retinal detachment. Surgical techniques such as laser beam coagulation of retinal vessels may improve vision for selected patients with early diagnosis.

Vascular changes in patients with diabetes, especially capillary changes, contribute to the development of renal sclerosis, often progressing to end-stage renal disease. Many of these patients have to undergo either peritoneal dialysis or hemodialysis as a result. Diabetes contributes to accelerated atherosclerotic changes in the blood vessels, resulting in myocardial infarction, stroke, and gangrene in the lower extremities. Many people with diabetes have to undergo amputation as a result of ischemia to the lower extremities. Additionally, nervous system manifestations (diabetic neuropathy) are commonly seen, which cause pain and decreased sensation in the extremities and contribute to the development of diabetic gangrene.

The patient has pain and paresthesias. The pain—described as burning, cramping, itching, or crushing—is usually worse at night and may occur only at that time. Complete or partial loss of sensitivity to touch and temperature is common. Foot injury and ulcerations may occur without the patient ever having pain. At times the skin becomes so sensitive (hyperesthesia) that even light pressure from bed sheets cannot be tolerated. Many men with diabetes experience problems with impotence or premature ejaculation. Reports of prevalence of impotence among men with diabetes vary from 30% to 60%. Impotence associated with DM is believed to result from damage to the sacral parasympathetic nerves. Patients of either gender may have orthostatic hypotension and bladder or bowel dysfunction.

Neuropathy affecting the autonomic nervous system may also result in gastropathy, a delayed gastric emptying that can produce anorexia, nausea, vomiting, early satiety, and a persistent feeling of fullness. These problems were previously referred to as gastroparesis, a term now reserved for the condition in which the stomach is severely affected and is very slow to empty solid foods. Metoclopramide (Reglan) stimulates gastric emptying and has been used in the treatment of gastroparesis.

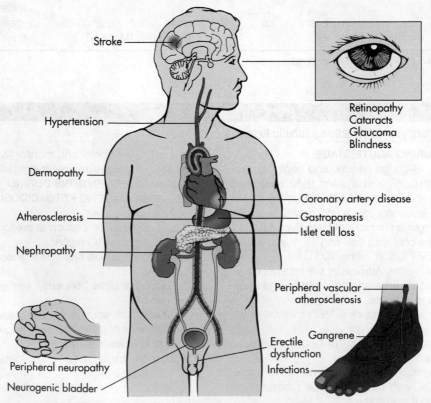

Stroke

Retinopathy
Cataracts
Glaucoma
Blindness

Hypertension

Dermopathy

Coronary artery disease

Atherosclerosis

Gastroparesis

Islet cell loss

Nephropathy

Peripheral vascular atherosclerosis

Gangrene

Peripheral neuropathy

Erectile dysfunction

Neurogenic bladder

Infections

FIGURE 11-18 Long-term complications of diabetes mellitus.

Nursing diagnoses and interventions for the patient with DM include but are not limited to the following:

Nursing Diagnoses	Nursing Interventions
Ineffective therapeutic regimen management, related to health beliefs	Instruct in proper self-injection of insulin; have patient perform return demonstration. Reinforce instructions regarding availability of glucose and glycogen sources. Remove potentially hazardous objects from environment.
Noncompliance (diabetic management, high risk for), related to patient's value system	Establish therapeutic relationship so patient can express negative feelings. Correct misconceptions about treatment regimen. Assist patient in setting long-term goals for lifetime optimal disease management. Involve significant others when possible, and encourage communication between them and the patient. Refer patient to appropriate agencies and services (local support groups, ADA).

Education for the person with diabetes has many important aspects, including the proper administration of insulin or oral hypoglycemic medications and their side effects (see Communication box); the signs and symptoms of hyperglycemia and hypoglycemia; methods of testing blood glucose levels and of urine testing for acetone; planning and preparing the prescribed diet; and personal hygiene, emphasizing skin and foot care. Stress the interrelationships of diet, medication, and exercise. Instruct the patient to visit the dentist regularly and an ophthalmologist annually. Because infections and illnesses of any kind could result in loss of diabetic control, instruct the patient to notify the physician at the first sign of any illness. Special plans for travel include taking extra insulin vials and syringes, carrying food and some form of concentrated carbohydrate, and arranging for SMBG or urine testing. Provisions for adequate rest time must be made, since exhaustion can lead to changes in the overall condition.

Before discharge from the hospital, the patient should verbalize an understanding of how to prevent complications and display an interest in maintaining optimal wellness (see Cultural Considerations box). Stress the importance of regular medical checkups. The social aspects of DM cannot be ignored. Patients need to learn about lifestyle adjustment and should wear medical-alert jewelry and carry medical information wallet cards at all times. Decisions such as whether to attempt pregnancy should be thoroughly explored by women with diabetes. Above all, the patient must accept the responsibility for self-care and recognize

---

 Communication

Importance of Proper Foot Care for Patients with Diabetes

Mr. Garcia is a 67-year-old Hispanic American who was diagnosed 18 months ago with type 2 diabetes mellitus. He has done well on a regimen of diet, exercise, and oral hypoglycemic medication (glyBURIDE [DiaBeta], 2.5 mg/day). Three days ago he dropped a brick on his right foot while remodeling his fireplace and was treated in the emergency department. He is being seen today for a follow-up visit with his internist. The office nurse, Mrs. Bloom, will first talk with him and assess his condition.

Nurse: Good morning, Mr. Garcia How are you doing this morning?

Patient: Much better, thank you. My foot still gives me a little trouble when I walk very far, but the swelling is down. I've been watching for red streaks, like they told me to in the emergency department, but so far there is only this scraped place and a bruise on the top of my foot (shows nurse the area).

Nurse: That's good. What kind of treatment are you using for your injured foot?

Patient: I'm washing my foot twice a day with soap and water, putting Neosporin ointment on the scrape, and then putting on a bandage.

Nurse: That sounds as if that should be adequate. Now let me get a close look at both feet (thoroughly examines the injured area, as well as the rest of the right foot, then examines the left foot). The skin on your feet looks a little dry, Mr.

Garcia, and your toenails are getting quite thick and long. Do you have any problems cutting them?

Patient: I sure do! It's pretty hard for me to see exactly where I need to clip them sometimes, and I'm afraid I'll cut my toe, so I usually just let them go until my wife can help me. She's scared of cutting me, so she usually doesn't get them short enough.

Nurse: I understand. Proper foot care is important for any patient with diabetes to prevent complications such as infection or tissue injury that could become serious. Dr. Mason usually refers his patients to a podiatrist when they are having problems such as yours. A podiatrist specializes in care of the feet, and can properly trim your toenails as needed, as well as care for any corns or calluses that may develop.

Patient: That sounds like a really good idea. I sure don't want to wind up like my cousin and some other people I've seen, having to have a toe or my whole foot amputated! Can you give me the name of a good podiatrist?

Nurse: Yes, I can (hands pamphlet to Mr. Garcia). This pamphlet stresses the importance of foot care, and on the back page has the names of four podiatrists Dr. Mason recommends. You can choose the one you prefer. Now, I'm going to get Dr. Mason so that he can examine you.

Patient: Thanks, Mrs. Bloom. It's really good not to have to worry about cutting those toenails anymore!

Cultural Considerations

Chronic Conditions

- When dealing with a patient with a chronic condition, identification of the patient's cultural background, values, and beliefs can assist the health care team in identifying appropriate regimens. This is particularly important in a condition such as diabetes mellitus, which may require major lifestyle changes for successful management.
- In assessing patients, it is important to consider the best way to communicate across cultures. For example, Asian and Mexican cultures consider asking a direct question and expecting a direct answer to be ill mannered and rude. Phrasing questions in a more indirect way will foster more effective communication.

Home Care Considerations

Diabetes Mellitus

- Considering the day of short hospitalization or no hospitalization and the overwhelming amount of information to be learned, home care is a high priority for people with diabetes mellitus.
- Frequently, older adults have difficulty with mobility and changes in vision that may hamper the drawing up of insulin.
- Often there is missing information as to why control cannot be obtained; that missing link may be found during a home visit.
- Diabetes caregivers and home care agencies often team up to provide good care for the older adult.
- Home care personnel network with other community resources to improve the older adult's quality of life or help deal with economic issues.
- Diabetic management should include education in:
  —Motivation
  —Self-monitoring of blood glucose
  —Exercise
  —Nutrition therapy
  —Medications
  —Written treatment plan

---

that making the right choices can affect life expectancy and quality. A current trend is for hospitals to employ a diabetes nurse specialist to develop and implement patient and staff education (see Home Care Considerations box).

Prognosis

Although the life expectancy for the person with diabetes is usually decreased, current research and recent advances have led to the hope of a much better prognosis. Early diagnosis and prompt, accurate treatment are essential in promoting longevity. Quality of life has been enhanced by better ways to control hyperglycemia and by earlier recognition of developing complications. Life expectancy and quality of life are directly related to glycemic control.

❖ NURSING PROCESS for the Patient with an Endocrine Disorder

The role of the licensed practical nurse/licensed vocational nurse (LPN/LVN) in the nursing process as stated is that the LPN/LVN will:

- Participate in planning care for patients based on patient needs
- Review patient's care plans and recommend revisions as needed
- Review and follow defined prioritization for patient care
- Use clinical pathways, care maps, or care plans to guide and review patient care

■ Assessment

Hormones affect every body tissue and system, causing diverse signs and symptoms of endocrine dysfunction. Endocrine disorders may have nonspecific or specific clinical manifestations. Some specific signs of endocrine dysfunction are the classic "polys" (**polyuria, polydipsia,** and **polyphagia**) in DM and exophthalmos in hyperthyroidism. Specific signs make the assessment easier, whereas nonspecific signs and symptoms, such as tachycardia, fatigue, and depression, are more problematic.

■ Nursing Diagnosis

Nursing diagnoses are determined from careful examination of patient data. Nursing diagnoses for the patient with an endocrine disorder may include but are not limited to the following:

- Deficient knowledge
- Risk for situational low self-esteem
- Disturbed sensory perception
- Risk for deficient fluid volume
- Risk for infection
- Risk for injury
- Sexual dysfunction
- Disturbed body image
- Ineffective coping
- Impaired home maintenance
- Noncompliance
- Imbalanced nutrition: less than body requirements
- Imbalanced nutrition: more than body requirements
- Activity intolerance

■ Expected Outcomes and Planning

The plan for management of patients with endocrine disorders must center on education to enable patients to understand their disorders, develop a healthy lifestyle, and prevent complications of their disease.

The care plan focuses on accomplishing individual goals and outcomes that relate to the identified nursing diagnoses. Examples of these include the following:

Goal 1: Patient will demonstrate safety in self-injections of insulin.

Evaluation: Patient independently administers insulin injection safely and accurately.

Goal 2: Patient will demonstrate SMBG.

Evaluation: Patient performs SMBG accurately.

■ Implementation

A major nursing responsibility is to help patients gain self-management skills for their chronic endocrine disorder through teaching and counseling. Self-management skills are probably the major factor in controlling the health problem and maintaining an optimal quality of life. Self-management skills are implemented through education in the disease process, the management of medications, the management of nutrition, and the role of exercise; SMBG; hygiene; the prevention of complications; and assistance with psychological adjustment.

■ Evaluation

During and after patient educational teaching on self-management skills, assist in evaluating the success of the teaching by noting patient progress based on stated goals and outcomes. For example, when the patient performs SMBG, observe the patient's skill, correct him or her as necessary, and evaluate the patient's technique to ensure accuracy. When patients are unable to meet expected outcomes, be ready to revise the care plan to promote success.

Get Ready for the NCLEX® Examination!

Key Points

- Endocrine glands are ductless glands that release chemicals (hormones) into the bloodstream to regulate body activities.
- The pituitary gland, located in the brain, is the master gland of the endocrine system.
- Hormones have a generalized effect on metabolism, growth and development, and reproduction.
- The endocrine glands regulate themselves by a series of negative feedback messages.
- The hormones secreted by the endocrine glands affect tissues of the entire body, and an imbalance in their levels may contribute to pathologic changes in many different systems.
- Acromegaly and gigantism, disorders of the pituitary gland, result in growth changes that may have a negative effect on the patient's self-image and self-esteem.
- Diabetes insipidus is a disorder of the posterior pituitary and must not be confused with DM, a disorder of the pancreas.
- Clinically, SIADH is characterized by hyponatremia and water retention that progresses to water intoxication. When caring for the patient with hyperthyroidism, provide for adequate rest periods and be sure that fluid and food intake meets the patient's nutritional needs.
- The emotions of the patient with hyperthyroidism are labile, so try to eliminate sources of stress from the environment, to help prevent emotional trauma.
- ^{131}I should not be administered to a pregnant patient because of the risk to the fetus; nurses who are pregnant should not care for these patients.
- The thyroidectomy patient faces three life-threatening postoperative complications: hemorrhage, tetany, and thyroid crisis.
- The patient with hypothyroidism may experience sluggish mental and physical functioning, so be patient and allow adequate time for nursing routines.
- The prognosis for papillary adenocarcinoma of the thyroid is excellent because few of these tumors metastasize.
- When administering IV calcium chloride to any patient, be careful that none of the drug extravasates because tissue sloughing may result.

- The extreme hypertension often seen in patients with pheochromocytoma may result in cerebrovascular accident.
- Depression is common in patients who suffer from Cushing's syndrome; be alert for suicidal thoughts and suicide attempts.
- The four main facets of medical treatment for the patient with DM are diet, SMBG, exercise, and medication.
- Type 1 DM is usually first diagnosed in people younger than 30 years of age; type 2 DM is more commonly found after age 35, and the incidence increases with age.
- As insulin resistance progresses, the pancreas secretes greater amounts of insulin to compensate. This in turn leads to progressive beta-cell failure and a lessening of insulin production. Both beta-cell dysfunction and insulin resistance are required for the development of hyperglycemia, the central metabolic characteristic of type 2 DM.
- The older person with diabetes may have a high blood glucose level before excreting any into the urine because of an increased renal threshold for glucose.
- The diabetic diet must be individualized, taking into consideration many factors, such as age, lifestyle, food preferences, and the ability to cook and store food.
- The person with type 1 DM must have access to a source of quick glucose at all times, in the event of a hypoglycemic reaction.
- Become familiar with the clinical manifestations of DKA, HHNC, and hypoglycemic reaction to properly assess diabetic patients, respond therapeutically, and educate them in self-care.
- Observe patients on insulin therapy and oral hypoglycemic medications during the time of peak action of the medication, and initiate treatment promptly if hypoglycemia develops.
- The nurse must be knowledgeable about the various insulin types and characteristics.
- Two new insulin-enhancing drugs given subcutaneously are pramlintide and exenatide.
- There are five classes of oral hypoglycemic drugs: sulfonylureas, meglitinides, biguanide, alpha-glucosidase inhibitors, and thiazolidinediones.
- DKA can result in seizures, brain damage, or death for the patient with type 1 DM.

Additional Learning Resources

Go to your companion CD for an audio glossary, animations, video clips, and more.

evolve Be sure to visit the Evolve site at http://evolve.elsevier.com/ Christensen/adult/ for additional online resources.

Review Questions for the NCLEX® Examination

1. Which of the following hormones is responsible for "fight or flight"?

   1. Estrogen and testosterone
   2. FSH and LH
   3. Epinephrine and norepinephrine
   4. Calcitonin and parathyroid hormone

2. The hormones responsible for blood calcium levels are:

   1. calcitonin and parathyroid hormone.
   2. estrogen and progesterone.
   3. melatonin and follicle-stimulating hormone (FSH).
   4. thyroxine and parathyroid hormone.

3. Which of the following is the master gland of the body?

   1. Thyroid gland
   2. Adrenal gland
   3. Pineal gland
   4. Pituitary gland

4. What hormone is responsible for male secondary sex characteristics?

   1. Estrogen
   2. Progesterone
   3. Testosterone
   4. Adrenaline

5. The patient received ^{131}I yesterday in an attempt to slow the progression of her hyperthyroid condition. For which personnel would participating in her direct bedside care be dangerous?

   1. A 19-year-old first-semester nursing student
   2. A 34-year-old staff nurse who is new to the unit
   3. A 22-year-old aide who is 6 weeks pregnant
   4. A 49-year-old RN just returning from sick leave

6. A 35-year-old patient had a total thyroidectomy. The first night she experienced signs and symptoms of postoperative tetany. The nurse should implement the physician's order and immediately administer:

   1. sodium iodide PO.
   2. potassium chloride IV.
   3. magnesium sulfate IM.
   4. calcium gluconate IV.

7. A 47-year-old mother of three had cranial surgery to remove a pituitary tumor 3 days ago, leaving her with partial left hemiparesis and diabetes insipidus. Which nursing diagnosis is of the greatest priority postoperatively?

   1. Risk for deficient fluid volume, related to excessive loss via the urinary system
   2. Hopelessness, related to development of chronic illness (hemiparesis and diabetes insipidus)

3. Risk for impaired oral mucous membrane, related to dehydration
4. Coping, ineffective family: compromised, risk for, related to chronic illness

8. A 34-year-old construction worker was recently diagnosed as having acromegaly. Given the pathophysiology of his condition, the patient's laboratory test results will probably show elevated levels of:

   1. FSH.
   2. LH.
   3. TSH.
   4. GH.

9. While assessing a postoperative thyroidectomy patient, the nurse checks for damage to the laryngeal nerve. Which is most likely to suggest that damage may have occurred?

   1. The patient complains of a slight sore throat.
   2. The patient's voice tone has changed slightly.
   3. The patient is unable to swallow fluids.
   4. The patient is becoming increasingly hoarse.

10. To help a patient newly diagnosed with type 1 diabetes mellitus meet the goal of maintaining blood glucose control, which is the greatest priority in the care plan?

    1. Teach the patient the effect of diet, exercise, and insulin on the blood glucose level.
    2. Refer the patient to the hospital dietitian for intense education about his dietary needs.
    3. Instruct the patient on SMBG, observe return demonstrations, and correct his technique as needed.
    4. Review with the patient the desired effects of his medication, as well as possible side effects.

11. A 22-year-old man has had type 1 diabetes for the past year. Which statement demonstrates his need for more teaching?

    1. "If I want to lose weight, all I have to do is increase my dose of insulin."
    2. "I can have an occasional beer if it's calculated into my diet."
    3. "I will maintain better control of my blood sugar if I eat regular meals."
    4. "It is important that I eat properly, exercise regularly, and take my insulin injections."

12. To meet the goal of preventing injury to a type 1 diabetic patient, which nursing intervention is most important to include in the care plan?

    1. Assess peripheral pulses and capillary refill in the lower extremities.
    2. Instruct the patient in the proper technique for self-injection of insulin.
    3. Stress the importance of keeping the skin on the feet soft and supple.
    4. Remove potentially hazardous objects from the patient's environment.

13. A 45-year-old has been admitted to the hospital unit with the primary medical diagnosis of Addison's disease (adrenal hypofunction). Assessment reveals postural hypotension, fatigue, nausea, vomiting, and

poor skin turgor. Which of these nursing diagnoses is of greatest priority at this time?

1. Risk for infection
2. Risk for imbalanced body temperature
3. Risk for injury
4. Risk for deficient fluid volume

14. A human insulin formula that begins to take effect in less than half the time of regular, fast-acting insulin and more closely mimics the body's own hormone action is:

1. Humulin R, Novolin R.
2. lispro (Humalog), aspart (NovoLog).
3. Humulin N, Novolin N.
4. Humulin 70/30, Novolin 70/30.

15. The polydipsia and polyuria related to diabetes are caused primarily by:

1. the release of ketones from cells during fat metabolism.
2. fluid shifts resulting from the osmotic effect of hyperglycemia.
3. damage to the kidneys from exposure to high levels of glucose.
4. changes in RBCs resulting from attachment of excessive glucose to hemoglobin.

16. In planning care for a 78-year-old patient with type 2 diabetes admitted to the hospital with pneumonia, the nurse recognizes that the patient:

1. must receive insulin therapy to prevent the development of ketoacidosis.
2. has islet cell antibodies that have destroyed the ability of the pancreas to produce insulin.
3. has minimal or absent endogenous insulin secretion and requires daily insulin injections.
4. may have sufficient endogenous insulin to prevent ketosis but is at risk for development of hyperosmolar coma.

17. A diabetic patient takes a combination of regular and NPH insulin twice a day for glucose control. The nurse teaches the patient to be alert for hypoglycemia:

1. immediately after breakfast and dinner.
2. immediately after lunch and dinner.
3. in the late afternoon and at bedtime.
4. immediately after dinner and at bedtime.

18. The nurse assists the patient with dietary management of diabetes with the knowledge that a diabetic diet is designed:

1. to be used only for type 1 diabetes.
2. for use during periods of high stress.
3. to normalize blood glucose by elimination of sugar.
4. to help normalize blood glucose through a balanced diet.

19. In teaching a newly diagnosed type 1 diabetic "survival skills," the nurse includes information about:

1. weight-loss measures.
2. elimination of sugar from the diet.

3. need to reduce physical activity.
4. capillary blood glucose monitoring.

20. An appropriate instruction for the patient with diabetes related to care of the feet is:

1. use heat to increase blood supply.
2. avoid softening lotions and creams.
3. inspect all surfaces of the feet daily.
4. use iodine to disinfect cuts and abrasions.

21. The oral hypoglycemic that works primarily by reducing hepatic glucose production and lowering fasting blood glucose levels is:

1. repaglinide (Prandin).
2. acarbose (Precose).
3. metformin (Glucophage).
4. rosiglitazone (Avandia).

22. The types of insulin used in an insulin pump are _____ or _____ insulin.

23. Circle all correct statements.

1. Regular insulin (Humulin R) has an onset of action of 30 minutes to 1 hour.
2. Lispro (Humalog) has an onset of action of 15 minutes.
3. NPH (Humulin N) has an onset of action of 2 hours.
4. Glargine (Lantus) has an onset of action of 6 to 10 hours.

24. The normal range of serum sodium is:

1. 10 mEq/L.
2. 8.9 to 10.1 mEq/L.
3. 135 to 145 mEq/L.
4. 8 to 23 mEq/L.

25. In syndrome of inappropriate antidiuretic hormone (SIADH) the body secretes:

1. too much antidiuretic hormone (ADH).
2. too little antidiuretic hormone (ADH).

26. Clinically, SIADH is characterized by what? *(Select all that apply.)*

1. Peripheral edema
2. Hyponatremia
3. Water retention
4. Brain cells becoming edematous

27. In the medical management of SIADH, the physician orders:

1. increased fluid intake to 3000 mL/day.
2. fluid restriction to 800 to 1000 mL/day.

28. Choose the correct nursing interventions for SIADH. *(Select all that apply.)*

1. Daily weight
2. I&O
3. Fluid restriction
4. Foods high in sodium

29. If the diabetic patient engages in increased exercise, his insulin requirement:
    1. increases.
    2. decreases.
    3. remains unchanged.

30. Chvostek's sign, Trousseau's sign, carpopedal spasms, and laryngeal spasms are postoperative complications of total thyroidectomy that indicate:
    1. low levels of serum calcium.
    2. high levels of serum calcium.
    3. low levels of serum sodium.
    4. high levels of serum sodium.

31. An appropriate nursing intervention for a patient admitted into the hospital with signs and symptoms of diabetic ketoacidosis is:
    1. obtain blood glucose immediately.
    2. administer NPH insulin intravenously.
    3. give intravenous glucagon.
    4. take vital signs every 4 hours.

32. Cushing's syndrome results from what? *(Select all that apply.)*
    1. Excessive levels of adrenocortical hormones in plasma
    2. Hyperplasia of adrenal tissue from overstimulation of ACTH
    3. Overuse of corticosteroid drugs
    4. Adrenocortical insufficiency when the adrenal glands do not secrete adequate amounts of glucocorticoids

33. Addison's disease results from:
    1. decreased production of parathyroid hormones.
    2. excessive secretion of epinephrine and norepinephrine.
    3. inadequate secretion of glucocorticoids and mineralocorticoids.
    4. overactivity of the parathyroid glands with decreased production of parathyroid hormone.

34. In a patient with pheochromocytoma, the principal clinical manifestation is:
    1. darkly pigmented skin and mucous membranes.
    2. moonface and buffalo hump.
    3. severe hypertension.
    4. carpopedal spasms.

35. This blood test measures the amount of glucose that has become incorporated into the hemoglobin within an erythrocyte. This test reveals the effectiveness of diabetes therapy for the preceding 8 to 12 weeks. It is called _____ or _____.

36. Good skin care, especially of the feet, is essential for the person with diabetes mellitus because. *(Select all that apply.)*
    1. poor circulation can lead to the development of skin problems.
    2. elevated glycosylated hemoglobin in RBCs impedes the release of oxygen to the tissues.
    3. low blood glucose levels make pathogens thrive and proliferate rapidly.
    4. vascular changes decrease blood oxygen and nutrient supply to the tissues and affect the supply of WBCs in the area and thus adversely affect phagocytosis.

Care of the Patient with a Reproductive Disorder

Barbara Lauritsen Christensen

Objectives

Anatomy and Physiology

1. List and describe the functions of the organs of the male and female reproductive tracts.
2. Discuss menstruation and the hormones necessary for a complete menstrual cycle.

Medical-Surgical

3. Discuss the impact of illness on the patient's sexuality.
4. Discuss nursing interventions for the patient undergoing diagnostic studies related to the reproductive system.
5. Discuss the importance of the Papanicolaou's test in early detection of cervical cancer and mammography as a screening procedure for breast cancer.
6. List nursing interventions for patients with menstrual disturbances.
7. Discuss the etiology and pathophysiology, clinical manifestations, assessment, diagnostic tests, medical management, nursing interventions, patient teaching, and prognosis for infections of the female reproductive tract.
8. Discuss four important points to be addressed in discharge planning for the patient with pelvic inflammatory disease.
9. List four nursing diagnoses pertinent to the patient with endometriosis.
10. Identify the clinical manifestations of a vaginal fistula.
11. Describe the common problems with cystocele and rectocele and the related medical management and nursing interventions.
12. Discuss the etiology and pathophysiology, clinical manifestations, assessment, diagnostic tests, medical management, nursing interventions, patient teaching, and prognosis for cancers of the female reproductive system.
13. Identify four nursing diagnoses pertinent to ovarian cancer.
14. Describe the preoperative and postoperative nursing interventions for the patient requiring major surgery of the female reproductive system.
15. Describe six important points to emphasize in teaching breast self-examination.
16. Compare four surgical approaches for cancer of the breast.
17. Discuss adjuvant therapies for breast cancer.
18. Discuss nursing interventions for the patient who has had a modified radical mastectomy.
19. List several discharge planning instructions for the patient who has undergone a modified radical mastectomy.
20. Discuss the etiology and pathophysiology, clinical manifestations, assessment, diagnostic tests, medical management, nursing interventions, patient teaching, and prognosis for inflammatory disorders of the male reproductive system.
21. Distinguish between hydrocele and varicocele.
22. Discuss the importance of monthly testicular self-examination beginning at 15 years of age.
23. Discuss patient education related to prevention of sexually transmitted infections.

Key Terms

amenorrhea (ă-měn-ŏ-RĒ-ă, p. 546)
candidiasis (kăn-dĭ-DĪ-ă-sĭs, p. 591)
carcinoma in situ (kăr-sĭ-NŌ-mă ĭn SĪ-tū, p. 565)
chancre (SHĂNG-kěr, p. 589)
Chlamydia trachomatis (klă-MĬD-ē-ă tră-KŌ-mă-tĭs, p. 591)
circumcision (sĭr-kŭm-SĬZH-ŭn, p. 584)
climacteric (klī-MĂK-těr-ĭk, p. 551)
colporrhaphy (kŏl-PŎR-ă-fē, p. 562)
colposcopy (kŏl-PŎS-kŏ-pē, p. 542)
cryptorchidism (krĭp-TŎR-kĭ-dĭz-ěm, p. 585)
culdoscopy (kŭl-DŎS-kŏ-pē, p. 542)
curettage (KŪ-rě-tăhzh, p. 544)
dysmenorrhea (dĭs-měn-ō-RĒ-ă, p. 546)
endometriosis (ěn-dō-mē-trē-Ō-sĭs, p. 560)
epididymitis (ěp-ĭ-dĭd-ě-MĪ-tĭs, p. 584)

fistula (FĬS-tū-lă, p. 561)
introitus (ĭn-TRŌ-ĭ-tŭs, p. 562)
laparoscopy (lă-pă-RŎS-kō-pē, p. 542)
mammography (măm-MŎG-ră-fē, p. 544)
menorrhagia (měn-ō-RĀ-jă, p. 546)
metrorrhagia (mě-trō-RĀ-jă, p. 546)
panhysterosalpingo-oophorectomy (păn-HĬS-těr-ō-SĂL-pĭng-gō-oof-ō-RĔK-tō-mē, p. 569)
Papanicolaou (Pap) test (smear) (pă-pě-NĬ-kō-lōu těst, smēr, p. 542)
phimosis (fĭ-MŌ-sĭs, p. 584)
procidentia (prō-sĭ-DĚN-shă, p. 562)
sentinel lymph node mapping (SĚN-tĭ-něl lĭmf nōd MĂP-ĭng, p. 574)
trichomoniasis (trĭk-ō-mō-NĪ-ă-sĭs, p. 590)

Conception and birth are made possible through the dynamics of the normally functioning male and female reproductive systems. Reproduction of like individuals is necessary for the continuation of the species. The male and female sex glands (gonads) produce the gametes (sperm, ova) that unite to form a fertilized egg (zygote), the beginning of a new life.

ANATOMY AND PHYSIOLOGY OF THE REPRODUCTIVE SYSTEM

MALE REPRODUCTIVE SYSTEM

The organs of the male reproductive system include the testes, the ductal system, the accessory glands, and the penis (Figure 12-1). These structures have various functions: (1) producing and storing sperm, (2) depositing sperm for fertilization, and (3) developing the male secondary sex characteristics.

Testes (Testicles)

The two oval **testes** (gonads) are enclosed in the **scrotum,** a saclike structure that lies suspended from the exterior abdominal wall. This position keeps the temperature in the testes below normal body temperature, which is necessary for viable sperm production and storage. Each testis contains one to three coiled seminiferous tubules that produce the sperm cells. After puberty, millions of sperm cells are produced daily. The testes also produce the hormone testosterone. Testosterone is responsible for the development of male secondary sex characteristics.

Ductal System
Epididymis

Sperm (Figure 12-2) produced in the seminiferous tubules immediately travel through a network of ducts called the **rete testis.** These passageways contain cilia that sweep sperm out of the testes into the **epididymis,** a tightly coiled tube structure that lies superior to the testes and extends posteriorly. With sexual stimulation smooth muscle within the walls of the epididymis contract, forcing the sperm along the seminiferous tubules of the testes to the vas deferens.

Ductus Deferens (Vas Deferens)

The **ductus deferens** is approximately 18 inches (46 cm) long and rises along the posterior wall of the testes. As it moves upward, it passes through the inguinal canal into the pelvic cavity and loops over the urinary bladder. The ductus deferens, the nerves, and the blood vessels are enclosed in a connective tissue sheath called the **spermatic cord.** If a man chooses to be sterilized for birth control, it is a simple procedure to make small slits on either side of the scrotum and sever the ductus deferens. This procedure is called a **vasectomy.** It renders the man sterile because sperm can no longer be expelled.

Ejaculatory Duct and Urethra

Behind the urinary bladder, the ejaculatory duct connects with the ductus deferens. The ejaculatory duct is only 1 inch (2.5 cm) long. It unites with the urethra to pass through the prostate gland. Each of the two ejaculatory ducts empties into the prostate urethra. The urethra extends the length of the penis with the urinary meatus. The urethra carries both sperm and urine, but, because of the urethral sphincter, it does not do so at the same time.

Accessory Glands

The ductal system transports and stores sperm. The accessory glands, which produce seminal fluid (semen), include the seminal vesicles, the prostate gland, and Cowper's glands. With each ejaculation (2 to 5 mL

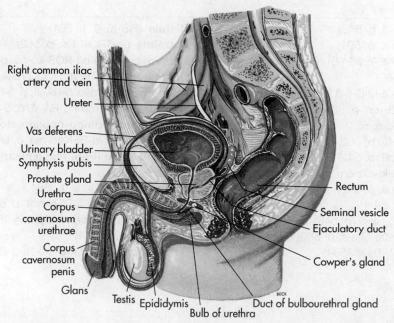

FIGURE 12-1 Longitudinal section of the male pelvis showing the location of the male reproductive organs.

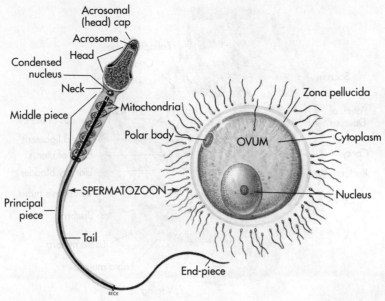

Acrosomal
(head) cap
Acrosome
Head
Condensed
nucleus
Neck
Middle piece
Mitochondria
Polar body
Zona pellucida
OVUM
Cytoplasm
Nucleus
←SPERMATOZOON→
Principal
piece
Tail
End-piece

FIGURE 12-2 Male sex cell (spermatozoon) greatly enlarged *(left)*. Female sex cell (ovum) surrounded by sperm at time of fertilization *(right)*.

of fluid), approximately 200 to 500 million sperm are released.

Seminal Vesicles

The **seminal vesicles** are paired structures that lie at the base of the bladder and produce 60% of the volume of semen. The fluid is released into the ejaculatory ducts to meet with the sperm.

Prostate Gland

The single, doughnut-shaped **prostate gland** surrounds the neck of the bladder and urethra. It is a firm structure, about the size of a chestnut, composed of muscular and glandular tissue. The prostate secretes alkaline fluid that contributes to motility of sperm. Smooth muscle of the prostate contracts during ejaculation, expelling semen from the urethra. The ejaculatory duct passes obliquely through the posterior part of the gland. The prostate gland often hypertrophies with age, expanding to surround the urethra and making voiding difficult.

Cowper's Glands

Cowper's glands are two pea-sized glands under the male urethra. They correspond to the Bartholin's glands in women and provide lubrication during sexual intercourse.

Urethra and Penis

The male **urethra** has two purposes: conveying urine from the bladder and carrying sperm to the outside. The cylindrical **penis** is the organ of copulation. The shaft of the penis ends with an enlarged tip called the **glans penis.** The skin covering the penis, called the **prepuce,** or foreskin, lies in folds around the glans. This excess tissue is sometimes removed in a surgical procedure called circumcision to prevent **phimosis**

(tightness of the prepuce of the penis that prevents retraction of the foreskin over the glans).

Three masses of erectile tissue, the corpus spongiosum and two copora cavernosa, contain numerous sinuses that fill the shaft of the penis. With sexual stimulation the sinuses fill with blood, causing the penis to become erect. Sexual stimulation concludes with ejaculation, which is brought about by peristalsis of the reproductive ducts and contraction of the prostate gland. After ejaculation, the penis returns to a flaccid state.

Sperm

Spermatogenesis (the process of developing spermatozoa) begins at puberty and continues throughout life. Mature sperm consist of three distinct parts: (1) the head; (2) the midpiece; and (3) the tail, which propels the sperm. Once deposited in the female reproductive system, mature sperm live approximately 48 hours (or in some cases up to 5 days). If they come in contact with a mature egg, the enzyme on the head of each sperm bombards the egg in an attempt to break down its coating (see Figure 12-2). It takes thousands of sperm to break the coating, but only one sperm enters and fertilizes the egg. The remaining sperm disintegrate. Once fertilization takes place, a chemical change occurs making the ova impenetrable for other sperm.

FEMALE REPRODUCTIVE SYSTEM

The organs of the female reproductive system include the ovaries, the uterus, the fallopian tubes, and the vagina (Figure 12-3). These organs, along with a few accessory structures, produce the ovum, house the fertilized egg, maintain the embryo, and nurture the newborn infant. The ability to conceive and nurture this new human being requires the intricate balance of many hormones and the menstrual cycle.

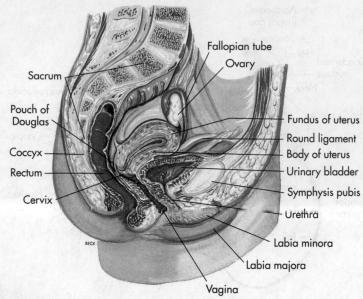

FIGURE 12-3 Longitudinal section of the female pelvis showing the location of the female reproductive organs.

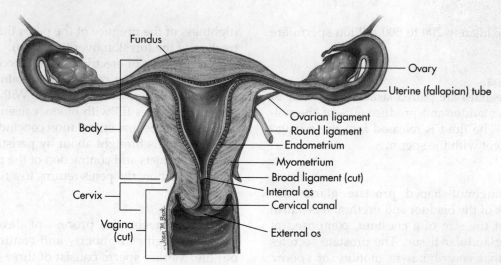

FIGURE 12-4 Sectioned view of the uterus showing relationship to the ovaries and the vagina.

Ovaries

The paired **ovaries** (gonads) are the size and shape of almonds. They are located bilateral to the uterus immediately inferior to the fallopian fimbriae. At puberty they release progesterone and the female sex hormone estrogen, and they release a mature egg during the menstrual cycle. Each ovary contains 30,000 to 40,000 microscopic ovarian follicles.

Fallopian Tubes (Oviducts)

The **fallopian tubes** are a pair of ducts opening at one end into the **fundus** (upper portion of the uterus) and at the other end into the peritoneal cavity, over the ovary. They are approximately 4 inches (10 cm) long with the fimbriae at the distal ends. The entire inner surface of the tubes is lined with cilia. When the graafian follicle of the ovary ruptures and releases the mature ovum, the fimbriae sweep the ovum into the fallopian tube. Fertilization takes place in the

outer third of this tube, and the fertilized ovum (**zygote**) is moved through the tube by a combination of muscular peristaltic movements and the sweeping action of the cilia. If the mature ovum is not fertilized, it disintegrates.

Uterus

The **uterus** is shaped like an inverted pear and measures $3 \times 2 \times 1$ inches ($7.5 \times 5 \times 2.5$ cm) in the nonpregnant state (Figure 12-4). It is located between the urinary bladder and the rectum and consists of three layers of tissue: (1) endometrium, the inner layer; (2) myometrium, the middle layer; and (3) perimetrium, the outer layer. The uterus is divided into three major portions (see Figure 12-4). The **fundus** (upper, rounded portion) is the insertion site of the fallopian tubes. The larger midsection is the **corpus** (body). The smaller, narrower lower portion of the uterus is the **cervix**, part of which actually descends into the vaginal vault. During pregnancy the uterus is capable of enlarging up to 500 times.

Vagina

The **vagina** is a thin-walled, muscular, tubelike structure of the female genitalia, approximately 3 inches (7.5 cm) long. It is located between the urinary bladder and the rectum. The superior portion articulates with the cervix of the uterus; the inferior portion opens to the outside of the body. The vagina is lined with mucous membrane, responsible for lubrication during sexual activity. The walls of the vagina normally lie in folds called **rugae.** This enables the vagina to stretch to receive the penis during intercourse and to allow passage of the infant during birth.

The external opening of the vagina is covered by a fold of mucous membrane, skin, and fibrous tissue called the **hymen.** For centuries the hymen was a symbol of virginity, but it is now known that rigorous exercise or the insertion of a tampon may tear the hymen. If the hymen does remain intact, it is ruptured by **coitus** (intercourse).

External Genitalia

The reproductive structures located outside the body are the external genitalia, or **vulva.** These structures include the mons pubis, labia majora, labia minora, clitoris, and vestibule (Figure 12-5).

Located superior to the symphysis pubis is a mound of fatty tissue, covered with coarse hair. This structure is the **mons pubis.** Extending from the mons pubis to the perineal floor are two large folds called the **labia majora** (large lips). These protect the inner structures and contain sensory nerve endings and an assortment of sebaceous (oil) and sudoriferous (sweat) glands. Directly under the labia majora lie the **labia minora** (small lips). These are smaller folds of tissue, devoid of hair, that merge anteriorly to form the prepuce of the

clitoris. The **clitoris** is comparable to the male penis and is composed of erectile tissue that becomes engorged with blood during sexual stimulation.

The space enclosing the structures located beneath the labia minora is called the **vestibule.** It contains the **clitoris,** the **urinary meatus,** the **hymen,** and the **vaginal opening.**

Accessory Glands

Bilateral to the urinary meatus lie the **paraurethral,** or **Skene's, glands,** the largest glands opening into the urethra. These glands secrete mucus and are similar to the male prostate gland. Bilateral to the vaginal opening are two small, mucus-secreting glands called the greater **Bartholin's glands (vestibular),** which lubricate the vagina for sexual intercourse.

Perineum

The area enclosing the region containing the reproductive structures is referred to as the **perineum.** The perineum is diamond shaped and starts at the symphysis pubis and extends to the anus.

Mammary Glands (Breasts)

The breasts are attached to the pectoral (chest) muscles. Breast tissue is identifiable in both sexes. During puberty, the female breasts change their size, shape, and ability to function. Each breast contains 15 to 20 lobes that are separated by adipose tissue. The amount of adipose tissue is responsible for the size of the breast. Within each lobe are many lobules that contain milk-producing cells; these lobules lead directly to the **lactiferous ducts** that empty into the nipple (Figure 12-6).

The nipple is composed of smooth muscle that allows it to become erect. The dark pink or brown tissue surrounding the nipple is called the **areola.** Milk production does not start until a woman gives birth. At this

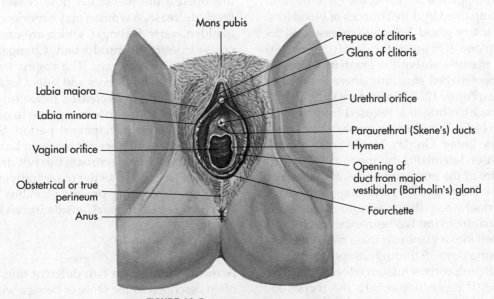

FIGURE 12-5 External female genitalia (vulva).

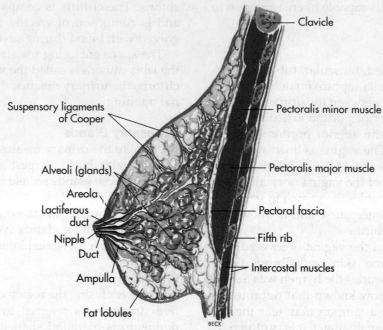

FIGURE 12-6 Lateral view of the breast (sagittal section). The gland is fixed to the overlying skin and the pectoralis muscles by the suspensory ligaments of Cooper. Each lobule of secretory tissue is drained by a lactiferous duct that opens through the nipple.

time, under the influence of prolactin, the milk is formed. The hormone oxytocin allows milk to be released.

Menstrual Cycle

Menarche, the first menstrual cycle, usually begins at approximately 12 years of age. Each month, for the next 30 to 40 years, an ovum matures and is released about 14 days before the next menstrual flow, which occurs on average every 28 days. If fertilization occurs, menstrual cycling subsides and the body adapts to the developing fetus.

Generally, the menstrual cycle is divided into three phases: (1) menstrual, (2) preovulatory, and (3) postovulatory. This discussion uses the example of a 28-day cycle. On days 1 through 5 of the cycle, the endometrium sloughs off, accompanied by 1 to 2 ounces of blood loss. The anterior pituitary gland begins to release follicle-stimulating hormone (FSH); as the level of FSH increases, the egg matures within the **graafian follicle** (a pocket or envelope-shaped structure where the ovaries prepare the ovum [Figure 12-7]). From days 6 through 13 (preovulatory phase), estrogen is released from the maturing graafian follicle. This estrogen causes vascularization of the uterine lining. On day 14, the anterior pituitary gland releases luteinizing hormone (LH), which causes the rupture of the graafian follicle and release of the mature ovum. The fingerlike projections of the fallopian tubes (fimbriae) sweep the ovum into the fallopian tube. Once this mature ovum has been expelled, the follicle is transformed into a glandular mass called the **corpus luteum.** During days 15 through 28 (postovulatory phase), the developing corpus luteum releases estrogen and progesterone. If pregnancy occurs, the corpus luteum continues to release estrogen and progesterone to maintain the uterine lining until the placenta is formed,

which then takes over the job of hormonal release. If pregnancy does not occur, the corpus luteum lasts 8 days and then disintegrates. Normally the corpus luteum shrinks and is replaced by scar tissue called **corpus albicans.** At this point the hormone level decreases over several days and menstruation starts again.

EFFECTS OF NORMAL AGING ON THE REPRODUCTIVE SYSTEM

Menopause usually occurs in women between 35 and 60 years of age. The average age is 51. Whether it occurs earlier or later, menopause should not be considered abnormal. Cigarette smoking and living at high altitudes are associated with early menopause. During menopause the menstrual flow ceases and hormone levels decrease. A woman may experience "hot flashes" (sudden warm feelings), which are caused by the decrease in estrogen production. Changes also occur in the reproductive organs. The vagina loses some of its elasticity, and the breasts and vulva lose some adipose tissue, resulting in decreased tissue turgor. The bones may also become brittle and prone to osteoporosis.

Men have no menopausal period. Sperm production decreases but does not cease. In later years, testosterone production decreases, but not dramatically.

Basically, as long as the older individual is healthy, nothing in the aging process prohibits normal sexual function (see Life Span Considerations box).

HUMAN SEXUALITY

Sexuality and sex are two different things. **Sexuality** is often described as the sense of being a woman or a man. It has biologic, psychological, social, and ethical dimensions. Sexuality influences life experiences, and sexual-

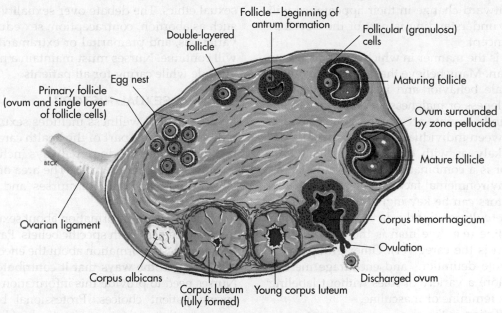

FIGURE 12-7 Mammalian ovary showing successive stages of ovarian (graafian) follicle and ovum development. Begin with the first stage (egg nest) and follow around clockwise to the final stage (corpus albicans).

 Life Span Considerations
Older Adults

Reproductive Disorders

WOMEN
- Many older women are reluctant to seek medical care for problems of the reproductive system. This may be related to cultural factors, embarrassment, or lack of knowledge. Routine gynecologic examination should continue as part of the overall physical examination, even after menopause.
- Certain forms of cancer of the reproductive tract are more common with aging. Any vaginal bleeding should be promptly reported to the physician, as should pelvic pain, pruritus, or skin lesions in the genital region.
- Decreased levels of estrogen and systemic diseases, such as diabetes, predispose older women to vaginitis.
- Breast cancer risk increases after 40 years of age. Breast examination should continue throughout the life span. The American Cancer Society (2009a, b) recommends an annual mammogram for women older than 40 years of age. Each

woman must make an individualized choice in consultation with her physician.

MEN
- Decreased production of testosterone results in changes in the male reproductive system, but the ability to procreate can continue into the eighth decade. Sexual interest often continues late in life.
- Chronic health problems, such as diabetes mellitus or hypertension, and many kinds of medication result in impotence in older men.
- Prostate enlargement is increasingly common with each decade after 40 years of age. Although this enlargement is usually benign, cancer of the prostate is a serious condition seen in older men. Ultrasonography of the prostate, when combined with rectal examination and prostate-specific antigen testing, is particularly useful in diagnosing prostate cancer.

ity is influenced by life experiences. The term **sex** has a more limited meaning. It usually describes the biologic aspects of sexuality such as genital sexual activity. Sex may be used for pleasure or reproduction. As a result of life's changes or by personal choice, sexual activity may be absent from a person's life for brief or prolonged periods. Some persons may choose to remain celibate.

The process by which people come to know themselves as women or men is not clearly understood. Being born with female or male genitalia and subsequently learning female or male social roles seem to be factors, though these do not explain differences of sexuality and sexual behavior. Such variations are more understandable if the nurse remembers that sexuality is intertwined with all aspects of self.

SEXUAL IDENTITY

Biologic identity, or the differences between men and women, is established at conception and further influenced at puberty by hormones. Gender identity is the sense of being feminine or masculine. As soon as the infant is born (and sometimes before), the outside world labels the child as a girl or boy. Adults adjust their behavior to relate to a female or male infant. These varied patterns of interaction influence the infant's developing sense of gender identity.

Children explore and seek to understand their own bodies. Combining this information with the way in which they are treated, they begin to create an image of themselves as a boy or as a girl. By 3 years of age, children are aware that they will remain boys or girls and that no outward change in their appearance will alter this. This understanding is part of the development of self-concept.

Gender role is the manner in which a person acts as a woman or man. Many believe that society influences female and male behavior and is thus the primary source of femaleness or maleness. Because society encourages certain behaviors according to one's gender, differences between individuals' sexual behaviors develop. Most likely, as with other human behaviors, sexual behavior is a combination of many interacting biologic and environmental factors.

Cultural factors can be key ingredients in defining sex roles. Some cultures tightly dictate roles as feminine or masculine (e.g., the man is the breadwinner, and the woman is the caregiver). Other groups have more flexible role definitions and encourage men or women to explore a variety of roles without labeling the behavior as feminine or masculine.

Sexual orientation is the clear and persistent erotic desire of a person for one sex or the other. There are heterosexual, homosexual, lesbian, and bisexual individuals, but the origins of sexual orientation are still not understood. Biologic theorists describe orientation in genetic terms, meaning it is determined at conception. Psychological theorists attribute orientation to early learning experiences, believing that cognitive processes are the determining factor. Still other theorists state that genetics and environment both play roles in the development of sexual preference.

For some people the inward sense of sexual identity does not match the biologic body. These people are known as transgenders. Researchers do not clearly understand how this mismatch occurs. Transgenders do not see their sexual identity as a choice; it is a clear and persistent orientation dating back to early childhood. In contrast, most homosexual men and women define themselves as satisfied with their gender and social roles; they simply have a persistent desire for their same sex.

A transvestite is most often a heterosexual man who periodically dresses like a woman; however, a transvestite may be a homosexual. Cross-dressing is usually done in private and kept secret even from those who are closest to him.

Because sexuality is linked to every aspect of living, any sexual choice involves personal, family, cultural, religious, and social standards of conduct. Ideas about ethical sexual conduct and emotions related to sexuality form the basis for sexual decision making. The range of attitudes about sexuality extends from a traditional view of sex only within marriage to a point of view that allows individuals to determine what is right. Sexual choices that overstep a person's ethical standard may result in internal conflicts.

Some people may judge sexual decisions as moral or immoral solely on religious standards; others view any private sexual act between consenting adults as moral. People will always have differing beliefs about sexual ethics. The debate over sexuality-related issues such as abortion, contraception, sex education, sexual variations, and premarital or extramarital intercourse will continue. Nurses must maintain a nonjudgmental attitude while caring for all patients.

TAKING A SEXUAL HISTORY

Because overall wellness includes sexual health, sexuality should be a part of the health care program. Yet health care services do not always include sexual assessment and interventions. The area of sexuality can be an emotional one for nurses and patients (see Health Promotion box).

Giving patients information about sexuality does not imply agreement with specific beliefs. Patients need accurate, honest information about the effects of illness on sexuality and the ways that it contributes to wellness. Nurses need to provide this information without influencing patient choices. Professional behavior must guarantee that patients receive the best health care possible without diminishing their self-worth. Promotion of self-education and honest examination of sexual beliefs and values can help in reducing sexual bias.

Although there is no single approach to taking a sexual history, certain principles make it more comfortable for both the patient and the nurse (Box 12-1):

- Obtain the sexual history early in the nurse-patient relationship, which indicates permission for patients to discuss sexual concerns.
- Avoid overreacting or underreacting to a patient's comments; this aids in truthful data collection.
- Use language that the patient understands; both the patient and the nurse may need to define their terms to ensure accurate data gathering.

Health Promotion

Factors that Can Interfere with the Promotion of Sexual Health

- Lack of information
- Conflicting values system (attitudes and beliefs)
- Anxiety (Are specific attitudes, feelings, and actions "normal"?)
- Guilt
- Lack of comfort with sexuality
- Invasion of privacy
- Lack of regard for hospitalized patient's need for time alone with significant other
- Manner in which the patient is touched
- Fear of being judged
- Lack of understanding of the effects of illness and treatment on sexual functioning

---

Box 12-1 Requirements for Taking a Sexual History

- Provision of privacy—a closed room
- An atmosphere of trust—ensure confidentiality
- Nurses' comfort with their own sexuality
- Nonjudgmental approach

- Move from the less sensitive to the more sensitive areas. This will promote nurse-patient comfort.
- At the end of the sexual history, ask if the patient has additional questions or concerns.

A brief sexual history assessment can be made and included in the nursing history through the use of three questions (Box 12-2). The questions may be adapted to address illness, hospitalization, life events, or any other relevant matter that influences or interferes with sexual health. The questions may also be adjusted to find out what the patient expects to happen as a result of procedures, medications, or surgery. Often the nurse does not need to ask the last two questions because many patients voice their concerns about masculinity, femininity, and sexual functioning without further encouragement.

Nurses may intervene in sexual problems among patient populations through four strategies: (1) educating patient groups likely to have sexual concerns, (2) providing anticipatory guidance throughout the life cycle, (3) promoting a milieu conducive to sexual health, and (4) validating normalcy about sexual concerns.

Several self-help groups and other organizations publish easy-to-read pamphlets on sexuality (see Health Promotion box). These pamphlets can often be purchased for a nominal fee and given to patients. Most pamphlets can be obtained directly from state or local chapters. Contact chapters of other self-help groups about the availability of resources for patients, such as newsletters that address sexuality.

Nurses can also write their own pamphlets for patients. Although this requires some effort, it may provide additional incentive for staff to address sexuality.

ILLNESS AND SEXUALITY

Illness may change a patient's self-concept and result in an inability to function sexually. Medications, stress, fatigue, and depression also affect sexual functioning.

⚡ Health Promotion

Self-Help Organizations that Publish Sexuality Pamphlets

- National Multiple Sclerosis Society (www.nationalmssociety.org): *Sexuality and MS*
- Arthritis Foundation (www.arthritis.org): *Living and Loving*
- American Cancer Society (www.cancer.org): *Sexuality for the Man with Cancer; Sexuality for the Woman with Cancer*
- American Diabetes Association (www.diabetes.org): several pamphlets and articles for men and women with diabetes mellitus

---

Box 12-2 | **Brief Sexual History**

- Has your (illness, pregnancy, hospitalization) interfered with your being a (husband, wife, significant other, father, mother)?
- Has your (abortion, heart attack) changed the way you see yourself as a (woman, man)?
- Has your (colostomy, mastectomy, hysterectomy) changed your ability to function sexually (or altered your sex life)?

Alcohol abuse can lead to a reduced sex drive and inadequate sexual functioning.

Lack of interest or desire for sexual activity often occurs when patients are preoccupied with symptoms of illness. Most often these sexual symptoms disappear as patients recover from the acute phase of illness and resume sexual activity. However, some illnesses—such as diabetes mellitus, end-stage renal disease, prostate cancer, certain types of prostate surgery, spinal cord injuries, and heart disease—may cause patients concern or may result in actual inabilities with sexual function.

Changes in the nervous system, circulatory system, or genital organs may lead to sexual health problems. Spinal cord injuries can interrupt the peripheral nerves and spinal cord reflexes that involve sexual responses. But spinal cord–injured men and women also have reported having satisfying orgasms in spite of complete denervation of all pelvic structures.

Sexual dysfunction of a patient with diabetes mellitus can occur when the disease is not well controlled, but the dysfunction generally disappears when the lack of control is diagnosed and treated. Approximately half of the men who have diabetes mellitus are impotent, generally because of poor control. Sexual counseling is important to (1) provide accurate information about the sexual aspects of the disorder, (2) dispel the patient's incorrect assumptions and expectations, and (3) give advice to improve the patient's sexual self-esteem and dispel the guilt frequently found in both partners.

A mastectomy results in both physical and emotional trauma. In addition to the resultant disfigurement, a patient must also grapple with (1) how to cope with cancer, (2) how the operation will affect her relationship with her spouse or significant other, (3) how to relate to the strangeness of her own body, and (4) how her sex life will be affected. Problems that arise with pelvic irradiation for cancer of the cervix are much harder to treat than those of mastectomy; the entire physiology of the vagina is altered by the radiation, causing a true loss of function. With a mastectomy the only function lost is the ability to nurse an infant. The goal for the patient and her partner is to face the issue in a straightforward manner, acknowledging the diagnosis and discussing their true feelings. If feelings are repressed rather than shared, both the patient and her significant other may suffer. Therapeutic counseling before surgery can aid the patient's and partner's acceptance and recovery after surgery.

LABORATORY AND DIAGNOSTIC EXAMINATIONS

DIAGNOSTIC TESTS FOR WOMEN

A physician performs the pelvic examination, which involves visualization and palpation of the vulva, the perineum, the vagina, the cervix, the ovaries, and the uterine surfaces. During the pelvic examination, specimens are frequently obtained for diagnostic purposes. The bimanual pelvic examination progresses from the visualization and palpation of the external genital organs for edema and irritations to an inspection for abnormalities of the internal organs. To visualize internal organs, the physician inserts a vaginal speculum. The physician may perform a rectovaginal examination to evaluate abnormalities or problems of the rectal area and the posterior internal organs (Box 12-3).

Colposcopy

Colposcopy (*colpo*, vagina or vaginal; and *scopy*, observation) provides direct visualization of the cervix and vagina. Prepare the patient for a pelvic examination and explain the purpose of the procedure. The physician inserts the vaginal speculum, followed by insertion of the colposcope for inspection of the area. The color of the tissue, presence of growths and lesions, and condition of the vascularity are observed and specimens obtained as necessary.

Culdoscopy

Culdoscopy is a diagnostic procedure that provides visualization of the uterus and adnexa (uterine appendages, i.e., the ovaries and fallopian tubes). Explain the purpose and the method of procedure. Prepare the patient for the vaginal operation with preoperative instructions. The patient is given a local, spinal, or general anesthetic. After the anesthetic is administered, the patient is assisted to a knee-chest position. The culdoscope is passed through the vaginal wall in back of the cervix. The area is examined for tumors, cysts, and endometriosis. During the procedure, **conization** (removal of eroded or infected tissue) may be done. This procedure is generally done on an outpatient basis. After the operation, assess for bleeding, assess vital signs, and monitor voiding.

Laparoscopy

Laparoscopy (examination of the abdominal cavity with a laparoscope through a small incision made beneath the umbilicus) provides direct visualization of the uterus and the adnexa. Preparation of the patient includes insertion of a Foley catheter to maintain blad-

der decompression for an open view. The procedure is done with a general anesthetic. The physician grasps the cervix with forceps and inserts a lighted laparoscope through the incision. Carbon dioxide may be introduced to distend the abdomen for easier visualization. If a biopsy is to be done or organs are to be manipulated, a second incision may be made in the lower abdomen to allow for instrument insertion. The ovaries and fallopian tubes are observed for masses, ectopic pregnancy, adhesions, and pelvic inflammatory disease (PID). Tubal ligations may be done using this procedure. Instruct the patient of the probability of shoulder pain afterward because of carbon dioxide introduced into abdomen.

Papanicolaou (Pap) Test (Smear)

Papanicolaou (Pap) test (smear) (a simple smear method of examining stained exfoliative peeling and sloughed-off tissue or cells) is most widely known for its use in the early detection of cervical cancer. Scrapings of secretions and cells are taken from the cervix and spread on a glass slide. The slide is sprayed with a fixative and sent to the laboratory for analysis. It is important that slides be properly labeled with the date, time of the last menstrual period, and whether the woman is taking estrogens or birth control pills. Instruct patients not to douche, use tampons, use vaginal medications, or have sexual intercourse for at least 24 hours before the examination. Collect careful menstrual and gynecologic history.

The American Cancer Society (ACS) (2009a) highly recommends that every woman begin annual Pap tests within 3 years after becoming sexually active or no later than 21 years of age. Women should be tested every year (regular Pap test) or every 2 years (thin prep Pap test). Women age 30 years or older who have had three normal Pap tests in a row may choose to be screened every 2 to 3 years instead of annually. Women age 70 years or older who have had three or more normal Pap tests in a row and no abnormal test results in the past 10 years may decide to stop having cervical screenings altogether. Also, women who have had a hysterectomy may stop having cervical cancer screenings (unless their surgery was done as a treatment for cervical cancer or precancerous cells).

Thin prep Pap tests may slightly improve the detection of cancers and greatly improve the detection of cervical precancers. Thin prep Pap tests also reduce the number of tests that need to be repeated.

The physician may recommend more frequent testing for women with a history of multiple sexual partners or sexually transmitted infections (STIs), a family history of cervical cancer, or those whose mothers used diethylstilbestrol (DES) during pregnancy.

Table 12-1 provides a comparison of interpretation classifications of the cytologic findings and treatment recommendations. The Bethesda system is preferred because it allows better communication between the

---

Box 12-3	**Endoscopic Procedures for Visualization of Pelvic Organs**

- **Colposcopy:** Visualization of vagina and cervix under low-power magnification
- **Culdoscopy:** Insertion of a culdoscope through posterior vaginal vault into Douglas's cul-de-sac for visualization of fallopian tubes and ovaries
- **Laparoscopy:** Insertion of a laparoscope (with patient under general anesthesia) through small incision in abdominal wall (inferior margin of umbilicus), then insufflation of abdomen with carbon dioxide; permits visualization of all pelvic organs

| Table 12-1 | Pap Test Interpretation Classifications and Action |

INTERPRETATION	NUMERICAL SYSTEM	DYSPLASIA CYTOLOGIC CLASSIFICATION	CERVICAL INTRAEPITHELIAL NEOPLASIA (CIN) CLASSIFICATION	BETHESDA SYSTEM*	ACTION
Negative (normal)	Class I	Negative squamous metaplasia	No designation	Negative (normal)	Repeat annually
Probably negative, may indicate infection	Class II	Atypical squamous cells	No designation	Infection Atypical squamous cells Reactive changes	Treat infection, repeat Pap
Suspicious, but not conclusive for malignancy	Class III	Mild dysplasia Moderate dysplasia	CIN I CIN II	Low-grade squamous intraepithelial lesion†	Treat infection, repeat Pap in 8-12 weeks; colposcopy
More suspicious, strongly suggestive of malignancy	Class IV	Severe dysplasia Carcinoma in situ	CIN III	High-grade squamous intraepithelial lesion†	Colposcopy, biopsy, treatment
Conclusive for malignancy	Class V	Invasive carcinoma	Invasive carcinoma	Invasive squamous cell carcinoma	Colposcopy, biopsy, treat with conization, hysterectomy

*The Bethesda system is the preferred system.
†The Bethesda Working Group suggests that "these two new terms encompass the spectrum of terms currently used to delineate the squamous cell precursors to invasive squamous carcinoma, including the grades of CIN, the degree of dysplasia, and carcinoma in situ."

cytologist and the clinician. The Bethesda system evaluates the adequacy of the sample (e.g., satisfactory or not satisfactory for interpretation) and provides a general classification of normal or abnormal and a descriptive diagnosis of the Pap smear. Although the classification system may vary, clinicians agree it is important to monitor Pap smears and ensure proper follow-up, including treatment of vaginal infections and colposcopy if necessary.

Pap tests have long been used to look for cervical cancer and precancerous cells. Cervista 16/18 and Cervista HPV HR are recently introduced tests for detecting the high-risk types of human papillomavirus (HPV) that are most likely to cause cervical cancer by looking for pieces of their deoxyribonucleic acid (DNA) in cervical cells. These DNA-based tests, in conjunction with the Pap test, have been approved by the U.S. Food and Drug Administration (FDA) (2009b) for women ages 30 and over with slightly abnormal Pap test results to find out if more testing or treatment may be needed.

Biopsy

Biopsies are procedures in which samples of tissue are taken for evaluation to confirm or locate a lesion. Tissue is aspirated by special needles or removed by forceps or through an incision.

A **breast biopsy** is performed to differentiate benign or malignant tumors. Breast biopsy is indicated for patients with palpable masses; suspicious areas appearing on mammography; and persistent, encrusted, purulent, inflamed, or sanguineous discharge from the nipples. The biopsy is performed by fine-needle aspiration (FNA); stereotactic or ultrasound core biopsy, under local anesthetic; or surgical biopsy, with general or local anesthetic. In an FNA, fluid is aspirated from the breast and expelled into a specimen bottle. Pressure is placed on the site to stop bleeding, then an adhesive bandage is applied. In an open surgical biopsy, an excisional biopsy is usually performed in a portion of the breast to expose the lesion and then remove the entire mass (Lewis et al., 2007). Another procedure called stereotactic and ultrasound core biopsy is a reliable diagnostic technique to obtain breast biopsy if an abnormal mass is seen on mammogram. A mammogram is used to find the lesion, the skin is anesthetized, and a small superficial incision is made. A biopsy gun device is fired into the lesion and removes a core sample of the mass. Compared with an open surgical biopsy, this procedure produces less scarring, uses only a local anesthesia, has reduced costs, and is done on an outpatient basis (Cleveland Clinic, 2009). Specimens of selected tissue may be frozen and stained for rapid diagnosis. The wound is sutured and a bandage applied. Observe the incision site for bleeding, tenderness, and erythema.

A **cervical biopsy** is done to evaluate cervical lesions and to diagnose cervical cancer. The biopsy is generally done without anesthesia. The colposcope is inserted through the vaginal speculum for direct visualization, the cervical site is selected and cleansed, and tissue is removed. The area is then packed with gauze or a tampon to check the blood flow.

An **endometrial biopsy** is performed to collect tissue for diagnosis of endometrial cancer and analysis for infertility studies. The procedure is generally performed at the time of menstruation when the cervix is dilated and cells are more easily obtained. The cervix is locally anesthetized, a curette is inserted, and tissue is obtained from selected sites of the endometrium.

Other Diagnostic Studies

Conization of the cervix is used to remove eroded or infected tissue or confirm cervical cancer. A cone-shaped section is removed when the mass is confined to the epithelial tissue. After surgery the area is packed with gauze to control bleeding. The patient is observed for bleeding and generally discharged from the hospital the same day.

Dilation and curettage (D&C) (scraping of material from the wall of a cavity or other surface; performed to remove tumors or other abnormal tissue for microscopic study) is a procedure used to obtain tissue for biopsy, to correct cervical stricture, and to treat dysmenorrhea. The patient is placed under general anesthesia, the cervix is dilated, and the inside of the uterus scraped with a curette. Packing may be inserted for hemostasis, and a perineal pad is applied for absorption of drainage. After vaginal packing is removed, instruct the patient to monitor for excessive vaginal bleeding or malodorous drainage.

Cultures and **smears** are collected to examine and identify infectious processes, abnormal cells, and hormonal changes of the reproductive tissue. Specimens collected for smears are prepared by spreading the collected smear on a glass slide and covering it with a second slide or spraying it with a fixative. Handle specimens with aseptic techniques and take care to avoid the transfer and spread of organisms. Cultures are taken from exudates of the breast, the vagina, the rectum, and the urethra. STIs and mastitis are diagnosed by isolation of the causative organisms. Treatment is prescribed according to the results of the culture.

Schiller's iodine test is used for the early detection of cancer cells and to guide the physician in doing a biopsy. An iodine preparation is applied to the cervix, and glycogen, which is present in normal cells, stains brown. Abnormal or immature cells do not absorb the stain. Unstained areas may be biopsied. This method of detection is valuable but not entirely reliable, since normal cells sometimes lack glycogen and malignant tissue sometimes contains glycogen. After the procedure the patient should wear a perineal pad to avoid stains on the clothing.

Radiographic examinations are performed to detect abnormal tissue, locate abnormal structures, and observe patency of ducts.

Hysterograms and **hysterosalpingograms** are studies for visualizing the uterine cavity to confirm (1) tubal abnormalities (adhesions and occlusions), (2) the presence of foreign bodies, (3) congenital malformations and leiomyomas (fibroids), and (4) traumatic injuries. The patient is placed in the lithotomy position. A speculum is inserted into the vagina, a cannula is inserted through the speculum into the cervical cavity, and a contrast medium is injected through the cannula. As the contrast medium progresses through the cavity, the uterus and fallopian tubes are viewed by a fluoroscope and films are taken.

Mammography is radiography of the soft tissue of the breast to allow identification of various benign and neoplastic processes, especially those not palpable on physical examination. **Digital mammography** is a newer technique that allows a clear and more accurate image; it involves digitally coding x-ray images into a computer (Lewis et al., 2007). It is believed that the average breast tumor is present for 9 years before it is palpable. Digital mammography is helpful as a screening procedure. The ACS (2009a, b) recommends baseline mammograms for women between ages 35 and 39, with annual mammograms after age 40.

When the mammography procedure is scheduled, advise the patient to refrain from using body powders, deodorants, and ointments on the breast areas, since this could cause false-positive results. Before the procedure give the patient a gown and ask her to remove jewelry and upper garments. The technician asks the patient to sit or stand in an upright position and rest one breast on the radiographic table. A compressor is placed on the breast, and the patient is asked to hold her breath as an anterior view is taken. The machine is rotated, the breast is again compressed, and a lateral view is taken. This procedure is repeated on the other breast. The patient may be asked to remain until the radiographic films are read.

Because of the greater density of breast tissue, mammography is less sensitive in younger women, which may result in more false-negative results. About 10% to 15% of all breast cancers can only be detected by palpation and cannot be seen on mammography. Even if mammogram findings are unremarkable, all suspicious masses should be biopsied.

Ultrasound is a helpful diagnostic tool to differentiate a benign tumor from a malignant tumor. It is useful in women who have dense breasts with fibrocystic changes. Unlike a mammogram, an ultrasound will not detect microcalcifications (Lewis et al., 2007).

The ACS (2007b) recommends, in addition to annual screening with mammography, the use of magnetic resonance imaging (MRI) for women with a 20% to 25% or greater lifetime risk of developing breast cancer. An MRI is not recommended as a routine screening for all eligible women due to its high cost and greater risk of false positives as compared to mammograms.

In **pelvic ultrasonography,** high-frequency sound waves are passed into the area to be examined, and images are viewed on a screen; this is similar to a radiographic film. Ultrasound is useful in detecting foreign bodies (such as intrauterine contraceptive devices [IUDs]), distinguishing between cystic and solid tumor bodies, evaluating fetal growth and viability, detecting fetal abnormalities, and detecting ectopic pregnancy. Generally it is noninvasive, safe, and painless. Encourage the patient to drink fluids beforehand. Explain that a full bladder is essential to the accuracy of the test.

Tubal insufflation (Rubin's test) involves transuterine insufflation of the fallopian tubes with carbon dioxide. The procedure enables evaluation of the patency of the fallopian tubes and may be part of a fertility study. Tubal insufflation takes approximately 30 minutes and is usually performed on an outpatient basis. If the tubes are open, the gas enters the abdominal cavity. A high-pitched bubbling is heard through the abdominal wall with a stethoscope as the gas escapes from the tubes. The patient may complain of shoulder pain from diaphragmatic irritation. In this case a radiographic film shows free gas under the diaphragm. If the tubes are occluded, gas cannot pass from the tubes, and the patient will not report pain.

All **pregnancy tests,** regardless of method, are based on detection of **human chorionic gonadotropin** (hCG), which is secreted in the urine after the fertilization of the ovum. Regardless of method, it is important to know that the tests do not indicate whether the pregnancy is normal. False-positive results may occur.

Serum CA-125 is a tumor antigen associated with ovarian cancer, since it is positive in 80% of such cases. CA-125 antigen levels in the blood decrease as the cancer cells decrease. CA-125 has been touted as a way to detect primary ovarian cancer, but unfortunately it *does not* do so. CA-125 is useful mainly to signal a recurrence of ovarian cancer and to follow the response to chemotherapy treatment. If chemotherapy causes a progressive decline in CA-125, it is an accurate indicator of a good response and is a good prognostic sign. Other conditions—such as endometriosis, PID, pregnancy, gynecologic cancers, and cancer of the pancreas—may result in an elevation of serum CA-125.

DIAGNOSTIC TESTS FOR MEN

Testicular Biopsy

Testicular biopsy is a means to detect abnormal cells and the presence of sperm. The testing can be done by aspiration or through an incision. The anesthetic used depends on the technique. Postbiopsy care measures consist of scrotal support, ice pack, and analgesic medications. Warm sitz baths for edema may also be helpful. Instruct the patient to call the physician if bleeding or elevated temperature occurs.

Semen Analysis

Semen analysis can be performed to substantiate the effectiveness of a vasectomy, to detect semen on the body or clothing of a suspected rape victim, and to rule out or determine paternity. The procedure is generally one of the first tests performed on men to evaluate fertility. Semen can be collected for testing by manual stimulation, coitus interruptus, or the use of a condom.

Prostatic Smears

Prostatic smears are obtained to detect and identify microorganisms, tumor cells, and even tuberculosis in the prostate. The physician massages the prostate by way of the rectum, and the patient voids into a sterile container prepared with additive preservative. The specimen is collected and a smear is prepared in the laboratory.

Cystoscopy

In **cystoscopy** a man's prostate and bladder can be examined by passing a lighted cystoscope through the urethra to the bladder. Before the procedure, obtain a signed consent form and educate the patient concerning the procedure. The procedure is usually performed without anesthesia, but a local anesthetic may be instilled into the bladder. After the cystoscopy the patient may have pink-tinged urine and frequency and burning on urination. Provide comfort by warm sitz baths, heat, and a mild analgesic (Lewis et al., 2007). Cystoscopy can be done for both men and women to detect bladder infections and tumors.

Other Diagnostic Studies

Other diagnostic studies for men include the rectal digital examination and the **prostate-specific antigen** (PSA), a highly sensitive blood test. PSA, which is normally secreted and disposed of by the prostate, shows up in the bloodstream in cancer of the prostate and in a harmless condition called **benign prostatic hyperplasia** or **prostate enlargement.** The normal PSA is less than 4 ng/mL. Elevated PSA levels in the bloodstream mean something needs to be checked. Even a slight increase in PSA level needs to be closely monitored; referral to a urologist for a biopsy is recommended. Still another study is the alkaline phosphatase (ALP) test. The normal ALP is 35 to 142 units/L for men, and 25 to 125 units/L for women. These specific tests are useful in diagnosing benign prostatic hypertrophy, prostatic cancer, bone metastasis in prostatic cancer, and other disease conditions (Box 12-4).

Box 12-4	Nursing Interventions for the Patient Undergoing Diagnostic Studies

- Explain the examination carefully.
- Provide privacy.
- Obtain a signed consent when necessary.
- Prepare the skin for surgery according to agency protocol.
- Assess the patient for allergies.
- If appropriate, request that the patient partially or completely disrobe and remove all jewelry. Provide gown or drape.
- Give preexamination instructions; instruct the patient to avoid food or drink, if appropriate.
- Encourage verbalization and discussion of fears.
- Administer preexamination medication as ordered by the physician.
- If necessary, advise patients to go without medications for 24 hours. Obtain a medication history.
- If the specimen is to be collected at home, stress the importance of handling all specimens precisely as directed.
- It may be necessary to monitor vital signs.
- Be attentive during examination. Offer support as necessary.

- If appropriate, relay any immediate concerns to the physician.
- Guide patients to follow any postexamination instructions.
- Inform the patient that some discomfort can be expected. Minor discomfort can be relieved by mild analgesics such as aspirin or acetaminophen, but if pain becomes more intense, notify the physician. Most discomfort is temporary.
- When pertinent, tell the patient to rest and to avoid any heavy lifting for 24 hours after the examination as directed by the physician.
- If relevant, advise the patient to avoid douching or intercourse until the site is healed. Consult the physician.
- Caution the patient to report any bleeding from an incisional area.
- Advise the patient to avoid the use of tampons as directed by the physician.
- Tell the patient how to obtain test results.

Health Promotion

Health Teaching for Menstruation

- Knowledge of the physiologic process
- Factors that may alter the menstrual cycle: stress, fatigue, exercise, acute or chronic illness, changes in climate or working hours, and pregnancy
- Personal hygiene
  —Wear pads during early period of heavy flow.
  —Change tampons frequently to decrease risk of toxic shock syndrome.
  —Consult physician if tampons cause discomfort.
  —Take a daily shower for comfort; warm baths may relieve slight pelvic discomfort.
  —Keep perineal area clean and dry; cleanse from anterior to posterior.
  —Wear cotton underwear; remember that nylon pantyhose and tight-fitting slacks retain moisture and should not be worn for extended periods.
  —Feminine hygiene products, such as vaginal sprays and suppositories, may contribute to a feeling of cleanliness.

  —A daily douche is not recommended because it changes the protective bacterial flora of the vagina and predisposes the woman to infection.
- Exercise
  —Exercise is not contraindicated and may help prevent discomfort.
  —Modify exercise if fatigue occurs.
- Diet
  —Restrict salt intake if fluid retention is present.
  —Consult a physician if fluid retention persists after menstruation.
- Discomfort
  —For mild discomfort, take aspirin, acetaminophen (Tylenol), or ibuprofen (Motrin); apply warmth; and rest.
  —For prolonged, severe discomfort, consult a physician.

THE REPRODUCTIVE CYCLE

Menarche

Menarche, the beginning of menses, designates the first menstrual cycle. Menarche occurs in late puberty and indicates that the body is capable of supporting pregnancy. Menarche occurs 2 to 2½ years after breast development (Hockenberry & Wilson, 2007), usually about 9 to 17 years of age, the average age being 12½ years. The menstrual cycle length varies from 24 to 32 days; the average cycle lasts 28 days. The flow lasts from 1 to 8 days; the average is 3 to 5 days. The amount of flow is from 10 to 75 mL; the average is 35 mL per cycle.

Help patients maintain their reproductive and sexual health by instructing or counseling women about personal hygiene. Personal cleanliness is a health habit that should be promoted for all patients and

implemented in each care plan. Cleanliness is especially important during menstruation (see Health Promotion box).

DISTURBANCES OF MENSTRUATION

Because of the relationship between the menstrual cycle and the body's mechanisms of hormonal secretion, a decrease or increase in the activity of the hormonal glands can disturb menstruation. The most common disturbances include the following:

- **Amenorrhea:** absence of menstrual flow
- **Dysmenorrhea:** painful menstruation
- **Abnormal uterine bleeding**
- **Menorrhagia:** excessive bleeding in amount and duration
- **Metrorrhagia:** bleeding between menstrual periods

Another disturbance of the menstrual cycle is premenstrual syndrome (PMS), which is discussed later.

Suggested nursing diagnoses are *anxiety, ineffective coping, fear, pain, deficient knowledge,* and *low self-esteem.* Nursing interventions are based on specific behaviors, symptoms, and treatments.

AMENORRHEA

Amenorrhea (absence of menstrual flow) is normal before puberty, after menopause, during pregnancy, and sometimes during lactation. Menstrual flow may also be absent or suppressed as a result of hormonal abnormalities or surgical interventions such as a hysterectomy (surgical removal of the uterus).

Etiology and Pathophysiology

Amenorrhea is classified as primary when menarche has not occurred by the age of 17 to 18 years. The cause may be a congenital defect. Secondary amenorrhea means menarche has occurred but flow has ceased for at least 3 months or there has been an absence of vaginal fluid for 12 months, coupled with a history of irregular bleeding. Secondary amenorrhea may be due to normal pregnancy; frequent, vigorous exercise, as in female athletes; or an emotional disorder such as depression, anorexia (lack of appetite), or bulimia (an insatiable craving for food, often resulting in episodes of continuous eating followed by purging).

Assessment

Early diagnosis and prompt management are necessary to prevent more serious reproductive and genital problems. Urge the sexually active woman to see a physician as soon as a menstrual period is missed. Maintaining health during pregnancy is vital for both the mother and the fetus. Women who suspect their amenorrhea is caused by menopause can be examined by a physician to confirm this.

Obtaining a family history is important. Assess emotional factors or behaviors that may influence the menstrual cycle. A menstrual history includes (1) the number of periods missed and (2) whether amenorrhea was previously present. Determine recent use of medications and drugs.

Diagnostic Tests

Beyond the preliminary workup and when pregnancy is not a possibility, the diagnostic study for primary and secondary amenorrhea is the same. This study includes a pelvic examination; blood, urine, and hormonal analysis; determination of existing tumors; and a Pap test.

Medical Management

Treatment is based on the underlying cause and must be determined on an individual basis. Hormonal therapy may be needed.

Nursing Interventions and Patient Teaching

A nursing diagnosis and interventions for women with amenorrhea include but are not limited to the following:

Nursing Diagnosis	Nursing Interventions
Ineffective coping, related to lack of menstrual flow	Acknowledge patient's feelings and provide emotional support. Refer to counseling as necessary. Explain diagnostic procedures. Provide information, privacy, and consultation as indicated for sexual concerns.

Encourage patients to comply with treatment, and emphasize the importance of follow-up visits with the physician for treatment, therapy, and evaluation of treatment efficacy.

DYSMENORRHEA

Dysmenorrhea is uterine pain with menstruation, commonly called "menstrual cramps." Primary dysmenorrhea that is not associated with pelvic disorders usually develops when ovulatory function is established (less than 20 years of age) and there is no underlying organic disease. Often it disappears or declines after pregnancy or by a woman's late 20s. Secondary dysmenorrhea is painful menstruation caused by organic disease such as PID or endometriosis and most often occurs in women older than 20 years of age.

Dysmenorrhea is the greatest single cause of absenteeism among women. It is one of the most common health problems for which women seek treatment.

Etiology and Pathophysiology

The causes of dysmenorrhea can be related to endocrine imbalance; an increase in prostaglandin secretions; or chronic illnesses, fatigue, and anemia. A recent theory proposes that dysmenorrhea may be caused by hypercontractility of the uterus resulting from higher-than-normal levels of prostaglandins. Conditions that cause general debilitation, such as inadequate diet and exercise, anemia, and fatigue, are often related to dysmenorrhea.

Assessment

Many women have systemic symptoms of breast tenderness, abdominal distention, nausea and vomiting, headache, vertigo, palpitations, and excessive perspiration. Assess the woman for colicky and cyclic pain and, infrequently, dull pain in the lower pelvis that radiates toward the perineum and back. This pain may be experienced 24 to 48 hours before menses or at the onset of menses. The family history is important, since dysmenorrhea has been reported to be significantly more common among mothers and sisters of women with dysmenorrhea. Secondary dysmenorrhea is suspected if the symptoms begin after 20 years of age. It has been described as a steady or cramping pain and may be specific to the site of pelvic disorder.

Diagnostic Tests

Diagnostic studies to rule out organic causes for dysmenorrhea include pelvic examination, laparoscopy, D&C, and hysterosalpingography.

Medical Management

Treatment of secondary dysmenorrhea is aimed at the cause. Surgical and medication intervention may be appropriate, depending on the severity and underlying causes of dysmenorrhea.

If no organic cause is found, instruct the woman to exercise and eat nutritious foods, especially those high in fiber, to avoid constipation. Local applications of heat and mild analgesics are prescribed. Medications for dysmenorrhea include prostaglandin inhibitors, such as ibuprofen (Motrin, Advil) and naproxen sodium (Anaprox). Oral contraceptives may be used to suppress ovulation by inhibiting prostaglandin levels (Table 12-2).

Nursing Interventions and Patient Teaching

Nursing diagnoses and interventions for women with dysmenorrhea include but are not limited to the following:

Nursing Diagnoses	Nursing Interventions
Deficient knowledge, related to lack of education concerning disease process and treatment	Present information on disease process, procedures to be performed, medications, and treatments. Prepare for informational question-and-answer sessions according to patient needs. Teach procedures patient must know how to perform. Obtain feedback. Be certain learning has taken place; reinforce teaching as needed. Develop a trusting relationship. Involve patient in care.
Pain, related to biologic agent	Assess nature of pain. Observe nonverbal cues. Encourage pain reduction techniques as appropriate.

Nursing Diagnoses	Nursing Interventions
	Explore best method for controlling pain (medication, positioning, comfort measures such as back rub or use of heat or cold). Monitor vital signs. Provide quiet environment, calm activities. Promote wellness; discuss with significant other ways in which he or she can assist patient.

Encourage a positive attitude and instruct women to maintain good posture, exercise, and practice good nutrition.

ABNORMAL UTERINE BLEEDING (MENORRHAGIA AND METRORRHAGIA)

Abnormal uterine bleeding may take many forms, including menorrhagia and metrorrhagia.

Menorrhagia is excessive bleeding at the time of the regular menstrual flow. The excessive bleeding can be characterized as an increased duration (more than 7 days), increased amount (more than 80 mL), or both. In younger women it may be attributed to endocrine disturbances, but in older women it usually indicates inflammatory disturbances or uterine tumors. Uterine fibroids (also called leiomyomas) and endometrial polyps are common causes of menorrhagia in women in their 30s and 40s. Emotional or psychological problems may also affect uterine bleeding. The severity of menorrhagia is usually estimated in terms of the number of pads or tampons used in excess of those used for regular menstrual flow.

Metrorrhagia is the appearance of uterine bleeding between regular menstrual periods or after menopause. It merits early diagnosis and treatment because it may indicate cancer or benign tumors of the uterus. Endometrial cancer must be considered for postmenopausal women experiencing spotting.

Diagnosis is made through a routine speculum and pelvic examination. Endometrial biopsy and ultrasonography are also used to diagnose gynecologic causes of menorrhagia and metrorrhagia. Endometrial ablation done by laser or electrosurgical technique has been successful with many patients with menorrhagia.

Nursing interventions include (1) assess for bleeding, pain, vaginal secretions, and psychosocial concerns; (2) encourage the woman to express her feelings; (3) explain the importance of recording dates, type of flow, and number of sanitary pads or tampons used; (4) teach the patient pain-relieving techniques; and (5) explain to the patient the importance of sharing her concerns with her partner.

Table 12-2   Medications for Reproductive Disorders

Generic (Trade)	Action	Side Effects	Nursing Implications
Oral contraceptives: estrogen-progesterone combinations (Ortho Novum, Norlestrin, Ovral, Triphasil)	Inhibits ovulation by suppressing gonadotropins, FSH and LH; alters genital tract to inhibit sperm penetration and inhibit implantation	Nausea, cramps, diarrhea, appetite change, acne, rash, increased BP, thrombophlebitis, edema, dysmenorrhea, bleeding irregularities, depression, fatigue, breast changes, cholestatic jaundice, optic neuritis	Monitor glucose, thyroid function, and liver function tests; check Homans' sign for clot detection; monitor BP; discontinue if patient is pregnant.
Conjugated equine estrogen (Premarin)	Needed for proper functioning of female reproductive systems; affects release of gonadotropins; inhibits ovulation; is involved in adequate calcium use in bone structure	Nausea, peripheral edema, enlargement of breasts, breast tenderness, anorexia, vomiting, diarrhea, headache, thrombophlebitis, dizziness, depression	Notify physician of weight gain of ≥5 lb/wk (patient may need diuretic); monitor BP; check liver function test; check Homans' sign for possible clots; give IV product slowly to prevent flushing.
Butoconazole (Femstat Cream)	Same as clotrimazole	Same as terconazole	Same as clotrimazole.
Clotrimazole (Mycelex-7m, Gyne-Lotrimin, Femcare)	Interferes with fungal DNA replication; binds sterols in fungal cell membrane	Rash, urticaria, stinging, burning, peeling, blistering skin fissures, abdominal cramps, bloating, urinary frequency	Watch for allergic reactions; note therapeutic response (decrease in size and number of lesions); use gloves for application; can be used through menstrual cycle; avoid use of other vaginal creams or suppositories during therapy.
Miconazole nitrate (Monistat-3, Monistat-7)	Same as clotrimazole	Vulvovaginal burning, itching, pelvic cramps, rash, urticaria, stinging, burning, contact dermatitis	Same as clotrimazole.
Tioconazole ointment (Vagistat-1)	Same as miconazole but two to eight times more potent	Vulvovaginal burning, itching, soreness, swelling	Same as clotrimazole.
Metronidazole (Flagyl, Protostat)	Direct-acting amebicide-trichomonacide; binds, degrades DNA in organism	Rash, headache, dizziness, fatigue, convulsions, blurred vision, nausea, vomiting, diarrhea, pseudomembranous colitis, albuminuria, neurotoxicity, metallic taste, disulfiram type of reaction with alcohol	Watch for allergic reactions and superinfection; check stool for parasites; give oral form with food; watch for vision problems; tell patient not to drink alcohol during therapy.
Nystatin (Mycostatin)	Same as clotrimazole	Rash, urticaria, stinging, burning	Same as clotrimazole.
Terconazole (Terazol-7, Terazol-3)	Same as clotrimazole	Vulvovaginal burning, itching, pelvic cramps, rash, urticaria, stinging, burning	Same as clotrimazole.
Topical Nystatin (Nilstat, Mycostatin, Bio-Statin)	Interferes with fungal DNA replication; causes fungal cell membrane permeability	Rash, stinging, burning, urticaria, nausea, vomiting, anorexia, diarrhea	Watch for allergic reaction; use gloves for topical application; for vaginal preparation, tell patient that she may need protective perineal pads.

BP, Blood pressure; *DNA,* deoxyribonucleic acid; *FSH,* follicle-stimulating hormone; *IV,* intravenous; *LH,* luteinizing hormone.   *Continued*

💊 **Table 12-2** Medications for Reproductive Disorders—cont'd

Generic (Trade)	Action	Side Effects	Nursing Implications
Topical amphotericin B (Fungizone cream, lotion, ointment)	Binds to ergosterol, altering cell membrane permeability in susceptible fungi	Urticaria, stinging, burning, dry skin, pruritus, contact dermatitis, staining of nail lesions	Cover lesions completely after cleansing and drying well; use gloves to prevent further infection; watch for allergic reactions; tell patient that it may discolor skin and clothing.
Medroxyprogesterone acetate (Provera, Amen, Cycrin, Depo-Provera)	Inhibits secretion of pituitary gonadotropins, which acts to prevent follicular maturation and ovulation; stimulates growth in mammary tissue	Irregular bleeding, breast tenderness, masculinization of fetus, edema, cholestatic jaundice, thrombophlebitis, anorexia, acne, mental depression, weight gain or loss	Notify physician of weight gain of ≥5 lb/wk; monitor BP at beginning of treatment and periodically thereafter; check liver function test; discontinue if patient is pregnant.
Estradiol transdermal system (Estraderm)	Same as conjugated equine estrogen	Same as conjugated equine estrogen	Same as conjugated equine estrogen.
Testosterone cypionate (Andro-Cyp)	Increases weight by building body tissue; increases potassium, phosphorus, chloride, and nitrogen levels; increases bone development	Acne, flushing, gynecomastia, edema, hypercalcemia, nausea, cholestatic hepatitis, aggressive behavior, headache, anxiety, mental depression, androgenic and anabolic activity	Check weight daily; monitor BP; monitor growth rate in children; check electrolyte (potassium-sodium, chloride, calcium) and cholesterol levels; monitor liver function test.
Danazol (Danocrine)	Synthetic androgen, causes atrophy of endometrial tissue; decreases FSH and LH, which leads to amenorrhea and anovulation	Fluid retention, virilization, androgenic effects, weight gain, amenorrhea, dizziness, headache, rashes, hepatic impairment	Check weight; monitor I&O; check for edema; give with food or milk to decrease gastrointestinal upset.
Acyclovir ointment (Zovirax)	Antiviral agent, interferes with DNA synthesis needed for viral replication	Mild pain with transient burning; stinging, pruritus, rash, vulvitis	Apply ointment q 3 hr or six times daily around the clock; cover all lesions; use gloves for self-protection when applying.

I&O, intake and output.

Women of all ages need to be educated about the importance of follow-up care when abnormal uterine bleeding is initially detected.

PREMENSTRUAL SYNDROME

PMS occurs in 30% to 50% of women between 25 and 45 years of age. It differs from dysmenorrhea because it has no relation to ovulation.

Etiology and Pathophysiology

The etiology and pathophysiology are not well understood. PMS is believed to be related to the neuroendocrine events occurring within the anterior pituitary gland. A loss of intravascular fluid into the body tissues causes water retention, bloating, and weight gain. PMS is thought to have a biologic trigger with compounding psychosocial issues. Some women have a genetic predisposition to PMS. Other proposed causes of PMS include estrogen and progesterone imbalances and nutritional deficiencies of

pyridoxine (vitamin B₆) or magnesium. **Premenstrual dysphoric disorder** (PMD-D) is the term applied to a type of PMS that includes a severe mood disorder.

PMS occurs 7 to 10 days before the menstrual period and usually subsides within the first 3 days after the onset of the menstrual flow. Evaluate sodium intake and the use of alcohol, tobacco, and caffeine as possible causes.

Clinical Manifestations

Symptoms are multiple and vary among individuals. Behavioral symptoms include anxiety, mood swings, irritability, lethargy (inactivity), fatigue, sleep disturbances, and depression. Physical symptoms—such as headache, vertigo, backache, breast tenderness, abdominal distention, acne, paresthesia (burning or tingling) of hands and feet, and allergies—appear or may become worse. Many symptoms appear alone or in combination with other symptoms. Some women accept the symptoms as being normal and only seek medical help after the symptoms become severe.

Assessment

Subjective data are specific symptoms experienced by each woman. Ask each patient to maintain a log for three consecutive menstrual cycles and to note symptoms and activities that relate to the menstrual period. The collected information can be analyzed and symptoms treated accordingly.

Objective data pertinent to the syndrome include the inability to perform activities of daily living (ADLs) in the multiple roles of a wife, a mother, and a career person.

Diagnostic Tests

PMS is diagnosed only after eliminating other possible causes for the symptoms. A focused health history and a physical examination are done to identify any underlying conditions, such as thyroid dysfunction, uterine fibroids, or depression, that may account for the symptoms. No definitive diagnostic test is available for PMS. When PMS or PMD-D is a possible diagnosis, a woman keeps a record of her symptoms for two or three menstrual cycles (Lewis et al., 2007). Tests include evaluation of estrogen and progesterone levels to rule out hormonal imbalances and determination of glucose levels; low levels may lead to irritability.

Medical Management

PMS has no single treatment and no specific medication. Some physicians prescribe analgesics, diuretics, and progesterone. Review the patient's diet. The patient should eat a diet high in complex carbohydrates, moderate in protein, and low in refined sugar and sodium, especially during the premenstrual interval. Supplements of vitamin B$_6$, calcium, and magnesium may be administered as prescribed. She should reduce or eliminate caffeine (in chocolate, tea, coffee, or other beverages), and alcohol and smoking. Encourage regular exercise three or four times a week for 30 minutes, especially during the premenstrual interval. Exercise results in release of endorphins, leading to mood elevation. Techniques for stress reduction include yoga, meditation, imagery, and biofeedback training. Because fatigue may exaggerate PMS symptoms, adequate rest, sleep, and relaxation are helpful. For reducing cramping pain, backache, and headache, prostaglandin inhibitors such as ibuprofen are used. For anxiety, buspirone (BuSpar) taken during the luteal phase of the menstrual cycle has helped some women. Women with PMD-D may benefit from antidepressants, including fluoxetine (Prozac, Sarafem) and tricyclic antidepressants such as amitriptyline (Elavil). Selective serotonin reuptake inhibitors (SSRIs) such as sertraline (Zoloft) have provided significant relief to women with severe PMS (Lewis et al., 2007).

Nursing Interventions and Patient Teaching

A nursing diagnosis and interventions for the woman with PMS include but are not limited to the following:

Nursing Diagnosis	Nursing Interventions
Anxiety, related to PMS	Encourage verbalization of feelings. Acknowledge existence of syndrome and its symptoms. Encourage patient to keep a menstrual symptom diary to document the cycle and nature of the symptoms. Encourage patient to plan activities during the symptom-free part of her cycle. Administer supplements of vitamin B$_6$, calcium, and magnesium as prescribed. Encourage attending self-help groups and reading self-help literature; group support tends to reduce stress. Provide emotional support in a nonjudgmental and caring manner. Assist in identifying possible sources of anxiety and coping mechanisms.

The patient should take responsibility for following a dietary plan of eating small meals and restricting or eliminating sugar, alcohol, caffeine, and nicotine; this may minimize the symptoms of PMS or PMD-D.

MENOPAUSE

The **climacteric** is the phase of the aging process of women and men who are making a transition from a reproductive phase to a nonreproductive stage of life. This phase occurs in middle adulthood and marks the onset of physical changes, a decrease in hormone secretion, and the cessation of ovulation and menses. The female climacteric is called **menopause**. Menopause is the normal cessation of menses; menstrual flow appears on an infrequent cycle for a time, usually less than 2 years. However, as long as the menstrual cycle occurs, no matter how infrequently, ovulation continues and the potential for conception exists.

Etiology and Pathophysiology

Menopause is the normal decline of ovarian function resulting from the aging process. Menopause begins in most women between 42 and 58 years of age (the average age being 51) and is characterized by infrequent ovulation, decreased menstrual function, and eventual cessation of the menstrual flow. Factors that have been linked to an earlier age at menopause include higher body mass index; cigarette smoking; and racial, ethnic, and socioeconomic factors (Santoro & Chervenak, 2004). Menopause is a milestone in a woman's life that is embedded in her own personality and her culture (Santoro & Chervenak, 2004).

Menopause may be artificially induced by such procedures as irradiation of the ovaries or surgical removal of both ovaries. Both cause menopause with all its physiologic changes, whereas ovaries left intact after a hysterectomy continue to function provided the woman has not yet reached the age of the climacteric. Menopause also may occur earlier due to illness, side effects of chemotherapy, or drugs.

Decline in ovarian function produces a variety of symptoms, including a decrease in the frequency, amount, and duration of the menstrual flow; spotting; amenorrhea; and **polymenorrhea** (increased number of menstrual periods). Symptoms can last from a few months to several years before menstruation ceases permanently. Menopause is not considered complete until 1 year after the last menstrual period.

Clinical Manifestations

Physical changes that occur in the body do not generally develop until after permanent cessation of menstruation. Changes of the reproductive system include shrinkage of vulval structures, atrophic vulvitis, shortening of the vagina, and dryness of the vaginal wall. A relaxation of supporting pelvic structures results from the decrease in estrogen. Cystitis and urinary frequency and urgency may appear as a result of changes in the urinary system. There is loss of skin turgor and elasticity; increased subcutaneous fat; decreased breast tissue; and thinning of hair of the axilla, the head, and the pubis. About 25% of postmenopausal women develop osteoporosis.

Assessment

Subjective data include a family history. Determine whether family members and significant others are aware of the transition and whether they are supportive. Note emotional illness, if present. Hot flashes caused by glandular imbalances may become prominent. Other symptoms may include fatigue, vertigo, headache, nausea, **dyspareunia** (painful intercourse), palpitations, and chest and neck pain. Some experience a feeling of being unwanted, and some may fear growing old; both feelings could cause depression.

Collection of **objective data** includes an awareness that some patients may display frequent crying spells or outbursts of anger. Explore the use of contraceptives. Assess frequency, amount, and duration of the menstrual flow. Diaphoresis, weight gain, vomiting, and tachycardia may occur.

Diagnostic Tests

Tests include analysis of hormonal levels. Other diagnostic testing may be indicated by specific symptoms. Some examinations are performed to rule out conditions such as cancer.

Medical Management

The status of hormone replacement therapy (HRT) for postmenopausal women has undergone a radical reversal in the past several years. The Women's Health Initiative (WHI), sponsored by the National Institutes of Health, has conducted extensive research on the effects of HRT on women's health. The findings demonstrated that long-term use of an HRT estrogen-progestin combination heightened the risk of ischemic stroke, coronary heart disease, breast cancer that is at a more advanced stage at the time of diagnosis (Chlebowski et al., 2003), ovarian cancer, and thromboembolism. In 2003 further analysis of WHI data found hormone use to increase the risk of cognitive decline in a small percentage of those who receive it (Yeh, 2007).

As a result of these studies, the American Congress of Obstetricians and Gynecologists, the National Institutes of Health (the study's sponsor), and the FDA recommend that women take the lowest effective dose of HRT for the shortest possible time to relieve menopausal symptoms (Akert, 2003).

Nurses are in a good position to apprise their patients of the benefits, risks, and appropriate uses of HRT. HRT is used for short-term treatment of moderate to severe symptoms of menopause, such as hot flashes, night sweats, and vaginal dryness. At present, there are no data that might indicate how long HRT can be taken without the risk of cardiovascular or other adverse effects, and it is not known whether lower dosages lessen the risk of complications. In women with moderate to severe menopausal symptoms, it is assumed that risk can be minimized by providing HRT therapy only until the severe symptoms disappear and using the lowest effective dosage. Low-dose alternatives in HRT include low-dose Prempro, containing either 0.45 mg conjugated estrogens and 1.5 mg medroxyprogesterone, or 0.3 mg conjugated estrogens and 1.5 mg medroxyprogesterone; or low-dose intravaginal estrogen products, such as estrogen topical vaginal cream (Premarin vaginal cream or Estrace) and low-dose vaginal rings. Because of the later diagnosis of breast cancer and colon cancer in women receiving combination HRT, closely scrutinize any abnormal mammogram and screen for colon cancer as part of the follow-up.

Most physicians recommend calcium and vitamin D supplements, which are available in many forms; the generic calcium carbonate products are the most cost effective.

Herbs such as soy or black cohash are used to decrease menopausal symptoms. Patients should consult their health care provider before taking these products (Ulbricht & Basch, 2005).

SSRIs, including the antidepressants paroxetine (Paxil), fluoxetine, and venlafaxine (Effexor), are an effective alternative to HRT in reducing hot flashes, even if the user is not depressed. Also known to relieve hot flashes are clonidine (Catapres), an antihypertensive drug, and gabapentin (Neurontin), an antiseizure drug (Lewis et al., 2007).

Nonhormonal Therapy

To relieve menopausal symptoms without the risks of HRT, several methods to decrease heat produced by the body and promote heat loss have been recommended. Reducing intake of caffeine and alcohol lowers the production of body heat. Suggestions to promote heat loss at night when hot flashes interfere with sleep include increasing air circulation, using light covers and loose-fitting clothing, and placing cool cloths on flushed areas. The daily use of 800 international units of vitamin E has been recommended to reduce hot flashes (Lewis et al., 2007).

Nursing Interventions and Patient Teaching

Education regarding menopause should occur before its onset. Many women appreciate opportunities to discuss menopause. Set up an exercise program that includes both movement and weight bearing to slow bone loss and modify coronary artery disease risk factors (Lewis et al., 2007). Walking is an excellent weight-bearing exercise. Other exercises include bicycling, stationary cycling, and aerobic dancing three or four times per week.

Nursing diagnoses and interventions for the menopausal patient include but are not limited to the following:

Nursing Diagnoses	Nursing Interventions
Situational low self-esteem, related to concerns about femininity, sexuality, and aging	Encourage patient and significant others to verbalize concerns.
	Confirm accurate information.
	Correct information related to self-concept issues.
	Avoid value judgments.
	Refer patient to couple, family, and sex therapy as appropriate.
	Provide understanding and support.
Deficient knowledge, regarding patient's physiologic and psychological changes, related to menopause	Explain the process of climacteric and menopause, at a level the patient can understand.

Nursing Diagnoses	Nursing Interventions
	Explain importance of keeping fit, eating a well-balanced diet, getting adequate rest and sleep, avoiding stress and fatigue, and continuing contraception until indicated by physician.
	If estrogen replacement therapy is ordered, inform patient about side effects.
	Instruct patient to report any vaginal bleeding occurring 6 months or more after last menstrual period.
	Inform patient of the availability of water-soluble lubricants if needed before coitus.

For patient teaching, emphasize that the climacteric is normal and self-limiting and that menopause is not the end of the patient's sex life. A nutritious diet and weight control will improve physical condition, and an exercise program will promote vitality. Interest and participation in various activities help decrease anxiety and tension. Skin creams and lotions can be used to prevent drying, pruritus, and cracking skin. Encourage the woman to perform breast self-examination (BSE) monthly and monitor calcium intake. Contraceptives should be used for 1 year after the last menstrual period. The patient can obtain a prescription for treatment of pruritus or burning of the vulva. Women can practice Kegel exercises regularly to strengthen pelvic muscles (see Health Promotion box). A water-soluble lubricant, such as KY Jelly, can be used to prevent dyspareunia. Explain the side effects of any medications or hormonal therapy. Emphasize that an annual physical examination is important for maintaining good health.

MALE CLIMACTERIC

Etiology and Pathophysiology

The climacteric is less pronounced in men and often may not even be apparent. The appearance of the climacteric phase is gradual and occurs between 55 and

---

🏃 Health Promotion

Kegel Exercises

Kegel exercises are performed to help strengthen and tighten muscles that support the pelvic organs. These muscles (pelvic floor) are used to stop the flow of urine. To perform Kegel exercises while standing or sitting, tighten the pelvic floor muscles as hard as you can. Hold for 5 seconds, then release. Repeat at least 10 times. This exercise can be done as many as 40 to 50 times each day.

70 years of age. There is a gradual decrease of testosterone levels and seminal fluid production. The impact is largely psychological, possibly because of the recognition of some reduction of sexual activity and interests.

Clinical Manifestations

Manifestations are mostly physiologic changes. Erections require more time and are not as full or firm. The prostate gland enlarges, and secretions diminish; seminal fluid decreases. The physical changes occur as the man grows older, and the most noticeable signs are loss or thinning of hair from the head, chest, axillae, and pubis. There may be some flushing and chilling. Muscle tone is decreased.

Assessment

Collection of **subjective data** reveals that the man is generally at the peak of his career or possibly considering retirement. He interprets his decreased sexual needs as a loss of productivity and sexual power. Therefore the assessment should invite verbalization of emotions with coping mechanisms.

Collection of **objective data** includes assessment of behaviors that may be causing the man stress and concern. Ask him to explore changes he has noted regarding his lifestyle and feelings of loss of self-worth.

Diagnostic Tests

Diagnostic tests include a complete physical examination to rule out abnormalities of structure and function.

Nursing Interventions and Patient Teaching

A nursing diagnosis and interventions for men experiencing male climacteric include but are not limited to the following:

Nursing Diagnosis	Nursing Interventions
Ineffective coping, related to situational crisis (climacteric)	Show understanding and concern.
	Assist patient in identifying how the problem affects his life and future, his family, and significant others.
	Encourage patient to talk about factors that could be influencing the way he sees the problem.
	Assist patient in identifying strengths and coping skills and the nature and strength of situational support.
	Collect data about current and potential sources of support.
	Assist patient in planning alternative solutions.
	Give positive reinforcement.

Inform the patient that the climacteric is normal. Encourage the patient to verbalize his fears and to seek counseling if stress increases.

ERECTILE DYSFUNCTION

Erectile dysfunction (ED) is a man's inability to attain or maintain an erect penis that allows satisfactory sexual performance. Several forms are recognized: (1) functional ED, which has a psychological basis; (2) anatomical ED, which results from a physical defect of genital structures; and (3) atonic ED, which involves disturbed neuromuscular function. Some neurologic abnormalities that affect erectile function are tabes dorsalis, caused by advanced syphilis; congenital spinal cord anomalies, such as spina bifida; spinal cord tumors; amyotrophic lateral sclerosis (Lou Gehrig's disease); multiple sclerosis; or cord compression caused by a herniated disk. Radical prostatectomy often leads to ED. Nerve-sparing surgery can decrease this occurrence.

ED can potentially interfere with a man's self-esteem, relationships, confidence, and sense of well-being. The prevalence alone makes ED a significant condition. About 20 million to 30 million men in the United States experience ED. ED may occur at any age; however, it is estimated that 50% of men between 40 and 70 years old have some degree of ED. ED in younger men is often a result of substance abuse, including alcohol or recreational drugs. Medical conditions that are associated with ED are diabetes mellitus, hypertension, renal disorders, cancer, coronary artery bypass surgery, and organ transplants. Men have a longer life expectancy than in past generations and expect to remain sexually active (Lewis et al., 2007). The nurse can best understand ED by developing a broad understanding of the factors that contribute to the condition.

Medical Management

Medical treatment is based on careful assessment of the causative factors. It is known that medications such as antihypertensives, antidepressants, antihyperlipidemics, diuretics, drugs for Parkinson's disease, marijuana, cocaine, antianxiety agents, and some cardiac agents may cause ED. Illicit or abused substances such as alcohol, cocaine, and nicotine are also known to cause ED. Disease conditions, such as diabetes mellitus or end-stage renal, heart, and chronic obstructive pulmonary disease, may also be causative factors.

A drug named sildenafil citrate (Viagra) is prescribed as an oral therapy for ED. The physiologic mechanism of erection of the penis involves release of nitric oxide in the corpus cavernosum during sexual stimulation. The drug enhances smooth muscle relaxation and the inflow of blood in the corpus cavernosum, thus allowing erection to occur. For most patients, the recommended dosage is 50 mg taken as needed approximately 1 hour before engaging in sexual activity. However, sildenafil may be taken anywhere from a half hour to 4 hours before sexual activity. Sildenafil has been shown to potentiate the hypotensive effects of nitrates; therefore its administration to patients who are using nitrates (either regularly or intermittently) in any form is contraindicated. Tadalafil (Cialis) is another antiimpotence agent for ED contraindicated for concurrent use with nitrates, nitric oxide, or alpha-adrenergic blockers. It should not be used in patients who have unstable angina, recent history of stroke, life-threatening heart failure, uncontrolled hypertension, or myocardial infarction within 90 days. For most patients, the recommended dosage is 10 mg before sexual activity (range 5 to 20 mg; not to exceed one dose in 24 hours). A third antiimpotence agent is vardenafil (Levitra) 10 mg, taken 1 hour before sexual activity (range 5 to 20 mg, no more than once daily). This drug is not to be used with nitrates because of an unsafe decrease in blood pressure, which could result in myocardial infarction or stroke (Skidmore-Roth, 2010).

Mechanical devices are available for the patient with ED. Surgical implantation of a penile prosthesis may be performed as a same-day procedure or may require hospitalization for 5 or more days, depending on the patient and the device used (Figure 12-8).

Nursing Interventions and Patient Teaching

The nurse is responsible for teaching the patient to administer hormonal medication (testosterone) and to watch for side effects. Advise the patient to take oral hormonal replacement drugs with meals to prevent nausea. Inform the patient about signs and symptoms of infection of the implant, including tenderness of the penis, fever, dysuria, and signs of urinary tract infection. Tell the patient to seek medical attention promptly if infection occurs.

INFERTILITY

Etiology and Pathophysiology

Infertility is defined as the inability to conceive after 1 year of sexual intercourse without birth control measures. Primary infertility refers to couples who have never conceived. Secondary infertility refers to couples who have conceived but are now unable to do so.

A woman's age has a significant bearing on her ability to conceive. Women are most fertile between 20 and 29 years of age, whereas men are most fertile in their late teens and early 20s. A man's fertility does not decrease much as he grows older, but a woman's fertility drops dramatically and decreases with menopause.

Infertility may be caused by impaired sperm or ova production or an occlusion in the reproductive system that prevents the sperm and ovum from meeting. Infections of the reproductive tract (such as PID) and STIs (such as syphilis) are frequently associated with infertility. Because the man may be the infertile partner in 40% of the cases of infertility, the quality and quantity of his sperm must be analyzed. The primary causes of infertility in women are tubal insufficiency and ovarian and uterine conditions, such as endometriosis or congenital defects.

Assessment

Collection of **subjective** and **objective data** includes physical examination and health histories for both partners to make the infertility assessment and prepare a treatment plan.

Diagnostic Tests

Specific testing is necessary to rule out systemic diseases such as diabetes mellitus, neoplasms, hepatic and renal diseases, and viral conditions. Genetic defects and disorders of the testes are explored. Diagnostic testing can produce a great deal of anxiety and stress. This testing may continue for fairly long periods with or without favorable results. Male testing is somewhat simpler and usually less expensive than female testing. If there is reason to suspect the man is infertile or sterile, it is appropriate to test him first. Male infertility testing includes semen analysis, which measures the quantity and quality of semen, volume of sperm cells, sperm motility, and sperm density; and endocrine imbalance testing, which explores possible disruption of the pituitary gonadotropins and testosterone production.

Female testing focuses on the ovulation process and function of the reproductive organs. The testing in-

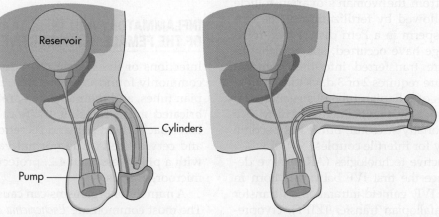

FIGURE 12-8 The Scott inflatable prosthesis has erect and flaccid positions designed to mimic normal erectile function.

cludes (1) basal body temperature to assess ovulation; (2) endometrial biopsy, which confirms ovulation and endometrial cyclic changes; (3) endocrine studies to assess the functioning of the adrenal and thyroid glands with anovulation cycles; (4) Rubin's insufflation test, which determines tubal patency; and (5) hysterosalpingography and hysterography to assess the position and alignment of the reproductive organs.

Male and female interaction studies include (1) Huhner's test, which examines the cervical mucus for motile sperm cells after intercourse, at midmenstrual cycle; (2) immunologic or immunoglobulin (antibody) testing for detection of spermicidal antibodies in the woman's sera; and (3) testing both the man and woman for normalcy of their sex chromosomes.

Medical Management

The management of infertility problems depends on the cause. If infertility is secondary to an alteration in ovarian function, supplemental hormone therapy may be attempted to restore and maintain ovulation. Drugs used to induce ovulation include clomiphene citrate (Clomid), and bromocriptine (Parlodel). These drugs increase the risk for multiple births. When an actual mechanical tubal blockage exists, a reparative microsurgical procedure can be done.

Poor cervical mucus may be a result of chronic cervicitis or inadequate estrogenic stimulation. Careful cauterization of the cervix may eradicate the chronic cervicitis, and the administration of estrogens can improve the quantity and quality of the cervical mucus.

Improving the patient's general health may help, especially when a debilitating or chronic illness is present. Eliminating or reducing psychological stress can improve the emotional climate, making it more conducive to achieving a pregnancy. Education of the couple regarding the probable time of ovulation and appropriate coital technique may also be indicated.

When a couple has not succeeded in conceiving even with infertility management, another option is intrauterine insemination with the partner's or a donor's sperm. If this technique does not succeed, **in vitro fertilization** (IVF) may be used. IVF is the removal of mature oocytes from the woman's ovarian follicle via laparoscopy, followed by fertilization of the ova with the partner's sperm in a Petri dish. When fertilization and cleavage have occurred, some of the resulting embryos are transferred into the woman's uterus. The procedure requires 2 or 3 days to complete and is used in cases of fallopian tube obstruction, decreased sperm count, and unexplained infertility. IVF is costly and emotionally stressful, but it has become an accepted therapy for infertile couples.

Assisted reproductive technologies (ARTs) have developed rapidly since the first IVF baby was born in 1978. ARTs include IVF, gamete intrafallopian transfer (GIFT), zygote intrafallopian transfer (ZIFT), cryopreserved embryo transfer (CPE), and donor oocyte programs. Current research could lead to a rapid expansion of these techniques in the next decade. With the increased knowledge of freezing techniques for embryos (CPE), couples will have increased pregnancy potential. Research is also investigating the replication of normal tubal secretions. This tubal factor is important because the pregnancy rate is higher with GIFT and ZIFT than with IVF. Finally, the development of embryo biopsy and genetic engineering may allow for preconception techniques for those couples with identified genetic abnormalities. It also raises the possibility of gender selection. Thus noncoital reproduction poses many ethical, legal, and social concerns. All decisions related to infertility are influenced by the couple's age, their wishes, and the length of time they have been attempting to conceive.

Nursing Interventions and Patient Teaching

The nurse has a major responsibility for teaching and providing emotional support throughout the infertility testing and treatment period. Feelings of anger, frustration, sadness, and helplessness between partners and between the couple and health care providers may increase as more tests are performed. Infertility can generate great tension in a marriage as the couple exhausts their financial and emotional resources. Few insurance carriers cover the cost of infertility testing or the therapeutic measures associated with infertility. Shame and guilt may arise when other people become involved in such an intimate area of a relationship.

Recognizing and dealing with the psychological and emotional factors that surface can assist the couple in coping with the situation. Encourage couples to participate in a support group for infertile couples and in individual therapy. Continue providing information and emotional support as therapeutic measures are attempted. Give couples ample opportunity to plan what is financially realistic; each GIFT and ZIFT attempt can exceed $10,000 and each IVF treatment costs $4500 to $6000.

Prognosis

Approximately 50% of couples who undergo assessment and treatment for infertility are likely to conceive.

INFLAMMATORY AND INFECTIOUS DISORDERS OF THE FEMALE REPRODUCTIVE TRACT

Infections of the female reproductive tract are most commonly found in the vagina, the cervix, the fallopian tubes, and their adjacent areas. The vagina is lubricated and protected by flora containing Döderlein's bacilli, acid pH, and secretions from the vaginal and cervical cells. The normal vaginal environment, with a pH of less than 4.2, protects against growth of microorganisms.

A number of organisms can cause vaginal infections. The most common are *Escherichia coli*, *Candida albicans*, and *Trichomonas vaginalis*. Infections are more likely to occur when the flora and the acidity of the vagina are disturbed by medications (birth control pills, antibiotics), stress, malnutrition, douching, aging, and disease. Yeast organisms grow best in an acid pH (−4.7), whereas *Trichomonas* and organisms causing nonspecific vaginitis flourish on a pH that is more alkaline (5+).

Organisms are often introduced from external sources by way of unclean douche nozzles, poor hygiene, inadequate handwashing, neglected nail care, soiled clothing, and intercourse. Vaginal infections can be sexually transmitted and will return unless both partners are treated. Predisposing factors include poor nutrition, inconsistent control of blood glucose levels in those with diabetes mellitus, stress, pregnancy, marked hormonal fluctuations, pH changes, and antibiotics (Lewis et al., 2007).

SIMPLE VAGINITIS

Etiology and Pathophysiology

Vaginitis is a common vaginal infection. It is usually caused by *E. coli,* an organism found in feces and the rectum. It may be caused by staphylococcal and streptococcal organisms, *T. vaginalis* (a flagellated protozoan), *C. albicans* (a yeastlike fungus), and *Gardnerella* bacillus.

Vaginitis is an inflammation of the vagina. If the patient changes perineal pads or tampons infrequently, the vaginal tract and inner groin become irritated. This creates a medium suitable for organism growth. Examination of the vaginal walls will show a profuse foamy (bubbly) exudate if the vaginitis is caused by *T. vaginalis.* If *C. albicans* is the causative agent, a thick, cheeselike discharge results. Bacterial vaginitis produces a malodorous milky discharge.

Clinical Manifestations

The exudate in vaginitis is yellow, white, or grayish white; curdlike; and generally accompanied by pruritus, burning, and edema of the surrounding tissue. Voiding and defecation generally intensify the symptoms.

Assessment

Subjective data include menstrual history, age at menarche, length of cycles, duration and nature of flow, dysfunctions, birth control methods, medications taken, family history of diabetes mellitus, previous vaginal infections, and STIs. Ask about sexual practices and signs of infection in the sex partner. Dysuria may occur as a consequence of local irritation of the urinary meatus.

Collection of **objective data** includes observation for excoriations of the skin caused by scratching, in which case secondary infection may result. Observe the specific type of exudate.

Diagnostic Tests

Diagnostic tests include direct visual examination of the vagina, culture of the organism, and bimanual examination to assess for inflammation of the vagina and its surrounding tissues.

Medical Management

Vaginal infection can be treated by a variety of methods. The major goals of treatment are to (1) cure the infection, (2) prevent reinfection, (3) prevent complications, and (4) prevent infection of the sexual partner(s). Douching is frequently prescribed for treatment, as are local applications of vaginal suppositories, ointments, and creams. Advise the patient to use the medication at bedtime and to remain recumbent for more than 30 minutes after insertion to allow absorption and prevent loss of any medication from the vagina. The patient may require oral medications appropriate to the organism. During treatment the patient should refrain from intercourse or request that her partner use a condom (see Table 12-2).

Nursing Interventions and Patient Teaching

Advise the patient of the importance of handwashing before and after vaginal application of medications. Heat may be applied in the form of douches, perineal irrigations, or sitz baths. Douching too frequently can alter normal vaginal flora. Discourage douching unless specifically prescribed by the health care provider.

Nursing diagnoses and interventions for the patient with vaginitis include but are not limited to the following:

Nursing Diagnoses	Nursing Interventions
Pain, related to vaginal discharge	Flush vagina with acid douche (15 mL white vinegar with 1000 mL water) as ordered. Apply antibiotic creams after douche as ordered. Provide sitz bath for edema.
Risk for infection, related to STIs	Administer medication and treatments as ordered. Teach preventive methods, such as use of condoms. Recommend that partner be checked for infection and treated as necessary to avoid reinfection.

Most patients with vaginal infections are directed to abstain from sexual intercourse during treatment. The male partner's use of a condom until the symptoms of infection disappear may be advised. Also inform the patient that her sexual partner should be treated.

Prognosis

With proper treatment, the prognosis is good.

SENILE VAGINITIS OR ATROPHIC VAGINITIS

This condition occurs in women after menopause and as they age. Low estrogen levels cause the vulva and vagina to atrophy and become susceptible to the invasion of bacteria. The exudate causes pruritus, edema, and skin irritations. Estrogen, vaginal suppositories, and ointments may be prescribed.

CERVICITIS

Cervicitis (infection of the cervix) is one of the most common diseases of the reproductive system. The infection is caused by vaginal infection or STIs, such as *Chlamydia trachomatis* infection, gonorrhea, herpes type 2, or trichomoniasis. The infection often follows childbirth or abortion in which lacerations occur. Therapy is specific to the causative organisms. Symptoms are backaches, whitish exudate, or pink-tinged menstrual discharge and dyspareunia. If cervicitis remains untreated, the tissues are continually irritated and the infection may spread to other pelvic organs. Personal hygiene and frequent warm tub baths can minimize odor and discomfort. Local applications of vaginal suppositories, ointments, and creams are usually prescribed. Drug therapy also includes azithromycin (Zithromax) 1 g orally as single dose or doxycycline (Vibramycin) 100 mg orally twice a day for 7 days; treat the partner with the same drugs (Lewis et al., 2007).

PELVIC INFLAMMATORY DISEASE

PID is any acute, subacute, recurrent, or chronic infection that may involve the cervix (cervicitis), uterus (endometritis), fallopian tubes (salpingitis), or ovaries (oophoritis) and may extend to the connective tissues lying between the broad ligaments.

Etiology and Pathophysiology

The most common causative organisms are *Neisseria gonorrhoeae*, streptococci, staphylococci, chlamydiae, and tubercle bacilli. PID can follow the insertion of a biopsy curette or an irrigation catheter, abortion, pelvic surgery, sexual intercourse, or pregnancy. The condition may occur with or without gonorrheal infection and may be mild or severe.

When conditions or procedures alter or destroy the cervical mucus, bacteria ascend into the uterine cavity. Pelvic examination and movement of the reproductive organs become painful. PID is serious because it may cause adhesions and sterility. Sexually active women with more than one partner are at increased risk for PID.

Clinical Manifestations

Signs and symptoms are temperature elevation, chills, severe abdominal pain, malaise, nausea and vomiting, and malodorous purulent vaginal exudate.

Assessment

Subjective data relate to the severity of the disorder, pain, time of onset, and frequency (primary infection or continuous reinfection). Sexual history, pelvic examinations, and pelvic procedures are important because they may reveal the origin of the pathogen. The patient may complain of lower abdominal and pelvic pain, dysmenorrhea, dysuria, and vulvar pruritus.

Objective data include the patient's knowledge, level of discomfort, and coping mechanisms. Assess the patient for fever and chills and the amount and characteristics of vaginal discharge. The vaginal discharge is purulent to thin and mucoid.

Diagnostic Tests

Diagnostic tests include Gram stains of secretions from the endocervix, urethra, and rectum. Culture and sensitivity testing identifies organisms and is helpful in selecting antibiotics for treatment. Laparoscopic visualization of the pelvic inflammation may be necessary to confirm the extent of infection. Vaginal ultrasonic examinations can aid in diagnosing abscesses and monitoring the treatment and healing process. The leukocyte count and erythrocyte sedimentation rate are elevated.

Medical Management

The goal of treatment is to control and eradicate the infection by preventing it from spreading to other body systems. Treatment includes systemic antibiotics administered intravenously or intramuscularly. The antibiotics of choice are usually cefoxitin (Mefoxin) and doxycycline to provide thorough coverage against the responsible pathogens. The patient must refrain from having intercourse for 3 weeks. The patient's partner(s) must be examined and treated as well. Pain control, rest, and adequate fluid intake are essential to the care. A corticosteroid is often added to the antibiotic treatment to aid in more rapid recovery and improvement in maintaining fertility (Lewis et al., 2007).

Nursing Interventions and Patient Teaching

The patient is usually hospitalized to isolate the organism and plan the treatment. Inform the patient and those assisting with the care of all specific precautions and observe standard precautions. Use goggles if any splashing is likely. Nursing interventions include (1) assessing pain and administering prescribed analgesics as needed; (2) monitoring vital signs and progress of treatment; (3) providing fluids to avoid dehydration; (4) performing palliative measures for comfort such as bathing, changing of perineal pads, personal hygiene, and warm douches; (5) providing patient support with a positive, nonjudgmental attitude; and (6) positioning the patient in Fowler's position to facilitate drainage.

Nursing diagnoses and interventions for the patient with PID include but are not limited to the following:

Nursing Diagnoses	Nursing Interventions
Pain, related to infection process	Manage pain with analgesics as ordered; assess effectiveness of pain-relief measures. Provide comfort measures.

Nursing Diagnoses	Nursing Interventions
Ineffective coping, related to condition	Provide emotional support. Encourage verbalization of feelings. Provide therapeutic environment for patient.
Ineffective health maintenance, related to insufficient knowledge of condition and complications	Teach patient about the significance of PID and the importance of complying with medication therapy.

Discharge planning should include patient teaching and instructions for (1) contacting the physician if a low-grade fever persists or purulent vaginal discharge occurs; (2) understanding the significance of the pelvic inflammatory condition; (3) complying with medication therapy; (4) observing handwashing technique and practices of personal hygiene, such as bathing, avoidance of tampons, frequent changing of perineal pads, and clean clothing; (5) understanding the importance of the sexual partner being examined and treated to avoid recurrence of the PID; and (6) recognizing that intercourse is sometimes painful after PID and that sexual activity should be avoided until advised by a physician.

Prognosis
Women with PID are usually of childbearing age. PID can lead to complications such as adhesions and strictures of the fallopian tubes, infertility, and increased risk of ectopic pregnancy (Lewis et al., 2007). With adequate treatment, the prognosis is good.

TOXIC SHOCK SYNDROME
Etiology and Pathophysiology
Toxic shock syndrome (TSS) is an acute bacterial infection caused by *Staphylococcus aureus*. It usually occurs in women who are menstruating and using tampons (particularly superabsorbent tampons). If the tampon is left in place too long, the bacteria may proliferate and release toxins into the bloodstream, causing TSS. Women at the greatest risk are those who insert tampons with their fingers instead of with inserters, women with chronic vaginal infections, and women with genital herpes. TSS can also occur in nonmenstruating women.

Clinical Manifestations
Often the patient has flulike symptoms for the first 24 hours. Between days 2 and 4 of the menstrual period, the patient may have an elevated temperature (up to 102° F [39° C]), vomiting, dizziness, headache, diarrhea, myalgia, hypotension, and signs suggesting the onset of septic shock. Sore throat, headache, and a red macular palmar or diffuse rash followed by desquamation of the skin, hands, and feet may de-

velop; urinary output is decreased, and the blood urea nitrogen (BUN) level is elevated. Disorientation may occur from dehydration and the release of toxins. Pulmonary edema and inflammation of mucous membranes may occur.

Assessment
Collection of **subjective data** includes determining whether the patient has recently used tampons and how long she used a single tampon before changing it. Obtain information about myalgia, sore throat, headache, and fatigue.

Collection of **objective data** includes assessing for edema. Assess the palms and soles for an erythematous rash. Desquamation and sloughing occur within 1 to 2 weeks after the rash. Note the patient's level of consciousness. Hypotension is a sign of TSS, as are nonpurulent inflammation of the conjunctiva and hyperemia of the oropharynx and vagina.

Diagnostic Tests
There is no definitive test for TSS. However, cervical-vaginal isolates of *S. aureus* are present 90% of the time. Blood tests demonstrate leukocytosis; thrombocytopenia; and elevated levels of bilirubin, BUN, creatinine, serum glutamic-pyruvic transaminase (alanine aminotransferase), serum glutamic-oxaloacetic transaminase (aspartate aminotransferase), and creatine phosphokinase. Blood and urine cultures should be taken along with throat cultures when appropriate.

Medical Management
Treatment of TSS varies because of the range in types and severity of symptoms. Antibiotic therapy is given according to the results of culture and sensitivity tests. Parenteral therapy is given to maintain proper fluid balance. Laboratory data are evaluated for electrolyte imbalance caused by vomiting and diarrhea, elevated BUN suggesting renal involvement, and elevated enzymes suggesting liver dysfunction.

Nursing Interventions and Patient Teaching
When the patient is hospitalized, bed rest is prescribed and antibiotics are administered. Closely monitor vital signs and fluid status. If there is respiratory distress, oxygen therapy is instituted.

Nursing diagnoses and interventions for the patient with TSS include but are not limited to the following:

Nursing Diagnoses	Nursing Interventions
Anxiety, related to TSS	Encourage patient to verbalize fears. Provide quiet, therapeutic environment. Provide support and understanding.

Continued

Nursing Diagnoses	Nursing Interventions
Deficient fluid volume, related to vomiting and diarrhea	Monitor amount, frequency, and characteristics of vomitus and diarrhea. Assess tissue turgor for evidence of dehydration. Assess patient for dry mucous membranes, and monitor parenteral fluids with electrolytes as ordered. Monitor intake and output (I&O).

Because the use of tampons during menstruation has been linked to TSS, advise patients not to use superabsorbent tampons. If tampons are used, they should be alternated with the use of pads. Before it is used, a tampon should be inspected for shedding and other flaws and discarded if any are noted. Tampons should be changed frequently (every 4 hours) and should be inserted carefully to avoid abrasions. Patients who have had TSS should not use tampons. Instruct the patient to wash hands thoroughly before inserting a tampon. Advise women who are menstruating and develop a sudden high fever accompanied by vomiting and diarrhea to seek immediate medical attention. If the woman is wearing a tampon, she should remove it immediately.

Prognosis

TSS is a rare and sometimes fatal disease. The effect of the toxin on the liver, kidneys, and circulatory system makes this a potentially life-threatening condition. Prognosis depends on the severity of the disease and how quickly therapeutic measures to combat shock and renal failure, if present, are instituted.

DISORDERS OF THE FEMALE REPRODUCTIVE SYSTEM

ENDOMETRIOSIS

Etiology and Pathophysiology

Endometriosis is a condition in which endometrial tissue appears outside the endometrial cavity. Endometrial tissue can be found on the ovaries, the fallopian tubes, and the uterus; within the abdominal cavity (the uterovesical peritoneum); and in the vagina (Figure 12-9). Tissue is believed to spread through lymphatic circulation, by menstrual backflow to the fallopian tubes and pelvic cavity, or through congenital displacement of the endometrial cells.

The tissue responds to the normal stimulation of the ovaries; bleeds each month; and forms an endometrial crust, which causes an endometrial cyst. This cyst may rupture and cause further reproduction of tissue.

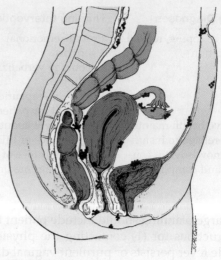

FIGURE 12-9 Common sites of endometriosis.

Clinical Manifestations

Symptoms are lower abdominal and pelvic pain with or without pain in the rectum. It may be unilateral or bilateral and may radiate to the lower back, legs, and groin. Symptoms are more acute during menstruation and subside after menstruation. Some evidence indicates that women have a greater chance (about seven times greater) of developing endometriosis if a sister or mother has it. The highest incidence of endometriosis is among white women 25 to 35 years of age who are in the higher socioeconomic classes and who postpone childbearing until the later reproductive years. Women who have not conceived or lactated are at greater risk.

Assessment

Subjective data include a history of the patient's symptoms, including pelvic pain with menstruation, aching, cramping, a bearing-down sensation in the pelvis, or lower back dyspareunia. The type of pain may indicate cysts that are about to rupture or infected tissue. The patient may reveal a history of menstrual irregularities such as amenorrhea.

Collection of **objective data** involves noting signs such as abnormal uterine bleeding, which appear 5 to 7 days before menses and last 2 or 3 days. Signs may also include infertility.

Diagnostic Tests

Laparoscopy with a biopsy of the lesions may confirm the diagnosis. Regular pelvic examinations are recommended to monitor progression.

Medical Management

Medical treatment consists of high-dose antiovulatory medications to inhibit ovulation and induce a state physiologically similar to pregnancy, thus suppressing menstruation. Synthetic androgens such as danazol (Danocrine) or a gonadotropin-releasing hormone agonist (e.g., leuprolide [Lupron]) may be prescribed to arrest proliferation of the endometrium and prevent ovulation, producing atrophy of the displaced endometrium (Lewis et al., 2007). Occasionally endometriosis spontaneously disappears. It is believed that an interruption of the menstrual cycle will slow the progress of the disorder. Some women who become pregnant are asymptomatic after pregnancy. When involvement is severe, surgery may be necessary. A laparoscopy may be performed to remove endometrial implants and adhesions. Lasers may be used to vaporize the small implants of endometrial tissue. A total hysterectomy, oophorectomy, and salpingectomy may also be done.

Nursing Interventions and Patient Teaching

Reinforce the physician's explanation of the expected results of treatment; instruct the patient regarding the dosage, frequency, and side effects of prescribed medications; and emphasize the importance of regular checkups and of reporting abnormal vaginal bleeding. Also encourage the patient to verbalize her concerns, and assist the patient with comfort measures.

Nursing diagnoses and interventions for the patient with endometriosis include but are not limited to the following:

Nursing Diagnoses	Nursing Interventions
Pain, related to displaced endometrial tissue	Institute comfort measures to cope with pain, such as medications and warm compresses to abdomen. Maintain bed rest when pain is most severe.
Sexual dysfunction, related to painful intercourse or infertility	Emphasize importance of communicating fears and concerns that lead to anxiety.

Prognosis

Approximately half of the women with endometriosis are infertile. If a young woman has endometriosis, advise her to have a family early, since the fertility rate is low. Menopause stops the progress of endometriosis.

VAGINAL FISTULA

Etiology and Pathophysiology

A fistula is defined as an abnormal opening between two organs. Vaginal fistulas are caused by an ulcerating process resulting from cancer, radiation, weakening of tissue by pregnancies, and surgical interventions. Vaginal fistulas are named for the organs involved (Figure 12-10). For example, a **urethrovaginal fistula** is an opening between the urethra and the vagina; a **vesicovaginal fistula** is an opening between the bladder and the vagina; and a **rectovaginal fistula** is an opening between the rectum and the vagina.

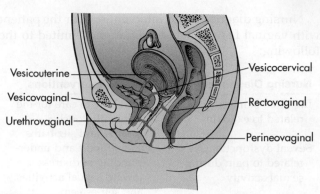

FIGURE 12-10 Types of fistulas that may develop in the vagina and the uterus.

Clinical Manifestations

Fistulas are recognized by their exudate, which has a distinct odor of urine or feces. Generally, a bladder infection is present. The vesicovaginal fistula causes a constant trickling of urine into the vagina; a rectovaginal fistula allows feces and flatus to enter the vagina.

Assessment

Subjective data include the patient's understanding of the exudate that occurs and of any causative factors. The patient reports the presence of urine or feces from the vagina.

Collection of **objective data** includes noting any behaviors that indicate stress, anxiety, and pain. The patient may express feelings of decreased self-esteem because of the condition. Observe for urine or feces on the perineal pad.

Diagnostic Tests

Diagnostic testing includes a methylene blue instillation in the bladder, and an intravenous (IV) pyelogram or cystoscopy to assist in locating the fistula. Pelvic examination is performed.

Medical Management

Healing is promoted by an increase in vitamin C and protein in the diet. The patient is given oral or parenteral antibiotics. If the organ tissue is healthy, a surgical approach is recommended. The surgical approach may be similar to anteroposterior colporrhaphy, which is discussed later in the chapter. Fistulas that are difficult to repair or very large may require urinary or fecal diversion.

Nursing Interventions

Soiling from leakage of urine or stool into the vagina is disturbing for the patient. Sitz baths, deodorizing douches, perineal pads, and protective undergarments are necessary. If the fistula is repaired surgically, insert a Foley catheter postoperatively to prevent strain on the suture line by a full bladder.

Nursing diagnoses and interventions for the patient with vaginal fistula include but are not limited to the following:

Nursing Diagnoses	Nursing Interventions
Impaired skin integrity, related to exudates	Teach how to care for the skin with douches, creams, and sitz baths.
Sexual dysfunction, related to pain during sexual activity	Offer support and understanding of distress toward sexual activities and self-esteem.

Prognosis

Vaginal fistulas may close spontaneously but frequently need to be repaired surgically. If so, 4 to 6 months are required for the inflammation to subside before surgery can be attempted.

RELAXED PELVIC MUSCLES

The most common problems resulting from relaxed pelvic muscles are displaced uterus with prolapse (downward displacement) and procidentia, cystocele, urethrocele, rectocele, enterocele, and malposition of the uterus.

Displaced Uterus

A displaced uterus is usually congenital, but may be caused by childbirth. Normally the uterus lies with the cervix at a right angle to the long axis of the vagina, and the body of the uterus is inclined slightly forward (see Figure 12-3). Backward displacement may be retroversion or retroflexion. Retroversion position places the cervix at the normal axis, but the body of the uterus is directed toward the sacrum. In retroflexion the angle of the body of the uterus is on the cervix. The patient has backache, muscle strain, leukorrheal discharge, and heaviness in the pelvic area. The patient also tires easily. Treatment consists of a pessary (a rubber or plastic doughnut-shaped ring placed in the vagina) and possibly uterine suspension.

Uterine Prolapse

Etiology and Pathophysiology

Prolapse of the uterus through the pelvic floor and vaginal outlet is traditionally rated as first degree (the cervix comes down to the introitus [an entrance to a cavity, as in the vaginal introitus]), second degree (the cervix protrudes through the introitus), or third degree (procidentia [the entire uterus protrudes through the introitus]) (Figure 12-11). Obstetric trauma, overstretching of the uterine muscle support system, multiple births, coughing, straining, the aging process, and lifting heavy objects contribute to uterine prolapse.

Clinical Manifestations

The patient complains of a feeling of "something coming down." She may have dyspareunia, a dragging or heavy feeling in the pelvis, backache, and bowel or bladder problems if cystocele or rectocele is also present. Stress

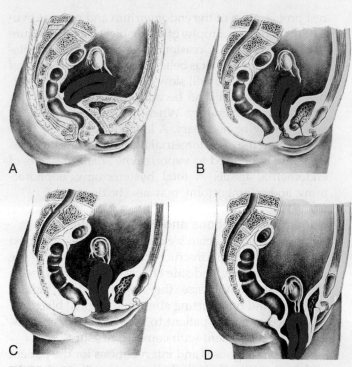

FIGURE 12-11 Uterine prolapse. **A,** Normal uterus. **B,** First-degree prolapse of the uterus. **C,** Second-degree prolapse of the uterus. **D,** Third-degree prolapse of the uterus (procidentia).

incontinence is a common and troubling problem. When second- or third-degree uterine prolapse occurs, the protruding cervix and vaginal walls are subjected to constant irritation, and tissue changes may occur.

Medical Management

Surgery generally involves a vaginal hysterectomy with anterior and posterior repair of the vagina and underlying fascia. It is also called an **anteroposterior colporrhaphy** (suture of the vagina) (also referred to as anterior posterior colporrhaphy or A&P repair).

When surgery is contraindicated, pessaries are used to provide uterine support. Before insertion of the vaginal pessary, the uterus is manually replaced in its normal position. Once inserted, the pessary holds the cervix in a posterior (anteflexed) position. When the pessary is properly placed, the woman is unaware of its presence and has no difficulty voiding or having intercourse. A variety of pessaries are available for the different degrees of prolapse. Every 3 to 4 months the pessary is cleaned and replaced by the woman, if possible, or by her health care provider. She is also checked for signs of irritation. Pessaries that are unattended for long periods are associated with erosion, fistulas, and an increased incidence of vaginal carcinoma.

Cystocele and Rectocele

Etiology and Pathophysiology

When the tissue, the muscles, and the ligaments that support the uterus and the perineum have been stretched and weakened by childbearing, multiple births, or cervical tears, the organs gradually move into other positions. The relaxation of the tissues, the

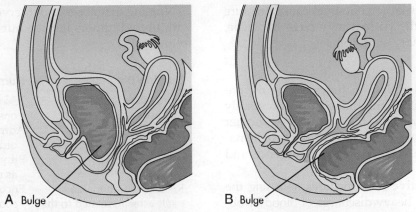

FIGURE 12-12 A, Cystocele. **B,** Rectocele.

muscles, and the ligaments of the bladder causes a displacement of the bladder into the vagina. This is referred to as a **cystocele** (Figure 12-12, *A*).

Clinical Manifestations
Clinical symptoms are urinary urgency, frequency, and incontinence; fatigue; and pelvic pressure. A large cystocele prevents complete emptying of the bladder, which leads to bacterial growth and infection.

The relaxation of the supporting tissues to the rectum causes the rectum to move toward the posterior vaginal wall and form a **rectocele** (Figure 12-12, *B*). The rectocele causes constipation, rectal pressure, heaviness, and hemorrhoids.

Medical Management
Cystocele and rectocele are corrected through anteroposterior colporrhaphy, a surgical repair involving shortening of the muscles that support the bladder and repair of the rectocele.

Nursing Interventions and Patient Teaching
An important aspect of preoperative care for colporrhaphy is ensuring as clean an operative area as possible. Patients may be given a cathartic followed by enemas to be sure the bowel is completely empty. A liquid diet for 48 hours before surgery will help keep the bowel empty. A cleansing vaginal douche is given the evening before and the morning of surgery. Postoperative care includes checking vital signs and observing for hemorrhage. A retention catheter is usually inserted into the bladder to keep it empty and prevent pressure on sutures. It is important to keep the fecal residue as soft as possible; some physicians order only liquids for several days, or they may order mineral oil to be given every night. An oil retention enema may be ordered, but cleansing enemas are not given. Carefully clean the patient's perineal area using surgical asepsis.

Encourage early ambulation. Advise the patient against standing for long periods or lifting heavy objects. Coitus must be avoided until healing occurs, usually after about 6 weeks.

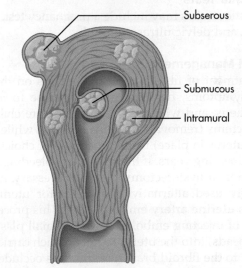

FIGURE 12-13 Leiomyomas. Uterine section showing whorl-like appearance and locations of leiomyomas, which are also called uterine fibroids.

Prognosis
With surgical correction, the prognosis is good.

LEIOMYOMAS OF THE UTERUS
Etiology and Pathophysiology
Leiomyomas (fibroids, myomas) are the most common benign tumors of the female genital tract (Figure 12-13). Fibroids are benign tumors arising from the muscle tissue of the uterus. The causes of leiomyomas is unknown. They seem to depend on ovarian hormones for their growth because of slow growth during reproductive years with atrophy occurring after menopause (Lewis et al., 2007). An estimated 20% to 25% of women over 30 years of age may develop uterine fibroid tumors. The size and number of leiomyomas vary. Most are found in the body of the uterus, but some occur in the cervix or involve the broad ligaments.

Clinical Manifestations
The symptoms are primarily pressure from an enlarging pelvic mass, pain (including dysmenorrhea), abnormal uterine bleeding, and menorrhagia. If the

fibroid tumor becomes large enough to cause pressure on other structures, the patient may have backache, constipation, and urinary symptoms.

Assessment
Collection of **subjective data** includes asking the patient about pain with menstruation or abnormally heavy menstrual flow. Have the patient describe her symptoms, which may include pelvic fullness or heaviness, constipation, urinary frequency or urgency, and menorrhagia.

Collection of **objective data** includes assessing the patient for excessively heavy discharge of blood by observing the number and saturation of perineal pads.

Diagnostic Tests
Diagnostic studies may include a pregnancy test, laparoscopy, and pelvic ultrasonography.

Medical Management
The treatment of fibroid tumors depends on the patient's symptoms, her age and how close to menopause she is, and whether she desires more children. **Myomectomy** (removal of uterine myomas while leaving the uterus in place) is the procedure of choice during childbearing years. If there is severe bleeding or an obstruction, a hysterectomy may be necessary. An increasingly used alternative treatment for uterine fibroids is **uterine artery embolization.** This procedure consists of injecting embolic material (small plastic or gelatin beads) into the uterine artery, which carries the material to the fibroid branches and thus occludes the arteries supplying blood to the tumor. Deprived of oxygen and nutrients, the tumor shrinks over time and symptoms diminish (McDaniel, 2007).

Six months after uterine artery embolization, fibroids are typically about 50% smaller in most women, and in 80% to 90% of women, the symptoms are considerably decreased or gone. About 5% of patients experience complications from the procedure, such as infection or permanent cessation of menstrual periods (McDaniel, 2007).

Nursing Interventions and Patient Teaching
Preoperative and postoperative nursing interventions are like those discussed for a patient who undergoes a hysterectomy. Reinforce the physician's explanation of the treatment plan—either a total hysterectomy or pelvic examination at regular intervals to monitor the status of the fibroid tumor. Instruct the patient about the dosage, frequency, and possible side effects of prescribed medications. Tell the patient with menorrhagia to include adequate iron in her diet to prevent iron deficiency anemia from the extra blood loss. Stress the importance of regular checkups to monitor the status of the fibroid tumor, and encourage the patient to express her feelings and assist her with coping mechanisms.

Nursing diagnoses and interventions for the patient with fibroid tumors include but are not limited to the following:

Nursing Diagnoses	Nursing Interventions
Pain, related to fibroid tumors	Assess pain location, onset, and duration. Administer analgesics as ordered. Provide comfort measures as needed.
Risk for situational low self-esteem, related to the presence of fibroid tumors	Encourage verbalization of concerns. Be an active listener.

Prognosis
Fibroid tumors of the uterus tend to disappear spontaneously with menopause. They rarely become malignant. Infertility may result from a myoma that obstructs or distorts the uterus or fallopian tubes. Myomas in the body of the uterus may cause spontaneous abortions; those near the cervical opening may make the delivery of a fetus difficult and may contribute to postpartum hemorrhage.

OVARIAN CYSTS
Etiology and Pathophysiology
Ovarian cysts are benign tumors that arise from dermoid cells of the ovary or from a cystic corpus luteum or graafian follicle.

Clinical Manifestations
Ovarian cysts enlarge and are palpable on examination. They may cause no symptoms, or they may result in a disturbance of menstruation, a feeling of heaviness, and slight vaginal bleeding.

Medical Management
The cysts may be removed by an ovarian cystectomy. Often ovarian cysts are not removed if the patient is not experiencing debilitating symptoms.

Nursing Interventions
If surgery is performed, nursing interventions are similar to those for the patient having an abdominal hysterectomy.

Prognosis
The prognosis is good; ovarian cysts do not become malignant.

CANCER OF THE FEMALE REPRODUCTIVE TRACT
Cancer is the second most common cause of death in women, and malignant tumors of the reproductive tract represent a significant portion of the total number

Cultural Considerations

Cancer of Female Reproductive System

- Ovarian cancer is seen more frequently among white women than among black women.
- Japanese women have a low incidence of ovarian cancer. However, second- and third-generation Japanese women in the United States have much higher rates, similar to those of white women born in the United States. Dietary practices may explain this difference.
- Endometrial cancer occurs more frequently among white women than among black women.
- Five-year survival rate for endometrial cancer (all stages combined) is 80% for white women and 55% for black women.
- Cervical cancer has a higher incidence among Hispanic, black, and Native American women than among white women. The mortality rate for cervical cancer is more than twice as high among black women as among white women.
- Jewish-American women have a low incidence of cervical cancer.

of deaths from cancer (see Cultural Considerations box).

Cervical cancer often affects women in their reproductive years. The cancer can be detected in its early stages with a diagnostic Pap test. Endometrial cancer is primarily a disease of women older than 50 years of age, but the incidence among younger women is increasing. Most cases of ovarian cancer occur in women older than 50, but malignant neoplasms of the ovaries may occur at all ages.

CANCER OF THE CERVIX

Cancer of the cervix is a neoplasm that can be detected in the early, curable stage by a Pap test. Cancer of the cervix is usually a squamous cell carcinoma. An estimated 11,270 cases of cervical cancer were diagnosed in 2009. As Pap screening has become more prevalent, preinvasive lesions are detected far more frequently than invasive cancer. An estimated 4070 cervical cancer deaths occurred in 2009. Mortality rates have declined sharply over the past several decades. The five-year relative survival rate for localized stage cervical cancer was 92%, and five-year relative survival rate for all stages of cervical cancer combined was 71% in 2009 (ACS, 2009c).

Etiology and Pathophysiology

Women who become sexually active in their teens are at an increased risk for cancer of the cervix, as are those who have had multiple sexual partners, had partners who had multiple sexual partners, and are of lower socioeconomic status. Cervical cancer risk is closely linked to sexual behavior, to STIs with several strains of HPV, and to smoking. Women who smoke have a 50% higher risk of developing cervical cancer than nonsmokers. Chronic infections and erosions of the cervix are most likely significant in the development of cancer.

Carcinoma in situ is a preinvasive, asymptomatic carcinoma that can only be diagnosed by microscopic examination of cervical cells. Once diagnosed, it can be treated early without radical surgery. Carcinoma in situ of the cervix is essentially 100% curable.

Clinical Manifestations

Most cervical cancer is silent in the early stages and offers few symptoms. The two primary symptoms are leukorrhea and irregular vaginal bleeding or spotting between menses. Bleeding often occurs after coitus or after menopause. Bleeding is slight at first but increases as the disease progresses. The vaginal exudate becomes watery, then increases and becomes dark and bloody with an offensive odor caused by necrosis (death of tissue) and infection of the tumor mass. As the cancer progresses, the bleeding may become constant and may increase in amount. With advanced stages the patient has severe pain in the back, upper thighs, and legs.

Assessment

Subjective data in the early stages of cancer of the cervix are not available, since the woman has no symptoms. If the tumor becomes more invasive, the patient experiences back and leg pain, weight loss, and malaise. Urge women to have regular health appraisals and pelvic examinations so that cancer of the cervix can be detected in its earliest stages.

Collection of **objective data** includes observing the sanitary pads for abnormal vaginal discharge. The vaginal exudate may be watery to dark red and malodorous. Note the number and saturation of the perineal pads. If the tumor becomes more invasive, assess the patient for anemia, fever, and lymphedema.

Diagnostic Tests

Cervical cancer is diagnosed with the following tests: (1) Pap test; (2) physical examination; (3) colposcopy and cervical biopsy; and (4) additional diagnostic studies, such as a computed tomography (CT) scan, chest radiographic evaluation, IV pyelogram, cystoscopy, sigmoidoscopy, or liver function studies to determine the extent of invasion. The ACS (2009a) recommends that cervical cancer screening begin approximately 3 years after a woman begins having vaginal intercourse, but no later than 21 years of age. Traditional Pap tests are less than 100% accurate in screening for cervical cell abnormalities, and false-positive and false-negative results do occur. A newer liquid-based technique, called ThinPrep, can reduce the number of inaccurate Pap tests results.

At or after age 30, women who have had three normal Pap test results in a row may get screened every 2 to 3 years, unless she has certain risk factors, such as human immunodeficiency virus (HIV) infection or a weak immune system. Women age 70 and older who have had three or more normal Pap tests and no abnormal Pap tests in the past 10 years may stop cervical cancer screening. Screening after a total hysterectomy (with removal of the cervix) is not necessary unless the surgery was done to treat cervical cancer or precancer. Women who have had a hysterectomy without removal of the cervix should continue cervical cancer screening at least until age 70 (ACS, 2009).

Medical Management

Gardisil is a vaccine that reduces the incidence of cervical cancer due to infection of HPV types 6, 11, 16, 18. To be effective, the vaccine should be given before a person becomes sexually active. The goal of these vaccines is to reduce the incidence of HPV-related genital disease, including precancerous cervical lesions and cervical cancer. Three injections are given over 6 months. The second dose is given 2 months after the first dose and the third dose 6 months after the first dose (Saslow et al., 2007).

The ACS recommends that the HPV vaccine be routinely given to girls ages 11 to 12 and as early as age 9 at the discretion of physicians. Vaccination is also recommended for females 13 to 18 to catch up on missed vaccine or to complete the vaccination series (Saslow et al., 2007).

Cervarix is a new 3-dose vaccine to prevent cervical cancer, cervical intraepithelial neoplasia (CIN) grades 1, 2, or worse, and adenocarcinoma in situ. It has been approved by the FDA for females 10 to 25 years old, and is undergoing pediatric testing for use in 9-year-old girls. Cervarix is effective against HPV types 16 and 18, but it does not offer coverage against all the other types of HIV infections nor is it effective after exposure to HPV (US FDA, 2009).

Carcinoma in situ is treated by removal of the affected area. A variety of techniques can be used, including electrocautery, cryosurgery (use of subfreezing temperature to destroy tissue), laser, conization, and hysterectomy. **Conization** is the surgical removal of a cone-shaped section of the cervix and is particularly useful in preserving childbearing function.

Early cervical carcinoma can be treated with a hysterectomy or intracavitary radiation (see Chapter 17).

A radical hysterectomy with pelvic lymph node dissection may be required for more extensive lesions. Invasive cervical cancers generally are treated by surgery, radiation, or both, as well as chemotherapy (cisplatin-based) in some cases. Radiation may be external or internal (e.g., cesium, radium). Brachytherapy, or internally implanted radiation into the cervix, is often done. The patient is hospitalized for 48 hours for treatment. The treatment plan is tailored to each patient based on the extent of the disease.

Nursing Interventions and Patient Teaching

Nursing interventions should include verbal reassurance. In advanced cervical cancer, position the patient comfortably; change her position slowly; maintain her body alignment; provide pain-relief measures;

change the patient's dressings and sanitary pads often; and assess color, odor, and amount of drainage. Assess the skin for impairment. See nursing interventions for a patient undergoing a hysterectomy.

Nursing diagnoses and interventions for the patient with cancer of the cervix include but are not limited to the following:

Nursing Diagnoses	Nursing Interventions
Impaired urinary elimination related to postsurgical sensorimotor impairment	Connect indwelling catheter to closed gravity drainage.
	Give meticulous catheter care as indicated.
	Record color and amount of urinary output.
	Promote micturition at regular intervals when catheter is removed.
	Catheterize for residual urine as ordered.
Risk for situational low self-esteem, related to body image change and value of reproductive organs	Encourage discussion with significant others.
	Relate importance of communicating anything that causes anxiety.
	Reinforce correct information to correct any misconceptions.
Ineffective tissue perfusion, peripheral, related to: • pelvic surgery • thrombophlebitis	Ensure that bed is not elevated in the knee gatch position.
	Assess proper placement of antiembolism stockings every 4 hours as ordered.
	Assist in passive and active leg exercises every shift.
	Encourage ambulation.
	Assess legs for erythema, increased tenderness, severe cramping, and positive Homans' sign every shift.

The key to preventing cervical cancer and treating it in the early stages is education. Educate and encourage patients to be responsible for their health by having a yearly Pap test. Education about the HPV vaccine for females is very important. Encourage patients to seek prompt medical assistance for any abnormal vaginal exudate.

Prognosis

The prognosis is good if the cancer is treated in the early stages. It usually takes 2 to 10 years for squamous cell carcinoma to become invasive beyond the basement membrane and metastasize. Therefore early diagnosis and treatment are vital. Survival for those with preinvasive lesions is nearly 100%; 92% of cervical cancer patients survive 1 year after diagnosis, and 71% survive

5 years (ACS, 2009c). When detected at an early stage, invasive cervical cancer has a 5-year survival rate of 92% for localized cancers.

CANCER OF THE ENDOMETRIUM

Etiology and Pathophysiology

Cancer of the endometrium usually affects postmenopausal women. An estimated 42,160 cases of cancer of the uterine corpus (body of the uterus) will be diagnosed in the United States in 2009 (ACS, 2009c). An estimated 7780 deaths were expected for 2009 (ACS, 2009c). Endometrial cancer is usually an adenocarcinoma. The tumor is more likely to be localized, but may spread to the cervix, bladder, rectum, and surrounding lymph nodes. It is the most common malignancy of the female genital tract. Women at increased risk are those with a history of irregular menstruation, difficulties during menopause, obesity, hypertension, or diabetes mellitus; those who have not had children; and those with a family history of uterine cancer. Obesity is a risk factor because adipose cells store estrogen. Women who used estrogen replacement therapy to treat menopausal symptoms are more likely to develop endometrial cancer. Progesterone plus estrogen replacement therapy (HRT) may largely offset the increased risk related to using only estrogen. Also at increased risk for developing endometrial cancer are women at high risk for developing breast cancer as well as those in an advanced stage of breast cancer who are taking tamoxifen (Nolvadex), an antiestrogen drug that blocks estrogen receptors.

The carcinoma in situ is slow growing. Invasion and metastasis occur later, with expansion to the cervix and the myometrium and ultimately to the vagina, the pelvis, and the lungs.

Clinical Manifestations

The first sign of endometrial cancer is abnormal uterine bleeding, usually in postmenopausal women. About 50% of patients with postmenopausal bleeding have cancer of the uterus. In premenstrual or postmenopausal women, any abnormal bleeding or spotting should be reported immediately.

Assessment

Collection of **subjective data** includes assisting the patient in identifying and reporting changes in reproductive or sexual health. The patient may report abdominal pressure, pain, and pelvic fullness. The patient will have a history of postmenopausal bleeding and leukorrhea. Pelvic and back pain and postcoital bleeding are late signs and symptoms.

Collection of **objective data** includes observing the color and amount of vaginal exudate on perineal pads. Assess the patient for enlarged lymph nodes.

Diagnostic Tests

Pelvic and rectal examination and endometrial biopsy are used to diagnose cancer of the endometrium. Any report of abnormal or unexpected bleeding in a postmenopausal woman requires a tissue sample to exclude endometrial cancer. The ACS recommends that an endometrial biopsy be performed at menopause and then periodically in women who are at risk for endometrial cancer (ACS, 2009c). The Pap test is not a reliable diagnostic tool for endometrial cancer, but it can rule out cervical cancer (Lewis et al., 2007).

Medical Management

Treatment of cancer of the endometrium depends on the stage of the tumor and the woman's health. Surgery, radiation, or chemotherapy may be used to remove the tumor and treat metastasis. For early cancer of the endometrium, total abdominal hysterectomy with bilateral salpingo-oophorectomy (TAH-BSO) is done. Intracavitary radiation followed by a TAH-BSO may be done for the early stage of endometrial cancer (stage I). Patients with stage II disease may receive pelvic irradiation to shrink the tumor and help prevent spread. Afterward the patient undergoes a hysterectomy. Patients with stages III and IV disease are uncommon, and treatment is based on the extent of the disease.

Nursing Interventions and Patient Teaching

See the section on interventions for the patient undergoing a hysterectomy; also see Chapter 17 for care of the patient through intracavitary radiation.

Health teaching and follow-up after discharge should emphasize the need for regular physical examination by the physician and the importance of compliance with the prescribed treatment plan.

Prognosis

Cancer of the endometrium is primarily a slow-growing adenocarcinoma. Metastasis occurs late, and the sign of irregular vaginal bleeding often appears early enough to allow for cure of the disease. The 5-year survival rate for all cases of endometrial cancer is about 83% (ACS, 2009c).

CANCER OF THE OVARY

Etiology and Pathophysiology

Ovarian cancer, the fourth most common cause of cancer death in women, is the leading cause of gynecologic death in the United States, following cancer of the uterine corpus. Risk for ovarian cancer increases with age; it occurs most frequently in women between 55 and 65 years of age.

The ACS (2009c) estimated that in 2009, 21,550 women would be diagnosed with ovarian cancer and nearly 14,600 would die of the disease.

In the early stages the tumors are asymptomatic; when detected, they usually have spread to other pelvic organs. Nothing alters the magnitude of risk for ovarian cancer more than genetics. Hereditary ovarian cancer accounts for 5% to 10% of ovarian cancers. In general, the closer the relative with ovarian cancer and the younger the relative at diagnosis, the higher the risk is. Women at increased risk are those who are infertile, anovulatory, nulliparous, and habitual aborters. Because they reduce the number of ovulatory cycles, thus reducing exposure to estrogen, the following practices can reduce the risk of ovarian cancer: oral contraceptive use (greater than 5 years), multiple pregnancies, breastfeeding, and early age of first birth. Other risk factors include a high-fat diet and exposure to industrial chemicals such as asbestos and talc. Ovarian cancer commonly spreads by peritoneal seeding of the cancer cells. Common sites of metastasis are the peritoneum, the omentum, and bowel surfaces.

Clinical Manifestations

In the early stages the symptoms may cause vague abdominal discomfort, flatulence, mild gastric disturbances, pressure, bloating, cramps, sense of pelvic heaviness, feeling of fullness, and change in bowel habits. Pain *is not* an early symptom. As the tumor progresses, abdominal girth enlarges from ascites, and there is flatulence with distention. Other symptoms may include urinary frequency, nausea, vomiting, constipation, menstrual irregularities, and weight loss. The Gynecologic Cancer Foundation, the Society of Gynecologic Oncologists, and the ACS issued the first national consensus statement on ovarian cancer symptoms in June, 2007. This statement mentions that certain symptoms such as bloating, pelvic or abdominal pain, difficulty eating, feeling full quickly, and urinary urgency or frequency are much more likely to occur in women with ovarian cancer than in women without ovarian cancer (ACS, 2007c). Women are strongly advised to see their gynecologist if they experience any of these symptoms almost daily for more than a few weeks.

Assessment

Collection of **subjective data** requires an awareness that cancer of the ovary is difficult to detect. The patient reports symptoms of abdominal discomfort, bloating, fullness, gastric disturbances (nausea, constipation), and urinary frequency.

Collection of **objective data** includes observing any increase in the abdominal girth. The patient may void at frequent intervals because of pressure on the bladder. The patient may be dyspneic due to ascites and pressure on the diaphragm.

Diagnostic Tests

Although detecting ovarian cancer early is difficult, an annual bimanual pelvic examination may help to identify pelvic masses. Because the ovaries are movable and therefore harder to assess, screening for ovarian tumors requires a thorough examination, including bimanual and rectovaginal examination. **Postmenopause palpable ovary syndrome** (a palpable ovary in a woman 3 to 5 years past menopause) may indicate

an early tumor. CT scan of the pelvis and abdomen is indicated if an ovarian mass is palpable. Definitive diagnosis of ovarian cancer is usually established by a tumor biopsy at the time of exploratory laparotomy, when staging and tumor debulking take place.

Ovarian cancer is diagnosed by palpation of a pelvic mass and aspiration of ascitic fluid and detection of cancer cells in the fluid. A blood test to determine CA-125 is used to identify women with ovarian cancer. High levels of CA-125 are found in the blood of 80% of women with epithelial ovarian cancer. But although the antigen test can help evaluate a woman's response to cancer treatment, it is controversial as an independent screening tool. Because of the test's lack of specificity and sensitivity, false-positive and false-negative results can occur. Many benign conditions, including endometriosis and fibroid tumors, can raise CA-125 levels above normal.

Vaginal ultrasonography, which also lacks specificity and sensitivity, may be used with pelvic examination and CA-125 antigen testing to follow a woman at increased risk.

Medical Management

Treatment often involves surgery alone or in conjunction with radiation or chemotherapy. Treatment depends on the stage of ovarian cancer (see Chapter 17). Surgery may be a TAH-BSO and omentectomy (excision of portions of the peritoneal folds). In some very early tumors, only the involved ovary is removed, especially in young women who wish to have children. The National Cancer Institute (NCI) issued a clinical announcement suggesting physicians use a combined modality approach after surgical debulking of the tumor: intraperitoneal chemotherapy, administered through a surgically implanted catheter, in addition to the standard IV chemotherapy (NCI, 2006). A gynecologic oncologist or surgical team with expertise in the staging and debulking of ovarian cancer should perform the surgery

Intraperitoneal chemotherapy employs two generic drugs already in widespread use for ovarian cancer: paclitaxel (Taxol) and cisplatin (Platinol). A list of facilities that provide intraperitoneal chemotherapy is available on the NCI website at http://ctep.cancer.gov/highlights/20060105_ovarian.htm.

Nursing Interventions

Nursing interventions for any patient with ovarian cancer include management similar to that for patients undergoing abdominal hysterectomy and receiving chemotherapy and external radiation (see Chapter 17). Because ovarian cancer is generally at an advanced stage when diagnosed, despite the woman's feeling well, support and encouragement to comply with the treatment regimen are important nursing interventions. As the disease progresses, become involved in activities to increase the patient's comfort.

Nursing diagnoses and interventions for the patient with cancer of the ovaries include but are not limited to the following:

Nursing Diagnoses	Nursing Interventions
Fear, related to diagnosis of cancer	Assist patient with recognizing and clarifying fears and with developing coping strategies for those fears. Be an active listener.
Situational low self-esteem, related to body image change and value of reproductive organs	Encourage patient's comments and questions about condition. Encourage discussion with significant others. Provide factual information to correct any misconceptions.

Prognosis
More than 75% of women with ovarian cancer are diagnosed with advanced disease. The 5-year survival rate for all stages is 46%. If diagnosed early and treated while the disease is localized, the 5-year survival rate is 93%. Relative survival rates for more advanced disease are 71% for regional disease and 31% for disease that has spread to distant sites (ACS, 2009c).

HYSTERECTOMY
A hysterectomy involves removal of the uterus, including the cervix. This procedure may be done for many conditions, such as dysfunctional uterine bleeding, endometriosis, malignant and nonmalignant tumors of the uterus and cervix, and disorders of pelvic relaxation and uterine prolapse.

Various terms are used to describe removal of the uterus. A total hysterectomy is removal of the entire uterus. The vagina remains intact, and intercourse is possible even though childbearing is not. Estrogens are still released. Menopause occurs naturally because the ovaries are still present. A total abdominal hysterectomy with bilateral salpingo-oophorectomy (TAH-BSO) is the removal of the uterus, fallopian tubes, and ovaries. It is sometimes called panhysterosalpingo-oophorectomy. A radical hysterectomy also includes removal of the pelvic lymph nodes. If the ovaries are removed in these surgeries, it induces menopause.

VAGINAL HYSTERECTOMY
A vaginal hysterectomy may be done for a prolapsed uterus. It is not used nearly as often as the abdominal approach. The vaginal approach is selected for the patient who cannot tolerate abdominal surgery or prolonged anesthesia. There is no abdominal incision. The patient is placed in a lithotomy position, and the uterus is removed through the vagina. Advantages of the vaginal entrance are that (1) there is no wound de-

hiscence, (2) there is less pain, (3) complications are less likely, (4) hospitalization is shorter, and (5) there is no abdominal scar. The most important disadvantage is a limited view of the operative field for visualizing intrapelvic and intraabdominal organs. Vaginal hysterectomy is not used in cases of uterine fibroids or enlarged uterine size. Other disadvantages are risk of bleeding and postoperative infection.

ABDOMINAL HYSTERECTOMY
An abdominal hysterectomy is preferred when there is a need to explore the pelvic cavity and when the fallopian tubes and ovaries are to be removed. The three procedures for an abdominal hysterectomy are named according to the extent of the surgery performed. A **subtotal hysterectomy** refers to the removal of the corpus (the midsection or body) of the uterus, leaving the cervical stump in place. Leaving the cervical stump in place may play a role in female sexual pleasure and orgasm. A **total hysterectomy** is the removal of the entire uterus, including the cervix, but leaving the fallopian tubes and ovaries in place. TAH-BSO involves the removal of the entire uterus, the fallopian tubes, and the ovaries.

Nursing Interventions
Preoperative Interventions
When the physician has explained the surgery to the patient, reinforce the explanation and answer any questions. Encourage verbalization of fears. Provide additional preoperative instructions to help the woman prepare for postoperative recovery. Instruct the patient how to turn, cough, and deep breathe.

Before a vaginal or abdominal hysterectomy, the colon is emptied to prevent postoperative distention. The patient may be on a low-residue diet for several days preoperatively. Enemas may be given the evening before surgery. The bladder may be decompressed to prevent trauma during surgery. The indwelling catheter generally remains in place for 1 or 2 days after surgery. An antiseptic vaginal douche may be ordered to decrease microbial invasion of the surgical site.

Surgical preparation of the skin on the abdomen, the pelvis, and the perineum often is performed in surgery. The patient signs a consent form, and oral intake after midnight is restricted. Occasionally, ureteral stents are placed in the ureters for identification and to prevent possible trauma to the ureters during surgery.

Postoperative Interventions
Postoperative nursing interventions focus on monitoring vital signs and preventing urinary retention, intestinal distention, and venous thrombosis. If a retention catheter was inserted, ensure it is kept patent and connected to closed drainage. Perform meticulous catheter care to prevent bladder infection. The indwelling catheter generally remains in place 1 or 2 days postoperatively. If no retention catheter is in place, check the patient frequently for bladder distention; accurately record

urinary output. The incidence of urinary retention after a hysterectomy is greater than after any other type of surgery, since some trauma to the bladder is unavoidable. If the patient does not have a catheter and is unable to void, catheterization every 8 hours may be necessary. Occasionally the patient has residual urine, and the physician may order catheterization to check for it; 50 mL or less is within the normal range.

A small up-and-down flush enema may be ordered to help relieve distention. Early ambulation is helpful to return the bowel to normal function. When bowel sounds have returned and flatus is being expelled, the patient is allowed liquids by mouth and a gradual return to solid foods.

Patients undergoing pelvic surgery are susceptible to venous stasis and thrombophlebitis because of trauma to blood vessels. The patient is usually permitted out of bed on the first postoperative day, but encourage the patient to dangle her legs and to sit on the side of the bed before standing and walking to avoid postural hypotension. Encourage the patient to cough, deep breathe, and use an incentive spirometer to prevent postoperative pneumonia and atelectasis. Antiembolism stockings may be used to prevent thrombus or embolus formation, and legs should be exercised frequently when the patient is in bed. Many physicians prescribe intermittent pneumonic compression cuffs for the calves to prevent venous stasis, deep-vein thrombosis, and pulmonary embolism. The patient should avoid bending her knees. This could cause pooling of blood in the pelvic cavity, resulting in stasis in the lower extremities. The patient at risk for thromboembolic disease may receive low-dose heparin or low-molecular-weight enoxaparin (Lovenox) to prevent thrombus formation.

Analgesics such as morphine may be ordered for relief of pain. Slight vaginal drainage may occur for 1 or 2 days, but report any unusual bleeding to the physician. Observe the abdominal dressing on the patient with an abdominal hysterectomy for evidence of hemorrhage. Use surgical asepsis for the dressing change. The patient usually receives IV feedings for _____ monitor the rate _____ for the patient _____ ut are not lim-

Nursing Diagnoses	Nursing Interventions
Chronic pain, related to metastatic process	Establish trusting relationship with patient. Monitor and document pain characteristics. Administer prescribed analgesics every 3 to 4 hours to control pain. Provide environment conducive to comfort and rest.

Nursing Diagnoses	Nursing Interventions
Excess fluid volume, related to ascites	Monitor IV fluids. Maintain accurate I&O. Weigh patient daily. Observe for signs of edema. Measure abdominal girth daily.
Compromised family coping, related to poor prognosis	Assess present coping abilities. Encourage and allow time for verbalization of feelings. Support patient's coping strengths, and discuss alternative coping measures. Involve patient and significant others in nursing interventions and procedures.

Patient Teaching

Before discharge, the physician explains to the woman and her partner that they should not have sexual intercourse for 4 to 6 weeks after surgery. With an abdominal incision, there may be further restrictions on heavy lifting (nothing greater than 10 pounds), walking up and down stairs, and prolonged riding in the car. Riding in the car may cause pelvic pooling and development of a thrombus in the legs.

Inform the patient that vaginal drainage is normal for about 2 to 4 weeks after an abdominal hysterectomy. Advise her to avoid wearing any tight clothing such as a girdle or knee-high hose, which might constrict circulation to the surgical site and cause venous stasis.

Several signs and symptoms of infection should be reported to the physician if they occur: (1) erythema, edema, exudate, or increased tenderness along the surgical incision; (2) increased malodorous vaginal exudate; (3) a temperature of 101° F (38.3° C) or more; and (4) any problems with urinating, such as difficulty in starting to void, voiding too often, voiding small amounts, or a burning sensation while urinating (indicative of a bladder infection).

DISORDERS OF THE FEMALE BREAST

FIBROCYSTIC BREAST CONDITION

Etiology and Pathophysiology

Fibrocystic breast condition involves benign tumors of the breasts. It usually occurs in women 30 to 50 years of age and is rare in postmenopausal women. This suggests that the occurrence is related to ovarian activity.

The cysts are characterized by numerous cellular changes, with an abnormal amount of epithelial hyperplasia and cystic formation within the mammary ducts. The cysts rarely become malignant, but the risk of breast cancer does increase for women who have fibrocystic breast condition; therefore observe the cysts carefully.

Clinical Manifestations

Cystic lesions are often bilateral and multiple. The cysts are soft, well differentiated, tender, and freely movable. The lumpiness and tenderness are more apparent before menses.

Diagnostic Tests

The disorder is diagnosed by mammography or ultrasound and confirmed by biopsy. As a therapeutic measure, the cyst is aspirated by needle and syringe to empty the secretions, and the fluid is sent to the laboratory for cytologic examination to rule out a malignancy. Aspiration produces a turbid, nonhemorrhagic, yellow, greenish, or brownish fluid.

Medical Management

When cysts recur in the same area and repeated aspirations are ineffective, surgical excision of the cyst may be done.

Conservative treatment is the usual approach to fibrocystic breast condition. The usefulness of eliminating methylxanthines (in coffee, tea, and cola) from the diet is still controversial, but it is the least expensive therapy. Many women have reported decreased symptoms after altering their diet, even though findings by palpation and mammogram were not significantly changed. Danazol may be prescribed to inhibit FSH and LH production, thereby decreasing ovarian production of estrogen. Danazol may cause weight gain, hot flashes, menstrual irregularities, hirsutism, and deepening of the voice. Vitamin E may also be prescribed, but its efficacy has not been proven.

Nursing Interventions and Patient Teaching

Instruct the patient to perform breast self-examination (BSE) 1 week after menses, to recognize the presence of cysts, and to note any changes.

ACUTE MASTITIS

Acute mastitis is an acute bacterial infection usually caused by *S. aureus* or streptococci. It is most often observed during lactation and late pregnancy. The infection may result from inadequate cleanliness of the breasts, a nipple fissure, or infection in the infant. The breasts are tender, inflamed, and engorged, obstructing the milk flow.

Treatment involves application of warm packs, support of the area with a well-fitting brassiere (which also supplies comfort), and systemic treatment with antibiotics.

CHRONIC MASTITIS

Chronic mastitis tends to develop in women between 30 and 50 years of age and is more common in those who have had children, have had difficulty with inverted and cracked nipples, and have had problems nursing their infants. A traumatic blow to the breasts allows the fat to necrose in the area and form abscesses. Increased fibrosis of the tissue causes cysts to

form. The cysts are tender, painful, and palpable on examination. The disorder is generally unilateral and benign and most frequently occurs in obese women. Treatment is the same as for acute mastitis.

BREAST CANCER

Breast cancer is the most common malignancy affecting women in the United States. Approximately 1 of every 8 women will develop breast cancer during her lifetime. The incidence of breast cancer in men is rare (less than 1%). Among men, there are about 1910 new cases of breast cancer and 440 deaths per year. The ACS (2009c) predicted that 194,280 women would be diagnosed with breast cancer in 2009 and that 40,610 would die. Breast cancer ranks second among cancer deaths in women (after lung cancer). Women consider this disease their most serious health problem. Women over 60 years of age have twice the incidence of breast cancer as women ages 45 to 60. In women older than 55, 50% more patients have metastatic disease at presentation than do younger women. Vital to the process of detection are monthly BSEs, breast imaging with digital mammography and MRI or ultrasound to differentiate a cyst from a lesion and to detect small tumors before they can be palpated, and periodic breast examinations by a physician.

Etiology and Pathophysiology

The cause of breast cancer is unknown. The high incidence in women implies a hormonal cause (Box 12-5).

Box 12-5   Predisposing Factors for Women at High Risk for Breast Cancer

- **Gender:** Being a female introduces a high risk.
- **Age:** Higher incidence occurs with women over 40 years of age and in the postmenopausal phase of life. After age 60 the incidence increases dramatically.
- **Race:** White women, in the middle or upper socioeconomic class, are at higher risk
- **Genetics:** The inherited susceptibility genes *BRCA1* and *BRCA2* account for approximately 5% of all cases and confer a lifetime risk in these women, ranging from 35% to 85%.
- **Family history:** This is especially important if diagnosed family member had ovarian cancer, was premenopausal, had bilateral breast cancer, or is a first-degree relative (mother, sister, daughter).
- **Parity** (total number of pregnancies): Risk is decreased for women if birth is before 18 years; it is increased for women who are not sexually active, infertile women, and women who become pregnant for the first time after 30 years of age.
- **Menopause:** Menopause after 55 years of age increases the risk.
- **Obesity:** Weight gain and obesity after menopause increase the risk.
- **Other cancer:** Risk is increased for women who had another cancer such as endometrial, ovarian, or colon; if cancer has appeared in one breast, it is more likely to occur in the other breast.

The primary risk factors are female gender, age older than 50, North American or Northern European descent, a personal history of breast cancer, atypical hyperplasia or carcinoma in situ, two or more first-degree relatives with the disease, and a first-degree relative with bilateral premenopausal breast cancer. Other risk factors include early menarche, a first pregnancy after age 30, natural menopause after age 55, and one or more breast cancer genes. The inherited susceptibility genes, *BRCA1* and *BRCA2*, account for approximately 5% of all cases and confer a lifetime risk in these women ranging from 35% to 85% (Hollingsworth et al., 2004). Recent findings suggest that prophylactic removal of the breasts and/or ovaries in *BRCA1* and *BRCA2* carriers decreases the risk of breast cancer considerably, although not all women who choose this surgery would have developed cancer. Women who consider this option should have an opportunity for counseling before reaching a decision (Hollingsworth et al., 2004). Results of a recent study suggest that women who are overweight are more likely to die from breast cancer. Current data indicate tamoxifen and raloxifene decrease breast cancer risk in women who are at increased risk (Kudachadkar & O'Regan, 2005). With the exception of advancing age and being female, though, most women who develop breast cancer do not have any risk factors for the disease. That is why it is so important to encourage even healthy women to undergo screening examinations.

Breast cancer is usually an adenocarcinoma, arising from the epithelium and developing in the lactiferous ducts; it infiltrates the parenchyma (the tissue of an organ other than the supporting or connective tissue). The cancer occurs most often in women who have not given birth or breastfed a child. It occurs most often in the upper outer quadrant of the breast because this is the location of most of the glandular tissue. A slow-growing breast cancer may take up to 10 or more years

to become palpable, or to reach the size of a small pea. Slow-growing lesions are often associated with a lower mortality rate. When referring to estimated growth rate of breast cancer, the term *doubling time* indicates the time it takes malignant cells to double in number. Assuming that the doubling is constant and that the neoplasm originates in one cell, a carcinoma with a doubling time of 100 days may not reach clinically detectable size (1 cm) for 8 years. Rapid-growing cancers have a much shorter preclinical course and a greater tendency to metastasize to regional nodes or more distant sites by the time a breast mass is discovered. In breast cancer, metastasis is by the lymphatic system and bloodstream (Figure 12-14). The most common sites for metastasis are, in order, bones, lungs, pleura, breast site, central nervous system, and liver.

Clinical Manifestations

Breast cancer is detected as a lump or mammographic abnormality in the breast. Breast tumors are usually small, solitary, irregularly shaped, firm, nontender, and nonmobile. There may be a change in skin color, feelings of tenderness, puckering or dimpling (peau d'orange—skin appearance of an orange peel) of tissue, nipple discharge, retraction of the nipple, and axillary tenderness.

More than 90% of breast cancers are detected by the patient. Women should perform BSEs monthly, preferably 1 week after menses. Postmenopausal women should perform a BSE on the same day each month (Figure 12-15). If there are questionable findings, the patient should immediately contact her physician (see Patient Teaching box).

Diagnostic Tests

The essential factors in the early detection of breast cancer are the regular performance of BSE, regular clinical breast examination (CBE), and routine mammography.

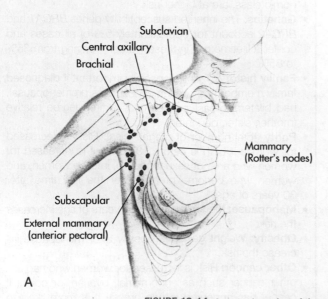

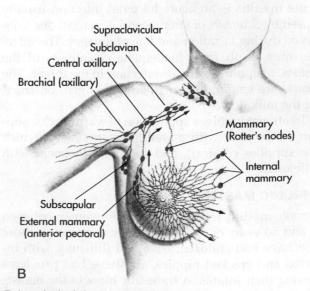

A

B

FIGURE 12-14 **A,** Lymph nodes of the axilla. **B,** Lymphatic drainage of the breast.

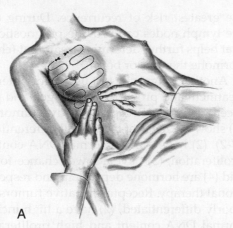

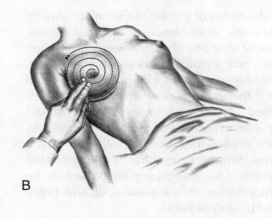

FIGURE 12-15 Methods for palpation. **A,** Back and forth. **B,** Concentric circles.

 Patient Teaching

Breast Self-Examination

- The majority of breast lumps are not cancer.
- Cancerous breast lesions are treatable.
- Breasts should be examined by premenopausal women each month, 7 or 8 days after conclusion of the menstrual period when they are least congested, and by postmenopausal women on the same day of each month.
- Visual inspection and palpation should be done.
- Visual inspection should be done when the woman is stripped to the waist and looking in a mirror, using the following arm positions: (1) arms at rest at sides, (2) hands on hips and pressed into hips, (3) contracting chest muscles, (4) hands over the head (torso in upright position), (5) hands over head (torso leaning forward).
- Palpation may be done in the shower when the soap and water help the hands glide over the skin. However, examination of large breasts and axillae is better done in a supine position rather than standing.
- The entire breast should be examined in a systematic way, moving clockwise, with a circular motion, or moving back and forth. Always include the axillae in the examination.
- Do not forget specific examination of the nipple, through compression for discharge, and the areola, through palpation.
- Report any changes to the physician.

The frequency of these examinations is determined by the woman's age, the presence of significant risk factors, and her medical history. Current guidelines accepted by the ACS (ACS, 2009a) regarding breast surveillance practices include the following:

- Monthly BSE starting at 20 years of age.
- Physical examinations of the breast by a trained health professional; CBE every 3 years between 20 and 40 years of age and every year for women 40 and older.
- Screening mammography annually beginning at 40 years of age. If first-degree family member has a history of breast cancer, screening mammogram is recommended at 35 years (ACS, 2007b).
- MRI screening for the following groups of women: women with 20% to 25% or greater lifetime risk

of breast cancer, women with a strong family history of breast or ovarian cancer, and women who were treated for Hodgkin's disease and received chest radiation.

New guidelines from the U.S. Preventative Services Task Force (USPSTF) (2009) recommend the following: (1) women age 40 to 49 should not receive routine screening mammography for breast cancer, but these women should decide for themselves when to begin mammography after weighing the risks and benefits; (2) women age 50 to 74 should receive screening mammography every 2 years (instead of annually); (3) routine breast self-examination (BSE) should no longer be taught. The Task Force states that this is not a recommendation against mammography for women in their 40s and BSE, but that there is not enough evidence to prove that women benefit from them. The ACS (2009b) and the American Congress of Obstetricians and Gynecologists (ACOG) (2009) state they will *not* be changing their guidelines.

Several techniques can be used to screen for breast disease or diagnose a suspicious physical finding. Mammography is a radiographic technique used to visualize the internal structure of the breast. Approximately 2 million women have mammograms annually. Mammography can detect tumors that cannot be felt by palpation. The minimum size detectable by physical examination is 1 cm. It takes 10 or more years to grow a tumor this size. Mammography can detect masses of 0.5 cm. Because tumors usually metastasize late in the preclinical course, earlier detection by mammography may prevent metastasis of smaller lesions.

Comparative mammography may show early cancer tissue changes. The diagnostic accuracy of mammography in combination with physical examination has significantly improved early and accurate detection of breast malignancies. In younger women, mammography is less sensitive because of the greater density of breast tissue, resulting in more false-negative results. Mammography will not reveal 10% to 25% of breast cancers. Masses should be biopsied, even if mammogram findings are unremarkable.

Definitive diagnosis of a mass can be made only by means of histologic examination of biopsied tissues. Biopsy technique may be either fine-needle aspiration (FNA) biopsy and cytologic examination or core-cutting needle biopsy, excisional biopsy, and incisional biopsy. Even if the lesion is nonpalpable, an FNA biopsy can be used. FNA and cytologic evaluation should be done only if an experienced cytologist is available, and all lesions read as negative are followed with a more definitive biopsy procedure. If the aspirated specimen is positive for malignancy, the patient can be given this information at the same visit and begin learning about treatment issues.

Improved imaging techniques have reduced the radiation exposure that accompanies mammography to insignificant levels. Therefore the benefits of mammography outweigh the risks from radiation exposure. Ultrasound (echogram, sonogram) can also be used to differentiate a benign cyst (fluid filled) from a malignant mass (solid). An ultrasound will not detect microcalcifications, which are often the only indicators of very small tumors.

Other methods used to help diagnose and stage breast cancer include MRI and positron emission tomography (PET). MRI and PET scans are used to help differentiate between malignant and benign disease in select patients.

A relatively new diagnostic tool used before therapeutic surgery is sentinel lymph node mapping, which identifies the first lymph node most likely to drain the cancerous cells. During this procedure a radioactive substance is injected around the breast biopsy site. The patient is then sent to the operating room, where a blue dye is injected as well. The area is then monitored to see which nodes take up the substances. The node that "lights up," containing the most radioactivity and blue dye, is considered the sentinel node and the one most likely to contain cancer cells. The identified node and at least two other nodes are then biopsied to see if they contain tumor cells. If they do not, it is likely that the more distant axillary nodes are cancer free. The nodes can be left intact, reducing the threat of complications such as edema, infection, pain, and loss of function of the arm. Sentinel lymph node dissection has been associated with lower morbidity rates and greater accuracy compared with complete axillary node dissection. National clinical research trials are evaluating whether standard lymph node dissection can be avoided if sentinel lymph node dissection is performed (Lewis et al., 2007). If one or more sentinel lymph nodes are positive for malignant cells, generally an axillary lymph node dissection is recommended (Lewis et al., 2007).

Axillary lymph node involvement is one of the most important prognostic factors in early-stage breast cancer. Metastasis in axillary nodes can be determined by pathologic examination of as few as 6 to 10 nodes. The more nodes involved, the greater the risk of recurrence. Patients with four or more positive nodes have the greatest risk of recurrence. During examination, the lymph nodes can provide prognostic information that helps further determine treatment (chemotherapy, hormone therapy, or both).

Another diagnostic test useful for determining both treatment and prognosis is estrogen and progesterone receptor status. Receptor-positive tumors commonly (1) show evidence of being well differentiated (see Box 17-2), (2) have a more normal DNA content and low proliferation, (3) have a lower chance for recurrence, and (4) are hormone dependent and responsive to hormonal therapy. Receptor-negative tumors (1) are often poorly differentiated, (2) have a high incidence of abnormal DNA content and high proliferation, (3) frequently recur, and (4) are usually unresponsive to hormonal therapy (Lewis et al., 2007).

Medical Management

The intervention for treatment of breast cancer depends on the tumor stage, the patient's age and health, the hormonal status, and the presence of estrogen receptors in the tumor. Radiation, chemotherapy, and surgery alone or in combination are the most common modes of treatment for breast cancer (see Chapter 17).

Staging

After breast surgery and axillary dissection, the staging process is completed. Axillary lymph node dissection or sentinel lymph node mapping is usually performed regardless of the treatment option selected. Examination of nodes provides the most powerful prognostic data currently available. Also, removal of axillary nodes is highly effective in preventing axillary recurrence, aids in decision making regarding adjuvant chemotherapy or hormonal therapy, and eliminates the need for axillary nodal radiation. Radiation of the axilla is equally effective in decreasing the incidence of axillary recurrence (see Figure 12-14).

The most widely accepted staging method for breast cancer is the American Joint Committee on Cancer's TNM system. This system uses tumor size (T), nodal involvement and size (N), and presence of metastasis (M) to determine the stage of disease (Box 12-6). Tumors are classified from stage I to stage IV.

Surgical Intervention

Surgery plays a vital role in the management of breast cancer. Tissue biopsy, inspection and biopsy of lymph nodes in the axillary areas, radiologic examinations, and laboratory reports aid in making the decision to perform surgery.

Because estrogen can affect a tumor's invasive ability, it is suggested to operate on premenopausal women during the menstrual phase, when estrogen levels are lower or opposed by progesterone.

Several surgical options are available for the removal of the breast carcinoma. **Breast conservation surgery**

Box 12-6	TNM System for Staging Breast Cancer

Breast cancer is staged using the TNM (tumor, node, metastasis) system, which categorizes the disease by tumor size and spread, lymph node involvement, and metastasis. The TNM system, which was developed by the American Joint Committee on Cancer and revised in 2003, works this way:

- **Tumor:** A number from **0** to **4** indicates the tumor's size and whether it has spread to nearby tissue. (**Tis** indicates a carcinoma in situ.) Higher numbers indicate a larger tumor or wider spread. For example, a tumor labeled **T1** is 2 cm or smaller; **T4** indicates a tumor of any size that has spread to the chest wall or the skin.
- **Nodes:** A number from **0** to **3** indicates whether the cancer has spread to surrounding lymph nodes and, if so, the number of nodes that are affected. For example, **N1** indicates a spread to one, two, or three lymph nodes under the arm on the same side as the breast cancer.
- **Metastasis:** **M0** means the cancer has not spread to distant organs; **M1** means the cancer has metastasized to other organs.

All of this information is combined to determine an overall stage of **0** to **IV.**

- **Stage 0:** Refers to carcinoma in situ, in which the tumor is confined to the milk duct or the lobule, no nodes have been affected, and no metastasis has occurred.
- **Stage I:** The tumor is 2 cm or smaller. Lymph nodes are negative. There is no distant cancer spread.
- **Stage IIA:** The tumor is 5 cm or smaller. It may have spread to one, two, or three axillary nodes. There is no distant cancer spread.
- **Stage IIB:** The tumor can be larger than 5 cm. Up to three lymph nodes may be involved, but there is no metastasis to other organs.
- **Stage IIIA:** The tumor may be more than 5 cm and has spread to more than 3 but fewer than 10 lymph nodes. No distant organs are involved.
- **Stage IIIB:** The tumor, regardless of size, has spread to the chest wall or the skin. There is lymph node involvement but no distant metastasis.
- **Stage IIIC:** Refers to any size tumor, including one that has spread to the chest wall or the skin. There is involvement of 10 or more lymph nodes, but no distant metastasis.
- **Stage IV:** The tumor can be any size. There is nodal involvement and metastasis to distant organs.

American Cancer Society (ACS). (2009). *How is breast cancer staged?* Available at www.cancer.org/docroot/CRI/content/CRI_2_4_3x_How_is_breast_cancer_staged_5.asp?mav=cri. Accessed November, 2009; and Lewis, S.L., et al. (2007). *Medical-surgical nursing: assessment and management of clinical problems.* (7th ed.). St. Louis: Mosby.

(termed **lumpectomy**), which conserves the breast, is the removal of a circumscribed area along with the tumor. This surgery is usually done when the tumor is small and located on the peripheral area of the breast. The breast contour and muscle support are preserved if possible. Research has shown that there is no survival advantage in taking the whole breast when the malignancy is confined to just one area and its size is less than 2 cm—as long as adjunctive radiation to the surrounding region, ending with a radiation boost to the tumor bed, is done to destroy any remaining microscopic disease (Mirshahidi, 2004). Axillary nodes are often removed in these breast-sparing procedures as well. Contraindications to lumpectomy or excisional biopsy include two or more separate tumors in separate quadrants of the breast, diffuse microcalcifications, a history of previous radiation to the region, a large tumor-to-breast ratio, a history of collagen vascular disease, large breasts, and a tumor located underneath the nipple.

One of the main advantages of breast conservation surgery and radiation is that it preserves the breast, including the nipple. The goal of the combined surgery and radiation is to maximize the benefits of both cancer treatment and cosmetic outcome while minimizing risks. Disadvantages of this surgery plus radiation include the increased cost over surgery alone and the possible side effects of radiation. Lumpectomy is followed by 6 weeks of radiation.

A **simple mastectomy** is the removal of the entire breast. The skin flap is retained to cover the incised area. Both pectoralis major and pectoralis minor muscles are left intact. The patient has the option of breast reconstruction.

A **modified radical mastectomy** may be performed if the tumor is 4 cm or larger, if it is invasive, or if the patient and physician decide this procedure is in the patient's best interest. In this operation all breast tissue, overlying skin, nipple, and pectoralis minor muscles are removed, as are samples of axillary lymph nodes and fascia under the breast. The pectoralis major muscle remains intact. The patient has the option of breast reconstruction, which can be performed immediately after the mastectomy or can be delayed until postoperative recovery is complete (about 6 months).

Most women diagnosed with early-stage breast cancer (tumors less than 5 cm) are candidates for either lumpectomy and radiation or modified radical mastectomy. Overall 10-year survival with lumpectomy and radiation is about the same as with modified radical mastectomy (Mirshahidi, 2004).

Adjuvant Therapies

Radiation therapy. Depending on the tumor's size, regional spread, and aggressiveness, radiation therapy is often prescribed. Radiation therapy may be used for breast cancer (1) as the primary therapy to destroy the tumor or as a companion to surgery to prevent local recurrence, (2) to shrink a large tumor to operable size, and (3) as the palliative treatment for pain caused by local recurrence and metastasis. Lumpectomy is almost always followed by radiation. Radiation therapy is usually started 2 to 3 weeks after surgery, when the wound is completely healed and the patient can comfortably raise her arm over her head. Contraindications include a diagnosis of breast cancer during the first or second trimester of pregnancy, delayed wound healing, collagen vascular disease, and previous radiation to the same breast.

In **external beam radiation,** the radiation procedure uses an external beam of high-energy protons. The treatments are usually done 5 days a week for 5 to 6 weeks. Adverse effects include fatigue and skin reactions such as burning, erythema, pruritus, dryness, infection, and pain.

Internal radiation, also known as implant radiation or **brachytherapy,** is a new procedure that is an alternative to traditional radiation treatment for early-stage breast cancer. The technique uses a balloon catheter to insert radioactive seeds into the breast after the tumor is removed (at the time of the lumpectomy or shortly thereafter into the tumor resection cavity). The seeds deliver a high dose of concentrated radiation directly to the site where the cancer is most likely to recur. Traditional radiation treatment can take 6 weeks; in contrast, high-dose brachytherapy may require only 5 days (Lewis et al., 2007).

Chemotherapy. Patients who require postsurgical chemotherapy—typically those with lymph node involvement or metastasis to distant organs—receive antineoplastic medications, hormones, a monoclonal antibody, or a combination of these medications. Regimens for node-negative disease (i.e., cancer that has not spread to the lymph nodes) include cyclophosphamide (Cytoxan, Neosar), methotrexate, and 5-fluorouracil (Adrucil, Efudex), referred to as CMF; cyclophosphamide, doxorubicin (Adriamycin), and 5-fluorouracil, or CAF; or doxorubicin and cyclophosphamide, commonly called AC. For those with node-positive disease, the regimens include CAF, AC followed by paclitaxel, doxorubicin followed by CMF, and CMF.

The most common adverse effects of traditional antineoplastic drugs are bone marrow suppression (which causes anemia, thrombocytopenia, and leukopenia), nausea and vomiting, alopecia, weight gain, mucositis, and fatigue. Agents such as filgrastim (Neupogen), which raise leukocyte counts, can combat the threat of infection that accompanies bone marrow suppression. Epoetin alfa (Procrit) is helpful in raising erythrocyte counts to help correct anemia. Other drugs typically ordered for chemotherapy patients are phenothiazines, such as prochlorperazine (Compazine), and serotonin antagonists such as granisetron (Kytril) and ondansetron (Zofran). These drugs prevent or lessen nausea and vomiting (Greifzu, 2004).

Hormonal therapy. Estrogen can promote the growth of breast cancer cells if the cells are estrogen-receptor positive. Hormonal therapy removes or blocks the source of estrogen, thus promoting tumor regression.

Two advances have increased the use of hormonal therapy in breast cancer. First, hormone receptor assays, which are reliable diagnostic tests, have been developed to identify women who are likely to respond to hormonal therapy. The tumor's estrogen and progesterone receptor status can be determined. These assays can predict whether hormonal therapy is a treatment option for women with breast cancer, either at the time of initial therapy or if the cancer recurs. Second, drugs have been developed that can inactivate the hormone-secreting glands as effectively as surgery or radiation. Premenopausal and perimenopausal women are more likely to have tumors that are not hormone dependent, whereas women who are postmenopausal are more likely to have hormone-dependent tumors. Chances of tumor regression are significantly greater in women whose tumors contain estrogen and progesterone receptors.

Estrogen deprivation can occur by destroying the ovaries by surgery or radiation or drug therapy. Hormonal therapy can block or destroy the estrogen receptors. Hormonal therapy is widely used to treat recurrent or metastatic cancer but may also be used as an adjuvant to primary treatment.

Tamoxifen is the hormonal agent of choice in postmenopausal, estrogen receptor–positive women with or without lymph node involvement. Tamoxifen, an antiestrogen drug, blocks the estrogen receptor sites of malignant cells and thus inhibits the growth-stimulating effects of estrogen. It is commonly used in advanced and early-stage breast cancer to prevent or treat recurrent disease. Tamoxifen may also be used to prevent breast cancer in high-risk individuals. Side effects of tamoxifen are minimal but include hot flashes, nausea, vomiting, vaginal discharge, and other effects commonly associated with decreased estrogen. It also increases the risk of blood clots, cataracts, and endometrial cancer in postmenopausal women. Tamoxifen is not used in women desiring continued fertility.

Toremifene (Fareston), an antiestrogen agent similar to tamoxifen, is indicated as first-line treatment for metastatic breast cancer in postmenopausal women with estrogen receptor–positive or estrogen receptor–unknown tumors. Fulvestrant (Faslodex) may be given to women with advanced breast cancer who no longer respond to tamoxifen. This drug slows cancer progression by destroying estrogen receptors in the breast cancer cells. Fulvestrant is given intramuscularly on a monthly basis.

Aromatase inhibitor drugs, which interfere with the enzyme that synthesizes endogenous estrogen, are used to treat advanced breast cancer in postmenopausal women with disease progression. These drugs include anastrozole (Arimidex), letrozole (Femara), vorozole (Rizivor), exemestane (Aromasin), and aminoglutethimide (Cytadren).

Research has shown that letrozole reduced the risk of recurrence of breast cancer among women by 43%. The women in the letrozole study had recently completed (after surgery) the standard 5-year course of tamoxifen, a powerful and widely used drug that eventually loses its effectiveness as, researchers believe, tumors become resistant to it. Until now, breast cancer patients who finished tamoxifen treatment could only wait and hope that their cancer would not recur; however, in up to 20% of such cases, it does recur within 5 years. Letrozole, previously approved by the FDA for advanced breast cancer, offers an exciting new option for extending treatment of early-stage disease (Kudachadkar & O'Regan, 2005). Letrozole, like tamoxifen, works by interfering with the hormone estrogen, which feeds breast cancer cells. Tamoxifen blocks estrogen receptors on the cells, whereas letrozole inhibits the creation of estrogen.

Bisphosphonates, such as pamidronate sodium (Aredia), are being used to delay bone metastases and reduce the occurrence of skeletal problems in patients with advanced breast cancer (Greifzu, 2004). Raloxifene (Evista), used to prevent bone loss, may also reduce the risk of breast cancer without stimulating endometrial growth. Raloxifene acts as an estrogen antagonist at the hormone-sensitive tissues of breast cancer and bone. Additional drugs that may be used to suppress hormone-dependent tumors include megestrol (Megace), DES, and fluoxymesterone (Halotestin) (Lewis et al., 2007).

Monoclonal antibody therapy. A recent drug treatment for breast cancer is the monoclonal antibody trastuzumab (Herceptin). It is used to treat metastatic breast cancer in women who overexpress (i.e., have an excess amount of) a breast cancer cell antigen called HER_2. Up to 30% of patients fall into this category.

Ovarian ablation. Another promising treatment option is **ovarian ablation** by means of a bilateral oopho-rectomy, which is used in combination with tamoxifen for metastatic disease.

Bone marrow and stem cell transplantation. Autologous (i.e., originating within self) bone marrow or stem cell transplantation combined with high-dose chemotherapy has been used to treat patients with advanced metastatic breast cancer. In this technique, patients donate their own bone marrow or peripheral blood, from which stem cells are harvested. Then they receive high doses of chemotherapy, which causes bone marrow suppression. The patient subsequently undergoes autologous bone marrow or stem cell transplantation to reconstitute or "rescue" their hematopoietic system to start producing hematopoietic blood cells.

Nursing Interventions

The physician discusses with the patient and the family the rationale for the specific surgical approach and the manner of coping with the cosmetic effects of and psychological response to the surgery. Patients will have questions about possible alternatives to standard or modified mastectomy.

The patient may be confused with so many options for therapy and surgical interventions. During this time, play an active role as listener, reinforce information provided by the physician, and encourage the patient to verbalize her concerns and recognize her feelings about the surgery. The emotional preparation of the patient may be more important than the physical preparation. Often she undergoes anticipatory grieving for the loss of a body part.

Preoperative preparation involves patient, support group, and nursing staff so that progressive care can run

---

⭐ **Nursing Care Plan 12-1** | **The Patient Undergoing Modified Radical Mastectomy**

Ms. Ceba, age 52, was diagnosed with ductal cell carcinoma of the left breast. She has undergone a left modified radical mastectomy

NURSING DIAGNOSIS *Fear, related to the cancer diagnosis and surgical intervention*

Patient Goals and Expected Outcomes	Nursing Interventions	Evaluation
Patient will be able to state fears Patient will state she has made improvement in coping	Encourage patient to talk about specific fears and feelings about each fear. Provide a calm, supportive environment. Provide information on coping mechanisms. Encourage consultation with resource persons (psychologist, clergy, nurse specialist, Reach to Recovery). Use support of family and significant others. Encourage use of comfort measures, such as music. Encourage patient's comments and questions about surgery and postoperative care.	Patient verbalizes fear, has support of significant others, and expresses confidence in ability to cope.

Continued

★ Nursing Care Plan 12-1 | The Patient Undergoing Modified Radical Mastectomy—cont'd

NURSING DIAGNOSIS *Infection, risk for, related to surgical incision and presence of drain*

Patient Goals and Expected Outcomes	Nursing Interventions	Evaluation
Skin will remain free of signs and symptoms of infection Vital signs and white blood cell (WBC) values will be maintained within normal limits	Assess skin integrity. Instruct patient on signs and symptoms of infection. Assess and report abnormal vital signs and elevated WBC; skin changes; and comfort level. Observe and record amount of exudate. Check drainage tubing for patency. Instruct patient to examine remaining breast once a month. Caution patient to avoid injections, vaccinations, taking of blood pressure, taking of blood samples, or insertion of intravenous line in affected area.	Incision has no erythema or purulent drainage. Temperature remains within normal. WBC remains normal.

NURSING DIAGNOSIS *Body image, disturbed, related to loss of breast through modified radical mastectomy*

Patient Goals and Expected Outcomes	Nursing Interventions	Evaluation
Patient will verbalize acceptance of altered body image as evidenced by absence of weeping, irritability, or verbalization of discomfort with present body; and by the attempting of difficult physical or mental tasks despite limitations Patient will demonstrate interest in her personal appearance Patient will verbalize plans to resume former activities	Encourage patient's comments and questions about surgery, progress, and prognosis. Encourage patient to discuss change in her body with husband or significant other. Reinforce correct information, and provide factual information to correct any misconceptions. Relate importance of communicating anything that causes anxiety. Encourage patient to verbalize and explore feelings regarding impact missing body part might have on patient's functioning as a sexual partner and in activities of daily living. Encourage patient to continue activities associated with femininity, such as fixing hair, using makeup, and wearing own apparel. Encourage patient to look at and touch the changed body part when she is ready. Encourage use of rehabilitation services (Reach to Recovery, Wellness Community).	Patient verbalizes feelings about surgery and change in body image; indicates beginning resolution of negative feelings toward self; and begins to accept altered body image.

Critical Thinking Questions

1. Ms. Ceba confides in her nurse that she feels ugly and unattractive and she refuses to look at her incision. What would be a helpful approach by the nurse?
2. In assessing Ms. Ceba, the nurse notes her holding her left arm guardedly in an adducted position. She does not use it for activities of daily living. What should effective patient teaching include?
3. What should be included in discharge teaching for Ms. Ceba to prevent trauma and infection of her left arm?

continuously from admission through surgery, recovery, and the postoperative period. The initial admission assessment provides data that are helpful for the nurse and patient in planning care. Nursing diagnoses can be developed and a care plan individualized according to the patient's needs (Nursing Care Plan 12-1).

Assess and identify members of the patient's support system to know their strengths and concerns about the pending treatment and interventions. Support does not always need to come from the immediate family and close friends. Outside support and resources can come from co-workers, religious groups, oncology clinicians, psychologists, and Reach to Recovery support groups. It is important to openly discuss the patient's fears; establishing a therapeutic relationship with the patient and family enables this to happen.

Reach to Recovery volunteers are a source of information, encouragement, and support for women with breast cancer. The organization is based on the premise that rehabilitation for the cancer patient should include communication with and support from another who was in a similar situation and learned to cope and resume her normal activities.

Nursing interventions for patients who undergo modified radical mastectomy include monitoring vital signs and observing for symptoms of shock or hemorrhage, since many large blood vessels are involved in the procedure. Drains such as Jackson-Pratt, Davol, or Hemovac may be placed in the axilla to facilitate drainage and prevent formation of a hematoma. Postoperative dressings are usually constrictive and bulky and may tend to impede respiratory effort and cause pain and discomfort. Assess for excessive exudates on the dressing and in the axillary region. Place a smaller, less bulky dressing over the incisional site for the first postoperative day. When the vital signs are stable, place the patient in a 45-degree Fowler's position to promote drainage. Change the position frequently, and encourage deep breathing and coughing.

Some patients may experience incisional pain for several days after surgery and when doing arm exercises. They may complain of numbness and referred pain in the arm of the operative area. The pain radiates to the shoulder and the back because of the severance of the peripheral nerves. Most of the nerves regenerate, but there are cases of residual numbness.

No matter what type of surgery the patient has, pain management and wound care are priorities. Typically a patient will have a patient-controlled analgesia pump with morphine for 12 to 24 hours. She then receives oral analgesics as needed.

Patient Teaching

It is important for the patient to deep breathe and cough to prevent postoperative atelectasis.

Physicians differ in opinion about the best position for the affected arm. Some physicians place the arm in the dressing and place it in a sling for a couple of days postoperatively. Some physicians prefer to avoid slings. If the arm is not restricted by dressings, it may be elevated on a pillow with the hand and wrist higher than the elbow and the elbow higher than the shoulder joint. This will facilitate the flow of fluids through the lymph and venous routes and prevent lymphedema (accumulation of lymph in soft tissues).

Usually the patient is allowed to ambulate on the first postoperative day. She needs assistance in moving out of bed as she learns to maintain balance because of breast removal and bulky dressings.

Instruct the patient not to have any procedures involving the arm on the affected side—blood pressure readings, injections, IV infusion of fluids, or the drawing of blood, which may cause edema or infection. She also needs to guard against infections from burns, needle pricks (sewing), and gardening injuries because defense mechanisms are lessened by the removal of lymph nodes. Removing lymph nodes and channels increases the risk of developing lymphedema, even years after surgery. Referral to physical therapy may be indicated to control lymphedema if it develops. An exercise regimen, built up gradually, can help decrease lymphedema. However, exercise should not be started until the incision has healed completely, which takes up to 2 weeks or at the physician's discretion. Tell the patient to avoid lifting heavy objects with the affected arm for 6 to 8 weeks. Instruct her to avoid sleeping on the involved arm. Clothing on the affected arm should be nonconstricting. Bracelets and watches should be worn on the unaffected arm (Box 12-7).

The longer the edema persists, the more difficult it is to manage. Diuretics and low-sodium diets are often prescribed. If the edema persists, an elastic stockinette is measured for precise fit to avoid venous flow constriction. The sleeve is applied from the wrist to the shoulder and worn when the patient is out of bed. When the patient is sleeping, position the arm to aid venous flow. If the lymphedema is severe, the physician may order Jobst extremity therapy. A pneumo-massage sleeve with automatic inflation and deflation can be placed on the arm. The compression pump is strictly contraindicated when there is evidence of acute phlebitis, perivascular lymphangitis, or cellulitis.

Isometric exercises are helpful for increasing the circulation and developing the collateral lymph system. The patient can open and clench fingers and squeeze a rubber ball in the first few postoperative days. This activity provides extension and flexion of the wrist and elbow; it is equivalent to sewing, knitting, typing, and playing piano when at home.

Preventing Muscle Contractures

Specific exercises may be ordered to restore the muscle strength and full range of motion of the affected area. Gentle exercises started early in the postoperative course help to decrease muscle tension and to regain

| Box 12-7 | Hand and Arm Care after Breast Surgery |

PREVENTION OF INFECTION
- Wear gloves when cleaning with harsh detergent.
- Wear gloves when gardening.
- Avoid injections, vaccinations, and venipuncture in involved arm.
- Use cuticle remover rather than cutting cuticles.
- Sew with a thimble.
- Avoid chapped hands; use lanolin cream daily.
- Take care when using equipment that might cut, scrape, or abrade.
- Shave underarms with an electric razor.
- Avoid insect bites; use insect repellent.

PREVENTION OF CONSTRICTING CIRCULATION
- Do not take blood pressure in involved arm.
- Wear loose clothing; avoid tight bra straps or tight sleeves.
- Wear watch or jewelry on uninvolved arm.
- Carry purse on uninvolved arm or shoulder.
- Prevent drag or pull:
  —Carry heavy packages on uninvolved arm.
  —Avoid motions that increase centrifugal force.

PREVENTION OF BURNS
- Wear padded mitts to reach into oven; use potholders.
- Prevent sunburn; use sunscreens with SPF of 15; cover arms during prolonged exposure.
- **Immediately report any signs of erythema, edema, warmth, or pain.**

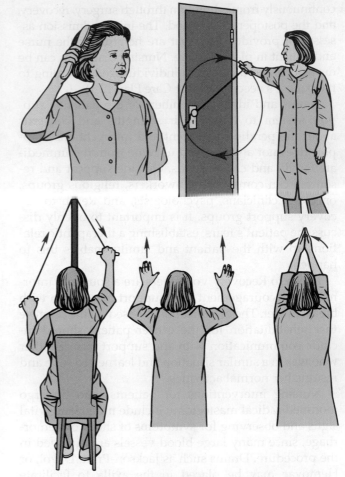

FIGURE 12-16 Exercises after mastectomy.

muscle function more quickly. The nurse or the therapist should instruct the patient and encourage the continuation of the exercises on discharge. Many of the exercises may be incorporated into ADLs as they are resumed (Figure 12-16; Box 12-8). Exercising can be painful, but the patient can meet the challenge with the encouragement of a support group.

Body Image Acceptance
After losing a breast, many patients experience grief over the loss of a body part. This acute grief is like a crisis and may last 4 to 6 weeks or longer. Grief makes the fact of loss real, and the process is essential for personal adaptation to the loss. Assist the patient in finding helpful coping mechanisms.

Initial coping mechanisms often begin to lose effectiveness at about 3 months, and a period of depression ensues. Provide anticipatory guidance for this eventuality. Special nursing interventions, in terms of both psychological support and self-care education, are necessary if the cancer recurs. Participation in a cancer support group is important and has been found to have a clinically significant impact on survival.

When deep breathing exercises are started immediately after surgery and the patient splints the area and exercises her arm, she will recognize the absence of the breast through touch. Dressing changes and incision cleansing with patient involvement make the absence

real. Being involved and responsible for the dressing and incision allows a more personal approach to the patient. At this time, the nurse's support is important. Provide a mirror or seat the patient in front of the mirror so she can see the operative site being cleansed and dressed. Be sensitive to the patient and be alert for signs of readiness to become involved in care and accept the loss of the body part. The incisional area may be erythematous and edematous, but the discoloration will gradually lessen and the site will become more comfortable. Encourage her to massage in cocoa butter or a cream to make the incisional line softer. Advise the patient that it takes time to accept the loss and heal both emotionally and physically.

Prosthesis
A breast prosthesis should not be worn unless authorized by the physician. Many breast forms are available. Forms are made of gels, molded silicone, and saline solution. Most forms are covered with soft fabric, are lightweight, and feel like breast tissue. There is a shape for each type of breast, since each body is different and each surgery is different. Forms have been developed that can be fitted for a right or left breast, slanted for the breast that was slanted, or formed with

Box 12-8   **Postmastectomy Arm Exercises**

CLIMBING THE WALL
1. Stand facing wall with toes 6 to 12 inches from wall.
2. Bend elbows and place palms of hands against wall at shoulder level.
3. Move both hands parallel to each other up the wall as far as possible until incisional pull or pain occurs.
4. Move both hands down to starting position.
5. Goal is complete extension with elbows straight.
6. Activities that use the same action include reaching top shelves, hanging out clothes, washing windows, hanging curtains, and setting hair.

ELBOW PULL-IN
1. Extend arms sideways to shoulder level.
2. Clasp hands behind neck.
3. Pull elbows forward until they touch.
4. Return to position 2.
5. Unclasp hands and extend arms sideways at shoulder level.
6. Lower arms to side.

BACK SCRATCH
1. Place hand of unoperated side on hip for balance.
2. Bend elbow of affected arm, placing back of hand on small of back.
3. Work hand up the back slowly until fingers reach opposite shoulder blade.
4. Lower arm and straighten both arms.

ROPE PULL
1. Attach a rope over a shower rod, a hook, or the top of an open door.
2. Sit on a chair (with door between legs If using a door) and grasp each end of rope.
3. Alternately pull on each end, raising affected arm to a point of incisional pull or pain.
4. The goal is to raise the affected arm almost directly overhead.

an outer curve that simulates the extension of a full breast under the axilla and upward on the chest. It is advisable to have a skilled fitter from a reliable company fit the prosthesis.

A well-fitted brassiere is essential before choosing the shape form. If the woman is active, she may desire a pocket or restraining cup. Some forms can be worn against the skin with no underpadding or bra cups. Most forms can be washed with water and mild detergent to keep them clean and supple. Many prostheses are waterproof and can be worn swimming; when wet, they do not "weigh down" the wearer.

When the patient is being fitted with a prosthesis, the best assurance that the fit is right is when each of the following is observed:

- The brassiere fits snugly around the rib cage.
- The prosthesis fills the bottom of the bra cup.
- The prosthesis projects the same as the remaining breast, with form bulk and nipples in position.
- The breasts are separated when the bra is centered.
- The top of the bra cup is filled and appears like the other breast.

Breast Reconstruction

The patient whose disease is limited to the breast may benefit from reconstructive surgery. The benefits of breast reconstruction include avoidance of an external prosthesis that has potential for slipping, greater choice of clothing (including lower necklines), and loss of self-consciousness about appearance. For many women, breast reconstruction is beneficial in improving self-esteem. Breast reconstruction can provide many women

with a renewed sense of wholeness and a return to a normal state. The most important indicators for reconstruction are the patient's motivation and desire for the procedure. The prime determinant for the procedure is the patient's clinical status. Goals for reconstruction are to select the simplest type that meets the patient's needs and expectations and to match the opposite breast in size, shape, and contour.

Breast reconstruction can be performed immediately after surgery or at a later time. An increasing number of women are electing immediate reconstruction; this may prolong the initial hospitalization but eliminates the need for a second hospitalization and contributes to self-esteem. Others wait until they have completed adjuvant chemotherapy or radiation to be certain the area is disease free.

Breast Implant

If the remaining skin is sufficient to cover an implant, surgery may consist of placing a permanent silicone implant under the pectoralis muscle. Possible complications of silicone implants include infection, deflation, a false mammography result, and silicone leaks.

Some researchers have suggested that the silicone filling or the implant covering can lead to autoimmune or connective tissue disease. Although most surgeries have not resulted in complications, differing opinions regarding the safety of breast implants led the FDA (2004) to issue some recommendations in early 1992. Breast implants were permitted after breast cancer surgery because of the offsetting positive contribution to recovery, but a moratorium was imposed on silicone implants solely for cosmetic purposes until data establishing safety could be provided. Many implants are now filled with saline or dextran instead of silicone.

Musculocutaneous Flap Procedure

Breast reconstruction. The musculocutaneous flap has made reconstruction possible for most patients who have undergone mastectomy, even when the pectoralis muscles have been removed or when nerve damage has resulted in muscle atrophy. The flap receives its blood supply from muscle, but it can include an overlying layer of skin. At the same time that this procedure is performed, a silicone or saline breast implant may be inserted; if enough pedicle tissue is available, no implant is needed.

Musculocutaneous flaps are most often taken from the back (latissimus dorsi muscle) or the abdomen (transverse rectus abdominis muscle). When the **latissimus dorsi musculocutaneous flap** is used for reconstruction, a block of skin and muscle from the patient's back is used to replace tissue removed during mastectomy (Figure 12-17, *E*). The **transverse rectus abdominis musculocutaneous (TRAM) flap** is the most frequently used flap operation for breast reconstruction. The rectus abdominis muscles are paired, flat muscles running from the ribcage down to the pubic bone. Arteries inside the muscle branch at many levels, and these branches supply blood to the fat and skin across a large expanse of the abdomen. In the TRAM technique, the surgeon elevates a large block of tissue from the lower abdominal area, but leaves it attached to the rectus muscle (Figure 12-17, *A* to *D*). This tissue is then tunneled under the skin or detached and placed as a "free flap" at the site of the breast reconstruction. The tissue is trimmed and shaped to form a breast mound similar to that of the opposite breast. An implant may be used in addition to the flap to achieve symmetry. The abdominal incision is closed in a fashion similar to that of an abdominal hysterectomy or a "tummy tuck." This surgical procedure can last 2 to 8 hours, with recovery taking 4 to 6 weeks. Complications include bleeding, hernia, and infection (Lewis et al., 2007).

Nipple reconstruction is usually performed as a separate procedure after the breast reconstruction has been completed. Nipple construction is generally from available tissue at the site or harvested tissue from the opposite breast. New techniques allow the nipple to be created from tissue and subcutaneous tissue of the breast mound. Areola reconstruction is provided by obtaining pigmented skin from the upper thigh or by using skin from the lateral chest area.

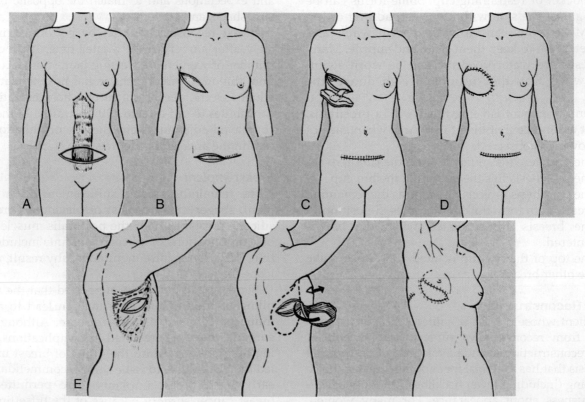

FIGURE 12-17 Transverse rectus abdominis musculocutaneous (TRAM) flap. **A,** TRAM flap is planned. **B,** The abdominal tissue, while attached to the rectus muscle, nerve, and blood supply, is tunneled beneath the abdomen to the chest. **C,** The flap is trimmed to shape the breast. The lower abdominal incision is closed. **D,** Nipple and areola are reconstructed after the breast has healed. **E,** In the latissimus dorsi musculocutaneous flap, a block of skin and muscle from the patient's back is used to replace tissue removed during mastectomy.

Table 12-3	Prognosis and Nodal Involvement in Breast Cancer	
LYMPH NODES INVOLVED	**METASTATIC RECURRENCE**	
1-3 nodes	50%-60% metastasis	
4-9 nodes	75%-85% metastasis	
10 nodes	Even worse prognosis	

🏠 Home Care Considerations

Cancer of the Breast

- Explain the follow-up routine to the patient and emphasize the importance of beginning and continuing breast self-examination and annual mammography.
- Symptoms that should be reported to the physician include new back pain, weakness, constipation, shortness of breath, and confusion.
- If adjuvant therapy is to be used, give the woman specific instructions about appointment times and treatment locations.
- If applicable, stress the importance of wearing a well-fitting prosthesis. The return of a normal external appearance is important to most women.
- Often the husband, sexual partner, or family member may need assistance in dealing with their emotional reactions to the diagnosis and surgery for them to effectively support the patient.
- If difficulty in adjustment or other problems develop, counseling may be necessary for women with breast cancer to deal with the emotional component of a modified radical mastectomy and the diagnosis of cancer.

Prognosis

The 5-year relative survival rate for localized breast cancer is 98%, with an 89% 5-year relative survival rate for all stages combined (ACS, 2007a). After the disease spreads beyond the breast, the survival rate drops dramatically. Breast cancer ranks second among cancer deaths in women. The most important prognostic factor is the stage of the disease (see Box 12-6; Table 12-3; Home Care Considerations box).

INFLAMMATORY AND INFECTIOUS DISORDERS OF THE MALE REPRODUCTIVE SYSTEM

PROSTATITIS

Etiology and Pathophysiology

Prostatitis is an acute or chronic infection of the prostate gland. Prostatitis is the most common problem involving the urinary system in men younger than 50 years. Bacterial invasion via the bloodstream and lymphatic channels, ascending from the urethra or descending from the bladder, commonly occurs (Lewis et al., 2007). The causative organisms include *E. coli, Klebsiella, Proteus, Pseudomonas, Streptococcus, N. gonorrhoeae,* and *C. trachomatis.*

Clinical Manifestations

Symptoms include sudden onset of chills and fever. There is urgency and frequency of urination, dysuria (pain when urinating), cloudy urine, perineal fullness,

perineal pain, lower back pain, arthralgia (pain in the joints), and myalgia (pain in the muscles). The patient may also have acute urinary retention caused by prostatic edema. On palpation, the gland is tender, edematous, and firm. In chronic prostatitis, many patients may appear asymptomatic, but generally the symptoms are the same as in the acute phase but less intense.

Diagnostic Tests

Diagnosis is based on culture and sensitivity tests of the urethra, prostatic fluid, and urine for organism identification and appropriate antibiotic therapy. Prostatic fluid is collected by prostate massage and expression of fluid. The pH of the fluid is generally elevated. A rectal examination done by the physician reveals gland tenderness and edema.

Medical Management

Medical management includes antibiotic therapy such as ofloxacin (Floxin), ciprofloxacin (Cipro) and sulfamethoxazole-trimethoprim (Bactrim). For patients who have multiple sex partners, doxycycline may be ordered. Oral antibiotics are given for up to 4 weeks for patients with acute prostatitis and 4 to 16 weeks for chronic prostatitis. The most common medications used for pain control are the antiinflammatory agents. Opioids should be used carefully because of the chronic nature of the pain (Lewis et al., 2007). Periodic digital massage of the prostate by the physician to increase the flow of infected prostatic secretions may be performed. Heat may be applied by means of sitz baths.

Nursing Interventions

Nursing interventions primarily focus on symptoms and include (1) a full explanation of antibiotic therapy and the need for compliance with treatment, which may be lengthy in chronic prostatitis; (2) supportive care such as bed rest to relieve strain and pain of the perineum and suprapubic area, sitz baths to promote muscle relaxation, and stool softeners to prevent straining on defecation; (3) monitoring of I&O; (4) bladder drainage with suprapubic catheterization if acute urinary retention develops into acute prostatitis (in acute prostatitis, passage of a catheter through an inflamed urethra is contraindicated); and (5) encouragement of follow-up for evaluation of the inflammation.

Nursing diagnoses and interventions for the patient with prostatitis include but are not limited to the following:

Nursing Diagnoses	Nursing Interventions
Acute pain, related to disease process	Assess type and location of pain; provide analgesics as ordered. Encourage bed rest to promote comfort.

Continued

Nursing Diagnoses	Nursing Interventions
Acute pain, related to disease process—cont'd	Provide nonpharmacologic comfort measures: • Assist patient with assuming comfortable position. • Provide diversional activity. • Provide a restful environment. Instruct patient in necessity of taking prescribed antibiotics and following orders for activity level.
Risk for situational low self-esteem, related to: • fear of impotence • embarrassment	Encourage patient to express feelings. Actively listen. Encourage adaptive coping behaviors.

Prognosis

Recurrent episodes of acute prostatitis may cause fibrotic tissue to form; such fibrosis causes a hardening of the prostate gland that may initially be confused with carcinoma.

EPIDIDYMITIS

Etiology and Pathophysiology

Epididymitis is an infection of the cordlike excretory duct of the testicle, usually secondary to an infectious process (sexually or nonsexually transmitted). It is one of the common infections of the male reproductive tract. The causative organisms are *S. aureus*, *E. coli*, streptococci, and *N. gonorrhoeae*. The inflammation is associated with urethral strictures, cystitis, and prostatitis.

Symptoms can occur after trauma to the genital area, after instrumentation of the urethra and cystoscopy, and after physical exertion or prolonged sexual activity.

Clinical Manifestations

Severe pain appears suddenly in the scrotum and radiates along the spermatic tube. Edema appears and the patient develops a "duck walk" or "waddling gait" because of the sensitivity and pain that walking stimulates. The scrotal area becomes tender. Pyuria (pus in urine) is present. Chills and fever are noted.

Diagnostic Tests

Diagnostic testing includes examination of the first daily flow of urine and delivery of a midstream specimen to the laboratory to check for pyuria. The epididymis is massaged by the physician, and a fluid expression specimen is sent to the laboratory. Physical examination of the scrotum is performed. Monitor the white blood cell count for leukocytosis.

Medical Management

Medical management includes a regimen of bed rest and support of the scrotum. The use of antibiotics is important for both partners, if the transmission is through sexual contact. Apply cold for relief of edema and discomfort, and administer the appropriate antibiotic. If abscess formation occurs, incision and drainage of the scrotum may be required.

Nursing Interventions

Nursing interventions for patients with epididymitis include (1) bed rest during the acute phase of illness; (2) support of the testicular area, with scrotal support by elevation of the scrotum on a folded towel during bed rest and athletic support when ambulatory; (3) ice compresses to the area in the initial phase to hasten recovery; (4) explanation of the need for compliance with antibiotic therapy until all signs of inflammation have disappeared; and (5) advice to refrain from sexual intercourse during the acute phase.

Prognosis

The infection can be bilateral and may recur. Bilateral epididymitis can cause sterility. Untreated epididymitis leads to necrosis of testicular tissue; in addition, abscesses can form, and septicemia can develop, which can be fatal.

DISORDERS OF MALE GENITAL ORGANS

PHIMOSIS AND PARAPHIMOSIS

Etiology and Pathophysiology

Phimosis is a condition in which the prepuce (foreskin) is too small to allow it to be retracted over the glans. Phimosis is often congenital but may be a result of local inflammation or disease. The condition is rarely severe enough to obstruct the flow of urine but may contribute to local infection because it does not permit adequate cleansing.

Paraphimosis is edema of the retracted uncircumcised foreskin, preventing normal return over the glans (Lewis et al., 2007). If the foreskin is not placed back in the forward position, an ulcer can develop. Paraphimosis can occur when the foreskin remains contracted during perineal cleansing, use of a urinary catheter, or intercourse. Treatment includes warm compresses; occasionally circumcision or dorsal slit of the prepuce is necessary. To prevent this problem, careful cleansing and replacement of the foreskin in the forward position are required (Lewis et al., 2007).

Medical Management

Circumcision may be performed, in which a part of the foreskin is removed, leaving the glans penis uncovered.

Nursing Interventions

After a circumcision a sterile petrolatum gauze dressing is applied and changed after each voiding. Observe the patient for unusual bleeding and obstruction of urine flow.

HYDROCELE

Etiology and Pathophysiology

A hydrocele is an accumulation of fluid between the membranes covering the testicle and the membrane enclosing the testicle. The scrotum slowly enlarges as the fluid accumulates. Diagnosis is fairly simple because the mass can be seen by shining a flashlight through the scrotum (transillumination). Pain occurs if the hydrocele develops suddenly. Most hydroceles occur in men older than 21 years of age, but it can occur in infants and children. The cause is not known, but it may develop as a result of trauma in the area, orchitis (inflammation of the testes), or epididymitis.

Medical Management

No treatment is indicated unless the edema becomes large and uncomfortable, in which case treatment includes aspiration of fluid from the sac or surgical removal of the sac to avoid constriction of the circulation of the testicles. After aspiration the pain is relieved and the scrotum can be examined more easily.

Nursing Interventions

Nursing interventions consist of maintaining bed rest, scrotal support with elevation, ice to edematous areas, and frequent changes of dressings to avoid skin impairment.

Prognosis

With treatment, prognosis is good.

VARICOCELE

Varicocele occurs when the veins within the scrotum become dilated. Obstruction and malfunctioning of the veins cause engorgement and elongation, which do not allow adequate drainage of the blood. The symptoms are a pulling sensation that causes a dull aching and pain accompanied by edema of the scrotal area. The treatment is surgical removal of the obstruction. Persistent varicoceles lead to infertility in 40% to 50% of cases (American Society for Reproductive Medicine Practice Committee, 2006). Nursing interventions include bed rest with scrotal support, ice on the incisional site, and medication for discomfort as ordered.

Ligation of the spermatic vein has been shown to improve semen quality.

CANCER OF THE MALE REPRODUCTIVE TRACT

The more common tumors of the male reproductive tract involve the testis, the prostate gland, and the penis. Most tumors of the male reproductive system are malignant. (See Chapters 10 and 17 for cancer of prostate gland.)

CANCER OF THE TESTIS (TESTICULAR CANCER)

Etiology and Pathophysiology

Testicular cancer is relatively uncommon, accounting for less than 1% of all cancers found in males. However, cancer of the testis is the most common malignancy in men 15 to 35 years of age (NCI, 2009b). The causes are unknown. The incidence of this cancer is higher in men with cryptorchidism (failure of testes to descend into the scrotum). Other associated factors are testicular atrophy, orchitis, and scrotal trauma. Most testicular cancers develop from embryonic germ cells. The two types of germ cell cancers are seminomas and nonseminomas. Although seminomas are the most common, they are the least aggressive. Nonseminoma testicular germ cell tumors are rare and very aggressive.

Clinical Manifestations

Testicular cancer may have a slow or rapid onset, depending on the type of tumor. The signs and symptoms of early disease include an enlarged scrotum and a firm, nontender, painless, smooth mass in the testicular area. Some patients complain of a dull ache or heavy sensation in the lower abdomen, perianal area, or scrotum. Acute pain is the presenting symptom in about 10% of patients.

Diagnostic Tests

Palpation of the scrotal contents is the first step in diagnosing testicular cancer. A cancerous mass is firm and does not transilluminate. Ultrasound of the testes is indicated when testicular cancer is suspected (e.g., a palpable mass) or persistent or painful testicular edema is present. If a testicular neoplasm is suspected, obtain blood to determine the serum levels of alpha-fetoprotein, lactate dehydrogenase, and hCG. A chest radiograph and CT scan of the abdomen and pelvis are obtained to detect metastasis.

Medical Management

Radical inguinal orchiectomy is usually the treatment of choice. This is the removal of the testis, epididymis, a portion of the gonadal lymphatics, and their blood supply. The remaining testis provides enough testosterone to maintain the man's sexual characteristics. He may have a lower sperm count and decreased sperm mobility. Surgery is generally followed by radiation or chemotherapy. Often a retroperitoneal lymph node dissection is performed to remove affected nodes and assist in determining the tumor stage. Staging a testicular tumor helps determine treatment.

Nursing Interventions and Patient Teaching

The most important aspect of care of patients who have or are at risk for a tumor of the testis is early detection by testicular self-examination (TSE). Young men should be taught to perform TSE monthly beginning at puberty. Video media and illustrations are available as teaching aids and ideally should be introduced during high school or college physical education classes. Information about TSE is available at the ACS and other websites (Lewis et al., 2007). The examination takes 3 minutes and should be done monthly. The best time to perform a TSE is after a warm shower when the scrotal skin is relaxed. The scrotum is checked for color, contour, and skin breaks. The left side is usually longer because the left testicle is suspended from a longer spermatic cord. Each testicle is gently palpated by grasping the scrotum in the center with the thumb and index finger (see Patient Teaching box; Figure 12-18). Normal testicles are firm but somewhat resilient, smooth, and mobile. If a testicle is indurated (hardened), carcinoma is suspected.

Prognosis

With the advent of tumor markers (which indicate the presence of disease and enable the physician to monitor its response to treatment), early detection, refined surgery, and effective chemotherapy, 99% of the patients obtain complete remission. Survival rates are re-

 Patient Teaching

Testicular Self-Examination

- Examine the scrotum once a month.
- Perform testicular self-examination after a bath or shower when scrotum is warm and most relaxed.
- Grasp testis with both hands and palpate gently between thumb and index finger. The testis should feel smooth and egg shaped and be firm to touch.
- The epididymis, found behind the testis, should feel like a soft tube (see Figure 12-1 and Figure 12-18).

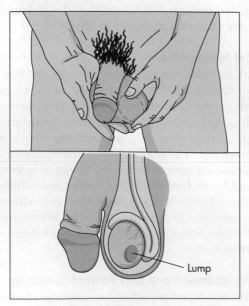

Lump

FIGURE 12-18 Testicular self-examination.

duced to 71% when cancer has spread to distant organs of the body, which emphasizes the need for early detection (ACS, 2009a).

CANCER OF THE PENIS

Etiology and Pathophysiology

Cancer of the penis is rare. It generally appears in men older than 50 years of age. Men who have not been circumcised, have not maintained good personal hygiene, or have had STIs are at risk.

Clinical Manifestations

The tumor is painless, and a wartlike growth or ulceration on the glans under the prepuce is present. It is common for metastasis to occur to the inguinal nodes and adjacent organs.

Diagnostic Tests

Biopsy confirms the diagnosis.

Medical Management

Surgical intervention requires removal of as little tissue as possible, but it may be necessary to do a partial or total amputation of the penis and to remove the adjacent tissue and inguinal lymph nodes. When metastasis involves the bladder and rectum, more radical surgery may be needed, and outlets for urinary or fecal elimination are provided by creating an ileal conduit and a colostomy. The surgeon may place a suprapubic catheter into the bladder to drain the urine.

Nursing Interventions

Nursing interventions include providing emotional support. If amputation of the penis is required, the patient faces the psychological trauma associated with the loss of sexuality and the ability to urinate naturally. Monitor urinary output by suprapubic catheter or, if an ileoconduit was performed, monitor urine in the urostomy bag. Elevation of the scrotum controls edema. Provide comfort measures to control pain.

SEXUALLY TRANSMITTED INFECTIONS

Today, despite sweeping advances in the diagnosis and treatment of communicable diseases, the incidence of infections transmitted through intimate or sexual activities continues to increase worldwide. STIs, previously called sexually transmitted diseases or venereal diseases, are infections that are usually transmitted during intimate sexual contact. They may have other routes of transmission (e.g., an infected mother to her newborn), occur with or without symptoms, and have long periods of asymptomatic infectivity.

Any sexually active person may be at risk for an STI. People who have frequent sexual contact with multiple partners are at increased risk. Commonly those most at risk are young, single, urban, poor, male, and homosexual. Because some STIs persist and are infectious for long periods (herpes genitalis, HIV), even people in mutually monogamous sexual relationships are at some risk. The proliferation of HIV since the late 1970s has produced an urgent reason to educate sexually active individuals about the risk of unprotected sexual contact.

Over one million people were living with HIV in the United States at the end of 2006, with an estimated 14,989 HIV-related deaths that year. Of those living with the infection, 278,400 (25%) were adolescent and adult women, and 11,000 were children under the age of 15. The number of new cases in the United States was 56,300, but the epidemic is growing at faster rates among women, people of color, people who live in poverty, and adolescents (CDC, 2006). In addition, treatment has provided major advances in the ability to keep HIV-infected people healthy for longer periods, and the death rate has fallen dramatically (Facts at a Glance, 2004) (see Chapter 16).

These are sobering statistics indeed. The number of people contracting the traditionally defined STIs (e.g., syphilis, gonorrhea) is even greater. Gonorrhea is estimated to infect 250 million people worldwide, and in 2004 more than 330,000 cases were reported in the United States. Annual syphilis incidence is about 50 million cases worldwide; in 2004, the total number of cases was 7980 in the United States. Since 2001, the incidence of syphilis has started to rise among women and men, particularly men who have sex with men (O'Rourke, 2007). No reliable statistics exist for the "new generation" STIs, such as trichomoniasis, herpes simplex virus (HSV), venereal warts, scabies, and others; these are probably even more prevalent now than in the past. In addition, bowel pathogens such as *Salmonella* organisms, amebas, hepatitis B, and hepatitis C may be sexually transmitted.

Despite the physical and emotional discomfort, the possibility of long-term disability (infertility, chronic infectivity), and advances in diagnosis and treatment that sharply decrease the period of infectivity, STIs continue to be among the world's most common communicable diseases. Four main factors are responsible: (1) unprotected sex, (2) antibiotic resistance, (3) treatment delay, and (4) sexual behavior patterns and permissiveness. The following is a discussion of some of the more commonly diagnosed STIs (see Safety Alert box).

GENITAL HERPES

Etiology and Pathophysiology
Genital herpes, or HSV, is an infectious viral disease characterized by recurrent episodes of acute, painful, erythematous, vesicular eruptions (blisters) on or in the genitalia or rectum. The two closely related forms are designated types 1 and 2. Most people are infected in infancy with type 1 during feeding or kissing by adults. There are infrequent recurrences around the

Safety Alert!
Sexually Transmitted Infections
- Teach "safe" sex practices including abstinence, monogamy with an uninfected partner, avoidance of certain high-risk sexual practices, and use of condoms and other barriers to limit contact with potentially infectious body fluids or lesions.
- All sexually active women should be screened for cervical cancer. Women with a history of STIs are at greater risk for cervical cancer than women without this history.
- Inform patients of the new HPV vaccine for girls and women ages 9 to 18 years to prevent HPV infection and the precancerous changes that lead to cervical cancer.
- Instruct patient in hygiene measures, such as washing and urinating after intercourse to destroy many causative organisms.
- Explain the importance of taking all antibiotics as prescribed. Symptoms improve after 1 or 2 days of therapy, but organisms may still be present.
- Teach patient about the need for treatment of sexual partners with antibiotics to prevent transmission of disease.
- Instruct patient to abstain from sexual intercourse during treatment and to use condoms when sexual activity is resumed to prevent spread of infection and reinfection.
- Explain the importance of follow-up examination and reculture at least once after treatment (if appropriate) to confirm complete cure and prevent relapse.
- Allow patient and partner to verbalize concerns to clarify areas that need explanation.
- Instruct patient about symptoms of complications and need to report problems to ensure proper follow-up and early treatment of reinfection.
- Explain precautions to take, such as being monogamous; asking potential partners about sexual history; avoiding sex with partners who use IV drugs or who have visible oral, inguinal, genital, perineal, or anal lesions; using condoms; and voiding and washing genitalia after coitus to reduce the occurrence of reinfection.
- Inform patient regarding state of infectivity to prevent a false sense of security, which might result in careless sexual practices and poor personal hygiene.

lips. HSV 2 is usually acquired sexually after puberty in the genital or anal regions.

Clinical Manifestations
Signs appear as fluid-filled vesicles after the incubation period. In women the vesicles usually occur on the cervix, which is considered the primary site, but may also be seen on the labia, rectum, vulva, vagina, and skin. In men vesicles are found on the glans penis, foreskin, and penile shaft (Figure 12-19). Other lesions may appear on the mouth and anus. Vesicles may rupture and develop into shallow, painful ulcers; they are erythematous with marked edema and tenderness. Lymph nodes may become involved. Initial lesions last from 3 to 10 days, and recurrent lesions have a duration of 7 to 10 days. The primary infection may be accompanied by fever; malaise; myalgia; dysuria; and, in women, leukorrhea. Sites are painful in the presence of fever, stress, or emotional upset or when exposed to

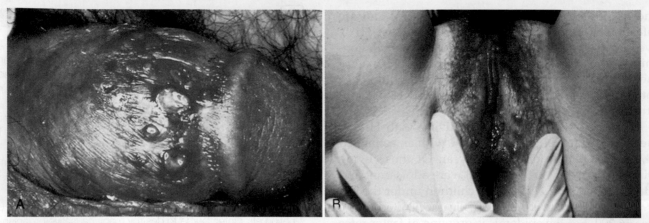

FIGURE 12-19 Herpes simplex virus type 2 in a male and female patient. Vesicular lesions on **A**, penis, and **B**, perineum.

intense heat. Urination may be painful from urine touching active lesions. Complications are rare.

Diagnostic Tests
Diagnosis is based on the physical examination and the patient history. The diagnosis is confirmed by appearance of the virus on tissue cultures. Cultures are more frequently positive when the lesions are from a primary infection versus recurrent infections. The Centers for Disease Control and Prevention (CDC, n.d.) recommend a serum serologic test for HSV 2 in addition to a viral tissue culture. These tests are highly accurate in diagnosing HSV 2 (Lewis et al., 2007).

Medical Management
The skin lesions of genital herpes heal spontaneously unless secondary infection occurs. Encourage symptomatic treatment such as practicing good genital hygiene and wearing loose-fitting cotton undergarments. The lesions should be kept clean and dry. Frequent sitz baths may soothe the area and reduce inflammation. Pain may require a local anesthetic such as lidocaine (Xylocaine) or systemic analgesics such as codeine and aspirin. Advise patients to abstain from sexual contact while lesions are present. However, sexual transmission of HSV has been documented even in the absence of clinical lesions; advise patients to use condoms.

Currently, acyclovir (Zovirax), which inhibits herpetic viral replication, is prescribed for primary infections or for suppression of frequent recurrences (more than six episodes per year). Although not a cure, acyclovir shortens the duration of viral shedding and the healing time of genital lesions and suppresses 75% of recurrences with daily use. Continued use of oral acyclovir for up to 5 years is safe and effective, but it should be interrupted after 1 year to assess the patient's rate of recurrent episodes. Adverse reactions to acyclovir are mild and include headache, occasional nausea and vomiting, and diarrhea. The safety of systemic acyclovir for treatment of pregnant women has not been established. Acyclovir ointment appears to be of no clinical benefit in the treatment of recurrent lesions, either in speed of healing or in resolution of pain. IV Acyclovir is reserved for severe or life-threatening infections in which hospitalization is required for the treatment of CNS infections (meningitis) or pneumonitis. Nephrotoxicity has been observed with high-dose IV use.

Two other antiviral agents are available for the treatment of HSV: valacyclovir (Valtrex) and famciclovir (Famvir). These purine analogs inhibit herpetic viral replication and are prescribed for primary and recurrent infections and to suppress frequent recurrences.

Nursing Interventions and Patient Teaching
Advise the patient to keep genital lesions clean and dry. Hands should be washed thoroughly after touching a lesion. Loose, absorbent underclothing is usually more comfortable than close-fitting clothing. Sitz baths decrease lesional discomfort and enhance urinary and bowel elimination. Teach the patient that sexual intercourse during the active lesion phase increases the risk of transmission and may also be painful. Patients should inform future sexual partners and health care providers of recurring or latent infections. Sexual transmission of HSV has been documented during asymptomatic periods; encourage the use of barrier methods, especially condoms. Inform the patient about the role of stress, poor nutrition, and insufficient rest in recurrences of signs and symptoms. Women patients need a yearly Pap test and should inform their physician in the event of pregnancy so that the disease can be monitored closely; there is a possibility of spontaneous abortion. Provide the patient with nonjudgmental support and with the contact number of the local herpes support group if one exists.

Prognosis
Genital herpes is a recurrent disease with no cure.

SYPHILIS
Etiology and Pathophysiology
The coiled spirochete *Treponema pallidum* causes syphilis. Congenital syphilis occurs in about 1 in 10,000 pregnancies, generally in minority populations. The

age-group with the highest incidence is 20 to 40 years. An increase in syphilis rates was noted from 2001 to 2007. In 2007 the total number of cases was 11,466. The increased incidence is mainly among men who have sex with men. The rates increased in whites, blacks, Hispanics, and Asians (CDC, 2007c).

Syphilis is the third most frequently reported communicable disease in the United States, exceeded only by varicella (chickenpox) and gonorrhea. Transmission occurs primarily through sexual contact during the primary, secondary, and latent stages of the disease. In addition to sexual contact, syphilis may be spread through contact with infectious lesions and sharing of needles among drug addicts. Prenatal infection from the mother to the fetus is possible. The organism thrives in the warm parts of the body and can be destroyed by soap and water. The spirochete penetrates intact skin and openings in the mucous membrane of the genital organs, rectum, and mouth.

Clinical Manifestations

Syphilis has four stages—primary, secondary, latent, and tertiary—each with its peculiar signs and symptoms. The signs and symptoms of syphilis include the clean-based chancre (painless erosion or papule that ulcerates superficially with a scooped-out appearance) of primary syphilis to the skin rashes of secondary syphilis. Moist, raised, gray to pink lesions of the genital or perirectal skin; enlarged lymph nodes; fever; fatigue; or infections of the eyes, bones, liver, or meninges may occur. In the late stages of syphilis, dementia, pain or loss of sensation in the legs, and destruction of the aorta occur. Destructive inflammatory masses can appear in any organ. In tertiary or late-stage syphilis the heart and blood vessels (cardiovascular syphilis) and the central nervous system (neurosyphilis) are frequently involved. Tabes dorsalis, paresis, and various psychoses may result.

Diagnostic Tests

Diagnostic tests include the Venereal Disease Research Laboratory (VDRL) slide test and rapid plasma reagin (RPR) test. All patients should be checked for gonorrhea as well.

Medical Management

Therapeutic management of syphilis is aimed at eradication of all syphilitic organisms. However, treatment cannot reverse damage that is already present in the late stage of the disease. Parenteral benzylpenicillin (penicillin G) remains the treatment of choice for all stages of syphilis. The parenteral route provides the highest concentration of antibiotic in the tissues (O'Rourke, 2007). To date, there is no evidence to suggest a decrease in the effectiveness of penicillin against *T. pallidum*. All stages of syphilis should be treated.

Appropriate antibiotic treatment of maternal syphilis before the eighteenth week of pregnancy prevents infection of the fetus. Appropriate treatment after 18 weeks

of pregnancy cures both mother and fetus because the antibiotics can cross the placental barrier. Treatment administered in the second half of pregnancy may pose a risk of premature labor. Some authorities recommend hospitalization and fetal monitoring of women at 20 weeks of gestation or later.

Carefully monitor all patients with neurosyphilis, with periodic serologic testing, clinical evaluation at 6-month intervals, and repeated cerebrospinal fluid examinations for at least 3 years. Specific therapeutic management is based on the specific symptoms.

Nursing Interventions

In addition to routine interventions for patients with STIs, monitor for drug reaction to penicillin, stress good handwashing technique, encourage follow-up visits with the physician, and inform the patient that he or she should absolutely not engage in sexual intercourse until cured.

Prognosis

Syphilis can be successfully treated at any stage of the disease, but treatment may be prolonged in latent and tertiary syphilis. Although syphilis can be cured in late stages, damage to the body is more difficult to manage. Untreated syphilis will go from primary to secondary, latent, and eventually tertiary stage.

GONORRHEA

Etiology and Pathophysiology

Gonorrhea is caused by *Neisseria gonorrhoeae*, a gram-negative diplococcoid bacterium, and almost exclusively follows sexual contact. It is the second most commonly reported STI in the United States. (Chlamydial infections are the most common.) Gonorrhea rates remained stable from 1997 to 2000 after a 74% decline from 1975 to 1997. From 2000 through 2004, reported cases of gonorrhea decreased 11.8%, but then the rate increased. More than 358,366 cases of gonorrhea were reported in the United States in 2006 (CDC, 2007b). The highest incidence of gonorrhea occurs in adolescents of all racial and ethnic groups, among blacks, and in persons living in the Southern United States. Most states have laws that permit examination and treatment of minors without the consent of parents (Lewis et al., 2007). Those at risk are sexually active individuals and those who are otherwise susceptible to infections. Gonorrhea is primarily an infection of the genital or rectal mucosa but is not limited to the genital organs; it can infect the mouth and the throat through oral sex with an infected partner. It may also infect the eyes. Three times as many men are infected as women. The incubation period of gonorrhea is 3 to 5 days.

Clinical Manifestations

Some infected men may be asymptomatic after the incubation period but in a short time develop signs and symptoms of urethritis, dysuria, infection with a profuse purulent discharge, and edema of the affected area. Most women remain asymptomatic but may show a greenish yellow discharge from the cervix. Other female signs and symptoms, depending on the infection site, are urinary frequency, purulent discharge from the urethra, pruritus, burning and pain of the vulva, vaginal engorgement and erythema, abdominal pain and distention, muscular rigidity, and tenderness. As the infection spreads, nausea, vomiting, fever, and tachycardia may develop. Other signs and symptoms are pharyngitis, tonsillitis, rectal burning, and purulent rectal discharge. PID, Bartholin's abscess, ectopic pregnancy, and infertility are the main complications of gonorrhea in women (Lewis et al., 2007).

Diagnostic Tests
Diagnosis is determined by cultures from the site of infection to isolate and identify the organism. Cultures of the discharge or secretion can provide a definitive diagnosis after incubation for 24 to 48 hours. An important concern in treatment for gonorrhea is coexisting chlamydial infection (see the discussion of chlamydia for more information). Chlamydia has been documented in up to 45% of gonorrhea cases. It is important to test for syphilis as well.

Medical Management
A history of sexual contact with a partner known to have gonorrhea is considered good evidence for the infection. Because of the short incubation period and high infectivity, treatment is instituted without awaiting culture results, even in the absence of signs or symptoms. Treatment of gonorrhea in the early stage is curative. Traditionally, the drug of choice for gonorrheal therapy was penicillin, but changes have been made because of (1) a rapid increase in the number of cases of gonorrhea caused by resistant strains of *N. gonorrhoeae* and (2) coexisting chlamydial infection.

There is no clinical distinction between infections caused by resistant or sensitive strains of *N. gonorrhoeae*. As a result, ceftriaxone (Rocephin), a penicillinase-resistant cephalosporin, has become part of the treatment plan. The most common treatment for gonorrhea is a single IM dose of ceftriaxone. Cefixime (Suprax) given orally one time is also effective. Other medications that may be used in the treatment of gonorrhea are ciprofloxacin, ofloxacin, and levofloxacin (Levaquin). The high frequency of coexisting chlamydial and gonococcal infections has led to the addition of doxycycline or tetracycline to the treatment plan. The expense of diagnosing chlamydial infection and the sequelae make this strategy cost effective. Patients with coincubating syphilis are likely to be cured by the same drugs.

All sexual contacts of patients with gonorrhea must be treated to prevent reinfection after resumption of sexual relations. The "Ping-Pong" effect of reexposure, treatment, and reinfection will cease only when infected partners are treated simultaneously. Additionally, advise the patient to abstain from sexual intercourse and alcohol for 2 to 4 weeks. Sexual intercourse allows the infection to spread and can retard complete healing as a result of vascular congestion. Alcohol irritates the healing urethral walls. Caution men against squeezing the penis to look for further discharge. Follow-up examination and reculture should be done at least once after treatment, usually in 4 to 7 days. Treat relapse, reinfection, and complications appropriately.

Nurses need to be alert to changes in CDC recommendations. Report the disease to infection control authorities as required by the local health agency.

Nursing Interventions and Patient Teaching
Advise patients that loose, absorbent underclothes, changed frequently after perineal or penile cleansing, enhance comfort. Sitz baths decrease lower abdominal discomfort and dysuria. Obtain laboratory specimens as ordered. Discuss alternative methods of birth control as appropriate. Encourage notification of present and past sexual partners of the diagnosis and stress the need for them to promptly seek medical care. Inform the female that sterility may occur as a result of gonorrhea.

Prognosis
With treatment, gonorrhea is curable. The inflammation may clear up without serious results, or it may become chronic and produce urethral stricture. Complications include prostatitis, epididymitis, orchitis, arthritis, and endocarditis. It can result in sterility in the female. No case of acute gonorrhea in the female should be considered cured until three consecutive negative smears of the cervix and Bartholin's and Skene's glands are obtained. The main cause for infections identified after completed treatment is reinfection, not treatment failure.

TRICHOMONIASIS
Etiology and Pathophysiology
Trichomoniasis is an STI caused by the protozoan *Trichomonas vaginalis*, which affects about 15% of sexually active women and 10% of sexually active men (CDC, 2007d). The incubation period is 4 to 28 days. Trichomoniasis is usually transmitted by sexual intercourse and, at times, by dirty douche nozzles, douche containers, and moist washcloths. Occasionally a newborn develops an infection from an infected mother. *T. vaginalis* thrives when the vaginal mucosa is more alkaline than normal. Frequent douching and use of oral contraceptives and antibiotics raise the normal pH of the vagina, making the woman more vulnerable to trichomoniasis.

Clinical Manifestations
Most men and approximately 70% of women are asymptomatic. The male signs and symptoms are mild to severe transient urethritis, dysuria, frequency of urination, pruritus, and purulent exudate. In women, signs and

symptoms include profuse, frothy, gray, green, or yellow malodorous discharge; pruritus; edema; tenderness of vagina; dysuria; frequency of urination; spotting; menorrhagia; and dysmenorrhea. Signs and symptoms may persist for a week to several months and may be more pronounced after menstruation or during pregnancy.

Diagnostic Tests

Diagnosis is based on the microscopic examination of the vaginal discharge that identifies *T. vaginalis.*

Medical Management

Treatment for both men and women is oral metronidazole (Flagyl) in small doses for 7 days or a single large dose. The patient should avoid alcoholic beverages, since alcohol can cause reactions such as disorientation, headache, cramps, vomiting, and possibly convulsions. Metronidazole can cause the urine to turn dark brown (see Table 12-2).

Nursing Interventions and Patient Teaching

Advise the patient to avoid alcohol during treatment; inform patients that their urine may turn dark orange or brown; and counsel patients to avoid douches, sprays, and powders during treatment. Teach the patient how to disinfect douche nozzles, applicators, diaphragms, and the toilet area. Encourage the patient to wear loose-fitting clothing and cotton underwear, to schedule follow-up visits with the physician, and to contact sexual partners so they can get treatment.

Prognosis

With treatment, trichomoniasis is curable. Reinfection is common if sexual partners are not treated simultaneously. Chronic infection may develop in untreated cases.

CANDIDIASIS

Etiology and Pathophysiology

Candidiasis (moniliasis) is a mild fungal infection that appears in men and women. Candidal infections are usually caused by *C. albicans* and *Candida tropicalis.* The fungi are a part of the normal flora of the gastrointestinal tract, mouth, vagina, and skin. The infection often occurs when the glucose level rises from diabetes mellitus or when resistance is lowered from diseases such as carcinoma. Radiation, immunosuppressant drugs, hyperalimentation, antibiotic therapy, and oral contraceptives may predispose individuals to candidiasis. Men and women display signs of scaly skin; erythematous rash; and occasional exudates that appear under the breasts, between the fingers, and in the axillae, groin, and umbilicus.

Clinical Manifestations

If the mother is infected, a newborn can contract thrush during delivery. The infant may display a diaper rash. The infant's nails become edematous and have a dark-ened, erythematous nail base with purulent exudate. Thrush may appear on the mucous membranes of the infant's mouth as pearly, bluish white "milk-curd" lesions and cause edema and engorgement. The infant may have an edematous tongue that can cause respiratory distress. The adult female patient may have a cheesy, tenacious white vaginal discharge accompanied by pruritus and an inflamed vulva and vagina. The adult male patient has signs of an infected penis with purulent exudate. Systemic infections are indicated by chills, fevers, and general malaise.

Diagnostic Tests

Diagnosis is based on evidence of the *Candida* species on a Gram stain of collected specimens from scraping of the vagina and penis, from pus, and from exudate from the mouth.

Medical Management

Treatment consists of managing any underlying condition, such as controlling diabetes mellitus, discontinuing antibiotics and oral contraceptives. Nystatin (Mycostatin) is effective for superficial candidiasis; topical amphotericin B is effective for skin and nail infections.

Nursing Interventions and Patient Teaching

Emphasize the use of prescribed ointments, sprays, and creams as indicated for each part of the body affected. Teaching includes the method for inserting vaginal suppositories (to be inserted high into the vagina when in a dorsal recumbent position) and remaining on the back for 30 minutes to allow suppository absorption. Patients should encourage sexual partners to have an examination and treatment. Teach good handwashing techniques to avoid reinfection or the transfer of the fungi. Encourage pregnant women to accept treatment to prevent infection of the newborn at the time of delivery.

Prognosis

Candidiasis is curable with the use of the prescribed treatment.

CHLAMYDIA

Etiology and Pathophysiology

Chlamydia trachomatis, a gram-negative, intracellular bacterium, causes several common STIs. Cervicitis and urethritis are most common, but like gonococci, chlamydial organisms also cause epididymitis in men and salpingitis in women. Chlamydial infections are the most commonly occurring STI in the United States. They are responsible for about 20% to 30% of diagnosed PID cases. In 2006 more than 1 million cases of genital chlamydial infections were reported in the United States (CDC, 2007a). It is estimated that about 11,000 women each year become involuntarily sterilized and 36,000 suffer ectopic pregnancies as a result of this organism. Chlamydia incidence is highest in young, promiscuous, indigent, unmarried women who live in the inner city and in those who have a prior history of STIs. Increases in chlamydia rates are more likely a result of better screening and use of more sensitive tests, rather than an increase of the total burden of the disease in the United States (CDC, 2007a). Chlamydia can be transmitted during vaginal, anal, or oral sex.

Although both men and women may have asymptomatic infection, women are more likely to be asymptomatic carriers even with deep pelvic infections, such as infection of the fallopian tubes and PID.

Clinical Manifestations

In men, signs and symptoms may include a scanty white or clear exudate, burning or pruritus around the urethral meatus, urinary frequency, and mild dysuria. Signs and symptoms of cervicitis in women may include one or more of the following: (1) vaginal pruritus or burning, (2) dull pelvic pain, (3) low-grade fever, (4) vaginal discharge, and (5) irregular bleeding. Symptoms of chlamydia may be absent or cause minor discomfort; therefore it has been called a silent disease. Females may develop a PID, which can result in infertility (Lewis et al., 2007). For this reason the CDC (2007a) recommends that all females younger than 25 years of age be routinely screened for chlamydia at their annual gynecologic examination. The CDC further advises annual screening of all women older than 25 years of age with one or more risk factors for the disease (CDC, 2007a).

Diagnostic Tests

The direct fluorescent antibody test provides a ready basis for diagnosis. However, this test is less specific than a culture and may produce false-positive results. Culturing for chlamydial organisms should be done if the laboratory facilities are available. New techniques using nucleic acid amplification promise to surpass culture as the gold standard of chlamydial testing. Treatment can be initiated promptly based on a confirmed diagnosis.

Medical Management

Chlamydial infections respond to treatment with tetracycline, doxycycline, azithromycin, or ofloxacin. For tetracycline, the dosage is 500 mg orally four times a day for at least 7 days. For doxycycline, the dosage is 100 mg two times a day. Doxycycline is more expensive than tetracycline. For ofloxacin, the dosage is 300 mg twice a day. Azithromycin (1 g in a single dose) offers the advantage of ease of administration, but safety for patients younger than 15 years of age has not been established. Alternative regimens include erythromycin, ofloxacin, and levofloxacin. Erythromycin is the drug of choice for use in pregnant patients. If this treatment is not tolerated, amoxicillin is an alternative. Follow-up care includes advising the patient to return if symptoms persist or recur, treating sexual partners, and encouraging the use of condoms during all sexual contact.

Box 12-9 **Prevention of Sexually Transmitted Infections**

- Reduce the number of sexual partners, preferably to one person.
- Avoid contact with individuals known to be infected or who are at risk of infection.
- Avoid contact with the genital area if signs and symptoms develop.
- Wash the hands and the genital-rectal area before and immediately after having intercourse.
- Pay special attention to washing the foreskin.
- A mouthwash or gargle with hydrogen peroxide (1 part peroxide to 3 parts of water) or Listerine antiseptic may slightly reduce the risk of oropharyngeal sexually transmitted infection (STI).
- Use barrier (condom) contraceptives with new partners.
- Use a water-based lubricant as opposed to an oil-based lubricant.
- Void after intercourse.
- Avoid excess douching.
- If an STI infection is suspected, seek medical help immediately.
- Individuals with multiple sexual partners should have an STI examination twice a year or more if needed.

Because chlamydial infections are closely associated with gonococcal infections, both infections are usually treated concurrently, even without diagnostic evidence.

Nursing Interventions and Patient Teaching

Patients' physical symptoms are often complicated by their emotional responses to STIs. Depression, anger, fear, and guilt need to be addressed if education and treatment are to be effective. Outcome is also influenced by educational and income levels, primary language, health insurance coverage, and support network. Patient education focuses on prevention (Box 12-9).

Prognosis

With treatment, chlamydial infection is curable. Reinfection occurs if sexual partners are not treated simultaneously. Chlamydial infections can be transmitted to infants during delivery, causing conjunctivitis and pneumonia. Poorly treated or untreated chlamydial infection can result in ectopic pregnancy or infertility.

ACQUIRED IMMUNODEFICIENCY SYNDROME

AIDS is the ultimately fatal, advanced stage of a chronic retroviral infection from the HIV virus that gradually destroys the cell-mediated immune system. (For a more detailed discussion on this STI, see Chapter 16.)

FAMILY PLANNING

Advances in drug therapy and family planning technology have made a range of options available for individuals wishing to prevent or plan conception. Birth control planning involves moral, religious, cultural, and personal values, and the nurse should be sensitive to these factors when discussing birth control with patients.

Numerous types of birth control procedures or devices can be employed. The selection of a method should be based on the patient's health, effectiveness of the method, cost, lifestyle, ease of use, and age and parity (total number of pregnancies) of the patient. The patient's willingness to comply with use and the

couple's preference are two additional factors taken into consideration when selecting a method of contraception. Reinforce the information given by the physician and encourage patients to seek more information, directing them to the source.

Contraceptive methods and products can be categorized as surgical (Figures 12-20 and 12-21), hormonal, barrier, and behavioral (Table 12-4).

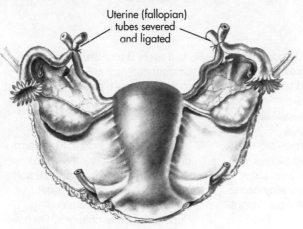

FIGURE 12-20 Tubal ligation. Oviduct ligated and severed.

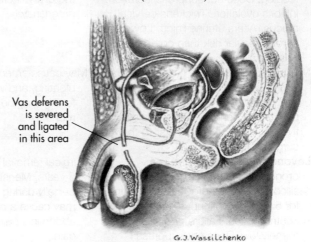

FIGURE 12-21 Vasectomy. Sperm duct severed (and ligated).

Table 12-4 Methods of Birth Control

DESCRIPTION	SIDE EFFECTS AND COMPLICATIONS	PATIENT EDUCATION
TEMPORARY METHODS **Combined** **Combination pill** contains both estrogen and progesterone (standard and low dose). Usually taken on 5th through 25th day of each cycle. Prevents ovulation; causes changes in endometrium; alterations in cervical mucus and tubal transport. Simple and unobtrusive in use. 99% effective. Failure from irregular or incorrect use.	Side effects of weight gain, nausea and vomiting, spotting and breakthrough bleeding, postpill amenorrhea, breast tenderness, headache, chloasma, irritability, nervousness, depression, and decreased libido. Complications of benign liver tumors, gallstones, myocardial infarction, thromboembolism, stroke (smokers >35 years of age at higher risk). Contraindications of history of cardiovascular or liver disease, hypertension, breast or pelvic cancer; use caution with diabetes mellitus, sickle cell anemia. Provides no protection against HIV transmission.	Instruct patient in correct use of pills. Tell patient to take pill same time each day; if forgotten one day, take two next day. Review side effects and contraindications. Explain that the patient should report cramps or edema of legs, chest pain. Discuss need for periodic (every 6-12 months), checkup that involves weight, BP, Pap smear, hematocrit. Review danger signs of drug. Take drug history, asking about use of phenytoin, phenobarbital, antibiotic (ampicillin), which decrease contraceptive action. Inform patient that method is usually not recommended for persons >35 years of age. Discourage smoking.
Morning-after pill (norgestrel and ethinyl estradiol [Ovral]) contains ethinyl estradiol 50 mcg and norgestrel 500 mg. Another use of combined hormonal contraception. 98.4% effective. Creates hostile uterine lining and alters tubal transport.	Nausea for 1-2 days. Does not prevent an ectopic pregnancy. At risk for usual hormonal complications of abdominal pain, chest pain, cough, shortness of breath, headache, dizziness, weakness, leg pain.	Take two Ovral within 72 hours of coitus. Repeat if vomiting occurs. Take second dose 12 hours later. Menses should begin within 2-3 weeks. Start an ongoing method of contraception immediately after menses.

Modified from Lewis S.L., et al. (2007). *Medical-surgical nursing: assessment and management of clinical problems.* (7th ed.). St. Louis: Mosby.   *Continued*
BP, Blood pressure; *HIV*, human immunodeficiency virus.

Table 12-4 Methods of Birth Control—cont'd

DESCRIPTION	SIDE EFFECTS AND COMPLICATIONS	PATIENT EDUCATION
TEMPORARY METHODS—cont'd		
Progestin Only		
Progestin-only pills (POPs or Minipills) are taken daily, with no pill-free days. Preferred for women who are breast-feeding. Does not suppress lactation. Inhibits ovulation. Thickens cervical mucus. Alters uterine lining. Lower cardiovascular risk than combined pills.	Menstrual changes, breakthrough bleeding, prolonged cycles or amenorrhea. Increase in functional cysts of the ovary. Increase in ectopic pregnancy.	Use alternate contraception when starting POPs or if pill is missed. Take pill at same time every day. Keep record of menses and get pregnancy test if 2 weeks late.
Medroxyprogesterone (Depo-Provera, DMPA) is a progestin-only drug given by injection every 3 months. A private, convenient, and highly effective method. Efficacy similar to that of surgical sterilization.	May cause amenorrhea, headaches, bloating, and weight gain. Return of fertility may be delayed for several months.	Return every 3 months for injection. Discontinue method for several months before planning to conceive.
Levonorgestrel (Norplant) is a progestin-only subdermal implant. Six silicone capsules provide protection for 5 years. Continuous, long-term contraception. Failure rate is extremely low. Does not suppress lactation. Pregnancy rate 0.8 per 100 users over 5 years.	Surgical removal of capsules after 5 years. Menstrual irregularities, especially during the first year. Later may cause amenorrhea. May cause abdominal pain, headaches, weight gain.	Is effective after 24 hours. Keep arm dry for 48 hours after insertion. Report arm pain. Implants are soft and flexible and cannot break. Expect some irregular bleeding. Report any other changes. Remove implants in 5 years. Continue to protect against STIs.
Barrier Method		
Diaphragms are dome-shaped latex caps with flexible metal ring (varies in size) covering cervix. Inner surface coated with spermicide before insertion. Provides mechanical barrier to sperm. Available by prescription, fitted by professional. Continuing motivation to use necessary. 87% effective. Failure from improper fitting or placement of device.	Allergy to latex or spermicide.	Demonstrate how to hold, insert, and remove device, using model. Allow for insertion and removal practice sessions. Advise patient that insertion may be just prior to coitus, but removal should be 6-8 hours after coitus. Tell patient to empty bowel and bladder before insertion. Give instructions for cleansing and storing, checking for holes or deterioration. Advise patient that diaphragm must be refitted after pregnancy, weight loss, or weight gain. Advise patient that it is not suitable if severe pelvic relaxation is present.
Cervical caps are rubber thimble-shaped shields covering cervix, held in place by suction. Spermicide in inner surface provides mechanical barrier to sperm. Fitted by professional. Effectiveness similar to that of diaphragm. Failure from dislodgment and improper fit.	Allergy to rubber; or spermicide, possible cervical irritation or erosion from suction.	Provide sufficient time for practice with insertion and removal (more time than for diaphragm). Give instructions for cleaning, storing, and inspecting for damage. Inform patient that it can be used with abnormalities of vaginal canal but not with cervical inconsistencies or PID.
Condoms		
Male: Thin rubber sheath fitting over erect penis, providing mechanical barrier to sperm. Simple method to use. No prescription necessary. 85% effective. Failure from tearing or slipping during coitus. Used with spermicide. Affords some protection against STIs and HIV transmission.	Possible allergy to rubber; possible decrease in sensation and interference with foreplay.	Advise patient to roll sheath along entire penis, leaving slack at end to receive semen. Inform patient that sharp objects (fingernails) may tear condom. Tell patient to hold sheath in place when penis is withdrawn to prevent emptying of sperm in or near vagina.

PID, Pelvic inflammatory disease; *STI,* sexually transmitted infection.

Table 12-4   Methods of Birth Control—cont'd

DESCRIPTION	SIDE EFFECTS AND COMPLICATIONS	PATIENT EDUCATION
TEMPORARY METHODS—cont'd		
Female: Double-ring system fitted into vagina up to 8 hours before intercourse. No prescription necessary. Affords protection against HIV, cytomegalovirus, and hepatitis B.	No significant side effects; generally acceptable to couple.	Discuss insertion, lubrication, and method of removal. More expensive than male condoms.
Other Methods		
Intrauterine devices (IUDs) are inserted Into uterus and are flexible objects made of plastic or copper wire (nonmedicated or medicated with substance to alter uterine environment), usually with attached string that protrudes into vagina. Contraception probably provided by inflammatory response in endometrium, preventing implantation. After insertion, no additional equipment necessary. 97% to 99% effective. Failure mainly from undetected expulsion. Most common type used today is Progestasert (contains progestins).	Increased menstrual flow, intramenstrual bleeding and cramping, especially during early months of use; possible complications of ectopic pregnancy, pelvic infection, perforation of uterus, infertility. Undetected expulsion of IUD resulting in pregnancy.	Discuss techniques and experience of insertion and removal. Inform patient that insertion may be more difficult and expulsion and complications greater in nulliparous patients. Instruct patient to check for string in vagina after each period; report to physician if unable to locate. Discuss need for annual pelvic examination and Pap test.
Rhythm method requires periodic abstinence during fertile portion of menstrual cycle. Requires strong motivation, self-control. Complies with all religious doctrines. 60% to 65% effective. Failure from difficulty in determining precise day of ovulation, irregularity of menses.	Inaccurate or incomplete knowledge of menstrual cycle.	Discuss methods to establish baseline menstrual patterns and identify ovulation. Give instructions in use of calendar or basal body temperature method to determine ovulation and fertile period.
PERMANENT		
Tubal sterilization includes a variety of abdominal and vaginal surgical procedures (laparotomy, laparoscopy, culdoscopy) that permanently prevent sperm and ovum from meeting. Crushing, ligating, clipping, or plugging of fallopian tubes (potentially reversible procedure). Nearly 100% (99.96%) effective. Failure due to recanalization of fallopian tubes, erroneous ligation (see Figure 12-20).	Bowel injury, hemorrhage, or infection.	Determine whether temporary contraceptives were used and reason for patient's dissatisfaction. Counsel regarding effects of procedure on physiology and sexual performance. Assist in obtaining written informed consent for procedure. Inform patient that procedure may require short-term hospitalization or can be done on outpatient basis.
Hysterectomy is surgical removal of uterus. 100% effective.	Bladder infection, vascular disorders, infection, hemorrhage, pain, psychological adjustment.	Assess or counsel regarding understanding of extent of surgery, altered physiology, complications, and sexual performance. Hysterectomy only performed for other reasons; sterility is secondary benefit when desired.
Vasectomy is bilateral surgical ligation and resection of ductus deferens.	Hematoma, edema, psychological adjustment (see Figure 12-21).	Inform patient that procedure is usually done as outpatient procedure and takes 15 to 30 minutes. Tell patient that alternative form of contraception is needed until no sperm are seen on examination. Explain that procedure does not affect masculinity.

❖ NURSING PROCESS *for the Patient with a Reproductive Disorder*

The role of the licensed practical nurse/licensed vocational nurse (LPN/LVN) in the nursing process as stated is that the LPN/LVN will:

- Participate in planning care for patients based on patient needs
- Review patient's care plan and recommend revisions as needed
- Review and follow defined prioritization for patient care
- Use clinical pathways, care maps, or care plans to guide and review patient care

▪ Assessment

People with reproductive disorders require skilled assessment by both the nurse and the physician. Assessment occurs through observation of the patient during the patient health history and while doing baseline and continuing assessment of the patient's objective and subjective data.

Health history data should be relevant to the patient's developmental age. Information about reproductive health and sexuality can form a large portion of the collected data. This history is as important as the physical and emotional data in determining appropriate nursing diagnoses and interventions. Data collected about sexual health, sexual relations, birth control methods, STIs, and the use of chemical substances provide an opportunity to clarify any misconceptions or myths revealed during history taking.

▪ Data Collection for Women

Data collection for adolescent and adult women focuses on the reproductive tract and the menstrual, gynecologic, and obstetric history.

The menstrual history encompasses menarche (onset of menstrual flow) through the climacteric (cessation of menstrual cycle), including: (1) age of onset; (2) date of last menstrual flow; (3) usual amount and volume of flow (number of pads used per day); (4) presence of **dysmenorrhea** (painful menstruation), **menorrhagia** (excessive flow), **amenorrhea** (absence of flow), or **metrorrhagia** (excessive spotting between cycles); and (5) other difficulties during menses.

The gynecologic assessment includes data on (1) vaginal discharge (odor, color, frequency, and duration), (2) vaginal pruritus (itching), (3) vaginal irritation with coital activity, (4) date and results of the last Pap test, (5) birth control methods or kinds of contraceptives used, and (6) any family history of cancer of the reproductive system.

If the adolescent or adult woman has conceived, information should be collected as to **gravidity** (number of pregnancies), **parity** (number of births), abortions, miscarriages, and stillbirths. Assessment of the breast includes (1) tenderness of the breast areas; (2) pain;

(3) masses in any specific areas; (4) presence of nipple discharge; (5) knowledge and frequency of BSE; and (6) date and results of last mammogram, if applicable.

▪ Data Collection for Men

The data collected from the male adolescent and the adult man include (1) urologic history of voiding difficulties and any discharge from the penis; (2) characteristics of the urine (odor, color, amount, and frequency); (3) information on prostate and testicular problems; (4) frequency of PSA testing, if applicable; (5) masses or lesions on genitalia; (6) frequency of TSE; (7) frequency of professional testicular examination; (8) measures to prevent infections; and (9) birth control method. In addition, note concerns about sexual health voiced by the patient.

▪ Nursing Diagnosis

Possible nursing diagnoses for the patient with a reproductive disorder include but are not limited to the following:

- Anxiety
- Disturbed body image
- Ineffective coping
- Fear
- Deficient fluid volume
- Ineffective health maintenance
- Risk for infection
- Deficient knowledge
- Acute pain
- Chronic pain
- Chronic low self-esteem
- Situational low self-esteem
- Sexual dysfunction
- Impaired skin integrity
- Ineffective tissue perfusion
- Impaired urinary elimination

▪ Expected Outcomes and Planning

Planning is a category of nursing behaviors in which patient-centered goals are established and strategies designed to achieve the goals and outcomes that relate to the identified nursing diagnosis (Table 12-5).

▪ Implementation

The implementation step for the patient with a reproductive disorder is the action-oriented phase of the nursing process in which the nurse initiates and carries out the objectives of the nursing care plan. See Complementary & Alternative Therapies box for additional treatment methods.

▪ Evaluation

Examples of goals and their corresponding evaluative measures include the following:

Goal 1: Patient will be able to cope effectively.
   Evaluative measure: Patient verbalizes fears and identifies two strategies for dealing with fear, such as

Table 12-5	Planning and Setting Goals for the Patient with a Reproductive Disorder		
NURSING DIAGNOSIS	**GOAL**	**OUTCOME**	
Coping, ineffective, related to fear of positive diagnosis of breast cancer	Patient will attend cancer support group weekly.	Patient expresses fears of unfavorable outcome.	
Knowledge, deficient, regarding postoperative care at home after modified radical mastectomy	Patient will state four postoperative risks before discharge.	Patient verbalizes signs and symptoms of infection.	
		Patient demonstrates exercises for affected arm.	
		Patient verbalizes need to avoid injections and taking of blood or blood pressure in affected arm.	
		Patient verbalizes need to examine remaining breast once a month.	

Complementary & Alternative Therapies

Male and Female Reproductive Disorders

MALE REPRODUCTIVE SYSTEM
- Yohimbine *(Pausinystalia yohimbe)* for erectile dysfunction and impotence

FEMALE REPRODUCTIVE SYSTEM
- Biofeedback, therapeutic touch, and acupuncture for primary dysmenorrhea
- Black cohosh *(Cimicifuga racemosa)* for menstrual irregularity, premenstrual syndrome (PMS), and menopausal problems

- Chamomile *(Matricaria recutita, Chamaemelum nobile)* for menstrual cramps
- Chaste tree *(Vitex agnus-castus)* for PMS
- Evening primrose *(Oenothera biennis)* for PMS
- Feverfew *(Tanacetum parthenium)* for menstrual problems
- Sage *(Salvia officinalis)* for menstrual irregularity
- Soybeans and other legumes for their phytoestrogens that may help prevent breast cancer

Modified from Black J.M., & Hawks, H.J. (2009). *Medical-surgical nursing: clinical management for positive outcomes.* (8th ed.). Philadelphia: Saunders.

questioning for clarification and relaxation breathing technique.

Goal 2: Patient will have adequate knowledge regarding postoperative care at home after modified radical mastectomy.

Evaluative measures: Patient states signs and symptoms of wound infection; lists proper arm exercises; verbalizes the need for BSE once per month; and states the need to avoid blood pressure checks, injections, and blood draws in affected arm.

Get Ready for the NCLEX® Examination!

Key Points

- Sperm are produced in the seminiferous tubules and stored in the epididymis.
- Testosterone, the male sex hormone, is responsible for male secondary sex characteristics.
- Seminal fluid is produced in the seminal vesicles, prostate gland, and Cowper's glands.
- The male urethra serves the twofold purpose of conveying urine from the bladder and carrying the reproductive cells and secretions to the outside.
- The uterus consists of three layers of tissue: (1) endometrium, the inner layer; (2) myometrium, the middle layer; and (3) perimetrium, the outer layer.
- In the ovulating female, an egg matures each month in the graafian follicle, which is located in the ovary.
- The menstrual cycle prepares the uterus and causes ovulation to occur each month.
- Because of the relationship between the menstrual cycle and the body's mechanisms of hormonal secretion, a decrease or increase in the activity of the hormonal glands can disturb menstruation.

- Early diagnosis and prompt management are necessary to prevent serious reproductive and genital problems.
- Health teaching for patients with menstrual disturbances includes a knowledge of the physiologic process, factors that alter menstruation, personal hygiene, exercise, diet, and pain management.
- Discharge planning is vital to prevent reinfection after PID.
- Pregnancy is encouraged in the patient with endometriosis, since it will slow the progress of the disorder; infertility is a complication as the condition continues.
- Menarche, the first menstrual cycle, usually begins around the age of 12 years.
- Serum CA-125 is useful mainly to signal a recurrence of ovarian cancer and in following the response to treatment.
- PSA is a highly sensitive blood test that is elevated in cancer of the prostate and in benign prostatic hyperplasia.
- There is no definitive test for TSS. However, cervical-vaginal isolates of *Staphylococcus aureus* are present 90% of the time with TSS.

- Vaginal fistulas are caused by an ulcerating process resulting from cancer, radiation, weakening of tissue from pregnancies, or surgical interventions.
- Correction of cystocele and rectocele is a surgical repair involving shortening of the muscles that support the bladder and repair of the rectocele. This is known as anteroposterior colporrhaphy.
- Screening tests for cervical abnormalities include routine Pap test; ThinPrep, a newer liquid-based technique for Pap tests; and testing for HPV.
- Vaccines are now available that reduce the incidence of cervical cancer due to infection of HPV (types 6, 11, 16, 18).
- A panhysterosalpingo-oophorectomy is the removal of the uterus, the fallopian tubes, and the ovaries.
- In breast cancer patients an axillary lymph node dissection is usually performed regardless of treatment options available. Examination of nodes provides the most powerful prognostic data currently available.
- A relatively new diagnostic tool used before therapeutic surgery for breast cancer is sentinel lymph node mapping, which identifies the first lymph node most likely to drain the cancerous cells.
- Overall 10-year survival with lumpectomy and radiation is about the same as with modified radical mastectomy.
- After losing a breast, many patients experience acute grief that may last 4 to 6 weeks or longer. Grief makes the fact of loss real.
- Caution patients who have undergone a modified radical mastectomy to avoid injections, vaccinations, taking of blood pressure or blood samples, or insertion of IV line in the affected arm.
- Phimosis is a condition in which the prepuce is too small to retract over the glans penis.
- Young men should be taught to perform TSE monthly beginning at 15 years of age for detection of testicular carcinoma.
- Oral acyclovir is prescribed for primary genital herpes to shorten the duration of the healing and suppress 75% of recurrence with daily use.
- Parenteral penicillin remains the treatment of choice for all stages of syphilis. All stages of syphilis should be treated.
- Because of penicillin-resistant strains of *N. gonorrhoeae*, penicillin, the former drug of choice for treatment of gonorrhea, has been changed to ceftriaxone.
- Chlamydial infections respond to treatment with tetracycline, doxycycline, azithromycin, or ofloxacin. Erythromycin is the drug of choice for use in pregnant patients.

Additional Learning Resources

Go to your companion CD for an audio glossary, animations, video clips, more.

evolve   Be sure to visit the Evolve site at http://evolve.elsevier.com/Christensen/adult/ for additional online resources.

Review Questions for the NCLEX® Examination

1. A patient visits her physician because of an increase in her abdominal girth and dyspnea during the past month as a result of pressure on her diaphragm. She is diagnosed as having cancer of the ovaries. These two clinical manifestations result from:
   1. development of ascites.
   2. metastasis to the bowel.
   3. dilation of the alveoli.
   4. bladder distention.

2. A 30-year-old premenopausal patient asks the nurse the most appropriate time of the month to do her self-examination of the breasts. The most appropriate reply by the nurse would be:
   1. during her menstruation.
   2. 7 to 8 days after conclusion of the menstrual period.
   3. the same day each month.
   4. the 26th day of the menstrual cycle.

3. A 52-year-old patient has ductal cell carcinoma of the left breast. After a modified radical mastectomy, a Davol drain is in place in the left axillary region. The main purpose of this drain is to:
   1. control numbness of her left incisional site.
   2. improve her ability to perform range-of-motion exercises on her affected side.
   3. facilitate drainage and prevent formation of a hematoma.
   4. prevent postoperative phlebitis in her affected arm.

4. A 35-year-old patient received a vasectomy. Teaching for this patient should include that:
   1. the procedure is reversible if he later changes his mind.
   2. he should abstain from sexual intercourse until the incision is completely healed.
   3. he should apply warm compresses to the scrotum four times a day.
   4. he should return to the physician at regular intervals for sperm counts.

5. A 44-year-old patient is admitted for an abdominal hysterectomy. She is instructed that she will have a Foley catheter in place postoperatively. She asks the nurse how many days she will have the catheter in place. The best response by the nurse would be that:
   1. the indwelling catheter will probably remain in place for 1 week.
   2. the indwelling catheter will be removed after you are fully awake from the anesthesia.
   3. the indwelling catheter will generally remain in place 1 to 2 days after surgery.
   4. the indwelling catheter will remain in place for a few days postdischarge.

6. A 60-year-old patient had a vaginal hysterectomy for a prolapsed uterus. The nurse is aware that patients undergoing pelvic surgery are more susceptible to certain postoperative complications, and thus adjusts postoperative interventions to prevent:
   1. wound dehiscence.
   2. wound infection.
   3. atelectasis and hypostatic pneumonia.
   4. venous stasis and thrombophlebitis.

7. A 49-year-old obese diabetic patient has had a total abdominal hysterectomy. On the second postoperative day, the patient complains of increased pain in the operative site. She states, "It feels like something suddenly popped." With the symptoms presented, it would be likely that when the nurse removes the abdominal dressing she may note that:

   1. the wound has purulent exudate.
   2. dehiscence has occurred.
   3. the wound is indurated and tender.
   4. the wound is well approximated.

8. A 20-year-old patient goes to the physician's office with vaginal pruritus, burning, dull pelvic pain, and purulent vaginal discharge. A diagnostic test reveals she has chlamydia. The nurse goes over the medication schedule carefully with the patient. Another important nursing intervention to achieve satisfactory patient outcome would be to:

   1. encourage her to have her sexual partner(s) seek medical care as soon as possible to avoid reinfection of the patient.
   2. recommend she abstain from sexual contact while lesions are present.
   3. provide social and emotional support because the edematous, draining lymph nodes may be disturbing to the patient's self-image.
   4. educate the patient that the causative organism is a spirochete that gains entrance into the body during intercourse.

9. A 40-year-old patient had a right modified radical mastectomy with wide resection of the axillary lymph nodes. Which interventions are encouraged in the postoperative care for the patient? *(Select all that apply.)*

   1. Encourage turning, coughing, deep breathing, and use of incentive spirometry.
   2. Take blood pressure readings on her right arm.
   3. Draw a circle around the drainage on the pressure dressing.
   4. Administer an oral analgesic every 4 hours as needed for pain.

10. A 23-year-old man is diagnosed with gonorrhea. Because of statements made in his patient interview, the nurse has established a nursing diagnosis of noncompliance. Which is the most effective way to overcome noncompliance for this patient?

    1. Telephone follow-up
    2. Case finding
    3. Single-dose treatment of ceftriaxone (Rocephin) IM
    4. Extensive patient education program

11. The nurse is teaching a group of teenagers about contraception and sexually transmitted infections (STIs). The nurse asks the students if they know which is the most prevalent STI. They are surprised to learn it is:

    1. syphilis.
    2. chlamydial infection.
    3. gonorrhea.
    4. herpes genitalis.

12. A 73-year-old patient comes to the physician's office with the complaint of constant seepage of feces from her vagina, causing her embarrassment due to soilage and odor. These are signs of:

    1. rectovaginal fistula.
    2. vesicovaginal fistula.
    3. urethrovaginal fistula.
    4. rectocele.

13. The American Cancer Society recommends that women have an annual screening mammography beginning at age:

    1. 21.
    2. 35.
    3. 40.
    4. 52.

14. The first lymph node most likely to drain the cancerous site in a breast cancer patient is known as the:

    1. axillary node.
    2. contaminated node.
    3. primary node.
    4. sentinal node.

15. While discussing risk factors for breast cancer with a group of women, the nurse stresses that the greatest risk factor for breast cancer is:

    1. being a woman over the age of 50.
    2. experiencing menstruation for 40 years or more.
    3. using estrogen replacement therapy during menopause.
    4. having a paternal grandmother with postmenopausal breast cancer.

16. A patient diagnosed with breast cancer has been offered the treatment choice of breast conservation surgery with radiation or a modified radical mastectomy. When questioned by the patient about these options, the nurse informs the patient that the lumpectomy with radiation:

    1. preserves the normal appearance and sensitivity of the breast.
    2. provides a shorter treatment period with fewer long-term complications.
    3. has about the same 10-year survival rate as the modified radical mastectomy.
    4. reduces the fear and anxiety that accompany the diagnosis and treatment of cancer.

17. Postoperatively the nurse teaches the patient with a modified radical mastectomy to prevent lymphedema by:

    1. using a sling to keep the arm flexed at the side.
    2. exposing the arm to sunlight to increase circulation.
    3. wrapping the arm with elastic bandages during the night.
    4. avoiding unnecessary trauma (e.g., venipuncture, blood pressure) to the arm on the operative side.

18. The nurse plans early and frequent ambulation for the patient who has undergone an abdominal hysterectomy to: *(Select all that apply.)*
    1. prevent urinary retention.
    2. prevent deep-vein thrombosis.
    3. relieve abdominal distention.
    4. maintain a sense of normalcy.

19. On the second postoperative day, a 63-year-old patient who had an abdominal hysterectomy complains of gas pains and abdominal distention. The patient has not had a bowel movement since surgery. Which nursing intervention will best stimulate peristalsis and relieve distention?
    1. Offering carbonated beverages
    2. Encouraging ambulation at least qid
    3. Administering a 1000 mL soapsuds enema
    4. Applying an abdominal binder

20. A 40-year-old patient has a history of multiple births in the past 15 years. She has been hospitalized for surgery to repair a cystocele. The nurse knows a cystocele presents symptoms of:
    1. rectal pressure.
    2. constipation.
    3. hemorrhoids.
    4. urinary frequency.

21. The Pap test is done as a diagnostic test for:
    1. cervical cancer.
    2. cancer of the breast.
    3. pelvic inflammatory disease.
    4. ovarian cancer.

22. The first significant sign of toxic shock syndrome that a patient will exhibit is:
    1. sudden high fever.
    2. vaginal hemorrhage.
    3. foul vaginal odor.
    4. sudden hypertension.

23. Lower abdominal and lower back pain that increases in severity during menstruation is a sign of the following disorder:
    1. cervical polyp.
    2. ovarian tumor.
    3. endometriosis.
    4. uterine cancer.

24. Osteoporosis is a disorder commonly seen in post-menopausal women; the dietary supplement recommended to retard this condition is:
    1. calcium and vitamin D.
    2. phosphorus and vitamin D.
    3. vitamins D and C.
    4. vitamins A and D.

25. The patient who has had a history of many pelvic inflammatory infections often seeks medical care for:
    1. vaginal discharge.
    2. infertility.
    3. hemorrhage.
    4. dyspareunia.

26. The woman at highest risk for toxic shock syndrome is the woman who:
    1. experiences multiple sexual contacts.
    2. inserts tampons with her fingers.
    3. suffers untreated chronic PID.
    4. experiences multiple abortions.

27. A 20-year-old patient goes to a neighborhood clinic because she has a purulent vaginal discharge. The physician suspects that the patient has gonorrhea. The nurse instructs the patient to empty her bladder before the pelvic examination. The chief purpose of this instruction is to:
    1. prevent possible rupture of a distended bladder.
    2. visualize the vaginal canal more easily.
    3. aid in assessment of the pelvic organs.
    4. enable the pelvic organs to resume their normal position.

28. The patient is to have a Pap smear. The nurse can prepare her for the test by educating her to:
    1. use a mild vinegar douche the night before the test.
    2. abstain from intercourse 24 hours before the test.
    3. take a warm tub bath the night before the test.
    4. save a first-voided AM urine specimen.

29. The patient's husband tells the nurse that his wife, who has been diagnosed with inoperable ovarian cancer, is talking about dying and fear of death. He asks the nurse for suggestions to help his wife. Which response by the nurse would be most helpful?
    1. "The patient will probably die of another disease before she dies of ovarian cancer."
    2. "Talk of death is normal at this time, but will diminish in the future."
    3. "The patient is expressing an acceptance of utilizing hospice care."
    4. "It is perfectly normal to want to talk about death. It is most helpful to support her by listening."

30. The American Cancer Society recommends that the human papillomavirus (HPV) vaccine against types 6, 11, 16, 18 be routinely given at what age to reduce the incidence of cervical cancer? *(Select all that apply.)*
    1. Ages 11 to 12 years
    2. Ages 13 to 18 years to catch up on mixed vaccine
    3. 24 to 26 years
    4. 30 to 35 years

Care of the Patient with a Visual or Auditory Disorder

Barbara Lauritsen Christensen

Objectives

Anatomy and Physiology

1. List the major sense organs and discuss their anatomical position.
2. List the parts of the eye and define the function of each part.
3. List the three divisions of the ear and discuss the function of each.
4. Describe the physiologic processes involved in normal vision and hearing.

Medical-Surgical

5. Describe two changes in the sensory system that occur as a result of the normal aging process.
6. Describe age-related changes in the visual and auditory systems and differences in assessment findings.
7. Describe the purpose, significance of results, and nursing responsibilities related to diagnostic studies of the visual and auditory systems.
8. Discuss the refractory errors of astigmatism, strabismus, myopia, and hyperopia, including etiology, pathophysiology, clinical manifestations, assessment, diagnostic tests, medical management, nursing interventions, and patient teaching.
9. Describe inflammatory conditions of the eye, including etiology, pathophysiology, clinical manifestations, assessment, diagnostic tests, medical management, nursing interventions, patient teaching, and prognosis.
10. Discuss Sjögren syndrome, ectropion, and entropion, including etiology, pathophysiology, clinical manifestations, diagnostic tests, medical management, nursing interventions, and prognosis.
11. Compare the nature of cataracts, diabetic retinopathy, macular degeneration, retinal detachment, and glaucoma, including the etiology, pathophysiology, clinical manifestations, assessment, diagnostic tests, medical management, nursing interventions, patient teaching, and prognosis.
12. Discuss corneal injuries, including etiology, pathophysiology, clinical manifestations, assessment, diagnostic tests, medical management, nursing interventions, patient teaching, and prognosis.
13. Describe the various surgeries of the eye, including the nursing interventions and prognosis.
14. Differentiate between conductive and sensorineural hearing loss.
15. Describe the appropriate care of the hearing aid.
16. List tips for communicating with hearing- and sight-impaired people.
17. Identify communication resources for people with visual and/or hearing impairment.
18. Describe major ear inflammatory and infectious disorders, including etiology, pathophysiology, clinical manifestations, assessment, diagnostic tests, medical management, nursing interventions, patient teaching, and prognosis.
19. Discuss noninfectious disorders of the ear, including etiology, pathophysiology, clinical manifestations, assessment, diagnostic tests, medical management, nursing interventions, patient teaching, and prognosis.
20. Describe the various surgeries of the ear, including the nursing interventions, patient teaching, and prognosis.
21. Describe home health considerations for people with eye or ear disorders, surgery, or visual and hearing impairments.
22. Provide patient instructions regarding care of the eye and ear in accordance with written protocol.

Key Terms

astigmatism (ă-STĬG-mă-tĭsm, p. 611)
audiometry (ăw-dē-ŎM-ĕ-trē, p. 632)
cataract (KĂT-ă-răkt, p. 617)
conjunctivitis (kŏn-jŭnk-tĭ-VĪ-tĭs, p. 614)
cryotherapy (krī-ō-THĔR-ă-pē, p. 620)
diabetic retinopathy (dī-ă-BĔT-ĭk rĕ-tĭn-NŎP-ă-thē, p. 618)
enucleation (ē-nū-klē-Ā-shŭn, p. 629)
exophthalmos (ĕk-sŏf-THĂL-mŏs, p. 607)
glaucoma (glăw-KŌ-mă, p. 623)
hyperopia (hī-pĕr-Ō-pē-ă, p. 611)
keratitis (kĕr-ă-TĪ-tĭs, p. 615)
keratoplasty (kĕr-ă-tŏ-PLĂS-tē, p. 629)
labyrinthitis (lăb-ĭ-rĭnth-Ī-tĭs, p. 639)
mastoiditis (măs-tŏy-DĪ-tĭs, p. 636)

miotics (mī-ŎT-ĭks, p. 625)
mydriatic (mĭd-rē-ĂT-ĭk, p. 608)
myopia (mī-Ō-pē-ă, p. 611)
myringotomy (mĭr-ĭn-GŎT-ŏ-mē, p. 645)
radial keratotomy (RĀ-dē-ăl kĕ-ră-TŎT-ŏ-mē, p. 612)
retinal detachment (RĔ-tĭ-năl dē-TĂCH-mĕnt, p. 622)
Sjögren syndrome (SHĔR-grĕnz SĬN-drōm, p. 615)
Snellen's test (SNĔL-ĕnz tĕst, p. 608)
stapedectomy (stā-pĕ-DĔK-tŏ-mē, p. 644)
strabismus (stră-BĬZ-mŭs, p. 611)
tinnitus (TĬ-nī-tĭs, p. 636)
tympanoplasty (tĭm-pă-nō-PLĂS-tē, p. 644)
vertigo (VĔR-tĭ-gō, p. 639)

ANATOMY AND PHYSIOLOGY OF THE SENSORY SYSTEM

The sensory system constantly gathers information through millions of receptors scattered throughout the body and delivers it to the brain for interpretation. This process enables humans to survive safely by enabling them to make appropriate responses to external stimuli. The five major senses are taste, touch, smell, sight, and hearing. The sense of balance (equilibrium) is linked with hearing, since the sensors are located within the ear.

ANATOMY OF THE EYE

The eye, which is only 1 inch (2.5 cm) in diameter, is a marvelous spherical structure that contains 70% of the sensory structures of the body. The optic tracts contain more than 1 million nerve fibers that carry messages from the eye to the brain, where they are interpreted. Only a small portion of the eye is visible externally; the remainder is enclosed in the skeletal bones of the face and cushioned in layers of fat. The bones surrounding the eyeball include the frontal, zygomatic, ethmoid, sphenoid, and lacrimal bones.

ACCESSORY STRUCTURES OF THE EYE

The accessory structures of the eye—eyebrows, eyelashes, eyelids, and lacrimal apparatus—function mainly as protective devices. In addition, six extrinsic eye muscles control gross eye movement and enable the eye to focus on any object in the visual field. The eye muscles are attached to the sclera (or white part of the eye) and move the eye laterally, medially, superiorly, and inferiorly.

The **lacrimal apparatus** (Figure 13-1) manufactures and drains tears to keep the eyeball moist and sweep away debris that might enter the eye. Tears are composed of a watery secretion that contains salt, mucus, and a bactericidal enzyme called **lysozyme.** The lacrimal glands are located superior and lateral to each eye. Blinking causes tears to flow medially to the lacrimal ducts, which empty into the nasolacrimal ducts and drain into the nasal cavity.

The **conjunctiva** is a thin mucous membrane that lines the inner aspect of the eyelids and the anterior surface of the eyeball to the edge of the cornea. Sometimes the blood vessels of the conjunctiva become dilated because of irritation or congestion, and the individual is said to have "bloodshot" eyes. The lower conjunctival sac is where eyedrops and eye ointment medication are usually administered.

STRUCTURE OF THE EYEBALL

The eyeball is composed of three layers, or tunics (Figure 13-2). The outermost layer of the eyeball is the fibrous tunic; it is composed of the sclera and the cornea. The **sclera,** or white of the eye, is a thick, white, opaque, connective tissue. The sclera gives shape to the eyeball and, because of its toughness, protects the inner eye structures. Posteriorly it is pierced by the optic nerve.

The **cornea** is the central anterior portion of the sclera. It is transparent and covers the iris, which is the colored portion of the eye. The cornea allows light rays to enter the inner portion of the eye. The cornea is the first part of the eye that refracts (bends) light rays. It is dense, uniform in thickness, and nonvascular, and it projects like a dome beyond the sclera. The cornea is one of the most highly developed, sensitive tissues in the body and is innervated by the trigeminal nerve (cranial nerve V). The avascular cornea obtains oxygen primarily through absorption from the tear film layer that bathes the epithelium. A small amount of oxygen is obtained from the **aqueous humor** (watery fluid in front of the lens in the anterior chamber of the eye) through the endothelial layers. The degree of corneal curvature varies in different individuals and in the same person at different ages. The curvature is more pronounced in youth than in advanced age.

At the junction of the sclera and cornea is a special structure called the canal of Schlemm. This tiny venous sinus at the angle of the anterior chamber of the eye drains the aqueous humor and funnels it into the bloodstream. This aids in controlling intraocular pressure (IOP; the pressure within the eyeball).

The middle layer of the eyeball is the vascular tunic. It contains the choroid, the ciliary body, and the iris. The posterior portion of the vascular tunic is the **choroid,** which is a thin, dark brown membrane that lines most of the internal area of the sclera. It is highly vascular and supplies nutrients to the retina. The anterior portion of the vascular tunic forms the ciliary body, which is an intrinsic muscular ring that holds the lens in place and changes its shape for near or distant vision. The ciliary body also attaches to the iris, a

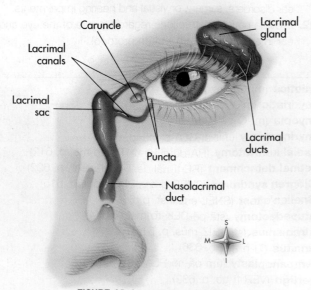

Caruncle

Lacrimal
gland

Lacrimal
canals

Lacrimal
sac

Lacrimal
ducts

Puncta

Nasolacrimal
duct

FIGURE 13-1 Lacrimal apparatus.

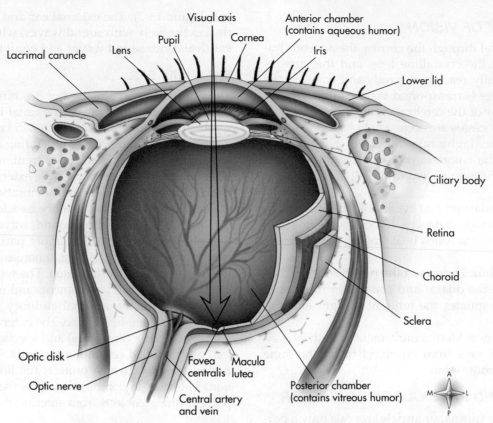

FIGURE 13-2 Horizontal section through the left eyeball. The eye is viewed from above.

pigmented intrinsic muscular ring that resembles a doughnut. Located slightly nasal to the center of the iris is a circular opening called the **pupil.** The iris lies between the cornea and the lens and regulates the amount of light entering the eye through the pupil, much like a camera shutter. Two sets of smooth muscle control the iris, which in turn controls the pupil. In bright light the circular muscle fibers of the iris contract and the pupil contracts; in dim light the radial muscles contract and the pupil dilates. Papillary constriction is a reflex that protects the retina from intense light or that permits more acute near vision.

The innermost tunic of the eye is the **retina,** a 10-layer, delicate, nervous-tissue membrane that receives images of external objects and transmits impulses through the optic nerve to the brain. It lies on the posterior portion of the eyeball. The retina contains specialized sensory cells called **rods** and **cones** (photoreceptors). The rods and cones are scattered throughout the retina except where the optic nerve exits the eye; this area is called the **optic disk** or **blind spot.** Rods are receptors for night vision and are also responsible for peripheral vision. Cones are responsible for day vision. The three kinds of cones are each sensitive to a different color: red, green, or blue. Color pigments that are sensitive to light enable the rods and cones to function. Rods detect only the presence of light, whereas cones detect different wave lengths of color.

The center of the retina is the **fovea centralis,** a pinpoint depression composed only of densely packed cones. The fovea centralis contains the greatest concentration of cones of any area in the retina. This area of the retina provides the sharpest visual acuity and most acute color vision. Surrounding the fovea is the **macula,** an area of less than 1 mm^2 that has a high concentration of cones and is relatively free of blood vessels. Vitamin A is responsible for the production of these color pigments. The absence of these three types of cones causes color blindness, which is an inherited condition found primarily in males.

CHAMBERS OF THE EYE

The eye is divided into the anterior and posterior chambers by the **crystalline lens,** a transparent, colorless structure that is biconvex, enclosed in a capsule, and held in place just behind the pupil by the suspensory ligament. The crystalline lens focuses light rays so that they form a perfect image on the retina. Anterior to the crystalline lens is the anterior chamber, which is filled with **aqueous humor,** a clear, watery fluid similar to blood plasma. The ciliary bodies of the choroid constantly secrete, drain, and replace aqueous humor to maintain normal IOP. Aqueous humor also helps maintain the eyeball's shape, keeps the retina attached to the choroid, and refracts light.

The posterior chamber is filled with **vitreous humor,** a transparent, jellylike substance that gives shape to the eyeball, keeps the retina attached to the choroid, and refracts light. It differs from the aqueous humor in that it is not continuously replaced.

PHYSIOLOGY OF VISION

Light must travel through the cornea, the aqueous humor, the pupil, the crystalline lens, and the vitreous humor and finally reaches the rods and cones of the retina. The image is transported via the optic nerve to the visual center of the cerebral cortex in the brain.

Four basic processes are necessary to form an image:
1. **Refraction:** Light rays are bent as they pass through the colorless structures of the eye, enabling light from the environment to focus on the retina.
2. **Accommodation:** The eye is able to focus on objects at various distances. It focuses the image of an object on the retina by changing the curvature of the lens.
3. **Constriction:** The size of the pupil, which is controlled by the dilator and constrictor muscles of the iris, regulates the amount of light entering the eye.
4. **Convergence:** Medial movement of both eyes allows light rays from an object to hit the same point on both retinas.

ANATOMY AND PHYSIOLOGY OF THE EAR

The external ear (**pinna,** or **auricle**) reveals only a portion of the complex organ of hearing. Within the ear are many structures that enable hearing and interpretation of sound and assist in maintaining equilibrium (balance). Anatomically, from the external structures to the internal structures, the ear has three distinct divisions: the external ear, the middle ear, and the inner ear (Figure 13-3). The external ear and the middle ear deal exclusively with sound waves, whereas the inner ear deals with sound waves and equilibrium.

EXTERNAL EAR

The external ear is composed of the auricle (pinna) and the external auditory canal. The canal is shaped like a small, curved tube (about 1 inch [2.5 cm] in length). It extends into the temporal bone, ending at the **tympanic membrane**—a thin, semitransparent membrane. The tympanic membrane separates the external ear from the middle ear and transmits sound vibrations to the internal ear by means of the auditory ossicles. The external ear is designed to collect sound waves and channel them to the middle ear. The upper part of the pinna is composed of elastic cartilage, whereas the lower part, the lobe, is mainly fleshy tissue. The whole structure is attached to the head by ligaments and muscles.

The walls of the external auditory canal are composed of cartilage-lined bone. The external auditory canal contains cilia (tiny hairs) and specialized sebaceous (oil) glands called **ceruminous glands.** They secrete **cerumen** (earwax), which protects the lining from infection. The cilia, in combination with the cerumen, also prevent foreign objects from entering the ear.

MIDDLE EAR

The middle ear, or tympanic cavity, is a small, air-filled chamber located within the temporal bone. The **eustachian tube,** or auditory canal, is lined with a mucous membrane that joins the nasopharynx and the middle-ear cavity. During swallowing or yawning, the tube

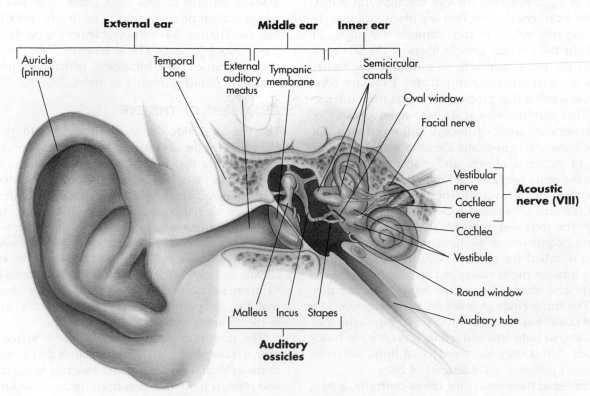

FIGURE 13-3 External, middle, and inner ear. (Not to scale.)

allows air to enter the middle ear, which equalizes the air pressure on either side of the tympanic membrane. Because the pharynx, the eustachian tube, and the middle ear are all covered with a continuous mucous membrane, infection can travel easily from the throat to the middle ear. This is often seen in young children. The posterior wall of the middle ear opens into the mastoid process, an area filled with air spaces, which also aids in equalizing air pressure. Infection of the middle ear, if untreated, can spread to the mastoid process.

Extending along the middle-ear chamber are three small bones (ossicles) that carry sound waves from the external ear to the inner ear. These ossicles are named according to their shape: the **malleus** (hammer), the **incus** (anvil), and the **stapes** (stirrup). The internal surface of the tympanic membrane is connected to the first of these three bones, the malleus. The malleus transfers sound waves to the incus, which in turn transfers them to the stapes. The stapes pushes against the oval window, a small membrane that marks the beginning of the inner ear. When sound waves cause the tympanic membrane to vibrate, that vibration is transmitted and amplified by the ear ossicles as it passes through the middle ear. Movement of the stapes against the oval window causes movement of fluid in the inner ear.

INNER EAR

A very important portion of the ear, the inner ear, or **labyrinth,** is a series of canals (Figure 13-4). Structurally, it contains the bony labyrinth, which is filled with

a fluid called **perilymph.** The bony labyrinth has three subdivisions called the **semicircular canal** (associated with the sense of balance), the **vestibule,** and the **cochlea.** The membranous labyrinth is a series of sacs and tubes that contain a thicker fluid called **endolymph.** Endolymph and perilymph conduct sound waves through the inner-ear system.

The **cochlea** resembles a snail's shell and contains the **organ of Corti,** the organ of hearing. It contains many hearing receptors, or hair cells. These cells respond to sound waves by stimulating the cochlear nerve (a branch of the eighth cranial nerve—the vestibulocochlear, or acoustic, nerve), which transmits the message to the brain. These hair cells may become damaged from noise pollution (i.e., high-intensity sounds such as those produced by jet engines, factory equipment, and rock bands). Once these cells are damaged or destroyed, hearing becomes permanently impaired.

Deeper in the inner ear, past the cochlea, is the **vestibule,** or the oval central portion of the bony labyrinth. The vestibule contains receptors that respond to gravity. They provide information on which way is up and which way is down, enabling an individual to remain in an upright position. Extending upward from the vestibule are three semicircular canals responsible for maintaining balance and equilibrium. They contain sensory hair cells and endolymph. The motion of the endolymph stimulates the hair cells, which stimulate the receptors; then the message is sent to the brain for interpretation (see Figure 13-4).

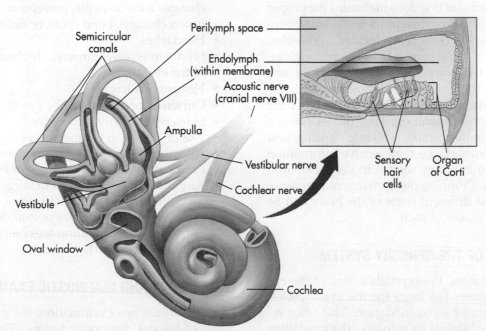

FIGURE 13-4 The inner ear. The bony labyrinth is the hard outer wall of the entire inner ear and includes semicircular canals, the vestibule, and the cochlea. Within the bony labyrinth is the membranous labyrinth *(purple)*, which is surrounded by perilymph and filled with endolymph. Each ampulla in the vestibule contains a crista ampullaris that detects changes in head position and sends sensory impulses through the vestibular nerve to the brain. *Inset* shows a section of the membranous cochlea. Hair cells in the organ of Corti detect sound and send the information through the cochlear nerve. Then vestibular and cochlear nerves join to form the eighth cranial nerve.

OTHER SPECIAL SENSES

TASTE AND SMELL

The tongue of the average adult contains approximately 10,000 taste buds; some are also located on the inner aspect of the cheeks. Certain locations on the taste buds are receptors for four taste sensations, as follow:

1. **Sweet:** Respond to sugar and other sweet substances; located on the tip of the tongue
2. **Sour:** Respond to acid content of foods; located on the sides of the tongue
3. **Salty:** Respond to metal ions within foods; located on the tip of the tongue
4. **Bitter:** Respond to alkaline or basic ions within foods; located on the posterior portion of the tongue

The receptors for the sense of smell (olfactory receptors) are located in the roof, or the upper part of the nasal cavity. On inhalation, an odor comes in contact with the olfactory receptors and the message is sent to the brain. Certain odors are remembered for a long time and stimulate certain memories (e.g., pine scent reminds people of Christmas; talcum powder reminds people of infants). The body is not able to regenerate olfactory cells; once they are damaged, the sense of smell is impaired.

TOUCH

The receptors for touch **(tactile receptors)** are located throughout the integumentary system. They respond to touch, pressure, and vibration.

POSITION AND MOVEMENT

Proprioception (sense of position) maintains the proper position of the body. **Proprioceptors** include any sensory nerve ending—such as those located in muscles, tendons, and joints—that responds to stimuli originating from within the body regarding movement and spatial position. They work in conjunction with the semicircular canals and the vestibule of the inner ear to maintain proper coordination. They orchestrate the body's movements in running, walking, dancing, and many other activities. Once they receive information from the environment, they send it to the cerebellum for interpretation. Proprioceptors enable one to sense the position of the different parts of the body and be aware of the movement of each.

NORMAL AGING OF THE SENSORY SYSTEM

As the individual ages, the crystalline lens of the eye hardens and becomes too large for the eye muscles, thus causing a loss of accommodation. This often results in a need for bifocals or trifocals. The crystalline lens loses some of its transparency and becomes more opaque, and glare begins to become a problem. The lens proteins are vulnerable to biochemical changes and exposure to ultraviolet (UV) light, resulting in cataract development. Hypertension and atherosclerosis lead to retinal vascular changes. Age-related macular degeneration (ARMD) contributes to impaired vision. The pupils become smaller and decrease the amount of light that reaches the retina, resulting in a need for brighter lighting for reading (Lewis et al., 2007).

Impaired hearing can result from age-related changes in the auditory system. A condition called **presbycusis,** a hearing deficit secondary to aging, can occur from numerous sources such as noise, vascular or systemic diseases, poor nutrition, ototoxic drugs, and pollution. These exposures occurring over the life span can damage the delicate hair cells of the organ of Corti, cause calcification of the ossicles of the middle ear, and interfere with sound conduction. Tinnitus (ringing in the ear) may also occur secondary to the aging process.

Visual and hearing losses in the older adult can result in physical and psychosocial problems. Early detection of these helps maintain a more productive lifestyle (Lewis et al., 2007). The remaining senses undergo slight changes that decrease their reaction or threshold time, which results in slower response or diminished sensation (see Life Span Considerations box).

NURSING CONSIDERATIONS FOR CARE OF THE PATIENT WITH AN EYE DISORDER

In caring for the patient with an eye disorder, review the following items:

- Eye pain, pruritus, photophobia, excessive tearing, dryness, floaters, light flashes, scotomas (defect of vision in a defined area of the visual field), halo around lights, diplopia, discharge, visual changes such as depth perception and peripheral vision changes, blind spots, or fading color vision
- Headaches
- Nystagmus (involuntary, rhythmic movements of the eyes)
- History of allergies
- Current medication for the eye disorder
- Side effects of any medications
- Use of glasses or contact lenses
- Adequacy of current eyewear prescription
- Personal habits related to care of eyewear
- Any previous eye injuries or surgeries

After gathering the information and reporting it to the physician, assist with the eye examination. The results of the initial examination are compared with normal findings (Table 13-1).

LABORATORY AND DIAGNOSTIC EXAMINATIONS

After the initial eye examination, the patient may require additional diagnostic testing. The major diagnostic eye tests, including Snellen's test, are explained in Table 13-2. **Amsler's grid test** is used to detect a defect of the macular area of the retina (see Table 13-2). The **tangent screen** evaluates central and peripheral

Life Span Considerations

Older Adults

Disorders of the Sensory System

- Multiple changes in vision that normally occur with aging include the following:
  —Changes in accommodation, resulting in increased difficulty focusing on close objects (presbyopia), which leads to difficulty reading or doing other close work
  —Decreased color perception and discrimination, particularly with shades of blue, green, and violet
  —Poor adaptation to changes in light, resulting in "night blindness" and increased sensitivity to glare due to increased opacity of the lens and decreased pupil size
  —Alterations in depth perception, leading to increased risk of falls
  —Decreased secretion of tears, resulting in complaints of dryness or pruritus, which leads to a high risk for irritation of the cornea
  —Increased incidence of moving particles or "floaters" that interfere with visually based tasks

- Older adults experience an increased incidence of eye disorders, including cataracts, retinal detachment, macular degeneration, and glaucoma.
- A third of all individuals older than 70 years of age have significant hearing loss.
- Hearing loss in older adults is most often sensorineural (presbycusis) and involves loss of the high frequencies. Hearing loss results in distortion of speech, which can lead to failure to respond to directions or inappropriate behaviors often misinterpreted as disorientation.
- Hearing loss can lead to social isolation when the person cannot understand and participate in normal conversation.
- A decreased number of receptors in the nasal cavities and papillae of the tongue results in changes in smell and taste. Most affected are the sweet and salty tastes.
- Medications often affect the taste of food and can contribute to altered nutrition.

Table 13-1 Normal Findings of the Adult Eye

AREA EXAMINED	FINDINGS
Eyelid	Blink reflex to light or touch intact. Lid margins just above the corneal borders.
Eyeball	Eyeball does not protrude beyond the supraorbital ridge of the frontal bone. The eyeball is usually moist; moisture may be diminished in the older adult.
Conjunctiva	**Palpebral** (eyelid): Pink, uniform blood vessels without discharge. **Bulbar:** Clear, tiny red vessels; in the older adult, the bulbar conjunctiva may lose luster.
Sclera	Generally white; may have yellow-tan dots in a dark-skinned individual.
Cornea	Transparent, smooth, convex. In the older adult, a gray ring around the cornea (**arcus senilis**) may be present as a result of lipid deposits.
Iris	Round, intact, bilateral coloration. In the older adult, color may be paler and shape less regular.
Pupil	Equal, round, reactive to light and accommodation. Response to light is equal bilaterally. In the older adult, constriction response may be slower.
Internal eye (including retina, vessels, and optic disk)	Retina is intact. Vessel structure is intact and bilaterally similar in pattern. Optic disk has well-defined border.
Visual acuity	
Distant vision	20/20 (able to read line 20 of eye chart at a distance of 20 feet)
Near vision	Able to read newspaper print at 14 inches
Peripheral vision	Side vision 90 degrees from central visual axis; upward 50 degrees; downward 70 degrees
Eye movement	Coordinated eye movement bilaterally
Color perception	Able to properly identify colors of major groups: red, blue, and green

fields of vision. The **Goldmann perimetry** test detects and evaluates the progression of glaucoma (an abnormal condition of elevated pressure within the eye because of obstruction of the outflow of aqueous humor), which affects peripheral vision. **Exophthalmometry** measures the degree of forward placement of the eye, known as exophthalmos (an abnormal condition characterized by a marked protrusion of the eyeballs). **Slit-lamp examination** is done to examine the conjunctiva, the lens, the vitreous humor, the iris, and the cornea. **Schirmer's tear** test evaluates the function of the major lacrimal glands (see Table 13-2). **Fluorescein angiography** is used to examine the microvascular structures of

the eye, to assess patency of the lacrimal system, and to assess for corneal abrasion.

DISORDERS OF THE EYE

BLINDNESS AND NEAR BLINDNESS

Etiology and Pathophysiology

Blindness is a loss of visual acuity that ranges from partial to total loss of sight. Total blindness is defined as no light perception and no usable vision. Functional blindness is present when the patient has some light perception but no usable vision. It may be congenital or acquired.

Table **13-2** Major Diagnostic Eye Tests

PURPOSE	EQUIPMENT	PROCEDURE	PATIENT TEACHING
Snellen's test* Assessment of visual acuity; used as screening test	Snellen's chart; eyepatch or cover	1. Patient stands or sits 20 feet from chart. 2. Patient covers one eye. 3. Ask patient to read above or below the 20/20 line. 4. Repeat step 3 using the other eye. 5. Document findings.	1. Explain test. 2. If findings are abnormal (i.e., other than 20 feet required to read the chart line), encourage patient to seek further eye testing.
Color vision Prerequisite for driver's license	Color chart or machine	1. Color dots are reflected on a background of mixed colors. 2. Patient identifies color patterns on the test field. 3. Document findings.	1. Explain procedure. 2. Encourage patient to seek further testing when results indicate inaccurate recognition of color patterns.
Refraction Measurement of visual acuity to determine refractory errors such as **myopia** (nearsightedness), **hyperopia** (farsightedness), **presbyopia** (inability to focus on close objects), and **astigmatism** (blurred vision)	Retinoscope or sample lenses	1. Ophthalmologist or optometrist asks patient to indicate clear or blurred vision with each lens change in the retinoscope.	1. Explain procedure. 2. Examiner discusses results with patient and encourages appropriate corrective measures.
Ophthalmoscopy Evaluation of underlying structures of the eye; routine screening	Ophthalmoscope; **mydriatic** (causing pupillary dilation) drops to dilate the pupil	1. Apply mydriatic drops (contraindicated in patients with closed-angle glaucoma). 2. As pupil dilation occurs, darken the room. 3. Instruct patient to remain still and focus on a stationary object. 4. Examiner uses ophthalmoscope to view internal eye structure. 5. Document findings.	1. Explain procedure. 2. Instruct patient that effects of the drops will last no longer than 1 hour. 3. Patient requires sunglasses when outside or in brightly lit room until pupils return to normal size. 4. Examiner discusses results with patient and encourages corrective measures.
Tonometry (see Figures 13-11 and 13-12) Measurement of intraocular pressure to detect tumors and glaucoma; pressure measured using a Schiøtz or Tono-Pen tonometer, but the most accurate readings are obtained by applanation tonometry	Tonometer (e.g., applanation [see Figure 13-11], Schiøtz [see Figure 13-12]); topical anesthetic may be used	1. Examiner places tonometer on cornea. 2. Obtain pressure readings. 3. Document findings. 4. In applanation tonometry, the surface of the anesthetized cornea is applanated by the tonometer, and the cornea is observed through the biomicroscope (see Figure 13-12). The normal intraocular pressure ranges from 10 to 22 mm Hg.	1. Explain procedure. 2. Encourage patient to relax to avoid false high readings. 3. Eyes are not to be rubbed for approximately 30 minutes to avoid corneal irritation. 4. Contact lenses may be reinserted 2 hours after completion of test.

*Eye chart test for visual acuity: letters, numbers, or symbols are arranged on the chart in decreasing size from top to bottom.

Table 13-2 Major Diagnostic Eye Tests—cont'd

PURPOSE	EQUIPMENT	PROCEDURE	PATIENT TEACHING
Amsler's grid test			
Used to diagnose and monitor macular problems	Handheld card printed with a grid of lines (similar to graph paper)	1. Patient fixates on center dot and records any abnormalities of the grid lines, such as wavy, missing, or distorted areas.	1. Explain test. 2. Regular testing is necessary to identify any changes in macular function.
Schirmer's tear test			
Measures tear volume produced throughout fixed time period; useful in diagnosing keratoconjunctivitis sicca	Strip of lacrimal filter paper	1. Place one end of strip of filter paper in lower cul-de-sac. 2. Measure area of tear saturation after 5 minutes.	1. Explain test. 2. Test may be done with closed or open eyes. 3. Normal results are 10-15 mm of wet paper. Less than 5 mm of wetting within 5 minutes is indicative of keratoconjunctivitis sicca.

The World Health Organization has determined that in the United States approximately 1.3 million people are legally blind (American Foundation for the Blind, 2009). The patient with either total or functional blindness is considered legally blind. Legal blindness refers to individuals with a maximum visual acuity of 20/200 with corrective eyewear and/or visual field sight capacity reduced to 20 degrees. (The normal visual field range is 180 degrees.)

Categories have been established to help determine the exact extent of the vision loss and what assistive measures are appropriate for the individual. These categories range from low vision loss (20/70 to 20/200) to three categories of blindness (20/400, 20/1200, and no light perception).

Congenital blindness results from various birth defects. Acquired blindness in adults occurs as a result of disorders such as diabetic retinopathy, glaucoma, cataracts, and retinal degeneration; acute trauma is also a common cause.

Clinical Manifestations

The degree of vision loss depends on the extent of trauma or disease. Symptoms may include diplopia, pain, presence of floaters and light flashes, and pruritus or burning of the eyes. Additional physical manifestations of the visually impaired patient include loss of peripheral vision; halos (rainbow colors seen around lights); a sense of orbital pressure; bulging of the eye(s); and any difference in the appearance of an eye structure, such as the pupil.

The wide variety of emotions associated with blindness range from fear, anxiety, disorientation, depression, helplessness, and hopelessness to acceptance. The patient may experience poor interpersonal communication skills and coping mechanisms. Because self-care skills may be impaired, a blind individual may prefer isolation, causing additional physical and emotional difficulties.

Assessment

Subjective data include patient complaints of blurred vision as an early symptom of an eye disorder. Determine the onset, the severity, and the duration of symptoms, as well as any factors that relieve them.

Collection of **objective data** may include observations of squinting and rubbing of the eyes. Note the patient's compensation measures, such as use of a magnifying glass. Also determine the use and effectiveness of assistive eyewear.

Medical Management

Corrective eyewear (contact lenses and glasses) is the first method of medical management for a partially sighted individual. If the visual defect results from an inflammatory disorder, medication appropriate to the causative agent is prescribed.

Additional assistive devices for a visually impaired patient include canes, guide dogs, magnifying systems, and telescopic lenses. The patient should be evaluated by an eye specialist to determine which devices are best suited. Some of the more technologically complex devices are expensive and may not be covered by insurance.

Canes are the most frequently used device for the partially or totally blind person. They are lightweight and portable and allow the patient simple maneuvering. The drawback is that canes do not usually help in detecting overhead objects. The newer laser canes provide more information about objects in front and at head and foot levels, but these are not readily available and are expensive. Guide dogs allow the blind person mobility that would otherwise be difficult. Trained dogs steer the patient away from obstacles, both aerial and stationary.

Surgical correction of the visual defect may provide eyesight. New laser surgeries provide excellent results in selected cases. Corneal transplants can restore vision in patients with corneal damage.

Nursing Interventions and Patient Teaching

The nurse might assume that patients who have been blind for years accept their condition, but this is not necessarily the case. Complications of long-term blindness may result in physical and emotional problems. Physically the patient may be malnourished from diminished cooking skills. The patient may also have secondary infections related to poor hygiene. Assistance with activities of daily living (ADLs) is a primary focus of patient care. Allow adequate time for the patient to assist in self-care. Emotional aspects of nursing interventions include appropriate communication (Box 13-1).

Vision loss affects not only the patient but also family, friends, and the community. Patients have different coping mechanisms. Be aware of the services and devices available for the partially sighted or blind person so you can make referrals. With proper rehabilitation, the visually impaired can develop independence and positive self-esteem (Lewis et al., 2007). The main resource for services for the legally blind patient is the state agency for rehabilitation of the blind (Brandt et al., 2008). The American Foundation for the Blind (www.afb.org) lists agencies to assist the partially sighted or blind patient.

For the patient with no functional vision, Braille or audiobooks for reading and a cane or guide dog for ambulation are examples of vision substitution techniques. If a patient has some remaining vision, vision enhancement techniques can help with walking, reading, and carrying out ADLs (Lewis et al., 2007). It is a nursing responsibility to educate, assist, counsel, and prevent complications. A comprehensive approach to care can help the patient successfully adjust to home, work, and society.

Nursing diagnoses and interventions for the patient with blindness or near blindness include but are not limited to the following:

Nursing Diagnoses	Nursing Interventions
Fear, related to blindness	Determine the patient's level of fear.
Risk for injury, related to new environment	Orient the patient to the environment.
	Use therapeutic touch.
	Avoid loud sounds that may startle the patient.
	Use protective devices, such as side rails and canes.
	Alter surroundings to afford safety (clear passageways, nonslip rugs, etc.).

The patient requires instruction on ambulatory safety. Advise the patient to walk slowly, get verbal

<table>
<tr><td>Box 13-1</td><td>Guidelines for Communicating with Blind People</td></tr>
</table>

- Announce your presence when entering the room.
- Talk in a normal tone of voice.
- Do not try to avoid common phrases in speech, such as "See what I mean?"
- Introduce yourself with each contact (unless well known to the person).
- Explain any activity occurring in the room.
- Announce when you are leaving the room so the blind person is not put in the position of talking to someone who is no longer there.

clues from the walking companion, and touch objects or borders. The walking companion should precede the patient by about 1 foot, with the patient's hand on the companion's elbow for security (Figure 13-5). For both short- and long-term blindness, describing the surroundings is appropriate.

Prognosis

Blindness and near-blindness disorders have been reduced as a result of emphasis on early diagnosis and treatment. Laser surgery treatment reduces and limits complications.

REFRACTORY ERRORS

Early childhood vision screening in schools has contributed to early diagnosis and treatment of refractory errors. Permanent visual loss may occur if strabismus and astigmatism are not treated at the preschool level

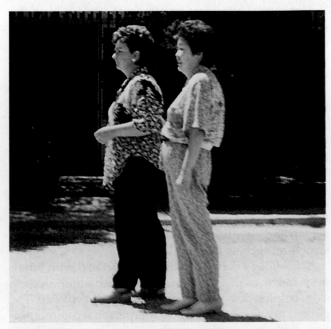

FIGURE 13-5 Sighted-guide technique. The walking companion serves as the sighted guide, walking slightly ahead of the patient with the patient holding the back of the companion's arm.

(Table 13-3). Physician monitoring of intermittent follow-up care is crucial until 10 years of age.

Astigmatism, Strabismus, Myopia, and Hyperopia

Common refractory errors (astigmatism, strabismus, myopia, and hyperopia) are described in Table 13-3.

Diagnostic Tests

Common tests used in the diagnosis of refractory errors include ophthalmoscopy, retinoscopy, visual acuity tests, and refraction tests.

Medical Management

New technology in eyewear significantly reduces refractory error problems in the adult. However, the preferred treatment is surgical correction.

Nursing Interventions and Patient Teaching

The hospitalized patient wearing corrective eyewear requires daily assistance in cleansing and maintenance. Eyeglass lenses are washed daily with a mild or diluted glass cleaner and rinsed before drying with a soft cloth. Check screw fittings to make sure they are secure. Contact lenses are cared for based on the man- ufacturer's directions. When not in use, place lenses in storage case per protocol. Take safety precautions when corrective eyewear is not worn.

A nursing diagnosis and interventions for the patient with astigmatism, strabismus, myopia, and hyperopia include but are not limited to the following:

Nursing Diagnosis	Nursing Interventions
Risk for injury, related to visual changes	Reinforce physician's instruction. Orient patient to the environment. Remove small, movable objects from the path of the visually impaired patient.

Encourage the patient to see an optometrist or ophthalmologist yearly to keep the eyewear prescription current. Instruct the patient on the use and care of eyewear; complications may result if the patient does not follow use and care instructions.

Myopia

See Table 13-3.

Table 13-3   Common Refractory Errors

DESCRIPTION	ETIOLOGY AND PATHOPHYSIOLOGY	CLINICAL MANIFESTATIONS	ASSESSMENT
Astigmatism			
Defect in the curvature of the eyeball surface	May be hereditary or a muscular deficit Occurs when the light rays cannot be focused clearly on a point on the retina because the spherical curve of the cornea is not equal in all meridians	Blurring of vision	**Subjective data:** Complaints of eye discomfort, difficulty in focusing, blurred vision
Strabismus			
Inability of the eyes to focus in the same direction: commonly called **cross-eyed**	May result from neurologic or muscular dysfunction or may be inherited	Eyeball position is not symmetrical	**Subjective data:** States difficulty in following objects
Esotropia: Eye turns in the direction of the nose **Exotropia:** Eye turns outward	Only one eye can fix on an object, because axes do not focus simultaneously		**Objective data:** Only one eye focuses or follows an object
Myopia			
Condition of nearsightedness	Elongation of the eyeball or an error in refraction so that parallel rays are focused in front of the retina	Inability to see objects at a distance	**Subjective data:** Difficulty seeing faraway objects **Objective data:** Snellen's test
Hyperopia			
Condition of farsightedness	May result from error of refraction in which rays of light entering the eye are brought into focus behind the retina	Inability to see objects at close range	**Subjective data:** Difficulty seeing near objects **Objective data:** Snellen's test

Diagnostic Tests

Diagnosis of myopia commonly follows a visit to the physician because of the patient's inability to see distant objects clearly. After routine examinations (see Table 13-3) the patient is assessed for corrective lenses or corrective refractory surgery.

Medical Management

The majority of patients are prescribed corrective eyeglasses or contact lenses. Patients who are unable or unwilling to wear corrective eyewear for occupational or cosmetic reasons may elect surgical correction.

Surgical Management

Refractory surgery is effective in treating the causes of visual problems instead of correcting symptoms. Myopia is the refractive error most commonly corrected by refractive surgery. Patients are selected based on the degree of myopia; the shape of the cornea; and the absence of medical conditions such as severe diabetes, glaucoma, or pregnancy. The usual age for correction is between 20 and 60 years. Radial keratotomy, photorefractive keratotomy, kerotorefractive surgery, and photorefractive keratectomy are procedures for myopia to markedly improve vision and are under continued study for long-term complications.

Keratorefractive surgery (surgery to alter the corneal curvature) is a new method of refractive correction. This surgical category includes a variety of procedures, including making cuts in the cornea or using a laser or a special microsurgical knife to open and replace a flap of corneal tissue.

Radial keratotomy (RK) is a technique in which the surgeon makes partial-thickness radial incisions in the patient's cornea, leaving an uncut optical zone in the center. The patient must evaluate the risk of serious complications, such as operative infection and corneal scarring, when considering this procedure.

Photorefractive keratectomy (PRK) is another procedure that uses an excimer laser to reshape the central corneal surface. It is used primarily to correct myopia but is also used for hyperopia and astigmatism. Evidence suggests that final visual acuity with this procedure is more predictable than with radial keratotomy, at least in the short term. Laser in-situ keratomileusis (LASIK) is a procedure in which first a corneal flap is folded back, and then an excimer laser removes some of the internal layers of the cornea. Afterward, the flap is returned to normal position and allowed to heal in place. Evidence supports claims that LASIK creates earlier visual stability in patients with a high degree of myopia than with PRK. Unlike RK, both PRK and LASIK procedures affect the central zone of the cornea (Lewis et al., 2007).

Intacs, which are corneal ring segments, are the newest innovation in refractive procedures. Intacs are two tiny half rings of plastic that are placed between the layers of the cornea around the pupil after the surgeon makes a tunnel-like pathway with a specially designed surgical knife. They can also be removed if necessary, and the effects on refractive error are completely reversed (Lewis et al., 2007).

Nursing Interventions and Patient Teaching

The patient leaves the hospital or clinic shortly after surgery. An eyepatch is placed on the operative site until the next morning. Patients can be up and around at home. Because of visual limitations, patients will need assistance. If the patient experiences pain, the physician prescribes oral analgesics. The patient is photosensitive and may complain of blurred vision initially. The patient is seen the next day for physician follow-up. Postoperative physician checkups are scheduled at 1 week and then monthly for 1 year. A nursing diagnosis and interventions for the patient with myopia are the same as for astigmatism and strabismus errors.

Instruct the patient preoperatively to stop wearing hard contact lenses 1 to 2 days before the surgical evaluation. Encourage rest the first day postoperatively. Inform the patient to notify the patient if pain persists after the first day. Instruct the patient that infection is a rare complication of the procedure. Tell the patient that vision is assessed regularly to evaluate functional vision without corrective eyewear. Advise patients that postoperative visual acuity is not always 20/20 without glasses. The goals of operative interventions are improving the patient's performance of ADLs and allowing him or her to drive a vehicle without glasses during the day. As a result of a slightly dilated pupil, the patient may experience a glare or halos from lights, which may require wearing glasses for night driving.

Hyperopia

Hyperopia is included in Table 13-3.

Diagnostic Tests

Common tests used in the diagnosis of hyperopia include ophthalmoscopy, retinoscopy, visual acuity tests, and refraction tests.

Medical Management

The main treatment for farsightedness is corrective eyewear, either contact lenses or glasses. A variety of lenses are available on the market, including hard, soft, and gas-permeable lenses.

Nursing Interventions and Patient Teaching

Emphasize the importance of proper care of contact lenses (see Health Promotion box). Eyeglasses should properly fit the bridge of the nose to eliminate slippage and an uneven level of each lens.

Health Promotion

Contact Lens Care

DO

- Wash and rinse hands thoroughly before handling a lens.
- Keep fingernails clean.
- Remove lenses from their storage case one at a time and place on the eye.
- Start with the same lens (left or right) at each insertion.
- Use lens-placement technique learned from eye specialist.
- Use proper lens care products and clean the lenses as directed by the manufacturer.
- Keep the lens storage kit clean.
- Wear lenses daily and follow the prescribed wearing schedule.
- Remove a lens if it becomes uncomfortable.
- Avoid potential corneal abrasions.
- Report any signs of photophobia, dryness, excessive burning, or tearing.
- Keep regular appointments with the eye specialist.
- Remove lenses during sunbathing, showering, or swimming.

DO NOT

- Use soaps that contain cream or perfume for cleansing lenses.
- Let fingernails touch lenses.
- Mix up lenses.
- Exceed prescribed wearing time.
- Use saliva to wet lenses.
- Use homemade saline solution or tap water to wet or clean lenses.
- Borrow or mix lens care solutions.

A nursing diagnosis and interventions for the patient with hyperopia include but are not limited to the following:

Nursing Diagnosis	Nursing Interventions
Deficient knowledge, related to lack of experience with corrective eyewear	Answer all questions the patient may have on eyewear maintenance. Obtain literature on lens care. Encourage physician follow-up as directed.

INFLAMMATORY AND INFECTIOUS DISORDERS OF THE EYE

Hordeolum, Chalazion, and Blepharitis

The most common infections and inflammatory disorders of the lid are listed in Table 13-4.

Diagnostic Tests

The eyelid margin is examined. Culture and sensitivity tests of any drainage may be ordered. Visual disturbances are also noted.

Medical Management

The physician prescribes antiinfective agents and may perform localized incision and drainage of a cyst or stye with the patient under local anesthesia. Warm normal saline compresses are ordered for 10 to 20 min-

Table 13-4   Common Infections and Inflammatory Disorders of the Lid

DESCRIPTION	ETIOLOGY AND PATHOPHYSIOLOGY	CLINICAL MANIFESTATIONS	ASSESSMENT
Hordeolum (stye) Acute infection of eyelid margin or sebaceous glands of the eyelashes	Frequently caused by the *Staphylococcus* organism One or more pustules may form	Abscess localized to base of eyelashes, with edema of lid	**Subjective data:** Localized tenderness and pain resulting from edema; pain diminished after pustule ruptures **Objective data:** Raised, erythematous area on eyelid; pustule exudate
Chalazion Inflammatory cyst on the meibomian gland at the eyelid margin; may require weeks to develop into a cyst	May be caused by infection; associated with diabetes mellitus, gout, and anemia	Discomfort, mass on eyelid, edema, visual disturbance	**Subjective data:** Pressure felt as eyelid closes over cornea; patient may describe vision changes **Objective data:** Cyst formation; eyelid edema
Blepharitis Inflammation of eyelid margins	Ulcerative: Caused by bacterial infection, usually staphylococcal organisms Nonulcerative: Caused by psoriasis, seborrhea, or allergic response	Pruritus, erythema of eyelid, eyelid pain, photophobia Excessive tearing	**Subjective data:** Eye pruritus; lids adhere together during sleep **Objective data:** Eyes erythematous; patient rubs eyes; sensitivity to light; tear spillage

utes two to four times a day. Lid scrubs using no-tear baby shampoo may be ordered.

Nursing Interventions and Patient Teaching

A primary objective of nursing care for the patient with an infectious or inflammatory process of the lids is prevention of the spread of infection. Take care when applying compresses. Hand hygiene is essential before contact with the eye.

Provide instructions on the use of prescribed drops or ointments. Teach the patient about the use of warm compresses and specific hygiene practices, such as keeping hands clean and away from the eyes and replacing mascara after 3 to 6 months because the oils decompose and may harbor bacteria. Caution the patient to avoid irritating fumes or smoke, which may cause rubbing of the eyes, leading to further infection. Discourage the use of eye makeup until all inflammation subsides.

Prognosis

In the majority of patients the inflammatory and infectious phases of these conditions respond favorably to topical antimicrobials. Incision and drainage of cyst-like formations result in minimal complications and risk to the patient.

Inflammation of the Conjunctiva
Etiology and Pathophysiology

Conjunctivitis is an inflammation of the conjunctiva caused by bacterial or viral infection, allergy, or environmental factors. It is commonly called **pinkeye**. Although this typically occurs initially in one eye, it spreads rapidly to the unaffected eye.

Acute bacterial conjunctivitis is usually transmitted by the hands after direct contact with a contaminated object. Pneumococcal, staphylococcal, streptococcal, *Haemophilus influenzae*, gonococcal, and chlamydial organisms are the major causative agents. Because of its warmth, moisture, and extensive vascularization, the eye provides the bacteria with an excellent medium for multiplication. Conjunctivitis represents about two thirds of the 1 million cases per year of eye inflammation and infection. The disease is usually self-limiting, leaving no permanent impairment.

Viruses of the respiratory or intestinal tract may result in a secondary infection of the eye. The two most common viral agents are *Chlamydia trachomatis* and type 1 herpes simplex virus (HSV). Trachoma, a highly contagious form of conjunctivitis, is caused by a strain of the *C. trachomatis* virus. Transmission is by direct contact with an ocular discharge. It is rare in the United States but is a major cause of blindness in Asia and in Mediterranean countries.

Clinical Manifestations

Contamination leads to an inflammatory process that produces erythema of the conjunctiva, edema of the lid, and a mucopurulent crusting discharge on the lids

and cornea. If untreated, this infection leaves the eyelid scarred with granulations that invade the cornea, resulting in loss of vision.

Assessment

Collection of **subjective data** requires an awareness that, during allergy seasons and exposure to environmental irritants, the patient may report pruritus, burning, and excessive tearing.

Collection of **objective data** includes observing eyes that are erythematous with edema of the lid. Also look for dried exudate.

Diagnostic Tests

The conjunctiva is scraped for bacteria and stained for microscopic examination.

Medical Management

Medical treatment is similar to that for blepharitis.

Nursing Interventions and Patient Teaching

The lid and lashes are cleansed of exudate with normal saline. Warm compresses are applied two to four times a day. When allergies are present, cold saline compresses may be ordered for control of edema and pruritus. Eye irrigations with normal saline or lactated Ringer's solution may be prescribed to remove secretions. Administer topical antibiotics and adrenocortical steroid medications. Eye pads are contraindicated because they enhance bacterial growth.

A nursing diagnosis and interventions for the patient with conjunctivitis include but are not limited to the following:

Nursing Diagnosis	Nursing Interventions
Pain, related to pruritus, secondary to inflammatory process	Apply warm or cold compresses. Administer prescribed eye medications; ensure proper instillation of eyedrops and ointments; administer eye irrigation as prescribed. Administer analgesics as ordered. Assess patient's limitations in visual perception. Implement safety measures as appropriate.

Instruct the patient and the family to avoid contact with the eyes or soiled materials when an infection is present. Individual washcloths and towels are to be used. Tell the patient to wash hands if contact is made with the eyes and before any treatments. Also teach the patient to perform and describe treatments such as irrigations, compresses, and medication administration. The patient should avoid noxious fumes or smoke and should not wear contact lenses during the suppuration period.

Prognosis

Conjunctivitis responds successfully to topical antimicrobials. Patient teaching reduces the risk of continued exposure and reinfection. Although highly contagious, the disease is self-limiting, leaving no chance of permanent visual impairment unless a chronic condition develops.

INFLAMMATION OF THE CORNEA

Etiology and Pathophysiology

Keratitis, an inflammation of the cornea, may result from injury; irritants; allergies; viral infection; or diseases such as congenital syphilis, smallpox, and some nervous disorders. It may be superficial and involve the epithelial layer only or may invade the subepithelial layer and the endothelial membrane. The layers of the eye are innervated, and thus inflammation causes acute pain. Ulcers may form in the eye membrane layers, resulting in scattered scarring of the corneal surface.

Pneumococcal, staphylococcal, streptococcal, and pseudomonal organisms are the most common bacterial causes of keratitis. The viral agent most often responsible for corneal inflammation is HSV. HSV keratitis is a growing problem, especially in immunocompromised patients. Keratitis can be triggered by stress, illness, and exposure to UV light. The condition may be associated with the use of ophthalmologic steroid medications. Overuse or abuse of topical steroids may injure epithelial cells.

Another form of keratitis is acanthamoebic keratitis. The *Acanthamoeba* organism is found in the soil, airborne dust, fresh water, and the noses and throats of healthy humans. This organism is often resistant to antimicrobial agents. Contact lens wearers are more susceptible because traditional cleaning agents for lenses include rinsing with clean or distilled water. People who swim frequently are at greater risk because the organism is not killed by usual methods of disinfection, such as chlorine.

Clinical Manifestations

Severe eye pain is the most common symptom that differentiates this disease from other eye inflammatory diseases. If uncontrolled, keratitis may result in blepharospasms and vision loss. Other symptoms include photophobia, tearing, edema, and visual disturbances.

Assessment

Subjective data include the severity and duration of the pain, the extent of light sensitivity, and any vision loss.

Collection of **objective data** includes assessing the patient for facial grimacing, lacrimation, and photophobia.

Diagnostic Tests

Depending on the causative agent, a variety of diagnostic tests may be ordered, including culture and sensitivity tests, fluorescein staining, and Gram staining. Ophthalmoscopic examination is also performed.

Medical Management

Medical management includes topical antibiotic therapy. Systemic antibiotics may be prescribed for severe cases. Cycloplegic-mydriatic drugs paralyze the ocular muscles of accommodation and dilate the pupil. For viral keratitis, therapy includes corneal debridement followed by topical therapy with vidarabine (Vira-A) or trifluridine (Viroptic) for 2 to 3 weeks. Corticosteroids are contraindicated because they contribute to a longer course, possible deeper ulceration of the cornea, and systemic complications. Drug therapy may also include acyclovir (Zovirax). Analgesics are used to control pain associated with acute inflammation. Pressure dressings may be ordered to relax the eye muscle and decrease discomfort. These dressings are often applied to both eyes because the eyes move together. Warm or cold compresses two to four times daily are prescribed for symptomatic relief. Epithelial debridement of loose tissue may be performed. Surgical management involves a corneal transplant, known as **keratoplasty.**

Nursing Interventions and Patient Teaching

Nursing interventions for keratitis include control of pain, safety, and prevention of complications. Nursing diagnoses and interventions for the patient with keratitis are the same for conjunctivitis. Provide information on self-care of a corneal abrasion. Also teach the patient to wash hands before instilling medication and to prevent infection by not rubbing the eyes. Instruct the patient to note any change in discharge or increase in pain and to notify the physician immediately.

Prognosis

Topical antibiotic, antiviral, or antifungal eyedrops, when begun promptly after diagnosis by culture, result in rapid healing and minimal visual impairment. Chronic keratitis may develop if treatment is delayed. Infection of the cornea can produce corneal ulcer and vision loss as a result of opaque scarring. Keratoplasty may then be indicated.

NONINFECTIOUS DISORDERS OF THE EYE

DRY EYE DISORDERS

Complaints of dry eye, caused by a variety of ocular disorders, are characterized by decreased tear secretion or increased tear film evaporation. Keratoconjunctivitis sicca (dry eyes) is caused by lacrimal gland dysfunction from an autoimmune mechanism. If the patient with keratoconjunctivitis sicca has associated dry mouth, the patient may have primary Sjögren syndrome (an immunologic disorder characterized by deficient fluid production by the lacrimal, salivary, and other glands, resulting in abnormal dryness of the mouth, eyes, and other mucous membranes) (*Mosby's Dictionary of Medicine, Nursing, and Health Professions, 2009*). If the patient has associated rheumatoid arthritis, scleroderma, or systemic lupus erythematosus, the patient has secondary Sjögren syndrome. The patient complains of a sandy or gritty sensation that typically worsens during the day and is better in the morning after eye closure with sleep. Treatment is directed at the underlying cause (Lewis et al., 2007).

Diagnostic Tests

The definitive test for dry eye, a noninfectious disorder of the lacrimal gland, is **Schirmer's test** (see Table 13-2). Normal results are 10 to 15 mm of wet paper.

Medical Management

Medical management for dry eye includes artificial tears replacement. Many nonprescription products are available. They should be used sparingly because preservatives in the drops or overuse can cause further irritation. Punctal plugs (temporary or permanent) may be inserted to close the tear ducts and keep the tears in the eyes longer.

If possible, limit medications that may cause dry eye as a side effect. If an infection accompanies the dry-eye syndrome, antibiotic therapy will be prescribed. Eliminate as many environmental irritants as possible. Filtering machines are available to control pollen and dust levels in the environment. If contact lenses cause local irritation and dry eye, a change in the prescription or type of lens is advised.

Surgical repair of an injured punctal sac by correctly aligning the eyelid margin or by probing an obstructed punctum (opening to the tear duct) to allow for tear reabsorption is the advised method of treatment.

Results of the fluorescein staining test for excessive tear disorder are considered normal if the dye disappears from the lacrimal cul-de-sac within 1 minute.

Nursing Interventions and Patient Teaching

The appropriate nursing diagnosis is *pain*, related to lack of natural eye moisture. Interventions are similar to those for conjunctivitis. Instruct the patient on instilling eye medications, practicing appropriate hygiene, and avoiding irritants.

Prognosis

Eyedrops alleviate the majority of symptoms caused by dry eye. Long-term use of artificial tears results in no adverse reactions. Control of medical conditions minimizes discomfort and complications. Surgical repair of the punctal sac is a safe procedure and has a good prognosis.

ECTROPION AND ENTROPION

Etiology and Pathophysiology

Ectropion and entropion are two noninfectious disorders of the lid causing an abnormal turning of the eyelid margins.

Ectropion is the outward turning of the eyelid margin. In the older patient it is common for the orbicularis oculi muscle to be relaxed. Paralytic ectropion occurs when orbicularis muscle function is disturbed, as with Bell's palsy. Other causes of ectropion are eyelid laceration and burns of the conjunctival tissue.

Entropion is an inward turning of the eyelid. The lower eyelid margin is the most frequently involved. The conjunctival membrane lining the eyelid and part of the eyeball are exposed. Entropion is caused by atrophy of the eyelid tissue, spasms of the orbicularis oculi muscle, or scarring of the tarsal plate (dense connective tissue that stiffens the eyelid) caused by congenital condition or trauma. Varying degrees of atonia commonly exist in the older adult orbicularis.

Clinical Manifestations

Ectropion and entropion are characterized by abnormal direction of the eyelid with tear spillage and corneal dryness.

Assessment

Collection of **subjective data** includes noting the degree of vision loss and determining tear loss and dryness of the cornea.

Collection of **objective data** includes observing the extent to which the patient can perform ADLs and the presence of any eyelid margin inflammation.

Diagnostic Tests

The physician diagnoses these conditions through a visual and ophthalmologic examination.

Medical Management

Medical intervention consists of topical medications to reduce conjunctival and corneal inflammation or drying. Surgery is the preferred treatment. Resection of the tarsal plate, removal of the scarred tissue, or tightening of the orbicularis oculi muscle is the choice for permanent repair.

Nursing Interventions

Interventions for ectropion and entropion involve monitoring the medical treatment and reporting its progress. A nursing diagnosis for the patient with ectropion or entropion is *disturbed sensory perception*, related to edema and exudate. Interventions include assistance in self-care activities, safety measures, observation for infection and inflammation, and medication and dressing treatments as prescribed.

Prognosis

Early diagnosis and treatment of eyelid disorders reduces the risk of conjunctival and corneal inflammation and scarring. Monitoring treatment reduces the need for surgical intervention and minimizes visual disturbances.

DISORDERS OF THE LENS

Cataracts

Etiology and Pathophysiology

A cataract is a crystalline opacity or clouding of the lens. The patient may have a cataract in one or both eyes. If they are present in both eyes, one cataract may affect vision more than the other. The lens is normally clear and transparent. As a person ages, opacification of the lens gradually occurs. About 50% of Americans between 65 and 74 years old have some degree of cataract formation. After 75 years of age, the statistic rises to about 70% of Americans. For Americans older than 65 years, cataract removal is the most common surgical procedure. When a cataract develops, the lens becomes foggy and vision decreases. If a large enough portion of the lens becomes opaque, light cannot reach the retina.

Cataracts may be congenital (e.g., from exposure to maternal rubella) or acquired from systemic disease, trauma, toxins (e.g., radiation or UV light exposure, certain drugs such as systemic corticosteroids or long-term topical corticosteroids), and intraocular inflammation. Most cataracts are age related (senile cataracts). The patient with diabetes mellitus tends to develop cataracts at a younger age than does the patient without diabetes. Smoking has been linked with the development of cataracts. Cataract development is mediated by a number of factors. In senile cataract formation, it appears that altered metabolic processes within the lens cause an accumulation of water and alterations in the fiber structure. These changes affect lens transparency, causing vision changes.

Clinical Manifestations

Cataract symptoms are painless, but include blurred vision, difficulty reading fine print, diplopia, photosensitivity, glare, abnormal color perception, and difficulty driving at night. Glare is due to light scatter caused by the lens opacities, and it may be significantly worse at night when the pupil dilates. The visual decline is gradual, but the rate of cataract development varies from patient to patient. The opacity can be seen in the center of the lens (Figure 13-6).

Assessment

Subjective data include blurred vision, often the first symptom to be expressed by the patient. Note any subjective complaints, such as "hazy" or "fuzzy" vision or abnormal color perception.

Collection of **objective data** involves observing the patient for difficulty in reading, such as noting whether

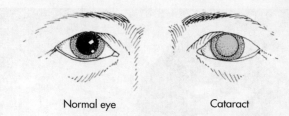

Normal eye   Cataract

FIGURE 13-6 Cataract, visible in the left eye as white opacity of the lens, is seen through the pupil.

the patient brings a newspaper close to the eyes. Also note sensitivity to light.

Diagnostic Tests

Diagnosis is based on decreased visual acuity or other complaints of visual dysfunction. The opacity is directly observable by ophthalmoscopic or slit-lamp microscopic examination. A totally opaque lens creates the appearance of a white pupil (see Figure 13-6).

Medical Management

Monitor the patient for changes in vision associated with increasing cataract size. For many patients the diagnosis is made long before they actually decide to have surgery. Often, changing the patient's eyewear prescription can improve the visual acuity, at least temporarily. If glare makes it difficult to drive at night, the patient can drive only during daylight hours and have a family member drive at night. When palliative measures no longer provide an acceptable level of visual function, the patient is an appropriate candidate for surgery. Surgery is the only definitive method of treatment and can be performed at any age. It can be done using a local, topical, or general anesthesia.

There are two methods of surgery: intracapsular and extracapsular extraction. Intracapsular surgery involves removing the lens and its entire capsule. Although some surgeons still perform intracapsular extraction (and it may be necessary in instances of trauma), the intracapsular technique has been largely replaced by extracapsular extraction. In the extracapsular method, the anterior capsule is opened and the lens nucleus and cortex are removed, leaving the remainder capsular bag intact. Healing is rapid with this method.

Phacoemulsification is the most common type of extracapsular cataract extraction (Figure 13-7). This technique uses ultrasound to break up and remove the cataract through a small incision, thereby reducing the healing time and decreasing the chance of complications.

During surgery the physician implants a synthetic (not from a human donor) intraocular lens in the posterior chamber behind the iris. At the end of the procedure, the patient receives injections of subconjunctival corticosteroid and antibiotic medications. Then an antibiotic and corticosteroid ointment is applied

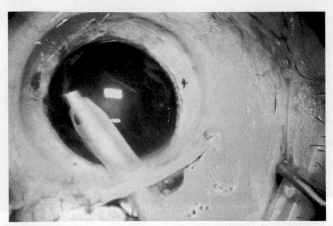

FIGURE 13-7 Phacoemulsification of a cataractous lens through a self-sealing, scleral-tunnel incision. Note the circular opening in the anterior lens capsule.

and the patient's eye is covered with a patch and protective shield. The patch is usually worn overnight and removed during the first postoperative visit. The patient receives a prescription for glasses after the eye is fully recovered (about 6 to 8 weeks postoperatively). Most of the postoperative refractive error is corrected with the intraocular lens, but the patient also needs corrective eyewear for near vision and for residual refractive error (Leyland & Zinicola, 2005). Special contact lenses provide the patient many options for comfort.

Nursing Interventions and Patient Teaching
Preoperative and postoperative nursing care is a primary nursing responsibility (Nursing Care Plan 13-1). Cataract symptoms usually develop slowly and can easily be detected. Encourage patients to have annual examinations, especially if they are age 40 or older. Surgery provides about a 90% success rate of acceptable levels of vision. Unless complications occur, the patient is usually ready to go home within a few hours after the surgery, as soon as the effects of sedative agents have worn off. Postoperative medications usually include antibiotic and corticosteroid drops to prevent infection and decrease the postoperative inflammatory response. Some evidence indicates that postoperative activity restrictions and nighttime eye shielding are unnecessary (American Society of Opthalmic Registered Nurses, 2004). However, many ophthalmologists still instruct the patient to avoid activities that increase IOP, such as bending, stooping, coughing, or lifting. Ophthalmologists may also recommend using an eyeshield over the operative eye at night for protection. Discuss safety measures appropriate to vision alterations, and instruct the patient to notify the physician of any complications such as pain, erythema, drainage, or sudden visual changes. If sudden pain occurs, call the physician (see Communication box and Patient Teaching box).

Prognosis
Gradual loss of lens transparency increases the risk of injury because of vision loss. Carefully monitor patients for degeneration of the lens. The condition may be accompanied by secondary glaucoma, which further reduces visual acuity. Surgical intervention is advised to improve vision. Postoperative complications of cataract surgery are uncommon, but may include infection, hemorrhage, or increased IOP (Lewis et al., 2007). Complications may recur years after cataract surgery and should be reported to the ophthalmologist.

DISORDERS OF THE RETINA

Diabetic Retinopathy
Etiology and Pathophysiology
Diabetic retinopathy is a disorder of retinal blood vessels characterized by capillary microaneurysms, hemorrhage, exudates, and the formation of new vessels and connective tissue. After 15 years with diabetes mellitus, nearly all patients with type 1 and 80% with type 2 have some degree of retinal disease accompanied by nephropathy. The incidence increases in relationship to how long the patient has the disease. The disorder occurs more frequently in patients with longstanding, poorly controlled diabetes mellitus (see Cultural Considerations box).

The initial stage of diabetic retinopathy may last several years. The earliest and most treatable stages often produce no changes in vision. Because of this, the patient with diabetes must have regular dilated eye examinations by an ophthalmologist or specially trained optometrist for early detection and treatment. The blood vessels in the retina begin to widen and become tortuous. Microaneurysms then develop at the periphery, and small hemorrhages develop. These may disappear, but they leave in their place scars that can decrease vision. Increased capillary permeability causes protein exudate.

⊕ Cultural Considerations

Hearing and Visual Problems

- Whites have a higher incidence of hearing impairment than blacks or Asian Americans.
- Incidence and severity of glaucoma are greater among blacks than among whites.
- Hispanics have an increased incidence of diabetic retinopathy.
- Native Americans have an increased incidence of otitis media when compared with whites.
- Whites have a higher incidence of macular degeneration than Hispanics, blacks, and Asian Americans.
- Eskimos are susceptible to primary closed-angle glaucoma, resulting from a thicker lens and a shallow chamber angle.
- Native Americans and blacks have a higher incidence of astigmatism than whites.

⭐ Nursing Care Plan 13-1 | The Patient with Cataracts

Ms. Jakobi is an 82-year-old who lives alone. She has developed bilateral cataracts and is admitted to same-day surgery for right cataract extracapsular procedure with intraocular lens implantation.

NURSING DIAGNOSIS *Risk for injury, related to altered visual acuity*

Patient Goals and Expected Outcomes	Nursing Interventions	Evaluation
Patient will not have any evidence of injury Patient will have a safe environment in which she will avoid injury	**PREOPERATIVE** Instill eyedrops as prescribed wearing clean latex or vinyl gloves. Administer preoperative medications or sedatives as ordered. Explain postoperative procedures to expect, such as patches and eyedrops. **POSTOPERATIVE** Instill mydriatic-cycloplegic and corticosteroid eyedrops as prescribed while wearing clean latex or vinyl gloves. Instruct patient to avoid moving head suddenly, heavy lifting, bending over, coughing, sneezing, vomiting, and straining with elimination, which cause increased intraocular pressure. Maintain prescribed eyepatch or shield in position during specified hours. Instruct patient to avoid lying on the side of the affected eye on the night after surgery. Remove environmental barriers to ensure safety. Keep side rails up at all times. Plan all care with patient: Explain routines of what will happen and when. Visit frequently and announce yourself on entering room. Assist with deep-breathing exercises every 1 to 2 hours while awake. Check with physician for any special positioning or precautions. (If turned, position patient on the unaffected side.) Elevate head of bed 30 degrees as ordered. Assist with and teach active and passive range-of-motion exercises every 4 hours. Provide increased activities and ambulation as ordered; assist as needed. Teach self-care activities, and assist as needed. Instruct family to remove unnecessary furniture and pick up objects that may be blocking pathways. Instruct patient that cataract surgery does not correct nearsightedness or farsightedness. Corrective lenses are still needed for these problems after surgery.	Patient feels secure about upcoming surgery. Patient uses measures to control complications from surgery.

NURSING DIAGNOSIS *Anxiety/fear, related to visual impairment*

Patient Goals and Expected Outcomes	Nursing Intervention	Evaluation
Patient will experience less anxiety and fear	Observe level of patient and family anxiety. Note patient's coping mechanism related to vision loss. Encourage patient and family to vent feelings and concerns. Support patient and family's positive actions toward adapting to visual limitations.	Patient and family display trust and security after venting feelings.

Critical Thinking Questions

1. Ms. Jakobi puts her call light on and tells the nurse that she has severe pain and pressure in her right eye. What should be the initial response by the nurse?
2. What should be included in Ms. Jakobi's discharge planning to minimize the risk of injury to her operative eye?
3. In visiting with Ms. Jakobi, the nurse finds that she enjoys embroidery and knitting. Ms. Jakobi states that she is looking forward to resuming her handiwork. What should be included as appropriate patient teaching?

Communication

Nursing-Patient Dialogue Regarding Postoperative Eye Surgery

Mrs. Betta, age 71, has been experiencing decreasing vision for the past 5 years. She seeks medical attention and is told that surgery is required to correct her condition. While talking to the patient, the nurse senses her reluctance to comply with postoperative treatment.

Patient: I'm too old to go through all the routines that the doctor wants me to. It involves too much.

Nurse: I know that surgery is a concern for you. You must have many emotions right now. It's understandable that you have concerns about your recovery.

Patient: There's so much to think about and remember.

Nurse: The doctor and our staff are here to help make your recovery as easy as possible for you. Tell me what bothers you the most.

Patient: What if I go home and fall? I could reinjure my eye or break something, like my hip.

Nurse: There are several things that you and your family can do to prevent any injury to yourself. The doctor and staff will explain these things very carefully to you.

Patient: I'm afraid I'm too old to learn.

 Patient Teaching

After Eye Surgery

- Teach patient and family proper hygiene and eye care techniques to ensure that medications, dressings, and surgical wound are not contaminated during necessary eye care.
- Teach patient and family about signs and symptoms of infection and when and how to report those to allow early recognition and treatment.
- Instruct patient to comply with postoperative restrictions on head positioning, bending, coughing, and Valsalva's maneuver to optimize visual outcomes and prevent increased intraocular pressure.
- Instruct patient to instill eye medications using aseptic techniques and to comply with prescribed eye medication routine to prevent infection.
- Instruct patient to monitor pain and take prescribed medication for pain as directed and to report pain not relieved by prescribed medications.
- Stress the importance of continued follow-up as recommended to maximize potential visual outcomes.

From Lewis, S.L., et al. (2007). *Medical-surgical nursing: Assessment and management of clinical problems.* (7th ed.). St. Louis: Mosby.

As the disease progresses, new blood vessels form on the retina and into the vitreous. These new vessels rupture, causing decreased vision. Some of the blood may be absorbed, which improves vision until another hemorrhage occurs. Significant vision loss eventually occurs as these hemorrhages continue. Vitreous contraction and full detachment can occur as the vessels and surrounding tissue become fibrous.

Clinical Manifestations

Symptoms include microaneurysms, which can only be identified by ophthalmoscopy in the initial stage. In the advanced stages the patient has progressive vision loss and the presence of "floaters," which are minute products of the hemorrhage.

Assessment

Collection of **subjective data** includes assessment of the duration and control of diabetes mellitus. The patient has varying degrees of vision loss, from decreased vision to blindness. Assess the patient's knowledge of therapy.

Collection of **objective data** involves noting that in the early stages there are no symptoms; as the disease progresses, vision is diminished.

Diagnostic Tests

Indirect ophthalmoscopy shows dilated and tortuous vessels and narrowing or obliteration of the arteries. Opacities, hemorrhages, and microaneurysms can be seen. Slit-lamp examination magnifies the lesions.

Medical Management

Surgical intervention includes early photocoagulation, cryotherapy (cryopexy) and/or vitrectomy (see pp. 630-631). Photocoagulation uses a laser beam to destroy new blood vessels, seal leaking vessels, and help prevent retinal edema. A vitrectomy or cryotherapy may be performed when photocoagulation is not possible. A topical anesthetic is used in cryotherapy so that a cryoprobe can be placed directly on the surface of the eye. When the probe is properly located, its tip creates a frozen area that extends through the external tissue, then through the eyeball until it reaches a specific point on the retina. Multiple points on the retina can be treated in this way (Lewis et al., 2007).

Nursing Interventions and Patient Teaching

A nursing diagnosis and interventions for the patient with diabetic retinopathy include but are not limited to the following:

Nursing Diagnosis	Nursing Interventions
Fear, related to unfamiliarity with procedure	Determine patient's knowledge of purpose and procedures of photocoagulation, cryotherapy, or vitrectomy.

Home care after surgery for the patient with diabetic retinopathy is the same as for any eye surgery.

Prognosis

The best treatment of diabetic retinopathy is early detection. Frequent eye examinations reduce the complication of vision loss, and modern laser technology is highly effective in reducing further damage to the retina and improving vision.

Age-Related Macular Degeneration

Etiology and Pathophysiology

Age-related macular degeneration (ARMD) of the aging retina is characterized by slow, progressive loss of central and near vision. ARMD is the most common cause of vision loss in people older than 60. A gene responsible for some cases of ARMD has been recently identified. Family history is a major risk factor. Additional risk factors are long-term exposure to UV light, hyperopia, cigarette smoking, and light-colored eyes (Johns Hopkins University, 2004). Nutrition may play a role in the progression of ARMD. The Age-Related Eye Disease Study (AREDS) revealed a dietary supplement of vitamin C, vitamin E, beta-carotene, and zinc slowed the development of advancing ARMD; however, it did not seem to have any effect on people with minimal ARMD or those with no ARMD (National Eye Institute [NEI], National Institutes of Health [NIH], 2008). Studies also indicate that consuming large amounts of dark green, leafy vegetables containing lutein (e.g., spinach, kale) may decrease the risk of developing ARMD (Lewis et al., 2007).

There are two types of macular degeneration. The first, called the **wet type** (also called neovascular macular degeneration), has sudden new vessel growth in the macular region. The macula becomes displaced, and scarring occurs. Because scarred cells no longer register light, vision loss is irreversible. Wet macular degeneration accounts for 10% of cases.

The second, known as the **dry type** (also called nonexudative or nonneovascular macular degeneration), occurs in 90% of cases of macular degeneration. Degenerative changes are the cause. Lipid deposits are followed by slow atrophy of the macular region, including the retina. People with dry ARMD notice that reading and other close-vision tasks become more difficult. In this form the macular cells have wasted or atrophied and simply do not function as well as previously. Patients report that "sometimes I see the image and sometimes it sort of blinks at me, like I have a short circuit."

Clinical Manifestations

The hallmark sign of ARMD is the appearance of drusen in the fundus found on ophthalmoscopic evaluation. Drusen appear as yellowish exudates beneath the retinal pigment of epithelium and represent localized or diffuse deposits of extracellular debris. The main symptom of macular degeneration is gradual and variable bilateral loss of **central vision.** One eye may have a greater loss than the other. Color perception may also be affected.

Assessment

Collection of **subjective data** includes noting that the patient may have difficulty distinguishing colors correctly. Assess for visual disturbances and coping mechanisms for the loss. Macular degeneration develops differently in each person, so the symptoms may vary. However, some of the most common symptoms include (1) a gradual loss of ability to see objects clearly; (2) distorted vision, with objects appearing to be the wrong size or shape or straight lines appearing wavy or crooked; (3) gradual loss of clear color vision; (4) scotomas (blind spots in the visual field); and (5) a dark or empty area appearing in the center of vision.

Collection of **objective data** includes noting the degree to which the patient can centrally view objects.

Diagnostic Tests

Ophthalmoscopy is used to detect opacity, hemorrhage, and new blood vessel formation. The examiner looks for retinal detachment, drusen, and other fundus changes associated with ARMD, and any other abnormalities. Using Amsler's grid test may help define the involved areas (see Table 13-2).

Medical Management

Previously, the treatment for wet ARMD was a laser macular photocoagulation to destroy abnormal blood vessels. Unfortunately, the laser beam also destroyed photoreceptor cells and retinal pigment epithelium, leaving a blind spot from the scarred area in the retina (Lewis et al., 2007). Photodynamic therapy is a new treatment for wet ARMD. This treatment uses intravenous verteporfin (Visudyne) and a "cold" laser. Verteporfin becomes active when exposed to the "cold" laser light wave. This procedure causes deconstruction of abnormal blood vessels but does not cause permanent damage to the retinal pigment epithelium and photoreceptor cells. The specific guidelines when this can be used by patients with wet ARMD are very strict and only about 10% of patients are eligible for treatment (Lewis et al., 2007). Caution patients to avoid direct exposure to sunlight and other intense forms of light for 5 days after treatment (Lewis et al., 2007). There is no treatment for the dry type.

Unfortunately, central vision damaged by macular degeneration cannot be restored. However, since macular degeneration does not damage peripheral vision, low vision aids such as telescopic and microscopic special lenses, magnifying glasses, and electronic magnifiers for close work can be prescribed to help make the most of remaining vision. Often people, with adaptation, can cope well and continue to do most things they were accustomed to doing. **High-dose nutritional supplements** of zinc, beta-carotene, and vitamins C and E have been shown to reduce the risk of progression to advanced ARMD by 25% (NEI, NIH, 2008). A diet rich in fruits and dark green leafy vegetables is also recommended (NEI, NIH, 2008).

Nursing Interventions and Patient Teaching

The patient needs patience and understanding to cope with the continuing loss of sight. Help the patient through the process of accepting loss of sight. Maintaining safety is important because only peripheral vision exists.

A nursing diagnosis and interventions for the patient with macular degeneration include but are not limited to the following:

Nursing Diagnosis	Nursing Interventions
Disturbed sensory perception (visual), related to disease process	Note the extent of visual loss and the level of difficulty with ADLs; assist the patient in developing ways of performing these activities. Determine the patient's support systems and elicit help if available.

Instruct the patient about the disease process, stressing that peripheral vision will be maintained. Provide ways for the patient to maintain as much independence as possible, and help family and friends determine the areas in which to assist.

Prognosis
Early diagnosis of macular degeneration is critical to prevent blindness. Watchful waiting is the only approach to dry macular degeneration. Ophthalmic laser surgery is of limited benefit because of the gradual and progressive course of the disorder. Photocoagulation is preventive, not curative.

Retinal Detachment
Etiology and Pathophysiology
Retinal detachment is a separation of the retina from the choroid in the posterior area of the eye (Figure 13-8). This usually results from a hole in the retina that allows vitreous humor to leak between the choroid and the retina. The immediate cause may be severe trauma to the eye, such as a contusion or a penetrating wound. In most cases, however, retinal detachment is the result of internal changes related to aging and sometimes inflammation of the eye. Retinal detachment may also occur in debilitated patients when there is sudden severe physical exertion. As the detachment progresses, it interrupts the transmission of visual images from the retina to the optic nerve. The result is a progressive loss of vision to complete blindness.

Clinical Manifestations
Symptoms include a sudden or gradual development of flashes of light, followed by floating spots, a "cobweb," a "hairnet," and loss of a specific field of vision.

Assessment
Subjective data include patient complaints of flashing lights unilaterally and floaters. Progressive vision restriction occurs in one area. If the tear is acute and extensive, the patient describes a sensation like a curtain being drawn across the eye. Because the retina does

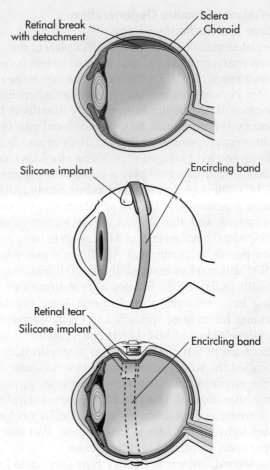

FIGURE 13-8 Retinal break with detachment: surgical repair by scleral buckling technique.

not contain sensory nerves that relay sensations of pain, the condition is painless.

Collection of **objective data** includes observing the patient for the ability to perform ADLs. Also assess the level of anxiety associated with coping.

Diagnostic Tests
Visual acuity measurements should be the first diagnostic procedure with any complaint of vision loss. Indirect and direct ophthalmoscopy is used to detect pallor of the retina and the detachment. Three-mirror gonioscopy provides a magnified view of any retinal lesions. Slit-lamp examination magnifies the lesions. Ultrasound may be useful to identify a retinal detachment if the retina cannot be directly visualized (e.g., when the cornea, lens, or vitreous humor is hazy or opaque).

Medical Management
The treatment of choice is early corrective intervention. One of four procedures may be performed.

Laser photocoagulation burns localized tears or breaks in the posterior portion of the eyeball, eventually sealing the tear or break.

Cryotherapy freezes the borders of a retinal hole with a frozen-tipped probe. The probe is applied to the scleral surface directly over the retinal hole area. The hole seals when the resultant inflammatory process produces scarring.

ElectroDiathermy burns a retinal break using an ultrasonic probe. The probe is applied to the scleral surface directly over the retinal break. Sealing occurs from the resultant inflammatory and scarring process.

Scleral buckling is an extraocular surgical procedure that involves indenting the globe so the pigment epithelium, choroid, and sclera move toward the detached retina. This not only helps seal retinal breaks, but also helps relieve inward traction on the retina. The retinal surgeon sutures a silicone implant against the sclera, causing the sclera to buckle inward. The surgeon may place an encircling band over the implant if there are multiple retinal breaks, if the surgeon cannot locate suspected breaks, or if there is widespread inward traction on the retina (see Figure 13-8). If present, subretinal fluid may be drained by inserting a small-gauge needle to facilitate contact between the retina and the buckled sclera. Scleral buckling is usually accomplished with the patient under local anesthesia. The patient may be discharged on the first postoperative day, or scleral buckling surgery may be performed as an outpatient procedure.

Pneumatic retinopexy. Pneumatic (pertaining to air or gas) **retinopexy** is an intraocular procedure that involves the injection of a gas into the vitreous cavity to form a temporary bubble that closes retinal breaks and places pressure on the separated retinal layers. This bubble is temporary and is combined with treatments of laser photocoagulation or cryotherapy. For several weeks the patient must position the head in a forward position so the bubble is in contact with the retinal break (Lewis et al., 2007).

Nursing Interventions and Patient Teaching

Postprocedure management includes cycloplegic, mydriatic, and antiinfective eyedrops. Eyepatches are applied over only the operative eye or both eyes, providing the required rest of the eye for 1 or 2 days. Safety measures are essential because the eyes are patched.

Depending on the procedures, the position of the head postoperatively may vary. If air is injected into the vitreous, the head is positioned with the unaffected eye upward and the patient lying on the abdomen or sitting forward for 4 to 5 days.

Dark glasses are prescribed after removal of the eye patches to decrease the discomfort of **photophobia** (abnormal sensitivity to light).

A nursing diagnosis and interventions for the patient with retinal detachment include but are not limited to the following:

Nursing Diagnosis	Nursing Interventions
Anxiety, related to visual alterations	Allow the patient the opportunity to discuss feelings and fears about the possible loss of vision. Answer questions honestly and correct any misunderstandings. Explain the reasons for restrictions of activities and for procedures.

Discuss with the patient temporary restrictions of reaching, work, and activity (see Patient Teaching box).

Prognosis

Retinal detachment requires treatment. Reattachment is successful in 90% of cases; the degree of sight restoration depends on the extent and duration of separation. Maximum vision is achieved within 3 months after surgery. Unless replaced, a detached retina slowly dies after several years. Blindness from retinal detachment is irreversible.

GLAUCOMA

Etiology and Pathophysiology

Glaucoma is not one disease, but rather a group of disorders characterized by (1) increased intraocular pressure (IOP) because of obstruction of the outflow of aqueous humor, (2) optic nerve atrophy, and (3) progressive loss of peripheral vision (Figure 13-9). Glaucoma is found in people who are middle-age and older. Approximately 12% to 15% of all blindness in the United States results from glaucoma. One in 50 white people is affected. However, 1 in 10 blacks develops glaucoma. It is seldom seen in people younger than 35 years of age but may occur in infancy.

Open-angle glaucoma, also known as **primary open-angle glaucoma (POAG),** represents 90% of the cases of primary glaucoma. In POAG the outflow of aqueous humor is decreased in the trabecular meshwork. In essence, the drainage channels become occluded, like a clogged kitchen sink. The course of the disease is slowly progressive and results from degenerative changes. It is often bilateral.

Patient Teaching

Retinal Detachment

- Return to sedentary activity in 2 weeks; no heavy lifting or active physical activity for 6 weeks, or as instructed by physician.
- Check with physician about shampooing hair.
- Limit reading for 3 weeks or as instructed by physician.
- Use correct technique for administration of eye medications.
- Report to ophthalmologist any signs of further detachment (flashes of light, increase in floaters, blurred vision).
- Report for medical follow-up visits as instructed.

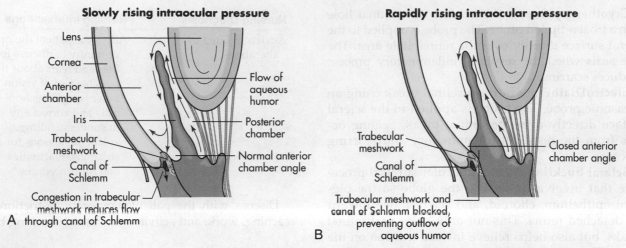

Slowly rising intraocular pressure

Lens
Cornea
Anterior chamber
Iris
Trabecular meshwork
Canal of Schlemm
Congestion in trabecular meshwork reduces flow
A through canal of Schlemm

Flow of aqueous humor
Posterior chamber
Normal anterior chamber angle

Rapidly rising intraocular pressure

Trabecular meshwork
Canal of Schlemm
Trabecular meshwork and canal of Schlemm blocked, preventing outflow of aqueous humor
B

Closed anterior chamber angle

FIGURE 13-9 A, Primary open-angle glaucoma (POAG). Congestion in the trabecular meshwork reduces the outflow of aqueous humor. **B,** Acute angle-closure glaucoma (AACG). Angle between the iris and the anterior chamber narrows, obstructing the outflow of aqueous humor.

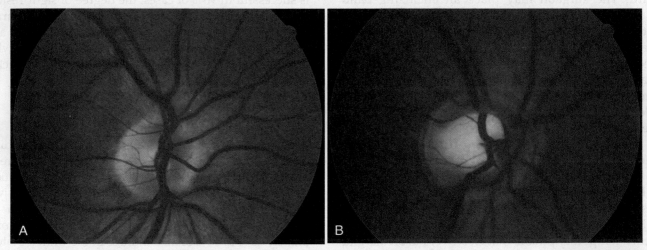

FIGURE 13-10 A, In the normal eye, the optic cup is pink with little cupping. **B,** In the glaucomatous eye, the optic disk is bleached and optic cupping is present. (Note the appearance of the retinal vessels, which travel over the edge of the optic cup and appear to dip into it.)

Closed-angle glaucoma, also known as **acute angle-closure glaucoma (AACG),** occurs if there is an abrupt angle change of the iris, causing rapid vision loss and dramatic symptoms. This type of glaucoma represents 10% of the total number of glaucoma cases in the United States.

Clinical Manifestations

In POAG the patient has no signs or symptoms during the early stages of the disease. As the symptoms become apparent, they include loss of peripheral vision (tunnel vision), eye pain, difficulty adjusting to darkness, halos around lights, and inability to detect colors. IOPs are elevated.

AACG produces excruciating pain in or around the eye, decreased vision, and nausea and vomiting. The sclera is erythematous, and the pupil is enlarged and fixed. The patient sees colored halos around lights and has an acute increase in the IOP.

As glaucoma progresses, **optic disk cupping** occurs. This is visible with direct or indirect ophthalmoscopy. The optic disk becomes wider, deeper, and paler (light gray or white). Optic disk cupping may be one

of the first signs of chronic open-angle glaucoma. Optic disk photographs are useful for comparison over time to demonstrate an increase in the cup-to-disk ratio and progressive blanching (Figure 13-10).

Assessment

Collection of **subjective data** includes noting the time of day that eye pain occurs. Also assess frequency, intensity, and duration of the pain. Note complaints of peripheral vision loss, maladaptation to darkness, and halos seen around lights. Determine the severity of headaches and presence of nausea and vomiting.

Collection of **objective data** includes noting a need for frequent eyeglass prescription changes. Elevated IOPs are also present.

Diagnostic Tests

Schiøtz tonometry is used to test for IOP (Figure 13-11). A patient with glaucoma would test above the normal range of 10 to 22 mm Hg. IOP is usually between 22 and 32 mm Hg in POAG. IOP may be 50 mm Hg or higher in AACG. Applanation tonometry is also used to measure IOP (Figure 13-12). Visual field studies show a decline in the patient's peripheral vision. Optic disk cupping occurs as glaucoma progresses. Optic disk cupping leads to optic nerve damage.

Medical Management

Keeping the IOP low enough to prevent the patient from developing optic nerve damage is the primary focus of glaucoma therapy.

POAG is medically treated by the use of beta blockers, **miotics** (agents that cause the pupil to constrict), and carbonic anhydrase inhibitors (Table 13-5). A beta blocker, such as betaxolol hydrochloride (Betoptic), reduces IOP. Miotics, such as pilocarpine, constrict the pupil and draw the iris away from the cornea, allowing aqueous humor to drain out of the canal of Schlemm (see Figure 13-9). Carbonic anhydrase inhibi-

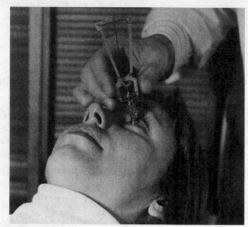

FIGURE 13-11 Measurement of intraocular pressure with the Schiøtz tonometer.

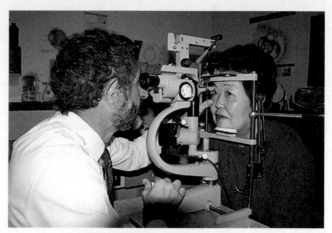

FIGURE 13-12 Applanation tonometry.

Table 13-5 Medications for Eye Disorders

Generic (Trade)	Actions and Uses	Side Effects	Nursing Implications
Sulfacetamide sodium (Sulamyd)	Broad-spectrum bacteriostatic antiinfective agent used in the treatment of ocular infections (conjunctivitis, corneal ulcers, trachoma, and chlamydial infections)	Pruritus, edema, erythema, other eye irritations	It is contraindicated in those with sulfonamide hypersensitivity; purulent exudate may inactivate drug; do not use silver preparations concurrently; comply with full course of treatment; store properly; discard solution if it discolors; warn patient to avoid sharing washcloths and towels with family members.
Betaxolol hydrochloride (Betoptic)	Beta-adrenergic blocking agent that reduces formation of aqueous humor; used for open-angle glaucoma	Insomnia, irritation of eyelids, stinging on instillation, occasional tears, photophobia, systemic effects, possible disorientation, bradycardia, weakness, dyspnea	Know pregnancy cautions; do not touch dropper on eye; keep container tightly closed; determine intraocular pressure 4 weeks after treatment; use cautiously in patients with history of heart failure or with diabetes mellitus.
Timolol maleate (Timoptic)	Beta-adrenergic blocking agent that reduces aqueous humor formation; used for open-angle glaucoma and hypertension; used with caution for patients who have heart conditions	Ocular sensitivity, severe irritation of eye or eyelid, systemic effect of cardiac failure, chest pain, disorientation, diarrhea, dizziness, exacerbation of asthma	It may mask hypoglycemia; measure intraocular pressure after 4 weeks of treatment; avoid abrupt cessation; use cautiously in patients with bronchial asthma and heart conditions; know pregnancy and breastfeeding cautions; keep container tightly closed.

Continued

Table 13-5 Medications for Eye Disorders—cont'd

Generic (Trade)	Actions and Uses	Side Effects	Nursing Implications
Dexamethasone (Decadron)	Decreases inflammation	Local irritation, retardation of corneal healing, blurred vision, eye pain, secondary eye infection	It may mask infection; use only for short term in children; tell patient not to wear contact lens during treatment; shake bottle before using; check with physician before using for future eye conditions; check with physician if condition does not improve in 5-7 days.
Acetazolamide (Diamox)	Lowers intraocular pressure; used for open-angle glaucoma	Diarrhea, weakness, discomfort, urinary frequency, loss of appetite, nausea, vomiting, numbness in hands; contraindicated with severe renal, hepatic, or adrenocortical impairment	Know pregnancy and lactation cautions; give with food; in diabetes, it may increase blood and urine glucose levels; caution patient about drowsiness; monitor intake and output (I&O) and weight daily.
Pilocarpine hydrochloride (Pilocar, Isopto, Carpine)	Reduces intraocular pressure; used for open-angle glaucoma	Muscle tremors, nausea and vomiting, dyspnea, wheezing, bronchial spasms, local irritation	Encourage patient to have periodic intraocular pressure determinations; monitor for blurred vision or changes in vision; use cautiously in bronchial asthma and hypertension; apply light finger pressure on lacrimal sac 1 minute after instillation of drops.
Cyclopentolate hydrochloride (Cyclogyl)	Anticholinergic drug that produces dilation of pupil and temporary paralysis of ciliary muscles; used in glaucoma; a diagnostic agent for angle-closure glaucomas	Ataxia, behavioral disturbances, tachycardia, disorientation, fever	Prevent contamination of dropper; warn patient of increased sensitivity to light and suggest sunglasses; contraindicated in closed-angle glaucoma; use cautiously in older adults.
Mannitol (Osmitrol)	Osmotic diuretic that reduces intraocular pressure; used for glaucoma	Fluid and electrolyte imbalance, chest pain, tachycardia, chills and fever, difficult urination	Administer by intravenous infusion; know pregnancy caution; duration of action is 1-3 hours; monitor vital signs at least hourly and I&O, weight, and potassium levels daily.
Polyvinyl alcohol (Liquifilm Forte)	Tearlike lubricant; used for dry eyes and eye irritations	Headache, burning, blurred vision, eye pain	Teach patient to instill; to avoid contamination of solution, warn patient not to touch tip of container to eye.
Gentamicin sulfate (Garamycin)	Bactericidal antibiotic; used for treatment of blepharitis and conjunctivitis	Pruritus, erythema, edema, ocular discomfort, blurred vision (may occur for few minutes after application)	Comply with full course of therapy; if no improvement occurs after a few days, check with physician.

Patient Teaching

Glaucoma

- Medical supervision is required for the rest of life.
- Eyedrops **must** be continued as long as prescribed even in the absence of symptoms; usually treatment is lifelong.
  —Blurred vision decreases with prolonged use.
  —Avoid driving for 1 to 2 hours after administration of miotics.
- To prevent complications:
  —Press lacrimal duct for 1 minute after eyedrop insertion to prevent rapid systemic absorption.
  —Have reserve bottle of eyedrops at home.
  —Carry eyedrops when away from home.
  —Carry card stating you have glaucoma and the eyedrop solution prescribed.

- Bright lights and darkness are not harmful.
- There is no apparent relationship between vascular hypertension and ocular hypertension.
- Report any reappearance of symptoms immediately to ophthalmologist.
- If admitted to the hospital for a different medical condition, alert the staff of continued need for prescribed eyedrops.
- Avoid the use of mydriatic or cycloplegic drugs (e.g., atropine) that dilate the pupils.

---

tors, such as acetazolamide (Diamox), decrease the production of aqueous humor. The result is a lowering of IOP. Surgery, which consists of a trabeculectomy or laser trabeculoplasty, is done when medications do not control the pressure. **Trabeculectomy** is the removal of corneoscleral tissue, usually the canal of Schlemm and trabecular meshwork. This produces an increase in the outflow of aqueous humor. Laser trabeculoplasty produces openings in the trabecular meshwork.

AACG is medically treated with osmotic diuretics, such as mannitol; carbonic anhydrase inhibitors; and miotics. Surgical treatment includes a peripheral iridectomy or an iridotomy. A peripheral iridectomy is the removal of part of the iris. The procedure is performed with the patient under local anesthesia. This procedure often restores drainage of the aqueous humor. Postoperatively observe the patient for signs and symptoms of local hemorrhage or excessive pain. An iridotomy is an incision into the iris of the eye to create an opening for aqueous flow. A local or general anesthetic may be used. Postoperatively observe the dressing for signs of drainage.

Nursing Interventions and Patient Teaching
Nursing interventions involve protecting the patient's safety, monitoring compliance to therapy, and reinforcing discharge instructions. Depending on the practice setting, educate individual patients and families, groups of patients, or entire communities about the risk of glaucoma. Let them know that the incidence of glaucoma increases with age and that a comprehensive ophthalmic examination is invaluable in identifying people with glaucoma or those at risk of developing glaucoma. Stress the importance of early detection and treatment in preventing visual impairment. The current recommendation is for an ophthalmologic examination every 2 to 4 years for people between 40 and 64 years of age, and every 1 to 2 years for people 65 years of age or older. Blacks in every age-group should have more frequent examinations because of the increased incidence and more aggressive course of glaucoma in these individuals.

Because of the chronic nature of glaucoma, encourage the patient to follow the therapeutic regimen and follow-up recommendations prescribed by the ophthalmologist (see Patient Teaching box). Provide accurate information about the disease process and treatment options, including the rationale underlying each option. Teach the patient about the purpose, frequency, and technique for administration of prescribed antiglaucoma agents. In addition to verbal instructions, give all patients written instructions that contain the necessary information without being overwhelming. Encourage the patient to comply with the medication regimen by (1) stressing the sight-saving nature of the drops, (2) helping the patient identify the most convenient and appropriate times for medication administration, and (3) advocating a change in therapy if the patient reports unacceptable side effects (Lewis et al., 2007).

Prognosis
Today's method of medical and surgical management provides the patient with an excellent prognosis for a full recovery. Complications are few if care is obtained early in the course of the condition. When the patient ignores glaucoma or is noncompliant with therapy, blindness may occur. Regular eye examinations are required to detect and monitor for increased IOP. Generally, once damage has occurred, the condition is irreversible. Surgery and medication help lessen the complications from glaucoma.

CORNEAL INJURIES

Etiology and Pathophysiology
The cornea is the convex, transparent outermost layer of the eye. It is composed of five layers of tissue and is uniform in nature. The cornea is nonvascular; therefore no bleeding occurs from injury unless subcorneal structures are involved. The cornea is kept moist by tear production and is protected from daily insult by the eyelid. Any wound causes the cornea to become abnormally hydrated and decreases the normal transparency (Lewis et al., 2007).

Foreign bodies are the most common cause of corneal injury. Dust particles, propellants, and eyelashes may lodge in the conjunctiva or cornea. The eyes blink in response to the irritant, and further irritation occurs from the upper lid closing frequently, thus moving the foreign body into deeper layers or a wider area of the cornea.

Burns often occur in the home and workplace. When burns affect the eye, it is a medical emergency. Depending on the chemical causing the burn, the damage may be superficial or deep. Chemical irritants such as acids and alkalis and metal flashes from acetylene blowtorches cause significant pain, depending on the depth of chemical erosion.

Abrasions and lacerations are usually superficial scratches caused by fingernails or clothing. They may be painful, depending on the depth of the abrasion.

Penetrating wounds are the most serious corneal injuries. Eye structures may be injured permanently, resulting in total blindness. Infection may result from the introduction of microorganisms on the penetrating object.

Clinical Manifestations

Foreign bodies produce pain when the eyeball moves or the eyelid moves over the eyeball during blinking. Excessive tearing, erythema of the conjunctiva, and pruritus may occur. Acute pain and burning are the primary symptoms with any topical burn to the eye. Abrasions and lacerations produce mild to severe pain, depending on the depth of corneal involvement. The pain may be transitory and slight, or spasmodic and deep. Penetrating wounds result in varying degrees of pain. If underlying structures are involved, pain may be absent because the nerves have been severed.

Assessment

Foreign Bodies

Subjective data include the time and type of injury. Assess the patient for the degree and severity of eye pain and vision loss. Ask about any first aid treatment provided.

Collection of **objective data** includes observation of the foreign body and extent of damage. When the intracapsular area has been penetrated, fluid leaks from the eye.

Burns

Subjective data include the degree of pain. It is important to assess the substance causing the burn and any first aid treatment that has been provided. Vision loss is determined by the physician.

Collection of **objective data** includes noting the extent of the burn in and around the eye, including eyelashes and eyebrows, and assessing the condition of the eyeball.

Abrasions and Lacerations

Subjective data include the degree of pain after the incident and how the injury occurred. Note treatments used at the time of injury.

Collection of **objective data** includes assessing the degree of damage of the eyeball and surrounding structures and noting any vision loss.

Penetrating Wounds

Subjective data include the time and causative factors related to the injury. Assess presence and severity of pain. Determine whether any first aid treatment was given.

Objective data include the type and size of the penetrating object. Note any fluid leakage from the eye and damage to surrounding structures.

Diagnostic Tests

Tests include visual and ophthalmoscopic examination, fluorescein staining, peripheral vision tests, and slit-lamp examination.

Medical Management

Foreign bodies are medically treated with a flush of normal saline when the object is near the sclera and conjunctiva; it can then be removed by a clean swab or tissue. Cotton is not used, since it may scratch the cornea. If the object is not easily flushed away, the individual must see an ophthalmologist to have the object removed. Antibiotic topical eye ointments are ordered.

Burns are medically treated with a 15- to 20-minute or longer tap water flush immediately after burn exposure. This will help prevent scar formation. Separate the eyelids during the flush procedure. The patient is then treated in a local emergency department or physician's office for follow-up care. Home remedy first aid treatment should not be done. Topical antiinfective agents are ordered for the eye. Abrasions and lacerations of the eye are medically cleaned with a normal saline solution. Antibiotic therapy, usually topical, is prescribed (see Safety Alert box).

Seek medical assistance immediately for eye injuries, chemical eye burns, and foreign bodies that remain in the eye. Immediately after a penetrating wound injury, both eyes should be covered while the patient is transported to the hospital. Both eyes work in synchrony, so covering the unaffected eye prevents it from involuntarily moving with the other eye. A shield reduces further injury but must not touch the foreign object. A Styrofoam cup provides adequate coverage and is readily available. The foreign object should not be removed except by a trained physician.

Nursing Interventions and Patient Teaching

Nursing interventions for foreign bodies include assisting with the required irrigation of the eye. For burns, assist with the flushing process and providing

Safety Alert!

Eye Safety Measures

- Avoid frequent rinsing of eyes with unprescribed solutions.
- Discard any ophthalmic solution that is cloudy or discolored, has been open for longer than 3 months, or contains particles.
- Do not self-treat an eye inflammation with a medication prescribed for a previous eye disorder.
- To avoid eye strain:
  - Use a good light for reading or doing work that requires careful visual focus.
  - When reading or focusing eyes for long periods, look at distant objects for a few minutes at repeated intervals to rest eyes.
- Avoid rubbing eyes.
- Wash hands before and after touching eyes.
- Wear safety glasses when engaging in activities that could injure the eyes. If injury occurs, apply cool compress if no laceration is present; cover if laceration is present.
- Wear dark glasses for prolonged exposure to bright light (such as sunlight, snow, or water).
- Flush eyes immediately for 15 to 20 minutes or longer with cool water when any irritating substances are introduced.
- Do not attempt to remove foreign bodies from the cornea; cover the eye with an eyeshield (e.g., small paper cup) to prevent excessive movement or touching of the eye. Seek medical attention immediately.
- If a speck of dust blows in the eye, pull upper lid over lower lid and let the tears wash the speck to the inner canthus or lower lid, where it may be safely removed. Irrigate the eye with cool tap water, if necessary.

eye medications as ordered. For abrasions and lacerations, assist with cleaning the eye as ordered and providing general first aid.

When a patient has a penetrating wound, note whether the pupil on the affected side becomes irregular in size. This results when the iris of the affected eye moves to occlude the wound area. Infection potential is high; therefore topical and systemic antibiotics are ordered. If the wound is small, self-healing occurs. If the wound is large or deep, enucleation of the eye may be necessary.

Effective and immediate therapy is crucial for any eye injury. If treatment is interrupted, ineffective, or not sustained, permanent eye damage will occur. The most frequent complications include infection, vision disturbances, and blindness. A nursing diagnosis for the patient with an eye injury would be *pain, acute*, related to inflammatory process. (See the discussion on conjunctivitis.)

Ensure that the patient can apply ointments and dressings, if ordered. Instruct the patient in the use of other therapy devices, such as warm or cool compresses. Teach proper handwashing techniques. The patient should wear dark sunglasses if cycloplegic or mydriatic eyedrops are used. Instruct the patient to avoid future episodes with chemical or environmental hazards. Ensure that the patient understands discharge instructions, including the need for follow-up physician visits and symptoms to report. Determine the patient's knowledge about the progress of therapy.

Prognosis

Immediate and appropriate treatment reduces the severity and complications of eye injuries. Monitor the chosen treatment to prevent permanent eye damage and vision problems. Superficial corneal abrasions usually heal without incident. Deeper abrasions or burns may result in permanent visual loss due to scarring.

SURGERIES OF THE EYE

ENUCLEATION

Eye enucleation is the surgical removal of the eyeball. It is often necessary after severe eye trauma but may be done for other reasons, such as malignant tumors. Surgical methods vary from removal of the entire eyeball or the eyeball contents to removal of the eyeball and all underlying structures.

Nursing Interventions

The loss of an eye is extremely traumatic for the patient even though the enucleation may be done after severe painful blindness. Be aware of the patient's grieving over the loss of an eye and provide emotional support to the patient and the family (Lewis et al., 2007). Other nursing responsibilities include facilitating a therapeutic dialogue between the physician and patient regarding the exact nature of the surgery.

Postoperatively apply a pressure dressing over the socket of the eye to control hemorrhage. Observe the dressing at least every hour for the first 24 hours. Ask the patient about any pain on the affected side of the head or any headache, which might indicate hemorrhage or infection. Report these findings to the physician immediately. Avoid routine postoperative procedures of coughing and turning on the affected side to prevent sutures from dislodging.

Prognosis

Patients who undergo enucleation surgery are excellent candidates for prosthetic replacements. The wound is adequately healed approximately 6 weeks after the enucleation. An ocularist fits a permanent prosthesis designed to match the remaining eye. The patient must be carefully educated in how to remove, cleanse, and insert the prosthesis (Lewis et al., 2007).

KERATOPLASTY (CORNEAL TRANSPLANT)

Keratoplasty is the removal of the full thickness of the patient's cornea followed by surgical implantation of a cornea from a human donor. It is done to replace a damaged cornea resulting from trauma, ulceration, or congenital deformities. Approximately 40,000 corneal transplants are performed in the United States each year. Improved methods of tissue procurement and preservation, refined surgical techniques, postoperative topical corticosteroids, and careful follow-up have decreased graft rejection. Medications to suppress rejection (e.g., cyclosporine) may be ordered.

Corneal grafts are usually taken within 4 hours after death. An ideal donor is between 25 and 35 years of age and died of injury or acute disease. The corneas of people with chronic or communicable diseases—such as hepatitis, acquired immunodeficiency syndrome, or cancer—are not appropriate for transplantation. The eye banks test donors for human immunodeficiency virus and hepatitis B and C. The donor's eye should have normal light perception and projection. The donor's tissue is best used within 5 days after removal.

The nurse often has the most access to the family when questions of organ donation occur. Responsibilities include notification of appropriate supervisory personnel when an organ donation from a deceased donor is occurring. Keratoplasty is performed with the patient under local or general anesthesia. The transplanted tissue is sutured into place to maintain graft alignment and a watertight wound.

Nursing Interventions

Before surgery encourage the patient to express fears related to surgery. Give instructions in the use of protective eyeglasses if dilation-causing eye medication is used. Prevent injuries by using safety devices and orienting the patient to each new environment. Cleanse and prepare the surgical areas as ordered, usually with an antiseptic solution. Preoperative teaching includes deep breathing and turning to reduce any complications associated with surgery. Coughing is discouraged, since sutures may break. Maintain dietary restrictions, if ordered; a light breakfast may be allowed if the surgery is done with the patient under a local anesthesia. Administer prescribed medications.

After surgery ensure that correct postoperative positioning is maintained; the patient is usually positioned on the back or nonoperated side until the physician allows turning to the operated side. Reinforce activity restrictions as ordered to prevent injury to the eye. Use safety measures until the patient is able to ambulate safely. Anyone coming into the room should announce his or her presence. The patient should avoid bending, lifting, and straining for approximately 1 month to prevent increases in IOP or suture tension.

Progressive activity should be prescribed by the physician. Encourage regular postoperative visits with the eye surgeon. Report any severe or progressive pain to the surgeon immediately, as well as any complaints of erythema, loss of vision, or photophobia that would occur with corneal rejection. Administer systemic and ophthalmic medications. Maintain strict surgical asepsis during dressing changes. Staff, the patient, and the family must wash hands thoroughly before any contact with the eye area. Instruct the patient to avoid the use of such irritants as powder, perfume, and propellants, which might cause sneezing and displacement of sutures. The patient should not rub the eye area to avoid contaminating the site or displacing sutures. Assess the patient's diversional activities; television is usually permitted, but reading is limited because the side-to-side movement of the eyes may loosen the sutures. If an eyepatch or metal eyecup shield is ordered, demonstrate its care. The eyepatch is applied snugly to inhibit the blink reflex and allow the eye to rest. The metal eyeshield is used at night to protect the eye from trauma. Obtain discharge instructions from the physician regarding use of eyewear.

Prognosis

The cornea is avascular; therefore healing is slow. Incidence of infection is increased as a result. The transplanted donor tissue may be rejected. The chances of rejection are reduced if the donor is a family member with similar tissue type.

PHOTOCOAGULATION

Using a laser, the physician directs a small, intense beam of light into a small spot on the retina. The light converts to heat energy, and coagulation of tissue protein occurs; this is called **photocoagulation**. Photocoagulation is a nonsurgical procedure usually performed on an outpatient basis. Without surgical intervention, the structures of the eye remain undisturbed and only the sealing of leaks and destruction of offending tissue occur.

Photocoagulation is useful in diabetic retinopathy to cauterize hemorrhaging vessels. It cannot increase visual acuity but can prevent further loss. Usually no hospitalization or postoperative medical management is required.

Nursing Interventions

Postoperative assessment for patients who have undergone photocoagulation therapy includes assessment of vision. They may have constriction of peripheral fields and a temporary decrease in central vision. A decrease in night vision and a headache from the laser's bright light may also occur.

Prognosis

Photocoagulation is used to prevent eye damage and is not curative. Minimal destruction of tissue occurs with photocoagulation. The procedure is nonsurgical; therefore infection risk is minimal.

VITRECTOMY

A vitrectomy is the removal of excess vitreous fluid caused by hemorrhage and replacement with normal saline. Any scar tissue may also be removed.

Postoperative management includes the prescription of topical eye medication for 4 to 6 weeks. Acetaminophen or acetaminophen with codeine is prescribed for pain management. A pressure patch to the operative eye is placed immediately after surgery. Ice packs to reduce inflammation are ordered.

Nursing Interventions and Patient Teaching

The patient is required to maintain a position on the abdomen or sitting forward resting the nonoperated side of the head on a table to allow air that is in the eye to float against the retina. This position is maintained for 4 to 5 days.

Dark glasses are prescribed postoperatively to decrease the discomfort of photophobia. Postoperative care includes assessing the eyepatch; applying ice packs; monitoring vital signs, especially for fever; and assessing the dressing for bleeding.

Prognosis

The procedure has limited benefits and continues to be investigated as to its benefits versus complications.

NURSING CONSIDERATIONS FOR CARE OF THE PATIENT WITH AN EAR DISORDER

Once the history and general assessment have been completed, focus on assessment of the ear. Additional information would include the following:

- Occurrence of ear drainage, tinnitus, vertigo, wax buildup, pressures, pain, and pruritus
- Other medical diagnoses
- Family history
- Exposure to loud noises
- Behavioral clues indicating hearing loss (Box 13-2)
- History of medications used for ear disorders, specifically those known to be ototoxic
- Current medications for the ear disorder
- Side effects of medications, if any
- Associated speech pattern abnormalities
- Use of assistive hearing devices
- Home remedies that cause ear trauma

Communicate the gathered data to the appropriate personnel and document the findings in the patient record. The next step in the assessment process is to prepare the patient for the initial otoscopic diagnostic evaluation.

LABORATORY AND DIAGNOSTIC EXAMINATIONS

OTOSCOPY

With an otoscope the examiner can visualize the external auditory canal and the eardrum, or tympanic membrane. Normally the tympanic membrane is disk shaped and pearl gray or pale pink. Otoscopy is the initial examination of the ear, performed before other testing. One of the nurse's responsibilities is to explain

---

Box 13-2	Behavioral Clues Indicating Hearing Loss

Any adult who:

- Is irritable, hostile, and hypersensitive in interpersonal relations
- Has difficulty hearing upper-frequency consonants
- Complains about people mumbling
- Turns up volume on television and radio
- Asks for frequent repetition and answers questions inappropriately
- Loses sense of humor, becomes grim
- Leans forward to hear better; face becomes serious and strained
- Shuns large- and small-group audience situations
- May appear aloof and uninterested
- Complains of ringing in the ears
- Has an unusually soft or loud voice
- Repeatedly asks, "What did you say?"

---

to the patient the purpose and procedure. Reassure the patient that otoscopy is a painless test requiring only about 1 to 2 minutes, with slight pulling of the ear upward and backward for an adult and down and back for a child.

WHISPERED VOICE TEST

General screening regarding the patient's ability to hear can occur with tests using the whispered and spoken voice. To conduct the whispered test, stand 12 to 24 inches (30 to 61 cm) to the side of the patient, exhale, and speak in a low whisper. Then repeat the test using a louder whisper and spoken voice, increasing in loudness. Test each ear, with the patient covering the other ear. Ask the patient to repeat words or numbers or answer questions (Lewis et al., 2007).

TUNING FORK TESTS

The two most common tests using tuning forks are Weber's test and the Rinne test. These tests are used to determine hearing loss and collect data related to the type of loss.

Weber's test is a method of assessing auditory acuity, especially useful in determining whether defective hearing in an ear is a conductive loss caused by a middle ear problem or a sensorineural loss, resulting from a disorder in the inner ear or auditory nerve system. The test is performed by placing the stem of a vibrating tuning fork in the center of the patient's forehead or on the maxillary incisors. The sound is equally loud in both ears if hearing is normal. If the person has a sensorineural loss in one ear, the unaffected ear perceives the sound as louder. When conductive hearing loss is present, the sound is louder in the affected ear, but it does not hear ordinary background noise conducted through the air and receives only vibrations by bone conduction (Figure 13-13).

The **Rinne test** is a method of distinguishing conductive from sensorineural hearing loss. The test is performed with tuning forks placed ½ inch (1.25 cm) from the external auditory meatus and the vibrating stem placed over the mastoid bone. While one ear is tested, the other is masked (Figure 13-14). In sensorineural loss the sound is heard longer by air conduction, whereas in conduction hearing loss the sound is heard longer by bone conduction.

Nursing responsibility in both Weber's test and the Rinne test includes explanation of the purpose and procedure of the tests. Stress that the patient needs to concentrate and use hand signals to indicate the ear in which the sound is heard in Weber's test and when it is no longer heard in the Rinne test. In addition, assure the patient that the test is painless and requires only a few minutes.

Audiometric Testing

Audiometry is a test of hearing acuity. Audiometry is beneficial as a diagnostic test for determining the degree and type of hearing loss and as a screening test for

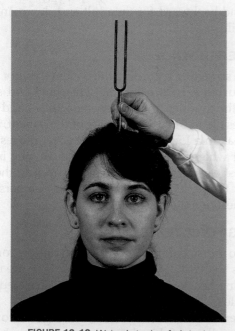

FIGURE 13-13 Weber's tuning fork test.

hearing acuity. Various audiometric tests determine the lowest intensity of sound at which an individual can perceive auditory stimulus (hearing threshold), hear different frequencies, and distinguish different speech tones.

Nursing responsibilities include explaining the purpose and procedure of each test and reviewing any required responses by the patient.

Vestibular Testing

The auditory and vestibular (balance and equilibrium) systems are closely related. Assess the patient's signs and symptoms carefully to determine whether they originate from balance or hearing loss. The patient needs to describe the symptoms in detail (Lewis et al., 2007).

Problems of the vestibular system may manifest as nystagmus or vertigo. Nystagmus is involuntary, rhythmic movements of the eye. The vibrations may be horizontal, vertical, rotary, or mixed (*Mosby's Dictionary of Medicine, Nursing, and Health Professions,* 2009). Vertigo is a feeling that the person or objects around the person are moving or spinning and is usually accentuated by movement of the head (Lewis et al., 2007). The Romberg and past-point tests are used for patients complaining of dizziness or disequilibrium.

The **Romberg test** measures the patient's ability to perform specific tasks with eyes open and then with eyes closed. The normal response is maintaining balance throughout the entire test. An abnormal response (in which the patient loses balance when standing erect, feet together, eyes closed) indicates loss of the sense of position.

Past-point testing measures the patient's ability to place a finger accurately on a selected point on the body. Inability to correctly perform the test indicates a lack of coordination in voluntary movements.

Explain the purpose and procedure of each test. Institute safety measures to prevent patient injury during the Romberg test if the patient cannot maintain balance.

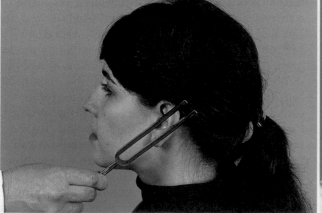
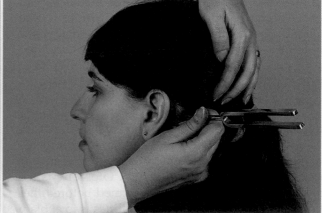

FIGURE 13-14 Rinne tuning fork test.

DISORDERS OF THE EAR

LOSS OF HEARING (DEAFNESS)

Hearing impairment is a state of decreased auditory acuity that ranges from partial to complete hearing loss. It is the most common disability in the United States: 28 million people have a hearing impairment. Among people older than 65 years of age, it is the third most common chronic condition. The quality of life for one third of the adults in the United States between 65 and 75 years of age is decreased because of hearing impairments. Recognition, diagnosis, and early treatment may help prevent further impairment and damage.

The implications of hearing loss are great. Hearing is needed to develop speech and conceptual ability; thus hearing loss may well affect personality development and intelligence-test responses when the hearing impairment is severe and congenital. This may have implications for the person's education and socialization. As hearing loss increases, the person may withdraw socially because of the inability to understand and be understood; this could lead to isolation and depression (see Health Promotion box).

Types of Hearing Loss

There are six types of hearing loss: conductive, sensorineural, mixed, congenital, functional (psychogenic), and central.

In **conductive hearing loss,** sound is inadequately conducted through the external or middle ear to the sensorineural apparatus of the inner ear. Common causes are buildup of cerumen and otitis media with effusion (escape of effusion). Other conditions that may result in conductive hearing loss are foreign bodies, otosclerosis, and stenosis of the external auditory canal. Sensitivity to sound is diminished, but clarity or interpretation of sound is not changed. When increased volume compensates for the loss, then hearing is normal; therefore a hearing aid can be helpful.

In **sensorineural hearing loss,** sound is conducted through the external and middle ear in a normal way, but a defect in the inner ear results in its distortion, making discrimination difficult. This type of hearing loss is usually caused by trauma, infectious processes, presbycusis (hearing loss caused by aging), congenital conditions, or exposure to ototoxic drugs. Destruction of cochlear hair by intense noise may also cause sensorineural loss. Amplifying sound, such as with a hearing aid, will help some people with this type of loss. Many people have an intolerance to loud noise and would not be helped by a hearing aid.

Mixed hearing loss is a combined conductive and sensorineural hearing loss.

Congenital hearing loss is present from birth or early infancy. It can be caused by anoxia or trauma during delivery, Rh incompatibility, or the mother's exposure during pregnancy to syphilis or rubella or use of ototoxic drugs.

Functional hearing loss has no organic cause. It is also known as **psychogenic** or **nonorganic hearing loss.** Functional hearing loss may be caused by an emotional or a psychological factor.

🚶 Health Promotion

Facilitating Communication for People with Impaired Hearing

- If the patient wears a hearing aid, make certain it is in place, turned on, and functioning properly.
- Get the person's attention by raising an arm or hand.
- Ask permission to turn off the television or radio or turn down volume.
- Start with the light on your face; this will help the person speech read.
- Face the person when speaking.
- Speech reading is a skill that not all hearing impaired are capable of achieving. Do not assume all hearing impaired can lip read.
- Speak clearly, but do not overaccentuate words.
- Speak in a normal tone; do not shout or raise the pitch of voice. Shouting overuses normal speaking movements and may cause distortion and be too loud for the person with sensorineural damage. If the person has conductive loss only, sometimes making the voice louder without shouting is helpful.
- If the person does not seem to understand what is said, express it differently. Some words are difficult to see in speech reading, such as *white* or *red*.
- Move closer to the person and toward the better ear if the person does not hear you.

- Write out proper names or any statement that you are not sure was understood.
- Do not eat, drink, chew gum, or cover the mouth when talking to a person with limited hearing.
- Observe for inattention that may indicate tiredness or lack of understanding.
- Use phrases rather than one-word answers to convey meaning. State the major topic of the discussion first and then give details.
- Do not show annoyance by careless facial expression; use normal facial expressions. People who are hard of hearing depend more on visual clues for acceptance.
- Encourage the use of a hearing aid if the person has one; allow the person to adjust it before speaking.
- If in a group, repeat important statements and avoid asides to others in the group.
- Avoid the use of the intercommunication system as this may distort sound and cause poor communication.
- Do not avoid conversation with a person who has hearing loss.

Modified from Conover, M., & Cober, J. (1970). Understanding and caring for the hearing impaired. *Nursing Clinics of North America, 5,* 497.

Central hearing loss occurs when the brain's auditory pathways are damaged, as in a stroke or a tumor.

Clinical Manifestations

Clinical manifestations vary, depending on the degree of deafness. Symptoms range from subtle clues, such as requests for repeating information, to more obvious signs of nonresponse.

Assessment

Collection of **subjective data** includes noting the onset and progression of the condition, deficit in one or both ears, family history, history of head trauma, exposure to noise, current medications, visual or speech disorders, and any other ear symptoms.

Collection of **objective data** must include an assessment of behavioral clues that indicate a hearing difficulty (see Box 13-2).

Diagnostic Tests

Conductive hearing loss produces lateralization of sound to the deaf ear in Weber's test. Results of the Rinne test show that sounds transmitted through bone conduction are heard longer than or equal to sounds transmitted through air conduction.

Sensorineural hearing loss produces lateralization of sound to the better ear in Weber's test. Results of the Rinne test show that air-conducted sounds are heard longer than bone-conducted sounds, but not twice as long.

Audiometric testing determines the type of hearing loss and the degree of impairment.

Medical Management

Medical management depends on the type of impairment. Surgical procedures may be required. Hearing aids or cochlear implants may be used when appropriate. Cochlear implantation is performed in individuals with profound bilateral sensorineural hearing loss who receive no measurable assistance from lip reading with a properly fitting hearing aid (see discussion of cochlear implants on p. 645 and Figure 13-15). The electrical activity of hearing is initiated by hair cells in the organ of Corti and sent to the brain along nerve fibers that make up the auditory nerve. In most deaf individuals, these hair cells are damaged. The goal of cochlear implantation is to bridge the gap created by the hair cell loss and directly stimulate the remaining neurons. Studies have shown that even with complete loss of hair cells, a percentage of cochlear neurons remains (Munson, 2006).

Nursing Interventions

Patients with partial hearing loss may benefit from a hearing aid. Help the patient care for the hearing aid as detailed in Box 13-3.

The hearing aid can only be useful if it is worn. Factors leading to nonuse may include the patient seeing the hearing aid as a sign of disability. Also, the magnification of sound may cause discomfort or irritability.

| Box 13-3 | Care of the Hearing Aid |

DO
- Handle with care.
- Wash earmold or plug daily in mild soap and water, using a pipe cleaner to cleanse the cannula.
- Dry earmold or plug thoroughly before reconnecting it to the receiver.
- Always keep an extra battery and cord available.
- When hearing aid is not in use, turn aid off and open battery compartment.
- If hearing aid whistles, reinsert earmold.
- If hearing aid fails to work:
  —Check the on-off switch.
  —Inspect earmold for cleanliness.
  —Examine battery for tightness of fit.
  —Examine cord plug for tightness of insertion.
  —Examine cord for breaks.
  —Replace battery or cord.
- Check for cracks in tubing or earmold.
- Check to see that earmold and hearing aid are inserted in the correct ear.
- Check that earmold or hearing aid is properly inserted.
- Check that volume control wheel is turned up to appropriate settings.

DON'T
- Put hearing aid on heated surface.
- Wash hearing aid.
- Drop hearing aid.
- Wear hearing aid in bath or shower.
- Wear hearing aid overnight.
- Ignore a hearing aid that is "whistling."
- Use in contact with cream, oil, or hair spray when hearing aid is on.

Therefore it is important to ensure that the hearing aid is used and works properly.

Nursing diagnoses and interventions for the patient with hearing loss include but are not limited to the following:

Nursing Diagnoses	Nursing Interventions
Disturbed sensory perception (auditory), related to disease process	Facilitate communication with the patient by following the interventions provided in the Health Promotion box (p. 633).
Social isolation, related to loss of hearing	Assess factors that contribute to social isolation. Identify support systems for patient. Identify patient concerns. Establish effective communication.

Patient Teaching

Assist the patient in learning to care for a hearing aid, if prescribed (see Box 13-3). Advise the patient to request that others speak slowly or more clearly and repeat if necessary.

Prognosis

Surgical repair of the injured structures increases the likelihood of restoring partial or complete hearing, especially when implants are used. Complications of surgery are rare. Technical advances have also improved the quality of hearing. Microtechnology has reduced the size of hearing aids until they are almost undetectable.

INFLAMMATORY AND INFECTIOUS DISORDERS OF THE EAR

External Otitis

Etiology and Pathophysiology

External otitis, or otitis externa, is an inflammation or infection of the external canal or the auricle of the external ear. It is sometimes called **swimmer's ear.** External otitis may be acute or chronic.

External otitis can be caused by allergy, bacteria, fungi, viruses, and trauma. Allergic reaction can stem from nickel or chromium in earrings. In addition, chemicals in hair sprays, cosmetics, hearing aids, and medications (especially sulfonamides and neomycin) are common sources of allergy. Common bacterial agents are *Staphylococcus aureus, Pseudomonas aeruginosa,* and *Streptococcus pyogenes.* Frequently the viruses herpes simplex and herpes zoster are implicated. The external ear may also be affected by eczema, psoriasis, and seborrheic dermatitis. Fungi such as *Aspergillus* and *Candida* may also be causes. External otitis is more prevalent during hot, humid weather.

Trauma from cleaning or scratching the ear canal with a foreign object (such as a cotton swab, bobby pin, or finger) may result in irritation and possible introduction of infectious organisms.

Cerumen in the older person becomes dry and hard. Because removal is more difficult, the cerumen may become impacted, causing discomfort and decreased hearing. Certain activities allow moisture to become trapped in the ear, creating a medium for infection; these include using earphones, hearing aids, earplugs, earmuffs, and stethoscopes. Excessive swimming may wash out the protective cerumen, remove skin lipids, and lead to secondary infection.

Malignant external otitis is a rare, lethal form caused by *Pseudomonas* organisms and occurring mostly in patients with diabetes. It is a bone-destroying infection that quickly involves all surrounding ear structures.

Clinical Manifestations

The acute inflammatory or infectious process produces pain with movement of the auricle or chewing, and often the entire side of the head aches. Erythema, scaling, pruritus, edema, watery discharge, and crusting of the external ear may occur. Drainage may be purulent or serosanguineous. If the *Pseudomonas* organism is the cause of the infection, the drainage is green and has a musty smell. Dizziness and decreased hearing may also be present if edema occludes the ear canal. With chronic external otitis there is usually pruritus,

but no pain with movement of the auricle. A discharge is also present.

Assessment

Collection of **subjective data** includes determining the onset, duration, and severity of pain, which is crucial to the assessment of inflammatory disease of the ear. An early indication of inflammation or infection of the ear is complaint of ear pain accompanied by patient gently pulling on the pinna. Ask the patient about any home remedies used to treat infections. Also assess knowledge of preventive measures.

Collection of **objective data** includes noting a discharge, which may be watery or yellow and tenacious with a fetid odor. The discharge is black if from a fungal infection. The patient may have a partial loss of hearing or feel like the ear is occluded if the ear canal is edematous or is obstructed by adenoids. Palpation of the external ear may produce pain.

Diagnostic Tests

Obtain a culture of the exudate to identify bacterial, viral, or fungal organisms.

Medical Management

Oral analgesics such as codeine may be used if the pain is severe. Corticosteroids (1% hydrocortisone) may be used to reduce edema to allow antibiotics to penetrate. Insert a wick into the ear canal to prevent loss of medication from the canal and to maintain continuous absorption of the medicine. The physician orders the frequency of the wick change. Antimicrobial agents such as antibiotic or antifungal eardrops may be used. The most commonly used contain 0.5% neomycin or 10,000 units/mL of polymyxin B. Systemic antibiotics are used only if the infection is severe. The specific antibiotic used depends on the results of the culture.

Nursing Interventions and Patient Teaching

Carefully cleanse the ear canal. Heat may be applied to the external ear for pain relief. Implement an adequate method of communication. Instill eardrops.

A nursing diagnosis and interventions for the patient with external otitis include but are not limited to the following:

Nursing Diagnosis	Nursing Interventions
Pain, related to inflammatory process	Apply warm compresses as ordered. Administer prescribed analgesics and instill ordered ear medications.

Ensure that the patient has the information to prevent further infection and can care for the infected ear.

Prognosis

External otitis responds favorably to topical antibiotic and corticosteroid eardrops. Systemic antibiotics are rarely required unless cellulitis is present. Acute external otitis may become a chronic problem. If the infection remains untreated and enters the brain, death can occur. The rare malignant external otitis media has a mortality rate of 50% to 75% unless the condition is treated.

Acute Otitis Media
Etiology and Pathophysiology

Acute otitis media, an inflammation or infection of the middle ear, is the most common disorder of the middle ear. Acute otitis media is most often caused by *Haemophilus influenzae* or *Streptococcus pneumoniae*. Chronic otitis media is usually caused by gram-negative bacteria, such as *Proteus*, *Klebsiella*, and *Pseudomonas* organisms. In addition, allergy, exposure to cigarette smoke, mycoplasma, and several viruses may be factors.

Otitis media occurs more frequently in children, especially at 6 to 36 months of age, and in the winter and early spring. Children's shorter and straighter eustachian tubes provide easier access of the organisms from the nasopharynx to travel to the middle ear. The patient usually has had a recent upper respiratory tract infection. The infection ascends via the eustachian tube and involves the lining of the entire middle ear. Usually only one ear is affected.

Viral infections frequently cause a serous otitis media. Retraction of the tympanic membrane occurs with a buildup of sterile serous exudate. If there is a secondary bacterial infection, purulent exudate collects behind the tympanic membrane, causing it to bulge. This is called **purulent otitis media.**

Clinical Manifestations

The patient experiences a sense of fullness in the ear and also has severe, deep throbbing pain behind the tympanic membrane. This severe pain may disappear if the tympanic membrane ruptures. Hearing loss, **tinnitus** (a subjective noise sensation heard in one or both ears; ringing or tinkling sounds in the ear), and fever may also be present.

Assessment

For information on collection of **subjective data,** refer to the discussion of external otitis.

Collection of **objective data** is the same as for external otitis, with the exception of noting pain on palpation of the external ear.

Diagnostic Tests

A culture of the purulent drainage is obtained to identify the causative organisms.

Medical Management

Antibiotic therapy is based on results of the culture. Amoxicillin for 10 days is the current therapy of choice in the United States. Analgesics are prescribed for severe pain. Sedatives may be prescribed for children to provide rest and pain relief. Local heat is used, and nasal decongestants are ordered (Table 13-6).

Needle aspiration of secretions collected behind the tympanic membrane may be necessary. Myringotomy—a surgical incision of the tympanic membrane to relieve pressure and release purulent exudate from the middle ear—may be required to prevent spontaneous rupture. A tympanostomy tube may be placed for short- or long-term use. Prompt treatment of an episode of acute otitis media generally prevents spontaneous perforation of the tympanic membrane.

Nursing Interventions and Patient Teaching

Inner-ear pressure may cause discomfort, requiring an analgesic. Sedatives may be ordered for young children.

Hearing loss may also occur. Effective communication is essential. Alert parents of young patients to this fact and enlist their help in monitoring the level of loss.

Chronic otitis media caused by repeated attacks of acute otitis media may result in a permanent perforation of the tympanic membrane. The result is a slight to moderate conductive hearing loss.

A growth called **cholesteatoma** (a mass of epithelial cells and cholesterol in the middle ear) occurs when a tympanic membrane perforation allows keratinizing squamous epithelium of the external auditory canal to enter and grow in the middle ear. Enlargement is slow, but the mass can expand into the mastoid antrum and destroy adjacent structures. Unless removed surgically, a cholesteatoma can cause extensive damage to the structures of the middle ear; erode the bony protection of the facial nerve; create a labyrinthine fistula; or even invade the dura, threatening the brain.

Mastoiditis, an infection of one of the mastoid bones, may develop. It is usually an extension of a middle-ear infection that was untreated or inadequately treated. Immediately report signs of mastoiditis, including earache, fever, headache, malaise, and large amounts of purulent exudate.

A nursing diagnosis and interventions for the patient with otitis media include but are not limited to the following:

Nursing Diagnosis	Nursing Interventions
Impaired skin integrity, related to edema and exudates	Note and report any purulent outer ear exudates. Keep ear clean and dry; use sterile cotton to absorb drainage, if ordered. Monitor temperature and report changes.

Table 13-6 Medications for Ear Disorders

Generic (Trade)	Actions and Uses	Side Effects	Nursing Implications
Carbamide peroxide (Debrox)	Cerumen removal	Contact dermatitis	Do not use if eardrum is perforated or if there is ear discharge; not recommended for children; avoid eyes; reevaluate if edema, erythema, or pain persists; use proper administration technique by allowing drops to enter ear canal; do not touch tip of dropper.
Colistin, neomycin, hydrocortisone, and thonzonium (Coly-Mycin S Otic)	Antibiotic-steroid-detergent used for susceptible disease of external auditory canal, mastoidectomy, and otitis media fenestration	Ototoxicity in prolonged use; contact dermatitis; hypersensitivity, including pruritus, skin rash, erythema, and edema	Do not heat bottle above body temperature; with herpes simplex, do not use if patient is infected; do not use if eardrum is perforated; use for 10 days only; keep dropper from touching skin; check with physician if signs and symptoms worsen or do not improve after 1 week; shake well before using; use cotton plug to keep moist; change plug daily.
Triethanolamine polypeptide oleate (Cerumenex)	Cerumen removal	Contact dermatitis	Fill ear canal; insert cotton plug after 15-30 minutes; irrigate ear canal with warm water.
Amoxicillin trihydrate (Amoxil)	Systemic penicillin antibiotic used in acute otitis media	Anaphylaxis, skin rash, diarrhea	Use caution during pregnancy and lactation; take for full treatment period; consult with physician if no improvement occurs in a few days; take on full or empty stomach; check with physician about treating diarrhea; do not give if patient has penicillin or cephalosporin allergy.
Cefaclor (Ceclor)	Second-generation cephalosporin used to treat amoxicillin-resistant otitis media	Anaphylaxis, skin rash, joint pain; fever, diarrhea, abdominal cramping	Store suspension in refrigerator; give full course of therapy; tell patient not to use alcohol; give on full or empty stomach; do not give if patient has penicillin or cephalosporin allergies.
Meclizine hydrochloride (Antivert)	Anticholinergic antihistamine that acts as antiemetic, antivertigo agent; treatment and prophylaxis; possibly effective for diseases affecting vestibular system	Drowsiness, blurred vision, dry mouth	Use caution during pregnancy and breastfeeding; give with food, water, or milk; tell patient to avoid alcohol and central nervous system (CNS) depressants; not recommended for children under 12.

Continued

Table 13-6 Medications for Ear Disorders—cont'd

Generic (Trade)	Actions and Uses	Side Effects	Nursing Implications
Dimenhydrinate (Dramamine)	Anticholinergic antihistamine used in treatment of vertigo	Blurred vision, drowsiness, shortness of breath, painful urination, disorientation	Antihistamines may inhibit lactation; give no CNS depressants; give with food or milk; use caution during pregnancy in early months.
Antipyrine and benzocaine (Auralgan)	Analgesic; local anesthetic; used for otitis media; adjunct to cerumen removal	Contact dermatitis	Use caution during pregnancy and lactation; date bottle and discard after 6 months from first use; do not use if eardrums are perforated; warm bottle; position patient on side and fill ear canal; use cotton plug; wash dropper before replacing in bottle.
Acetic acid (VoSol hydrochloride otic)	Antibacterial, antifungal, astringent; used for superficial infections of external auditory canal	Contact dermatitis, transient stinging	Clean ear first; use cotton plug for first 24 hours; contact physician if condition worsens or no improvement occurs after 5-7 days; do not wash dropper—doing so may dilute medication.
Trimethoprim-sulfamethoxazole (Bactrim)	Systemic antibacterial; used for acute otitis media; no sulfonamide allergy	Fever, itching, skin rash, photosensitivity, dizziness	Not recommended during lactation or pregnancy; emphasize importance of proper dental care; blood glucose levels may be affected in patients using oral antidiabetic agents; maintain adequate fluid intake; advise patient to avoid sun exposure; complete treatment; with pediatric suspension, shake well.
Polymyxin B, neomycin, bacitracin, and hydrocortisone (Cortisporin)	Antibiotic and steroid used in the same way as Coly-Mycin S; used to treat swimmer's ear	Ototoxicity in prolonged use, contact dermatitis, pruritus, erythema, edema	Use caution during pregnancy and lactation; do not use if eardrum is perforated; keep dropper from touching skin; shake well before using; use cotton plug to keep moist; change plug daily.

Ensure that the patient and parents (if appropriate) are aware of the necessity to complete the entire course of antibiotic therapy. Children are fed upright to prevent nasopharyngeal flora from entering the eustachian tube. Instruct the patient to blow the nose gently, not forcefully. If a myringotomy has been performed, instruct the patient or the parents to change the cotton in the outer ear at least twice a day (see Patient Teaching box).

Prognosis

Middle-ear infections usually resolve completely with antibiotic therapy. Since the advent of treatment with antibiotics, the incidence of severe and prolonged infections of the middle ear has been greatly reduced. Chronic or untreated otitis media may lead to sound transmission hearing loss, which is successfully treated with tympanoplasty.

Patient Teaching

Ear Infection

PREVENTION OF FURTHER INFECTION
- Protect ear canal during showers (use cotton with petrolatum in external canal or physician-approved earplugs; wear a shower cap over ears).
- Avoid swimming during infection or after a perforated eardrum; avoid swimming in contaminated water when infection is healed.
- Continue antibiotic therapy for prescribed number of days, even when symptoms disappear.
- Get adequate and early treatment of upper respiratory tract infections and allergic conditions.

CARE OF INFECTED EAR
- Use correct eardrop insertion or ear irrigations, as prescribed.
- Wash hands before and after changing cotton plugs to prevent secondary infection.
- Keep external ear clean and dry to protect skin from drainage.

SIGNS REQUIRING MEDICAL ATTENTION
- Fever
- Return of ear pain or discharge

Mastoiditis is difficult to treat and may require antibiotic therapy intravenously for several days. Because children are most often affected, immediate treatment of the infection is crucial. Residual hearing loss may follow the infection. If early decalcification is present, intense antibiotic therapy and myringotomy can usually cure mastoiditis; if it has progressed to further destruction, simple mastoidectomy is necessary.

Labyrinthitis

Etiology and Pathophysiology
Labyrinthitis is an inflammation of the labyrinthine canals of the inner ear. Labyrinthitis is the most common cause of vertigo (the sensation that the outer world is revolving about oneself or that one is moving in space). A common cause is a viral upper respiratory tract infection that spreads into the inner ear; other causes include certain drugs and foods. The vestibular portion of the inner ear may be destroyed by streptomycin. Tobacco and alcohol may also be causative factors. A rarer form of labyrinthitis is caused by bacteria. It is usually associated with middle-ear and mastoid infections. Since the advent of antibiotics, bacterial labyrinthitis occurs infrequently.

Clinical Manifestations
Severe and sudden vertigo is the most common symptom of labyrinthitis. Also present are nausea and vomiting, nystagmus, photophobia, headache, and ataxic gait.

Assessment
Subjective data include the frequency and duration of the vertigo and any safety measures taken by the patient during an attack. Assess other symptoms such as hearing ability, ringing in the ears, and nausea. Because fear is associated with the attacks, explore the patient's feelings.

Collection of **objective data** includes noting vomiting and any jerking movement of the eyeballs, unilaterally or bilaterally. Assess the color and moisture of skin to determine the extent of autonomic response.

Diagnostic Tests
Electronystagmography may show a diminished or absent nystagmus with stimulation. Audiometric testing shows a low-tone sensorineural hearing loss.

Medical Management
Labyrinthitis has no specific treatment. Usually antibiotics and dimenhydrinate (Dramamine) or meclizine (Antivert) for vertigo are prescribed. If nausea and vomiting persist, administer parenteral fluids.

Nursing Interventions and Patient Teaching
It is important to note the frequency and degree of vertigo. Administer antibiotics and medications and assess fluid intake to ensure that dehydration does not occur.

Nursing diagnoses and interventions for the patient with labyrinthitis include but are not limited to the following:

Nursing Diagnoses	Nursing Interventions
Risk for injury, related to altered sensory perception (vertigo)	Keep side rails up. Note presence of vertigo before patient ambulates. Supervise ambulation. Caution the patient not to attempt ambulation alone and to call for assistance.
Fear, related to altered sensory perception (vertigo)	Explore patient's feelings about attack. Teach patient concerning actions during an attack (see Patient Teaching box). Reinforce physician's treatment orders.

Instruct the patient about vertigo and how it is treated (see Patient Teaching box).

Prognosis
Labyrinthitis usually resolves itself, with little or no hearing impairment.

Obstructions of the Ear

Etiology and Pathophysiology
Ear canal obstruction is usually caused by impaction or excessive secretion of cerumen or by foreign bodies, including insects. Children often place beans, beads,

Patient Teaching

Vertigo

- Nature of the disorder
  - Physiologic basis for the vertigo
  - Avoidance of any known precipitating factors
  - Rationale for a low-salt diet
- Actions to take during an attack
  - Lie down immediately, and call for help if necessary at the first signs of an attack.
  - If driving when an attack occurs, pull over immediately to the curb.
  - Lie immobile and hold head in one position until vertigo lessens.
- Ask for assistance when ambulating if dizzy.
- Take prescribed medications as instructed even if no recent attacks have occurred; check with physician before discontinuing any medication.
- Seek medical attention for changes in symptoms or in the nature of attacks.

pebbles, and small toys in their ears. Usually those objects are found on routine examination. Obstruction by cerumen can be caused when excessive amounts are produced by overactive glands or from impaction of cerumen in narrow or tortuous ear canals.

Clinical Manifestations

The obstruction may cause the ear to feel occluded. The patient may have tinnitus or buzzing, pain in the ear, and slight hearing loss.

Assessment

Collection of **subjective data** includes interviewing the patient about any possible foreign bodies being introduced into the ear and any home remedies used to remove the object. If the patient is a child, determine risk factors related to ear obstructions, such as beads or nuts.

Collection of **objective data** involves noting any presence of a foreign body in the external ear canal. Observe children for tugging of the pinna.

Diagnostic Tests

Otoscopic examination provides visualization of the cause of the obstruction.

Medical Management

Medical management includes removal of cerumen by irrigation or cerumen spoon. Remove foreign objects with forceps, if possible. Smother insects with drops of an oily substance and remove them with forceps. Medications, such as carbamide peroxide 6.5%, may be used to soften cerumen. Surgical removal of the foreign object may be necessary.

Nursing Interventions and Patient Teaching

Assist with the irrigation of the ear. Instill medications into the ear as ordered.

A nursing diagnosis and interventions for the patient with obstructions of the ear include but are not limited to the following:

Nursing Diagnosis	Nursing Interventions
Disturbed sensory perception (auditory), related to presence of foreign body causing obstruction	Note the presence and amount of hearing impairment and tinnitus. Assure the patient (or parents) that once the obstruction is removed, any hearing loss or tinnitus should disappear.

Inform the patient and parents about the danger of placing objects in the ears. Also reinforce the method for preventing cerumen obstruction by instilling one or two drops of an oily substance at night. This is followed by hydrogen peroxide in the morning and cleaning with a soft cotton wick.

Prognosis

Ear canal obstructions caused by cerumen and foreign bodies resolve completely with treatment. Vertigo may be experienced temporarily until the ear canal dries. The older adult may become disoriented from the cerumen impaction and temporary loss of hearing.

NONINFECTIOUS DISORDERS OF THE EAR

Otosclerosis

Etiology and Pathophysiology

Otosclerosis is a condition characterized by chronic progressive deafness caused by the formation of spongy bone, especially around the oval window, with resulting ankylosis (immobility of a joint) of the stapes. Formation of new bone in adolescence or early adulthood progresses slowly. Gradual replacement of normal bone in the otic capsule by highly vascular otosclerotic bone occurs. This replacement bone is described as spongy. Calcification of the area follows, and the fixation of the footplate of the stapes in the oval window causes tinnitus and then deafness.

Otosclerosis is an autosomal dominant genetic disease. Women are affected twice as often as men. Otosclerosis is bilateral in about 80% of patients. Frequently pregnancy triggers a rapid onset of this condition. Previous ear infections are not believed to be related to otosclerosis.

Clinical Manifestations

The patient with otosclerosis experiences a slowly progressive conductive hearing loss and a low- to medium-pitched tinnitus. The deafness is usually first noted between the ages of 11 and 20.

Assessment

Subjective data include the degree and progression of hearing loss or tinnitus and mild dizziness to vertigo. Assess family history for the disease.

Collection of **objective data** includes assessment of behavioral clues related to hearing loss (see Box 13-2).

Diagnostic Tests

Otoscopy reveals a normal eardrum. A pink blush called **Schwartz's sign** may be seen through the ear; this indicates a high degree of vascularity in active otosclerotic bone. The result of the Rinne test shows sounds transmitted by bone conduction lasting longer than by air conduction in the affected ear. Weber's test results are the reverse from those of normal hearing. Both Weber's test and audiometric testing show a lateralization of sound more to the affected ear. Audiometric testing may show minimal to total hearing loss. Tympanometry may reveal evidence of stiffness in the sound conduction system. Hearing loss ranges from mild in the early stages to total loss in the later stages.

Medical Management

Sodium fluoride with vitamin D and calcium carbonate may be used to stabilize the hearing loss that results from otosclerosis. These agents help retard bone resorption and promote calcification of bony lesions. There is normal inner ear function; therefore amplification of sound by using a hearing aid can be effective (Lewis et al., 2007). Surgical treatment with stapedectomy restores hearing. The ear with poorer hearing is repaired first, and the other ear may be operated on 6 months to a year later. When a stapedectomy is not indicated, an air conduction hearing aid may be prescribed.

Nursing Interventions and Patient Teaching

Nursing diagnoses and interventions of otosclerosis are specific to poststapedectomy care. For patient teaching, see the discussion on ear surgery.

Prognosis

Patients report varying degrees of success with hearing after stapedectomy surgery. For some patients, stapedectomy is successful in permanently restoring hearing. A hearing aid may further enhance sound conduction to more normal levels.

Ménière's Disease

Etiology and Pathophysiology

Ménière's disease is a chronic disease of the inner ear characterized by recurrent episodes of vertigo, progressive unilateral nerve deafness, and tinnitus. Ménière's disease is most common in women between 30 and 60 years of age. The cause is unknown, although occasionally the condition follows middle-ear infection or trauma to the head.

There is an increase in endolymph fluid, either from increased production or decreased absorption. This causes increased pressure in the inner-ear labyrinth. Attacks of severe vertigo, tinnitus, and progressive deafness result from this increased pressure. Usually one ear only is involved.

Clinical Manifestations

The patient experiences recurrent episodes of vertigo with associated nausea, vomiting, diaphoresis, tinnitus, and nystagmus. A sense of fullness in the ear and hearing loss may be present. These attacks last from a few minutes to several hours. Attacks may occur several times a year. Sudden movements often aggravate the symptoms.

Assessment

Collection of **subjective data** includes noting the frequency and severity of the vertigo attack. The patient may complain of tinnitus. Note the patient's history and knowledge of the disorder and circumstances that precipitate an attack. Assess actions taken by the patient during an attack and the degree of relief those actions provide.

Collection of **objective data** includes determining unilateral or bilateral hearing loss. Observe the patient for associated signs during an attack.

Diagnostic Tests

Diagnostic tests are ordered to rule out central nervous system disease. The audiogram demonstrates a mild low-frequency sensorineural hearing loss. Audiologic tuning fork tests show a sensorineural deficit. Vestibular testing shows lack of balance. A glycerol test is performed, in which the patient is given a dose of glycerol orally followed by audiograms over the next 3 hours. A diagnosis of Ménière's disease is made if the patient's speech and hearing improve after taking the glycerol. The improvement is due to the osmotic effect of glycerol that pulls fluid from the inner ear (Lewis et al., 2007).

Medical Management

There is no specific therapy for Ménière's disease. Fluid restriction, diuretics, and a low-salt diet are prescribed in an attempt to decrease fluid pressure. Advise the patient to avoid caffeine and nicotine.

Dimenhydrinate, meclizine, diazepam (Valium), diphenhydramine (Benadryl) and fentanyl with droperidol (Innovar) may be prescribed for use between attacks to reduce the vertigo. In acute attacks the medications may be given intravenously. Atropine is also given for its anticholinergic effect during these acute attacks.

For preservation of hearing, surgical procedures may be performed. Approximately 5% to 10% of the patients with Ménière's disease require surgery. These surgeries and subsequent nursing interventions are discussed in Table 13-7.

| Table 13-7 | Surgery for Ménière's Disease |

TYPE	DESCRIPTION	RESIDUAL	POSTOPERATIVE NURSING INTERVENTIONS
Surgical destruction of labyrinth	Extraction of membranous labyrinth by suction; access to inner ear through external canal (stapes and incus removed)	Destroys remaining hearing	Keep patient on bed rest and NPO until vertigo subsides in 1-3 days. Avoid sudden movement of head for 1-2 weeks. Take action to prevent falls from unsteadiness for 1-3 weeks.
Endolymphatic subarachnoid shunt	Insertion of drain tube from endolymphatic sac into subarachnoid space; access through mastoid	Preserves hearing in 60%-70% of patients	Monitor for vertigo (rare).
Cryosurgery	Application of intense cold to lateral semicircular canals to decrease sensitivity or to create an otic-periotic shunt; access through mastoid	Preserves hearing in 80% of patients	Monitor for dizziness for 2 days. Take action to prevent falls from unsteadiness for 2-3 weeks.
Vestibular nerve section	Dissection of cranial nerve VIII (vestibular portion); access through mastoid or through cranial drilling over roof of internal auditory canal	Preserves hearing in 90% of patients	Same as for surgical destruction of labyrinth.

NPO, Nothing by mouth.

Nursing Interventions and Patient Teaching

Maintain the prescribed low-salt diet and administer diuretics as ordered. Acute vertigo is treated symptomatically with bed rest, sedation, and antiemetics or medications for motion sickness. Nursing interventions are planned to minimize vertigo and provide for patient safety. During an acute attack keep the patient in a quiet, darkened room in a comfortable position. The patient may have some auditory deficit, which requires alternate methods of communication. If the patient's tinnitus becomes distressing, an increase in background noise, such as music, may provide relief. Fluorescent or flickering lights or watching television may exacerbate symptoms and should be avoided. Have an emesis basin available because vomiting is common.

Nursing diagnoses and interventions for the patient with Ménière's disease include but are not limited to the following:

Nursing Diagnoses	Nursing Interventions
Risk for injury, related to sensory-perceptual alterations (vertigo)	Keep side rails up. Assist with ambulation and instruct the patient to call for assistance before attempting to ambulate. Have the patient sit or lie down when vertigo occurs. Have the patient move slowly and avoid turning the head suddenly.

Nursing Diagnoses	Nursing Interventions
	Administer medications as prescribed. Position patient on unaffected side. Stand in front of patient and prevent head turning. Avoid bright or glaring lights around patient. Place all needed supplies so that patient does not have to turn head.
Social isolation, related to unpredictable vertigo attacks	Assess factors that contribute to social isolation. Assess feelings of loneliness and abandonment. Identify support systems for patient. Identify patient concerns. Establish effective communication.

Provide information about a low-salt diet and taking diuretics. Warn the patient to avoid reading when vertigo or tinnitus is present. Instruct the patient to avoid smoking to prevent vasoconstriction. The patient should learn to identify precipitating factors and the proper actions to take when an attack occurs: (1) sit or lie down immediately, (2) stop the car and pull over to the side of the road, and (3) keep medication available at all times (Nursing Care Plan 13-2).

⭐ **Nursing Care Plan 13-2**   **The Patient with Ménière's Disease**

Ms. Luison is a 66-year-old patient admitted with Ménière's disease. She complains of severe dizziness, nausea, vomiting, ringing in the ears, hearing loss, and an unsteady gait. She is accompanied by her husband of 35 years.

NURSING DIAGNOSIS *Anxiety, related to effect of disorder*

Patient Goals and Expected Outcomes	Nursing Interventions	Evaluation
Patient will experience decreased signs and symptoms of anxiety Patient will control her anxiety	Encourage patient to explore concerns about decreased hearing and effects of vertigo attacks and to take action in relation to the concerns. Explore patient's knowledge of the disorder and correct misunderstandings. Educate patient on strategies that can give her back some control over her life. Suggest keeping an emesis basin, a pillow, a blanket, a car phone, and a large sign with the words "HELP, POLICE" in the car in case of a sudden Ménière's attack. Encourage realistic hope about expected hearing ability as described by physician. Refer patient to necessary support services, such as social worker or audiologist. Refer patient for more information to Vestibular Disorders Association (VEDA; www.vestibular.org).	Patient states that level of anxiety has decreased.

NURSING DIAGNOSIS *Risk for injury, related to vestibular auditory alterations*

Patient Goals and Expected Outcomes	Nursing Interventions	Evaluation
Patient will describe actions to avoid vertigo Patient will remain free of injury Patient will remain safe from falls	Help patient identify avoidable actions that precipitate vertigo attacks. Encourage patient to move slowly and not turn head suddenly when vertigo is present. If tinnitus is distressing, increase background noises, such as music. If hearing is decreased: • Use measures to facilitate communication with hearing impaired. • Carry wax earplugs; even after losing some hearing, ears are often sensitive to loud noises, which can trigger vertigo. • Refer patient to audiologist, if appropriate. Keep side rails up when patient with vertigo is in bed. Assist with ambulation as needed. Encourage patient to sit or lie down and to remain immobile if signs of dizziness occur. Teach patient to stop car at side of road immediately at first signs of dizziness while driving.	Patient avoids physical environment that could cause injury. Patient does not manifest evidence of injury.

Critical Thinking Questions

1. Ms. Luison states that she would prefer going to the bathroom without the assistance of a nurse. What is an appropriate response by the nurse?
2. Ms. Luison tells the nurse that she is depressed because of her unpleasant symptoms and wonders if she will ever feel well again. What would be a therapeutic reply?
3. The nurse notes an unpleasant odor from Ms. Luison; her hair is unkempt, and she has poor oral hygiene. The nurse is preparing to give her a warm, therapeutic bed bath. Ms. Luison states, "I feel too dizzy to take a bath." What nursing interventions would help promote personal hygiene and patient compliance?

Prognosis

Approximately 75% to 85% of patients experience improvement with medical management and supportive therapy. The remainder of patients may, in time, require surgical intervention. Usually several yearly attacks occur until the disease either resolves itself or progresses to complete deafness in the affected ear.

SURGERIES OF THE EAR

STAPEDECTOMY

Stapedectomy is the removal of the stapes of the middle ear and insertion of a graft and prosthesis, performed to restore hearing in cases of otosclerosis. The stapes that has become fixed is replaced so that vibrations can again transmit sound waves through the oval window to the fluid of the inner ear.

Using a local anesthetic and an operating microscope for visualization, the surgeon removes the stapes and covers the opening into the inner ear with a graft of body tissue. One end of a small plastic tube or piece of stainless steel wire is attached to the graft, while the other end is attached to the two remaining bones of the middle ear, the malleus and the incus.

Nursing Interventions

Postoperative management consists of external ear packing to ensure healing; the packing is left in place for 5 or 6 days. Depending on physician preference, the patient remains in bed for approximately 24 hours and resumes activity gradually. Keep the patient flat with the operative side facing upward to maintain the position of the prosthesis and graft; make certain that the patient is not turned. Headache, nausea, vomiting, and dizziness are expected early in the postoperative period as a result of stimulation of the labyrinth intraoperatively. The patient's hearing does not improve until the edema subsides and the packing is removed by the physician (see Patient Teaching box).

Possible complications of the stapedectomy include infection of the external, middle, or inner ear. Displacement or rejection of the prosthesis or graft may occur, or perilymph fluid may leak around the prosthesis into the middle ear, causing ringing in the ears and vertigo.

Prognosis

During surgery the patient often reports an immediate improvement in hearing in the operative ear. Because of the accumulation of blood and fluid in the middle ear, the hearing level decreases postoperatively but does return to near-normal levels. After stapedectomy, 90% of patients experience an improvement in hearing, in many instances to near-normal levels.

TYMPANOPLASTY

Tympanoplasty is any of several operative procedures on the eardrum or ossicles of the middle ear to restore or improve hearing in patients with conductive hear-

 Patient Teaching

After Ear Surgery

- Change cotton in ear daily as prescribed.
- Open mouth when sneezing or coughing and blow nose gently one side at a time for 1 week (to prevent increased ear pressure and infection).
- Keep ear dry for 6 weeks (to prevent infection).
  —Do not wash hair for 1 week.
  —Protect ear when outdoors using two pieces of cotton (use petrolatum jelly on outer ball).
  —Protect ear with shower cap when bathing.
- Wear ear protectors as necessary to prevent exposure to loud noises.
- Follow activity guidelines:
  —No physical activity for 1 week.
  —No exercises or active sports for 3 weeks.
  —Return to work in 1 week (3 weeks for strenuous work).
- Avoid exposure to people with upper respiratory tract infections.
- Avoid airplane flights for at least 1 week (to prevent effects of pressure changes).

ing loss. These operations may be used to repair a perforated eardrum, for otosclerosis, or for dislocation or necrosis of a small bone of the middle ear.

Nursing Interventions

Postoperative management consists of bed rest until the next morning. Elevate the head of the bed 40 degrees, and have the operative side facing upward. Medications include opioid analgesics, otic and oral antibiotics, and meclizine for vertigo.

Postoperatively monitor and report the presence of bleeding; the amount, color, and consistency of drainage; and temperature. Note complaints of vertigo when the patient is getting out of bed; with sudden movements, nausea and vertigo may occur. Possible complications include infection and displacement of the graft.

Nursing diagnoses and interventions for the patient after a tympanoplasty include but are not limited to the following:

Nursing Diagnoses	Nursing Interventions
Impaired physical mobility, related to surgical procedure	Note patient's ability to comply with bed rest order. Keep the patient's operative side up; do not allow the patient to be turned.
Risk for activity intolerance, related to pain and vertigo	Keep side rails up. When movement is allowed, begin gradually. Administer prescribed medications for pain and vertigo as needed. Assist with ambulation to prevent injury.

Prognosis

Hearing will improve if there is no involvement of the ossicles.

MYRINGOTOMY

Myringotomy, also called tympanotomy, is a surgical incision of the eardrum. It is performed to relieve pressure and release purulent exudate from the middle ear. The procedure is done with the patient under either local or general anesthesia. A myringotomy may be performed in one of two ways: (1) using a myringotomy knife, the surgeon makes a curved incision in the drumhead; or (2) a heated wire loop is touched for about 1 second to the drumhead, producing a 2-mm hole.

Nursing Interventions and Patient Teaching

Purulent exudate and fluid may drain immediately, requiring suctioning. Cotton placed in the ear absorbs drainage, which may continue several days. Change the cotton frequently to avoid recontamination of the surgical area. The incision usually heals quickly with little scarring. Hearing is not usually disrupted.

Medications commonly used are tetracycline (Achromycin V) and polymyxin B (Neosporin) eardrops as antiinfective agents. Tylenol with codeine may be used for pain. Monitor for signs of bleeding and reports any occurrence. Note incisional pain or hearing impairment.

Patient teaching involves providing the information in the Patient Teaching box (p. 644) and ensuring the patient understands.

Prognosis

Once pressure is relieved, hearing is restored to more normal levels unless scarring is present.

COCHLEAR IMPLANT

The cochlear implant is a hearing device for the profoundly deaf. The system consists of a surgically implanted induction coil beneath the skin behind the ear and an electrode wire placed in the cochlea (Figure 13-15). The implanted parts interface with an externally worn speech processor. The system stimulates auditory nerve fibers by an electric current so that signals reach the brainstem's auditory nuclei and ultimately the auditory cortex. The implant is intended for the patient whose sensorineural hearing loss is either congenital or acquired. A small computer changes the spoken words into electrical impulses that are transmitted to the implanted cochlear coil. The ideal candidate is one who became deaf after acquiring speech and language. The adult who was born deaf or became deaf before learning to speak may be considered a candidate for a cochlear implant if she or he has followed an aural-oral educational approach.

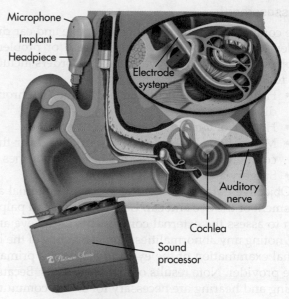

FIGURE 13-15 Cochlear implant.

The implant offers the profoundly deaf the ability to hear environmental sounds, including speech, at comfortable loudness levels. Multichannel cochlear implants also aid in speech production. Extensive training and rehabilitation are essential to receive maximum benefit from these implants. The positive aspects of a cochlear implant include providing sound to the person who heard none, improving the sense of security, and decreasing the feelings of isolation. With continued research, the cochlear implant may offer the possibility of hearing rehabilitation for a wider range of hearing-impaired individuals.

The deaf community is concerned with cultural pride. They believe that life without hearing is healthy and functional and that deafness is not a disease that needs to be cured. The National Association of the Deaf originally opposed use of cochlear implants; it now endorses their use, stating, "cochlear implantation is a technology that represents a tool to be used in some forms of communication, and not a cure for deafness" (Munson, 2006).

❖ NURSING PROCESS for the Patient with a Visual or Auditory Disorder

The role of the licensed practical nurse/licensed vocational nurse (LPN/LVN) in the nursing process as stated is that the LPN/LVN will:

* Participate in planning care for patients based on patient needs
* Review patient's care plan and recommend revisions as needed
* Review and follow defined prioritization for patient care
* Use clinical pathways, care maps, or care plans to guide and review patient care

■ **Assessment**

The complexity of the assessment for eye and ear disorders depends on the patient's disease or problem. Subjective data for both eye and ear disorders include the following:

- Health history, including any acute or chronic disease
- History of current complaint
- Medications, including prescription, over-the-counter, and home remedies or folk medicines
- Surgery and other treatments

Objective data include the external and internal assessment of the eye and ear. Use inspection and palpation to assess the external components of the eye and ear, noting any abnormalities. Review results of the internal examination of the eye and ear by the primary care provider. Note results of diagnostic tests. Because seeing and hearing are necessary for safety, communication, self-care, and psychosocial interaction, assess these areas as well.

■ **Nursing Diagnosis**

Nursing assessment identifies the patient's needs. Care is based on the nursing diagnoses that have been identified. Possible nursing diagnoses include the following:

- Ineffective health maintenance
- Anxiety
- Self-care deficit (specify)
- Fear
- Impaired environmental interpretation syndrome
- Impaired home maintenance
- Impaired social interaction
- Risk for injury
- Risk for loneliness
- Disturbed sensory perception: auditory
- Disturbed sensory perception: visual
- Social isolation

■ **Expected Outcomes and Planning**

Impairment of vision or hearing requires a major adjustment in the life of an individual. The patient must adjust to the loss and changes in lifestyle, whether the loss is permanent or temporary. The care plan focuses on achieving specific goals and outcomes that relate to the identified nursing diagnoses. Examples of these include:

Goal 1: Patient will remain free of injury.
Outcome: Patient and family inspect environment for potential hazards related to loss of vision or hearing.
Goal 2: Patient will remain socially active.
Outcome: Patient displays interest in social and recreational activities.

■ **Implementation**

Measures used in the care of a patient with vision or hearing loss center around helping the patient remain physically and emotionally safe and secure and ensuring that the patient's needs are communicated and met while adjusting to the loss. Nursing interventions include promoting safety, assisting with ADLs, facilitating communication, and encouraging diversional activity. Also assess readiness to learn and teach health promotion practices (see Patient Teaching boxes throughout this chapter). Consider the patient's culture, beliefs, values, and habits and the special needs of the older adult.

■ **Evaluation**

Systematic evaluation requires determining whether expected outcomes have been met. Refer to the goals and outcomes identified when assisting in planning care and evaluating the achievement of the goals. Examples of goals and their evaluative measures include:

Goal 1: Patient will remain free of injury.
Evaluative measure: Ask patient and family to describe what environmental changes need to be made to ensure safety.
Goal 2: Patient will remain socially active.
Evaluative measure: Observe patient participating in social activities.

Get Ready for the NCLEX® Examination!

Key Points

- The five major senses are taste, touch, smell, sight, and hearing and balance.
- The accessory structures of the eye are the eyebrows, the eyelids, the eyelashes, and the lacrimal apparatus.
- The three tunics of the eyeball are the fibrous tunic (sclera), the vascular tunic (choroid), and the retina.
- The two chambers of the eye are the anterior chamber, which contains aqueous humor, and the posterior chamber, which contains vitreous humor.
- Image formation at the retina requires four basic processes: refraction, accommodation, constriction, and convergence.
- The photoreceptors of the retina are the rods and cones. The rods control vision in dim light, and the cones control vision in bright light. The cones are also responsible for color vision.
- Light entering the eye must travel through the cornea, the aqueous humor, the pupil, the crystalline lens, the vitreous humor, and finally the retina.
- The ear is divided into external, middle, and inner ears.
- The external ear flap is called the pinna (auricle); it extends into the external ear canal.
- The middle ear contains the ossicles and the entrance of the eustachian tube and ends with the tympanic membrane.
- The inner ear contains the vestibule, the cochlea, and the semicircular canals.
- The organ of Corti is the organ of hearing; it is located within the cochlea.
- The semicircular canals are responsible for the sense of balance and equilibrium.
- The taste buds differentiate four basic tastes: sweet, sour, salty, and bitter.
- Normal aging causes decreased hearing and sight as a result of normal changes of the structures.
- Individuals who have chronic disease or are older than 40 years of age should be examined yearly to detect eye abnormalities or prescribe changes in therapy.
- Refractory errors include hyperopia (farsightedness), presbyopia (farsightedness related to the aging process), and astigmatism (objects waver).
- Ranges of 20/20 to 20/40 vision are considered normal, whereas 20/200 with correction is defined as legal blindness.
- ARMD is divided into two classic forms: dry (atrophic) and wet (exudative). In dry ARMD, which accounts for 90% of patients with ARMD, the macular cells have wasted or atrophied. Wet ARMD is characterized by the development of abnormal blood vessels in or near the macula.
- Cataracts are an opacity of the lens and may be removed by intracapsular or extracapsular extraction.
- Glaucoma is not one disease, but rather a group of disorders characterized by (1) increased IOP and the consequences of elevated pressure, (2) optic nerve atrophy, and (3) peripheral visual field loss.

- Loss of hearing may result from cerumen buildup, infection, trauma, or use of ototoxic drugs, or it may be a congenital condition.
- Conductive hearing loss is a decrease in amplification, whereas sensorineural hearing loss is interference within the inner ear.
- Prevention of serious complications of ear disorders, such as infections, mastoiditis, and brain abscess, requires early detection and treatment.
- *Injury, risk for,* is the primary nursing diagnosis for the patient experiencing vertigo, which occurs in labyrinthitis and Ménière's disease.
- An essential communication tip for speaking to the hearing impaired is to face the patient and to speak clearly without shouting.
- A cochlear implant is a hearing device for the profoundly deaf. The implanted device is intended for the patient with sensorineural hearing loss.

Additional Learning Resources

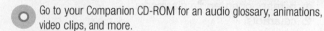 Go to your Companion CD-ROM for an audio glossary, animations, video clips, and more.

evolve   Be sure to visit the Evolve site at http://evolve.elsevier.com/Christensen/adult/ for additional online resources.

Review Questions for the NCLEX® Examination

1. The patient is to have a laser treatment to cauterize hemorrhaging vessels caused by diabetic retinopathy. The name of the procedure is:
   1. enucleation.
   2. scleral buckle.
   3. photocoagulation.
   4. trabeculoplasty.

2. The parents of an 11-year-old patient want to know more about their child's conductive hearing loss. The nurse would explain that:
   1. sound is delivered through the external and middle ear, but a defect in the inner ear results in distortion of sound.
   2. sound is inadequately delivered through the external or middle ear to the inner ear.
   3. there is no organic cause, but a functional problem exists.
   4. the brain's auditory pathways are damaged.

3. The patient has impaired hearing. To facilitate communication, the nurse would:
   1. face the patient when speaking.
   2. overaccentuate words to make the communication more effective.
   3. shout to allow the patient to hear.
   4. use one-word answers when speaking.

4. The patient tells the nurse he has dizziness. He states that the doctor used another term. The medical term is:

1. tinnitus.
2. labyrinthitis.
3. sensorineural.
4. vertigo.

5. The patient is diagnosed with an inner ear problem. The major symptom would be:

1. echoing.
2. intense pain.
3. vertigo.
4. loss of hearing.

6. Evaluation of the eye as it adjusts to seeing objects at various distances is called:

1. PERRLA.
2. refraction.
3. focusing.
4. accommodation.

7. The patient has tunnel vision, eye pain, difficulty in adjusting to darkness, halos seen around lights, and failure to detect colors. These indicate:

1. primary open-angle glaucoma.
2. cataracts.
3. entropion.
4. detached retina.

8. Which of the following would be a safety hazard in the home of a patient who is visually impaired?

1. Area rug
2. Room carpeting
3. Tile floor
4. Concrete flooring

9. An older adult falls at home, resulting in a blunt injury of an eyeball. The eye is tearing excessively, and the patient complains of a severe stabbing pain as if "something is in my eye!" First aid measures would include:

1. applying a cool compress three times a day (tid).
2. lightly covering the eye with a sterile gauze pad.
3. removing any particles that may be embedded in the eye.
4. irrigating the eye with tap water.

10. The patient has just had cataract surgery. Important discharge instructions would include: (Select all that apply.)

1. wearing an eyeshield at night on the operative eye.
2. avoiding bending, stooping, coughing, or lifting.
3. instilling prescribed eyedrops into the conjunctival sac.
4. administering an analgesic every 4 hours on a regular basis.

11. Which assessment finding would indicate a need for possible glaucoma testing?

1. Presence of "floaters"
2. Colored halos around lights
3. Intermittent loss of vision
4. Pruritus and erythema of the conjunctiva

12. While communicating with a patient, you notice a possible hearing deficit in one ear. Which nursing intervention would be appropriate?

1. Shout in the affected ear.
2. Speak clearly and in a slightly louder voice toward the patient's face.
3. Plug the affected ear and shout in the unaffected ear.
4. Speak more softly than usual in the affected ear.

13. What is the most likely cause of hearing loss in the older adult?

1. Cerumen buildup
2. Ossification of the pinna
3. Low batteries in the hearing aid
4. Fluid in the ear

14. Patients with permanent visual impairment:

1. feel most comfortable with other visually impaired people.
2. may experience the same grieving process that is associated with other losses.
3. may feel threatened when others make eye contact during a conversation.
4. usually need others to speak loudly so they can communicate appropriately.

15. A 32-year-old construction worker suffered a penetrating wound to the eye. The best intervention for anyone at the scene to take is to:

1. gently remove the object.
2. wipe away the blood and tears.
3. cover the object with a paper cup and tape.
4. do nothing; rush to the hospital.

16. A 71-year-old patient complains of being severely dizzy. The nurse should encourage the patient to:

1. avoid sudden movements.
2. avoid noises.
3. increase fluid intake.
4. lie on affected side.

17. The patient has been blind for the past 10 years. He is hospitalized with heart failure. In the care of a long-term blind individual, it is important to:

1. keep all items at a distance so he won't bump into them.
2. schedule a consultation with an occupational therapist to teach activities of daily living.
3. announce when you enter and leave the room.
4. initiate a referral to the Department of Health and Human Services.

18. The patient has a family history of cataracts. He asks what symptom would be present if he begins to develop them. The nurse might respond that the first symptoms of a cataract are usually:

1. pain in the eyes.
2. blurred vision.
3. loss of peripheral vision.
4. dry eyes.

19. The patient has had cataract surgery. Discharge teaching would include:

    1. lifting light objects is acceptable.
    2. wearing eyepatches for the first 72 hours.
    3. bending at the knees and keeping the head straight.
    4. bending at the waist is acceptable if done slowly.

20. The patient is scheduled for a stapedectomy. Appropriate postoperative teaching should include:

    1. changing cotton from external ear canal hourly.
    2. gently blowing both nares simultaneously.
    3. teaching patient to open mouth when sneezing or coughing.
    4. limiting activities for 3 weeks.

21. A 15-year-old hearing-impaired patient is having problems communicating with the staff. Which behavior would improve communication? *(Select all that apply.)*

    1. Overaccentuating words
    2. Facing the patient when speaking
    3. Speaking in conversational tones
    4. Asking permission to turn off television or radio

22. A 76-year-old patient is partially blind. His physician has diagnosed primary open-angle glaucoma. The goal of treatment in glaucoma is to:

    1. decrease aqueous humor.
    2. increase aqueous humor.
    3. decrease discomfort.
    4. restore vision.

23. The priority nursing responsibility while caring for a patient with vertigo is:

    1. safety.
    2. comfort.
    3. hygiene.
    4. quiet.

24. While cleaning the garage the patient splashed a chemical in his eyes. The initial priority following the chemical burn is to:

    1. transport to a physician immediately.
    2. cover the eyes with a sterile gauze.
    3. irrigate with water for 15 minutes or longer.
    4. irrigate with normal saline for 1 to 5 minutes.

25. The patient visits the physician for a routine physical examination that involves testing distance vision. As she faces the Snellen's chart, the nurse instructs the patient to:

    1. use both eyes to read the chart.
    2. read the chart from right to left.
    3. cover one eye while testing the other.
    4. use either eye because they will be the same.

26. A 49-year-old patient recently was blinded as a result of an automobile accident. This is her initial ambulation to the bathroom. What precautions should the nurse take when ambulating the patient?

    1. Precede the patient with patient's hand on the nurse's elbow.
    2. Follow the patient with the patient's hand on the nurse's elbow.
    3. Walk in front of the patient, telling of any obstacles.
    4. Walk behind the patient with the nurse's hand on the patient's shoulder.

27. The patient comes into the clinic complaining of progressive loss of vision in the center of his visual field. His physician would probably diagnose this condition as:

    1. macular degeneration.
    2. primary open-angle glaucoma.
    3. color blindness.
    4. retinal degeneration.

28. After cataract surgery the patient complains of sudden sharp pain in the operative eye. The nurse should immediately:

    1. remove the metal eyeshield to relieve pressure.
    2. call the physician.
    3. administer an analgesic.
    4. document complaint of pain on chart.

29. A surgical procedure for the treatment of retinal detachment is:

    1. punctal sac repair.
    2. radial keratotomy.
    3. vitrectomy.
    4. scleral buckling.

30. The _____ is a surgically implanted hearing device for the profoundly deaf person whose sensorineural hearing loss is either congenital or acquired.

31. The patient is asked to sign a surgical consent for treatment of otosclerosis. Which statement indicates correct understanding of the procedure?

    1. "It involves surgical repair of the external ear."
    2. "It means cutting the nerve in my ear."
    3. "It cleans the ear canal of wax."
    4. "It will help me hear sounds again."

32. The area of most acute vision in which there is the greatest concentration of rods and cones in the retina is the:

    1. fovea centralis.
    2. optic chiasm.
    3. optic disk.
    4. ora serrata.

33. Two drugs used in treating open-angle glaucoma are:

    1. atropine, Sulamyd.
    2. Betoptic, pilocarpine.
    3. Decadron, Liquifilm.
    4. mannitol, Cyclogyl.

34. The triad of symptoms in Ménière's disease includes:

    1. vertigo, sensorineural hearing loss, tinnitus.
    2. sensorineural hearing loss, vomiting, nystagmus.
    3. tinnitus, headache, vision changes.
    4. headache, vertigo, vomiting.

Objectives

Anatomy and Physiology

1. Name the two structural divisions of the nervous system and give the functions of each.
2. List the parts of the neuron, and describe the function of each part.
3. Explain the anatomical location and functions of the cerebrum, the brainstem, the cerebellum, the spinal cord, the peripheral nerves, and cerebrospinal fluid.
4. Discuss the parts of the peripheral nervous system and how the system works with the central nervous system.
5. List the 12 cranial nerves and the areas they serve.

Medical-Surgical

6. List physiologic changes that occur in the nervous system with aging.
7. Explain the importance of prevention in problems of the nervous system, and give several examples of prevention.
8. Identify the significant subjective and objective data related to the nervous system that should be obtained from a patient during assessment.
9. Differentiate between normal and common abnormal findings of a physical assessment of the nervous system.
10. Discuss the Glasgow coma scale
11. List common laboratory and diagnostic examinations for evaluation of neurologic disorders.
12. List five signs and symptoms of increased intracranial pressure, why they occur, and nursing interventions that decrease intracranial pressure.

13. Discuss various neurologic disturbances in motor function and sensory-perceptual function,
14. List four classifications of seizures, their characteristics, clinical signs, aura, and postictal period.
15. Give examples of six degenerative neurologic diseases and explain the etiology, pathophysiology, clinical manifestations, assessment, diagnostic tests, medical management, nursing interventions, and prognosis for each.
16. Discuss the etiology, pathophysiology, clinical manifestations, assessment, diagnostic tests, medical management, nursing interventions, and prognosis for a stroke patient.
17. Differentiate between trigeminal neuralgia and Bell's palsy.
18. Discuss the etiology, pathophysiology, clinical manifestations, assessment, diagnostic tests, medical management, nursing interventions, and prognosis for GBS, meningitis, encephalitis, and AIDS.
19. Explain the mechanism of injury to the brain that occurs with a stroke and traumatic brain injury.
20. Discuss the etiology, pathophysiology, clinical manifestations, assessment, diagnostic tests, medical management, nursing interventions, and prognosis for intracranial tumors, brain trauma, and spinal trauma.
21. Discuss patient teaching and home care planning for the patient with stroke, multiple sclerosis, Parkinson's disease, and myasthenia gravis.

Key Terms

agnosia (ăg-NŌ-zhă, p. 675)
aneurysm (ĂN-ūr-ĭ-zĭm, p. 696)
aphasia (ă-FĀ-zē-ă, p. 659)
apraxia (ă-PRĂK-sē-ă, p. 689)
ataxia (ă-TĂK-sē-ă, p. 681)
aura (ĂW-ră, p. 676)
bradykinesia (brā-dē-kĭ-NĒ-zē-ă, p. 683)
deep brain stimulation (DBS) (p. 685)
diplopia (dĭ-PLŌ-pē-ă, p. 669)
dysarthria (dĭs-ĂHR-thrē-ă, p. 659)
dysphagia (dĭs-FĀ-jē-ă, p. 672)
flaccid (FLĂK-sĭd, p. 660)
Glasgow coma scale (GLĂS-gō KŌ-mă skāl, p. 658)

global cognitive dysfunction (GLŌ-băl KŎG-nĭ-tĭv dĭs-FŬNK-shŭn, p. 706)
Guillain-Barré syndrome (GBS) (GĒ-yă bă-RĀ, p. 703)
hemianopia (hĕm-ē-ă-NŌ-pē-ă, p. 661)
hemiplegia (hĕm-ē-PLĒ-jă, p. 673)
hyperreflexia (hī-pěr-rĕ-FLĔK-sē-ă, p. 710)
nystagmus (nĭs-TĂG-mŭs, p. 681)
paresis (pă-RĒ-sĭs, p. 660)
postictal period (pōst-ĬK-tăl PĒ-rē-ŏd, p. 676)
proprioception (prō-prē-ō-SĔP-shŭn, p. 661)
spastic (SPĂS-tĭk, p. 660)
stroke (strōk, p. 694)
unilateral neglect (ū-nĭ-LĂT-ěr-ăl nĕ-GLĔCT, p. 661)

ANATOMY AND PHYSIOLOGY OF THE NEUROLOGIC SYSTEM

The nervous system is responsible for communication and control within the body. It interprets or processes the information received and sends it to the appropriate area of the brain or spinal cord, where the response is generated. The nervous system is the body's link with the environment. It works in conjunction with the endocrine system to maintain the body's homeostasis. The nervous system reacts in split seconds, whereas the hormones secreted by the endocrine glands work more slowly in initiating a response. The clinical picture for the patient with neurologic problems is often complex. Understanding these conditions requires knowledge of the anatomy and physiology of the nervous system.

STRUCTURAL DIVISIONS

The nervous system has two main structural divisions. The first division, the central nervous system (CNS), is made up of the brain and the spinal cord. It occupies a medial position in the body and is responsible for interpreting incoming sensory information and issuing instructions based on past experiences. The second component is the peripheral nervous system, which lies outside the CNS.

The peripheral nervous system contains two main divisions: the somatic nervous system and the autonomic nervous system. The somatic nervous system sends messages from the CNS to the skeletal muscles (voluntary muscles). The autonomic system transmits messages from the CNS to the smooth muscle, the cardiac muscle, and certain glands. The autonomic system is sometimes called the **involuntary nervous system** because its action takes place without conscious control.

CELLS OF THE NERVOUS SYSTEM

Two broad categories of cells exist within the nervous system. The first category, the neurons, are the transmitter cells (Figure 14-1). They carry messages to and from the brain and spinal cord. The second category, the neuroglial or glial cells, are the support cells to the neurons. They support and protect the neurons while producing cerebrospinal fluid (CSF), which continuously bathes the structures of the CNS.

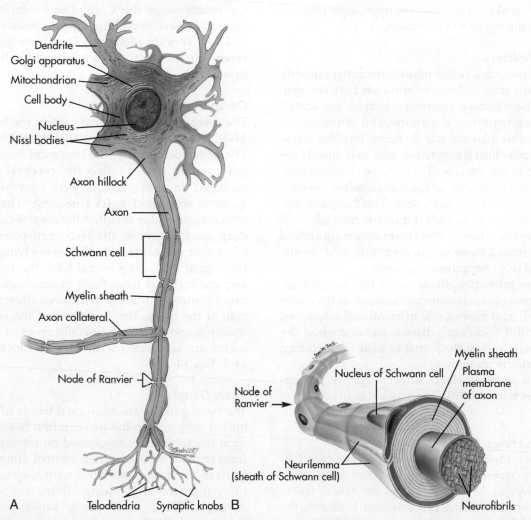

FIGURE 14-1 A, Diagram of a typical neuron showing dendrites, cell body, and axon. **B,** Myelinated axon, showing a cross-section of concentric layers of the Schwann cell filled with myelin.

Neuron

A neuron (nerve cell) is the basic cell of the nervous system. It is a separate unit composed of three main structures: the cell body, the axon, and the dendrites. The cell body contains a nucleus surrounded by cytoplasm. The axon is a cylindric extension of a nerve cell that conducts impulses away from the neuron cell body. The dendrites are branching structures that extend from a cell body and receive impulses. Between each neuron is a gap (space) called the synapse, defined as the region surrounding the point of contact between two neurons or between a neuron and an effector organ, across which nerve impulses are transmitted through the action of a neurotransmitter.

All neurons are governed by the "all or none law," which means there is never a partial transmission of a message; the impulse is either strong enough to elicit a response or too weak to generate the message.

Neuromuscular Junction

The area of contact between the ends of a large myelinated nerve fiber and a fiber of skeletal muscle is called the neuromuscular junction. This area of contact is necessary for the body to function. The neurotransmitters act to make certain that the neurologic impulse passes from the nerve to the muscle.

Neurotransmitters

Numerous chemicals called neurotransmitters modify or result in the transmission of impulses between synapses. The best-known neurotransmitters are acetylcholine, norepinephrine, dopamine, and serotonin.

Acetylcholine plays a role in nerve impulse transmission; it spills into the synapse area and speeds the transmission of the impulse. The enzyme cholinesterase is then released to deactivate the acetylcholine once the message or impulse has been sent. This happens rapidly and continuously as each impulse is relayed.

Norepinephrine has an effect on maintaining arousal (awakening from a deep sleep), dreaming, and regulation of mood (e.g., happiness, sadness).

Dopamine primarily affects motor function; it is involved in gross subconscious movements of the skeletal muscles. It also plays a role in emotional responses. A person with Parkinson's disease has decreased dopamine levels and suffers tremors, or involuntary, trembling muscle movements.

Serotonin induces sleep, affects sensory perception, controls temperature, and has a role in control of mood.

Neuron Coverings

Many neuron fibers (axons and dendrites) (see Figure 14-1) are covered with a white, waxy, fatty material called myelin. Myelin increases the rate of transmission of impulses and protects and insulates the fibers. Axons leaving the CNS are wrapped in layers of myelin with indentations called the nodes of Ranvier. These nodes further increase the rate of transmission because the impulse can jump from node to node.

In the peripheral nervous system the myelin is produced by Schwann cells (see Figure 14-1). The outer membrane of the Schwann cells gives rise to another layer called the neurilemma. The neurilemma is important because it helps regenerate injured axons. Thus regeneration of nerve cells occurs only in the peripheral nervous system. Cells damaged in the CNS result in permanent damage (paralysis) because they do not have neurilemma and are not able to regenerate.

CENTRAL NERVOUS SYSTEM

The **CNS**—one of the two main divisions of the nervous system, composed of the brain and the spinal cord—functions somewhat like a computer but is much more complex. The cranium protects the brain, and the vertebral column protects the spinal cord.

Brain

Specialized cells in the brain's mass of convoluted, soft, gray or white tissue coordinate and regulate the functions of the CNS. The brain is one of the largest organs, weighing approximately 3 pounds (1.4 kg). It is divided into four principal parts: the cerebrum, the diencephalon, the cerebellum, and the brainstem.

Cerebrum

The cerebrum is the largest part of the brain (Figure 14-2). It is divided into the left and right hemispheres. The outer portion of the cerebrum is composed of gray matter and is called the **cerebral cortex.** It is arranged in folds, called **gyri** (convolutions); the grooves are called **sulci** (fissures). The connecting structure or bridge is called the corpus callosum. Two deep sulci subdivide the two hemispheres into four lobes that are named for the bones lying over them: the frontal lobe, the parietal lobe, the temporal lobe, and the occipital lobe. Each hemisphere of the cerebrum controls initiation of movement on the opposite side of the body. The functions of the cerebrum are multiple and complex. Specific areas of the cerebral cortex are associated with specific functions (Figure 14-3, Box 14-1).

Basal Ganglia

The basal ganglia are additional bands of gray matter buried deep within the two cerebral hemispheres that form the subcortical associated motor system (the extrapyramidal system). They control automatic movement of the body associated with skeletal muscle activity (e.g., the arms swing alternating with the legs during walking; swallowing; saliva; and blinking) (Lewis et al., 2007).

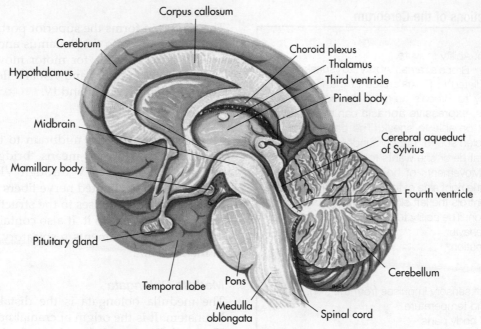

FIGURE 14-2 Sagittal section of the brain (note position of midbrain).

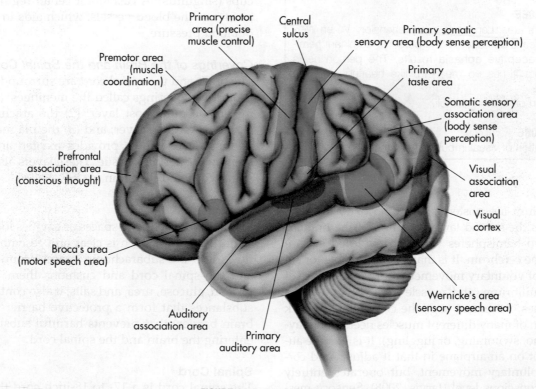

FIGURE 14-3 Cerebral cortex.

Diencephalon

The diencephalon is often called the **interbrain**. It lies beneath the cerebrum and contains the thalamus and the hypothalamus. The thalamus serves as a relay station on the way to the cerebral cortex for some sensory impulses; it interprets other sensory messages, such as pain, light touch, and pressure. The hypothalamus, which lies beneath the thalamus, plays a vital role in the control of body temperature; fluid balance; appetite; sleep; and certain emotions, such as fear, pleasure, and pain. Both the sympathetic and parasympathetic divisions of the autonomic system are under the control of the hypothalamus, as is the pituitary gland. Thus the hypothalamus influences the heartbeat, the contraction and relaxation of the walls of the blood vessels, hormone secretion, and other vital body functions (see Figure 14-2).

Box 14-1	Functions of the Cerebrum

FRONTAL LOBE
- Written speech: Ability to write.
- Motor speech, Broca's area: Ability to speak. Motor speech is mediated in Broca's area in the frontal lobe. When an injury to Broca's area (or the hemisphere in general) occurs, **expressive aphasia** can result and the patient will not be able to speak. The patient can only produce a garbled sound, but can understand language and knows what he or she wants to say.
- Motor ability: Movements of body. The left side of the brain controls the right side of the body, and the right side of the brain controls the left side of the body.
- Intellectualization: The ability to form concepts, personality, emotion, behavior.
- Judgment formation.

PARIETAL LOBE
- Interpretation of sensory impulses from the skin, such as touch, pain, and temperature.
- Recognition of body parts.
- Determination of left from right.
- Determination of shapes, sizes, and distances.

TEMPORAL LOBE
- Wernicke's area: Language comprehension. When Wernicke's area is damaged in the person's dominant hemisphere, **receptive aphasia** results. The person hears sound, but it has no meaning, like hearing a foreign language.
- Integration of auditory stimuli.

OCCIPITAL LOBE
- Interpretation of visual impulses from the retina.

Cerebellum

The cerebellum lies posterior and inferior to the cerebrum and is the second largest portion of the brain. It contains two hemispheres with a convoluted surface much like the cerebrum. It is mainly responsible for coordination of voluntary movement and maintenance of balance, equilibrium, and muscle tone. It coordinates and smoothes movement (e.g., the complex and quick coordination of many different muscles needed in playing the piano, swimming, or juggling). It is like the automatic pilot on an airplane in that it adjusts and corrects the voluntary movement, but operates entirely below the conscious level (Jarvis, 2008). Sensory messages from the semicircular canals in the inner ear send their messages to the cerebellum (see Figure 14-2).

Brainstem

The brainstem is located at the base of the brain and contains the **midbrain,** the **pons,** and the **medulla oblongata** (see Figure 14-2). These structures connect the spinal cord and the cerebrum. The brainstem carries all nerve fibers between the spinal cord and the cerebrum.

Midbrain

The midbrain forms the superior portion of the brainstem. It merges into the thalamus and the hypothalamus. It is responsible for motor movement, relay of impulses, and auditory and visual reflexes. It is the origin of cranial nerves III and IV.

Pons

The pons connects the midbrain to the medulla oblongata; the word pons means "bridge." It is the origin of cranial nerves V through VIII. The pons is composed of myelinated nerve fibers and is responsible for sending impulses to the structures that are inferior and superior to it. It also contains a respiratory center that complements respiratory centers located in the medulla.

Medulla Oblongata

The medulla oblongata is the distal portion of the brainstem. It is the origin of cranial nerves IX and XII. The medulla controls heartbeat, rhythm of breathing, swallowing, coughing, sneezing, vomiting, and hiccups (singultus). A vasomotor center regulates the diameter of the blood vessels, which aids in the control of blood pressure.

Coverings of the Brain and the Spinal Cord

The brain and the spinal cord are surrounded by three protective coverings called the meninges: (1) the dura mater, the outermost layer; (2) the arachnoid membrane, the second layer; and (3) the pia mater, the innermost layer, which provides oxygen and nourishment to the nervous tissue. These layers also bathe the spinal cord and the brain in CSF.

Ventricles

The four ventricles are spaces or cavities located in the brain. The CSF, which is clear and resembles plasma, flows into the subarachnoid spaces around the brain and the spinal cord and cushions them. It contains protein, glucose, urea, and salts; it also contains certain substances that form a protective barrier (the blood-brain barrier) that prevents harmful substances from entering the brain and the spinal cord.

Spinal Cord

The spinal cord is a 17- to 18-inch cord that extends from the brainstem to the second lumbar vertebra. It has two main functions: conducting impulses to and from the brain and serving as a center for reflex actions such as a knee jerk (Figure 14-4). A sensory neuron sends the information to the cord, a central neuron (located within the cord) interprets the impulse, and a motoneuron sends the message back to the muscle or organ involved. Thus a message is sent, interpreted, and acted on without traveling to the brain.

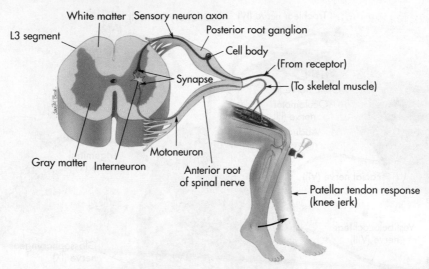

FIGURE 14-4 Neural pathway involved in the patellar reflex.

PERIPHERAL NERVOUS SYSTEM

The **peripheral nervous system** is made up of the motor nerves, the sensory nerves, and ganglia outside the brain and the spinal cord. It is composed of 31 pairs of spinal nerves, 12 pairs of cranial nerves, and the autonomic nervous system.

Spinal Nerves

The 31 pairs of spinal nerves are all mixed nerves. This means that they transmit sensory information to the spinal cord through afferent neurons and motor information from the CNS to the various areas of the body through efferent neurons. The spinal nerves are named according to the corresponding vertebra (e.g., C1, C2).

Cranial Nerves

There are 12 pairs of cranial nerves, which attach to the posterior surface of the brain, mainly the brainstem. Eleven of the pairs conduct impulses between the head, the neck, and the brain; the vagus nerve (X) also serves organs in the thoracic and abdominal cavities (Figure 14-5). Table 14-1 lists the cranial nerves, their impulses, and functions.

Autonomic Nervous System

The autonomic nervous system controls the activities of the smooth muscle, the cardiac muscle, and all glands. The autonomic nervous system is not a separate nervous system but a subdivision of the peripheral nervous system.

It is misleading to think of this system as the automatic system, although most activity is performed on an unconscious level. Its primary function is to maintain internal homeostasis; for example, it strives to maintain a normal heartbeat, a constant body temperature, and a normal respiratory pattern.

To maintain this homeostasis, the autonomic system has two divisions: the **sympathetic nervous system** and the **parasympathetic nervous system.** These two divisions are antagonistic: one slows an action, and the other accelerates the action. These systems function simultaneously, but they are able to dominate each other as the need arises. In times of stress the sympathetic system takes over to prepare the body for "fight or flight." Heartbeat accelerates, blood pressure rises, and adrenal glands increase their secretions. To calm the body after a crisis, the parasympathetic system becomes dominant, slowing the heartbeat and decreasing the blood pressure and adrenal hormone output.

EFFECTS OF NORMAL AGING ON THE NERVOUS SYSTEM

The effects of aging on the nervous system are variable. The changes that occur include a loss of brain weight and a substantial loss of neurons (1% a year after age 50), with the cortex losing cells faster than the brainstem. The remaining cells undergo structural changes. Aging also brings about a general decline in interconnections of dendrites, a reduction in cerebral blood flow, and a decrease in brain metabolism and oxygen utilization. The neurons may contain senile plaques, neurofibrillary tangles, and the age pigment lipofuscin. Older adults often have an altered sleep/wakefulness ratio, a decrease in the ability to regulate body temperature, and a decrease in the velocity of nerve impulses. The blood supply to the spinal cord is decreased, resulting in slower reflexes.

Normal changes in the nervous system associated with aging are *not* the same as senility, organic brain disease, or Alzheimer's disease (AD). Many older people reach old age with no functional deterioration of the nervous system. However, these normal changes may make care or rehabilitation of the older patient a challenge (see Life Span Considerations box).

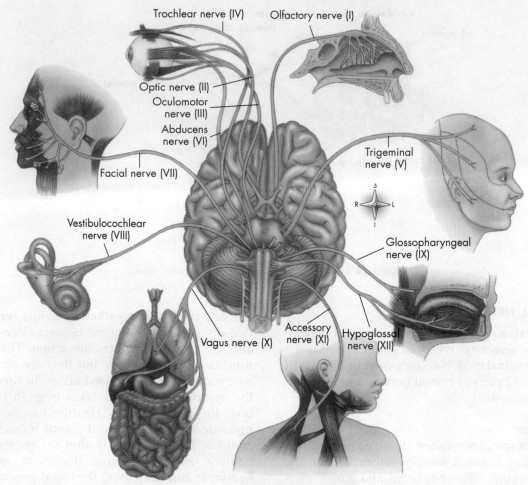

FIGURE 14-5 Cranial nerves.

Life Span Considerations

Older Adults

Neurologic Disorder

- As neurons are lost with aging, neurologic function deteriorates, resulting in slowed reflex and reaction time.
- Tremors that increase with fatigue are commonly observed.
- The sense of touch and fine motor coordination diminish with aging.
- Most older people possess the ability to learn, but the speed of learning is slowed. Short-term memory is more affected by aging than long-term memory.
- The incidence of physiologic dementia or organic brain syndrome—including Alzheimer's disease, Pick's disease, and multiinfarct dementia—increases with age.
- The incidence of stroke increases with age. The prognosis is affected by the location and extent of the cerebral damage. Rehabilitation potential after a stroke is often reduced by advanced age and coexisting medical problems.
- Nerve irritation from arthritis, joint injuries, or spinal-cord compression can cause chronic pain or weakness.
- Dementia is not a normal consequence of aging but may be a result of many reversible conditions, including anemia, fluid and electrolyte imbalance, malnutrition, hypothyroidism, metabolic disturbances, drug toxicity, a drug reaction or idiosyncrasy, and hypotension.

PREVENTION OF NEUROLOGIC PROBLEMS

Many conditions of the nervous system have no known cause. Other neurologic problems can be prevented or their effects reduced by modifying lifestyle factors. Neurovascular diseases are in part associated with defined risk factors—the same factors that increase the risk of cardiac disease, including high blood pressure, high blood cholesterol levels, cigarette smoking, obesity, stress, and lack of exercise.

Avoidance of cigarette smoking has been found to decrease the incidence of lung cancer. This is significant for the nervous system, because cancer of the lung often metastasizes to the brain.

Prevention of neurologic problems resulting from trauma is a major challenge. These injuries include spinal cord injury and head injury, which occur frequently in young people. Patient teaching on avoiding such injuries should include avoidance of drug and alcohol use, safe use of motor vehicles (e.g., using automobile seatbelts; wearing helmets with bicycles, motorcycles, and snowmobiles), safe swimming practices (e.g., not diving in shallow water), safe handling and storage of firearms, use of hardhats in dangerous construction areas, and use of protective gear as needed for sports (see Safety Alert box).

Table 14-1	Cranial Nerves		
NERVE*		**CONDUCTS IMPULSES**	**FUNCTIONS**
I	Olfactory	From nose to brain	Sense of smell
II	Optic	From eye to brain	Vision
III	Oculomotor	From brain to eye muscles	Eye movements, extraocular muscles, pupillary control (pupillary constriction)
IV	Trochlear	From brain to external eye muscles	Down and inward movement of eye
V	Trigeminal Ophthalmic branch Maxillary branch Mandibular branch	From skin and mucous membrane of head to brain; from teeth to brain; from brain to chewing muscles	Sensations of face, scalp, and teeth; chewing movements
VI	Abducens	From brain to external eye muscles	Lateral movement of eye
VII	Facial	From taste buds of tongue to brain; from brain to facial muscles	Sense of taste on anterior two thirds of tongue; contraction of muscles of facial expression
VIII	Acoustic (vestibulocochlear)	From ear to brain	Hearing; sense of balance (equilibrium)
IX	Glossopharyngeal	From throat and taste buds of tongue to brain; from brain to throat muscles and salivary glands	Sensations of throat, taste, swallowing movements, gag reflex, taste posterior one third of tongue, secretion of saliva
X	Vagus	From throat, larynx, and organs in thoracic and abdominal cavities to brain; from brain to muscles of throat and to organs in thoracic and abdominal cavities	Sensations of throat, larynx, and thoracic and abdominal organs; swallowing, voice production, slowing of heartbeat, acceleration of peristalsis
XI	Spinal accessory	From brain to certain shoulder and neck muscles	Shoulder movements (trapezius muscle) and turning movements of head (sternocleidomastoid muscles)
XII	Hypoglossal	From brain to muscles of tongue	Tongue movements

*The first letter of the words in the following sentence are the first letters of the names of cranial nerves: "On Old Olympus's Towering Tops A Finn And German Viewed Some Hops." Many generations of students have used this or a similar mnemonic to help them remember the names of cranial nerves.

⚠ Safety Alert!

Preventing Neurologic Injuries

- One of the best ways to prevent head injuries is to prevent car and motorcycle accidents.
- Become active in campaigns that promote safe driving. Speak to driver's education classes regarding the danger of unsafe driving and driving after drinking alcohol or taking drugs.
- The use of seatbelts in cars and the use of helmets for riding on motorcycles are the most effective measures for increasing survival after accidents.
- Individual states have legislation requiring the use of automobile safety devices for both children and adults.
- Recommend the wearing of protective helmets by lumberjacks, construction workers, miners, horseback riders, bicycle riders, snowboarders, and skydivers.
- Encourage swimmers of all ages to refrain from diving into shallow water or areas in which water depth is unknown.

Neurologic diseases, such as meningitis or brain abscess, that occur as a result of infection can sometimes be prevented by prompt treatment of ear and sinus infections. The practice of safe and responsible sex is important, since some neurologically related dis-

eases, such as syphilis and human immunodeficiency virus (HIV) disease, are spread by sexual contact. Safe practices include abstinence, monogamy, and the use of condoms. Treatment for drug abuse, especially intravenous (IV) use, is important, as is the prevention of HIV disease.

ASSESSMENT OF THE NEUROLOGIC SYSTEM

HISTORY

A comprehensive history is essential for diagnosing neurologic disease. This includes specifics about symptoms experienced and the patient's understanding and perception of what is happening. Obtaining information from family members or significant others may also be helpful. Follow the same format routinely to make certain information is complete.

For patients with suspected neurologic conditions, the presence of many symptoms or subjective data may be significant. These include the following.

- Headaches, especially those that first occur after middle age or those that change in character (e.g., headaches that are worse in the morning or awaken a person from sleep)

Table 14-2 | **Levels of Consciousness**

LEVEL	DESCRIPTION
Alert	Responds appropriately to auditory, tactile, and visual stimuli
Disorientation	Disoriented; unable to follow simple commands; thinking slowed; inattentive, flat affect
Stupor	Responds to verbal commands with moaning or groaning, if at all; seems unaware of the surroundings
Semicomatose	Is in impaired state of consciousness, characterized by obtundation and stupor, from which a patient can be aroused only by energetic stimulation
Comatose	Unable to respond to painful stimuli; cornea and pupillary reflexes are absent
Cannot swallow or cough
Is incontinent of urine and feces
Electroencephalogram pattern demonstrates decreased or absent neuronal activity

- Clumsiness or loss of function in an extremity
- Change in visual acuity
- Any new or worsened seizure activity
- Numbness or tingling in one or more extremities
- Pain in an extremity or other part of the body
- Personality changes or mood swings
- Extreme fatigue or tiredness

MENTAL STATUS

Assessment of the neurologic patient's mental status generally includes orientation (person, place, time, and purpose), mood and behavior, general knowledge (such as the names of U.S. presidents), and short- and long-term memory. The patient's attention span and ability to concentrate may also be assessed.

It is important to document mental status in specific terms. For instance, it is better to note "oriented to name, date, hospital, and purpose" than to note simply "oriented." Record actual patient statements. Vary orientation questions because some patients may learn the correct answers through repetition.

Level of Consciousness

Level of consciousness (LOC) is the earliest and most sensitive indicator of the patient's neurologic status. Changes in LOC are a result of impaired cerebral blood flow, which deprives the cells of the cerebral cortex and the reticular activating system (RAS) of oxygen. The RAS is located in the brainstem with neural connections to many parts of the nervous system (Lewis et al., 2007). The RAS is a functional system in the brain essential for wakefulness, attention, concentration, and introspection (*Mosby's Dictionary of Medicine, Nursing, and Health Professions*, 2006). A decreasing LOC is the earliest sign of increased intracranial pressure (ICP). LOC has two components: *arousal* (or wakefulness) and *awareness*. Wakefulness is the most fundamental part of LOC. If the patient can open the eyes spontaneously to voice or to pain, the wakefulness center in the brainstem is still functioning. Awareness, a higher function controlled by the RAS in the brainstem, is the ability to interact

with and interpret the environment. Awareness has four components, which are assessed as follows:

1. **Orientation:** Ask questions about orientation to person, place, time, and purpose.
2. **Memory:** Assess short-term memory; do not ask yes or no questions.
3. **Calculation:** Ask a simple math problem (e.g., "If you had $2 and your apple costs $1.25, how many quarters would you get back?").
4. **Fund of knowledge:** Ask the patient to name the president and to tell you what's on the national news.

Restlessness, disorientation, and lethargy may be seen first. Record observations in terms of behavior and signs—not labels such as "disoriented." See Table 14-2 for one method of classifying LOC.

Glasgow Coma Scale

The Glasgow coma scale (Table 14-3) is a quick, practical, and standardized system for assessing the degree of consciousness impairment in the critically ill and for predicting the duration and ultimate outcome of coma, particularly with head injuries. The Glasgow coma scale was developed in 1974 and consists of a three-part neurologic assessment: eye opening, best motor response, and best verbal response.

The stronger the stimulus needed to obtain a response, the lower the patient's score. The number value assigned to each part of the scale is added to yield an objective score. The score for a patient who is not neurologically impaired is 15; the lowest possible score is 3. Generally, any score of 8 or less is commonly accepted as a definition of coma. The scale has a high degree of consistency even when used by staff of varied experience.

FOUR Score Coma Scale

A recently developed scale for assessing coma is the FOUR (Full Outline of UnResponsiveness) Score coma scale (Wijdicks & Bamlet, 2005). It is used to assess patients with neurologic conditions that affect cognitive function such as stroke, craniotomy, and traumatic brain injury. It assesses eye response, motor response,

Table 14-3	Glasgow Coma Scale: Demonstrating Measurement of Level of Consciousness		
CATEGORY OF RESPONSE	**APPROPRIATE STIMULUS**	**RESPONSE**	**SCORE**
Eyes Open	• Approach to bedside • Verbal command • Pain	Spontaneous response	4
		Opening of eyes to name or command	3
		Lack of opening of eyes to previous stimuli but opening to pain	2
		Lack of opening of eyes to any stimulus	1
		Untestable	U
Best Verbal Response	• Verbal questioning with maximum arousal	Appropriate orientation, conversant; correct identification of self, place, year, and month	5
		Confusion; conversant, but disorientation in one or more spheres	4
		Inappropriate or disorganized use of words (e.g., cursing), lack of sustained conversation	3
		Incomprehensible words, sounds (e.g., moaning)	2
		Lack of sound, even with painful stimuli	1
		Untestable	U
Best Motor Response	• Verbal command (e.g., "raise your arm, hold up two fingers") • Pain (pressure on proximal nailbed)	Obedience of command	6
		Localization of pain, lack of obedience but presence of attempts to remove offending stimulus	5
		Flexion withdrawal,* flexion of arm in response to pain without abnormal flexion posture	4
		Abnormal flexion, flexing of arm at elbow and pronation, making a fist	3
		Abnormal extension, extension of arm at elbow usually adduction and internal rotation of arm at shoulder	2
		Lack of response	1
		Untestable	U

From Lewis, S.L., et al. (2007). *Medical-surgical nursing: Assessment and management of clinical problems.* (7th ed.). St. Louis: Mosby.
*Added to the original scale by many centers.

brainstem reflexes, and respiration (Table 14-4). Each component is graded on a scale of 0 (worst response) to 4 (best response). The scores are not totaled; therefore there is not a *sum* score in this scale.

The FOUR Score scale may be used as a complementary grading scale, along with the Glasgow coma scale (Wolf & Wijdicks, 2007). The Glasgow coma scale and FOUR Score scale are usually implemented in the intensive care unit.

LANGUAGE AND SPEECH

It is important to assess the language and speech capability of the neurologic patient (see Box 14-1 and Figure 14-3). Speech is a function of the dominant hemisphere, which is on the left side of the brain for all right-handed people and most left-handed people. Aphasia is an abnormal neurologic condition in which the language function is defective or absent because of an injury to certain areas of the cerebral cortex—Broca's area in the frontal lobe and Wernicke's area in the posterior part of the temporal lobe.

Aphasia includes all areas of language, including speech, reading, writing, and understanding. Aphasia has been subdivided as follows:

- **Sensory aphasia, or receptive aphasia:** Inability to comprehend the spoken word or written word. Wernicke's area in the temporal lobe is associated with language comprehension. Pathologic conditions in this area result in receptive aphasia.
- **Motor aphasia:** Inability to use symbols of speech (also called *expressive aphasia*). Broca's area in the frontal lobe mediates motor speech. Pathologic conditions in this area result in expression aphasia.
- **Global aphasia:** Inability to understand the spoken word or to speak. Pathologic conditions in Broca's and Wernicke's areas result in global aphasia.

Anomia is a form of aphasia characterized by the inability to name objects. Dysarthria is difficult, poorly articulated speech that usually results from interference in control over the muscles of speech. The general cause is damage to a central or peripheral nerve.

CRANIAL NERVES

Assessment of cranial nerve function is another important part of the neurologic assessment (see Figure 14-5). The 12 pairs of nerves emerge from the cranial cavity through openings in the skull (see Table 14-1 for specifics of cranial nerve classification and assess-

Table 14-4	FOUR Score Coma Scale	
CATEGORY OF RESPONSE	**RESPONSE**	**SCORE**
Eye response (E)	Eyelids open or opened, tracking, or blinking to command	4
	Eyelids open but not tracking	3
	Eyelids closed, open to loud noise, not tracking	2
	Eyelids closed, open to pain, not tracking	1
	Eyelids remain closed with pain	0
Brainstem reflexes (B)	Pupil and corneal reflexes present	4
	One pupil wide and fixed	3
	Pupil or corneal reflexes absent	2
	Pupil and corneal reflexes absent	1
	Absent pupil, corneal, and cough reflex	0
Motor response (M)	Thumbs up, fist or peace sign, to command	4
	Localizing to pain	3
	Flexion response to pain	2
	Extensor posturing	1
	No response to pain or generalized myoclonus status epilepticus	0
Respiration (R)	Not intubated, regular breathing pattern	4
	Not intubated, Cheyne-Stokes breathing pattern	3
	Not intubated, irregular breathing pattern	2
	Breathes above ventilator rate	1
	Breathes at ventilator rate or apnea	0

From Wijdicks, E.J., et al. (2005). Validation of a new coma scale, the FOUR score coma scale. *Annals of Neurology, 58*(4), 585.

ment). The cranial nerves are tested in the following ways:

I (olfactory)	Identification of common odors
II (optic)	Testing of visual acuity and visual fields
III (oculomotor)	Testing of ability of eyes to move together in all directions, testing pupillary response
IV (trochlear)	Tested with oculomotor; testing eye movements
V (trigeminal)	Jaw strength and sensation of face, corneal reflex
VI (abducens)	Tested with oculomotor; testing eye movements
VII (facial)	Ability of face to move in symmetry, identification of tastes
VIII (acoustic, or vestibulocochlear)	Testing of hearing through whisper or other means and checking equilibrium and balance
IX (glossopharyngeal)	Identification of tastes
X (vagus)	Gag reflex, movement of uvula and soft palate
XI (spinal accessory)	Shoulder and neck movement
XII (hypoglossal)	Tongue motion

MOTOR FUNCTION

Evaluation of the neurologic patient's motor status detects abnormalities in the normal functioning of nerves and muscles. Motor function disturbances are the most commonly encountered neurologic symptom. In general, the motor status examination includes gait and stance, muscle tone, coordination, involuntary movements, and the muscle stretch reflexes.

Reflexes that are usually tested include biceps, triceps, brachioradialis, quadriceps, gastrocnemius, and soleus muscles. The examiner taps briskly over the muscle with a reflex hammer. The response is noted and graded on a scale, usually from 0 to 4+, with 4+ being hyperreflexic. The most important feature of any reflex pattern is not the absolute value on the scale, but the comparison of one side of the body with the other. Stick figures are commonly used to record the bilateral values.

Damage to the nervous system often causes a serious problem in mobility. A loss of function is called **paralysis;** a lesser degree of movement deficit from partial or incomplete paralysis is called paresis.

Injury or disease of motoneurons causes alterations of muscle strength, tone, and reflex activity. The specific signs and symptoms vary according to whether the lesion involves an upper motoneuron or a lower motoneuron. Muscles may be flaccid (weak, soft, and flabby and lacking normal muscle tone), with absent deep tendon reflexes, or spastic (involuntary, sudden movement or muscular contraction), with increased reflexes. With some muscle problems, the affected muscle shows small, rapid, continuous twitching, called **fasciculations.** Fasciculations are localized, spontaneous, and involuntary without movement of limb. With other problems, clonus (a forced series of alternating contractions and partial relaxation of a muscle) may occur.

SENSORY AND PERCEPTUAL STATUS

The sensory examination is the most difficult part of the neurologic evaluation. Specific alterations in sensation that should be assessed include pain; touch; temperature; and proprioception, the sensation pertaining to spatial-position and muscular-activity stimuli originating from within the body or to the sensory receptors that those stimuli activate. This sensation enables one to know the position of the body without looking at it and to recognize objects by the sense of touch.

Unilateral neglect, a condition in which an individual is perceptually unaware of and inattentive to one side of the body, may also occur. Another perceptual problem is hemianopia, which is characterized by defective vision or blindness in half of the visual field.

In most clinical settings it is usually not feasible or necessary to complete the total neurologic examination during shift-to-shift assessments of the patient. However, in many settings, such as intensive care units, the neurologic checks may be done as frequently as every 15 minutes. The most important factors include orientation, LOC, bilateral muscle strength, speech, involuntary movements, ability to follow commands, and any abnormal posturing.

LABORATORY AND DIAGNOSTIC EXAMINATIONS

BLOOD AND URINE TESTS

Assessment of the neurologically impaired patient includes a variety of blood and urine tests. A culture of the urine may rule out infection involving the urinary tract. Other urine testing may indicate the presence of diabetes insipidus. Urine drug screens may be done to rule out drug use as a cause of lethargy or to identify specific drugs ingested.

Arterial blood gas (ABG) values may be an important diagnostic tool in monitoring the oxygen content of the blood. The gases may be altered with neurologic diseases such as Guillain-Barré syndrome (GBS), which may affect breathing patterns. Blood tests that are routinely done may help narrow the diagnosis of neurologic disorder.

CEREBROSPINAL FLUID

Examination of the CSF can yield information about many neurologic conditions. Normally CSF contains up to 10 lymphocytes per milliliter. An increase in the number of cells may indicate an infection, such as tuberculosis or a viral infection. Bacterial infections such as tuberculous meningitis often lower the CSF glucose level and chloride levels. A culture or smear examination is done to determine the causative organism in meningitis. Spinal-fluid protein is elevated when a degenerative disease or a brain tu-

mor is present. Blood in the spinal fluid indicates hemorrhage from somewhere in the ventricular system. A protein electrophoresis evaluation may give evidence of neurologic diseases such as multiple sclerosis (MS) (Table 14-5).

Lumbar Puncture

A lumbar puncture is often performed as part of the diagnostic workup of the patient who may have a neurologic problem. It is contraindicated in patients who might have increased ICP, since the withdrawal of fluid may cause the medulla oblongata to herniate downward into the foramen magnum.

A lumbar puncture is done to obtain CSF for examination, to relieve pressure, or to introduce dye or medication. It is a common procedure, done in the patient's room or in the diagnostic imaging department. The procedure takes 10 to 15 minutes. Slight pain and pressure may be felt as the dura is entered. A sharp, shooting pain down one leg may be caused by the needle coming close to a nerve.

The patient is usually positioned on the side with the knee and head flexed at an acute angle. This allows for maximal lumbar flexion and separation of the interspinous spaces. After anesthetizing the area with a local anesthetic, the physician inserts the needle below the level of the spinal cord, at the L4-L5 or L5-S1 interspace (Figure 14-6). The inner needle is removed to allow for drainage and measurement of spinal fluid. The level-of-fluid column in the manometer is used to measure the pressure. The first specimen of spinal fluid may contain blood from slight bleeding at the site of the puncture. This specimen should not be sent for cell count.

Table 14-5	Normal Characteristics of Cerebrospinal Fluid
DETERMINATION	**VALUE**
Specific gravity	1.007
pH	7.35-7.45
Chloride	120-130 mEq/L
Glucose	50-75 mg/dL
Pressure	80-200 mm H$_2$O
Total volume	80-200 mL (15 mL in ventricles)
Total protein	15-45 mg/dL (lumbar)
	10-25 mg/dL (cisternal)
	5-15 mg/dL (ventricular)
Gamma globulin	6%-13% of total protein
Cell count	
Red blood cells	None
White blood cells	0-10 cells (all lymphocytes and monocytes)
Culture and sensitivity	No organisms present
Serology for syphilis	Negative

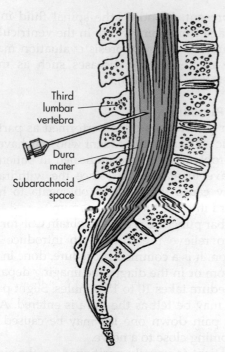

Third
lumbar
vertebra

Dura
mater

Subarachnoid
space

FIGURE 14-6 Position and angle of the needle when lumbar puncture is performed. Note that the needle is in the fourth lumbar interspace below the level of the spinal cord.

After the procedure the patient lies flat in bed for several hours. Assess the site of the puncture for any leakage, as evidenced by moisture on the bandage or around the puncture site. Headache is fairly common and is thought to be caused by the loss of spinal fluid through the dura mater. If a headache develops, bed rest, analgesics, and ice to the head may help. Opioids are usually not helpful.

OTHER TESTS

Routine skull radiographs of the head and vertebral column are useful in ruling out fractures of the skull and cervical vertebrae. Since the development of the computed tomography (CT) scan, skull radiographs are not used as extensively as before.

Computed Tomography Scan

The purpose of the CT scan, also called the **CAT scan,** is to detect pathologic conditions of the cerebrum and spinal cord using a technique of scanning without radioisotopes. No special physical preparation is required for the test. A CT scan takes 20 to 30 minutes if done without contrast medium and about 60 minutes with contrast. The procedure is painless, except for the slight discomfort when an IV line is started for the injection of the contrast dye. The patient may also have some discomfort in lying still and possible feelings of claustrophobia from being positioned in the head holder. If contrast medium is used, document and report to the physician any history of allergy to iodine and seafood, since iodine is present in the contrast medium.

During the procedure the patient lies supine with the head positioned within a rubber head holder to prevent air gaps between the machine and the scalp. The head is scanned in two planes simultaneously and at various angles. Each image that appears is a specific layer of brain tissue. The computer displays a printout that indicates areas of increased density (e.g., tumors or thrombi).

Brain Scan

Like the CT scan, the brain scan's purpose is detecting pathologic conditions of the cerebrum. It uses radioactive isotopes and a scanner. No special physical preparation is required. The procedure takes approximately 45 minutes for the actual scan. The patient is injected with a radioisotope and then lies still while a scanner passes over the brain area. Concentrated areas of uptake are reflected. There are generally no adverse effects from the procedure and only minimal discomfort associated with the IV administration of the radioactive isotopes. If mercury is used as the isotope indicator, a mercurial diuretic (meralluride [Mercuhydrin]) is administered several hours before the procedure to allow a greater concentration of the mercury to circulate to brain tissue, since meralluride minimizes the uptake of mercury by the kidneys. Brain scans are being used less frequently than in the past because of the excellent results obtained from CT scan and magnetic resonance imaging (MRI).

Magnetic Resonance Imaging

MRI uses magnetic forces to image body structures. It is used to detect pathologic conditions of the cerebrum and the spinal cord and in detection of stroke, MS, tumors, trauma, herniation, and seizure. Because MRI yields greater contrast in the images of soft tissue structures than does the CT scan, it is the diagnostic test of choice for many neurologic diseases. Recent advances in MRI techniques include diffusion-weighted imaging and magnetic resonance spectroscopy. Because the scan involves a magnetic force, caution the patient to remove watches, credit cards, and any metal from the clothing before entering the scanning room. Ask the patient about the presence of any metal in the body that would preclude the use of the scan, such as orthopedic appliances, aneurysm clips, and pacemakers.

During the procedure the patient lies supine with the head positioned in a head holder. The test takes 45 to 60 minutes. The procedure is painless, except for the discomfort in lying still and possible feelings of claustrophobia. Warn the patient that the machine makes different and loud noises during the scanning procedure.

Magnetic Resonance Angiography

Magnetic resonance angiography (MRA) uses differential radio waves and magnetic field signals to visualize flowing blood to evaluate extracranial and intra-

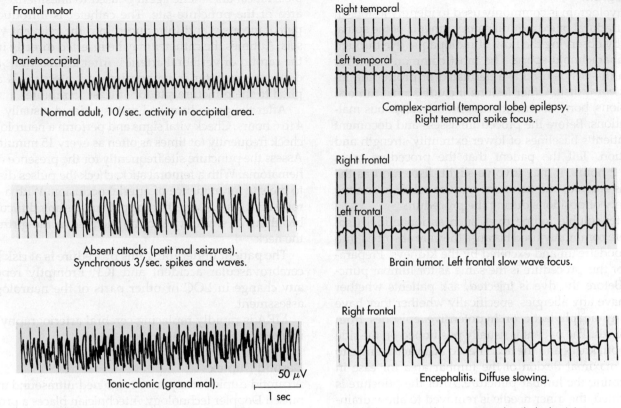

FIGURE 14-7 Tracings of electroencephalogram. The normal tracing is demonstrated, as are several pathologic states.

cranial blood vessels. It is a noninvasive procedure for viewing possible occlusions in arteries. It provides both anatomical and hemodynamic information. It can be used in conjunction with contrast media (contrast-enhanced MRA). MRA is rapidly replacing cerebral angiography in diagnosing cerebrovascular diseases. MRA has been useful in evaluation of the cervical carotid artery and large-caliber intracranial arterial and venous structures.

Positron Emission Tomography Scan

Another evaluative measure that is similar to CT and MRI scans is the positron emission tomography (PET) scan. In this procedure the patient receives an injection of deoxyglucose with radioactive fluorine. The area in question is scanned, and a color composite picture is obtained. Shades of color indicate the level of glucose metabolism, suggestive of a pathologic state. PET scanning provides a noninvasive means of determining biochemical processes that occur in the brain. It is increasingly being used to monitor patients who had a stroke or who have AD, Huntington's disease, tumors, epilepsy, and Parkinson's disease. As with the CT scan, discomfort is minimal. Inform the patient of the need to lie still for the duration of the scan, which is usually about 45 minutes.

Electroencephalogram

The electroencephalogram (EEG) provides evidence of focal or generalized disturbances of brain function by measuring the electrical activity of the brain. Among the cerebral diseases assessed by EEG are epilepsy, mass lesions (e.g., tumors, abscess, hematoma), cerebrovascular lesions, and brain injury. The test requires no special preparation, but encourage the patient to be quiet and rest before the procedure. An exception is a sleep-deprived EEG, where the patient is kept awake the night before the test and the EEG is usually done first thing in the morning. The EEG usually takes about 1 hour to complete. The patient's hair and scalp should be clean. The electrodes are placed on the scalp with collodion in a set pattern to cover all scalp areas. An EEG is painless.

The basic resting rhythm of the EEG is affected by opening the eyes or altering attention. Recordings are sometimes made while the patient is asleep or sleep deprived, when the seizure threshold may be lowered. Comparisons are made of different patterns of the recordings (Figure 14-7). After the test allow the patient to rest. Assist the patient if necessary in washing the hair and removing the collodion from the scalp.

Myelogram

The myelogram is commonly used to identify lesions in the intradural or extradural compartments of the spinal canal by observing the flow of radiopaque dye through the subarachnoid space. The most common lesion for which this test is used is a herniated or protruding intervertebral disk. Other lesions include spinal tumors, adhesions, bony deformations, and arteriovenous malformations. Before the procedure assess and document the patient's baselines of lower-extremity strength and sensation. Tell the patient that the procedure takes about 2 hours, it may involve slight discomfort as the dura is entered, and he or she may be asked to assume a variety of positions during the procedure.

Water-soluble iodine dyes such as iopamidol (Isovue) are commonly used because they are absorbed into the bloodstream and excreted by the kidneys. Preparation for this procedure is the same as for lumbar puncture. Before the dye is injected, ask patients whether they have any allergies, specifically whether they have had any anaphylactic or hypotensive episodes from other dyes. The patient is usually positioned on the side with both knees and the head flexed at an acute angle to allow maximal flexion of the lumbar area for ease in performing the lumbar puncture. After the puncture is performed, the inner needle is removed to allow drainage of CSF, measurement of pressure, and collection of specimens. The dye is instilled and the needle is removed. The patient is then turned to various positions so the spinal cord can be visualized while fluoroscopic and radiopaque films are taken. The patient usually undergoes a CT scan 4 to 6 hours after a myelogram.

After the procedure, observe the puncture site for any leakage of CSF, and assess the strength and sensation of the lower extremities. Headache is fairly common. It may be accompanied by nausea and occasionally by vomiting. The patient should be flat for a few hours.

Angiogram

The angiogram (cerebral arteriography) is a procedure used to visualize the cerebral arterial system by injecting radiopaque material. It allows detection of arterial aneurysms, vessel anomalies, ruptured vessels, and displacement of vessels by tumors or masses.

Before the procedure the patient is usually given clear liquids, although in some institutions all oral intake is restricted. Assess the patient for any allergy to iodine because the dye contains iodine. If the femoral approach is to be used, mark the locations of the bilateral pedal pulses. If the carotid artery is used, measure the neck circumference as part of the baseline data. Immediately before the procedure, measure baseline vital signs and pulses and perform a neurologic check.

The test takes approximately 2 to 3 hours. The patient may experience discomfort in lying still for that time. When the dye is injected, most patients complain of feeling extremely hot and seeing flashes of light. The patient is positioned supine on the radiograph ta-

ble. A local anesthetic agent is used to anesthetize the area of the puncture site. The catheter is introduced percutaneously and introduced into the relevant vessels. At times the catheter may be inserted directly into the carotid or vertebral arteries. After all injections are done, the catheter is withdrawn and pressure is applied to the puncture site for at least 15 minutes.

After the procedure, bed rest is ordered, usually for 4 to 6 hours. Check vital signs and perform a neurologic check frequently (at times as often as every 15 minutes). Assess the puncture site frequently for the presence of a hematoma. With a femoral stick, check the pulses distal to the site for evidence of arterial occlusion. With a carotid stick, assess whether the patient has any difficulty breathing or swallowing or an increase in the girth of the neck.

The patient undergoing this procedure is at risk for cerebrovascular accident and ICP. Promptly report any change in LOC or other parts of the neurologic assessment.

MRA is rapidly replacing cerebral arteriography in many facilities.

Carotid Duplex

A carotid duplex study uses combined ultrasound and pulsed Doppler technology. A technician places a probe on the skin over the carotid artery and slowly moves the probe along the course of the common carotid to the bifurcation of the external and internal carotid arteries. The ultrasound signal emitted from the probe reflects off the moving blood cells within the vessel. The frequency of the reflected signal corresponds to the blood velocity. This response is amplified and is registered on a graphic record and also as sound. The graphic record registers blood velocity. Increased blood flow velocity can indicate stenosis of a vessel. Carotid duplex scanning is a noninvasive study that evaluates carotid occlusive disease. This study is often ordered when a patient has a transient ischemic attack (TIA).

Electromyogram

An electromyogram (EMG) measures the contraction of a muscle in response to electrical stimulation. It provides evidence of lower motoneuron disease; primary muscle disease; and defects in the transmission of electrical impulses at the neuromuscular junction, such as in myasthenia gravis (MG). There is no special preparation for the test. The test takes approximately 45 minutes for one muscle study. Inform the patient that it is uncomfortable when the electrode is inserted into the muscle and when the electrical current is used. The muscle may ache for a short time after the procedure.

During the test an electrode is inserted into selected skeletal muscles. An electric current is passed through the electrode, and the machine graphs the variations of muscle potentials (voltage). After the procedure assess the patient for signs of bleeding at the site of the electrode insertion. The patient may need an analgesic for discomfort and a rest period.

Echoencephalogram

An echoencephalogram uses ultrasound to depict the intracranial structures of the brain. It is especially helpful in detecting ventricular dilation and a major shift of midline structures in the brain as a result of an expanding lesion. The preparation of the patient, the actual procedure, and aftercare are similar to those of the brain scan.

COMMON DISORDERS OF THE NEUROLOGIC SYSTEM

HEADACHES

Etiology and Pathophysiology

Headache is a common neurologic complaint; its significance and its causes vary. The source of recurring headache should be determined through careful physical examination with appropriate neurologic assessment. Some tumors may produce no symptoms except for headache for a long period.

The exact mechanism of head pain is not known. Although the skull and brain tissues are not able to feel sensory pain, pain arises from the scalp, its blood vessels and muscles, and the dura mater and its venous sinuses. Pain also arises from the blood vessels at the base of the brain and from cervical cranial nerves. Blood vessels may dilate and become congested with blood. Headaches can be classified as vascular, tension, and traction-inflammatory. Vascular headaches include migraine, cluster, and hypertensive headaches. Tension headaches may arise from psychological problems of tension or stress or from medical problems such as cervical arthritis. Traction-inflammatory headaches include those caused by infection, intracranial or extracranial causes, occlusive vascular structures, and temporal arteritis.

Clinical Manifestations

Headache pain may be made worse by stress or tension. Knowledge of the patient's perception of the effect of stress on the pain is important in planning effective interventions.

Migraine headaches are unusual in that prodromal (early signs and symptoms of a developing condition or disease) signs and symptoms occur before the acute attack. These may include visual field defects; unusual smells or sounds; disorientation; paresthesias; and, in rare cases, paralysis of a part of the body. During a migraine headache, signs and symptoms may include nausea, vomiting, sensitivity to light, chilliness, fatigue, irritability, diaphoresis, edema, and other signs of autonomic dysfunction. Abnormal metabolism of serotonin, a vasoactive neurotransmitter found in platelets and cells of the brain, plays a major role. A history of migraine with aura in young women is now known to

 Communication

Nurse-Patient Therapeutic Communication Concerning Patient's Headache

Nurse: Can you describe your problem to me?
Patient: It's a pain in my head.
Nurse: When did this pain start?
Patient: About a month ago.
Nurse: Did anything else happen at that same time?
Patient: My daughter left home for college.
Nurse: How did you feel about that?
Patient: I was really upset. She was my baby. I can't believe that she's gone.
Nurse: Was there anything else that you noticed at the same time? Like an increased temperature or nasal drainage?
Patient: No, I don't think so.
Nurse: What made the headache worse?
Patient: Thinking about my loneliness.
Nurse: What made the headache better?
Patient: Sleeping or taking a Valium.
Nurse: Have you had trouble sleeping or noticed that your appetite was worse?
Patient: I wake up early in the morning. I don't feel much like eating.
Nurse: Have you lost weight?
Patient: About 10 pounds in the last month.
Nurse: Can you tell me what the pain feels like?
Patient: It's a pain that goes through my whole head. It throbs and gets worse in the evening.
Nurse: What do you think is the cause of the headache?
Patient: I guess maybe I'm upset that my daughter left.

cause atherosclerosis (deposits, or plaques, containing lipids and lipophages that form within the intima and inner media of large and medium-size arteries). Because each migraine episode decreases cerebral blood flow, damage to the cerebral endothelium from repeated episodes of vasospasm increases the patient's risk for atherosclerosis and stroke (Phillips, 2007).

Assessment

Subjective data include the patient's understanding of the headache, possible causes, and any precipitating factors. Determine what measures relieve the symptoms and the location, frequency, pattern, and character of the pain. This includes the site of return of the headache, time of day, and intervals between headaches. Also assess the initial onset of the headache, any symptoms that occur before the headache or associated symptoms, the presence of allergies, and any family history of similar headache patterns.

Objective data include any behaviors indicating stress, anxiety, or pain. Changes in the ability to carry out activities of daily living (ADLs), an abnormally raised body temperature, and sinus drainage may be important. Also document abnormalities noted during the physical examination (see Communication box).

Diagnostic Tests

It is important to evaluate headaches that are not transient. Usual testing includes a neurologic examination, a CT scan (MRI or PET scan may also be done), a brain scan, skull radiographs, and a lumbar puncture. A lumbar puncture is not done, however, if there is evidence of increased ICP or if a brain tumor is suspected because quick reduction of pressure produced by removal of the spinal fluid may cause brain herniation. In these situations a CT scan is done first.

Medical Management

Dietary Counseling

Some foods may cause or worsen headaches. These include foods containing tyramine, nitrates, or glutamates (e.g., monosodium glutamate [MSG], often used in the preparation of Chinese foods and on salad bars). Other substances that may provoke headaches include vinegar, chocolate, yogurt, alcohol, fermented or marinated foods, ripened cheese, cured sandwich meat, caffeine, and pork.

Psychotherapy

Patients with headaches may respond to psychotherapy. This does not mean that the headache pain is not physiologic, but counseling can help the patient develop awareness of stress factors and deal with the pain. The patient may need help expressing feelings about intractable headache pain.

Medications

Medications are often used to treat headaches.

Migraine headaches. Acetylsalicylic acid (aspirin) or acetaminophen may help relieve mild or moderate migraine pain. For moderate to severe headaches, the triptans have become the first line of the therapy. Triptans are thought to act on receptors in the extracerebral, intracranial vessels that become dilated during a migraine attack. Stimulating these receptors constricts cranial vessels, inhibits neuropeptide release, and reduces nerve impulse transmission along trigeminal pain pathways.

Eletriptan (Replax) is the seventh triptan to be marketed for treatment of migraine, joining almotriptan (Axert), frovatriptan (Frova), naratriptan (Amerge), rizatriptan (Maxalt), sumatriptan (Imitrex), and zolmitriptan (Zomig). Classified as selective serotonin receptor agonists, these drugs are all indicated to treat acute migraine (with or without aura) in adults. In addition to relieving headache pain, the triptans also relieve the nausea, vomiting, and photophobia associated with acute migraine attack.

Evidence is growing for the role of preventive treatment in the management of migraine headaches (Brandes, 2005; Loder & Biondi, 2005). The decision to initiate prophylactic treatment is individually determined based on frequency and severity of headaches and on any disability due to headaches. Topiramate (Topamax), taken daily, has been shown to be an effective therapy for migraine prevention in adults. Not all patients become pain free on this medication (Lewis et al., 2007). Other preventive drugs for migraine headaches include beta-adrenergic blockers (e.g., propranolol [Inderal], atenolol [Tenormin]), tricyclic antidepressants (e.g., amitriptyline [Elavil]), selective serotonin reuptake inhibitors (e.g., fluoxetine [Prozac]), calcium channel blockers (e.g., verapamil [Isoptin]), divalproex (Depakote), clonidine (Catapres), and thiazides.

Cluster headaches. Because the pain associated with vascular cluster headaches is often severe, narcotic analgesics, sometimes given intramuscularly, are used. Patients with cluster headaches usually feel fine between attacks, so no analgesic is needed during these times.

Tension headaches. Nonnarcotic analgesics are often used to treat tension headaches. These include acetaminophen, propoxyphene, phenacetin, ibuprofen, and aspirin. Narcotics are avoided because these drugs are often subject to abuse; it is much better to counsel patients to develop other ways to relieve headaches.

Nursing Interventions and Patient Teaching

Because stress and emotional upsets may precipitate some headaches and worsen others, the patient requires relaxation and rest. Help the patient with relaxation techniques, planned sleeping hours, and regular rest periods. Alcohol should not be used to relieve tension because it may become addicting and has been found to be a significant cause of cluster headaches. Regular physical exercise may also help prevent headaches, especially ones caused by tension.

If a patient is suffering from a severe headache, plan nursing interventions so that only essential activities take place. Group interventions so that the patient has adequate time to rest.

Comfort Measures

Other treatments that may help a patient with a headache include cold packs applied to the forehead or base of the skull and pressure applied to the temporal arteries. People with migraine headaches are usually most comfortable lying in a dark, quiet room.

Identifying Triggering Factors

Triggering factors associated with severe and recurring headaches may include fatigue, alcohol, stress, seasonal climate changes, hunger, allergies, and menstruation. Help the patient identify these factors, if necessary, through ongoing observation or assessment of the patient's personality, habits, ADLs, career plans, work habits, family relationships, coping mechanisms, and relaxation activities. The patient may keep a diary or journal to help collect this information.

Nursing diagnoses and interventions for the patient with headache include but are not limited to the following:

Nursing Diagnoses	Nursing Interventions
Anxiety, related to pain	Provide quiet environment. Encourage verbalization of concerns. Provide diversional activities.
Acute or chronic pain, related to disease process	Administer prescribed medications. Provide comfort measures. Maintain nonstressful environment. Encourage pain reduction techniques as appropriate: rocking movements, external warmth, breathing patterns.

Teaching is an important part of the nursing intervention of the patient with headaches. Topics include (1) avoidance of factors that trigger headaches; (2) relaxation techniques, including biofeedback; (3) maintenance of regular sleep patterns; (4) medications to be used (including dosage, actions, and side effects); and (5) the importance of follow-up care.

Prognosis
With proper treatment the person with headaches can expect to live a normal life. Changes in lifestyle may need to occur, especially during acute episodes of headache pain. The person may have to adjust to periodic headaches and rest until the headache resolves.

NEUROPATHIC PAIN

Etiology, Pathophysiology, and Clinical Manifestations
Neuropathic pain other than headache is common. Examples include postherpetic neuralgia, phantom limb pain, diabetic neuropathies, and trigeminal neuralgia (Lewis et al., 2007). The transmission of pain is not fully understood, but patients may experience disabling pain either caused by a disorder within the nervous system or caused at a distant part of the body. Neuropathic pain may arise from lesions involving the peripheral cutaneous nerves, the sensory nerve roots, the thalamus, and the central pain tract (lateral spinothalamic) at some level. Each produces characteristic pain. Pain receptors are not adaptable—they are specific for pain only—and pain impulses continue at the same rate as long as the stimulus is present. Pain receptors can be activated by

cellular damage, certain chemicals such as histamine, heat, ischemia, muscle spasm, and sensations of cold and pruritus that go beyond a specific level of intensity.

Pain that is described as unbearable and does not respond to treatment is classified as **intractable.** It is chronic and often debilitating and may prevent the patient from functioning in ADLs.

Assessment
The perception of pain is highly subjective. Pain may vary from mild to excruciating. **Subjective data** include the patient's understanding of the pain; any precipitating factors; and measures that relieve stress, including medication. The site, frequency, and nature of the pain are important, as is the patient's usual coping patterns when under stress. Associated symptoms and measures that make the pain worse are important subjective data.

Objective data may be limited when assessing neuropathic pain. Objective factors to assess are behavioral signs indicating pain or stress, a change in the ability to carry out ADLs, muscle weakness or wasting, vasomotor responses (such as flushing), abnormalities of spinal reflexes, and abnormalities noted during the sensory examination.

Diagnostic Tests
Diagnostic tests for the patient in pain may include electrical stimulation, used to define the pain to a greater degree. Psychological testing may be part of the workup. If back or neck pain is present, a myelogram is usually performed.

Medical Management
Nonsurgical Methods of Pain Control
Neuropathic pain sometimes responds to other methods of pain control. These include transcutaneous electrical nerve stimulation and spinal cord stimulation. Both techniques use electrodes applied near the site of pain or on or around the spine (see Chapter 2). The stimulator modifies the sensory input by blocking or changing the painful sensation with a stimulus that is perceived to be less painful or nonpainful. Acupuncture is also used to treat patients with neuropathic pain.

Nerve Block
A nerve block is used to control intractable pain. It involves injecting a local anesthetic, alcohol, or phenol close enough to a nerve to block the conduction of impulses. Sources of pain often treated with a nerve block include trigeminal neuralgia, cancer, and peripheral vascular disease. The effect lasts from several months to several years. Pain and spasticity may also be controlled by means of an epidural catheter. Medication is usually administered continuously.

Medications

Medications are often used to treat patients with neuropathic pain. Anticonvulsant medications such as gabapentin (Neurontin) and carbamazepine (Tegretol) are often useful. Other medications include nonopioid analgesics such as acetaminophen, nonsteroidal antiinflammatory drugs, and acetylsalicylic acid. Opioids do not appear as helpful for neuropathic pain although they are still sometimes used. Antidepressants—such as amitriptyline, doxepin (Sinequan), imipramine (Tofranil-PM), and nortriptyline (Pamelor)—appear to be effective in treating neuropathic pain. The emphasis should be on helping the patient learn various other measures to control the pain.

Surgical Methods of Pain Control

In cases of intractable pain that does not respond to more conservative measures, surgery may be necessary to reduce or eliminate pain. Neurosurgical procedures include neurectomy, rhizotomy, cordotomy, and percutaneous cordotomy. These procedures all have potential complications that need to be considered before the decision is made to perform surgery. For example, a patient who undergoes a cordotomy may have difficulties with postural hypotension, ability to feel hot or cold, and possibly motor and bowel function. Temporary edema of the cord from the procedure may lead to temporary paralysis or leg weakness.

Nursing Interventions and Patient Teaching
Comfort Measures

A patient with neuropathic pain may be uncomfortable and should be assisted to assume a position of comfort. For example, the patient with back pain should avoid movements that cause direct or indirect movement of the spinal cord. The patient may find lying in a supine position uncomfortable. Help the patient find a comfortable position and, if necessary, actively assist the patient in turning or moving. Straining when having a stool can intensify pain, and a stool softener may be needed. Offer prune juice and a high-fiber diet and encourage the patient to drink up to 2000 mL/day or more of fluids.

Promotion of Rest and Relaxation

As with headache, stress and emotional upsets may precipitate or exacerbate neuropathic pain. Facilitate rest and relaxation, with planned sleeping hours and rest periods as needed.

Some patients with pain, especially intractable pain, may respond well to psychotherapy. This does not mean that the pain does not have a physiologic basis, but counseling can help the patient develop awareness of what makes the pain worse and how to cope with the discomfort.

Nursing diagnoses and interventions for the patient with neuropathic pain are the same as those listed previously for headache, with the addition of the following:

Nursing Diagnoses	Nursing Interventions
Risk for disuse syndrome, related to lack of use of a body part as a result of pain	Explain need for regular exercise program to maintain joint mobility; provide range-of-motion (ROM) exercises to all body joints every 2 to 4 hours. Be positive and reassuring in approach.
Feeding, bathing/hygiene self-care deficit, related to pain	Assist with basic ADL needs as necessary, but encourage patient to participate as much as possible. Provide sufficient time for ADLs. Facilitate use of self-help devices as needed. Provide for total hygiene as indicated.

Teaching is an important part of the nursing interventions of the patient with neuropathic pain. Include the factors taught to the patient with headache, and help patient become aware of physical methods such as positioning the body to increase comfort and structuring the home and work setting to minimize stress.

Prognosis

As with headache pain, neuropathic pain can in most cases be treated adequately. Lifestyle changes may be helpful in allowing the person to have a better quality of life.

INCREASED INTRACRANIAL PRESSURE
Etiology, Pathophysiology, and Clinical Manifestations

Increased ICP is a complex grouping of events that occurs because of multiple neurologic conditions. It often occurs suddenly, progresses rapidly, and requires surgical intervention. It is a potential complication in many neurologic conditions and can rapidly lead to death if not treated and reversed.

Increased ICP occurs in patients with acute neurologic conditions such as a brain tumor, hemorrhage, anoxic brain injury, and toxic or viral encephalopathies; it is most commonly associated with head injury. An increase in any one of the contents of the cranium is usually accompanied by a reciprocal change in the volume of one of the others. This is be-

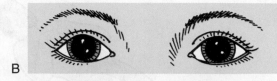

A, Unequal pupils, also called anisocoria. B, Dilated and fixed pupils, indicative of severe neurologic deficit.

FIGURE 14-8

cause the cranial vault is rigid and nonexpandable. Pressure may build up slowly over weeks or rapidly, depending on the cause. Usually one side of the brain is more involved, but both sides of the brain eventually become involved.

As the pressure increases within the cranial cavity, it is first compensated for by venous compression and CSF displacement. As the pressure continues to rise, the cerebral blood flow decreases and inadequate perfusion of the brain occurs. This inadequate perfusion starts a vicious cycle that causes the Pco_2 to increase and the Po_2 and pH to decrease. These changes cause vasodilation and cerebral edema. The edema further increases the ICP, which causes increased compression of neural tissue and an even greater increase in ICP.

When the pressure buildup is greater than the brain's ability to compensate, pressure is exerted on surrounding structures where the pressure is lower. This movement of pressure is called **supratentorial shift** and can result in herniation. As a result of herniation of the brain, the brainstem is compressed at various levels, which in turn compresses the vasomotor center, the posterior cerebral artery, the oculomotor nerve, the corticospinal nerve pathway, and the fibers of the ascending RAS. The life-sustaining mechanisms of consciousness, blood pressure, pulse, respiration, and temperature regulation are all impaired. A rise in systolic pressure and an unchanged diastolic pressure, resulting in a widening pulse pressure, bradycardia, and abnormal respiration, are late signs of increased ICP and indicate that the brain is about to herniate.

Assessment

Increased ICP must be detected early while it is still reversible. The ability to make accurate observations, interpret observations intelligently, and record observations carefully is most important for the nurse working with patients with increased ICP.

Subjective data for a diagnosis of increased ICP include the patient's understanding of the condition, any visual changes such as diplopia (double vision), a change in the patient's personality, and a change in the ability to think. The diplopia usually results from paralysis or weakness of one of the muscles that controls eye movement. It often occurs fairly early in the process. Nausea or pain, especially headache, is also important. The headache is thought to result from venous congestion and tension in the intracranial blood vessels as the cerebral pressure rises. Headache that oc-

curs with increased ICP usually increases in intensity with coughing, straining at stool, or stooping. It is usually present in the early morning and may awaken the patient from sleep.

Objective data include a change in the LOC, which is the earliest sign of increased ICP. During assessment, it takes more stimulation to get the same response from the patient. Manifestations of a change in the LOC include disorientation, restlessness, and lethargy. Record observations in terms of behaviors and signs and symptoms, not in terms of labels. Pupillary signs may also change with increased ICP. Pupillary responses are controlled by cranial nerve III (oculomotor nerve). The pupils usually change on the same side as the lesion. The first and most subtle clue to trouble is that the pupil reacts, but sluggishly. As the brain herniates, the nerve is compressed—with the top part of the nerve being affected first. The **ipsilateral** pupil (when the lesion is in one hemisphere) remains dilated and is incapable of constricting. The pupil appears larger than that of the affected side and does not react to light. As the ICP increases and both halves of the brain become affected, bilateral pupil dilation and fixation occur. Dilating pupils that respond slowly to light are a sign of impending herniation. A pupil that is fixed and dilated, sometimes called a **blown pupil,** is an ominous sign that *must* be reported to the physician immediately (Figure 14-8).

Changes in the blood pressure and pulse are seen with increasing ICP. Herniation causes ischemia of the vasomotor center, which excites the vasoconstrictor fibers, causing the systolic blood pressure to rise. If the ICP continues to increase, a widening pulse pressure occurs.

Pressure in the vasomotor center also increases the transmission of parasympathetic impulses through the vagus nerve to the heart, causing a slowing of the pulse. A widened pulse pressure, increased systolic blood pressure, and bradycardia are together called **Cushing's response.** It is considered an important diagnostic sign of late-stage brain herniation.

Brain herniation produces respiratory problems that are variable and related to the level of the brainstem compression or failure. The breathing pattern may be deep and stertorous (snorelike) or periodic (Cheyne-Stokes) respirations. **Ataxic** breathing may also occur; this is an irregular and unpredictable breathing pattern with random, shallow, and deep breaths and occasional pauses. It is seen in patients

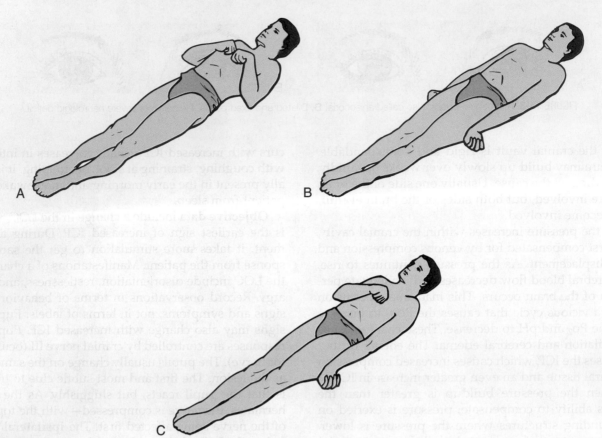

FIGURE 14-9 Decorticate and decerebrate responses. **A,** Decorticate response. Flexion of arms, wrists, and fingers with adduction in upper extremities. Extension, internal rotation, and plantar flexion in lower extremities. **B,** Decerebrate response. All four extremities in rigid extension, with hyperpronation of forearms and plantar extension of feet. **C,** Decorticate response on right side of body and decerebrate response on left side of body.

with medulla oblongata damage. As ICP increases to fatal levels, respiratory paralysis occurs.

Failure of the thermoregulatory center because of compression occurs later with increased ICP. It results in high, uncontrolled temperatures. This hyperthermia increases the metabolism of brain tissue.

Compression of the upper motoneuron pathway (corticospinal tract) interrupts transmission of impulses to the lower motoneuron, and progressive muscle weakness occurs. Babinski's reflex, hyperreflexia, and rigidity are additional signs of decreased motor function. Seizures may occur. Herniation of the upper part of the brainstem may produce characteristic posturing when the patient is stimulated (Figure 14-9). The worsening of motor problems is significant, because it means that the ICP is continuing to increase.

Vomiting and singultus (hiccups) are two objective signs of increased ICP. The vomiting is often projectile and usually not preceded by nausea; this is called unexpected vomiting. Singultus is caused by compression of the vagus nerve (cranial nerve X) as brainstem herniation occurs.

One last objective sign is papilledema, which is detected with the use of an ophthalmoscope (usually by

the physician). As ICP increases, the pressure is transmitted to the eyes through the CSF and to the optic disk. As the optic disk becomes edematous, the retina is also compressed. The damaged retina cannot detect light rays. Visual acuity is lessened as the blind spot enlarges. **Papilledema** is also called a **choked disk.**

Diagnostic Tests

Diagnostic studies are aimed at identifying the presence and the underlying cause of increased ICP. The diagnosis of increased ICP is made with CT or MRI, which can show actual structural herniation and shifting of the brain. Because of CT and MRI, the diagnosis of increased ICP has been completely revolutionized and the therapeutic options greatly increased (Lewis et al., 2007).

Most of the time, acute increased ICP is a medical emergency, and diagnostic tests must be done quickly. Other tests include ICP measurement, EEG, cerebral angiography, transcranial Doppler studies, and PET. In general, lumbar puncture is not performed when increased ICP is suspected because of the possibility of cerebral herniation from the sudden release of the pressure in the skull from the area above the lumbar puncture. This can lead to pressure on cardiac and respiratory centers in the brainstem and potentially death (Lewis et al., 2007).

In postoperative or critically ill patients, internal measuring devices are used to diagnose increased ICP. One of the most common measuring devices requires the placement of a hollow screw through the skull into the subarachnoid space. The device is connected to a transducer and oscilloscope for continuous monitoring. Waveforms are produced that indicate the ICP.

Medical Management

The goals of treatment are to identify and treat the underlying cause of increased ICP. Preventing increased ICP may not be possible, but preventing further increases in pressure with resulting damage to the brain is crucial. The medical treatment depends on the cause of the pressure. For example, surgery may be done to remove a tumor. If surgery is not possible, efforts are made to reduce the pressure through drug therapy or other measures.

Ensuring adequate oxygenation to support brain function is the first step in management of increased ICP. Endotracheal intubation may be necessary. Arterial blood gases analysis guides the oxygen therapy. With controlled ventilation, the Pco_2 can be lowered to below normal, which causes a slightly alkalotic pH. The decrease in the Pco_2 and the increase in pH will decrease vasodilation and decrease ICP. The goal is to maintain the Pao_2 at 100 mm Hg.

Mechanical Decompression

Rapidly rising ICP can be relieved by mechanical decompression. This may include a craniotomy, in which a bone flap is removed and then replaced, or a craniectomy, in which a bone flap is removed and not replaced. The craniectomy is often done when pressure is high. Other means of decompression include drainage of the ventricles or any subdural hematoma.

Internal monitoring devices are being used more frequently to diagnose and monitor increased ICP. Three basic monitoring systems are used: the ventricular catheter, the subarachnoid bolt or screw, and the epidural sensor. These monitoring devices produce pressure waves that can be evaluated to indicate the status of ICP.

Medications

Three types of medications are usually administered to patients with increased ICP: osmotic diuretics, corticosteroids, and anticonvulsants. Osmotic diuretics are also called hyperosmolar drugs. They draw water from the edematous brain tissue. An example of this type of medication is mannitol. It begins to reduce increased ICP within 15 minutes, and its effects last for 5 to 6 hours. Loop diuretics such as furosemide (Lasix), bumetanide (Bumex), and ethacrynic acid (Edecrin) may also be used in the management of increased ICP.

Continuous midazolam (Versed) and atracurium besylate (Tracrium) infusions are also used.

The corticosteroid that may be given is dexamethasone (Decadron). Corticosteroids are thought to control edema surrounding cerebral tumors and abscesses but appear to have limited value in managing head-injured patients (Lewis et al., 2007). With this drug, monitor blood glucose levels because steroids can affect carbohydrate metabolism and glucose utilization and result in elevated blood glucose levels.

To prevent gastrointestinal ulcers and bleeding, patients receiving corticosteroids should concurrently be given antacids, histamine-receptor blockers (e.g., cimetidine [Tagamet], ranitidine [Zantac]), or proton pump inhibitors (e.g., omeprazole [Prilosex], pantoprazole [Protonix, Protonix I.V.]).

Anticonvulsants are given to prevent seizures. Phenytoin (Dilantin) is the most commonly given drug. It can be given intravenously but usually not intramuscularly because of poor absorption. Fosphenytoin (Cerebyx) is a short-term IV or intramuscular anticonvulsant in current use. Opioids and other drugs that cause respiratory depression are avoided.

Nursing Interventions and Patient Teaching

Therapeutic measures to reduce venous volume include the following:

- Elevate the head of the bed to 30 to 45 degrees to promote venous return.
- Place the neck in a neutral position (not flexed or extended) to promote venous drainage.
- Position the patient to avoid flexion of the hips, the waist, and the neck and rotation of the head, especially to the right. Avoid extreme hip flexion because this position causes an increase in intraabdominal and intrathoracic pressures, which can produce a rise in ICP.
- Instruct the patient to avoid isometric or resistive exercises.
- Restrict fluid intake.
- Implement measures to help the patient avoid the Valsalva maneuver (any forced expiratory effort against a closed airway, such as straining to have a stool). Avoid enemas and laxatives if possible.
- Have a Foley catheter in place if the patient is not alert because of the large amount of urine that is produced.
- Perform suctioning only as necessary and for no longer than 10 seconds with administration of 100% oxygen before and after to prevent decreases in the Pao_2.
- Administer oxygen via mask or cannula to improve cerebral perfusion.
- Use a hypothermia blanket to control body temperature (increased body temperature increases brain damage).

Nursing diagnoses and interventions for the patient with increased ICP may include but are not limited to the following:

Nursing Diagnoses	Nursing Interventions
Ineffective breathing pattern, related to neuromuscular impairment	Maintain patent airway; avoid flexion of neck. Administer oxygen and humidification as ordered. Provide oral nasopharyngeal airway as indicated for managing secretions; suction oropharynx as needed.
Risk for injury, related to physiologic effects of sustained elevation in ICP	Elevate head of bed 30 degrees. Maintain body position; avoid semiprone or prone position. Avoid compression of neck veins. Check blood pressure, pulse, and respiration every 30 minutes. Perform neurologic check every 30 minutes using Glasgow coma scale; report any findings below 8 to physician.

The patient with increased ICP is often unresponsive. Share information about procedures that are being done with the patient and the family. This may help both be as cooperative as possible.

Prognosis

The prognosis for the patient with increased ICP depends on the cause and the speed with which it is treated. The nurse assumes an important role in monitoring the patient for signs and symptoms of increased pressure. After herniation of the brain has begun as a result of pressure, there is little chance for complete reversal without significant brain damage.

DISTURBANCES IN MUSCLE TONE AND MOTOR FUNCTION

Etiology and Pathophysiology

Motor function disturbances are the most commonly encountered neurologic signs and symptoms. Damage to the nervous system often causes serious problems in mobility. An example of this is the patient with cerebral palsy.

Clinical Manifestations

Injury or disease of motoneurons results in alterations of muscle strength, tone, and reflex activity. Muscle tone may be described as **flaccid** (weak, soft, flabby, and lacking normal muscle tone) or **hyperreflexic** (increased reflex actions). The specific clinical manifestations differ according to the location of the neurologic lesion.

Assessment

Subjective data for patients with motor problems include the patient's understanding of the problem and possible causes. Ask about the initial onset of the symptoms; measures that improve symptoms; and the presence of clumsiness, incoordination, or abnormal sensation. If the lesion occurs suddenly, as in traumatic spinal cord injury, subjective symptoms may be minimal. If the motor deficit develops slowly, subjective symptoms may be so subtle that they are at first ignored.

Objective data include coordination, muscle strength, muscle tone, and muscle atrophy. Reflexes are often checked, as well as the presence of clonus or fasciculations and the ability to move muscles. Any abnormal gait is significant, as is a change in the ability to carry out ADLs.

Diagnostic Tests

One of the most common procedures for detecting pathologic conditions of muscle is the EMG. It detects the various types of electrical activity and abnormal patterns that may appear in resting muscle in the presence of disease.

Medical Management

Patients with motor problems may have spasticity. Muscle relaxants may be used to decrease tone and involuntary movements. Some commonly prescribed medications include baclofen (Lioresal), dantrolene (Dantrium), and diazepam (Valium). Baclofen has been used intrathecally to reduce spasticity. Common side effects of these drugs include drowsiness and vertigo. These side effects are increased by the use of alcohol or other depressants.

Some patients may have severe swallowing difficulty (dysphagia). This commonly results from obstructive or motor disorders of the esophagus and is commonly associated with neurologic problems. The patient with dysphagia often requires prefeeding and feeding exercises.

In patients at severe risk for aspiration, a video fluoroscopy with barium may be done when aspiration is suspected. The procedure requires the patient to swallow a small amount of liquid or semisolid barium while a fluoroscopic examination is being done.

For patients with paralysis, the eye on the affected side of the body may need to be protected if the lid remains open and there is no blink reflex. The patient is at high risk for corneal scratches or irritation. Irrigation with a physiologic solution of sodium chloride may be used, followed by eyedrops. An eye pad may be used to keep the eye closed, although an eyeshield is preferable.

Nursing Interventions

Safety Needs

Patients with paralysis have significant safety needs. This includes protection from falling, including the use of side rails when the patient is in bed and a chair restraint when the patient is in a chair, especially if balance cannot be maintained. If the patient also has a sensory problem, which often accompanies paralysis, he or she may not realize when part of the body is in danger. For example, a patient with a stroke may not be aware that a hemiplegic arm is hanging over the side of the wheelchair.

The eye on the affected side of the body should be cleaned and assessed for signs of infection on a regular basis, usually three times a day or more. Also inspect affected body parts for injury.

Regularly inspect the skin over bony prominences for signs of pressure. Paralyzed people are at risk for skin impairment, so teach them to turn themselves in bed and to reposition themselves in the bed or chair independently, if possible. If the patient is unable to turn independently, the nurse carries out this function. Usually the patient is turned from one side to another or from one side to the back to the other side. Repositioning also includes weight shifts, done by the patient or by staff. These weight shifts may include controlled leaning from one side to another or push-ups. If the patient is not able to do the activity, have him or her take responsibility for reminding staff when it is time to do the weight shift.

Inspect paralyzed or weakened areas at least daily for any signs of skin impairment. A mirror is often used to help the patient assess the skin so that he or she is not as dependent on staff or family.

Activity Needs

The extremities of a person who has an acute motor problem may be flaccid at first. Spasticity of muscles develops gradually. The joints then become flexed and fixed in useless, deformed positions unless preventive measures are taken.

Carefully place the extremities in a normal anatomical position to prevent deformity. Counterpositioning may be helpful. In hemiplegia (paralysis of one side of the body) the affected upper extremity is pulled inward at the shoulder joint and the wrist drops; in the lower extremity the knee flexes and the foot drops. In counterpositioning, position the patient so that the shoulder and upper arm are in abduction, the elbow is flexed, the wrist is dorsiflexed, the knee is in neutral position, and the foot is dorsiflexed. If the person is supine, place a pillow between the upper arm and the body to hold the arm in abduction. Physical therapists and occupational therapists can provide splints and braces that can aid in positioning (Figure 14-10).

Footboards may be used to prevent footdrop, although some believe that these contribute to in-

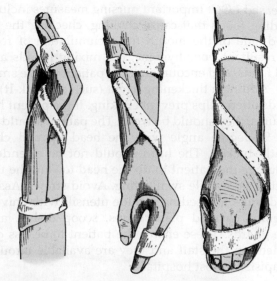

FIGURE 14-10 Volar resting splint provides support to wrist, thumb, and fingers of patient after cerebrovascular accident (stroke), maintaining them in position of extension.

creased spasticity and should not be used routinely for patients who have muscle spasms. High-topped tennis shoes or other devices, such as splints or braces, can help prevent footdrop, if therapy is initiated early. In some hospitals, casts are applied to patients' lower extremities to prevent footdrop or to reverse contractures. The presence of the cast impedes spasticity. A sling or hook hemiharness may be useful to support the affected arm to prevent shoulder subluxation.

The prone position is excellent for patients who are able to tolerate it. Not only does this position decrease the chance of skin impairment, but it also causes extension of the hip, the knee joints, and the ankles by means of gravity. A pillow placed under the chest may help patients comfortably assume this position.

Positioning of the paralyzed person is extremely important. Complications such as footdrop and flexion contractures of the knee seriously limit mobility. As a result, the level of self-care and independence is diminished. Most joint deformities in a paralyzed person are preventable with early and continuing nursing interventions.

In addition to positioning, interventions for the person with paralysis include ROM exercises to all joints. These may be passive (carried out by the nurse) or active (carried out by the patient). Passive ROM is indicated at least three times daily for all joints that the patient cannot voluntarily move.

Nutritional Needs

Patience and persistence are often necessary in giving food and fluids to the patient with hemiplegia. Aspiration can occur and is related to loss of pharyngeal sensation, loss of oropharyngeal motor control, and decreased LOC. Important nursing measures include avoiding foods that cause choking, checking the affected side of the mouth for accumulation of food and resultant poor hygiene, not mixing liquids and solid foods, and encouraging the patient to take small bites. Adding a thickening agent (such as Thick-It) to liquids often helps prevent choking. If the patient has dentures, they should be worn. The patient should sit at a 90-degree angle with the head up and chin slightly tucked. The head should not be extended; encourage the patient to tip the head toward the unaffected side while swallowing. Avoid straws Assistive devices for feeding include utensils with universal cuffs, covered plastic cups, scoop dishes, and plate guards. These enable the patient to be less dependent on the staff and they are available through therapists in most hospitals.

Activities of Daily Living

During the acute rehabilitative phases of a motor problem, teach patients with paralysis how to carry out ADLs to the extent that they are able. A variety of devices are available to assist with dressing and grooming (Figures 14-11 and 14-12). The occupational therapist becomes involved in many of these activities, including homemaking. Stress the concept of the rehabilitative team in managing these patients. Teach the patient to compensate for weakness or paralysis. Give the patient the time to do activities on his or her own if able. It is often easier and faster to do things for the patient, but this defeats the purpose of rehabilitation.

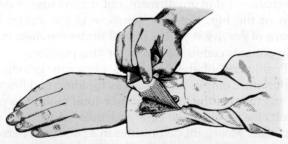

FIGURE 14-11 Velcro shirtsleeve to facilitate closure.

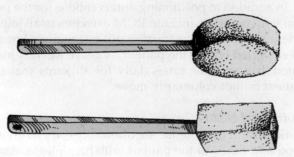

FIGURE 14-12 Long-handled bath sponges.

Psychological Adjustments

The person with paralysis may need assistance in adjusting to body changes. The loss of the ability to function independently is traumatic, and the patient may have fears of rejection, loss of self-esteem, and concerns about the future. A grief reaction similar to that described for a death may occur. At times the patient may relate to the paralyzed part of the body as though it were not a part of him or her and may have nicknames for the body part. To help the patient cope with the loss of function and change in body image, praise the patient for achievements, encourage expression of fears and grief, and help him or her see that there is life after disability. It might be helpful to arrange a visit by someone with the same disability who has been successfully rehabilitated.

Nursing diagnoses and interventions for the patient with alterations in muscle tone and motor function include but are not limited to the following:

Nursing Diagnoses	Nursing Interventions
Impaired physical mobility, related to neuromuscular impairment	Perform active or passive ROM exercise every 4 hours, to all extremities, neck, hands, fingers, wrists, elbows, and knees.
	Provide physical therapy as ordered (massage and stretching exercises).
	Maintain planned rest periods.
	Encourage ambulation to tolerance.
	Arrange for necessary assistive devices for home care needs.
Risk for disuse syndrome, related to impaired functioning of body part	Perform hand, finger, foot exercises; assist in active and passive ROM exercises every 2 to 4 hours.
	Assist patient with using supportive devices as indicated (overhead trapeze, braces, walker, cane).
	Encourage use of involved side when possible.
	Instruct patient to use unaffected extremity to support weaker side (e.g., lift involved left leg with right leg or lift involved left arm with right arm).
	Turn every 2 hours.

The Patient with a Neurologic Disorder

- **Nutritional-metabolic pattern:** Neurologic problems can result in inadequate nutrition. Problems related to chewing, swallowing, facial nerve paralysis, and muscle coordination could make it difficult for the patient to ingest adequate nutrients.
- **Elimination pattern:** Bowel and bladder problems are often associated with neurologic problems, such as stroke, head injury, spinal cord injury, multiple sclerosis, and dementia. It is important to determine whether the bowel or bladder problem was present before the neurologic event to plan appropriate interventions.
- **Activity-exercise pattern:** Many neurologic disorders can cause problems in the patient's mobility, strength, and coordination. These problems can change the patient's usual activity and exercise patterns.
- **Sleep-rest pattern:** Sleep can be disrupted by many neurologically related factors. Discomfort from pain and inability to move and change to a position of comfort because of muscle weakness and paralysis could interfere with sound sleep.
- **Cognitive-perceptual pattern:** Because the nervous system controls cognition and sensory integration, many neuro-

logic disorders affect these functions. Assess memory, language, calculation ability, problem-solving ability, insight, and judgment.
- **Self-perception–self-concept pattern:** Neurologic disease can drastically alter control over one's life and create dependency on others for daily needs.
- **Role-relationship pattern:** Ask the patient if neurologic problems have led to changes in roles, such as spouse, parent, or breadwinner. These changes can dramatically affect both the patient and significant others.
- **Sexuality-reproductive pattern:** Assess the ability to participate in sexual activity, since many nervous system disorders can affect sexual response.
- **Coping–stress tolerance pattern:** The physical sequelae of a neurologic problem can seriously strain a patient's ability to cope. Often the problem is chronic and may require the patient to learn new coping skills.
- **Value-belief pattern:** Many neurologic problems have serious, long-term, life-changing effects. These effects can strain the patient's belief system and should be assessed

Data from Lewis, S.L., et al. *Medical-surgical nursing: Assessment and management of clinical problems.* (7th ed.). St. Louis: Mosby.

Patient Teaching

Teaching is an extremely important part of caring for the person with motor problems. Appropriate teaching activities include safety needs, skin care, activity (ROM and positioning), medications (dosage, action, times, and side effects), good nutrition, ADLs, bowel and bladder care, and follow-up care. Written instructions reinforce teaching and give the patient something to refer to at home (see Health Promotion box). Prepare family members to assume some of the care for the patient.

DISTURBED SENSORY AND PERCEPTUAL FUNCTION

Etiology and Pathophysiology

The presence of a lesion anywhere within the sensory system pathway, from the receptor to the sensory cortex, alters the transmission or perception of sensory information. The parietal cortex is of major importance in interpretation of sensation. Loss of, decrease in, or increase in sensation of pain, temperature, touch, and proprioception results in difficulty in daily functioning. Any alteration lessens the patient's protection from inadvertent injury.

One specific loss is proprioception, or the ability to know the position of the body and its parts without directly looking at the part. **Agnosia** is a total or partial loss of the ability to recognize familiar objects by sight, touch, or hearing or to recognize familiar people through sensory stimuli as a result of organic brain damage.

Assessment

Subjective data include the patient's understanding of the sensory disturbance, measures that relieve symptoms (including medications), and symptoms that occur with the sensory problem. An example is the person who experiences weakness of a hand and at the same time feels numbness and tingling. Collect information on the onset of the sensory problem and the specific site in the body.

Collection of **objective data** includes noting the patient's ability to perform purposeful movements or to recognize familiar objects.

Medical Management

Refer to medical management for alterations in the patient's muscle tone and motor function.

Nursing Interventions and Patient Teaching

The most important nursing intervention for the patient with sensory dysfunction is teaching the patient protective measures. This includes helping the patient learn to inspect parts of the body that have no feeling or protect sensitive body parts from the discomfort of linen rubbing over them. If a patient has a deficit in one sense, he or she should learn to compensate with another (e.g., the patient who learns to lip read because of a hearing deficit; the patient with hemianopia who is taught to scan the printed page).

A nursing diagnosis and interventions for the patient with a sensory or perceptual problem are the same as those for the patient with a motor problem, with the addition of but not limited to the following:

Nursing Diagnosis	Nursing Interventions
Risk for injury, related to sensory or perceptual disturbances	Maintain safe environment. Teach patient to protect body parts that have decreased sensation. Teach patient to inspect body parts for possible injury. Protect patient from sustaining injury from hot liquid or heating pads.

The teaching for a patient with a sensory deficit is essentially the same as that for the patient with a motor deficit.

OTHER DISORDERS OF THE NEUROLOGIC SYSTEM

Functioning of the neurologic system can be interrupted for a variety of reasons. These include conduction abnormalities, degenerative diseases, vascular problems, infection, tumors, trauma, and cranial and peripheral nerve disorders. Selected disorders in each area are discussed.

CONDUCTION ABNORMALITIES

EPILEPSY OR SEIZURES

Etiology and Pathophysiology

Epilepsy is a group of neurologic disorders characterized by recurrent episodes of convulsive seizure, sensory disturbances, abnormal behavior, LOC, or all of these.

Cases of epilepsy have been recorded throughout history. Seizures occur in all races and affect men and women equally. There is no apparent geographic distribution. In the United States it is estimated that approximately 2.7 million people suffer from active epilepsy, with 200,000 new cases being diagnosed each year (Epilepsy Foundation, 2009). The incidence rates are higher in the first year of life, decline through childhood and adolescence, plateau in middle age, and rise sharply again among older adults. The population within highest prevalence of new-onset epilepsy is those over the age of 60 (Tian et al., 2005).

Clinical Manifestations

Seizures can be classified according to the features of the attack. The types include generalized tonic-clonic (grand mal), absence (petit mal), psychomotor (automatisms), jacksonian (focal), and miscellaneous (myoclonic and akinetic) seizures (Table 14-6).

Epilepsy is associated with paroxysmal, uncontrolled electrical discharges in the neurons of the brain that re-

sult in the sudden, violent, involuntary contraction of a group of muscles. The patterns or forms of seizures vary and depend on the area of the brain from which the seizure arises (see Figure 14-7). Seizures occur for a variety of reasons, including cerebral trauma, intracranial infection, brain tumor, vascular disturbances, alcohol intoxication, hypoglycemia, electrolyte imbalance, barbiturate withdrawal, and water intoxication. Although many causes of seizure disorders have been identified, three fourths of all cases are considered idiopathic (without a known cause) (Lewis et al., 2007).

The excessive neuronal discharges may result in a tonic convulsion, with alternate contraction and relaxation of opposing muscle groups. This gives the characteristic tonic-clonic jerking movements of the body. Seizures are followed by a rest period of variable length, called the postictal period (after a seizure). During this period the patient usually feels groggy and acts disoriented. Complaints of headache and muscle aches are common. Usually the patient sleeps after a seizure and may experience amnesia for the event.

When recurrent, generalized seizure activity occurs at such frequency that full consciousness is not regained between seizures, it is called status epilepticus. This is a medical emergency and requires medical and nursing interventions. Repeated seizures cause the brain to use more energy than can be supplied; the neurons become exhausted and cease to function, which may result in permanent brain damage or death (Lewis et al., 2007). The nursing interventions always involve ensuring that there is a patent airway and protecting the patient from injury. Medications to stop the seizure activity may be given in high doses that render the patient unconscious. The nurse must then assume total care of the patient's needs. Insert a Foley catheter and an IV line. Intubate the patient if necessary for ventilatory support. Protect the skin from injury. Take care with safety reminder devices if the patient is awake and active so that they do not cause injury if the patient begins to have a seizure.

Assessment

Subjective data include the patient's awareness of the disorder and any precipitating factors. Assess whether an aura preceded the seizure. An aura occurs in about 50% of all patients with generalized tonic-clonic seizures. Aura is a sensation (such as of light or warmth) or emotion (such as fear) that may precede an attack of migraine or an epileptic seizure. An epileptic aura may be psychic, or it may be sensory with olfactory, visual, auditory, or taste hallucinations. The exact character of the aura varies from person to person. Awareness of an aura warns the person of the impending seizure and allows him or her to seek safety and privacy.

Objective data include the number of seizures occurring within a specific time, the character of the seizure, and any behaviors noted and injuries suffered.

Table 14-6   Characteristics of Seizures

INCIDENCE	CHARACTERISTICS	CLINICAL SIGNS	AURA	POSTICTAL PERIOD
GENERALIZED TONIC-CLONIC (FORMERLY KNOWN AS GRAND MAL)				
Most common	Generalized; characterized by loss of consciousness and falling to the floor or ground if patient is upright, followed by stiffening of the body (tonic phase) for 10-20 seconds and subsequent jerking of the extremities (clonic phase) for another 30-40 seconds	Aura Cry Loss of consciousness Fall Tonic-clonic movements Incontinence, cyanosis, excessive salivation, tongue or cheek biting	Yes Flashing lights Smells Spots before eyes (scotomata) Vertigo	Yes Need for 1-2 hours' sleep Headache, muscle soreness commonly felt May not feel normal for several hours or days after a seizure No memory of a seizure
ABSENCE (FORMERLY KNOWN AS PETIT MAL)				
Occurs during childhood and adolescence Frequency decreases as child gets older Rarely continues beyond adolescence	Sudden impairment in or loss of consciousness with little or no tonic-clonic movement Occurs without warning Has tendency to appear a few hours after arising or when person is quiet	Sudden vacant facial expression with eyes focused straight ahead (staring spell) that lasts only a few seconds All motor activity ceases except perhaps for slight symmetric twitching about eyelids Possible loss of muscle tone May have an extremely brief loss of consciousness	No	No
PSYCHOMOTOR (AUTOMATISMS; ALSO CALLED PARTIAL SEIZURES)				
Occur at any age	Sudden change in awareness associated with complex distortion of feeling and thinking and partially coordinated motor activity Longer than absence seizures	Behaves as if partially conscious; may continue an activity that was initiated before the seizure, such as counting out change or picking items from a grocery shelf, but after the seizure does not remember the activity Often appears intoxicated May do antisocial things, such as exposing self or carrying out violent acts Autonomic complaints, such as shivering, lip smacking, repetitive movements that may not be appropriate Urinary incontinence	Yes Complex hallucinations or illusions	Yes Confusion Amnesia Need for sleep
JACKSONIAN-FOCAL (LOCAL OR PARTIAL)				
Occur almost entirely in patients with structural brain disease	Depends on site of focus May or may not be progressive	Commonly begin in hand, foot, or face May end in tonic-clonic seizure	Yes Numbness Tingling Crawling feeling	Yes

Continued

Table 14-6	Characteristics of Seizures—cont'd				
INCIDENCE	**CHARACTERISTICS**	**CLINICAL SIGNS**	**AURA**	**POSTICTAL PERIOD**	
MYOCLONIC					
May antedate tonic-clonic by months or years	May be very mild or may have rapid, forceful movements	Sudden, excess jerk of the body or extremities; may be forceful enough to hurl the person to the floor or ground Brief seizures that may occur in clusters No loss of consciousness	No		
AKINETIC					
Not common	Peculiar generalized tonelessness	Falls in flaccid state Unconscious for minute or two	Rarely	No	

Describe the seizure as completely as possible, including duration, the patient's movements, whether the patient was incontinent, any cries or sounds that were made, and the level of alertness.

Diagnostic Test

The most common test used to evaluate seizures is the EEG (see Figure 14-7). It allows a specific diagnosis of the seizure.

Medical Management

Medications

In 70% of patients, seizure disorders are controlled by one or more antiseizure drugs (Table 14-7). Therapy is aimed at preventing seizures because cure is not possible. Drugs generally act by stabilizing nerve cell membranes and preventing spread of the epileptic discharge. The choice of medication depends on the type of seizure. Failure to take the prescribed medication or an adequate dose is often the cause of treatment failure. Blood levels may be checked to determine the therapeutic level of the medications taken. The primary goal of antiseizure drug therapy is to obtain maximum seizure control with minimum toxic side effects.

Surgical Therapy

Many patients with epilepsy are unable to control their seizures with medications and are candidates for surgical intervention. All types of epilepsy do not benefit from surgery. Three requirements must be met before surgical intervention can occur: (1) the diagnosis of epilepsy must be confirmed; (2) an adequate trial with drug therapy without therapeutic results must occur; and (3) the type of seizure disorder must be defined. Surgical treatments include removal of small areas of the hippocampus, anterior temporal lobe resection, and disconnective surgery incising through nerve pathways that allow the spread of the seizures. The benefits of surgery are the reduction or cessation of seizures (Lewis et al., 2007).

Activities of Daily Living

Until seizures are controlled, patients should avoid activities such as driving a car, operating machinery, or swimming. Maintaining adequate rest and good nutrition is also important. Alcohol use should be avoided. If the patient is receiving long-term phenytoin therapy, good hygiene practices for the mouth and teeth are important because of the side effect of edematous and enlarged gums (gingival hyperplasia). The patient should wear a medical-alert bracelet or tag (see Patient Teaching box).

Patient Teaching

The Patient with Seizures

* Explain the need for the patient to continue taking medications even when seizure activity has stopped.
* Teach the patient about medications prescribed, including expected results, time and dosage, and side effects.
* Inform the patient that medical-alert bracelets, necklaces, and identification cards are available. However, the use of these medical identification tags is optional. Some patients have found them beneficial, but others prefer not to be identified as having a seizure disorder.
* Caution the patient to avoid the use of alcohol if taking antiseizure medications.
* Explain the need for good oral hygiene for people taking phenytoin (Dilantin) (a side effect is gingival hyperplasia).
* Stress the importance of adequate rest and a balanced diet.
* Educate about available community resources.
* Explain restrictions concerning driving.
* Explain the importance of follow-up care.
* A tonic-clonic seizure can be treated with first aid; it is not necessary to send the patient to the hospital (or call an ambulance) after a single seizure unless the seizure is prolonged, another seizure immediately follows, or extensive injury has occurred.
* In the event of an acute seizure, protect the patient from injury. This involves supporting and/or protecting the head, turning the patient to one side, loosening any constricting garments, and, if the patient is seated, easing him or her onto the floor.

Table 14-7 Medications for Preventing and Controlling Seizures

Generic (Trade)	Use Related to Seizure Type	Toxic Effects
Phenytoin sodium (Dilantin)	Generalized tonic-clonic, focal, psychomotor	Ataxia, vomiting, nystagmus, drowsiness, rash, fever, gum hypertrophy, lymphadenopathy
Divalproex (Depakote)	Generalized tonic-clonic and myoclonic seizures	Sedation, drowsiness, behavior changes, visual disturbances, hepatic failure
Oxcarbazepine (Trileptal)	Generalized tonic-clonic and partial seizures	Feeling abnormal, headache, dizziness, vertigo, anxiety, burred vision
Phenobarbital (Luminal)	Generalized tonic-clonic, focal, psychomotor	Drowsiness, rash
Primidone (Mysoline)	Generalized tonic-clonic, focal, psychomotor	Drowsiness, ataxia
Ethosuximide (Zarontin)	Absence seizures, psychomotor, myoclonic, akinetic	Drowsiness, nausea, agranulocytosis
Trimethadione (Tridione)	Absence seizures	Rash, photophobia, agranulocytosis, nephrosis
Diazepam (Valium)	Generalized tonic-clonic and status epilepticus, mixed	Drowsiness, ataxia
Carbamazepine (Tegretol)	Generalized tonic-clonic, psychomotor	Rash, drowsiness, ataxia
Valproic acid (Depakene)	Absence seizures	Nausea, vomiting, indigestion, sedation, emotional disturbance, weakness, altered blood coagulation
Clonazepam (Klonopin)	Absence seizures, akinetic, myoclonic, generalized tonic-clonic seizures	Drowsiness, ataxia, hypotension, respiratory depression
Mephenytoin (Mesantoin)	Tonic-clonic, focal, psychomotor	Ataxia, nystagmus, pancytopenia, rash
Gabapentin (Neurontin)	Focal, generalized tonic-clonic in adults	Somnolence, fatigue, ataxia, dizziness, anorexia
Lamotrigine (Lamictal)	Focal, generalized tonic-clonic in adults	Rash, dizziness, tremor, ataxia, diplopia, headache, gastrointestinal upset, Stevens-Johnson syndrome (rare)
Felbamate (Felbatol)	Seizures in children, generalized tonic-clonic seizures in adults; may be used to treat patients whose seizure disorders are refractory to other drugs	Irritability, insomnia, anorexia, nausea, headache; can cause aplastic anemia and hepatic failure
Fosphenytoin sodium (Cerebyx)	Short-term parenteral (IV or IM) in acute generalized tonic-clonic seizures; used for status epilepticus and for preventing and treating seizures during neurosurgery	Dizziness, paresthesia, tinnitus, pruritus, headache, somnolence, ataxia, muscular incoordination, nystagmus, double vision, slurred speech, nausea, vomiting, and hypotension
Topiramate (Topamax), tiagabine (Gabitril), levetiracetam (Keppra), zonisamide (Zonegran)	Indicated for partial seizures and for secondary generalized seizures; currently used as adjunctive therapy	Topiramate: somnolence, dizziness, ataxia, speech disorders and related speech problems, difficulty with memory, paresthesia, diplopia; tiagabine: dizziness, lightheadedness, asthenia (lack of energy), somnolence, nausea, nervousness, irritability, tremor, thinking abnormally, difficulty with concentration or attention

Nursing Interventions and Patient Teaching
Care during a Seizure

The primary goals of the nurse and the family caring for a patient having a seizure are protection from aspiration and injury and observation and recording of the seizure activity. Never leave the patient alone. If the patient is sitting or standing, lower him or her to the floor in an area away from furniture and equipment. Support and protect the head; if possible, turn the head to the side to maintain the airway. If there is time, loosen clothing around the neck. Do not try to restrain the patient during the seizure. Do *not* try to pry open the jaw to place a padded tongue blade. No objects should be placed in the mouth. After the seizure the patient may require suctioning and oxygen. Padded side rails may be used, especially if seizures often occur during sleep.

When a seizure occurs, carefully observe and record details of the event because the diagnosis and subsequent treatment often rest solely on the seizure description. Note all aspects of the seizure: What events preceded the seizure? When did the seizure occur? How long did each phase (aural [if any], ictal, postictal) last? What occurred during each phase?

Nursing diagnoses and interventions for the patient with seizures may include but are not limited to the following:

Nursing Diagnoses	Nursing Interventions
Ineffective airway clearance, related to mucus accumulation in oropharyngeal area during seizure	Place patient in side-lying position to prevent aspiration and ensure airway patency. Suction secretions as needed.
Risk for injury, related to rapid onset of altered state of consciousness and seizure activity	If patient is out of bed during seizure activity, assist to the floor and remove objects that may harm him or her. Provide privacy. Maintain patent airway. After the seizure, inform patient of seizure and reorient if necessary.

Prognosis

Seizure disorders can affect a patient's emotional, economic, and social well-being. Society's attitude has improved, but epilepsy still carries a social stigma. Most states have legal sanctions against driving if one has epilepsy. The inability to maintain a driver's license can negatively affect one's lifestyle (Lewis et al., 2007).

The majority of patients with seizures are able to control them with medications and can lead a fairly normal life. With most seizure disorders, the number and intensity of seizures stay constant. However, in patients who experience a first seizure as a result of a brain tumor or another brain pathologic condition, the prognosis is more uncertain.

DEGENERATIVE DISEASES

The term **degenerative diseases** refers to neurologic disorders in which there is a premature aging of nerve cells, which is caused by suspected metabolic disturbance or for which the cause is unknown. Six diseases are discussed: multiple sclerosis (MS), Parkinson's disease, Alzheimer's disease (AD), myasthenia gravis (MG), amyotrophic lateral sclerosis (ALS), and Huntington's disease.

MULTIPLE SCLEROSIS

Etiology and Pathophysiology

MS is a chronic, progressive, degenerative neurologic disease that affects many people. The cause is unknown, although genetics have been implicated, since there is a higher rate of the disease among relatives. Patients with the first signs and symptoms of MS have a proliferation of a certain type of immune cell called **gamma delta T cells** in their spinal fluid. These cells are not found in patients who have had the disease for a long time. T cells, the "field commanders" of the immune system, usually defend the body from outside attackers. In MS, however, something goes wrong and induces the T cells to attack the body. Myelin damage occurs. The beginning mechanism may be a viral infection early in life that becomes apparent as an immune process later in life. A defective immune response also seems to have an important role in the pathology of MS.

The onset of signs and symptoms is usually between 15 and 50 years of age. Women are affected more often than men. The highest number of people with MS live in the Great Lakes area, the Pacific Northwest, and the North Atlantic states. MS is five times more prevalent in temperate climates between 45 and 66 degrees of latitude.

Multiple foci of **demyelination** are distributed randomly in the white matter of the brainstem, the spinal cord, optic nerves, and the cerebrum. During the demyelination process, the myelin sheath and the sheath cells are destroyed, causing an interruption or distortion of the nerve impulse so that it is slowed or blocked (Figure 14-13). Areas of degeneration show evidence of partial healing, which explains the transitory nature of early signs and symptoms.

Clinical Manifestations

The onset is often insidious and gradual, with vague symptoms that occur intermittently over months or years, thus the disease may not be diagnosed until long after the onset of the first symptom. Because of the wide distribution of areas of degeneration, the variety of signs and symptoms in MS is greater than in other neurologic diseases. These include visual problems, urinary incontinence, fatigue, weakness or incoordination of an extremity, sexual problems such as impotence in men, and swallowing difficulties. The majority of people have early remissions that may last for a year or more. The disease is characterized by chronic, progressive deterioration in some persons and by remissions and exacerbations in others. Exacerbations may be related to fatigue, chilling, or emotional disturbances. With repeated exacerbations, progressive scarring of the myelin sheath occurs, and the overall trend is progressive deterioration in neurologic function.

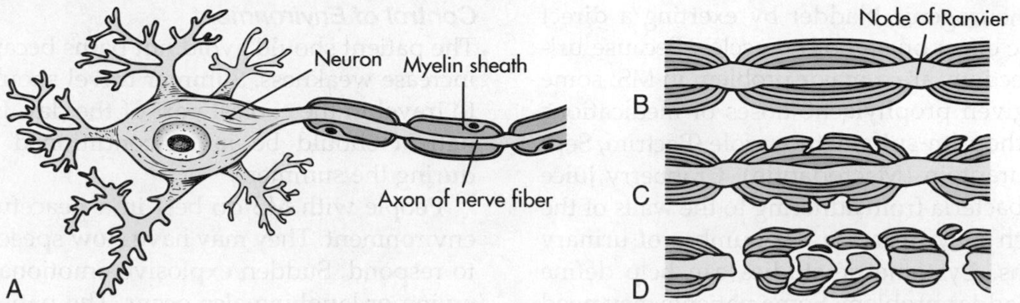

FIGURE 14-13 Pathogenesis of multiple sclerosis. **A,** Normal nerve cell with myelin sheath. **B,** Normal axon. **C,** Myelin breakdown. **D,** Myelin totally disrupted; axon not functioning.

Assessment

Subjective data include the patient's understanding of the disease. Eye problems such as diplopia, scotomata (spots before the eyes), and blindness may be present. The patient may also talk about weakness or numbness of a part of the body, fatigue, emotional instability, bowel and bladder problems, vertigo, or loss of joint sensation. Involvement of the cerebellum can result in ataxia (impaired ability to coordinate movement) and tremor. In men, impotence is significant. Pain is not a common symptom.

Objective data include documented abnormalities in neurologic testing; these may include nystagmus (involuntary, rhythmic movements of the eye; the oscillations may be horizontal, vertical, rotary, or mixed); muscle weakness and spasms; changes in coordination; or a spastic, ataxic gait. Cerebellar signs include ataxia, dysarthria, and dysphagia. There may be evidence of behavior changes such as euphoria, emotional lability, or mild depression. Urinary incontinence and intention tremors of the upper extremities may be present.

Diagnostic Tests

MS has no definitive diagnostic test; diagnosis is based primarily on history and clinical manifestations and the presence of multiple lesions over time as measured by MRI. Examination of the CSF in patients with MS may show elevated gamma globulin, a proliferation of gamma delta T cells in the initial phase, and increased number of lymphocytes and monocytes. A CT scan may show enlargement of the cerebral ventricles. MRI scanning has been helpful in diagnosing MS over time in the presence of multiple lesions; sclerotic plaques as small as 3 to 4 mm in diameter can be detected.

Medical Management
Medications

No specific treatment exists for MS, although many different remedies have been tried. Symptoms are controlled with the use of adrenocorticotropic hormone (ACTH) and corticosteroids such as prednisone (Deltasone) or dexamethasone. These may be given orally, intramuscularly, or intravenously. The effects of ACTH and the steroids on the demyelinating process are unknown, although they probably help by reducing edema and acute inflammation at the site of demyelination. If steroids are used in high doses at the start of an exacerbation, the episode seems to resolve more rapidly. However, these drugs do not affect the ultimate outcome or degree of residual neurologic impairment from the exacerbation. If spasticity is a problem, drugs such as diazepam, dantrolene, and baclofen may help prevent or decrease the spasms. Immunomodulating drugs modify the disease process. Interferon beta-1b (Betaseron), given subcutaneously every other day, is indicated for use in ambulatory patients with relapsing-remitting MS to reduce the frequency of clinical exacerbations. Interferon beta-1a (Avonex) is similar to interferon B-1b in efficacy and is used in similar patient groups with MS. It is given intramuscularly once a week. Interferon beta-1a (Rebif) is administered subcutaneously three times weekly. A new immunomodulator is glatiramer acetate (Copaxone), approved for use in relapsing-remitting MS. Glatiramer is not an interferon, but it is believed to help MS patients by interrupting the inflammatory cycle and preventing the body's immune system from attacking the myelin coating that protects the nerve fiber. It is given subcutaneously daily. Mitoxantrone (Novantrone) is a drug for the treatment of primary-progressive and progressive-relapsing MS. It is an immunosuppressant drug that reduces both B and T lymphocytes. It is given intravenously monthly. Because of cardiac toxicity, it cannot be used for more than 2 to 3 years (Lewis et al., 2007). Many research studies are being conducted in the search for more effective medications to use in the treatment of MS.

Elimination

Urinary frequency and urgency may respond to propantheline (Pro-Banthine). Cholinergic drugs such as bethanechol (Urecholine) can sometimes help the patient with a neurogenic bladder by exerting a direct antispasmodic effect on smooth muscles. Because urinary tract infections are a major problem in MS, some patients are given prophylactic doses of medications such as trimethoprim-sulfamethoxazole (Bactrim, Septra) or nitrofurantoin (Macrodantin). Cranberry juice may prevent bacteria from adhering to the walls of the bladder, which may decrease the number of urinary tract infections. Cystometric studies can help define the specific bladder problem. Some patients may need to be taught self-catheterization.

Encourage the patient to drink adequate fluids (at least 2000 mL/day). If the patient suffers from constipation, a stool softener such as docusate sodium (Colace) may be used, as well as prune juice.

Nursing Interventions
Nutrition
A well-balanced diet with high-fiber foods and adequate fluids is important. Although there is no standard prescribed diet, a high-protein diet with supplemental vitamins is often recommended. Obesity makes it more difficult for the patient to meet daily needs and maintain mobility. The patient who is obese should be referred to the dietitian and be placed on a calorie-restricted diet that will help the patient lose weight slowly, while receiving adequate nutrition.

Skin Care
Teach the patient with MS and/or the caregiver frequent turning to avoid skin impairment. Devices to relieve pressure, such as eggcrate or air mattresses, may be helpful. Because of sensory involvement, the patient may not feel discomfort that signals the need to change position.

Activity
Encourage patients with MS to exercise regularly, but not to the point of fatigue. Physical therapy sometimes improves neurologic dysfunction. Exercise also helps daily functioning for patients with MS not experiencing an exacerbation. Exercise decreases spasticity, increases coordination, and retrains unaffected muscles to substitute for impaired ones (Rietberg et al., 2005). Water exercise is an especially beneficial type of physical therapy. Because of the buoyancy water gives to the body, the patient has more control over the body and is able to perform activities that would be impossible on land (Lewis et al., 2007).

Daily rest periods may be helpful. During an acute exacerbation, patients are often kept as quiet as possible; this includes bed rest.

One side of the body is often more affected than the other. The patient must learn to stabilize the gait by leaning toward the less-involved side. If the foot slaps forward while the patient is walking, teach him or her to put the foot down in a pronounced fashion and roll the weight forward on the side of the foot.

Control of Environment
The patient should avoid hot baths because they often increase weakness. Summer travel should be planned to travel in the coolest part of the day. If possible, the patient should be in air-conditioned surroundings during the summer.

People with MS do best in a peaceful and relaxed environment. They may have slow speech and be slow to respond. Sudden explosive emotional outbursts of crying or laughing also occur. The patient and family need support in dealing with this behavior.

Nursing diagnoses and interventions for the patient with MS may include but are not limited to the following:

Nursing Diagnoses	Nursing Interventions
Risk for powerlessness, related to physical limitations imposed by progressive physical deterioration, loss of body control, and threat to physical integrity	Provide emotional support, thorough explanations, and reassurance. Be alert to emotional changes and mood swings. Encourage the patient's participation and expression of needs and feelings. Maintain planned rest periods. Encourage self-care as indicated. Provide physical care as indicated.
Bathing/hygiene, feeding, toileting self-care deficit, related to limitations in physical mobility imposed by disease process	Administer oral hygiene before meals. Assist with or provide physical hygiene as indicated by physical ability. Maintain appropriate bathing temperatures. Administer oral hygiene every 4 hours and as needed. Catheterize intermittently as indicated; teach self-catheterization when possible. Plan bladder dysfunction program as appropriate for spasticity or flaccidity. Institute bowel control program (establish regular bowel routine, avoid constipation). Assist in dressing and grooming as indicated. Provide nutritious, attractive meals.

Patient Teaching

Teaching is important for both the patient with MS and significant others. In late stages of the disease, the care functions usually are assumed by someone other than the patient. Important points include those for the patient with motor and sensory problems (see pp. 672-676). In addition, stress the importance of spacing activities and avoiding temperature extremes and the potential for emotional lability. Make certain that the patient or the family has the address of the nearest MS society or support group.

Prognosis

The prognosis is variable. Some patients have MS for many years with few deficits, whereas other patients quickly become debilitated. The patient's ability to conserve energy and avoid stress may help prevent exacerbations. Exacerbations are treated and may resolve. The average life expectancy after the onset of symptoms is more than 25 years.

PARKINSON'S DISEASE

Etiology and Pathophysiology

Parkinsonism is a syndrome that consists of a slowing down in the initiation and execution of movement (bradykinesia), increased muscle tone (rigidity), tremor, and impaired postural reflexes. Parkinson's disease, a form of parkinsonism, is named after James Parkinson, who, in 1817, wrote a classic essay on "shaking palsy," a disease whose cause is still unknown today. Many other disorders resemble this disease, but their causes are known. These include drug-induced parkinsonism, postencephalitic parkinsonism, and arteriosclerotic parkinsonism. The pathophysiology of these disorders, with the exception of drug-induced parkinsonism, is the same. Damage or loss of the dopamine-producing cells of the substantia nigra in the midbrain leads to depletion, in the basal ganglia, of dopamine that influences the initiation, modulation, and completion of movement and regulates unconscious autonomic movements. In cases of drug-induced parkinsonism, the dopamine receptors in the brain are blocked.

According to the American Parkinson Disease Association, Parkinson's disease affects more than 1 million people in the United States. Symptoms commonly occur after 50 years of age. Peak onset of Parkinson's disease is in the 60s. The average age of the patient with Parkinson's disease is 65 years. There is apparent genetic cause and no known cure. The disease rarely occurs in blacks. Parkinson's disease is more common in men by a ratio of 3:2.

Parkinsonism has many causes. Encephalitis lethargica, or type A encephalitis, has been clearly associated with the onset of parkinsonism. However, the incidence of postencephalitic parkinsonism has dwindled since the 1920s, when there was a large outbreak of this infectious illness. Parkinsonian-like symptoms have occurred after intoxication with a

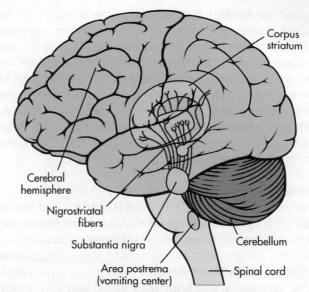

FIGURE 14-14 Nigrostriatal disorders produce parkinsonism. Left-sided view of the human brain showing the substantia nigra and the corpus striatum *(shaded area)* lying deep within the cerebral hemisphere. Nerve fibers extend upward from the substantia nigra, divide into many branches, and carry dopamine to all regions of the corpus striatum.

variety of chemicals, including carbon monoxide and manganese (among copper miners) and a product of meperidine-analog synthesis. Drug-induced parkinsonism can follow therapy with reserpine (Hydropres), methyldopa (Aldomet), haloperidol (Haldol), and phenothiazine (Thorazine).

Although patients with cerebrovascular disease may have parkinsonian-like symptoms, there is little evidence that parkinsonism is caused by arteriosclerosis. Distinguishing arteriosclerosis from true Parkinson's disease is important for prognostic purposes. Patients with arteriosclerosis do not respond as well to treatment and are more likely to experience side effects of drug therapy. Most patients with parkinsonism have the degenerative or idiopathic form, for which the term *Parkinson's disease* is usually reserved.

Other factors linked to Parkinson's disease include reduced estrogen levels and exposure to pesticides, herbicides, industrial chemicals, and metals (mercury, copper, and manganese). Menopausal women who have not received hormone therapy are at risk (McCarron, 2006).

The pathology of Parkinson's disease is associated with the degeneration of the dopamine-producing neurons in the substantia nigra of the midbrain, which in turn disrupts the normal balance between dopamine and acetylcholine in the basal ganglia (Figure 14-14). Major signs and symptoms, such as tremors, muscle rigidity, slowed movements, and impaired balance and coordination, occur when approximately 60% to 80% of dopamine-producing cells have been destroyed. It is believed that there is normally a balance between acetylcholine and dopamine in the basal ganglia. Any shift in the balance of activity (an increase in acetylcholine or a decrease in dopamine) seems to lead to parkinson-like symptoms. Dopamine is a neurotransmitter that is essential for normal functioning of the extrapyramidal motor system, including control of posture, support, and voluntary motion. In Parkinson's disease the levels of dopamine-synthesizing enzymes and metabolites are reduced, and postmortem analysis of cross-sections of the midbrain shows loss of the normal melanin pigment in the substantia nigra and loss of neurons. In addition, deficient amounts of gamma-aminobutyric acid, serotonin, and norepinephrine have been found in basal ganglia and in the substantia nigra.

Clinical Manifestations

The onset of Parkinson's disease is gradual and insidious, with a gradual progression and a prolonged course. In the beginning stages, only a mild tremor, handwriting changes, a slight limp, or a decreased arm swing may be evident. Later in the disease the patient may have a shuffling, propulsive gait with arms flexed and loss of postural reflexes (Figure 14-15). Some patients may have a slight change in speech patterns. None of these alone is sufficient evidence for a diagnosis of the disease.

Because Parkinson's disease has no specific diagnostic test, the diagnosis is based solely on the history, a thorough neurologic examination, and clinical features. A firm diagnosis can be made only when the patient has at least two signs of the classic triad: tremor, rigidity, and bradykinesia (slow or retarded movement). In the early stage of the disease there are subtle changes in cognitive function that can progress to dementia. The ultimate confirmation of Parkinson's disease is a positive response to a low-dose trial of an antiparkinsonian medication, such as carbidopa-levodopa (Sinemet).

Tremor

Tremor, often the first sign, may be minimal initially, so the patient is the only one who notices it. This tremor can affect handwriting, causing it to trail off, particularly toward the ends of words. Parkinsonian tremor is more prominent at rest but disappears when the patient moves; it is aggravated by emotional stress or increased concentration. The hand tremor is described as "pill rolling" because the thumb and forefinger appear to move in a rotary fashion, as if rolling a pill, coin, or other small object. Tremor can involve the hands, diaphragm, tongue, lips, and jaw but rarely causes shaking of the head. Eventually tremors can become so pronounced that the patient cannot hold a newspaper steady enough to read or make a call on a push-button telephone. Unfortunately, in many people a benign essential tremor has mistakenly been diagnosed as Parkinson's disease. Essential tremor occurs during voluntary movement, has a more rapid frequency than parkinsonian tremor, and is often familial.

Rigidity

Rigidity, the second sign of the triad, is the increased resistance to passive motion when the limbs are moved through their range of motion. Parkinsonian rigidity is typified by a jerky quality when the joint is moved, like

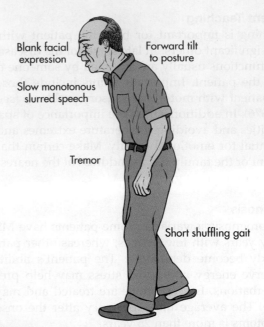

Blank facial expression

Forward tilt to posture

Slow monotonous slurred speech

Tremor

Short shuffling gait

FIGURE 14-15 Characteristic appearance of a patient with Parkinson's disease.

intermittent catches in the movement of a cogwheel. This is termed *cogwheel rigidity*. The rigidity is caused by sustained muscle contraction and consequently elicits a complaint of muscle soreness; fatigue and achiness; or pain in the head, the upper body, the spine, or the legs. Another consequence of rigidity is slowness of movement, since it inhibits the alternating contraction and relaxation of opposing muscle groups (e.g., the biceps and triceps). Simple movements such as tying shoes and rising from a chair become a challenge.

Bradykinesia

Bradykinesia is particularly evident in the loss of automatic movements, which is secondary to physical and chemical alteration of the basal ganglia and related structures in the extrapyramidal portion of the CNS. In the unaffected patient, automatic movements are involuntary and occur subconsciously. They include blinking the eyelids, swinging the arms while walking, swallowing saliva, expressing oneself with facial and hand movements, and making minor postural adjustment. The patient with Parkinson's disease does not execute these movements and lacks spontaneous activity. This accounts for the stooped posture, masked face (deadpan expression), drooling, and shuffling gait (festination) that are characteristic of a person with this disease (see Figure 14-15). The voice softens and loses modulation too, further contributing to communication problems. One may see evidence of bradykinesia in the patient's handwriting. The words become tiny and different from earlier handwriting samples. This is referred to as micrographia (McCarron, 2006). The patient often has a shuffling, propulsive gait that he or she is unable to stop until meeting an obstruction. In addition, there is difficulty initiating movement. Movements such as getting out of a chair cannot be executed unless they are consciously willed.

Assessment

Parkinson's disease starts with subtle symptoms and progresses slowly. **Subjective data** include fatigue, incoordination, judgment defects, emotional instability, anxiety, depression, and heat intolerance. Assess the patient's understanding of the disease.

Objective data include tremor, which is the outstanding sign of the disease. This has been described as a pill-rolling motion of the fingers or a resting tremor. Bradykinesia is present with rigidity and loss of postural reflexes. Muscle rigidity leads to a masklike appearance of the face; slowed, monotonous speech; and drooling. Dysphagia, or difficulty swallowing, is a common late complication of neurologic degeneration, which poses the risk of choking and aspiration pneumonia. The patient may be constipated. There may be a scaly, erythematous rash, particularly near the ears and eyebrows and in the scalp and nasolabial folds. Moist, oily skin is usually noted. Postural hypotension is prevalent and may be caused by failure of the arterial baroreceptors located in the aortic arch and the internal carotid arteries (McCarron, 2006).

Diagnostic Tests

Parkinson's disease has no firm diagnostic tests. If there is a history of chronic dementia, the CT scan may show cerebral atrophy. The EEG may show minimal slowing, and the upper gastrointestinal evaluation may show decreased motility.

Medical Management
Medications

Treatment for Parkinson's disease is based on easing the signs and symptoms of the disease. Several different drugs have had a dramatic effect on the course of the disease: trihexyphenidyl hydrochloride (Artane), benztropine mesylate (Cogentin), levodopa (Dopar) (the most commonly prescribed medication for Parkinson's disease), amantadine hydrochloride (Symmetrel), carbidopa-levodopa (for 35 years, the gold standard of therapy), selegiline hydrochloride (Eldepryl), ropinirole (Requip), tolcapone (Tasmar), pramipexole (Mirapex), pergolide (Permax), rasagiline (Azilect), and rotigotine (Neupro).

After prolonged treatment with some of the drugs, side effects such as dyskinesia (abnormal involuntary movements) may occur and the medication's effectiveness may decrease. Hospitalization may be helpful, during which time all drugs are withdrawn for a time. This is called a **drug holiday**. The medications are then restarted, and often smaller doses produce favorable results. Complications such as aspiration can occur during this time because withdrawal of the drugs causes immobility and rigidity (Table 14-8). To combat these problems, newer drug classes have been developed.

Surgery

Surgery that involves destroying portions of the brain that control the rigidity or tremor—so-called ablation surgery—has been used for Parkinson's disease for more than 50 years. However, it has been replaced by deep brain stimulation (DBS). DBS involves placing an electrode in either the thalamus, globus pallidus, or subthalamic nucleus and connecting it to a generator placed in the upper chest (like a pacemaker). The device is programmed to deliver a specific current to the targeted brain location. DBS can be adjusted to control symptoms and is reversible (the device can be removed). The procedure is nonablative and relatively safe and can improve dyskinesias (an impairment of the ability to execute voluntary movements), gait, rigidity, and tremors. This procedure is often reserved for patients who have developed severe side effects to drug therapy or severe motor complications.

Medications are discontinued several days preoperatively so that signs and symptoms will be at their maximum at the time of surgery.

Another treatment approach for Parkinson's disease involves human fetal dopamine cell transplants into the basal ganglia in an attempt to provide viable dopamine-producing cells to the brain.

Nursing Interventions
Activity Needs

Pay special attention to posture. Lying on a firm bed without a pillow may help prevent the spine from bending forward. Holding the hands folded behind the back when walking may help keep the spine erect and prevent the arms from falling stiffly at the sides. Problems secondary to bradykinesia can be alleviated by relatively simple measures. Advise patients who tend to "freeze" while walking to consciously think about stepping over imaginary or real lines on floor, drop rice kernels and step over them, rock from side to side, lift the toes when stepping, and take one step backward and two steps forward. A patient who has difficulty rising from a sitting position can use a chair that gently propels him or her to an upright position (McCarron, 2006). Do not hurry the patient because it will make the bradykinesia worse.

Nutrition

Diet is of major importance to the patient with Parkinson's disease to avoid malnutrition and constipation. Patients with dysphagia and bradykinesia need appetizing foods that can be easily chewed and swallowed. Food should be cut into bite-sized pieces before it is served. Eating six small meals a day may be less exhausting than eating three large meals. Allow ample time for eating to avoid frustration and encourage independence. When the disease is advanced, aspiration is a real concern. Take care during feeding. Unless the disease is well controlled by medication, drooling can be a problem and increases with general excitement.

Table 14-8 Medications for Disorders of the Neurologic System

Generic (Trade)	Action	Side Effects	Nursing Implications
Amantadine hydrochloride (Symmetrel)	Treats some cases of Parkinson's disease and drug-induced extrapyramidal reactions, although its action in treatment of Parkinson's disease is unknown	Nausea, vomiting, vision changes, dysrhythmias, disorientation, orthostatic hypotension, depression, fatigue	Tell patient to drink no alcohol; administer no CNS depressants; know pregnancy cautions; tell patient not to cease taking medication without conferring with physician and not to deviate from prescribed dosage; for best absorption, instruct patient to take after meals; if orthostatic hypotension occurs, instruct patient not to stand or change positions too quickly.
Baclofen (Lioresal)	Reduces transmission of impulses from spinal cord to skeletal muscles; is antispasticity agent for treatment of spinal spasticity resulting from multiple sclerosis or spinal cord injury	Drowsiness, dizziness, disorientation, lightheadedness, hypotension, urinary frequency, possible increase in blood glucose level	Be aware of pregnancy cautions; give oral form with meals or milk to prevent gastrointestinal distress; watch for increased incidence of seizures in patients with epilepsy; tell patient to avoid activities that require alertness until CNS effects of drugs are known.
Trihexyphenidyl hydrochloride (Artane)	Blocks central cholinergic receptors, helping to balance cholinergic activity of basal ganglia; is antidyskinetic and antiparkinsonian; controls some mild cases as an adjunct to more potent drugs; controls extrapyramidal reactions caused by drugs	Skin rash, eye pain, nervousness, headaches, tachycardia, urinary hesitancy, urine retention, dry mouth, disorientation	Do not give antacids or antidiarrheal agents within 1 hour of giving medication; give with food; caution patient to rise slowly; use cautiously in patients with narrow-angle glaucoma and hypertension; warn patient to avoid activities that require alertness until CNS effects of drugs are known; tell patient to relieve dry mouth with cool drinks, ice chips, and hard candy.
Pyridostigmine bromide (Mestinon)	Inhibits destruction of acetylcholine released from parasympathetic and somatic efferent nerves; causes acetylcholine to accumulate, promoting increased stimulation of receptor; is used in myasthenia gravis and by the oral route for senility associated with Alzheimer's disease	Headache, seizures, bradycardia, hypotension, bronchospasm, increased bronchial secretions	Judging optimum dosage is difficult; monitor and document patient's response after each dose when using for myasthenia gravis; stress importance of taking drug exactly as ordered, on time, and in evenly spaced doses.
Benztropine mesylate (Cogentin)	Blocks central cholinergic receptors, helping to balance cholinergic activity in basal ganglia; is indicated in treatment of mild cases of Parkinson's disease and control of extrapyramidal reactions	Dizziness, drowsiness, depression, orthostatic hypotension, palpitation, tachycardia	Stress importance of following prescribed dosage; discontinue drug slowly; tell patient not to drink alcohol; advise patient of breast-feeding warnings; give with food; tell patient to rise slowly and notify physician of severe allergic reactions; do not give with antacids.
Tacrine hydrochloride (Cognex)	Acts as reversible cholinesterase inhibitor, used for treatment of mild to moderate dementia of Alzheimer's type	Bradycardia, nausea and vomiting, loose stools, ataxia, CNS disturbance, anorexia, agitation, increased serum transaminase levels, jaundice	Know risk of ulcers; monitor liver enzyme weekly for first 18 weeks; increase dosage at 6-week intervals; do not use NSAIDs concomitantly; be aware that it potentiates theophylline.

CNS, Central nervous system; *I&O,* intake and output; *NSAIDs,* nonsteroidal antiinflammatory drugs.

Table 14-8	Medications for Disorders of the Neurologic System—cont'd		
Generic (Trade)	**Action**	**Side Effects**	**Nursing Implications**
Levodopa (Dopar, Larodopa)	Antiparkinsonian agent (mechanism of action is unknown); increases balance between cholinergic and dopaminergic activity to allow more normal body movements and alleviate signs and symptoms	Aggressive behavior, involuntary grimacing, head and body movements, depression, suicidal tendencies, orthostatic hypotension, nausea, vomiting, darkened urine, excessive and inappropriate sexual behavior	Do not give to patients with narrow-angle glaucoma; monitor patients receiving antihypertensive and hypoglycemic agents; advise patient to change positions slowly and dangle legs; protect drug from heat, light, moisture.
Carbidopa-levodopa (Sinemet)	Increases levels of dopamine and levodopamine; is antiparkinsonian agent; improves modulation of voluntary nerve impulses transmitted to the motor cortex (lower dosage is needed than with single-dose therapy; efficiency may increase 75% when carbidopa and levodopa are used in combination)	Mental depression, mental changes, nausea and vomiting, orthostatic hypotension, dizziness, uncontrollable body movements	Give with food; give only as directed; effectiveness may take months; warn patient of breastfeeding and pregnancy cautions; caution patient about drowsiness and getting up too fast; lying down may affect control of blood glucose and darken urine.
Selegiline hydrochloride (Eldepryl)	Monoamine oxidase (MAO) inhibitor used as treatment adjunct to levodopa and carbidopa-levodopa; may slow Parkinson's disease and need for increased medication; may prolong life span of people with Parkinson's disease	Severe orthostatic hypotension, increased tremors, chorea, restlessness, grimacing, nausea and vomiting, slow urination, increased sweating, alopecia	Advise patient not to take more than 10 mg/day (there is no evidence that a greater amount improves effectiveness and it may increase adverse reactions); warn patient not to drink alcohol and drink only a little coffee; give with food; tell patient to rise slowly and notify physician of side effects; tell patient not to take over-the-counter cold remedies; monitor blood pressure and respirations.
Donepezil (Aricept)	Improves cholinergic function by inhibiting acetylcholinesterase; anti-Alzheimer's agent; may temporarily lessen some of the dementia associated with Alzheimer's disease, but does not alter the course	Diarrhea, nausea, vomiting, fatigue, headache, ecchymoses, atrial fibrillation, vasodilation	Monitor heart rate (may cause bradycardia); assess cognitive function periodically during therapy; administer in the evening just before bed; may be taken without regard for food.
Memantine (Namenda)	Believed to act as an *N*-methyl-D-aspartate receptor antagonist to decrease glutamate, which is an excitatory neurotransmitter in the CNS; approved for the treatment of moderate to severe Alzheimer's disease; does not prevent or slow neurodegeneration, but found in clinical studies to slow symptom progression	Dizziness, headache, constipation, hypertension, urinary frequency	Monitor I&O; Do not give to patients with severe renal impairment; use cautiously in those with moderate renal impairment; be aware that conditions that increase urine pH, including severe urinary tract infections, lead to decreased excretion and increased serum levels.

When patients are dressed, garments with generous pockets for an ample supply of tissues will help them to be less conspicuous.

Elimination

The patient with Parkinson's disease may feel urgency and hesitancy in voiding. Measures appropriate for the patient with MS also apply to these patients. Chronic constipation may be a real concern. The patient should be on a diet high in fiber and roughage for bulk. Encourage oral fluid intake, and use stool softeners, suppositories, and prune juice if necessary. Mild cathartics such as milk of magnesia are used if required.

Nursing diagnoses and interventions for the patient with Parkinson's disease are the same as those for the patient with MS, with the addition of but not limited to the following:

Nursing Diagnoses	Nursing Interventions
Impaired physical mobility, related to: • rigidity • bradykinesia • akinesia	Assist with ambulation to assess degree of impairment and to prevent injury. Perform active ROM exercises to all extremities to maintain joint ROM, prevent atrophy, and strengthen muscles. Consult physical therapist or occupational therapist for aids to facilitate ADLs and safe ambulation. Teach techniques to assist with mobility by instructing patient to step over imaginary line and rock from side to side to initiate leg movements; these techniques help deal with "freezing" (akinesia) while walking.
Risk for aspiration, related to disease process	Ensure that, when eating, the patient sits at 90-degree angle with head up and chin slightly tucked, avoiding extending the head. Provide soft-solid and thick-liquid diet because these consistencies are more easily swallowed. Consult a speech therapist and a dietitian because they can provide specific plans to improve swallowing. Encourage patient to take small bites. Avoid use of straws.

Patient Teaching

Education for the patient with Parkinson's disease should include the importance of taking medications on the prescribed time schedule. Stress the need for good skin care and keeping active so that the patient remains as mobile as possible. Demonstrate proper ambulation and positioning to the patient and to the family if they will be taking care of the patient. Also teach proper feeding techniques to reduce the risk of aspiration (see Nursing Diagnoses box).

Prognosis

There is no cure for Parkinson's disease. Parkinson's disease is a chronic degenerative disorder with no acute exacerbations. If the patient takes medication as prescribed, signs and symptoms can be controlled for a long period.

Most patients with Parkinson's disease have their needs provided for by family caregivers (e.g., spouse, children). The burden of caregiving increases as the disease progresses. Many caregivers, especially if they are older adults, suffer from deteriorating physical and mental health. Eventually long-term care is often required for the patient with Parkinson's disease (Lewis et al., 2007).

ALZHEIMER'S DISEASE

Etiology and Pathophysiology

AD is a chronic, progressive, degenerative disorder that affects the cells of the brain and causes impaired intellectual functioning. It is a common cause of dementia in the older person and affects men and women in equal numbers. Approximately 4.5 million Americans suffer from AD. It is estimated that 5% of people older than 65 and 50% of those older than age 85 have AD. Alzheimer's may strike people in their 40s and 50s. The cause is unknown, although research has shown a genetic link.

The changes in the brain of patients with AD include plaques in the cortex, neurofibrillary tangles (a tangled mass of nonfunctioning neurons), and loss of connections between cells and cell death (Figure 14-16). This neuronal damage occurs primarily in the cerebral cortex and causes a decrease in brain size. These changes were first discovered in 1907 by the German neurologist Alois Alzheimer.

Homocysteine is a simple amino acid. Research is presenting evidence that, in older adults, elevated plasma levels of homocysteine are associated with a significantly increased risk for AD or another type of dementia. Put in practical terms, the investigators observed that a 5-mmol increment in the plasma homocysteine level increased the risk of AD by 40% (Seshadri et al., 2002). Blood homocysteine levels may be lowered by eating foods rich in folic acid, such as fruits and green leafy vegetables. Clinical trials are under way to determine whether the risk of AD can be reduced by dietary supplements and vitamins that control free radicals (e.g., folic acid, vitamins C and E) and

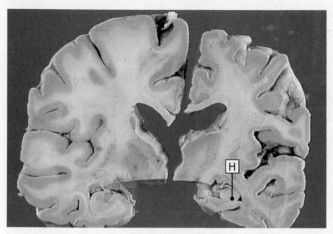

FIGURE 14-16 Effects of Alzheimer's disease on the brain.

those that reduce homocysteine levels (e.g., vitamins B_6 and B_{12}) (National Institute on Aging, 2007).

Studies have shown that individuals who engage in activities that require information processing (e.g., reading, learning a new language, doing crossword puzzles) have a lower risk of developing AD. Dietary patterns, physical activity, leisure activities, and educational achievements may decrease AD risk (National Institute on Aging, 2007).

Clinical Manifestations

The progression of AD is commonly divided into four stages. In the early stage a person with Alzheimer's has relatively mild memory lapses and may have difficulty using the correct word. The attention span is decreased, and there may be disinterest in surroundings. Depression may occur at this time. In the second stage the person has more obvious memory lapses, especially with short-term memory, and usually is disoriented to time. Loss of personal belongings is common, as is confabulating (making up stories) to explain the loss of memory. Patients may lose their ability to recognize familiar faces, places, and objects and may get lost in a familiar environment. Loss of impulse control is common. Behavioral manifestations of AD (e.g., agitation, repetitiveness, wandering, resisting care) result from changes in the brain. A specific type of agitation is termed **sundowning,** in which the patient becomes more confused and agitated in the late afternoon or evening.

The AD patient's behavior is neither intentional nor subject to self-control. Some patients develop psychotic manifestations (i.e., delusions, illusions, hallucinations). By the time a person reaches the third stage, he or she has total disorientation to person, place, and time. Motor problems such as apraxia (an inability to carry out learned sequential movements on command, perform purposeful acts, or use objects properly), **visual agnosia** (inability to recognize objects by sight), and **dysgraphia** (difficulty communicating via writing) interfere with the ability to carry out daily functions. Wandering is common. In the terminal stage, se-

vere mental and physical deterioration is present. Total incontinence is common.

These stages may have some variations. However, all people with AD experience a steady deterioration in their physical and mental status, usually lasting 5 to 20 years until death occurs (Box 14-2).

Assessment

Memory loss is the first symptom usually noticed in AD, combined with the inability to carry out normal activities. Other evidence may be agitation or restlessness. It is important to rule out other conditions such as pernicious anemia, drug reactions, depression, or hormonal imbalances.

Diagnostic Tests

The diagnosis of AD is primarily a diagnosis of exclusion. AD has no specific diagnostic test. A CT scan, EEG, MRI, and PET may be used to rule out other pathologic conditions. A family history of AD is significant. At times the diagnosis can only be confirmed at the time of autopsy.

Medical Management

The care of the patient with AD can be frustrating for the caregiver and the physician because the treatment options are so limited. Often medications make the condition worse. Lorazepam (Ativan) or haloperidol in small doses may be necessary to lessen agitation and unpredictable behavior. Treatment of depression in patients with AD may improve cognitive ability. Depression is treated most often with selective serotonin reuptake inhibitors such as fluoxetine, sertraline (Zoloft), fluvoxamine (Luvox), and citalopram (Celexa). Trazodone (Desyrel), an antidepressant, may help with problems related to sleep but may also cause hypotension. Some antiseizure drugs (neuroleptics), including valproic acid (Depakene) and carbamazepine, tend to act as mood stabilizers and are used to manage behavioral problems (Lewis et al., 2007). Donepezil (Aricept), rivastigmine (Exelon), and galantamine (Razadyne) may have short-term benefit for mild cognitive impairment. Memantine (Namenda) is the first drug approved for the treatment of moderate to severe AD. Memantine does not prevent or slow neurodegeneration, but it was found in clinical studies to slow symptom progression. Many clinical drug trials are trying to find drugs that manage the signs and symptoms of AD while limiting the rate of disease progression. Research shows that the simple addition to a normal diet of large doses of folic acid and vitamin B_{12} will substantially reduce homocysteine levels (Seshadri et al., 2002).

Nursing Interventions and Patient Teaching

Nursing interventions are directed toward maintaining adequate nutrition. This can be a challenge because often the patient will not sit still long enough to eat. Providing finger foods and letting the patient eat while walking may help. Frequent feedings with high

| Box 14-2 | Early Warning Signs of Alzheimer's Disease |

- Memory loss that affects job skills
  —Frequent forgetfulness or unexplainable confusion at home or in the workplace may signal that something is wrong.
  —This type of memory loss goes beyond forgetting an assignment, colleague's name, deadline, or phone number.
- Difficulty performing familiar tasks
  —Most people occasionally become distracted and forget something (e.g., leave something on the stove too long).
  —People with Alzheimer's disease (AD) may cook a meal but then forget not only to serve it but also that they made it.
- Problems with language
  —Most people have trouble with finding the "right" word from time to time.
  —People with AD may forget simple words or substitute inappropriate words, making their speech difficult to understand.
- Disorientation to time and place
  —Most people occasionally forget the day of the week or what they need from the store.
  —People with AD can become lost on their own street, not knowing where they are, how they got there, or how to get back home.
- Poor or decreased judgment
  —Many individuals from time to time may choose not to dress appropriately for the weather (e.g., not bringing a coat or sweater on a cold evening).

- People with AD may dress inappropriately in more noticeable ways, such as wearing a bathrobe to the store or a sweater on a hot day.
- Problems with abstract thinking
  —For the person with AD, this goes beyond challenges such as balancing a checkbook. They may have difficulty recognizing numbers or doing even basic calculations.
- Misplacing things
  —For many individuals, temporarily misplacing keys, purses, or wallets is a normal albeit frustrating event.
  —The person with AD may put items in inappropriate places (e.g., eating utensils in clothing drawers) but have no memory of how they got there.
- Changes in mood or behavior
  —Most individuals experience mood changes.
  —People with AD tend to exhibit more rapid mood swings for no apparent reason.
- Changes in personality
  —As most individuals age, they may demonstrate some change in personality (e.g., become less tolerant).
  —People with AD can change dramatically, either suddenly or over time. For example, someone who is generally easygoing may become angry, suspicious, or fearful.
- Loss of initiative
  —People with AD may become and remain uninterested and uninvolved in many or all of their usual pursuits.

Adapted from Alzheimer's Association. (2007). Early warning signs. Chicago: Alzheimer's Association. From Lewis, S.M., et al. Medical-surgical nursing: Assessment and management of clinical problems. (7th ed.). St. Louis: Mosby.

nutritive value are important. Encourage fluids of at least 2000 mL/day (Nursing Care Plan).

Safety demands a special mention. Because of memory problems, patients with AD often do dangerous things, such as walking outside while undressed, turning on stoves, wandering away, and setting fires. Measures that the family can take include removing burner controls from the stove at night, double-locking all doors and windows, and keeping the person under constant supervision. Disruptive behavior—including aggressive, agitated behavior—may occur. One frustrating part of the disease is that many patients sleep for only short periods and are awake most of the night.

Most of the time, education is directed at the family, because by the time the condition is diagnosed there is usually serious mental impairment. Help the family set a realistic schedule that also allows them time for rest and relaxation. If necessary, the family may need to consider placing the patient in a long-term care facility. Put the family in touch with the local support group for AD.

Prognosis

Currently no effective treatment is available to stop the progression of AD, which occurs at a variable rate. The course of the disease can span 5 to 20 years. The eco-

nomic costs of AD in the United States range from approximately $19,000 annually for the care of the person with early disease to $37,000 and more for the person with late disease. Ultimately, most patients die from complications such as pneumonia, malnutrition, and dehydration. Special Alzheimer's units and family and nursing approaches may help the patient stay as productive and safe as possible. The burden on the individual, the family, caregivers, and society as a whole is staggering. Support groups for caregivers and family members have been formed throughout the United States to provide an atmosphere of understanding and to give current information about the disease and related topics such as safety, legal, ethical, and financial issues. Nurses often receive personal and professional satisfaction in participating in such support groups.

MYASTHENIA GRAVIS

Etiology and Pathophysiology

MG is an autoimmune disease of the neuromuscular junction characterized by the fluctuating weakness of certain skeletal muscle groups. MG is an unpredictable neuromuscular disease with lower motoneuron characteristics. MG can occur at any age, but most commonly occurs between the ages of 10 and 65 years. The

Nursing Care Plan 14-1   The Patient with Alzheimer's Disease

Ms. Andrea is a 65-year-old who has been a seamstress. She has a history of progressive memory loss, paranoia, disorientation, and agitation. She was diagnosed as having Alzheimer's disease 2 years ago. Her family kept her at home until 6 months ago, when she was admitted to a long-term care institution. The nursing history indicates that she is incontinent of urine about 50% of the time and expresses a great deal of anxiety, especially around new situations or people. She cries frequently and at times attempts to hit the staff.

NURSING DIAGNOSIS *Anxiety, related to cognitive impairments*

Patient Goals and Expected Outcomes	Nursing Interventions	Evaluation
Patient will demonstrate decreased anxiety as evidenced by decreased outbursts of agitation or crying, the ability to sleep through most of the night, and cooperation with care	Continue to assess presence of anxiety. Comfort patient when she is crying. Provide simple explanation for all procedures. Use calm, undemanding, unhurried approach. Keep nursing interventions consistent and simple. Assist patient in doing relaxation techniques. Maintain consistency of caregiver when able. Minimize patient's choices in care. Encourage patient to exercise. Offer snack at bedtime.	Patient sleeps 5 to 6 hours per night. Patient remains calm with care. Patient experiences decreased episodes of crying or striking out at others.

NURSING DIAGNOSIS *Functional urinary incontinence, related to condition and cognitive impairment*

Patient Goals and Expected Outcomes	Nursing Interventions	Evaluation
Patient will be continent Patient will be free of urinary tract infection	Take patient to bathroom on regular schedule. Encourage adequate fluid intake (at least 2000 mL/day). Determine patient's preference for fluid. Place sign on door indicating "Toilet" or "Bathroom," or with a picture. If patient has urgency, ensure closeness to bathroom. Simplify closures on clothing. Avoid fluids just before bed. Use disposable protective perineal garments (Attends) only as needed.	Patient is free of episodes of incontinence. Patient is free of infection. Patient will void when taken to the bathroom.

Critical Thinking Questions
1. Ms. Andrea continually wanders about the long-term care facility. She is unable to sit at the table for an entire meal. She has lost approximately 20 pounds in the past 3 months. What are some helpful measures to improve her nutritional status?
2. What are some helpful interventions to help Ms. Andrea obtain a better sleep pattern?
3. Ms. Andrea has difficulty in maintaining good personal hygiene. What are some methods for assisting Ms. Andrea in maintaining personal hygiene?

peak age of onset in women is 20 to 30 years. In young people, women are more affected than men, but among older people the distribution between the genders is about equal. Occurrence within families is rare; however, infants of affected mothers may have symptoms at birth. These symptoms usually disappear within several weeks. The incidence is about 14 in every 100,000 population.

With MG, no observable structural change occurs in the muscle or nerve. Nerve impulses fail to pass at the myoneural junction (the space between the nerve ending and muscle fiber), resulting in muscle weakness. MG is caused by an autoimmune process. It is thought to be triggered by antibodies that attack acetylcholine receptor sites at the neuromuscular junction. This attack damages and reduces the number of receptor sites, preventing conduction along the normal pathway at normal conduction speeds. Patients with MG have only about one third as many acetylcholine receptors at the neuromuscular junction as is normal.

About 25% of the patients with MG have been found to have a thymoma, and almost 80% have changes in the cellular structure of the thymus gland.

Clinical Manifestations

MG occurs in both ocular and generalized terms. In ocular MG the signs and symptoms include ptosis (eyelid drooping) and diplopia (double vision). In about 15% of cases, MG remains confined to the eye muscles. The generalized variety may vary from mild to severe signs and symptoms. The patient may complain initially of ptosis and diplopia. Skeletal weakness involving the muscles of the extremities, the neck, the shoulders, the hands, and the diaphragm; dysarthria; and dysphagia may follow. The vocal cords can become weak, and the voice can sound nasal. As the disease progresses, it affects the trunk and lower limbs, leading to difficulty with walking, sustained sitting, and raising the arms over the head. Usually the distal muscles are not as affected as the proximal muscles. Muscle weakness may become so severe that the person cannot breathe without mechanical ventilation. Bowel and bladder sphincter weakness occurs with severe loss of muscle control. Exacerbations of the disease may be initiated by upper respiratory tract infections, emotional tension, and menstruation.

Assessment

Subjective data include the patient's understanding of the disease; complaints of weakness or double vision; difficulty chewing or swallowing; and any bowel or bladder incontinence.

Objective data include any documented muscle weakness on neurologic testing. Nasal-sounding speech may be noted; the voice often fades after a long conversation and breath sounds diminish. Note ptosis of the eyelids and weight loss if there are swallowing problems.

Diagnostic Tests

Because of the slow, insidious onset and occurrence of symptoms with stress, MG sometimes is misdiagnosed as hysteria or neurosis. The diagnosis of MG can be made on the basis of history and physical examination. The simplest diagnostic test for MG is to have the patient look upward for 2 to 3 minutes. If the problem is MG, the eyelids will droop so that the person can barely keep the eyes open. The diagnosis can be made partly on the basis of EMG. The IV anticholinesterase test is a reliable diagnostic test. Edrophonium (Tensilon), a short-acting cholinesterase inhibitor, which decreases the amount of cholinesterase at the neuromuscular junction while making acetylcholine available to muscles, is administered intravenously. The patient response is carefully evaluated. Muscle function improves dramatically after IV injection with Tensilon in a short time with patients who have the illness. Another diagnostic test is serum testing for antibodies to

acetylcholine receptors. Acetylcholine receptor antibodies are present in 80% to 90% of patients with generalized myasthenia, so their presence can be used to diagnose the disease.

Medical Management

Medical management includes the use of anticholinesterase drugs such as neostigmine (Prostigmin) and pyridostigmine (Mestinon). These medications promote nerve impulse transmission and effectively alleviate symptoms. Usually the patient is taught how to adjust the dosage depending on symptoms. Corticosteroids may be used as an adjunct therapy. Immunosuppressive medications, including azathioprine (Imuran), cyclosporine (Sandimmune), and cyclophosphamide (Cytoxan), are used because of MG's immune component. Many classes of drugs are contraindicated or must be used with caution in patients with MG; these include anesthetics, antidysrhythmics, antibiotics, quinine, antipsychotics, barbiturates, sedatives, hypnotics, opioids, tranquilizers, and thyroid preparations (Fisher, 2004).

Plasmapheresis as a therapy for MG was first reported in 1976. This procedure involves separation of plasma from blood by a machine called a cell separator, which can be connected to the patient by a vascular cannula. This process removes the antibodies produced by the autoimmune response. Plasmapheresis can yield short-term improvement in symptoms and is indicated for patients in crisis or in preparation for surgery when corticosteroids need to be avoided.

Thymectomy is indicated for almost all patients with a thymoma. For some patients without thymoma, thymectomy may result in improvement in symptoms. Excision of the thymus reduces symptoms of MG in many patients. A thymectomy is a complex surgery, and patients with MG are at high risk for complications from anesthesia.

Another treatment option is the administration of IV immune globulin to reduce the production of acetylcholine antibodies. IV immune globulin is used for a severe relapse of MG.

During exacerbations of the disease, and when the respiratory status is compromised, the patient may require intubation and mechanical ventilation. A tracheostomy may be necessary.

Nursing Interventions and Patient Teaching

Respiratory problems typically occur in patients with MG. Upper respiratory tract infections occur because the patient may not have the energy to cough effectively, and pneumonia or airway obstruction may develop. Aspiration often occurs. During acute episodes of the disease, the patient may require hospitalization. Serial determination of vital capacity, minute volumes, and tidal volumes is made to assess the need for respiratory assistance. The patient may also be taught airway protective techniques during swallowing (e.g.,

Patient Teaching

Myasthenia Gravis

- Teach the importance of taking medication at the time prescribed and taking it early enough before eating or engaging in activities to obtain maximum relief.
- Explain how to adjust medication dose to maintain muscle strength.
- Caution about medications to avoid.
- Teach importance of seeking medical attention at first sign of an upper respiratory tract infection.
- Explain importance of eating only when sitting up to prevent aspiration.
- Caution patient to avoid crowds in flu and cold season.
- Explain how to adjust to daily activities to allow for leisure activities and rest periods.
- Explain planning to use minimal energy in activities that are essential so that energy may be conserved for activities that the patient enjoys.
- Advise patient to wear a medical-alert bracelet that identifies the patient as having myasthenia gravis.

chin tuck, double swallow). Suctioning is done as needed, and if swallowing becomes impaired, a feeding tube may be necessary.

People with MG may have to change daily patterns of activity. Help the patient and the family plan so that minimal energy is used in activities that are essential to remaining relatively self-sufficient, with energy left for leisure activities. Physical therapy such as ROM exercises may be beneficial for maintaining muscle function.

The patient with MG is usually able to adjust the medication depending on the symptoms. Also, the patient can have much control over preventing respiratory complications. Therefore teaching is important and should include those topics listed in the Patient Teaching box.

Prognosis

MG is a chronic disease. The course is variable with periods of exacerbation and remission. Some cases are mild, but others are severe, with death resulting from respiratory failure. Patients with a thymoma may experience improvement after a thymectomy.

AMYOTROPHIC LATERAL SCLEROSIS

Loss of both upper and lower motoneurons is the major pathologic change in ALS, a rare, progressive neurologic disease that usually leads to death in 2 to 6 years. This disease became known as Lou Gehrig's disease when the famous baseball player was stricken with it in 1939. The onset is between 40 and 70 years of age, and two times as many men as women are affected.

For unknown reasons, motoneurons in the brainstem and spinal cord gradually degenerate in ALS. The dead motoneuron cannot produce or transport vital signals to muscle. Consequently, electrical and chemical messages originating in the brain do not reach the muscles to activate them.

The primary symptoms are weakness of the upper extremities (the hands are often affected first), dysarthria, and dysphagia. However, weakness may begin in the legs. Muscle wasting and fasciculations (muscle twitching) result from the denervation of the muscles and lack of stimulation and use. Death usually results from respiratory tract infection secondary to compromised respiratory function.

Unfortunately there is no cure for ALS. A drug called riluzole (Rilutek) slows the progression of ALS. The drug helps protect motoneurons damaged by the disease and can add 3 months or more to a patient's life.

Multidisciplinary ALS teams at large academic centers such as Johns Hopkins Medical Center and Allegheny University of the Health Sciences are offering renewed hope to these patients. Usually coordinated by a nurse, these programs provide experimental drugs; physical, occupational, and speech therapy; nutritional regimens; and psychological support. Patients in these programs may live 15 years or more after diagnosis—three times the typical life expectancy (Robert Packard Center of ALS Research at Johns Hopkins, 2009).

This illness is devastating because the patient remains cognitively intact while wasting away. The challenge of nursing interventions is to guide the patient in use of moderate intensity, endurance type exercises for the trunk and limbs, since this may help reduce ALS spasticity (Palmieri, 2007c). Support the patient's cognitive and emotional functions by facilitating communication, providing diversional activities such as reading and human companionship, and helping the patient and the family with advanced care planning and anticipatory grieving related to loss of motor function and ultimate death. About 30% of patients with ALS live up to 5 years after diagnosis, and 10% to 20% survive for more than 25 years. However, some patients may die in the first year after diagnosis (Palmieri, 2007c).

HUNTINGTON'S DISEASE

Huntington's disease is a genetically transmitted autosomal dominant disorder that affects both men and women of all races. The offspring of a person with this disease have a 50% risk of inheriting it. The diagnosis often occurs after the affected individual has children. The onset of Huntington's disease is usually between 30 and 50 years of age. In the United States, approximately 25,000 people have Huntington's disease and another 150,000 have a 50/50 chance of developing it.

Diagnosis is based on family history, clinical symptoms, and the detection of the characteristic deoxyribonucleic acid (DNA) pattern from blood samples. People who are asymptomatic but who have a positive family history of Huntington's disease face the dilemma of whether to get tested. If the test is positive, the person will develop Huntington's disease, but at what age and to what extent cannot be determined (Lewis et al., 2007).

Like Parkinson's disease, the pathology of Huntington's disease involves the basal ganglia and the extrapyramidal motor system. However, instead of a deficiency of dopamine, Huntington's disease involves an overactivity of the dopamine pathway. The net effect is an excess of dopamine, which leads to symptoms that are the opposite of those of parkinsonism. The clinical manifestations are characterized by abnormal and excessive involuntary movements (chorea). These are writhing, twisting movements of the face, limbs, and body. The movements get worse as the disease progresses. Facial movements involving speech, chewing, and swallowing are affected and may cause aspiration and malnutrition. The gait deteriorates, and ambulation eventually becomes impossible. Perhaps the most devastating deterioration is in mental functions, which include intellectual decline, emotional lability, and psychotic behavior. Death usually occurs 10 to 20 years after the onset of symptoms.

Because there is no cure, therapeutic management is palliative. Antipsychotic (e.g., haloperidol), antidepressant (fluoxetine, sertraline), and antichorea (clonazepam [Klonopin]) medications are prescribed and have some effect. However, they do not alter the course of the disease.

This disease presents a great challenge to health care professionals. Transplantation of fetal striatal neural tissues into the brain is an experimental treatment that may be effective (Kim, 2004). The goal of nursing management is to provide the most comfortable environment possible for the patient and the family by maintaining physical safety, treating the physical symptoms, and providing emotional and psychological support. Because of the choreic movements, caloric requirements are as high as 4000 to 5000 calories/day to maintain body weight. As the disease progresses, meeting caloric needs becomes a greater challenge when the patient has difficulty swallowing and holding the head still. Depression and mental deterioration can also compromise nutritional intake. Genetic counseling is important. DNA testing can be done on fetal cells obtained by amniocentesis or chorionic biopsy. Genetic testing can determine whether a person is a carrier. No test is available to predict when symptoms will develop.

VASCULAR PROBLEMS

Interference with function because of vascular conditions is a common neurologic impairment.

STROKE

Etiology and Pathophysiology

Stroke (or "brain attack") is an abnormal condition of the blood vessels of the brain, characterized by hemorrhage into the brain or the formation of an embolus or thrombus that occludes an artery, resulting in ischemia of the brain tissue normally perfused by the damaged vessels. The term *brain attack* is increasingly used to

 Cultural Considerations

Stroke

A high mortality rate from strokes exists among black men, possibly as a result of the high frequency of hypertension, obesity, and diabetes mellitus in this group. Thrombotic strokes are twice as common among blacks as among whites. Hemorrhagic strokes are three times more common among blacks than among whites. Hispanics, Native Americans, and Asian Americans have a higher stroke incidence than whites.

describe stroke. This term communicates the urgency of recognizing the clinical manifestations of a stroke and treating a medical emergency, just as one would with a heart attack.

After the onset of a stroke, immediate medical attention is crucial to reduce disability and death (Lewis et al., 2007). Stroke is the most common disease of the nervous system. It is estimated that 700,000 people in the United States suffer a stroke annually. It is ranked as the third leading cause of death in the United States, with about 160,000 deaths annually. Strokes affect people in all age-groups, but most are between 75 and 85 years of age. Strokes leave many people with serious, long-term disability. Of those who survive, 50% to 70% are functionally independent, and 15% to 30% live with permanent disability. Common long-term disabilities include hemiparesis, inability to walk, complete or partial dependence in ADLs, aphasia, and depression (see Cultural Considerations box).

Strokes are classified as ischemic or hemorrhagic, based on the underlying pathophysiologic findings. Ischemic strokes are thrombotic and embolic. These account for 85% of strokes. The remaining 15% are hemorrhagic strokes, which result from bleeding into the brain tissue itself (Figure 14-17). Many underlying factors also contribute: atherosclerosis, heart disease, hypertension, kidney disease, peripheral vascular disease, and diabetes mellitus. Other risk factors include family history of stroke, obesity, high serum cholesterol, cigarette smoking, stress, cocaine use, and a sedentary lifestyle. Newer low-dose oral contraceptives have lower risks for stroke than early forms of birth control pills, except in those individuals who are hypersensitive and smoke. Hypertension is the single most important modifiable risk factor. Stroke risk can be reduced by up to 42% with appropriate treatment of hypertension. Atrial fibrillation is the most important treatable cardiac-related risk factor (Phillips, 2007). Atrial fibrillation is responsible for about 15% to 20% of all strokes. The risk for stroke in people with diabetes mellitus is four to five times higher than the general population. Carotid artery stenosis, also called carotid artery disease, is defined as the narrowing of the carotid arteries that supply blood to the brain, usually from plaque buildup (atherosclerosis) in the inner lining of the artery. It is responsible for 80% of the 500,000

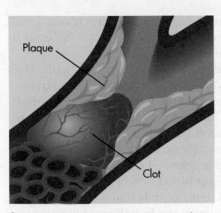

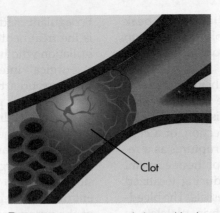

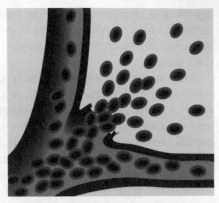

A Thrombotic stroke. Cerebral thrombosis is a narrowing of the artery by fatty deposits called *plaque*. Plaque can cause a clot to form, which blocks the passage of blood through the artery.

B Embolic stroke. An embolus is a blood clot or other debris circulating in the blood. When it reaches an artery in the brain that is too narrow to pass through, it lodges there and blocks the flow of blood.

C Hemorrhagic stroke. A burst blood vessel may allow blood to seep into and damage brain tissues until clotting shuts off the leak.

FIGURE 14-17 Three types of stroke.

TIAs that affect patients annually (Phillips, 2007). In 2002 data from the Women's Health Initiative (longitudinal intervention trial in middle-age women) showed an increased risk of stroke in women taking estrogen plus progestin compared with those not receiving hormone replacement therapy. These data suggest that postmenopausal hormone replacement therapy does not protect against stroke (Women's Health Initiative, 2002).

Clinical Manifestations

A stroke can have an effect on many body functions, including motor activity, elimination, intellectual function, spatial perception, personality, affect, sensation, and communication. The functions affected are directly related to the artery involved and the area of brain it supplies. Permanent damage can result from a stroke because of anoxia of the brain. The vessel most commonly affected is the middle cerebral artery. The patient may be unconscious and may experience seizures as a result of generalized ischemia and the brain's response to abrupt hypoxia.

Ischemic Stroke

Deficient blood flow to the brain from a partial or complete occlusion of an artery results in an ischemic stroke. Ischemic strokes are divided into **thrombotic** and **embolic** and account for about 80% of all strokes (National Institute of Neurological Disorders and Stroke, n.d.).

Thrombotic Stroke

Thrombosis is the most common cause of stroke, and the most common cause of cerebral thrombosis is atherosclerosis. Additional disease processes that cause thrombosis are hypertension or diabetes mellitus, both of which accelerate the arteriosclerotic process. Additional risk factors associated with thrombotic strokes include coagulation disorders, polycythemia vera, arteritis, chronic hypoxia, and dehydration. In 30% to 50% of individuals, thrombotic strokes have been preceded by a TIA. Stroke resulting from thrombosis is seen most often in the 60- to 90-year-old age-group. Thrombosis occurs in relation to injury of a blood vessel wall and formation of a blood clot. The lumen of the blood vessel becomes narrowed, and if it becomes occluded, infarction occurs. Thrombosis develops readily where atherosclerotic plaques have already narrowed blood vessels. Thrombi usually occur in larger vessels, especially the internal carotid arteries.

Symptoms of this type of stroke tend to occur during sleep or soon after arising. This is thought to result partly because recumbency lowers blood pressure, which can lead to brain ischemia. Postural hypotension may also be a factor. Neurologic signs and symptoms frequently worsen for the first few hours after a stroke and peak in severity within 72 hours as edema increases in the infarcted areas of the brain.

Embolic Stroke

Embolism is the second most common cause of stroke. People who have a stroke resulting from embolism are usually younger. The emboli most commonly originate from a thrombus in the endocardial (inside) layer of the heart, often caused by rheumatic heart disease, mitral stenosis and atrial fibrillation, myocardial infarction, infective endocarditis, valvular prostheses, and atrial septal defects. Less common causes of emboli include air, fat from long bone (femur) fractures, amniotic fluid after childbirth, and tumors. The embolus travels upward to the cerebral circulation and lodges where a vessel narrows or bifurcates. They most frequently occur in the midcerebral artery.

Hemorrhagic Stroke

Hemorrhagic stroke accounts for approximately 15% of all strokes and result from bleeding into the brain tissue or subarachnoid space. The bleed causes damage by destroying and replacing brain tissue. The peak incidence of aneurysms occurs in people who are 35 to 60 years of age. Women are more frequently affected than men.

An aneurysm is often the cause of hemorrhage. An aneurysm is a localized dilation of the wall of a blood vessel usually caused by atherosclerosis and hypertension or, less frequently, by trauma, infection, or a congenital weakness in the vessel wall. It ruptures as a result of a small hole that occurs in a part of the aneurysm. The hemorrhage spreads rapidly, producing localized damage and irritation to the cerebral vessels. The bleeding usually stops when a plug of fibrin platelets is formed. The hemorrhage begins to absorb within 3 weeks. Recurrent rupture is a risk 7 to 10 days after the initial hemorrhage. The patient with intracerebral hemorrhage has no forewarning; has rapid, severe symptoms; and has a poor prognosis for recovery. Fifty percent of patients die soon after the stroke. Only about 20% are functionally independent after 6 months.

Transient Ischemic Attack

TIA refers to an episode of cerebrovascular insufficiency with temporary episodes of neurologic dysfunction lasting less than 24 hours and often less than 15 minutes. Most TIAs resolve within 3 hours. TIAs may be caused by microemboli that temporarily occlude the blood flow. TIAs often occur in patients with carotid artery stenosis. The most common deficits are contralateral weakness of the lower face, hands, arms, and legs; transient dysphasia; numbness or loss of sensation; temporary loss of vision of one eye; or a sudden inability to speak. Other symptoms may include tinnitus, vertigo, blurred vision, diplopia, eyelid ptosis, and ataxia. Between attacks the neurologic status is normal.

A TIA should be considered a forerunner of a stroke. After a TIA the health care provider orders a complete workup to rule out carotid artery stenosis. Duplex ultrasonography is the primary noninvasive test for carotid artery stenosis. If a patient is symptomatic and duplex ultrasound findings are abnormal, MRA or contrast-enhanced CT angiography (CTA) may be ordered to confirm the diagnosis and classify the severity of the carotid artery stenosis (Phillips, 2007). Evaluation must be done to confirm that the signs and symptoms of a TIA are not related to other brain lesions, such as a developing subdural hematoma or an increasing tumor mass. CT of the brain without contrast media is the most important initial diagnostic study.

The major importance of TIAs is that they warn the patient of an underlying pathologic condition. At least one third of patients who experience TIAs will have a stroke in 2 to 5 years. The patient is given medications that prevent platelet aggregation, such as aspirin, ticlopidine (Ticlid), dipyridamole (Persantine), and clopidogrel (Plavix). Aspirin is the most frequently used antiplatelet agent, commonly at a dose of 81 to 325 mg/day. An an-

ticoagulant medication (e.g., oral warfarin [Coumadin]) is the treatment of choice for individuals with atrial fibrillation who have had a TIA.

Surgical interventions for the patient with TIAs from carotid artery disease include carotid endarterectomy (CEA) or percutaneous transluminal angioplasty and stenting. In CEA the atheromatous lesion is removed from the carotid artery to improve blood flow. CEA surgery causes a reduction in stroke and vascular death. This surgery is reserved for patients with occlusions of 70% to 99% of blood flow. The long-term benefit of carotid endarterectomy is based on the severity of the preoperative stenosis. In patients with stenosis of 30% or less, surgery actually increases the risk for an ipsilateral stroke in the first 5 years postoperatively. There has been no proven effect within 5 years when the stenosis is 31% to 40% and only a marginal improvement in patients with 50% to 69% stenosis. However, the greatest benefit occurs when the stenosis is 70% or more (Phillips, 2007).

Percutaneous transluminal angioplasty is the insertion of a balloon to open a stenosed artery to permit increased blood flow. This procedure is used to treat patients with clinical manifestations related to stenosis in the vertebrobasilar or carotid arteries and their branches. The risk of the angioplasty procedure is the possibility of dislodging emboli, which can travel to the brain or retina.

Assessment

Subjective data include the description of the onset of symptoms; the presence of headache; any sensory deficit, such as numbness or tingling; the inability to think clearly; and visual problems. In the case of a hemorrhage, the headache may be described as sudden and explosive. Assess the patient's ability to understand the condition.

Objective data include hemiparesis or hemiplegia, any change in the LOC, signs of increased ICP, respiratory status, and aphasia. The exact clinical picture varies, depending on the area of the brain affected (Figure 14-18). A lesion on one side of the brain affects motor function on the opposite (contralateral) side of the brain. When the middle cerebral artery is affected, as is most common, the signs and symptoms seen include contralateral paralysis or paresis, contralateral sensory loss, dysphasia or aphasia if the dominant hemisphere is involved, spatial-perceptual problems, changes in judgment and behavior if the nondominant hemisphere is involved, and **contralateral (homonymous) hemianopia** (Figure 14-19).

In right-handed people and in most left-handed people, the left hemisphere is dominant for language skills. Language disorders affect expression and comprehension of written and spoken words. When a stroke damages the dominant hemisphere of the brain, the patient may experience **aphasia** (total loss of comprehension and use of language). Strokes affecting

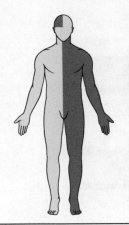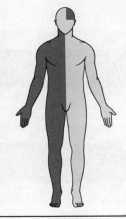

Right brain damage
(Stroke on right side of
the brain)

- Paralyzed left side: hemiplegia
- Left-sided neglect
- Spatial-perceptual deficits
- Tends to deny or minimize problems
- Rapid performance, short attention span
- Impulsive, safety problems
- Impaired judgment
- Impaired time concepts

Left brain damage
(Stroke on left side of
the brain)

- Paralyzed right side: hemiplegia
- Impaired speech/language aphasias
- Impaired right/left discrimination
- Slow performance, cautious
- Aware of deficits: depression, anxiety
- Impaired comprehension related to language, math

FIGURE 14-18 Manifestations of right-sided and left-sided stroke.

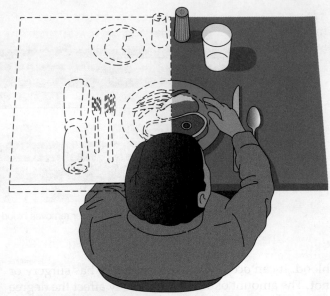

FIGURE 14-19 Spatial and perceptual deficits in stroke. Perception of a patient with homonymous hemianopsia shows that food on the left side is not seen and thus is ignored.

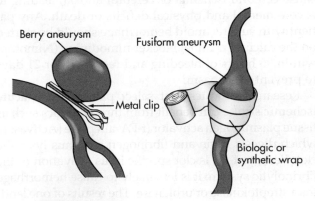

FIGURE 14-20 Clipping and wrapping of aneurysms.

Broca's areas of the brain cause difficulty in speaking and writing, or **expressive aphasia** (Lewis et al., 2007) (see Figure 14-3 and Box 14-1). If a patient has a stroke that affects Wernicke's center in the brain, he or she will have **receptive aphasia,** that is, difficulty comprehending the spoken and written language (Lewis et al., 2007).

A stroke patient may experience **dysarthria,** which is difficult or poorly articulated speech. Dysarthria is a result of deficits in the muscular control of speech and not in a pathologic condition of the Broca's area that is involved in speech production (Lewis et al., 2007). Some stroke patients experience a combination of aphasia and dysarthria.

Diagnostic Tests

Noncontrast CT is the primary test used to diagnose a stroke. CT can indicate the size and location of the lesion and differentiate between ischemic and hemorrhagic stroke. For optimal results, the CT scan should be obtained within 25 minutes and read within 45 minutes of arrival at the emergency department. If the stroke is ischemic and is less than 3 hours old, the CT will appear normal because the brain structure with or without blood flow appears the same in a noncontrast CT scan. If the CT scan appears normal with no sign of hemorrhage, the patient qualifies for fibrinolytic therapy (Lewis et al., 2007). CTA provides visualization of

vasculature. MRI is used to determine the extent of brain injury. MRI has greater specificity than CT. PET is also useful in assessing the extent of tissue damage by showing the brain's metabolic activity. After TIAs, a cerebral angiogram may be done. Doppler, CTA, or MRA studies of the carotid arteries should be performed. The results of these noninvasive carotid artery studies determine whether the more invasive cerebral angiogram is performed.

Medical Management

If the patient has had a hemorrhagic stroke as a result of an aneurysm, surgery may be necessary to prevent a rebleed. The surgery consists of performing a craniotomy; tying off or clipping the aneurysm; and removing the clot to prevent rebleeding into the brain (Figure 14-20). An aneurysm often causes vasospasm in the brain as blood in the subarachnoid space becomes an irritant. Vasospasm narrows blood vessels in the brain, decreasing perfusion to the areas they supply with

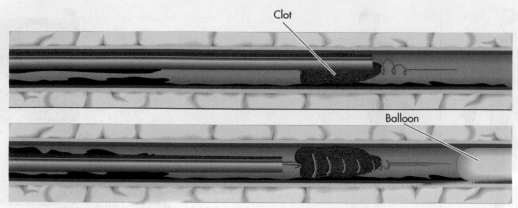

FIGURE 14-21 The MERCI Retriever removes blood clots in patients who are experiencing ischemic stroke.

blood. It can occur whether the patient has surgery or not. The amount of blood can directly affect the degree of vasospasm.

Vasospasm typically occurs in 30% to 60% of cases between postoperative days 4 and 12. The mortality rate is as high as 50%. If it is not treated rapidly, it can cause cerebral ischemia or cerebral anoxia, leading to severe mental and physical deficits or death. Any patient with subarachnoid hemorrhage should be started on the calcium channel blocker nimodipine (Nimotop) within 96 hours of bleeding and receive it for 21 days to prevent vasospasm.

Research indicates that select patients with **acute ischemic stroke** can benefit from thrombolytics such as tissue plasminogen activator (t-PA, alteplase [Activase]), which digests fibrin and fibrinogen and thus lyses the clot. Because t-PA is clot specific in its activation of the fibrinolytic system, it is less likely to cause hemorrhage than streptokinase or urokinase. The results of one landmark study have revealed that selected patients who are treated within 3 hours of the onset of symptoms are at least 30% more likely than patients who do not receive timely treatment to recover with little or no disability after 3 months. **Time lost is brain lost.** Although thrombolysis improves the chance of recovery by up to 30%, only 2% to 3% of ischemic stroke patients receive it. That is largely because of the limited therapeutic window (Barker, 2006).

In the summer of 2004, the U.S. Food and Drug Administration approved the first mechanical device for endovascular embolectomy: Mechanical Embolus Removal in Cerebral Ischemia (MERCI) Retriever. This device is used to remove blood clots inside the brain and can be used up to 8 hours after acute stroke onset (Barker, 2006). The MERCI Retriever is a tiny corkscrew device that uses a microcatheter inserted through a femoral artery balloon catheter (Figure 14-21). Under x-ray guidance, the balloon catheter is maneuvered until it reaches the clot in the artery in the brain. Once the clot is entrapped, the balloon catheter is inflated to temporarily prevent forward flow while the blood clot is

withdrawn. The clot is enclosed in the balloon catheter and removed from the body. The balloon is deflated and blood flow is restored to the brain (Lewis et al., 2007).

It is important to educate patients about the risk factors associated with stroke and to instruct them to dial 911 immediately if they or someone else shows signs of stroke. Immediate treatment in the nearest hospital gives patients the best chance for improved outcomes—whether treatment is within 3 hours for t-PA or within 8 hours for the MERCI Retriever (Barker, 2006).

Patients with stroke symptoms need to be triaged, transported, and treated as rapidly as patients experiencing an acute myocardial infarction. In administration of thrombolytic drugs, the single most important factor is timing. Patients are screened carefully before treatment is initiated. This includes blood tests for coagulation disorders, recent history of gastrointestinal bleeding, and a CT or MRI scan to rule out hemorrhagic stroke. In patients with acute ischemic stroke, thrombolytic therapy increases short-term mortality, increases (but not a statistically significant amount) symptomatic or fatal intracranial hemorrhage, decreases long-term death rate, and decreases dependence in terms of ADLs. The decision to use thrombolytic therapy should be based on a discussion of the risks and benefits with the patient and the family. Some patients would accept a high risk of death from hemorrhage in an attempt to improve their chances of escaping permanent aphasia or dependency. Others prefer to avoid interventions that carry significant risk (Lewis et al., 2007). Patients with stroke caused by thrombi and emboli (ischemic strokes) may also be treated with platelet inhibitors and anticoagulants (after the first 24 hours if treated with t-PA) to prevent the formation of more clots. Common anticoagulants include heparin, enoxaparin (Lovenox), and warfarin. Platelet inhibitors include aspirin, ticlopidine, clopidogrel, and dipyridamole.

Drugs to reduce ICP, such as dexamethasone, may be given. Suppositories such as bisacodyl (Dulcolax) are generally prescribed to be given daily or every other day. However, some physicians order stool softeners, laxatives, or enemas.

Fluids may be restricted for the first few days after a stroke in an effort to prevent edema of the brain. The patient is fed IV fluids, or a nasogastric or gastrostomy tube may be inserted and tube feedings begun.

The length of time the patient remains in bed depends on the type of stroke suffered, deficits noted, and the physician's judgment in regard to early mobilization. Some physicians prescribe fairly long periods of rest after strokes, whereas others believe in early mobilization—1 or 2 days after the accident occurred.

Nursing Interventions

Carefully monitor the patient's neurologic status. The neurologic assessment includes the Glasgow coma scale (see Table 14-3), LOC, pupillary responses, extremity movement and strength, facial symmetry, speech, and vital signs. A decrease in the LOC may indicate increasing ICP (Lewis et al., 2007). Interventions in the initial phase are directed toward preventing neurologic deficits (see Clinical Pathway 14-1 on Evolve).

Because nutrition is a concern and the patient may have difficulty swallowing at first, tube feedings and IV fluids may be necessary. See the section on motor and sensory problems for a discussion of techniques to assist in feeding the patient with dysphagia.

If the patient is responsive after the onset of the stroke, help the patient assume as much self-care as possible. This includes teaching the patient one-handed dressing techniques and one-handed feeding techniques if motor deficits have occurred. It is important to reinforce teaching by other members of the patient's health team.

The patient with a stroke may be incontinent at first. Remove the urinary catheter (if there is one) as soon as possible to prevent urinary tract infection and delayed bladder retraining. Because of the lower incidence of urinary tract infections, an intermittent catheterization program may be used for patients with urinary retention. Place the patient on a bladder training program to assist in regaining continence. This usually includes taking the patient to the bathroom every few hours and encouraging fluids (at least 2000 mL/day), with the majority given between 8 AM and 7 PM. Assess the patient's normal bowel pattern before the stroke and include this in the nursing care plan if possible. If the patient has difficulty with communication, a picture of a bathroom or toilet can be useful.

Return of motor impulses and movement in involved extremities occurs in stages, lasting from hours to months. Recovery may also halt at a specific stage and progress no further. Return of function is significant for functional use of extremities but also increases the possibility of contractures. Appropriate nursing interventions to prevent contractures include passive exercise, active exercise, strength building of the unaffected side, and early ambulation to promote the return of muscle function.

One way to position the patient with a stroke is the **Bobath approach,** designed to normalize muscle tone by providing as many sensations of normal muscle tone, posture, and movement as possible. The goal of the treatment is to redirect short-term memory toward an appreciation of normal movement of the paralyzed side by incorporating techniques of weight bearing, counterrotation, and protraction of the shoulder girdle and pelvis. The reader is referred to a rehabilitation nursing text for further description of this technique. Nurses in rehabilitation settings are often taught this approach.

Patients may experience a loss of proprioception with a stroke. Neurologic deficits of apraxia and agnosia (a total or partial loss of the ability to recognize familiar objects or people) may also occur. Assist the patient with activities by repeating directions and demonstrating care. If the patient has hemianopia, which is common, approach the patient from the nonparalyzed side for care. Teach the patient to scan past midline to the side with the deficit. These patients may also fail to recognize that they have a paralyzed side. This is called **unilateral neglect** (described earlier). Teach the patient to inspect this side of the body for injury and to protect it from harm. These patients often show poor judgment and may move impulsively or unsafely. Observe for this and take safety precautions if needed until the patient can learn to compensate for this lack of judgment. Patients who have had a stroke may have difficulty controlling their emotions. Emotional responses may be exaggerated or unpredictable. Depression and feelings associated with changes in body image and loss of function can make this worse. Patients may also be frustrated by mobility and communication problems.

To foster the patient's self-esteem, always treat the patient as an adult, not as a child. Praise and reinforce the patient's successful efforts and gains in self-care.

Communication Problems

Many stroke patients have speech problems, including dysarthria and aphasia. A speech pathologist evaluates and treats the patient with language disorders. The patient may be frustrated and should be approached in an unhurried manner. Often the patient does much better with communication when not feeling pressured to speak. Giving the patient a communication board may be helpful. Wait for the patient to communicate, rather than prompting or finishing the sentence before the patient has a chance to find the appropriate word. Inability to articulate does not mean that the patient has decreased cognitive abilities.

Nursing diagnoses and interventions for the patient who has had a stroke include but are not limited to the following:

Nursing Diagnoses	Nursing Interventions
Impaired verbal communication, related to ischemic injury	Speak slowly and distinctly. Ask questions that can be answered by yes or no (or by signals). Try to anticipate patient needs. Provide a call signal within reach of the unaffected hand. Begin speech therapy as soon as possible.
Imbalanced nutrition: less than body requirements, related to impaired ability to swallow	Provide IV fluids and tube feedings as prescribed during the initial period. Refer to speech therapist for assessment of swallowing problems. Assess ability to swallow before initiating feedings. Position patient with head elevated and turned to unaffected side during feedings. Provide foods initially that are easier to swallow (soft foods, except for mashed potatoes). Thin liquids are often difficult to swallow and may promote coughing. Thicken liquids with a commercially available thickening agent (Thick-It). Do not use milk products because they tend to increase the viscosity of mucus and increase salivation. Use a training cup for fluids as necessary. Do not use a straw. Inspect mouth for food trapped in cheek pockets. Be patient when feeding patient and provide directions for swallowing as needed. Ensure that meals are unrushed and nonstressful. Encourage patient to feed self as soon as possible; provide self-help devices as necessary. Provide scrupulous oral hygiene after meal because food may collect on the affected side of the mouth.

Patient Teaching

Teaching for a patient with a stroke should include techniques to compensate for the deficits suffered as a result of the stroke. In this the nurse functions as part of the rehabilitation team. Begin rehabilitation at the time of admission to the acute care facility. The patient will probably attend occupational and physical therapy and perhaps speech therapy. Depending on the patient's status, the patient's rehabilitation potential, and available resources, the patient may be transferred to a rehabilitation facility or unit.

If the patient is receiving medications (e.g., for hypertension or anticoagulation), teach the patient and the family about side effects and the dosing schedule. Discuss plans for follow-up. Also teach the patient's family techniques to enhance safety and communication. If the patient has a problem with dysphagia, teach the family appropriate communication techniques. Because of the chronicity of caring for the stroke patient, caregivers are at high risk for stress. Referral to an appropriate stroke support group is needed. Write instructions for the patient or the family to refer to after discharge. Most rehabilitation centers also include therapeutic leaves as a way to test the family's skills and knowledge. Each pass or leave has specific goals; obtain feedback from the family about additional teaching that may be needed. Also educate the family and the patient about perceptual problems associated with stroke and techniques to compensate for these deficits (e.g., writing down instructions for the patient who has trouble carrying out an activity alone).

Prognosis

The prognosis for patients with a stroke depends on the size of the lesion in the brain and the patient's premorbid status. More than 160,000 deaths occur in the United States each year as a result of strokes. Of those who survive, 50% to 70% are functionally independent; however, 15% to 30% have a permanent disability. The most frequent long-term disabilities include hemiparesis, inability to ambulate, aphasia, depression, and complete or partial dependence in ADLs. In 2005 the cost of stroke was estimated to be $56.8 billion per year in the United States (Lewis et al., 2007). With therapy, significant functional gains can be made, even when paralysis or weakness continues. Many patients are able to return home and remain independent after a stroke. With new medical treatment for selected patients, using t-PA for thrombolysis or mechanical clot removal, the prognosis is greatly improved.

CRANIAL AND PERIPHERAL NERVE DISORDERS

TRIGEMINAL NEURALGIA

Etiology and Pathophysiology

Trigeminal neuralgia is one specific kind of peripheral nerve problem. It is caused by degeneration of or pressure on the trigeminal nerve (cranial nerve V), and its etiology is unknown. It is also called **tic douloureux.** It

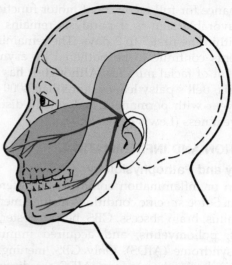

FIGURE 14-22 Pathway of trigeminal nerve and facial areas innervated by each of the three main divisions of this nerve.

usually affects people in middle or late adulthood and is slightly more common in women. The pathophysiology is not fully understood.

Clinical Manifestations

Trigeminal neuralgia is characterized by excruciating, knifelike, or lightninglike shock in the lips, upper or lower gums, cheek, forehead, or side of the nose. The pain radiates along one or more of the three divisions of the fifth cranial nerve (Figure 14-22). The fifth cranial nerve has both motor and sensory branches. In trigeminal neuralgia the sensory (or afferent) branches, primarily the maxillary and mandibular branches, are involved. The pain typically extends only to the midline of the face and head because this is the extent of the tissue supplied by the offending nerve. The attacks are usually brief, lasting only seconds to 2 to 3 minutes, and are generally unilateral. Recurrences are unpredictable; they may occur several times a day or weeks or months apart. Areas along the course of the nerve are known as **trigger points,** and the slightest stimulation of these areas may initiate pain. People with trigeminal neuralgia try desperately to avoid triggering them. Precipitating stimuli include chewing, toothbrushing, a hot or cold blast of air on the face, washing the face, yawning, or even talking.

Medical Management

Antiseizure medications such as carbamazepine, phenytoin, valproate, gabapentin, oxcarbazepine (Trileptal), lamotrigine (Lamictal), and topiramate are the drugs of choice for the treatment of trigeminal neuralgia pain. Absolute alcohol injected into the peripheral branches of the trigeminal nerve provides relief for weeks to months. Biofeedback, acupuncture, and megavitamins are other therapies used.

Permanent relief of pain is obtained only by surgery that involves inserting a fine needle through the cheek and injecting an alcohol solution or surgically resecting the sensory root of the trigeminal nerve. This is not always successful. Within 24 hours after a fifth nerve resection, many patients develop herpes simplex of the lips (cold sores). Usually these lesions heal in approximately 1 week.

Nursing Interventions

It is common for patients with trigeminal neuralgia not to have eaten properly for some time because eating causes pain. They may be undernourished and dehydrated. They may not have washed, shaved, or combed the hair for some time. Oral hygiene often has been neglected. Measures to increase comfort for patients before surgery or for patients being treated nonsurgically are listed in Box 14-3.

Prognosis

The acute pain seldom lasts more than a few seconds or 2 or 3 minutes, but it is excruciating. The onset of pain can occur at any time during the day or night and may recur several times daily for weeks at a time. Some patients have more or less continuous discomfort and sensitivity of the face. Although this condition is considered benign, the severity of the pain and the disruption of lifestyle can result in almost total physical and psychological dysfunction or even suicide. Permanent relief of pain is obtained only by surgery.

BELL'S PALSY (PERIPHERAL FACIAL PARALYSIS)
Etiology and Pathophysiology

Bell's palsy is thought to be caused by an inflammatory process involving the facial nerve (cranial nerve VII) anywhere from the nucleus in the brain to the periphery. Although the exact etiology is not known, there is evidence that reactivated herpes simplex virus (HSV) may be involved in the majority of cases. The reactivation of the HSV causes inflammation, edema, ischemia, and eventual demyelination of the facial nerve, creating pain and disturbances in motor and sensory function. Any of the three branches of the facial nerve may be affected. The disorder can be unilateral or bilateral. It can affect any age-group, but is more common in the 20- to 60-year-old age range.

Clinical Manifestations

With Bell's palsy there is usually an abrupt onset of numbness, stiffness, or drawing sensation of the face. Unilateral weakness of the facial muscles usually occurs, resulting in a flaccidity of the affected side of the face with inability to wrinkle the forehead, close the eyelid, pucker the lips, smile, frown, whistle, or retract the mouth on that side. The face appears asymmetric, with drooping mouth and cheek. Other symptoms include loss of taste, altered chewing ability, reduction of saliva on the affected side, pain behind the ear on the affected side, and ringing in the ear or other hearing loss.

Medical Management

Bell's palsy has no specific therapy. Electrical stimulation or warm moist heat along the course of the nerve may help. Stimulation may maintain muscle tone and prevent atrophy. Corticosteroids, especially prednisone, are started immediately, preferably before paralysis is complete. When the patient improves to the point that the corticosteroids are no longer necessary, they should be tapered off over a 2-week period. Because HSV is implicated in approximately 70% of cases of Bell's palsy, treatment with acyclovir (Zovirax), alone or in conjunction with prednisone, is used. Additional antiviral agents to treat HSV, including valacyclovir (Valtrex) and famciclovir (Famvir), have also been used in the management of Bell's palsy.

Nursing Interventions

Protection of the eye when the eyelid does not close is important. To prevent drying of the cornea, instill artificial tears frequently while the patient is awake. Apply an ointment with use of an impermeable eyeshield at night to facilitate retention of moisture (Lewis et al., 2007). Massage of the affected areas is sometimes recommended. Active facial exercises may be prescribed for 5 minutes three times a day. These include wrinkling the brow and forehead, closing the eyes, and puffing out the cheeks.

Prognosis

Some 85% of patients recover fully in weeks or months, although recovery may take as long as a year. Recovery of taste is the first sign of improvement; if it occurs within the first week, it signals a good chance for full recovery of motor function. Another favorable sign is if paralysis remains incomplete within the first 5 to 7 days. The remaining 15% of patients continue to be bothered by asymmetric movement of facial muscles. Although it has a good prognosis, Bell's palsy leaves more than 8000 Americans a year with permanent, potentially disfiguring facial weakness (Lewis et al., 2007).

INFECTION AND INFLAMMATION

Etiology and Pathophysiology

Infection or inflammation commonly interferes with function. Some specific conditions include meningitis, encephalitis, brain abscess, GBS, herpes zoster, neurosyphilis, poliomyelitis, and acquired immunodeficiency syndrome (AIDS). Only GBS, meningitis, encephalitis, brain abscess, and AIDS are discussed in this chapter.

The nervous system may be affected by a variety of organisms and may suffer from toxins of bacteria and viruses. These toxins reach the nervous system from a variety of sources, including adjacent bones, blood, or lymph. Meningitis can occur as a result of an invasive procedure such as surgery.

Assessment

Subjective data include a history of infection, such as an upper respiratory tract infection, and discomfort such as headache or stiff neck. The initial onset of symptoms, difficulty in thinking, and weakness may be important. Assess the patient's understanding of the condition.

Objective data include behavioral signs indicating discomfort or disorientation and an inability to carry out ADLs. Physical assessment may reveal abnormalities; fever, vomiting, abnormal CT results, seizures, altered respiratory patterns, tachycardia, or meningeal irritation. Also assess the patient's LOC and orientation.

Diagnostic Tests

Many of the infections of the nervous system can be diagnosed by examining the CSF. A CT scan or an EEG may also be done.

Nursing Interventions and Patient Teaching

Nursing diagnoses and interventions for the patient with an infection or inflammation are the same as those for the patient who has had a stroke, with the addition of but not limited to the following:

Nursing Diagnoses	Nursing Interventions
Hyperthermia, related to inflammatory response to CNS infection	Assess temperature every 2 hours and as needed. Provide cooling measures as needed; avoid cooling to point of shivering.

Nursing Diagnoses	Nursing Interventions
	Administer antipyretics and antibiotics as ordered.
	Monitor parenteral fluids as ordered.
	Control exposure to extremes in temperature.
	Assess temperature, pulse, and respiration every 2 hours as indicated.
Acute confusion, related to neurophysiologic response to infection	Introduce self to patient and establish rapport to prevent agitation.
	Relate date, time of day, and recent activities.
	Speak in kind tone, using short, simple sentences.
	Maintain a therapeutic environment.

Education for the patient with an infection includes teaching about the disease process, the treatments involved, and the expected outcomes. If the patient is seriously ill, the initial teaching involves the family. Other aspects of teaching for motor and sensory problems may also be relevant for the patient with an infection or inflammation, depending on the signs and symptoms demonstrated.

GUILLAIN-BARRÉ SYNDROME (POLYNEURITIS)
Etiology and Pathophysiology
Guillain-Barré syndrome (GBS) is also called acute inflammatory polyradiculopathy or postinfectious polyneuritis. It is an acute, rapidly progressing, and potentially fatal form of polyneuritis. It results in widespread inflammation and demyelination of the peripheral nervous system. The disease affects people of all ages and is seen equally in men and women. It affects 1.5 people in 100,000 each year. The etiology is unknown, but it is thought to be an autoimmune reaction involving the peripheral nerves. GBS often follows a viral infection, trauma, surgery, viral immunizations, or HIV infection. Other pathogens include *Campylobacter jejuni* (precedes the syndrome in about 30% of cases), mycoplasma, pneumoniae, cytomegalovirus, Epstein-Barr virus, and varicella-zoster virus (Lewis et al., 2007).

The peripheral nervous system is composed of 31 pairs of spinal nerves, 12 pairs of cranial nerves, and various plexuses and ganglia. Each nerve cell, or neuron, is composed of several parts, including the axon. Responsible for transmitting nerve impulses, axons are wrapped in segments of insulation called the myelin sheath, which is composed of Schwann cells.

In GBS the antibodies attack the Schwann cells, causing the sheath to break down (a process called de-

myelination) and the uninsulated portion of the nerve to become inflamed. Nerve conduction is interrupted, causing the classic signs of muscle weakness, tingling, and numbness. These signs begin in the legs or feet and work their way upward, perhaps because the signals to and from the legs are most vulnerable because they have to travel the longest distance. The demyelination is self-limiting. Once it stops, the Schwann cells rebuild the lost insulation. Remyelination, and therefore recovery, occurs in reverse; it starts at the top of the body and proceeds downward.

Clinical Manifestations
There is variation in the pattern of the onset of weakness and in the rate of progression of signs and symptoms. The progression may stop at any point. The patient may have difficulty swallowing, breathing, and speaking if cranial nerves VII, IX, and X are involved. Symmetric muscle weakness and lower motoneuron paralysis are present. The paralysis usually starts in the lower extremities and moves upward to include the thorax, the upper extremities, and the face. Respiratory failure may occur if the intercostal muscles are affected. Fluctuating blood pressure may occur as a result of effects on the autonomic nervous system.

Diagnostic Tests
GBS is diagnosed by elimination of other reasons for the signs and symptoms and by the characteristic muscle weakness. A CT scan may be ordered to rule out tumors or stroke. Changes in the respiratory status may aid in the diagnosis. A lumbar puncture is done. CSF in patients with GBS commonly has elevated protein levels. The physician may order a nerve conduction velocity study to test for slow impulse transmission. Electromyography and nerve conduction studies are markedly abnormal. A history of a recent infection is considered important.

Medical Management
Once GBS is suspected, hospitalization is essential. The patient's condition can rapidly deteriorate into paralysis that affects the respiratory muscles.

Adrenocortical steroids are used to treat the signs and symptoms of GBS. It has also been found that therapeutic plasmapheresis (the removal of unwanted or pathologic components from the patient's blood serum by means of a continuous-flow separator) in the first 2 weeks of GBS leads to decreased severity and length of symptoms. An alternative to plasmapheresis is IV immunoglobulin (Sandoglobulin). Patients receiving high-dose immunoglobulin need to be well hydrated and have adequate renal function.

Patients who develop respiratory failure require mechanical ventilation and may require a tracheostomy. ABG monitoring and pulmonary function tests are used to assess the respiratory status. If the patient has severe paralysis and is expected to have a long recovery period, a gastrostomy tube may be placed to provide adequate nourishment.

Nursing Interventions

Closely monitor respiratory function. If the patient requires mechanical ventilation, be aware that cognition (the mental faculty or process by which knowledge is acquired) is not impaired and that the patient requires reassurance. The patient may also need to be fed intravenously or through a nasogastric tube. Attention to the prevention of complications, such as contractures, pressure ulcers, and loss of ROM, is important to allow complete recovery. Initiate physical therapy early in the course of the disease to prevent contractures. Administer medication to help reduce neuropathic pain, such as gabapentin or a tricyclic antidepressant such as amitriptyline. Assess the patient's vital signs and motor strength frequently. Monitor the patient for signs of hypoxia.

Prognosis

Of the people suffering from GBS, 85% regain complete function. Only 20% of patients have weakness at 1 year and only 5% have severe permanent disability. The recovery period may vary from weeks to years. Those not recovering completely have some degree of permanent neurologic deficit. Generally, recovery from the disease occurs in the reverse order of how the paralysis or weakness occurred.

MENINGITIS

Etiology and Pathophysiology

Meningitis is an acute infection of the meninges. It is usually caused by one of several organisms, including pneumococci, meningococci, *Neisseria meningitidis*, staphylococci, streptococci, *Haemophilus influenzae*, and viral aseptic agents. The bacteria in the subarachnoid space cause an inflammatory reaction in the pia mater, arachnoid and pus accumulation in the CSF and possible injury to nervous tissue.

Meningitis can be classified as bacterial (septic), or viral (aseptic). The incidence of bacterial meningitis is higher in fall and winter when upper respiratory tract infections are common. Pathologic changes that can occur include hyperemia of the meningeal vessels, edema of brain tissue, increased ICP, a generalized inflammatory reaction with exudation of white blood cells into the subarachnoid spaces, and associated hydrocephalus (in infants) caused by exudate occluding the ventricles.

Clinical Manifestations

Two abnormal signs that occur with meningitis are **Kernig's sign** (the inability to extend the legs completely without extreme pain) and **Brudzinski's sign** (flexion of the hip and knee when the neck is flexed). The onset of meningitis is usually sudden and is characterized by severe headache, stiffness of the neck, irritability, malaise, and restlessness. The patient develops nausea and vomiting; delirium; and increased temperature, pulse rate, and respirations.

Diagnostic Tests

A CT of the head is ordered to rule out increased ICP. A lumbar puncture to obtain CSF is performed, unless ICP is increased. The CSF is sent to the laboratory to identify the pathogen responsible for causing the meningitis.

Medical Management

Rapid diagnosis and treatment are crucial in caring for the patient with bacterial meningitis. When meningitis is suspected, cultures are collected and diagnosis is confirmed. Treatment of meningitis includes multiple antibiotics given intravenously over a 2-week period. Medication options include ampicillin, penicillin, piperacillin, and third-generation cephalosporin (usually ceftriaxone [Rocephin] or cefotaxime for treating bacterial meningitis). Corticosteroids (dexamethasone) are given intravenously to decrease ICP. Anticonvulsants are given to prevent seizures. Aseptic (viral) meningitis is treated with supportive therapy, such as maintaining bed rest, ensuring fluid and electrolyte balance, and providing rest and comfort measures (Lower, 2007).

Nursing Interventions

Respiratory isolation is required until the pathogen can no longer be cultured from the nasopharynx. This is usually accomplished after 24 hours of effective antibiotic therapy. Other nursing interventions include the general care given a critically ill patient who may be irritable, disoriented, and unable to take fluids. Dehydration is common, and the patient almost always has an IV line. Keep the room darkened and noise to a minimum because any increase in sensory stimulation may cause a seizure. If the patient is disoriented, take safety precautions. Vigorously manage fever because it increases cerebral edema and the frequency of seizures. In addition, neurologic damage may result from an extremely high temperature over a prolonged time. Acetaminophen may be used to reduce fever. However, if the fever is resistant to acetaminophen, more vigorous means are necessary, such as an automatic cooling blanket (Lewis et al., 2007).

Prophylactic antibiotic therapy for family and friends in close contact with a patient with bacterial meningitis may be recommended to destroy the causative bacteria that may have colonized in the nasopharynx.

Some forms of bacterial meningitis can be prevented by vaccination. The pneumococcal vaccine may be given to adults age 65 and older and other high-risk adults. The meningococcal vaccine is effective against *N. meningitidis* and is recommended for patients ages 11 to 12 and college freshmen living in dormitories. The *H. influenzae* vaccine has significantly decreased meningitis caused by this organism in children (Lewis et al., 2007).

Prognosis

With most cases of meningitis, the prognosis for complete recovery is good. The prognosis depends on the speed with which antibiotics are administered. With severe cases of meningitis, residual neurologic damage or death may occur.

ENCEPHALITIS

Encephalitis is an acute inflammation of the brain and is usually caused by a virus. Many different viruses have been implicated in encephalitis; some are associated with certain seasons of the year and endemic to certain geographic areas. Epidemic encephalitis is transmitted by ticks and mosquitoes. Nonepidemic encephalitis may occur as a complication of measles, chickenpox, or mumps.

Encephalitis is a serious, sometimes fatal disease. Overall mortality rate ranges from 5% to 20%, with the highest mortality rate in encephalitis caused by HSV and the eastern and Venezuelan equine viruses. Unfortunately, HSV encephalitis is the most common form of viral encephalitis. Cytomegalovirus encephalitis is a common complication in patients with AIDS.

Manifestations resemble those of meningitis, but they have a more gradual onset. They include headache, high fever, seizures, and a change in LOC. Early diagnosis and treatment of viral encephalitis are essential for favorable outcomes. Brain imaging techniques such as MRI and PET, along with viral studies of CSF, allow for earlier detection of viral encephalitis.

Medical management and nursing interventions are symptomatic and supportive. Cerebral edema is a major problem, and diuretics (mannitol) and corticosteroids (dexamethasone) are used to control it. The disease is characterized by diffuse damage to the nerve cells of the brain, perivascular cellular infiltration of glial cells, and increasing cerebral edema. The sequelae of encephalitis include mental deterioration, amnesia, personality changes, and hemiparesis.

Acyclovir or vidarabine (Vira-A) are used to treat encephalitis caused by HSV infection. Acyclovir has fewer side effects than vidarabine and is often the preferred treatment. Use of these antiviral agents has been shown to reduce mortality rates from 70% to 30%, although neurologic complications may not be reduced. Long-term symptoms include memory impairment, epilepsy, anosmia, personality changes, behavioral abnormalities, and dysphasia. For maximal benefit, antiviral agents should be started before the onset of coma.

WEST NILE VIRUS

West Nile virus (WNV) has been commonly found in humans and birds and other vertebrates in Africa, Eastern Europe, western Asia, and the Middle East, but it was not documented in the United States until 1999. The virus can infect humans, birds, mosquitoes, horses, and some other animals.

The principal route of human infection with WNV is through the bite of an infected female mosquito. Mosquitoes become infected when they feed on infected birds. When the virus is injected into humans by a mosquito, it can multiply and possibly cause illness. The incubation period ranges from 3 to 14 days. Most people who become infected with the virus do not have any type of illness. Those who develop West Nile fever have flulike manifestations of fever, headache, back pain, myalgia, and anorexia, lasting only a few days and without any long-term health effects. It is estimated that 1 in 150 people infected with WNV develops encephalitis or meningitis, a more severe form of the disease. **WNV meningitis** is usually associated with a sudden onset of febrile illness, headache, chills, neck pain, and sometimes confusion. Patients with **WNV encephalitis** often have fever; headache; altered LOC; disorientation; behavioral and speech disturbances; and other neurologic signs such as hemiparesis, seizures, and coma. Advanced age is the most significant risk factor contributing to death from infection; conditions such as immunosuppression are also contributing factors (Bender, 2003). Even in areas where the virus is circulating, however, few mosquitoes are infected with the virus. The chances of becoming severely ill from any one mosquito bite are extremely small.

The current standard for diagnosing WNV is by testing blood or CSF with the immunoglobulin M (IgM) antibody capture enzyme-linked immunosorbent assay (ELISA) and immunoglobulin G indirect ELISA. The IgM test may not be positive when symptoms first occur; however, it becomes positive in most infected people within days of symptom onset. Someone recently vaccinated against yellow fever or Japanese encephalitis also will have a positive IgM antibody test result.

WNV cannot be transmitted through casual contact such as touching or kissing a person who has the disease. However, in a small number of cases, the virus has been transmitted through blood transfusion, organ transplantation, breastfeeding, and pregnancy (from mother to fetus).

One can reduce the risk of becoming infected with WNV by applying insect repellent to exposed skin. Choose an insect repellent that contains *N,N*-diethyl-3-methylbenzamide (DEET) and one that provides protection for the amount of time to be spent outdoors. Also spray clothing because mosquitoes can bite through thin clothing. Wearing long-sleeved shirts, long pants, and socks while outdoors can reduce the risk. Take special precautions from April to October, the months when mosquitoes are most active.

DEET is the gold standard in currently available over-the-counter insect repellents. DEET was developed in 1946 by the U.S. Army for use by military personnel in insect-infested areas. It has been used worldwide for more than 40 years and has a remarkable safety profile. Toxic reactions can occur, and they are usually linked to misuse of the product, such as massive exposure due to chronic use. Reports of greatest concern involve encephalopathy caused by DEET exposure. Most adverse reactions, though, are less serious, involving eye irritation and inhalation irritation (related to spraying repellent in the eyes or inhaling it).

DEET has been classified as a group D carcinogen (not classifiable as a human carcinogen). For casual use, a 10% to 35% concentration provides adequate protection. The American Academy of Pediatrics recommends limiting DEET repellents to a 30% maximum concentration when used on infants and children. DEET is not recommended for use in children younger than 2 months (Centers for Disease Control and Prevention, 2008).

Other means of decreasing the mosquito population and thus decreasing the possibility of transmission of the WNV include the following (Overstreet, 2004):

- Limit outdoor activities between dusk and dawn.
- Place mosquito netting over infant carriers or strollers when outdoors.
- Keep swimming pools, outdoor saunas, and hot tubs clean and properly chlorinated. Remove standing water from pool covers.
- Store any containers that may become filled with standing water, such as cans, flowerpots, or trash cans, indoors.
- Install or repair window and door screens so that mosquitoes cannot get indoors.

If WNV infection is confirmed, treatment is supportive, intended to manage symptoms, such as headache, fever, and nausea. In more severe cases, patients may need intensive therapy, often involving hospitalization for IV fluids, airway management, respiratory support, and prevention of secondary infections such as pneumonia. To manage WNV encephalitis, the patient may receive interferon alfa-2$_b$, steroids, antiseizure medications, or osmotic diuretics.

Approximately 80% of WNV infections are asymptomatic. Infected people have a transient viremia, making transmission of the virus via donated blood, organs, or tissue possible. As with many viruses, contact with the blood of an infected person could lead to transmission of the virus; therefore use the same standard precautions as with all patients.

Since July 2003, more than 2.5 million blood donations have been screened for WNV. As of September 16, 2003, the Centers for Disease Control and Prevention's surveillance system reported that 601 viremic donations had been identified. Two cases of blood transfusion–associated WNV infection were detected in the United States in 2003—one in Texas and one in Nebraska. Both people were receiving care, including blood transfusions, for other serious health conditions.

They developed encephalitis from the WNV infection; both recovered (Goldrick, 2003).

BRAIN ABSCESS

Brain abscess is an accumulation of pus within the brain tissue that can result from a local or a systemic infection. Direct extension from ear, tooth, mastoid, or sinus infection is the primary cause. Other causes for brain abscess formation include septic venous thrombosis from a pulmonary infection, infective endocarditis, skull fracture, and a nonsterile neurologic procedure. Streptococci and staphylococci are the primary infective organisms.

Clinical manifestations are similar to those of meningitis and encephalitis and include headache and fever. Signs of increased ICP may include drowsiness, confusion, and seizures. Focal symptoms may be present and reflect the local area of the abscess. For example, visual field deficits or psychomotor seizures are common with a temporal lobe abscess, whereas an occipital abscess may be accompanied by visual impairment and hallucinations.

Antimicrobial therapy is the primary treatment for brain abscess. Other manifestations are treated symptomatically. If drug therapy is not effective, the abscess may need to be removed if it is encapsulated. In untreated cases the mortality rate approaches 100%. Seizures occur in approximately 30% of the cases. Nursing interventions are similar to those for management of meningitis or increased ICP. If the abscess is removed surgically, nursing interventions are similar to those described under intracranial tumors.

Other infections of the brain include subdural empyema, osteomyelitis of the cranial bones, epidural abscess, and venous sinus thrombosis after periorbital cellulitis.

ACQUIRED IMMUNODEFICIENCY SYNDROME

Etiology and Pathophysiology

AIDS is a disease that has serious implications for the nervous system, with more than 80% of advanced HIV disease patients having neurologic signs and symptoms. Patients develop neurologic signs and symptoms either from infection with HIV itself or as a result of associated infections. See Chapter 16 for a discussion of advanced HIV disease (AIDS).

Clinical Manifestations

Patients with AIDS may have AIDS dementia complex (ADC), which is known as subacute encephalitis. They may exhibit difficulty concentrating or a recent memory loss, which may progress to a global cognitive dysfunction (generalized impairment of intellect, awareness, and judgment). Patients may also experience opportunistic infections such as meningitis, HSV, cytomegalovirus, toxoplasmosis, and cryptococcal meningitis. Primary malignant lymphomas of the CNS may also develop.

Diagnostic Tests

The diagnostic tests used to determine whether a neurologic problem is related to AIDS include serologic studies, analysis of CSF through a lumbar puncture, CT scan, and MRI. At times, a cerebral biopsy may be necessary to make the differential diagnosis.

Medical Management

Treatment of the patient with neurologic problems related to AIDS depends on the infection. Methods of treatment include administration of antiviral, antifungal, and antibacterial agents. Radiation has been used on the affected part of the brain. Experimental therapies, including iron dextran (DexFerrum), have been tried. Dehydration or shock is treated with fluid volume expanders. Seizures are controlled with diazepam, phenytoin, or fosphenytoin. Mortality remains high despite aggressive therapy.

Nursing Interventions

The patient is likely to be disoriented and may need to be reoriented frequently. Safety measures such as padded side rails may be necessary to prevent injury to the patient, who may have seizures. The patient may experience pain and have difficulty sleeping. Administer medications as needed and structure activities to avoid waking the patient. Visual problems may also be associated with the disease; be careful to orient the patient to nursing interventions.

Most patients with AIDS experience depression and a sense of powerlessness about the disease. They may isolate themselves from others. Encourage patients to talk about their fears and concerns, help them find emotional support, and refer them to a support group. Above all, maintain a nonjudgmental attitude, regardless of how the patient contracted the disease.

The patient may be incontinent of bowel and bladder. Encourage an active bowel and bladder program. If the patient has diarrhea, keep the rectal area as clean and dry as possible and administer antidiarrheals if ordered. The patient may also have nausea. Offer foods that the patient likes in small, frequent meals. Tube feedings or total parenteral nutrition may be needed if the patient agrees.

Prognosis

The prognosis for the patient with AIDS is terminal, often within a short time. Currently, little can be done to substantially lengthen life. After a patient experiences neurologic complications, AIDS is usually fairly well advanced.

BRAIN TUMORS

Etiology and Pathophysiology

Brain tumors include both benign and metastatic lesions. All areas and structures of the brain can be affected. Primary brain tumors, or **neoplasms,** form when changes occur in the genetic structure of normal brain cells (neurons and glial cells). Changes may be caused by a genetic predisposition, an environmental trigger, or both; the causes of most primary brain tumors are unknown. Most benign tumors affect the meninges, whereas most malignant tumors affect the glial cells (Palmieri, 2007b). These tumors include gliomas, meningiomas, pituitary tumors, and neuromas. Metastatic tumors also occur frequently in the brain. Brain tumors are named for the tissues from which they arise.

Assessment

Subjective data include the patient's understanding of the diagnosis, changes in personality or judgment, and abnormal sensations or visual problems. The patient may complain of unusual odors with tumors of the temporal lobe. Also assess headache, nausea or hearing loss, or the inability to carry out daily activities. Patients with brain tumors usually experience headaches as a prominent early symptom. The headache is usually intermittent, moderate to severe, associated with nausea or vomiting, and typically worse in the morning. The patient may also have paresis, diplopia, or weakness (Palmieri, 2007c).

Objective data include motor strength, gait, the level of alertness and consciousness, and orientation. Assess the pupils for response and equality. In some patients, the initial sign of a brain tumor is new-onset seizures; about half of patients have seizure activity at some time during their illness. Other troubling signs of a brain tumor are cognitive changes in memory, speech, concentration, and communication. The patient's family may notice changes in intellectual function, personality, and behavior (Palmieri, 2007b). Speech impairments, cranial nerve abnormalities, and signs and symptoms of increased ICP are also significant.

Diagnostic Tests

No one procedure is entirely diagnostic of brain tumors, but a CT scan is often the basis for the diagnosis. Other tests that may be performed include the brain scan, MRI, PET scans, and the EEG. Arteriography may also be done.

Medical Management

The general method of treatment for brain tumors includes surgical removal when feasible, radiation, and chemotherapy. The choice of therapy is determined by the tumor type and site. A combination of methods is often used. The blood-brain barrier may limit the effectiveness of chemotherapy when used as adjuvant therapy or to treat tumor recurrence (Palmieri, 2007c).

Surgery

A surgical opening through the skull is called a **craniotomy.** After removing the bone, the surgeon makes an incision into the meninges and removes the tumor. The removed bone is carefully preserved and may be replaced at the end of surgery if there is no indication of infection or increased ICP. The removal of part of the skull without replacement is called **craniectomy**. Recent advances have been made in the use of intracranial endoscopy.

Nursing Interventions

Preoperative preparation of both the patient and the family is important. Specific fears may be related to a permanent change in appearance, dependency, and possible death. A baseline neurologic assessment is important. Explain treatments and procedures, including shaving the hair. Usually hair is shaved in the operating room. It is then given to the patient, who may choose to have it made into a wig. Prepare the family for the patient's appearance after surgery.

Postoperative care is determined by the patient's condition. Most patients spend one or two nights in an intensive care unit under close nursing observation with frequent neurologic checks. Assess the patient carefully for indications of increased ICP. The patient may have residual motor or sensory problems as a result of the tumor or surgery.

Nursing diagnoses and interventions for the patient with a brain tumor are the same as those for the patient who has had a stroke, with the addition of but not limited to the following:

Nursing Diagnoses	Nursing Interventions
Disturbed sensory perception: visual, auditory, kinesthetic, tactile, related to compression or displacement of brain tissue	Maintain method of communication. Provide for social environment. Provide orientation and appropriate level of stimuli.
Acute confusion, related to: • altered circulation • destruction of brain tissue	Protect patient from self-injury. Provide soft safety reminder devices as indicated. Assist patient in self-care activities. Speak in kind tone using short, simple sentences. Give one direction at a time. Relate date, time of day, and recent activities. Maintain a therapeutic environment. Keep equipment and personal possessions in same place. Encourage socialization.

Prognosis

The outlook for the patient with a brain tumor depends on whether the tumor is benign or malignant and on its size and location. Tumors that infiltrate the brain usually result in a decreased life span. With radiation and chemotherapy, patients with malignant tumors may live longer.

TRAUMA

Interference with neurologic function can occur as a result of trauma. Parts of the nervous system commonly subjected to trauma include the brain, the spinal cord, and peripheral nerves. Only the first two are discussed in this chapter.

HEAD INJURY

Etiology and Pathophysiology

The term *head trauma* is used primarily to signify craniocerebral trauma, or head injury, which includes an alteration in consciousness, no matter how brief. Head injury is the second most common cause of neurologic injuries and the major cause of death between ages 1 and 35. Previously, the most common causes of head injury in the United States were motor vehicle collisions and falls. Deaths from motor vehicle collisions and falls have decreased; however, firearm-related head injury death rates have increased. Head injury can result from recreational injuries, sports-related trauma, and assaults. The incidence of traumatic brain injury is twice as high in males as in females (Lewis et al., 2007).

Craniocerebral trauma may result in injury to the scalp, skull, and brain tissues. Injuries vary from minor scalp wounds to concussions and open fractures of the skull with severe damage to the brain. The amount of obvious damage is not indicative of the seriousness of the trouble. Effects of severe head injury include cerebral edema, sensory and motor deficits, and increased ICP.

Injuries to the brain can result from direct or indirect trauma to the head. Indirect trauma is caused by tension strains and shearing forces transmitted to the head by stretching the neck. Direct trauma occurs when the head is directly injured. Indirect trauma results in an **acceleration-deceleration** injury, with rotation of the skull and its contents. Bruising or contusion of the occipital and frontal lobes, the brainstem, and the cerebellum may occur.

Clinical Manifestations

Head injuries may be open or closed. Open head injuries result from skull fractures or penetrating wounds. The amount of injury with this type of wound is determined by the velocity, mass, shape, and direction of the impact. A skull fracture (linear, comminuted, depressed, or compound) may also occur. Fractures of the base of the skull are more serious because they are near the medulla.

Closed head injuries include concussions (a violent jarring of the brain against the skull), contusions, and lacerations. Lacerations of the scalp bleed profusely because of the vascularity in the region. Hemorrhage resulting from craniocerebral trauma may occur in the scalp or the epidural, subdural, intracerebral, and intraventricular areas. Epidural and subdural hematomas require careful and continuous observation. Epidural hematomas resulting from arterial bleeding form as blood collects rapidly between the dura and skull. If lethargy or unconsciousness develops after the patient regains consciousness, an epidural hematoma may be suspected and needs immediate treatment.

A subdural hematoma forms as venous blood collects below the dura. Because the bleeding is under venous pressure, the hematoma formation is relatively slow. The clot causes pressure on the brain surface and displaces brain tissue. If a patient who has been conscious for several days after head injury loses consciousness or develops neurologic signs and symptoms, suspect a subdural hematoma. Subdural hematomas may be classified as acute, subacute, or chronic.

Assessment

Subjective data include the patient's understanding of the injury and the resulting pathologic processes. Determine how the injury happened and whether the patient has headache, nausea, or vomiting. Note abnormal sensations and a history of LOC and of bleeding from any orifice.

Objective data include the status of the respiratory system, level of alertness and consciousness, and size and reactivity of the pupils; check these frequently. Also assess the patient's orientation, motor status, vital signs, bleeding or vomiting, and abnormal speech patterns. The presence of **Battle's sign** (a small hemorrhagic spot behind the ear) usually indicates a fracture of a bone of the lower skull (Figure 14-23).

Diagnostic Tests

CT, MRI, and PET scans are the primary diagnostic imaging examinations in assessing soft tissue injuries.

Medical Management

Immediate care of the patient with a head injury is directed toward lifesaving measures and the maintenance of normal body function until recovery is ensured. It is extremely important to maintain a patent airway and ensure adequate oxygenation. Suctioning may be necessary (but never through the nose because of the possibility of a skull fracture), along with the administration of oxygen. Check ABG levels. Stabilize the cervical spine; assume neck injury with head injury until diagnostic examination proves otherwise.

Medications are used to reduce cerebral edema and increased ICP, which are common problems in patients with head injuries. Medications include mannitol and dexamethasone. Pegorgotein, a scavenger of oxygen-derived free radicals, has been used experimentally. Codeine or other analgesics that do not de-

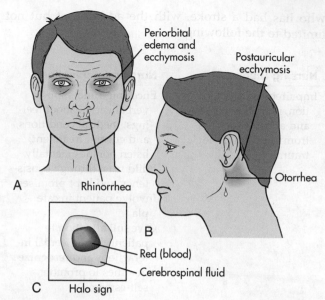

FIGURE 14-23 **A,** Raccoon eyes and rhinorrhea. **B,** Battle's sign (postauricular ecchymosis) with otorrhea. **C,** Halo or ring sign.

press the respiratory system are used for pain control. Anticonvulsants may be given to prevent seizures. Take measures to control elevated temperatures, since hyperthermia increases brain metabolism, resulting in brain damage.

Nursing Interventions

Check the patient's ears and nose carefully for signs of blood and serous drainage, which indicate that the meninges are torn and spinal fluid is escaping. *Do not attempt to clean out the orifice.* If there is evidence of drainage from the nose, the patient should not cough, sneeze, or blow the nose. If there is a question about whether drainage is CSF, Tes-Tape will show a positive reaction for glucose. Meningitis is a possible complication when communication with the meninges and the nose or ears occurs.

The patient with a head injury often shows a loss of memory and loss of initiative. Behavioral problems associated with a lack of judgment and restlessness may also occur. Restlessness may be caused by the need for a change of position, pain, or the need to empty the bladder. These patients require firm but gentle care, with specific guidelines for what behavior is allowed. Medications to decrease agitation may be needed. It is not helpful to argue with patients, but redirecting their attention may help. Memory aids such as a log book or written schedule can assist with orientation.

The length of convalescence depends on the amount of brain damage and how rapid the recovery is. Many patients with head injury recover physically but have behavioral and psychological problems that make it difficult for them to function independently.

A nursing diagnosis and interventions for the patient with a head injury are the same as for the patient who has had a stroke, with the addition of but not limited to the following:

Nursing Diagnosis	Nursing Interventions
Impaired social interaction, related to cognitive and affective deficits from neurophysiologic trauma	Encourage and support verbalization about feelings, medical conditions, and current treatment; listen nonjudgmentally. Build trust through consistency and kept promises. Involve patient in care plan. Give full attention to patient during verbal interactions and recognize qualities to promote self-esteem.

Patient Teaching

A patient with a mild head injury may be seen in the emergency department but not be admitted to the hospital. Teach the patient about observations for complications such as increased drowsiness, nausea, vomiting, worsening headache or stiff neck, seizures, blurred vision, behavioral changes, motor problems, sensory disturbances, or decreased heart rate. Teaching for patients with a head injury who have residual deficits severe enough to require rehabilitation is similar to that needed for patients with motor or sensory problems.

Prognosis

The outcome for a patient with a head injury is often unpredictable. The extent of damage or recovery is not positively correlated with the amount of damage seen in surgery or on CT scan. Even minor head injuries can have residual effects. The person with a head injury is more prone to injuries and problems related to the brain damage.

SPINAL CORD TRAUMA

Etiology and Pathophysiology

Spinal cord injury from accidents is a common and increasing cause of serious disability and death. Approximately 10% of traumatic injuries to the nervous system involve the spinal cord. Most people involved with spinal cord injuries are men between 18 and 25 years of age. Automobile, motorcycle, diving, surfing, and other athletic accidents and gunshot wounds are major causes of spinal cord injury.

The soft tissue of the spinal cord is protected by the vertebral column. Injuries to this column include a simple fracture, compressed or wedge fracture, comminuted or burst fracture, or dislocation of the vertebrae (Figure 14-24). As a result, the cord is often damaged. Severe traumatic lesions of the spinal cord may result in total transection of the spinal cord or tearing

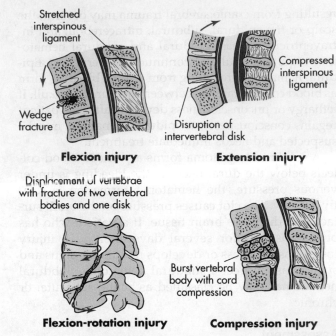

FIGURE 14-24 Mechanisms of spinal injury.

of the cord from side to side at a particular level, with a complete loss of spinal cord function. This total transection is also called a **complete cord injury.** With this type of injury, all voluntary movement below the level of the trauma is lost. A partial transection, or **incomplete injury,** of the cord may also occur. Tetraplegic patients (formerly referred to as quadriplegic) are those who sustain injuries to one of the cervical segments of the spinal cord. Paraplegic patients are those whose lesions are confined to the thoracic, lumbar, or sacral segments of the spinal cord. The signs and symptoms of an incomplete injury vary (Table 14-9).

Clinical Manifestations

Initially, in most spinal cord injuries, there is a period of flaccid paralysis and a complete loss of reflexes below the level of trauma. Sensory and autonomic functions are also lost. The loss of systemic sympathetic vasomotor tone may result in vasodilation, increased venous capacity, and hypotension. This is called areflexia, or spinal shock, and is temporary. During this time the patient may need temporary respiratory support.

One important complication of spinal cord injury is autonomic dysreflexia or hyperreflexia, a neurologic condition characterized by increased reflex actions. It occurs in patients with cord injuries at the sixth thoracic vertebra or higher and most commonly in patients with cervical injuries. Autonomic dysreflexia is an abnormal cardiovascular response to stimulation of the sympathetic division of the autonomic nervous system; the condition occurs as a result of stimulation of the bladder, large intestine, or other visceral organs (Figure 14-25). The clinical signs include severe bradycardia, hypertension (systolic blood pressure up to 300 mm Hg),

Table 14-9 Functional Level of Spinal Cord Injury and Rehabilitation Potential

LEVEL OF INJURY	MOVEMENT REMAINING	REHABILITATION POTENTIAL
TETRAPLEGIA **C1-C3** Often fatal injury, vagus nerve domination of heart, respiration, blood vessels, and all organs below injury	Movement in neck and above, loss of innervation to diaphragm, absence of independent respiratory function	Ability to drive electric wheelchair equipped with portable ventilator by using chin control or mouth stick, headrest to stabilize head; computer use with mouth stick, head wand, or noise control; 24-hour attendant care, able to instruct others
C4 Vagus nerve domination of heart, respirations, and all vessels and organs below injury	Sensation and movement in neck and above; may be able to breathe without a ventilator	Same as C1-C3
C5 Vagus nerve domination of heart, respirations, and all vessels and organs below injury	Full neck, partial shoulder, back, biceps; gross elbow, inability to roll over or use hands; decreased respiratory reserve	Ability to drive electric wheelchair with mobile hand supports; indoor mobility in manual wheelchair; able to feed self with setup and adaptive equipment; attendant care 10 hr/day
C6 Vagus nerve domination of heart, respirations, and all vessels and organs below injury	Shoulder and upper back abduction and rotation at shoulder, full biceps to elbow flexion, wrist extension, weak grasp of thumb, decreased respiratory reserve	Ability to assist with transfer and perform some self-care; feed self with hand devices; push wheelchair on smooth, flat surface; drive adapted van from wheelchair; independent computer use with adaptive equipment; attendant care 6 hr/day
C7-C8 Vagus nerve domination of heart, respirations, and all vessels and organs below injury	All triceps to elbow extension, finger extensors and flexors, good grasp with some decreased strength, decreased respiratory reserve	Ability to transfer self to wheelchair; roll over and sit up in bed; push self on most surfaces; perform most self-care; independent use of wheelchair; ability to drive car with powered hand controls (in some patients); attendant care 0-6 hr/day
PARAPLEGIA **T1-T6** Sympathetic innervation to heart, vagus nerve domination of all vessels and organs below injury	Full innervation of upper extremities, back, essential intrinsic muscles of hand; full strength and dexterity of grasp; decreased trunk stability, decreased respiratory reserve	Full independence in self-care and in wheelchair; ability to drive car with hand controls (in most patients); independent standing in standing frame
T6-T12 Vagus nerve domination only of leg vessels, GI and genitourinary organs	Full, stable thoracic muscles and upper back; functional intercostals, resulting in increased respiratory reserve	Full independent use of wheelchair; ability to stand erect with full leg brace, ambulate on crutches with swing (although gait difficult); inability to climb stairs
L1-L2 Vagus nerve domination of leg vessels	Varying control of legs and pelvis, instability of lower back	Good sitting balance; full use of wheelchair; ambulation with long leg braces
L3-L4 Partial vagus nerve domination of leg vessels, GI and genitourinary organs	Quadriceps and hip flexors, absence of hamstring function, flail ankles	Completely independent ambulation with short leg braces and canes; inability to stand for long periods

From Lewis, S.L., et al. (2007). *Medical-surgical nursing: assessment and management of clinical problems.* (7th ed.). St. Louis: Mosby.
GI, Gastrointestinal.

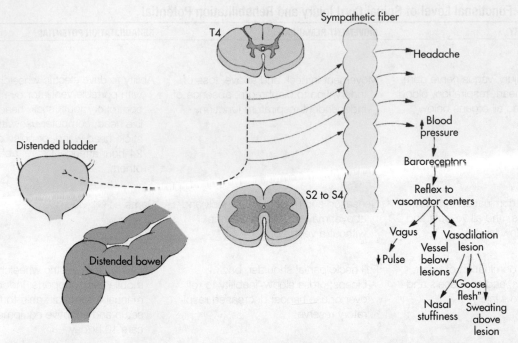

FIGURE 14-25 Pictorial diagram of cause of autonomic hyperreflexia (dysreflexia) and results.

diaphoresis, "goose flesh," flushing (above the level of the lesion), dilated pupils, blurred vision, restlessness, nausea, severe headache, and nasal stuffiness. Patients tend to develop individual signs and symptoms of this condition and are soon able to recognize them. The most common causes of this condition include a distended bladder or a fecal impaction. It is a medical emergency that requires immediate treatment to prevent a stroke, blindness, or death (Box 14-4).

In most cases of spinal cord injury, men experience impotence, decreased sensation, and difficulties with ejaculation. Impaired fertility is common. The experience of orgasm is described as different than before the injury. Women with spinal cord injury are able to continue to perform sexually, although perception of sexual pleasure is usually altered.

Assessment

Subjective data include information about the nature of the injury, any dyspnea, and unusual sensations. The presence of pain, any loss of consciousness, and the absence of sensation on sensory examination are important to assess.

Objective data include the level of alertness and consciousness; orientation; pupil size and reactivity; motor strength; skin integrity; and bowel and bladder status, including distention. Assess for other injuries, such as fractured bones or head injury.

Diagnostic Tests

Radiographs are often taken first to detect any cervical vertebra fracture or displacement. A spinal tap or myelogram may also be done to detect occlusion. A CT scan and MRI may help rule out spinal cord injury.

Box 14-4 **Emergency Care for Autonomic Dysreflexia or Hyperreflexia**

- Unless contraindicated, place patient in sitting position to decrease blood pressure.
- Check patency of catheter for kinking. If catheter is occluded, insert new catheter immediately.
- Check rectum for impaction.
- If it is necessary to remove impaction, use an anesthetic ointment.
- Administer ganglionic blocking agent such as hexamethonium or a vasodilator such as nitroprusside (Nipride) as ordered if conservative measures are not effective.
- Continue monitoring blood pressure.
- Send urine for culture if no other cause is found; urinary tract infection can lead to symptoms of autonomic dysreflexia.

Medical Management

Immediate care after spinal cord injury is directed toward realignment of the bony column in the presence of fractures or dislocations. This may involve simple immobilization, skeletal traction, or surgery for spinal decompression. Skeletal traction may include Crutchfield tongs (Figure 14-26), halo traction (see Chapter 4), or a Stryker or Foster frame. Bracing may be used for thoracic or lumbar injuries. Often surgical decompression is not performed until after a period of skeletal traction if the injury involves the cervical region. In patients seen within 8 hours of injury, high-dose methylprednisolone is given.

Nursing Interventions and Patient Teaching

Throughout all stages of hospitalization of the patient with a spinal cord injury, nursing and medical interventions are directed toward restoring structural or body

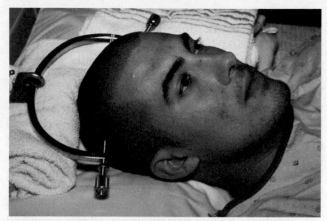

FIGURE 14-26 Patient with Crutchfield tongs inserted into skull to hyperextend.

integrity. All efforts are taken to ensure that the skin is intact, that contractures do not develop, and that ROM is maintained. Early mobilization is important. When patients, especially those with tetraplegia, begin to sit up, it may be necessary to wrap the legs with thromboembolism stockings to encourage venous return. Slowly increasing the angle of sitting up is essential to prevent hypotension. A recliner wheelchair is usually necessary.

Usually a Foley catheter is inserted initially; later bladder training is started (see Chapter 10). Chronic indwelling catheterization increases the risk of infection. Intermittent catheterization should begin as early as possible. This helps maintain bladder tone and decreases the risk of infection. Encourage fluid intake of more than 2000 mL/day. Encourage cranberry juice to decrease renal calculi formation.

Patients are usually started on a bowel program early in their hospital stay. At first, bisacodyl suppositories are given at regular intervals (usually every other night). This is followed by digital stimulation to promote peristalsis. The goal is to eliminate the need for suppositories. Other aids to bowel programs are the use of adequate fluids (usually at least 3000 to 4000 mL/day, unless contraindicated), stool softeners, and prune juice.

Nursing diagnoses and interventions for the patient with a spinal cord injury are the same as those for the patient with a motor or sensory problem, with the addition of but not limited to the following:

Nursing Diagnoses	Nursing Interventions
Autonomic dysreflexia, related to neurophysiologic trauma to spinal cord above sixth thoracic vertebra	See Box 14-4 for emergency interventions.
Impaired urinary elimination, related to sensory-motor impairment	Check carefully for voiding and for distention of bladder. Teach patient intermittent self-catheterization if indicated. Teach patient Crede's maneuver as indicated.

Nursing Diagnoses	Nursing Interventions
	Use Foley catheter if indicated; administer meticulous aseptic technique in changing catheters. Teach patients signs of infection. Encourage patient to have a genitourinary checkup at least yearly. Maintain fluid intake of 3000 to 4000 mL/day unless contraindicated. Use adult perineal protector for incontinency, if necessary.

Teaching of the patient with a spinal cord injury includes education about autonomic dysreflexia and about sexual functioning after spinal cord injury. Other teaching points are found in the sections of this chapter dealing with the patient with motor or sensory problems.

Prognosis

In cases of a complete spinal cord injury, there is almost no chance of return of any function. However, the paraplegic or tetraplegic patient can live a satisfying life with adaptations and assistance. Today, with improved treatment strategies (specifically, intermittent catheterization), even the very young patient with a spinal cord injury can anticipate a long life. The prognosis for life is generally only about 5 years less than for people of the same age without spinal cord injury. Take care to prevent infections, such as urinary tract or respiratory tract infections. With patients with incomplete cord lesions, the amount of function regained is variable and often unpredictable.

❖ **NURSING *PROCESS* for the Patient with a Neurologic Disorder**

The role of the licensed practical nurse/licensed vocational nurse (LPN/LVN) in the nursing process as stated is that the LPN/LVN will:

- Participate in planning care for patients based on patient needs
- Review patient's plan of care and recommend revisions as needed
- Review and follow defined prioritization for patient care
- Use clinical pathways, care maps, or care plans to guide and review patient care

■ **Assessment**

People with neurologic deficits require skilled assessment by both a nurse and a physician. Assessment includes observing the patient during the patient history. Nursing assessment is an ongoing process and should be tailored to meet the patient's needs. For example, hourly neurologic checks will not be as detailed as the initial assessment.

While interviewing the patient, obtain data about subjective complaints, such as pain, dizziness, or vision difficulties. Also assess the ability to speak and reason. Observations may also include vital signs, data about gait, symmetry of body parts, evidence of pain, or seizure activity. During ongoing assessments, data are usually obtained about pupil size, level of alertness, ability to perform motor tasks, changes in LOC, and ability to speak. Because subtle changes in neurologic status can often be the first sign of a complication, be alert for small changes in the neurologic assessment and report these to the proper person.

■ **Nursing Diagnosis**

Nursing assessment helps identify the patient's needs for care and observation. The actual care of the patient is then based on the nursing diagnoses that have been identified. Possible nursing diagnoses for a patient with a neurologic disorder include but are not limited to the following:

- Autonomic dysreflexia
- Impaired verbal communication
- Compromised family coping
- Risk for disuse syndrome
- Risk for falls
- Grieving
- Risk for infection
- Deficient knowledge
- Impaired memory
- Impaired physical mobility
- Imbalanced nutrition: less than body requirement
- Acute pain
- Chronic pain
- Bathing/hygiene self-care deficit
- Feeding self-care deficit
- Toileting self-care deficit
- Impaired swallowing
- Acute confusion
- Ineffective tissue perfusion (cerebral)

■ **Expected Outcomes and Planning**

The plan for providing neurologic assessment and care should focus on the type of deficit the patient is experiencing and possible complications. Consider a patient's preferences and mental status. The type of care required determines the supplies and equipment needed. Schedule necessary care around tests and procedures and the patient's need for rest.

The care plan focuses on achieving specific goals and outcomes that relate to the identified nursing diagnosis. Examples of these include the following:

Goal 1: Patient's cerebral perfusion will be maintained.

Outcome: Patient remains awake, alert, and oriented; coma scale score remains the same or improves.

Goal 2: Patient will maintain optimal nutrition.

Outcome: Patient maintains or attains optimal weight, and laboratory values indicating nutritional health are within normal limits.

■ **Implementation**

Nursing interventions for the patient with a neurologic disorder include those that maintain cerebral perfusion and other functioning, as well as those that prevent complications such as decubitus, falls, or contractures. Certain principles guide nurses in providing neurologic care:

- The neurologic system is a complex system that produces a wide variety of neurologic signs and symptoms.
- Identical disorders may result in different sets of signs and symptoms in different patients.
- The maintenance of cerebral perfusion is of utmost importance.
- The patient with a neurologic illness is prone to complications.
- Disorders of the nervous system produce physical problems and a wide variety of cognitive difficulties.

While providing care to meet the patient's specific challenges, also assess the patient's readiness to learn. At times the family must receive the primary teaching because the patient is unable to understand. Consider the patient's preferences and background in delivering care. Encourage the patient to be as independent as possible and give appropriate feedback. Preserve the patient's dignity and privacy whenever possible. Also consider the special needs of older patients (see Life Span Considerations box, p. 656).

■ **Evaluation**

Evaluate the success of planned interventions during and after care is given. The process is ongoing and dynamic because the patient's condition often changes. Always be ready to revise the care plan as needed. For example, if a patient has new episodes of confusion after surgery, notify the physician, increase safety measures, and assess more frequently.

Ongoing systematic evaluation requires determining whether specific outcomes have been met. The evaluation is specific to measure the goals identified. Examples of goals and their corresponding evaluative measures include the following:

Goal 1: Patient will be free of infection.

Evaluative measure: Assess patient for any signs of infection such as increased temperature, frequency of urination, erythematous incision, elevated white blood cell count, or confusion.

Goal 2: Patient will remain clear and oriented in thought processes.

Evaluative measure: Ask patient to respond to orientation questions. Observe ability to engage in conversation and to carry out care activities.

Get Ready for the NCLEX® Examination!

Key Points

- The nervous system is the body's link with the environment. It allows the interpretation of information and appropriate action.
- The two main structural divisions of the nervous system are the CNS and the peripheral nervous system.
- The CNS is composed of the brain and the spinal cord.
- The peripheral nervous system is composed of the nerve cells lying outside of the CNS. It is divided into the somatic nervous system and the autonomic nervous system.
- A nerve cell is composed of three parts: the dendrite, the cell body, and the axon.
- The brain and the spinal cord are protected by the bony coverings (skull and vertebral column), the CSF, and the three meninges (pia mater, arachnoid, and dura mater).
- The cerebrum is the largest part of the brain and contains five major areas: motor, sensory, visual, speech, and auditory. The cerebrum governs the ability to reason and make judgments.
- The diencephalon lies beneath the cerebrum and contains the thalamus and hypothalamus. The thalamus serves as a relay station. The hypothalamus has several roles, such as temperature control, water balance, and appetite.
- The cerebellum is the second largest portion of the brain and is responsible for coordination of skeletal muscles and maintenance of balance and equilibrium.
- The peripheral nervous system is composed of the cranial nerves, the spinal nerves, the somatic nervous system and the autonomic nervous system.
- The autonomic nervous system contains two subdivisions: the sympathetic nervous system and the parasympathetic nervous system. The sympathetic nervous system speeds things up, and the parasympathetic nervous system slows things down.
- Normal changes of aging are not the same as senility, AD, or organic brain damage.
- The source of any headache should be determined through neurologic testing because it may be a symptom of a serious pathologic condition.
- A lumbar puncture should not be done if there is evidence of increased ICP because of the danger of brain herniation.
- Any increase in the volume of one of the contents of the cranium (brain, blood vessels, and CSF) results in increased ICP because the cranial vault is rigid and does not expand.
- Classic signs of increased ICP include restlessness, disorientation, headache, contralateral hemiparesis, an ipsilaterally dilated pupil, and visual changes that include blurring and diplopia.
- Nursing intervention measures can significantly influence ICP.

- Epilepsy is a transitory disturbance in consciousness or in motor, sensory, or autonomic functions with or without loss of consciousness, caused by sudden, excessive, and disorderly electrical discharges of the brain.
- Early signs and symptoms of MS are usually transitory.
- Stroke, or "brain attack," is the most common disease of the nervous system and can be caused by thrombus, embolus, or hemorrhage. The term *brain attack* is used to describe stroke and communicates the urgency of recognizing stroke signs and symptoms and treating their onset as a medical emergency, just as one would with a myocardial infarction.
- The MERCI device can be used for up to 8 hours after acute stroke onset to remove blood clots from arteries deep inside the brain.
- Helpful nursing interventions for the patient with AD include using nonverbal cues or demonstrations as adjuncts to verbal cues, providing few choices, and not hurrying the patient.
- Trigeminal neuralgia (tic douloureux) is characterized by excruciating, burning pain that radiates along one or more of the three divisions of the fifth cranial nerve.
- With Bell's palsy, there is usually an abrupt onset of numbness, a feeling of stiffness, or a drawing sensation of the face.
- Of the people suffering from GBS, 85% regain complete function.
- Approximately 80% of patients with advanced HIV disease (AIDS) have neurologic symptoms that result from infection from HIV itself or from associated complications of the disease.
- Many patients with head injury may recover physically, but they will have behavioral and psychological problems that make it difficult for them to function independently.
- The signs and symptoms of intracranial tumors result from both local and general effects of the tumor.
- Autonomic dysreflexia in the patient with spinal cord injury is a medical emergency that demands quick nursing interventions.
- The first sign of increased ICP may be a declining state of consciousness.
- It is important to document patients' behaviors in terms of what is seen, not what is inferred.
- It is estimated that 1 in 150 people infected with WNV will develop encephalitis or meningitis, a more severe form of the disease.

Additional Learning Resources

Go to your Companion CD for an audio glossary, animations, video clips, and more.

evolve   Be sure to visit the Evolve site at http://evolve.elsevier.com/Christensen/adult/ for additional online resources.

Review Questions for the NCLEX® Examination

1. A patient is admitted to the hospital with the diagnosis of transient ischemic attack. What normal change of aging would the nurse expect to see in this 90-year-old man?

   1. Increased sense of touch
   2. Diminished long-term memory
   3. Increased reflex time
   4. Decreased fine motor coordination

2. A 35-year-old patient is being seen for complaints of headache, which she has experienced for the past month. Her physician wants to rule out a brain tumor. In this case, what diagnostic test is contraindicated?

   1. Brain scan
   2. PET scan
   3. Lumbar puncture
   4. Electroencephalography

3. A nurse in the emergency department of her community hospital is teaching a group of sixth graders how to prevent head and spine injuries. Teaching would include all but:

   1. use of helmets for bicycles, motorcycles, and skateboarding.
   2. use of a lumbar support for sports activities.
   3. safe handling and storage of guns.
   4. use of seatbelts and shoulder harnesses in a car.

4. A 70-year-old with back pain is scheduled to have a myelogram in the morning to rule out a pathologic condition of the spine. In preparing him for the procedure, what information is important to share?

   1. That mental status will be assessed frequently
   2. That the patient will lie completely supine and still during the procedure
   3. That the patient will be able to ambulate immediately after the test
   4. That strengths of the lower extremities will be assessed frequently

5. The nursing assessment of an 80-year-old who has had a stroke found that she had difficulty swallowing. A videofluoroscopy with barium was performed to rule out aspiration. The rehabilitation team in the skilled nursing facility determined that she can eat a soft diet with one-to-one supervision. Which is important to prevent aspiration?

   1. Tipping the head toward the unaffected side while swallowing
   2. Extending the head during swallowing
   3. Mixing solids and liquids to facilitate swallowing
   4. Encouraging the patient to take large bites to make swallowing easier

6. A 12-year-old student has a history of generalized tonic-clonic seizures. The school nurse educates his classmates about his seizure activity by telling them:

   1. he will be normal immediately after the seizure.
   2. it is important to place a tongue blade in his mouth during the seizure.

3. his desk should be placed in a corner of the room by himself.
4. he may cry out at the beginning of a seizure.

7. The patient was involved in a snowmobile accident. On admission to the emergency department, he is receiving oxygen and is intubated. His Glasgow coma scale score is 6. About 10 minutes after arrival, he is noted to have a widened pulse pressure, increased systolic blood pressure, and bradycardia. These signs are considered an important diagnostic sign of late stage increased ICP. Together they are known as:

   1. anisocoria.
   2. supratentorial shift.
   3. Cushing's response.
   4. medullary reflex.

8. A 76-year-old who has had Parkinson's disease for the past 6 years has now been admitted to a nursing home. The nurse doing the admission interview and assessment notices which characteristic sign of the disease?

   1. Bradykinesia
   2. Increased postural reflexes
   3. Sensory loss
   4. Intention tremor

9. A 13-year-old student is admitted to the pediatric unit with possible meningitis. The nurse finds that the patient cannot extend her legs completely without experiencing extreme pain. The nurse knows that this is an indication of meningitis and is called:

   1. Brudzinski's sign.
   2. Battle's sign.
   3. Kernig's sign.
   4. Cosgrow's sign.

10. A patient is diagnosed with Bell's palsy as indicated by a feeling of stiffness and a drawing sensation of the face. What is important to teach her about the disease?

    1. There is a heightened awareness of taste, so foods must be bland.
    2. There may be an increased sensitivity to sound.
    3. The eye is susceptible to injury if the eyelid does not close.
    4. Drooling from increased saliva on the affected side may occur.

11. What is the first nursing intervention for a patient with autonomic dysreflexia?

    1. Sit the patient upright, if permitted.
    2. Check for bowel impaction.
    3. Give medication as ordered.
    4. Place the patient in supine position.

12. When teaching the patient with Parkinson's disease, which response would indicate the need for further education?

    1. "If I miss an occasional dose of the medication, it doesn't matter much."
    2. "I need to exercise at least some every day."

3. "I need to be sitting straight up with my chin slightly tucked so I won't choke when I eat or drink."

4. "I should eat a diet high in fiber and roughage to decrease my constipation."

13. Important nursing interventions for a patient with sensory dysfunction are: *(Select all that apply.)*

1. teaching the patient protective measures in relation to the sensory deficit.

2. inspecting parts of the body that have no feeling to ascertain any impairment of skin integrity.

3. having the patient practice scanning the printed page.

4. keeping the patient warm with the use of heating pads.

14. When injury to the spinal cord is in the cervical region, the resultant complication would be:

1. tetraplegia.

2. hemiplegia.

3. paraplegia.

4. paresthesia.

15. The nurse determines that a patient is unconscious when the patient:

1. has cerebral ischemia.

2. responds only to painful stimuli.

3. is unaware of self or environment.

4. does not respond to verbal stimuli.

16. The nurse plans care for the patient with increased intracranial pressure with the knowledge that the best way to position the patient is to:

1. keep the head of the bed flat.

2. maintain the head of the bed at 30 degrees.

3. increase the head of the bed's angle to 30 degrees with patient on left side.

4. use a continuous-rotation bed to continuously change patient position.

17. During admission of a patient with a severe head injury to the emergency department, the nurse places the highest priority on assessment for:

1. patency of airway.

2. presence of a neck injury.

3. neurologic status with the Glasgow coma scale.

4. cerebrospinal fluid leakage from the ears or nose.

18. The primary goal of nursing interventions after a craniotomy is:

1. preventing infection.

2. ensuring patient comfort.

3. avoiding need for secondary surgery.

4. preventing increased intracranial pressure.

19. A right-handed patient with right-sided hemiplegia and aphasia resulting from a stroke most likely has a lesion in the:

1. left frontal lobe.

2. right brainstem.

3. motor areas of the right cerebrum.

4. medial superior area of the temporal lobe.

20. A patient experiencing TIAs is scheduled for a carotid endarterectomy. The nurse explains that this procedure is done to:

1. promote cerebral flow to decrease cerebral edema.

2. reduce the brain damage that occurs during a stroke-in-evolution.

3. prevent a stroke by removing atherosclerotic plaques obstructing cerebral blood flow.

4. provide a circulatory bypass around thrombotic plaques obstructing cranial circulation.

21. A 69-year-old patient has been admitted to the medical floor with a diagnosis of Parkinson's disease. His nursing interventions will include: *(Select all that apply.)*

1. encouraging activities to increase his speed for doing ADLs.

2. care during feeding to prevent aspiration.

3. providing means for disposal of facial tissues.

4. diet high in fiber and generous fluid intake.

Matching

Column A	Column B
22. _____ MRI	a. Optic disk is edematous "choked disk"
23. _____ Myelography	b. Involuntary rhythmic movement of the eyes; oscillations that are horizontal, vertical, or mixed
24. _____ Babinski's sign	
25. _____ Nystagmus	
26. _____ Papilledema	c. Use of magnetic forces to image body structures
	d. Backward flexion of the great toe due to an abnormal CNS condition
	e. Diagnostic procedure done to identify tumors of the spinal cord or herniated nucleus pulposus by observing flow of Amipaque dye

27. Which sign or symptom of late-stage increased intracranial pressure should the LPN/LVN be aware of? *(Select all that apply.)*

1. Increase in systolic blood pressure

2. Widening of pulse pressure

3. Bradycardia

4. Unequal pupils that react slowly to light

5. Tachycardia

28. The nursing interventions that would be appropriate and beneficial to a patient who has had a stroke with right-sided hemiplegia and expressive aphasia include: *(Select all that apply.)*

1. stating questions so that the patient can verbalize freely to articulate his needs.

2. encouraging self-help, such as bathing.

3. remaining calm and conversing in an intelligent manner.

4. performing ROM to all extremities every shift.

29. The nurse is teaching patients with potential aspiration problems airway protective techniques during swallowing. Which procedures should be taught? *(Select all that apply.)*

    1. Chin tuck
    2. Double swallow
    3. Full Fowler's position
    4. Use of a straw
    5. Soft or pureed foods

30. The pathophysiology of myasthenia gravis is caused by:

    1. myelin sheath breakdown.
    2. degeneration of the dopamine-producing neurons in the midbrain.
    3. antibodies attacking the acetylcholine receptors, damaging them, and reducing their number.
    4. inflammation of cranial nerve VII.

31. A graphic recording of the electrical conduction activities of the brain that is a helpful diagnostic tool for a patient with seizures is called:

    1. ECG.
    2. MRI.
    3. PET.
    4. EEG.

32. The condition that involves cranial nerve VII that results in tenderness to the posterior ear, followed by paralysis of the facial muscles unilaterally with ptosis of the eyelid and mouth pulled to the opposite side of the face, is:

    1. trigeminal neuralgia.
    2. Bell's palsy.
    3. Romberg.
    4. proprioception.

33. Two of the more effective therapies that lead to faster recuperation for the patient with Guillain-Barré syndrome are:

    1. Avonex and Betaseron.
    2. thymectomy and Zarontin.
    3. Depakote and Zarontin.
    4. plasmapheresis and intravenous immune globulin.

34. Select patients with acute ischemic stroke can benefit from:

    1. IV Tensilon in the first 3 hours.
    2. anticholinesterase in the first 3 hours.
    3. thrombolytics such as t-PA in the first 3 hours.
    4. intravenous immune globulin in the first 3 hours.

35. The primary goals of the nurse and the family caring for a patient having a seizure do not include: *(Select all that apply.)*

    1. protection from aspiration.
    2. protection from injury.
    3. recording of seizure activity.
    4. gently restraining to prevent injury.

36. Parkinson's disease is caused by:

    1. myelin sheath pathologic condition.
    2. damage or loss of the dopamine-producing cells of the midbrain, leading to dopamine depletion in the basal ganglia.
    3. depletion of the neurotransmitter acetylcholine resulting in muscular weakness.
    4. presence of atheroma in arterial walls.

37. A nonablative surgical treatment in selected patients with Parkinson's disease in which stimulation wires are placed in the thalamus, globus pallidus, or subthalamic nucleus to improve dyskinesias, rigidity, bradykinesia, tremor, and overall motor function is:

    1. deep brain stimulation.
    2. MERCI retriever.
    3. vagal nerve stimulation.
    4. disconnection surgery.

Care of the Patient with an Immune Disorder

Barbara Lauritsen Christensen

Objectives

1. Differentiate between natural and acquired immunity.
2. Compare and contrast humoral and cell-mediated immunity.
3. Explain the concepts of immunocompetence, immunodeficiency, and autoimmunity.
4. Review the mechanisms of immune response.
5. Discuss five factors that influence the development of hypersensitivity.
6. Identify the clinical manifestations of anaphylaxis.
7. Outline the immediate aggressive treatment of systemic anaphylactic reaction.
8. Discuss the two types of latex allergies and recommendations for preventing allergic reactions to latex in the workplace.
9. Discuss selection of blood donors, typing and crossmatching, storage, and administration in preventing transfusion reaction.
10. Explain an immunodeficiency disease.
11. Discuss the cause of autoimmune disorders.
12. Explain plasmapheresis in the treatment of autoimmune diseases.

Key Terms

adaptive immunity (ă-DĂP-tĭv ĭ-MŪ-nĭ-tē, p. 720)
allergen (ĂL-ĕr-jĕn, p. 722)
anaphylactic shock (ăn-ĕ-flăk-tĭc, p. 727)
antigen (ĂN-to-jĕn, p. 721)
attenuated (ă-TĔN-ū-āt-ĕd, p. 723)
autoimmune (ăw-tō-ĭ-MŪN, p. 730)
autologous (ăw-TŎL-ŏ-gĕs, p. 729)
cellular immunity (SĔL-ū-lĕr ĭ-MŪ-nĭ-tē, p. 722)
humoral immunity (HŪ-mŏr-ĕl ĭ-MŪ-nĭ-tē, p. 721)
hypersensitivity (hī-pĕr-sĕn-sĭ-TĬV-ĭ-tē, p. 724)
immunity (ĭ-MŪ-nĭ-tē, p. 720)

immunization (ĭm-ū-nĭ-ZĀ-shŭn, p. 721)
immunocompetence (ĭm-ū-nō-KŎM-pĕ-tĕns, p. 719)
immunodeficiency (ĭm-ū-nō-dĕ-FĬSH-ĕn-sē, p. 730)
immunogen (ĭm-Ū-nō-jĕn, p. 722)
immunology (ĭm-ū-NŎL-ŏ-jē, p. 720)
immunosuppressive (ĭm-ū-nō-sū-PRĔ-sĭv, p. 729)
immunotherapy (ĭm-ū-nō-THĔR-ă-pē, p. 723)
innate immunity (ĭ-NĀT ĭ-MŪ-nĭ-tē, p. 720)
lymphokine (LĬM-fō-kīn, p. 721)
plasmapheresis (plăz-mă-fĕ-RĒ-sĭs, p. 731)
proliferation (prō-lĭf-ĕ-RĀ-shŭn, p. 721)

NATURE OF IMMUNITY

The human body exists in an environment of antagonistic forces that are constantly attacking and threatening its integrity. In response to these onslaughts, the body exhibits a wide array of adaptations to protect against external and internal harmful agents. This chapter deals with those mechanisms.

The word *immune* is derived from the Latin word *immunis,* meaning "free from burden." Immunology is an evolving science that essentially deals with the body's ability to distinguish self from nonself. The body makes this distinction through a complex network of highly specialized cells and tissues that are collectively called the **immune system.** The immune system (also called the **host defense system**) is critical to our survival.

The immune system has three main functions: (1) to protect the body's internal environment against invading microorganisms by destroying foreign antigens and pathogens thus preventing the development of infections (Lewis et al., 2007); (2) to maintain homeostasis by removing damaged cells from the circulation, thereby maintaining the body's various cell types in an unchanged and uniform form (Lewis et al., 2007); and (3) to serve as a surveillance network for recognizing and guarding against the development and growth of abnormal cells. Abnormal cells (mutations) are constantly being formed in the body but are recognized as abnormal cells and are destroyed (Lewis et al., 2007). When the immune system responds appropriately to a foreign stimulus, the body's integrity is maintained; this is called immunocompetence.

Immunocompetence is the immune system's ability to mobilize and use its antibodies and other responses to stimulation by an antigen. If the immune response is too weak or too vigorous, homeostasis is disrupted, causing a malfunction in the system. This is called **immunoincompetence.** With disruption of the homeostatic balance of the immune system, a number of diseases develop. Inappropriate immune responses are classified into four categories: (1) hyperactive responses against environmental antigens (e.g., allergy); (2) inability to protect the body, as in immunodeficiency disorders (e.g., acquired immunodeficiency syndrome [AIDS]); (3) failure to recognize the body as self, as in autoimmune disorders (e.g., systemic lupus erythematosus); and (4) attacks on beneficial foreign tissue (e.g., organ transplant rejection or transfusion reaction).

Immunity is the quality of being insusceptible to or unaffected by a particular disease or condition. Immunity has two major subclassifications: innate (natural) and adaptive (acquired) (Figure 15-1). Innate immunity is nonspecific, whereas adaptive immunity is specific. The study of the immune system is immunology.

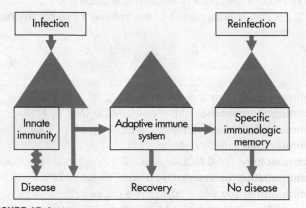

FIGURE 15-1 When an infectious agent enters the body, it first encounters elements of the innate immune system. These may be sufficient to prevent disease; if not, a disease will result and the adaptive immune system is activated. The adaptive immune system helps the patient recover from the disease and establishes a specific immunologic memory. After reinfection with the same agent, no disease results. The individual has acquired immunity to the infectious agent.

INNATE, OR NATURAL, IMMUNITY

The body's first line of defense, innate immunity, provides physical and chemical barriers to invading pathogens and protects against the external environment. The innate system is composed of the skin and mucous membranes, cilia, stomach acid, tears, saliva, sebaceous glands, and secretions and flora of the intestine and vagina. These organs, tissues, and secretions provide biochemical and physical barriers to disease. The first line of defense provides nonspecific immunity to the individual (Table 15-1).

ADAPTIVE, OR ACQUIRED, IMMUNITY

If the components of innate or natural immunity fail to prevent invasion or to destroy a foreign pathogen, the adaptive, or acquired, immune response assists in the battle. This is the body's second line of defense against disease. Adaptive immunity provides a specific reaction to each invading antigen and has the unique ability to remember the antigen that caused the attack. The adaptive immune system is composed of highly specialized cells and tissues, including the thymus, the spleen, bone marrow, blood, and lymph (Figure 15-2). Adaptive immunity includes both humoral and cell-mediated immunity. The adaptive immune system's specificity (i.e., being specific) results from the production of antibodies in the cells. Antibodies develop naturally after infection or artificially after vaccinations.

The cells of the immune system are the macrophages (any phagocytic cell involved in defense against infection) and the lymphocytes. When organisms pass the epithelial barriers, phagocytes become activated. Phagocytes also migrate through the bloodstream to the tissues for the body's second line of defense against disease. Phagocytes engulf and destroy microorganisms that pass the skin and mucous membrane barri-

Table 15-1	Innate (Natural) and Adaptive (Acquired) Immunity	
CHARACTERISTICS	**INNATE (NATURAL)**	**ADAPTIVE (ACQUIRED)**
Physical barriers	Physical defense: skin and mucous membranes Mucous membranes line body cavities such as the mouth and stomach. These cavities secrete chemicals (saliva and hydrochloric acid) that destroy bacteria. Cilia, tears, and flora of the intestine and vagina also provide natural protection.	None
Response mechanisms	Nonspecific: Mononuclear phagocytic system; inflammatory response	Specific immune response: Humoral immunity, cellular immunity
Soluble factors	Chemical defense: Lysozyme, complement, acute phase proteins, interferon	Antibodies, lymphokines
Cells	Phagocytes, natural killer (NK) cells	T cells, B cells
Specificity	None	Present
Memory	None	Present

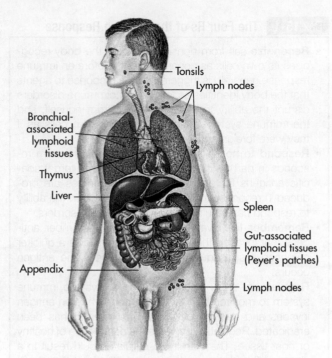

FIGURE 15-2 Organization of the immune system.

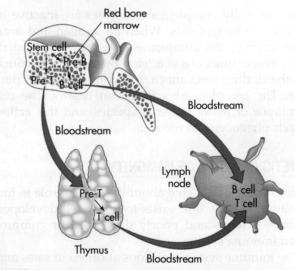

FIGURE 15-3 Origin and processing of B and T cells. B and T cells originate in red bone marrow. B cells are processed in the red marrow, whereas T cells are processed in the thymus. Both cell types circulate to other lymph tissues. B cells produce antibodies to destroy specific foreign antigens (humoral immunity). T cells attack and destroy antigens (cell-mediated immunity).

ers. These cells also assist in the immune response by carrying antigens to the lymphocytes.

Lymphocytes include the T and B cells (Figure 15-3) and the large, granular lymphocytes also known as **natural killer,** or NK, cells. Approximately 70% to 80% of the lymphocytes are T-cell lymphocytes. When activated, T cells release a substance called lymphokine. Lymphokine attracts macrophages to the site of infection or inflammation and prepares them for attack. T cells cooperate with the B cells to produce antibodies but do not produce antibodies themselves. T cells are

responsible for cell-mediated immunity and protect the body against viruses, fungi, and parasites. T cells also provide protection in allografts (transfer of tissue between two genetically dissimilar individuals of the same species) and against malignant cells.

B cells make up approximately 20% to 30% of the lymphocyte population. B cells trigger the production of antibodies and proliferate (increase in number) in response to a particular antigen (a substance recognized by the body as foreign that can trigger an immune response). An antigen is usually a protein that causes the formation of an antibody and reacts specifically with that antibody. B cells migrate to the peripheral circulation and tissues and eventually are filtered from the lymph and stored in the lymphoid tissue of the body.

The initial formation of B cells does not require antigen stimulation or any other environmental stimulus. However, B-cell proliferation (reproduction or multiplication of similar forms) depends on antigen stimulation. B cells are responsible for humoral immunity. B cells produce antibodies and protect against bacteria, viruses, and soluble antigens.

HUMORAL IMMUNITY

Humoral immunity (one of the two forms of immunity that respond to antigens, such as bacteria and foreign tissue) is mediated by the B cells. B cells produce antibodies in response to antigen challenge. On first exposure to a given antigen, a primary humoral response is initiated. This response is generally slow compared with subsequent antigen exposures. When a second exposure occurs, memory B cells cause a quick response, regardless of whether the first exposure was to an antigen or to immunization. Immunization is a process by which resistance to an infectious disease is induced or increased.

Antigen is presented to the T-helper cell population by the macrophages. T lymphocytes can be categorized into T-helper (CD_4) and T-suppressor (CD_8) cells. An antigen is taken to the B cells and, assisted by T-helper cells, the B cells initiate production of antibodies. T-suppressor cells maintain the humoral response at a level appropriate for the stimulus.

Antibodies produced by one's own body are said to provide active immunity. An example of active immunity is a person who has been vaccinated against rubeola (red measles). In contrast, temporary, or passive, immunity is provided by antibodies that are formed by one person in response to a specific antigen and administered to another person. An example of passive immunity is hepatitis B immune globulin administered after exposure to hepatitis B virus in a nonimmune person.

Even though humoral immunity is mediated by the B-cell population, T-helper cells and T-suppressor cells are vital to the immunocompetent person. **Immunocompetence** is the ability of an immune system to mobilize and deploy its antibodies and other responses to stimulation by an antigen. Both the number and functions of the helper and T-suppressor cells help determine the strength and persistence of an immune response. The normal ratio of T-helper cells to T-suppressor cells in the body is 2:1. When this ratio is disrupted, autoimmune and immunodeficient diseases occur. Factors that may weaken immunocompetence include the aging process, viruses, radiation, and chemotherapeutic drugs (*Mosby's Dictionary of medicine, nursing, and health professions*, 2009).

Exposure to antigen and response with antibody may activate either (1) the humoral complement (one of the 25 complex enzyme serum proteins) system, which results in breakdown of the bacteria and release of lysosomes to destroy bacteria; or (2) the antigen-antibody reaction, which results in mast cells releasing histamine, which produces the symptoms of allergy. When symptoms of allergy occur, antigen is referred to as allergen (a substance that can produce a hypersensitive reaction in the body but may not be inherently harmful). When immunity results, antigen is referred to as immunogen (any agent or substance capable of provoking an immune response or producing immunity).

CELLULAR IMMUNITY

Cellular immunity, also called **cell-mediated immunity** (the mechanism of acquired immunity characterized by the dominant role of small T cells), results when T cells are activated by an antigen. Whole cells become sensitized in a process similar to that which stimulates the B cells to form antibodies. Once these T cells have been sensitized, they are released into the blood and body tissues, where they remain indefinitely. On contact with the antigen to which they are sensitized, they attach to the organism and destroy it. Cellular immunity is involved in resistance to infectious diseases caused by viruses and some bacteria.

Cellular immunity is of primary importance in (1) immunity against pathogens that survive inside cells, including viruses and some bacteria (e.g., *Mycobacterium* organisms); (2) fungal infections; (3) rejection of transplanted tissues; (4) contact hypersensitivity reactions; (5) tumor immunity; and (6) certain autoimmune diseases (Box 15-1).

Hypersensitivity reactions are cell-mediated responses of the body (Box 15-2).

COMPLEMENT SYSTEM

The word *complement* became part of the terminology of immunology at the turn of the nineteenth century, when researchers recognized that blood plasma contained a substance necessary to complete the destruction of bacteria. The complement system includes approximately 25 serum enzymatic proteins that interact with one another and with other components of the innate (natural) and adaptive (acquired) immune sys-

---

Box 15-1	The Four Rs of the Immune Response

- **Recognize** self from nonself: Normally the body recognizes its own cells as nonantigenic; therefore an immune response generally is triggered only in response to agents that the body identifies as foreign. Autoimmune disorders disrupt the ability to differentiate self from nonself, and the immune system attacks the body's own cells as if they were foreign antigens.
- **Respond** to nonself invaders: The immune system responds in part by producing antibodies that target specific antigens for destruction. New antibodies are produced in response to new antigens. Deficits in the ability to respond can result in immunodeficiency disorders.
- **Remember** the invader: The ability to remember antigens that invaded the body in the past allows a quicker response if subsequent invasion by the same antigen occurs.
- **Regulate** its action: Self-regulation allows the immune system to monitor itself by "turning on" when an antigen invades and "turning off" when the invasion has been eradicated. Regulation prevents the destruction of healthy or host tissue. The inability to regulate could result in a chronic inflammation and damage to the host tissue.

---

tems. Normally, complement enzymes are inactive in plasma and body fluids. When an antigen and antibody interact, the complement system is activated. Complement functions in a "step-by-step" series much like the clotting mechanism, but with a different purpose. The complement system can destroy the cell membrane of many bacterial species, and this action attracts phagocytes to the area.

GENETIC CONTROL OF IMMUNITY

More is being discovered about the genetic role in immunity. A genetic link exists to both well-developed immune systems and poorly developed or compromised immune systems.

The immune system develops at different rates and at different times in fetal and early life. Bone marrow serves as an important mechanism of producing stem cells and all the other cells involved in the immune response.

EFFECTS OF NORMAL AGING ON THE IMMUNE SYSTEM

With advancing age, there is a decline in the immune system. The primary clinical evidence for this immunosenescence is the high incidence of tumors in older adults. Older adults are also more susceptible to infections (such as influenza and pneumonia) from pathogens that they were relatively immunocompetent against earlier in life.

Aging does not affect all aspects of the immune system. The bone marrow is relatively unaffected by increasing age. However, aging has a pronounced ef-

Review of the Mechanisms of Immune Response

- The skin and mucous membranes are natural barriers to infectious agents. When these barriers are crossed, the immune response begins in the immunocompetent host.
- The first time an antigen enters the body, the antigen is processed by macrophages and presented to lymphocytes. Responses of B cells to the antigen in humoral immunity require interaction with T-helper cells, which assist B cells in responding to the antigen by proliferating, synthesizing, and secreting the appropriate antibody. Antigens are then neutralized by antibodies or can form immune complexes or be phagocytosed by macrophages or neutrophils.
- Humoral immunity responds to antigens such as bacteria and foreign tissue. Humoral immunity is the result of the development and continuing presence of circulating antibodies in the plasma. Humoral immunity consists of antibody-mediated immunity. *Humoral* means body fluid, and antibodies are proteins found in plasma. Therefore the term *humoral immunity* is used.
- Cellular immunity is the primary defense against intracellular organisms, including viruses and some bacteria (e.g., mycobacteria).

- In cellular immunity the antigen is processed by macrophages and recognized by T cells. T cells produce lymphokines, which further attract macrophages and neutrophils to the site for phagocytosis, or cytotoxic killer T cells can respond directly.
- Immunodeficiency is an abnormal condition of the immune system in which cellular or humoral immunity is inadequate and resistance to infection is decreased. The immunodeficiency diseases are sometimes classified as B-cell (antibody) deficiencies, T-cell (cellular) deficiencies, and combined T- and B-cell deficiencies.
- Hypersensitivity reaction is an inappropriate and excessive response of the immune system to a sensitizing antigen. The antigen stimulant is an allergen. Humoral reactions, mediated by the circulating B lymphocytes, are immediate such as anaphylactic hypersensitivity. Cellular reactions, mediated by the T lymphocytes, are delayed cell-mediated hypersensitivity reactions.

fect on the thymus, which decreases in size and activity. These changes in the thymus are probably a primary cause of immunosenescence. Both T and B cells show deficiencies in activation, transit time through the cell cycle, and subsequent differentiation. However, the most significant alterations seem to involve T cells. As thymic output of T cells diminishes, the differentiation of T cells in peripheral lymphoid structures increases. Consequently, there is an accumulation of memory cells rather than new precursor cells responsive to previously unencountered antigens.

Delayed hypersensitivity response, as determined by skin testing with injected antigens, is frequently decreased or absent in older adults. The clinical consequences of a decline in cell-mediated immunity are evident. Older adults have an increased risk of death from cancer (see Life Span Considerations box).

IMMUNE RESPONSE

There are two ways of helping the body to develop immunity: **immunization** and **immunotherapy**. The theory behind immunization is that controlled exposure to a disease-producing pathogen develops antibodies while preventing disease. The first immunization is credited to Edward Jenner (1796), who observed that individuals who had had cowpox became immune to the disease. The idea of administering "attenuated [weakened] microbes" developed, and the scientific approach was applied by Louis Pasteur. Vaccines and toxoids are altered, or attenuated (the process of weakening the virulence of a disease organism), to reduce their power without affecting their ability to stimulate the production of antibodies. After immuni-

 Life Span Considerations

Older Adults

Immune Disorder

- Older adults are at increased risk for inflammation and infections resulting from changes in natural defense mechanisms.
- Pathogens are able to enter through breaks in fragile, dry skin, increasing the risk of skin infections.
- Decreased movement of respiratory secretions increases the risk of respiratory tract infections.
- Decreased production of saliva and gastric secretions increases the risk of gastrointestinal infections.
- Decreased tear production increases the risk of eye inflammation and infections.
- Structural changes in the urinary system that lead to urinary retention or stasis increase the risk of urinary tract infection.
- Signs and symptoms of infection tend to be more subtle than in younger individuals. Because older adults have decreased body temperature, fever may be more difficult to detect. Changes in behavior such as lethargy, fatigue, disorientation, irritability, and loss of appetite may be early signs of infection.
- Immune system functioning declines with advanced age. Research is continuing.
- The older adult's immune system continues to produce antibodies; therefore immunization for diseases such as pneumonia and influenza is recommended.
- Older adults who have chronic illnesses are generally at increased risk for infection.

zation the immune system mounts a greater response to a second encounter with an antigen. The vaccine, or toxoid, stimulates humoral immunity, which provides protection from disease for months to years.

Immunotherapy (a special treatment of allergic responses that administers increasingly large doses of the offending allergens to gradually develop immunity) consists of injecting a person with a very diluted antigen (allergen) to which the patient has a type I hypersensitivity. The strength of the dilution is increased as weekly injections are given over a 1- to 3-year period. The theory is that immunotherapy assists the individual in building tolerance to the allergen without developing fever or increased signs and symptoms. *Desensitization* is another term used for immunotherapy. It is indicated for patients with clinically significant disease for whom avoidance of the allergen or treatment with medication is inadequate. It is considered safe in properly selected patients but is a lengthy, expensive process with a potential for severe anaphylaxis.

Immunotherapy may be co-seasonal, preseasonal, or perennial. Perennial therapy is most widely accepted because it allows for a higher cumulative dose, which produces a better effect. Perennial therapy usually begins with 0.05 mL of a 1:10,000 dilution and increases to 0.5 mL in a 6-week period. In the next series the amount given again decreases to 0.05 mL while the dilution lessens to 1:1000. The amount increases each week until a 0.5-mL dose is given. The next cycle begins with a 0.05-mL dose of 1:100 dilution, increasing to 0.5 mL over another 6-week period. Perennial therapy is administered subcutaneously. Observe the patient for at least 20 minutes after administration because a hypersensitivity reaction or anaphylaxis may occur.

The treatment protocol for anaphylaxis with immunotherapy is generally accepted to be 0.2 to 0.5 mL of 1:1000 epinephrine hydrochloride (Adrenalin Chloride) subcutaneously every 20 minutes for three doses.

Most patients begin immunotherapy at the physician's office, and subsequent weekly injections are given until the maintenance level is reached. Home administration by the patient or a family member is acceptable once maintenance level is reached. Interrupted regimens because of illness may place the patient at risk for reaction. Consult the physician before administering a dose of diluted allergen if the patient's maintenance immunotherapy was interrupted by illness or other factors.

DISORDERS OF THE IMMUNE SYSTEM

Immune system failure occurs in several ways and expresses itself in mild to severe form. The system can malfunction at many points while attempting to provide the body with protective defense. It is thought that failures occur because of genetic factors, developmental defects, infection, malignancy, injury, drugs, or altered metabolic states.

The severity of altered immune response disorders ranges from mild to chronic to life threatening. The disorders are categorized as follows:

1. **Hypersensitivity** disorder involves allergic response and tissue rejection.

2. **Immunodeficiency** disease involves altered and failed immune response.

3. **Autoimmune** disease involves extensive tissue damage resulting from an immune system that seemingly reverses its function to one of self-destruction.

See Box 15-1 for the four Rs of the immune response.

HYPERSENSITIVITY DISORDERS

Etiology and Pathophysiology

Hypersensitivity is an abnormal condition characterized by an excessive reaction to a particular stimulus. **Hypersensitivity reaction** is an inappropriate and excessive response of the immune system to a sensitizing antigen. **Hypersensitivity disorders** arise when harmless substances (such as pollens, danders, foods, and chemicals) are recognized as foreign. The body mounts an immune response in much the same way it does to any foreign protein. The result, however, differs. The host becomes sensitive after first exposure and on subsequent exposure exhibits a hypersensitivity reaction. Chronic exposure leads to chronic allergy response, which ranges from mild to incapacitating signs and symptoms.

Hypersensitivity disorders are believed to be caused by a genetic defect that allows increased production of immunoglobulin E (IgE; a humoral antibody) with release of histamine and other mediators from mast cells and basophils. Humoral reactions, mediated by the circulating B lymphocytes, are immediate. Cellular reactions, mediated by the T lymphocytes, are delayed hypersensitivity reactions. Exposure to antigen may occur by inhalation, ingestion, injection, or touch (contact). Signs and symptoms caused by histamine release include vasodilation, edema, bronchoconstriction, mucus secretion, and pruritus. Reaction may be local (gastrointestinal, skin, respiratory, conjunctival) or systemic (anaphylaxis). The exact mechanism and pathway of these inflammatory responses are not clearly understood.

A combination of interrelated factors occurs that increases the severity of symptoms (Box 15-3). The disorders that result from hypersensitivity, which are discussed in other chapters, are urticaria, angioedema, allergic rhinitis, allergic conjunctivitis (hay fever), atopic dermatitis, and asthma. Approximately 40% of all cases of asthma are related to an allergic response (Global Institute of Asthma, 2004).

Assessment

Assessment should involve predominantly the integumentary, gastrointestinal, respiratory, and cardiovascular systems. Be aware of the seasonal nature of the complaints.

Subjective data include pruritus, nausea, and uneasiness.

Box 15-3   Factors Influencing Hypersensitivity

- **Host response to allergen:** The more sensitive the individual, the greater the allergic response is.
- **Exposure amount:** Generally, the more allergen the individual is exposed to, the greater the chance of severe reaction is.
- **Nature of the allergen:** Most allergic reactions are precipitated by complex, high-molecular–weight protein substances.
- **Route of allergen entry:** Most allergens enter the body via gastrointestinal and respiratory routes. Injections of venoms and medications hold a more severe threat of allergic response.
- **Repeated exposure:** Generally, the more the individual is exposed, the greater the response is.

 Health Promotion

Assessing the Patient with Allergies

- Obtain a comprehensive history that covers family allergies, past and present allergies, and social and environmental factors, especially the physical environment.
- Identify the allergens that may have triggered a reaction.
- Determine the time of year that an allergic reaction occurs as a clue to a seasonal allergen.
- Obtain information about any over-the-counter or prescription medications used to treat allergies.
- In addition to identification of the allergen, find out about the clinical manifestations and course of allergic reaction.
- Ask about pets, trees, and plants on the property; air pollutants; and floor coverings, houseplants, and cooling and heating systems in the home and workplace.
- Have the patient keep a daily or weekly food diary with a description of any untoward reactions.
- Screen for any reaction to medication.
- Review questions about the patient's lifestyle and stress level in connection with allergic symptoms.

Objective data include sneezing, excessive nasal secretions, lacrimation, inflamed nasal membranes, skin rash or areas of raised inflammation, diarrhea, cough, wheezes, impaired breathing, and hypotension.

Hypersensitivity illnesses are diagnosed largely through patient history and physical examination. The most important diagnostic tool is a detailed history, listing (1) onset, nature, and progression of signs and symptoms; (2) aggravating and alleviating factors; and (3) frequency and duration of signs and symptoms. Assess environmental, household, and occupational factors. Common offenders include pollens, spores, dusts, food, drugs, and insect venoms. Many but not all offenders are seasonal. Signs and symptoms generally vary from mild upper respiratory tract manifestations, such as sneezing and excessive nasal secretions, to watery, itching eyes. Skin signs and symptoms are often eczema-like or urticarial (hives). Diarrhea may be a gastrointestinal complaint in some individuals. More severe signs and symptoms include those of the lower respiratory tract, such as coughing, wheezing, chest discomfort, breathing difficulties, and shock, which could be followed by cardiovascular collapse and respiratory arrest. The complete history assists in an accurate diagnosis (see Health Promotion box).

The physical examination should include a thorough assessment of the skin, the middle ear, the conjunctiva, the nasooropharynx, and the lungs.

Diagnostic Tests

Laboratory studies are usually not necessary unless allergic signs and symptoms are severe and protracted. A complete blood count (with differential to identify the type of white blood cells that are elevated), skin testing, total serum IgE levels, and a specific IgE level for a particular allergen may be ordered. The latter test is called radioallergosorbent test (RAST).

Medical Management

Treatment of hypersensitivity disorders includes (1) symptom management with medications, (2) environmental control, and (3) immunotherapy.

The most effective treatment is environmental control, which includes avoidance of the offending allergen. Pollens are seasonal and can be avoided at season peaks with air conditioning and limited time spent outdoors. Mold spores can be reduced by maintaining dry conditions and using air filters. House dust can be controlled by damp dusting, use of air filters, and decreased use of carpet and overstuffed furniture. Most other offending allergens (food, drugs, chemicals, and stinging insects) can simply be avoided.

Medications are used to treat and alleviate signs and symptoms. Antihistamines compete with histamine by attaching to the cell surface receptors and blocking histamine release. Antihistamines therefore must be initiated soon after exposure or taken on a regular basis. Drowsiness, mucous membrane dryness, and occasionally central nervous system excitation are side effects of the earlier antihistamines. Examples of these include pseudoephedrine (Actifed), diphenhydramine (Benadryl) chlorpheniramine (Chlor-Trimeton), and brompheniramine (Brovex). Nonsedating antihistamines include cetirizine (Zyrtec), loratadine (Claritin), and fexofenadine (Allegra). The nonsedating antihistamines are more desirable for those who experience drowsiness with antihistamine use (Table 15-2).

Leukotriene inhibitors are agents that significantly reduce symptoms of an allergic reaction caused by the release of leukotrienes from mast cells and basophils. Three are currently available in the United States: montelukast (Singulair) and zafirlukast (Accolate) act

Table 15-2 Medications for Immune Disorders

Generic (Trade)	Action	Side Effects	Nursing Implications
Diphenhydramine (Benadryl)	Antihistamine	Drowsiness, confusion, nasal stuffiness, dry mouth, photosensitivity, urine retention	Use cautiously with central nervous system depressants, including alcohol; give with food; it is a safe hypnotic for older adults; tell patient to avoid driving or hazardous activity due to drowsiness.
Loratadine (Claritin)	Nonsedating antihistamine	Slight sedation (more common with increased doses)	Store in tight container at room temperature. Teach patient and family to avoid driving or other hazardous activities if drowsiness occurs.
Fexofenadine (Allegra)	Nonsedating antihistamine	Headache, drowsiness, blurred vision, hypotension, bradycardia, tachycardia, dysrhythmias (rare), urinary retention, pancytopenia	
Dexamethasone (Decadron)	Corticosteroid		Do not use for extended period; use cautiously with patients with diabetes or peptic ulcers.
Flunisolide (AeroBid)	Corticosteroid (inhaled)	Headache, transient nasal burning, epistaxis, nausea, vomiting	Not effective for acute episodes; use regularly; teach care and cleaning of inhaler; if symptoms do not improve in 3 weeks, consult physician.
Epinephrine (Adrenalin Chloride, Sus-Phrine, EpiPen)	Bronchodilator	Nervousness, tremor, headache, hypertension, tachycardia, ventricular fibrillation, stroke	Do not use with monoamine oxidase inhibitor; use cautiously in patients with hyperthyroidism, hypertension, diabetes, and heart disease.

as leukotriene-receptor blockers, and zileuton (Zyflo) inhibits the production of leukotrienes.

Nursing Diagnoses

Nursing diagnoses for patients with hypersensitivity include (1) *risk for injury,* related to exposure to allergen; (2) *activity intolerance,* related to malaise; and (3) *risk for infection,* related to inflammation of protective mucous membranes.

Patient Teaching

Patient teaching should revolve around the specific diagnosis. Advise the patient with seasonal allergies to avoid offending allergens, and ensure he or she understands the therapeutic medication plan. Focus on health promotion and health teaching for self-care management (see Safety Alert box).

Safety Alert!

Treating the Patient with a Hypersensitivity Reaction

- List all of a patient's allergies on the chart, the nursing care plan, and the medication record.
- After an allergic disorder is diagnosed, therapeutic treatment is aimed at reducing exposure to the offending allergen; treating the symptoms; and, if necessary, desensitizing the person through immunotherapy.
- All health care workers must be prepared for the rare but life-threatening anaphylactic reaction, which requires immediate medical and nursing interventions.
- Instruct the patient to wear a medical-alert bracelet listing the particular drug allergy.
- For a patient allergic to insect stings, commercial bee sting kits contain epinephrine and a tourniquet. Teach the patient to apply the tourniquet and self-inject the subcutaneous epinephrine. The patient should wear a medical-alert bracelet and carry a bee sting kit whenever going outdoors.

ANAPHYLAXIS

Etiology and Pathophysiology

The most severe IgE-mediated allergic reaction is anaphylaxis, or systemic reaction to allergens. **Anaphylaxis,** or anaphylactic shock, is an acute and potentially fatal hypersensitivity (allergic) reaction to an allergen (Lewis et al., 2007). The allergens causing anaphylaxis include (1) venoms; (2) drugs, such as penicillin and aspirin; (3) contrast media dyes; (4) insect stings (such as bees and wasps); (5) foods such as eggs, shellfish, and peanuts; (6) latex; and (7) vaccines.

The hypersensitivity reaction results in a sudden severe vasodilation as a consequence of the release of certain chemical mediators from mast cells. The vasodilation causes an increase in capillary permeability, which causes fluid to seep from the vascular space into the interstitial space (Lewis et al., 2007).

Clinical Manifestations

In anaphylaxis the reaction occurs rapidly after exposure, from seconds to a few minutes. A massive release of mediators initiates events in target organs throughout the body. Skin and gastrointestinal signs and symptoms may occur, although respiratory and cardiovascular signs and symptoms predominate. Fatal reactions are associated with a fall in blood pressure, laryngeal edema, and bronchospasm, leading to cardiovascular collapse, myocardial infarction, and respiratory failure. Anaphylactic reactions are classified as mild, moderate, and severe.

Assessment

Early recognition of signs and symptoms and early treatment may prevent severe reactions and even death. Generally, the more rapid the onset, the more severe the outcome is. The patient may have a feeling of uneasiness that increases to a sense of foreboding and then a fear of impending death. The skin may or may not be involved. Urticaria, pruritus, and angioedema may be present in mild and moderate anaphylaxis, whereas cyanosis and pallor may be seen in severe reactions. Upper respiratory signs and symptoms range from congestion and sneezing to edema of the lips, the tongue, and the larynx with stridor and occlusion of the upper airways. Lower respiratory signs and symptoms occur soon thereafter and include bronchospasm, wheezing, and severe dyspnea. Gastrointestinal signs and symptoms increase from nausea, vomiting, and diarrhea to dysphagia and involuntary stools. The patient may have cardiovascular signs and symptoms, such as tachycardia and hypotension. Signs and symptoms may worsen, and the patient may display coronary insufficiency, vascular collapse, dysrhythmias, shock, cardiac arrest, respiratory failure, and death.

Medical Management

Immediate aggressive treatment is the goal in anaphylaxis. At the first sign, 0.2 to 0.5 mL of epinephrine 1:1000 is given subcutaneously for mild symptoms. It may be repeated at 20-minute intervals as prescribed by the physician. Epinephrine produces bronchodilation and vasoconstriction and inhibits the further release of chemical mediators of hypersensitivity reactions from mast cells. The effects of epinephrine take only a few minutes (Lewis et al., 2007). Epinephrine 1:10,000, 0.5 mL IV at 5- to 10-minute intervals, may be administered for severe reaction as prescribed by the physician. Diphenhydramine 50 to 100 mg may be given intramuscularly or intravenously as indicated for allergic signs and symptoms. If moderate to severe signs and symptoms occur, IV therapy with volume expanders and vasopressor agents such as dopamine (Intropin) may be initiated to prevent vascular collapse, and the patient may be intubated to prevent airway obstruction. Oxygen may be administered by nonrebreather mask. Intubation or a tracheostomy may be required for oxygen delivery if progressive hypoxia exists. Place the patient in a recumbent position and elevate the legs. Keep the patient warm.

Nursing Interventions and Patient Teaching

Nursing interventions begin with assessing respiratory status, including dyspnea, wheezing, and decreased breath sounds. Also assess circulatory status, including dysrhythmias, tachycardia, and hypotension. Monitor vital signs continually. Other assessments include (1) intake and output (I&O); (2) mental status, including anxiety, malaise, confusion, and coma; (3) skin status, including erythema, urticaria, cyanosis, and pallor; and (4) gastrointestinal status, including nausea, vomiting, diarrhea, and incontinence.

The diagnosis is most often made by a history of signs and symptoms. Looking at and listening to the anxious patient should be leading clues in suspecting anaphylaxis. Question the patient about recent exposure to known antigens that cause anaphylaxis (Box 15-4). Most laboratory studies are not beneficial.

Box 15-4	Common Allergens Causing Anaphylaxis	
DRUGS	**VENOMS**	**FOODS**
Vaccines	Honeybees	Milk
Allergen extracts	Wasps	Peanuts
Enzymes	Hornets	Brazil nuts
Penicillins		Cashew nuts
Sulfonamides		Shellfish
Cephalosporins		Egg albumin
Dextrans		Strawberries
Hormones		Chocolate
Contrast media		
Anesthetic agents		

Nursing diagnoses and interventions for the patient with anaphylaxis include but are not limited to the following:

Nursing Diagnoses	Nursing Interventions
Ineffective breathing pattern, related to: • edema • bronchospasm • increased secretions	Maintain airway. Administer high-flow oxygen via nonrebreather mask. Endotracheal intubation or a tracheostomy will be established for oxygen delivery if progressive hypoxia exists. Administer prescribed medications. Keep the patient warm. Monitor vital signs. Suction if necessary. Anticipate intubation with severe respiratory distress.
Decreased cardiac output, related to: • increased capillary permeability • vascular dilation	Monitor IV fluid infusions as ordered. Monitor vital signs. Monitor I&O. Obtain complete allergy history. Document signs and symptoms, interventions, and response.

Reassure the patient during procedures. After the event, teach the patient about avoidance of the allergen, advise him or her to wear or carry medical-alert identification, and teach the patient to prepare and administer epinephrine subcutaneously.

Prognosis

If the signs and symptoms are left untreated, anaphylaxis can lead to death in a relatively short time.

LATEX ALLERGIES

Allergies to latex products have become an increasing problem, affecting patients and health care professionals. The increase in allergic reactions has coincided with the sharp increase in glove use after the introduction of universal precautions against infectious diseases in 1987. It is estimated that 8% to 17% of health care workers regularly exposed to latex are sensitized. The more frequent and prolonged the exposure, the greater likelihood of developing a latex allergy. In addition to gloves, latex-containing products used in health care include blood pressure cuffs, stethoscopes, tourniquets, IV tubing, syringes, electrode pads, oxygen masks, tracheal tubes, colostomy and ileostomy pouches, urinary catheters, anesthetic masks, and adhesive tape.

Latex proteins can become aerosolized through powder on gloves and can result in serious reactions when inhaled by sensitized individuals; therefore all health care agencies are advised to use powder-free gloves. Certain food proteins are similar to some proteins in rubber; therefore an allergic reaction to latex may also result in an allergic reaction to some foods. Bananas, avocados, kiwi, tomatoes, water chestnuts, peaches, grapes, and apricots are the most common foods to result in an allergy if one is allergic to latex (Lewis et al., 2007).

Types of Latex Allergies

Two types of latex allergies that can occur are **type IV allergic contact dermatitis** and **type I allergic reactions.** Type IV contact dermatitis is caused by the *chemicals used in the manufacturing process of latex gloves.* It is a delayed reaction that occurs within 6 to 48 hours. Typically the person first has dryness, pruritus, fissuring, and cracking of the skin, followed by erythema, edema, and crusting at 24 to 48 hours. Chronic exposure can lead to thickening and hardening of the skin, scaling, and hyperpigmentation. The dermatitis may extend beyond the area of physical contact with the allergen.

A type I allergic reaction is a response to the *natural rubber latex proteins* and occurs within minutes of contact with the proteins. These types of allergic reactions can range from skin erythema, urticaria, rhinitis, conjuctivitis, or asthma to full-blown anaphylactic shock. Systemic reactions to latex may result from exposure to protein via various routes, including the skin, mucous membranes, inhalation, or blood.

Nursing Interventions

The identification of patients and health care workers sensitive to latex is crucial in preventing adverse reactions. Collect a thorough health history and history of any allergies, especially for patients with any complaints of latex contact symptoms. However, not all latex-sensitive individuals can be identified, even with a thorough history. Risk factors include long-term exposure to latex products (e.g., health care personnel, individuals who have had multiple surgeries, rubber industry workers) and a history of hay fever, asthma, and allergies to certain foods (e.g., avocados, guava, kiwi, bananas, water chestnuts, hazelnuts, tomatoes, potatoes, peaches, grapes, apricots, peanuts).

The National Institute for Occupational Safety and Health (NIOSH) has published recommendations for preventing allergic reactions to latex in the workplace.* In summary, they include the following:

- Use nonlatex gloves for activities that are not likely to involve contact with infectious materials (e.g., food preparation, housekeeping).
- Use powder-free gloves with reduced protein content.

---

*U.S. Department of Health and Human Services, National Institute for Occupational Safety and Health. (1997). *Preventing allergic reactions to natural rubber latex in the workplace.* US DHHS/NIOSH Pub. No. 97-135.

- Do not use oil-based hand creams or lotions when wearing gloves.
- After removing gloves, wash hands with mild soap and dry thoroughly.
- Frequently clean work areas that are contaminated with latex-containing dust.
- Know the signs and symptoms of latex allergy, including skin rash; hives; flushing; itching; nasal, eye, or sinus symptoms; asthma; and shock.
- If symptoms of latex allergy develop, avoid direct contact with latex gloves and products.
- People who have a latex allergy should wear a medical-alert bracelet and carry an epinephrine pen.

Use latex precaution protocols for patients identified as having a positive latex allergy test or a history of signs and symptoms related to latex exposure. Many health care facilities have created latex-free product carts that can be used for patients with latex allergies (Lewis et al., 2007).

TRANSFUSION REACTIONS

Transfusion reactions are a hypersensitivity disorder, best illustrated by reactions that occur with mismatched blood. Preventing transfusion reaction requires careful selection of blood donors, followed by careful typing and crossmatching of blood from donor to recipient. Storage of blood and administration protocol are critical. Refrigerate blood and blood components at specific temperatures until a half hour before administration. Administer blood within 4 hours of removal from refrigeration, and blood components within 6 hours. Donor and recipient numbers are specific and must be thoroughly checked and the patient identified with an armband. Administer all blood and blood products through microaggregate filters. Monitor for adverse effects.

Transfusion reactions are labeled mild, moderate, and severe. The most severe reactions occur within the first 15 minutes, moderate reactions occur within 30 to 90 minutes, and mild reactions may be delayed to late in the transfusion or hours to several days after transfusion.

Mild transfusion reaction signs and symptoms include dermatitis, diarrhea, fever, chills, urticaria, cough, and orthopnea. Treatment includes (1) stopping the transfusion; and (2) administering saline, steroids, and diuretics as ordered. Transfusion may continue at a slower rate. In moderate reactions—in which fever, chills, urticaria, and wheezing occur after the first 30 minutes of administration—stop the transfusion and continue with saline. Antihistamines and epinephrine may be given. The physician decides whether to continue the transfusion. With severe reaction stop the transfusion and give saline to provide venous access. Return the blood or blood product and tubing to the laboratory for immediate testing if any type of reaction occurs. Further nursing responsibilities after a blood transfusion reaction include (1) following hospital protocol for collecting required

blood and urine specimens to assess for hemolysis, (2) filling out a transfusion reaction record, and (3) documenting the transfusion reaction on the appropriate form on the patient's chart (Lewis et al., 2007).

The best method for preventing transfusion reaction is autologous (pertaining to a tissue occurring naturally and derived from the same individual) transfusion, or use of one's own blood, for replacement therapy. The blood can be frozen and stored for as long as 3 years. Usually the blood is stored without being frozen and is given to the person within a few weeks of donation.

DELAYED HYPERSENSITIVITY

Delayed hypersensitivity reactions occurring 24 to 72 hours after exposure are mediated by T cells accompanied by release of lymphokines. Delayed reaction contact dermatitis, such as after contact with poison ivy, is one example. Tissue transplant rejection, another example, is discussed here.

Transplant Rejection

Transfer of healthy tissue or organs from a donor to a recipient has been done for many years. The immune process that protects the body from foreign protein is the same process at work in tissue transplant rejection. Knowledge of the function of the immune system enabled medical experts to find a way to control the rejection process. Now the body is prepared before tissue transplant to decrease the chances of rejection.

Autograft, or transplantation of tissue from one site to another on an individual, is successful. It is used after trauma, especially on full-thickness burns, and in reconstructive surgery. Isograft is transfer of tissue between genetically identical individuals (e.g., identical twins). Allograft is transplantation of tissue between members of the same species. Because few humans are born with an identical sibling, allograft is the most common form of tissue transplant.

Antigenic determinants on the cells lead to graft rejection via the immune process. Therefore antigenic determinants in recipient tissue and donor tissue are matched as closely as possible before transplantation. Tissue matching leads to a better chance of success.

Tissue rejection does not occur immediately after transplantation. It takes several days for vascularization to occur. Seven to 10 days after blood supply is adequately established, sensitized lymphocytes appear in sufficient numbers for sloughing to occur at the site.

Graft rejection is slowed through use of chemical agents that interfere with the immune response. Included are corticosteroids, cyclosporine (Neoral, Sandimmune), and azathioprine (Imuran). This is referred to as immunosuppressive therapy (the administration of agents that significantly interfere with the immune system's ability to respond to antigenic stimulation by inhibiting cellular and humoral immunity).

Infection is a threat to the immunosuppressed patient. Meticulous aseptic technique is required when caring for these individuals. Prophylactic antibiotic therapy may be advisable, and good skin care is necessary. Limit the frequency of bedside visits for both staff and family. Do not allow people with infection near the patient.

IMMUNODEFICIENCY DISORDERS

The first evidence of immunodeficiency (an abnormal condition of the immune system in which cellular or humoral immunity is inadequate and resistance to infection is decreased) disease is an increased susceptibility to infection. The problem can manifest as recurrent or chronic infection. Unusually severe infection with complications or incomplete clearing of an infection may also indicate an underlying immunodeficiency.

Defects in genes leading to immunodeficiency provide a hereditary link to the diseases. Many diseases are believed to be associated with immunodeficiency. These diseases include AIDS, agammaglobulinemia, and multiple myeloma, which are discussed elsewhere in the text.

When the immune system does not adequately protect the body, an immunodeficient state exists. The immunodeficiency disorders involve an impairment of one or more immune mechanisms: (1) phagocytosis, (2) humoral response, (3) cell-mediated response, (4) complement, and (5) a combined humoral and cell-mediated deficiency. Immunodeficiency disorders are primary if the immune cells are improperly developed or absent, and secondary if the deficiency is caused by illnesses or treatment. Primary immunodeficiency disorders are rare and often serious, whereas secondary disorders are more common and may be less severe.

PRIMARY IMMUNODEFICIENCY DISORDERS

The basic categories of primary immunodeficiency disorders include (1) phagocytic defects, (2) B-cell deficiency, (3) T-cell deficiency, and (4) a combined B-cell and T-cell deficiency.

SECONDARY IMMUNODEFICIENCY DISORDERS

Drug-induced immunosuppression is the most common type of secondary immunodeficiency disorder. Immunosuppressive therapy is prescribed for patients to treat a wide variety of chronic diseases, including inflammatory, allergic, hematologic, neoplastic, and autoimmune disorders. Immunosuppressive therapy is also used to prevent rejection of a transplanted organ. Some of these immunosuppressive drugs are cyclosporine, mycophenolate mofetil (CellCept), and azathioprine. Immunosuppression is also a serious side effect of cytotoxic drugs used in cancer chemotherapy. Generalized leukopenia often results, leading to a decreased humoral and cell-mediated response. Therefore secondary infections are common in immunosuppressed patients.

Stress may alter the immune response. This effect involves interrelationships between the nervous, endocrine, and immune systems.

A hypofunctional immune system exists in young children and older adults. Immunoglobulin levels decrease with age and therefore lead to a suppressed humoral immune response in older adults. Thymic involution occurs with aging, along with decreased numbers of T cells. The incidence of malignancies and autoimmune diseases increases with aging and may be related to immunologic deterioration.

Malnutrition also alters cell-mediated immune responses. When protein is deficient over a prolonged period, the thymus gland atrophies and lymphoid tissue decreases. In addition, susceptibility to infections increases.

Radiation destroys lymphocytes either directly or through depletion of stem cells. As the radiation dose is increased, more bone marrow atrophies, leading to severe pancytopenia and severe suppression of immune function.

Surgical removal of lymph nodes, thymus, or spleen can suppress the immune response. Splenectomy in children is especially dangerous and may lead to septicemia from simple respiratory tract infections.

Hodgkin's lymphoma greatly impairs the cell-mediated immune response, and patients may die from severe viral or fungal infections. Viruses, especially rubella, may cause immunodeficiency by direct cytotoxic damage to lymphoid cells. Systemic infections can place such a demand on the immune system that resistance to a secondary or subsequent infection is impaired.

AUTOIMMUNE DISORDERS

Autoimmune disorders entail the development of an immune response (autoantibodies or cellular immune response) to one's own tissues; thus these disorders are failures of the tolerance to "self." Autoimmune disorders may be described as an immune attack on the self and result from the failure to distinguish "self" protein from "foreign" protein.

For some unknown reason, immune cells that are normally unresponsive (tolerant to self-antigens) are activated. Both T cells and B cells can have tolerance to self-antigens. Therefore an alteration in T cells alone or in both B cells and T cells can produce autoantibodies and autosensitized T cells to cause pathophysiologic tissue damage. The particular autoimmune disease depends on which self-antigen is involved.

Autoimmune diseases tend to cluster so that a given person may have more than one (e.g., rheumatoid arthritis and Addison's disease), or the same or related autoimmune diseases may be found in other members of the family. This observation has led to the concept of genetic predisposition to autoimmune disease.

As a person ages, the probability of failure in any system occurs. The pathophysiology of autoimmune responses is not clearly understood. Nevertheless, many illnesses are now believed to be in this classification. Included are pernicious anemia, Guillain-Barré syndrome, scleroderma, Sjögren's syndrome, rheumatic fever, rheumatoid arthritis, ulcerative colitis, male infertility, myasthenia gravis, multiple sclerosis, Addison's disease, autoimmune hemolytic anemia, immune thrombocytopenic purpura, type 1 diabetes mellitus, glomerulonephritis, and systemic lupus erythematosus. These conditions are discussed elsewhere in the text.

PLASMAPHERESIS

Plasmapheresis is the removal of plasma that contains components causing, or thought to cause, disease. When plasma is removed, it is replaced by substitution fluids such as saline or albumin. Therefore the term *plasma exchange* more accurately describes this procedure.

Plasmapheresis has been used to treat autoimmune diseases such as systemic lupus erythematosus, glomerulonephritis, myasthenia gravis, thrombocytopenic purpura, rheumatoid arthritis, and Guillain-Barré syndrome. The rationale is to remove pathologic substances present in plasma. Many disorders for which plasmapheresis is being used are characterized by circulating autoantibodies (usually of the immunoglobulin G [IgG] class) and antigen-antibody complexes. Immunosuppressive therapy prevents recovery of IgG production, and plasmapheresis prevents antibody rebound.

In addition to removing antinuclear antibodies (an autoantibody that reacts to nuclear material) and antigen-antibody complexes, plasmapheresis may also remove inflammatory mediators (e.g., complement) that are responsible for tissue damage. In the treatment of systemic lupus erythematosus, plasmapheresis is usually reserved for the patient in an acute attack who is unresponsive to conventional therapy.

Plasmapheresis involves the removal of whole blood through a needle inserted in one arm and circulation of the blood through a cell separator. The separator divides the blood into plasma and its cellular components by centrifugation or membrane filtration. Plasma, platelets, white blood cells, or red blood cells can be separated selectively. The undesirable component is removed, and the remainder is returned to the patient through a needle in the opposite arm. The plasma is generally replaced with normal saline, lactated Ringer's solution, fresh frozen plasma, plasma protein fractions, or albumin. When blood is manually removed, only 500 mL may be taken at one time. However, with the use of apheresis procedures, more than 4 L of plasma can be pheresed in 2 to 3 hours.

As with administration of other blood products, be aware of side effects associated with plasmapheresis. The most common complications are hypotension and citrate toxicity. Hypotension is usually the result of vasovagal reaction or transient volume changes. Citrate is used as an anticoagulant and may cause hypocalcemia, which may manifest as headache, paresthesias, and dizziness. See text for complete coverage of various autoimmune disorders.

Get Ready for the NCLEX® Examination!

Key Points

- The two major forms of immunity are innate (natural) and acquired (adaptive).
- T lymphocytes, B lymphocytes, and macrophages are the three major cells active in acquired immunity.
- B lymphocytes produce antibodies. T lymphocytes do not produce antibodies, but assist the B cell. T lymphocytes release lymphokines.
- Macrophages trap, process, and present antigen to T lymphocytes.
- Autoimmune disorders are failures of the tolerance to "self."
- Plasmapheresis is used to treat autoimmune diseases such as systemic lupus erythematosus, glomerulonephritis, myasthenia gravis, thrombocytopenic purpura, rheumatoid arthritis, and Guillain-Barré syndrome.
- Infection is a primary threat to the immunosuppressed patient. Aseptic technique is required when caring for these patients. Good skin care is necessary.
- Careful selection of blood donors and careful typing and crossmatching of blood are important to prevent transfusion reaction.

- Early recognition of signs followed by early treatment may decrease the severity of allergic reaction.
- The five factors influencing hypersensitivity response are host response to allergen, exposure amount, nature of the allergen, route of allergen entry, and repeated exposure.
- Two types of latex allergies are type IV allergic contact dermatitis and type I allergic reactions. Type IV is caused by the chemicals used in the manufacturing process of latex gloves, whereas type I allergic reaction is a response to the natural rubber latex proteins.

Additional Learning Resources

 Go to your Companion CD for an audio glossary, animation, video clips, and more.

evolve Be sure to visit the Evolve site at http://evolve.elsevier.com/Christensen/adult/ for additional online resources.

Review Questions for the NCLEX® Examination

1. Immune disorders that result from failure of the tolerance to "self" responding immunologically to one's own antigens are known as:

   1. immunodeficiency disorders.
   2. hypersensitivity disorders.
   3. desensitization disorders.
   4. autoimmune disorders.

2. A nurse is caring for a patient who had a kidney transplant. What should be included in the care of a patient with a suppressed immune system?

   1. Prophylactic antibiotic therapy
   2. Meticulous aseptic technique
   3. Restriction of all visitors
   4. Antineoplastic medication administration

3. Which statement describes innate, or natural, immunity?

   1. The body's first line of defense against disease, which protects locally against the external environment
   2. The body's second line of defense against disease, which protects the internal environment
   3. Mediated by B cells to produce antibodies in response to antigenic challenge
   4. An immunity that is specific

4. The nurse is caring for a patient with a history of numerous allergies. What is the most important teaching concept?

   1. Immunotherapy regimen
   2. Avoidance of the allergen
   3. Antihistamine administration
   4. Adrenaline administration

5. Humoral immunity is mediated by:

   1. T cells.
   2. B cells.
   3. macrophages.
   4. myeloblasts.

6. Cellular immunity develops when which cells are activated by an antigen?

   1. T cells
   2. B cells
   3. Neutrophils
   4. Monoblasts

7. Desensitization is another term for:

   1. autoimmune disorders.
   2. adaptive immunity.
   3. immunotherapy.
   4. immunodeficiency disease.

8. After a bee sting, the patient's face becomes edematous and she begins to wheeze. Based on this assessment, the nurse would be prepared to administer:

   1. aminophylline.
   2. Benadryl.
   3. epinephrine.
   4. Valium.

9. The nurse gave an intramuscular penicillin injection to a patient. What would be a sign of a systemic anaphylactic response?

   1. Increased blood pressure
   2. Bradycardia
   3. Urticaria
   4. Wheezing

10. A 38-year-old patient is receiving 2 units of packed red blood cells at 125 mL/hr. Fifteen minutes after the start of the blood transfusion, the nurse notes the following vital signs: pulse 110 bpm, respirations 28 breaths/min, blood pressure 98/58 mm Hg, and temperature 101° F. The patient is shivering. The nurse's next action would be to:

    1. slow the infusion rate.
    2. stop the infusion.
    3. administer aspirin as ordered for elevated temperature.
    4. report the findings to the nurse manager.

11. A 72-year-old patient is admitted to the hospital with a diagnosis of immunodeficiency disease. The primary nursing goals would be to:

    1. reduce the risk of the patient developing an infection.
    2. encourage the patient to provide self-care.
    3. plan nutritious meals to provide adequate intake.
    4. encourage the patient to interact with other patients.

12. The patient tells the nurse he is overwhelmed. There is so much he must do to keep his new kidney functioning, and then rejection may still occur. Which nursing diagnosis is appropriate?

    1. Ineffective coping
    2. Disturbed body image
    3. Impaired adjustment
    4. Situational low self-esteem

13. What is the correct nursing intervention for anaphylaxis? *(Select all that apply.)*

    1. Assess vital signs every 4 hours.
    2. Assess respiratory status frequently.
    3. Maintain patent airway.
    4. Administer epinephrine 1:1000, 0.2 to 0.5 mL subQ, as ordered.

14. The patient comes to the clinic for his weekly allergy injection. He missed his appointment the week before because of a family emergency. Which action is appropriate in administering the patient's injection?

    1. Administer the usual dosage of the allergen.
    2. Double the dosage to account for the missed injection the previous week.
    3. Consult with the physician about decreasing the dosage for this injection.
    4. Reevaluate the patient's sensitivity to the allergen with a skin test.

15. The nurse advises a friend who asks him to administer his allergy injections that:
    1. it is illegal for nurses to administer injections outside of a medical setting.
    2. he is qualified to do it if the friend has epinephrine in an injectable syringe provided with his extract.
    3. avoiding the allergens is a more effective way of controlling allergies and allergy shots are not usually effective.
    4. immunotherapy should only be administered in a setting where emergency equipment and drugs are available.

16. A patient is undergoing plasmapheresis for treatment of systemic lupus erythematosus. The nurse explains that plasmapheresis is used to:
    1. remove T lymphocytes in her blood that are producing antinuclear antibodies.
    2. remove normal particles in her blood that are being damaged by autoantibodies.
    3. exchange her plasma that contains antinuclear antibodies with a substitute fluid.
    4. replace viral-damaged cellular components of her blood with replacement whole blood.

17. Type I allergic reaction to latex is a response to the
    _____ _____ _____ _____.

18. The most common allergens that cause an anaphylactic reaction include: (Select all that apply.)
    1. leafy green vegetables.
    2. bees, wasps.
    3. shellfish.
    4. peanuts.

19. Which illness is believed to be an autoimmune disorder? (Select all that apply.)
    1. Rheumatoid arthritis
    2. Lung cancer
    3. Systemic lupus erythematosus
    4. Guillain-Barré syndrome

Care of the Patient with HIV/AIDS

*e*volve

http://evolve.elsevier.com/Christensen/adult/

Craig E. Nielsen

Objectives

1. Describe the agent that causes HIV disease.
2. Provide the definition of AIDS given in January 1993 by the Centers for Disease Control and Prevention.
3. Explain the differences between HIV infection, HIV disease, and AIDS.
4. Describe the progression of HIV infection.
5. Discuss how HIV is and is not transmitted.
6. Describe patients who are at risk for HIV infection.
7. Discuss the pathophysiology of HIV disease.
8. List signs and symptoms that may be indicative of HIV disease.
9. Discuss the laboratory and diagnostic tests related to HIV disease.
10. Discuss the issues related to HIV antibody testing.
11. Describe the multidisciplinary approach in caring for a patient with HIV disease.
12. List opportunistic infections associated with advanced HIV disease (AIDS).
13. Discuss the nurse's role in assisting the HIV-infected patient with coping, grieving, reducing anxiety, and minimizing social isolation.
14. Implement a care plan for the patient with AIDS.
15. Discuss the importance of adherence to HIV treatment.
16. Discuss the use of effective prevention messages in counseling patients.
17. Define the nurse's role in the prevention of HIV infection.

Key Terms

acquired immunodeficiency syndrome (AIDS) (ĭm-ū-nō-dĕ-FĬSH-ĕn-sē, p. 744)
adherence (ăd-HĔR-ĕns, p. 760)
CD₄⁺ lymphocyte (LĬM-fō-sīt, p. 742)
Centers for Disease Control and Prevention (CDC) (p. 734)
enzyme-linked immunosorbent assay (ELISA) (ĭm-ū-nō-ZŌR-bĕnt, p. 747)
HIV disease (p. 744)
HIV infection (p. 744)
human immunodeficiency virus (HIV) (p. 734)
Kaposi's sarcoma (kă-PŌS-sĕz săr-KŌ-mă, p. 734)

opportunistic (ŏp-pŏr-tū-NĬS-tĭk, p. 736)
phagocyte (făg-ō-SĬT-ĭk, p. 744)
***Pneumocystis jiroveci* (formerly *carinii*) pneumonia (PCP)** (nū-mō-SĬS-tĭs kă-RĬN-ē, p. 734)
retrovirus (rĕ-trō-VĪ-rŭs, p. 742)
seroconversion (sĕr-ō-kŏn-VĔR-zhŭn, p. 740)
seronegative (sĕr-ō-NĔG-ă-tĭv, p. 747)
vertical transmission (p. 739)
viral load (p. 739)
virulent (VĬR-ū-lĕnt, p. 735)
Western blot (p. 747)

NURSING AND THE HISTORY OF HIV DISEASE

As early as 1979, physicians in New York and California were noting cases of *Pneumocystis jiroveci* (formerly *carinii*) pneumonia (PCP), an unusual pulmonary disease caused by a fungus and primarily associated with people who have suppressed immune systems. These physicians also noted an increase in the number of people with **Kaposi's sarcoma**, a rare cancer of the skin and mucous membranes characterized by blue, red, or purple raised lesions seen mainly in Mediterranean men. The interesting thing was that these two diseases were occurring at alarming rates in clusters of young homosexual men whose immune systems were failing. Researchers at the **Centers for Disease Control and Prevention (CDC)**, a division of the U.S. Public Health Service in Atlanta that investigates and controls various diseases, soon learned that this immune disorder was also affecting injecting drug users and hemophiliacs. They later learned that it also affected heterosexual men and women.

The origins of **human immunodeficiency virus (HIV)** remain somewhat obscure, and why HIV gave rise to the acquired immunodeficiency syndrome (AIDS) pandemic only in the twentieth century has not yet been determined. The earliest case of HIV infection has been dated to 1959. It was identified in the Democratic Republic of Congo by using different methods of molecular clock analysis. It has also been estimated that HIV began to radiate from its source around the 1930s (Buonaguro et al., 2007). The escalating pandemic likely resulted from the combination of significant cultural and sociobehavioral changes, the use of nonsterile needles for parenteral injections and vaccinations, and the unintended contamination of products used for medical treatments.

HIV/AIDS has been recognized as a clinical syndrome since the early 1980s. But several researchers have identified patients who might have fit the CDC's Case Surveillance definition before this time. For example, the unusual and rapid death of a 15 year-old black boy from aggressive disseminated Kaposi's sarcoma suggests he might be the first confirmed case of HIV infection in the United States (Garry et al., 1988). This patient from St. Louis had no international travel experience, which suggests that other individuals were HIV infected as well. This also suggests that HIV has existed in some form in the United States since at least the 1960s.

HIV is known as **zoonotic,** an organism that has been able to cross from an animal species to humans. A similar virus was noted in primates (called simian immunodeficiency virus) and likely crossed into humans with the hunting and consumption of these animals in Africa. Other examples of zoonotic transmission include severe acute respiratory distress syndrome, anthrax, and Hantavirus and West Nile virus (World Health Organization [WHO], 2009). HIV began to spread in the middle to late 1970s, but because of the long incubation period, in most countries the viral epidemic progressed undetected. When the virus began causing widespread disease in the 1980s, it provoked fear among laypeople and health care providers alike. It was also an exciting time for health care workers because they knew they were seeing a new pathogen with a route of transmission not completely understood. In spite of the stigmas and fears that emerged (which still exist to some extent today), nurses were at the forefront providing care. Nurses met the challenges of providing and coordinating services, organizing community-based organizations, teaching about prevention, and helping patients deal with a terminal disease.

In June 1981, the CDC published a notation about some patients with signs and symptoms that later would be attributed to AIDS (CDC, 1981). The signs and symptoms listed were related to the development of opportunistic infections (OIs). Since that time, AIDS has become known as one of the most challenging infectious diseases of the twentieth and twenty-first centuries. In 1982, the CDC stated that blood and other body fluids may transmit the disease, and they issued a statement about using precautions with other people's body fluids.

In 1983 French researchers isolated the virus believed to be responsible for AIDS, and they called it lymphadenopathy-associated virus (Barré-Sinoussi et al., 1983). One year later an American scientist claimed the discovery of the etiologic agent and named it the human T-cell lymphotropic virus type III (Gallo et al., 1984). Other researchers discovered viruses that ap-

peared to be the same or close members of the same family. In 1986 the International Committee on Taxonomy of Viruses renamed the virus, calling it the human immunodeficiency virus (HIV). In that same year a second and distinctly different strain of the virus was discovered in West Africa. Researchers believed that this strain may have been present in West Africa for many years. The scientific names assigned to distinguish the two viruses are HIV-1 and HIV-2.

The discovery of a second HIV strain was both major and alarming, since it was the first clue that HIV could change its appearance and mutate rapidly. This capability for rapid mutation, often referred to as genetic promiscuity, has become the trademark of this virus. It represents an immense challenge for scientists as they search for treatment and vaccine strategies. HIV-1 is found worldwide and is the prevalent strain in most places, including the United States, Europe, and Central Africa. HIV-1 and HIV-2 are both spread in the same ways and have similar signs and symptoms. Both of these viral strains also result in OIs. Whereas most HIV-1 infected people develop profound immunodeficiency and high viral loads, resulting in death, most HIV-2 infected people act as long-term nonprogressors (Rowland-Jones & Whittle, 2007). Patients diagnosed with HIV-2 tend to be less infectious during the initial stage of the infection than those diagnosed with HIV-1. As the HIV-2 infection progresses, the patient's ability to infect other people increases. The prevalence rate of HIV-2 is higher in parts of Africa and in the countries surrounding Africa. This is thought to be related to commercial trading relationships and immigration. There are increased reports of cases in the United States of HIV-2, mainly in refugees and immigrants from countries with HIV-2.

HIV-1 is much more virulent (toxic) than HIV-2. People diagnosed with HIV-2 tend to have a normal life span when compared with their uninfected population cohort. Also, in contrast to HIV-1, HIV-2 does not result in higher mortality risks in patients between the ages of 55 and 80 years old (Rowland-Jones & Whittle, 2007). Patients infected with HIV-2 develop problems with immunodeficiency more slowly. However, HIV-2 patients who are malnourished, without adequate access to health care, and without clean water have an increased mortality risk when compared with a healthier HIV-2 infected patient.

Since the first cases of AIDS were reported in 1981, the CDC has revised the case definition three times in response to improved laboratory and diagnostic methods (CD_4^+ and viral test results), additional clinical conditions, increased knowledge of the natural history of HIV disease, and improved clinical management (CDC, 2006). The current definition (Table 16-1), used by all states and U.S. territories, allows the disease to be consistently monitored for public health purposes. Because HIV selectively infects and destroys cells that display

Table 16-1 Diagnostic Criteria for AIDS

1993 CLASSIFICATION SYSTEM FOR HIV INFECTION IN ADOLESCENTS AND ADULTS

	CLINICAL CATEGORIES		
CD_4^+ CELL CATEGORIES*	A: ASYMPTOMATIC, PGL, ACUTE HIV INFECTION	B: SYMPTOMATIC, NOT (A) OR (C) CONDITIONS	C: AIDS-INDICATOR CONDITIONS
1. $\geq$500/mm³	A1	B1	C1
2. 200-499/mm³	A2	B2	C2
3. <200/mm³	A3	B3	C3

CLINICAL CATEGORY A CONDITIONS	CLINICAL CATEGORY B CONDITIONS	CLINICAL CATEGORY C CONDITIONS
• Asymptomatic HIV infection • Persistent generalized lymphadenopathy (PGL) • Acute primary HIV illness (acute retroviral or seroconversion illness)	• Bacillary angiomatosis • Candidiasis, oropharyngeal (thrush) • Candidiasis, vulvovaginal; persistent, frequent, or poorly responsive to therapy • Cervical dysplasia (moderate or severe) or cervical carcinoma in situ • Constitutional symptoms, e.g., severe fever (101.3° F [38.5° C]) or diarrhea lasting more than 1 month • Herpes zoster (shingles) involving at least two distinct episodes or more than one dermatome • Idiopathic thrombocytopenic purpura • Listeriosis • Oral hairy leukoplakia • Pelvic inflammatory disease, particularly if complicated by tubo-ovarian abscess • Peripheral neuropathy	• Candidiasis of bronchi, trachea, or lungs • Candidiasis, esophageal • Cervical cancer, invasive • Coccidioidomycosis, disseminated or extrapulmonary • Cryptococcus, extrapulmonary • Cryptosporidiosis, chronic intestinal (>1 month's duration) • Cytomegalovirus (CMV) disease (other than liver, spleen, or nodes) • CMV retinitis • Encephalopathy, HIV related • Herpes simplex; chronic ulcer(s) (>1 month's duration); or bronchitis, pneumonitis, or esophagitis • Histoplasmosis, disseminated or extrapulmonary • Isosporiasis, chronic intestinal (>1 month's duration) • Kaposi's sarcoma • Lymphoma, Burkitt's (or equivalent term) • Lymphoma, primary of brain • *Mycobacterium avium* complex or *Mycobacterium kansasii*, disseminated or extrapulmonary • *Mycobacterium tuberculosis,* any site • *Mycobacterium*, other identified or unidentified species, disseminated or extrapulmonary • *Pneumocystis jiroveci* (formerly *carinii*) pneumonia • Pneumonia, recurrent • Progressive multifocal leukoencephalopathy • Salmonella septicemia, recurrent • Toxoplasmosis of brain • Wasting due to HIV

People with AIDS-indicator conditions (A3, B3, C1, C2, and C3) are currently reportable to local health departments in every state and U.S. territory. The red categories incorporate the AIDS surveillance case definition; these categories are AIDS indicators.
*According to the lowest, most accurate count, not the most recent count.

CD_4^+ molecules on their surface (primarily lymphocytes), the new definition includes all HIV-infected people who have CD_4^+ counts of 200 cells/mm³ or fewer (as opposed to the normal 600 to 1200 cells/mm³). These revisions to the AIDS surveillance case definition took into account the advances in diagnostic methods and treatment to provide more accurate information on

the numbers of life-threatening **opportunistic** (caused by normally nonpathogenic organisms in a host whose resistance has been decreased by such disorders as HIV disease) illnesses and deaths among HIV-infected individuals.

It was not until 1987, after the CDC reported three cases of occupationally acquired HIV infection in health care providers, that guidelines called universal blood and body fluid precautions, or standard precautions, were developed for the prevention of occupational exposure. This forever changed the way health care personnel protect themselves and others from the spread of bloodborne pathogens. That same year, the Association of Nurses in AIDS Care was established to address the needs of individuals with HIV disease and to provide a professional forum for nurses, who often faced discrimination for providing care to HIV-infected patients.

By now, a broad spectrum of individuals, including children and adults and people from all socioeconomic groups, is affected by this disorder (see Life Span Considerations box). Nurses have been instrumental in establishing education and treatment standards, in collaboration with community-based organizations. Today, nurses comprise the largest group of health care providers who care for individuals with HIV disease, stressing the importance of prevention and influencing policymakers. HIV nursing has imparted lessons that can be useful in other patient populations as well: the importance of patient education, adherence to medical regimens, prevention, and health-promoting behaviors.

SIGNIFICANCE OF THE PROBLEM

Disease Burden

Throughout the world, HIV is one of the leading causes of death and results in more deaths than any other disease caused by infection. As of 2007, approximately 33.2 million people were infected with HIV. Approximately 2.5 million living with this infection were children, and 2.5 million new diagnoses were made that year—7400 new cases each day. More than 2 million people die every year due to AIDS. Almost all of those people living with HIV reside in countries with low or middle incomes.

Sub-Saharan Africa has been hit especially hard (WHO, 2008). This region contains more than 65% of the world's HIV population and accounts for 76% of the total mortality rate attributed to AIDS (Henry J.

 Life Span Considerations

Older Adults

HIV Disease

- Approximately 7.5% of the total AIDS cases reported through the end of 2006 were people age 55 or older at the time of diagnosis (CDC, 2006). This figure does not include individuals who are HIV positive. Although still a relatively small percentage, the number of individuals in the older adult population with HIV/AIDS is increasing steadily.
- Improved treatments and prophylactic medications are contributing to individuals with HIV disease living longer, making the disease one of a chronic nature.
- A decrease in the immune system's ability to fight infection as efficiently in older adults leads to faster progression of HIV disease and increased complications.

Kaiser Family Foundation, 2007). It is estimated that by the year 2010, 18 million children in that region will lose both of their parents to AIDS. Death related to AIDS is largely associated with poor health care access for prevention and treatment services (Henry J. Kaiser Family Foundation, 2007). During the past 2 years the number of people infected with HIV has declined. This decreasing infection rate is thought to be related to increased access to antiretroviral treatments. Managing and treating this disease will remain a challenge for years to come, especially in the sub-Saharan region of Africa.

In the United States approximately 56,000 new cases of HIV are diagnosed each year (Hall et al., 2008). More than 1 million people in the United States are currently living with HIV/AIDS (Henry J. Kaiser Family Foundation, 2007). Between 2003 and 2006, the number of new HIV/AIDS cases in the United States stabilized, while the number of people who were living with the disease increased. At the end of 2006, almost 500,000 people were infected and living with HIV/AIDS (CDC, 2008). California, Florida, and New York accounted for most of the patients with AIDS diagnoses (CDC, 2008).

TRENDS AND MOST AFFECTED POPULATIONS

Beginning in 1996 the use of *highly active antiretroviral therapy* (HAART) greatly increased among persons with HIV infection in the United States. Since that time, fewer people have developed AIDS (CDC, 2009a). New HIV and AIDS cases affect varied racial groups, ethnic groups, geographic areas, and demographic populations. This epidemic has affected non-white people, women, heterosexuals, and intravenous drug users. However, people with HIV are living longer (CDC, 2008).

Men who have sex with other men (MSM) comprise the biggest proportion of HIV/AIDS patients, accounting for 71% of the total number of HIV infections in adult and adolescent males (CDC, 2007). The HIV infection rates of MSM decreased from 71% in 1983 to 44% in 1996. A prediction was made that this rate would continue to decrease to approximately 25% (Holmberg, 1996). Instead of decreasing, however, new HIV infections for MSM have stayed about the same. Despite media campaigns to educate MSM about high-risk behaviors, many believe that HIV is now a chronic and treatable disease, and this has led to an increase in high-risk sexual behaviors (Holmberg, 1996).

During the first 25 years of this epidemic, the distribution of new cases based on ethnicity and race changed (see Cultural Considerations box). Hispanics and blacks have been disproportionately infected with HIV. In 2006, although blacks made up only 13% of the population in the United States, they accounted for almost half of the total number of HIV/AIDS cases that were diagnosed. Black adults and adolescents are 10 times more likely to be diagnosed with AIDS than

---

Cultural Considerations

HIV Disease

- Since 1990 the number of Hispanics living in the United States has increased by 58%. This population increase is not the result of immigration, but of increases in fertility because the population is young. Future population growth is taking place in areas with the highest rates of HIV seroprevalence. Hispanics experience a higher seroprevalence rate than whites, and as a result, HIV prevention education is important. Although Hispanics comprise only 13% of the total U.S. population, they represented 19% of the AIDS cases diagnosed in 2006—almost three times that of whites.
- Barriers to prevention include difficulty providing care in a nonthreatening environment where health care providers are viewed as authorities.
- Undocumented residents, including Hispanics, are reluctant to seek HIV care because this condition disqualifies them for U.S. legal residency and they fear deportation. Additionally, nearly 80% of Hispanics are members of the Catholic church, which has historically been opposed to sex outside marriage, men having sex with men, and artificial birth control. These beliefs complicate prevention efforts that stress the use of condoms.
- Because of the deportation threat, recognize that Hispanic-American patients may not share important health information.
- Assessment and interventions should be sensitive to language and cultural differences.
- Provide a safe, supportive environment for assessment and treatment, and advocate for patients who need treatment, regardless of ability to pay for services or residency status.

---

white adults and adolescents. The primary risk factor for black men who developed HIV is sexual contact. In 2005, black MSM were much more likely to be infected with HIV. Another risk factor is when black men engage in high-risk heterosexual behavior (CDC, 2009a).

Some black men who engage in sex with other men identify themselves as heterosexuals because of the stigma and homophobia issues. Many black MSM are secretive about their homosexuality or choose not to identify their sexual orientation. This phenomenon is known as keeping it on the "down low." Prevention programs are challenged when people do not identify themselves as engaging in risky behaviors or having increased risk factors.

The number of women who have been infected is growing. In 2005 females accounted for 26% of new HIV/AIDS diagnoses, and most of the females were black (CDC, 2007c). HIV was the leading cause of mortality in black women between 25 and 34 years of age. Black women are 23 times more likely to be diagnosed with AIDS than white women. Young people between 15 and 24 years old make up 40% of the new diagnoses (CDC, 2007d). Most people are diagnosed between 25 and 44 years of age. In 2007, an estimated one half of all people infected with HIV/AIDS did not receive appropriate health care, and 25% were not yet diagnosed (Henry J. Kaiser Family Foundation, 2007).

During 2006, Hispanics accounted for almost 20% of the total number of HIV/AIDS cases in the United States (CDC, 2007b). Many socioeconomic and cultural factors have contributed to this epidemic and associated prevention challenges in the U.S. Hispanic and Latino communities. The primary risk factor for developing HIV in Hispanic men and women is sex with men. Hispanics also have higher rates than non-Hispanic whites of other sexually transmitted infections (STIs), including chlamydia, gonorrhea, and syphilis (CDC, 2007b). Transient Hispanic populations often have difficulty receiving access to health care because of social structure, language barriers, and migration patterns (CDC, 2008). The predicaments caused by poverty lead to limited access to appropriate health care, housing, and HIV prevention. All of these factors may directly or indirectly increase risk factors for HIV infection in the Hispanic population.

In 1996 researchers falsely predicted that HIV cases would increase for injecting drug users (Holmberg, 1996). The biggest increase in new HIV cases has occurred in heterosexual populations. In 1983 heterosexuals made up 5% of new HIV cases. In 2006 that number grew to 36% (CDC, 2008). Drugs that are not injected also affect the spread of HIV because drug users often engage in high-risk behaviors when they are under the influence (CDC, 2008).

As treatment for HIV has advanced, the progression from HIV to AIDS has slowed, resulting in a decreased mortality rate for those infected with HIV. Data from 2006 indicates that, although AIDS cases have remained stable, the death rate has decreased (CDC, 2008). Advanced treatment options mean that people are living longer after their AIDS diagnoses. Unfortunately, in countries where HIV-infected people are without adequate access to health care, HIV infection is still one of the leading causes of death.

TRANSMISSION OF HIV

Despite significant research into the modes of transmission of HIV, considerable fear and misinformation about HIV transmission, perhaps more than for any other disease, still exists. It is imperative that health care providers and patients be knowledgeable about modes of transmission and behaviors that put them at risk for HIV infection. Modes of transmission have remained constant throughout the course of the HIV pandemic. Health care providers also need to remember that transmission of HIV occurs through sexual **practices,** not sexual **preferences.**

The patterns in the spread of HIV changed considerably during the first two decades of the epidemic in the United States. Worldwide, sexual intercourse is by far the most common mode of HIV transmission, but in the United States, as many as one half of all new HIV infections are now associated either directly or indirectly with injection drug use—that is, using

HIV-contaminated needles to inject drugs or having sexual contact with an HIV-infected drug user. Overall, compared to the 1980s, HIV infection is spreading fastest in the United States among young people, injecting drug users, women, blacks, and Hispanics. The number of estimated pediatric AIDS cases diagnosed each year has declined since 1992. This decline is associated with the increased compliance with universal counseling and testing of pregnant women and the use of zidovudine (Retrovir, ZDV, AZT) by HIV-infected pregnant women and their newborn infants.

HIV is an **obligate virus,** meaning it must have a host organism to survive. The virus cannot live long outside the human body. HIV transmission depends on the presence of the virus, the infectiousness of the virus, the susceptibility of the uninfected host, and any conditions that may help put the person at risk. HIV is transmitted from human to human through infected blood, semen, cervicovaginal secretions, and breast milk. If these infected fluids are introduced into an uninfected person, the potential for HIV transmission exists. In addition to the aforementioned body fluids, HIV is also found in pericardial, synovial, cerebrospinal, peritoneal, and amniotic fluids. Vertical transmission of HIV, or transmission from a mother to a fetus, can occur during pregnancy, during delivery, or through postpartum breastfeeding (transmitted in the breast milk). Conditions that affect the likelihood of infection include the duration and frequency of exposure, the amount of virus inoculated, the virulence of the organism, and the host's defense capability (immune system). Although HIV has been found in other body fluids such as saliva, urine, tears, and feces, there has been no evidence that these substances are capable of transmission, unless the fluids contain visible blood.

HIV is generally transmitted by **behaviors** and not by casual contacts, such as hugging, dry kissing, shaking hands, or sharing food and utensils. HIV is not transmitted by animals or insects; coughing or sneezing; or sharing objects such as pencils, computer keyboards, or telephones. The three most common modes of HIV transmission are anal or vaginal intercourse, contaminated injecting drug equipment and paraphernalia, and transmission from mother to child.

Once infected, an individual is capable of transmitting HIV to others at any time throughout the disease spectrum, even when the host appears healthy and has no obvious signs of immune destruction. In HIV infection the viral load (amount of measurable HIV virions in the blood) is highest immediately after infection and during the later stages of the disease (Figure 16-1). During these periods, unprotected exposure (through sexual behaviors or blood) to an infected individual increases the likelihood that transmission will occur. However, it is important to remember that HIV can be transmitted during the entire disease spectrum.

SEXUAL TRANSMISSION

Sexual transmission of HIV remains the most common mode of transmission in the world today and is responsible for the majority of the world's total AIDS cases. Sexual activity provides the potential for the exchange of semen, cervicovaginal secretions, and blood. The sexual orientation or sexual practices of an individual are irrelevant in HIV transmission. Factors that are important are the presence of HIV in one or both partners and the occurrence of behaviors that puts one or both partners at risk for transmission. Some individuals become infected with HIV after a single unprotected sexual encounter, whereas others remain free from infection after hundreds of such encounters.

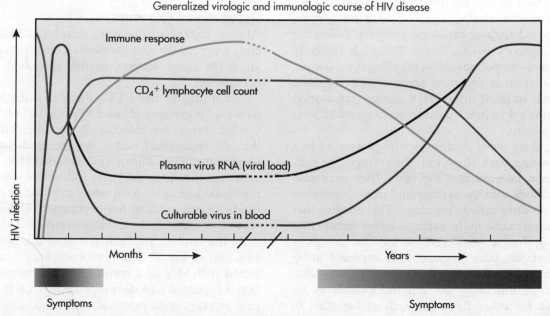

Generalized virologic and immunologic course of HIV disease

FIGURE 16-1 Viral load in the blood and the relationship to CD_4^+ lymphocyte cell count over the spectrum of HIV disease. *RNA,* Ribonucleic acid.

Although the majority of HIV transmissions in the United States occur in the MSM category via receptive anal intercourse, heterosexual transmission via anal intercourse is becoming increasingly prevalent. Heterosexual couples may prefer this method of sexual expression or use it because it eliminates the risk of pregnancy. Unfortunately, the most risky sexual activity is unprotected receptive anal intercourse. Because the rectum is generally tighter and less well lubricated than the vagina, the rectal mucosa may be torn, providing an excellent portal for the virus to enter the bloodstream.

During any form of sexual intercourse (anal, vaginal, oral), the risk of infection is considerably higher for the receptive partner, although infection can be transmitted to an insertive partner as well. The receptive partner generally has prolonged exposure to semen (National Institute of Allergy and Infectious Diseases, 2006). Other factors that may increase the risk of sexual transmission include ulcerating genital diseases, such as herpes simplex virus (HSV) and syphilis; chancres secondary to STIs; intact (uncircumcised) foreskin; sex that is "rough"; and immunosuppression due to drug use, including the use of nicotine and alcohol. Infection risk for HIV can also be increased during intercourse when the infected partner has a high viral load. An increased viral load is often found in the primary and late stages of infection (Klimas et al., 2008). Oral-genital transmissions have been reported but are considered rare, and experts disagree on whether this constitutes an actual mode of transmission.

PARENTERAL EXPOSURE

Injecting Drug Use

HIV may be transmitted by exposure to contaminated blood through the accidental or intentional sharing of injecting equipment and paraphernalia. Such equipment includes syringes, needles, cookers (spoons or bottle caps used for mixing the drug), and filtering devices (such as cotton balls). Injecting drug users represent the second highest exposure category, following the MSM category (CDC, 2006). Although typically seen in large metropolitan areas, injecting drug use occurs in smaller cities and rural areas as well. Injection is not limited to illicit drugs; HIV can be transmitted via contaminated "works" used to inject steroids, vitamins, and insulin.

Injecting drug users confirm needle placement in a vein by drawing back blood into the syringe; the substance is then injected into the vein. They may also draw blood back into the syringe and inject numerous times, a procedure called "booting." This ensures that no substance remains in the syringe. Other factors that put injecting drug users at risk for HIV include poor nutritional status, poor hygiene, and impaired judgment due to mood-altering substances. The long-term effects of injecting drug use put individuals at increased risk for other diseases, such as hepatitis B, hepatitis C, and other bloodborne illnesses.

Blood and Blood Products

Since 1985, blood banks in the United States have screened all donated blood for HIV-1 antibodies, and since 1992 they have also screened for HIV-2. Blood banks have also implemented procedures to find blood donors who might be at high risk for being infected with HIV. Blood from donors who are deemed high risk or that tests positive for HIV is discarded. In addition to HIV, blood is currently screened for HTLV-1, HTLV-2, hepatitis B virus, syphilis, and hepatitis C virus.

Every year, a small number of blood donations come from donors who are Infected with HIV but in whom the HIV antibody was undetected. When a blood donor has not yet undergone seroconversion (a change in serologic test results from negative to positive as antibodies develop in reaction to an infection), the current HIV antibody test is unable to detect the infection. In the past there was a 22-day window where the donor could donate HIV-infected blood that would not be detected by the HIV-1 and HIV-2 antibody test. Since 1995, however, blood has also been screened for HIV-1 p24 antigen. With this addition, this window has been reduced to 16 days. In 1999, another test called the nucleic acid amplification test was introduced. This test detects HIV-1 ribonucleic acid (RNA) and has reduced the window again to only 11 days. By 2003, after 25 million donations, only three people were infected with HIV after receiving a blood product transfusion. The blood came from two separate donors, and the blood tested negative for HIV with all currently available HIV tests (Donnegan, 2003).

Before 1985, people who received replacement clotting factors for blood coagulation difficulties had an increased risk of contracting HIV. Since 1985, a recombinant technique is used to manufacture the clotting factors or the clotting factors are treated with chemicals or heated to kill the HIV.

Occupational Exposure

Almost 25,000 adults who developed AIDS before 2003 were health care workers. This represents 5% of all AIDS cases among adults who had a known occupation.

According to the CDC, there is a distinction between a "documented" and a "possible" HIV seroconversion. When the infection is documented, it means that the individual had a documented exposure related to the occupation and developed HIV. A possible infection indicates that the individual worked in a high-risk setting with exposure to blood or other body fluids related to his or her occupation. However, there was no documented exposure event.

In the United States at the time this was written, 46% (26) of the 57 health care workers who were infected with HIV as a result of a documented occupational exposure had developed AIDS. Of those health care workers with possible exposures, 121 of 138 developed AIDS (Sepkowitz & Eisenberg, 2005). Of all health care workers with HIV, most did not have a documented exposure, and the source of their infection is thought to be from high-risk sexual behavior.

Most of the health care workers who have been infected with HIV are nurses. The second largest group is laboratory clinicians, and the third largest group is physicians (nonsurgical). Other health care workers with possible exposures included emergency medical technicians, health care aides, housekeepers, and maintenance workers. Most of the infections occurred after a needlestick injury with resulting puncture wound. There is thought to be some underreporting of exposures because it is voluntary. If a health care worker does have a needlestick resulting in exposure to a known HIV-infected person, the risk for contracting HIV is low, at just about 0.3%.

As of this writing, the last new HIV case involving a possible exposure to an HIV/AIDS patient was in 2000 (CDC, 2007f). Some cases are still being investigated.

Needlesticks that occur when a health care worker is exposed to known HIV-infected persons are known as percutaneous exposure. If the exposure involves a hollow-bore needle filled with blood that is placed in the patient's vein or artery, then the transmission risk of HIV is increased. Also, the transmission risk is increased if the health care worker suffers a deep injury at the time of the exposure. Scalpels, suture needles, and smaller gauge injection needles also pose a risk for transmission, but it is much smaller. If only the mucous membranes are exposed during the incident, then the risk for seroconversion is only 0.09%. There is a small risk for seroconverting if the health care worker's skin is not intact and is exposed to blood or body fluids.

Unfortunately, postexposure antiviral therapy given to health care workers after a documented exposure may result in severe hepatitis that may require a liver transplant. Some health care workers have died after documented or possible exposure to HIV, but that number has not been reported at this time.

PERINATAL (VERTICAL) TRANSMISSION

HIV infection can be transmitted from a mother to her infant during pregnancy, at the time of delivery, or after birth through breastfeeding. In the United States, it is estimated that approximately 30% of infected mothers will transmit HIV to their infants, with approximately 50% to 70% of the transmissions occurring late in utero or intrapartum. For unknown reasons, the rate of vertical transmission varies around the world; the rate in France is around 11%, but it is nearly 50% in parts of Africa. Factors such as the stage of maternal HIV disease (it is more likely to be transmitted during the initial and later stages of infection, when more of the virus is circulating in the mother's blood and body fluids), a decreased CD_4^+ count or high viral load, the presence or absence of STIs, and the mother's nutritional status all play a role in vertical transmission. Factors that increase the risk of transmission during

delivery include extreme prematurity; complicated pregnancies leading to extended labor; the mixing of maternal and fetal blood; newborn ingestion of maternal blood, amniotic fluid, or vaginal secretions; skin excoriation in the newborn; and being the first child born in a multiple gestation.

In 1994 the AIDS Clinical Trials Group (ACTG) 076 study demonstrated that a plan of zidovudine therapy started after the 14th week of gestation, given intravenously to the mother during delivery and including zidovudine syrup given to the infant after birth, reduces the risk of HIV transmission by 67% (Perinatal HIV Guidelines Working Group, 2001). The long-term effects of zidovudine or combination therapy are not known, but anecdotal evidence suggests that polydactyly (the congenital presence of more than the normal number of fingers and toes) and ventricular septal defect may be caused by zidovudine. It is difficult to determine whether these defects are caused by in utero exposure to the drug or whether the incidence is the same as in the general population. Children who received zidovudine in the womb and for the first 6 weeks of life are closely monitored by authorities to document any long-term side effects.

In addition to drug therapy, substantial advances have been made in understanding the pathophysiology, treatment, and monitoring of HIV infection. These advances have resulted in changes in the standard of care for individuals, including pregnant women, with HIV infection. More aggressive combination drug regimens that provide maximal viral suppression are now recommended. Although pregnancy alone is not a reason to defer treatment, the use of anti-HIV drugs during pregnancy requires special consideration. Unfortunately, no long-term data regarding the long-term effects on the fetus exist. Because of this, offering antiretroviral therapy (ART) to HIV-infected women—whether to primarily treat HIV infection or to reduce the likelihood of perinatal transmission—should be accompanied by a discussion of the known and unknown short- and long-term benefits and potential risks. Because of the findings of ACTG 076, zidovudine should be a part of this treatment regimen.

An HIV-positive pregnant woman should be given this information to make an informed decision about treatment options. Current recommendations call for routine HIV counseling and voluntary HIV testing of pregnant women and those women considering pregnancy. However, there are no legal requirements that a woman take zidovudine during pregnancy or that she be tested for HIV antibodies.

The HIV transmission rates from mother to child have been reduced due to several recommended interventions. This includes ART, formula feeding, and cesarean section. In developed countries, this number has decreased from 25% (without interventions) to less than 2%. In countries where ART is not available and mothers continue to breastfeed, by age 2 the infection rate for babies born to HIV-infected mothers can be as high as 25%. Infants born to HIV-infected mothers have positive HIV antibody results as long as 15 to 18 months after birth. This is caused by maternal antibodies that cross the placenta during gestation and remain in the infant's circulatory system. An earlier diagnosis of HIV infection can be made by doing an HIV viral culture or by measuring the amount of HIV RNA or viral load through a technique called polymerase chain reaction (PCR) or branched chain DNA testing (bDNA).

PATHOPHYSIOLOGY

HIV is classified as "slow" retrovirus or a lentevirus. After infection with these types of viruses, a long time passes before specific signs and symptoms appear. HIV requires cells for replication. The virus takes over the host cell and reproduces viral copies of itself. Retroviruses are made of RNA. Most organisms' genetic material is made up of deoxyribonucleic acid (DNA). The retrovirus uses an enzyme called reverse transcriptase to make its RNA change to DNA. This process allows the virus to be incorporated into the host's genetic material (Smith & Daniel, 2006).

HIV can cross over into the host at the dendritic immune cells that are located in the mucosal layer of the vulva, the vagina, the rectum, and the penis. The exterior layer of the dendritic cell passes the virus into the interior portion of the cell. The HIV virus is released into the lymphatic system via tissue or lymph nodes. Then the virus binds to a CD_4^+ lymphocyte (a type of white blood cell; a protein on the surface of cells that normally helps the body's immune system combat disease), where it can travel farther into the lymphatic system and begin the initial infectious cycle (Lekkerkerker et al., 2006).

When the viral particle attaches to the host cell's CD_4^+ receptor and coreceptor (CCR5 or CXCR4), this is the first step in replication of the virus (see Figure 16-1). The HIV virion enters the host cell when the virus binds with the cell. After binding to the cell, coreceptors are needed to continue the fusion process and to allow the viral particle to eject two copies of the virus's RNA. Inside the cell, HIV reverse transcriptase changes the viral RNA into DNA. A full copy of this DNA is created and broken down into smaller more functional pieces that are moved to the nucleus of the cell (Smith & Daniel, 2006). The HIV DNA moves into the nucleus of the cell, where viral integrase helps insert it into the DNA of the host. The inserted virus is called a provirus. After activation, the cell makes a new copy of HIV by using viral proteins. Afterward, there is an abnormal amount of immune activation, and this perpetuates the progress of the HIV infection because it creates more CD_4^+ cells that will be under attack by HIV and will eventually exhaust the immune system (Potter et al., 2007). The number of CD_8^+ T cells that are activated at this time is directly related to an increased risk of developing advanced HIV

infection, or AIDS. However, the HIV can remain dormant for years if the CD_4^+ cell remains inactivated (Potter et al., 2007). It has been difficult to completely control HIV because of its ability to remain undetected. Patients with HIV are advised to continue taking their antiretroviral medications.

New viral proteins are created when the infected CD_4^+ cell converts DNA into RNA. This process is called transcription. The process relies on the host cell and the viral genetic material. The new RNA is called messenger RNA (mRNA), and it is returned from the nucleus back into the cytoplasm. In the cytoplasm, mRNA is used as a template to begin making HIV protein. This process is called translation. The protein sequence of the mRNA is changed back into RNA, and this makes up the outer envelope and inner core of HIV. After translation the genetic materials become smaller and smaller pieces of viral material. The viral protease chunks the genetic products into smaller pieces so that they can infect more CD_4^+ host cells. This HIV protease is specific to this virus and is targeted by a class of medications called protease inhibitors that is used to manage HIV. The envelope's viral proteins are joined together inside the host cell's membrane, with the core proteins, RNA, and enzymes just inside the membrane.

HIV then "buds" by pinching off this cell (Smith & Daniel, 2006). One infected CD_4^+ cell has the ability to quickly make thousands of cell copies. The CD_4^+ cell dies due to this replication process. As time goes on, so many CD_4^+ cells are destroyed that the immune system becomes dysfunctional and OIs develop within the host.

INFLUENCES ON VIRAL LOAD AND DISEASE PROGRESSION

HIV replicates quickly after entering the host body. It can rapidly produce billions of copies, which infect CD_4^+ cells and the lymphatic system. The viral load of the host during the early stage of the infection can be extremely high and increases transmission risk to others who are exposed. The severity and progression of the infection are related to the host's infection with other STIs, age, and immune response (Fletcher & Klimas, 2007). Basic host immune defenses (cellular and humoral) help limit replication and slow progression of HIV. Unfortunately, these immune responses cannot completely eliminate HIV from the host. The host can remain healthy appearing even when infected with the virus (Table 16-2). Some patients live with the virus for at least 10 years without any treatment and appear healthy. They are referred to as long-term nonprogressors. When HIV patients who were also coinfected with another type of virus took ART, their CD_4^+ count was low (Cheng et al., 2007). When older people do not use ART, their rate of disease progression is much faster than in younger people. It is thought to be related to more pathogen exposure over their life, an increased number of memory CD_4^+ cells (which are tar-

Table 16-2   Types of White Blood Cells and their Involvement in HIV Disease

WHITE BLOOD CELL (WBC) TYPE	DESCRIPTION OF FUNCTION	ROLE IN HIV DISEASE
Neutrophils	Neutrophils normally constitute 50%-75% of all circulating leukocytes and are capable of phagocytosis. Important in the inflammatory response and the first line of defense against infection. Short life span.	Neutropenia (decreased WBC) commonly occurs in advanced HIV disease. Drug-induced neutropenia is common, especially with drugs used to treat PCP, toxoplasmosis, CMV retinitis or colitis, and with NRTI usage.
Monocytes, macrophages	Constitute about 3%-7% of all WBCs. Macrophages are distributed throughout tissue and are capable of phagocytosis. Involved in the inflammatory response. Capable of processing antigens for presentation to T cells. They have CD_4^+ receptors.	Monocytes and macrophages serve as a reservoir for HIV. When activated by stimulation with interferon (inflammatory response), they produce neopterin. Neopterin levels are increased in HIV disease.
Basophils, mast cells	Basophils and mast cells are involved in acute inflammation; breakdown of mast cells releases histamine and other factors.	In HIV infection, may inhibit leukocyte migration.
T-helper cells (CD_4^+ or T_4 cells)	T-helper cells contain CD_4^+ receptors. They are considered the "conductor" of the immune system because of their secretion of cytokines, which control most aspects of the immune response.	Major target of HIV. Progressive infection gradually destroys the available pool of T-helper cells so that the overall CD_4^+ cell count drops. Lower CD_4^+ cell counts correspond with more immunodeficiency and the onset of opportunistic infections. Infection with HIV can impair T-helper cell function without killing the cell.
Cytotoxic T cells or cytotoxic T lymphocytes (CTL, CD_8^+ cell)	Cytotoxic T cells contain CD_8^+ receptors and produce cytokines in a more limited fashion than CD_4^+ cells. They regulate viral and bacterial infections and are involved in direct killing of target cells by binding to them and releasing a substance that can perforate the cell membrane.	Increase in HIV infection. Represent the cellular response to infection. The strength of this initial cellular response has been shown to predict progression to AIDS (i.e., better cell response equals slower disease progression). Cytotoxic T cells kill T-helper cells infected with HIV.
Natural killer (NK) cells	Large granular lymphocytes involved in cell-mediated immune response. Target cells are coated with antibody that binds to receptors on the surface of NK cells, allowing the NK cell to attach to the target cell and kill them. NK cells kill target cells by releasing a substance that triggers lysis (breakdown of cell wall) of cell.	Retain normal counts and normal structure in patients with HIV infection, but they are functionally defective.
B cells	B cells produce antibodies specific to an antigen. They are capable of being stimulated by T-helper cells.	B cells are involved in the humoral response to HIV infection and produce a variety of antibodies against HIV. Present throughout the course of HIV disease.

CMV, Cytomegalovirus; *NRTI,* nucleoside reverse transcriptase inhibitor; *PCP, Pneumocystis jiroveci* (formerly *carinii*) pneumonia.

geted by HIV), and fewer numbers of naïve CD_4^+ cells. Older people tend to have a harder time keeping up with the demand to produce more CD_4^+ cells.

Many factors can increase HIV disease progression. People who use drugs and engage in high-risk sexual behavior are less likely to employ prevention methods. Depression may impair their use of resources to help manage their infection (Kalichman, 2008). Poor coping mechanisms and high levels of emotional stress have a negative impact on HIV disease progression (Ironson & Hayward, 2008; Leserman, 2008; Temoshok et al., 2008).

The virus can make amazing numbers of copies of itself daily (Ho et al., 1995; Wei et al., 1995). HIV contained in the plasma of blood has a half-life of less than 2 days. While the virus continues to replicate, many millions of CD_4^+ cells are produced and destroyed each day. The viral load in the patient's blood determines how quickly the CD_4^+ cells are destroyed.

The HIV viral load in the blood can remain low or difficult to detect for weeks or even months after the initial exposure and infection (Figure 16-2). When the immune system responds, the viral load decreases

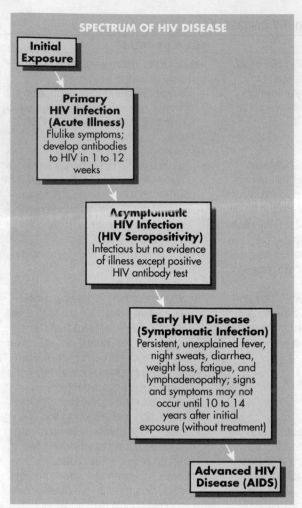

FIGURE 16-2 Spectrum of HIV disease and associated signs and symptoms at various stages of the disease process.

quickly as the body effectively contains the infection. Normally, antigens that are deemed as foreign intermingle with B cells. At this stage, antibodies are produced. T cells start a cellular-based immune response. In the early stages of the infection, the antibodies are able to reduce the viral load. T cells are beckoned to the lymph nodes where the virus is trapped (see Table 16-2). The virus replicates in the lymph system (nodes, tissue, spleen, and tonsils).

The lymphatic system carries the infection from one site to another. During this time, the HIV-infected person does not have any signs or symptoms. Over time, the lymphatic system is damaged by the HIV. The virus enters the blood, which increases the rate of disease progression. The body is not able to mount an adequate response to new infections. The immune system damage can be seen when examining B-cell dysfunction, but more important CD_4^+ cells are destroyed and their levels depleted (see Figure 16-1).

As the CD_4^+ cells are destroyed, the immune system fails. Immune dysfunction can occur when the CD_4^+ lymphocytes fall below 500 cells/mm^3 of blood. When the level falls below 200 cells/mm^3, severe immune system dysfunction is apparent. This results in the development of possibly fatal OIs in the host.

Monocytes can be infected by HIV because some of them also have CD_4^+ receptors. When the monocyte is infected, it can change into a phagocyte. When a phagocyte (cell that ingests and digests bacteria) is infected with HIV, it merely works as a factory to create more HIV. This infected phagocyte can rupture due to a normal local inflammatory response. When this happens, the HIV is spread even deeper into the body. In this way, the skin, the lungs, bone marrow, the central nervous system, and lymph nodes become directly infected.

SPECTRUM OF HIV INFECTION

The term HIV disease (the state in which HIV enters the body under favorable conditions and multiplies, producing injurious effects), encompasses the immune system progressive dysfunction that HIV infection produces within the host. HIV disease replaces the previous term *AIDS-related complex* (ARC). Acquired immunodeficiency syndrome (AIDS) (the end stage of HIV infection, in which the infected person has a CD_4^+ count of 200 cells/mm^3 or fewer) occurs as the disease progresses and the body is severely damaged by OIs (Table 16-3). At this stage, the host can no longer protect itself and the body is injured (see Figure 16-2). The CD_4^+ count is less than or equal to 200 cells/mm^3. People can live for years with the infection before they develop any signs or symptoms of HIV. The signs and symptoms include night sweats, weight loss, diarrhea, unexplainable fevers, and fatigue. The viral course of HIV depends on host factors. The host has an increased risk of morbidity and mortality when he or she has inadequate health care access, is of lower socioeconomic status, or is under the care of a health care provider with minimal experience dealing with HIV.

Progression from the early stages of HIV to end-stage HIV varies greatly. Three patterns have been found: typical progressors, long-term nonprogressors, and rapid progressors. In the typical progression pattern, people develop signs and symptoms several years after seroconverting. Many do not know they have been infected with HIV and can infect others. Long-term nonprogressors develop signs and symptoms at least 10 years after seroconverting. Long-term nonprogressors are rare. Their illness progression is thought to take longer because their immune response is very intense, so their viral load is lower. Also, there are genetic differences in their receptors (CCR5) on CD_4^+ lymphocytes that make it difficult for the HIV to attach. This allows their CD_4^+ and CD_8^+ cells to be maintained at near normal levels.

Approximately 5% to 10% of people who are infected with HIV are rapid progressors. These people move from being infected with HIV to an AIDS diagnosis within 3 years. Several common factors are found in rapid progressors: their cytotoxic T cells (CD_8^+) are dysfunctional and unable to contain HIV, the level of virus remains very high throughout the infection, and HIV antibodies are minimal.

Table 16-3	Proper Terms Related to HIV and AIDS

MISLEADING PHRASES	MORE ACCURATE PHRASES
High-risk groups	High-risk behaviors
Infected with AIDS	HIV infection
AIDS test	HIV antibody test
AIDS positive	HIV positive
AIDS victim or patient	Person living with HIV or AIDS
AIDS carrier	HIV-infected person

The term *AIDS* has been defined for surveillance and reporting purposes; it is not used alone to diagnose serious disease caused by HIV infection (see Table 16-3).

ACUTE RETROVIRAL SYNDROME

Viral replication occurs during the acute infection period. The viral load peaks in millions of copies of virus per milliliter of plasma. The decline of virus occurs right before the appearance of detectable antibodies that can be measured in the blood. The viral set point, or stabilizing of the viral load, is then reached 4 to 6 months after exposure. This viral set point is important, and some researchers believe it to be a prognostic indicator of long-term survival; that is, the lower the viral set point, the longer the individual will survive with HIV disease. Postexposure prophylaxis (PEP), begun as soon as possible after exposure, may help lower this viral set point. This theory is demonstrated in health care personnel who initiate PEP medications after an exposure and do not seroconvert.

Seroconversion is the development of antibodies from HIV, which takes place approximately 5 days to 3 months after exposure (generally within 1 to 3 weeks). This process is accompanied by a flulike or mononucleosis-like syndrome consisting of fever, night sweats, pharyngitis, headache, malaise, arthralgias, myalgias, diarrhea, nausea, and a diffuse rash prominent on the trunk. These symptoms last approximately 1 to 2 weeks, although some symptoms may last for several months. Seroconversion illness occurs in approximately 89% of HIV-infected people. HIV antibodies appear in 95% of people within 3 months, and 99% seroconvert within 6 months. The viral load during the period of seroconversion is extremely high, with a short-term drop in CD_4^+ cells. The CD_4^+ level quickly returns to normal as the immune system mounts an attack against the viral infection, resulting in viral loads existing at nearly undetectable levels in the blood. In most people the acute retroviral illness is mild and may be mistaken for a cold or other minor viral infection (Table 16-4).

EARLY INFECTION

The median time between HIV infection and the development of end-stage HIV disease, or AIDS, in an untreated individual is anywhere from 10 to 14 years (Figure 16-3). This phase of HIV disease is sometimes called the asymptomatic phase, because the HIV-infected individual looks and feels healthy. Some individuals have

Table 16-4	Primary HIV Infection: Signs and Symptoms

SIGNS AND SYMPTOMS	% OF PATIENTS EXPERIENCING
Fever	96
Adenopathy	74
Pharyngitis	70
Rash*	70
Myalgias	54
Diarrhea	32
Headache	32
Nausea and vomiting	27
Hepatosplenomegaly	14
Weight loss	13
Thrush	12
Neurologic symptoms†	12

*Erythematous maculopapular rash on face and trunk, sometimes extremities, including palms and soles. Some have mucocutaneous ulceration involving mouth, esophagus, or genitalia.
†Aseptic meningitis, meningoencephalitis, peripheral neuropathy, facial palsy, Guillain-Barré syndrome, brachial neuritis, cognitive impairment, or psychosis.

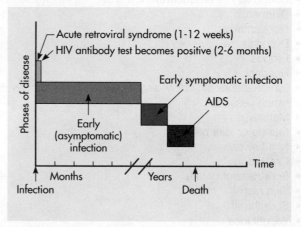

FIGURE 16-3 Timeline for the spectrum of HIV infection. This timeline represents the course of the illness from the time of infection to the clinical manifestations of it in an untreated individual.

vague symptoms indicative of a viral infection, including fatigue, headaches, low-grade fever, and night sweats. Because many of the symptoms of early infection are nondescript, a diagnosis of HIV infection might not be made. Consequently, individuals may continue to engage in risky sexual and drug-using behaviors. Although seemingly healthy, the HIV-infected individual is capable of transmitting HIV to others. Lack of knowledge of one's HIV antibody status puts one at risk for earlier development of more advanced disease, since changes in behaviors, such as those that promote health, are not instituted. Furthermore, if an individual is aware of the virus, early intervention with antiretroviral medications may prolong the asymptomatic phase and prevent progression to AIDS.

EARLY SYMPTOMATIC DISEASE

The early symptomatic phase of HIV infection occurs when the CD_4^+ cell count drops below 500 cells/mm³. Early symptoms include constitutional problems such as persistent, unexplained fevers; recurrent drenching night sweats; chronic diarrhea; headaches; and fatigue. These signs and symptoms become severe enough to affect activities of daily living (ADLs). A physical examination may reveal persistent generalized lymphadenopathy (PGL); recurrent or localized infections; and neurologic manifestations, such as numbness and tingling or weakness in the extremities (Box 16-1).

One of the most common infections seen in individuals with early symptomatic disease is oral candidiasis (thrush), a fungal infection rarely seen in healthy adults (Figure 16-4). Other infections that signal immune dysfunction include varicella-zoster virus, or shingles; persistent vaginal candidiasis (yeast infections); and increased frequency of oral or genital HSV outbreaks. Oral hairy leukoplakia (OHL), a condition related to the

Box 16-1 Signs and Symptoms of HIV Infection

- Abdominal pain
- Chills and fever
- Cough (dry or productive)
- Diarrhea
- Disorientation
- Dyspnea
- Fatigue
- Headache
- Lymphadenopathy (any disorder of the lymph nodes or lymph vessels)
- Malaise
- Muscle or joint pain
- Night sweats
- Oral lesions
- Shortness of breath
- Skin rash
- Sore throat
- Weight loss

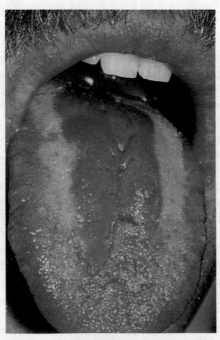

FIGURE 16-4 Oral candidiasis, or thrush, manifests with a whitish, curdlike substance on the tongue or inside the mouth.

Epstein-Barr virus, and oral thrush are early indicators of HIV disease and prognostic markers for disease progression. Because of this, dental health professionals are key individuals in case finding for early HIV disease.

PGL is defined as two or more enlarged lymph nodes (1 cm or greater), located in places other than the inguinal region, that persist for at least 3 months. PGL may be present for many years before an individual progresses to an AIDS diagnosis.

Neurologic manifestations of HIV disease occur in more than 90% of individuals who are infected. Neurologic symptoms include peripheral neuropathies, headaches, aseptic meningitis, cranial nerve palsies, and myopathies. These conditions may be caused by the HIV infection itself or may be side effects related to antiretroviral medications.

Several cofactors may influence a more rapid progression of HIV disease. Very young children and very old adults progress more quickly. Concurrent infections such as HSV, cytomegalovirus (CMV), or Epstein-Barr virus affect progression. Drug and alcohol use, including smoking, may suppress the immune system. Malnutrition is also known to affect immune function, but further study relative to HIV is needed.

AIDS

AIDS is the term used to describe the end stage, or terminal phase, of the spectrum of HIV infection. The CDC has developed specific diagnostic criteria that must be applied to make this diagnosis (see Table 16-1). These conditions are more likely to occur with severe immunosuppression. As HIV disease progresses, the CD_4^+ lymphocyte cell count decreases, and the ratio of CD_4^+ to CD_8^+ cells (T-helper cells to T-suppressor cells), which is normally 2 to 1, gradually shifts, resulting in more CD_8^+ than CD_4^+. The amount of virus detectable in the blood increases rapidly and remains high despite pharmacologic interventions. The number of white blood cells (WBCs) may also decline, and the person's reactivity to skin tests, such as purified protein derivative tuberculin, is decreased or absent. An individual is said to be anergic if no skin response is noted.

Without treatment, the median time from an AIDS diagnosis to death averages 1⅓ years, although this varies greatly. With the advent of more effective antiretroviral and opportunistic disease prophylaxis, the life span of an HIV-infected individual is unpredictable. Morbidity in people with advanced HIV disease also varies widely. Some people are severely ill and become terminal rather quickly, whereas others only have to make minor adjustments in their lifestyle to cope with medical regimens or physical symptoms, such as fatigue or pain. Significant advances in the management of HIV disease have made it resemble a chronic illness. The effects of therapy on mortality have been significant, with a leveling off of new AIDS cases reported to the CDC every year. This can be attributed to effective prophylaxis for OIs and to the development of HAART.

LABORATORY AND DIAGNOSTIC EXAMINATIONS

Strong evidence shows that early intervention postpones the onset of severe immunosuppression. Encourage individuals at risk for HIV infection to seek HIV antibody testing, and educate them in how to decrease the risk of HIV transmission.

HIV ANTIBODY TESTING

Patients need to understand the implications of an HIV antibody test (Box 16-2):

- The individual's blood is tested with enzyme-linked immunosorbent assay (ELISA) or enzyme immunoassay (EIA), antibody tests that detect the presence of HIV antibodies. If the EIA is positive for HIV, then the same blood is tested a second time. If the second EIA is positive, a more specific confirming test such as the Western blot is done. Blood that is reactive or positive in all three steps is reported to be HIV positive.
- Tests with indeterminate results are repeated at a later date, generally in 4 to 6 weeks. Consistently indeterminate results require the use of a viral culture or the measurement of viral load using a bDNA, a reverse transcriptase–polymerase chain reaction (RT-PCR), or nucleic acid sequence–based amplification (NASBA) laboratory measures.
- The series of laboratory tests confirms the presence of antibodies to HIV but does not mean the person has AIDS. The tests are not diagnostic of

AIDS. AIDS is diagnosed according to the 1993 CDC definition.

- A seronegative (the state of lacking HIV antibodies as confirmed by blood test) test is not an assurance that the individual is free of HIV infection, since seroconversion may not yet have occurred.
- A seronegative test does not mean that an individual is free from risk of infection. If an individual continues to engage in risky behaviors, such as unprotected sexual intercourse or use of contaminated needles or drug paraphernalia, transmission may occur (Box 16-3).

CD$_4$$^+$ CELL MONITORING

Monitoring CD$_4$$^+$ cells is one of the laboratory parameters used to track the progression of HIV disease. As the disease progresses, the number of CD$_4$$^+$ cells decreases. The more significant the loss, the more severe immunosuppression becomes. The CD$_4$$^+$ count is the best marker for the immunodeficiency associated with HIV infection. As such, the CD$_4$$^+$ count is used in making decisions about antiretroviral and prophylactic drug therapy and in evaluating specific complaints relative to the risk for contracting particular OIs. For example, *Mycobacterium avium* complex and CMV infections are rare in patients with CD$_4$$^+$ counts greater than 50 cells/mm^3. PCP and cryptococcosis are unusual in patients with CD$_4$$^+$ counts greater than 200 cells/mm^3. The CD$_4$$^+$ count is not a perfect surrogate marker of immunodeficiency, and factors such as the patient's clinical status must always be taken into account.

The CD$_4$$^+$ cell count reflects the number of CD$_4$$^+$ cells per cubic millimeter (or per microliter) of blood. It does not indicate the total number of CD$_4$$^+$ cells in the body. Millions of new CD$_4$$^+$ cells are produced daily and cleared by normal body processes (unrelated to the virus). The absolute CD$_4$$^+$ count can vary greatly in the same individual depending on the time of day the blood is drawn; which laboratory is used; and the presence of acute illness or other factors, such as alcohol. Therefore continue to use the same laboratory, draw blood at the same time of day, and avoid testing on days when the patient is acutely ill or under abnormal stress. When using the CD$_4$$^+$ count to make important treatment decisions, such as initiating prophylaxis for OIs, draw two separate samples a few weeks apart.

VIRAL LOAD MONITORING

The ability to detect HIV viral load measurements in plasma is a significant advancement in the monitoring of HIV disease. Viral load or burden refers to a quantitative measure of HIV viral RNA in the peripheral circulation, or the level of virus in the blood.

At present, three quantitative assay tests are available to measure viral load levels: NASBA, RT-PCR, and bDNA. Even very small numbers of infected cells can be detected by identifying virions. These tests can only be used to identify HIV. These tests are helpful

---

Box 16-2   **Tests Used to Detect HIV Infection**

ANTIBODY DETECTION TESTS
Screening Tests
- Enzyme-linked immunosorbent assay (ELISA)
- Agglutination assays
- Oral fluid test
- Urine screening test

Confirmatory Test
- Western blot (interpreted by a pathologist)
- Indirect immunofluorescent antibody assay
- Radioimmunoprecipitation assay (RIPA)

ANTIGEN DETECTION TESTS (P24 ANTIGEN)
HIV Viral Load Tests/
Nucleic Acid Determination Assays
- Reverse transcriptase–polymerase chain reaction (RT-PCR)
- Branched chain DNA (bDNA)
- Nucleic acid sequence–based amplification (NASBA)

Viral Culture Method
- HIV culture

ACTIVATED IMMUNE MARKERS
- Neopterin
- β$_2$-microglobulin
- Absolute CD$_4$$^+$ cell count
- CD$_4$$^+$ percentage
- CD$_8$$^+$ percentage
- CD$_4$$^+$/CD$_8$$^+$ ratio

Box 16-3   Pretest and Posttest Counseling Associated with HIV-Antibody Testing

GENERAL GUIDELINES
- People who are being tested for HIV are commonly fearful of the test results; therefore carry out the following steps:
  —Establish rapport with the patient.
  —Assess patient's ability to understand counseling.
  —Determine the patient's access to support systems.
- Explain the following benefits of testing:
  —Testing provides an opportunity for education that can decrease the risk of new infections.
  —Infected patient can be referred for early intervention and support programs.
- Discuss the following negative aspects of testing:
  —Breaches of confidentiality have led to discrimination.
  —A positive test affects all aspects of the patient's life (personal, social, economic) and can raise difficult emotions (anger, anxiety, guilt, thoughts of suicide).

PRETEST COUNSELING
- Determine the patient's risk factors and when the last exposure risk occurred. Individualize counseling according to these parameters.
- Provide education to decrease future risk of exposure.
- Provide education that will help the patient protect sexual and drug-sharing partners.
- Discuss problems related to the delay between infection and an accurate test:
  —Testing needs to be repeated at intervals for 6 months after each possible exposure.
  —The patient needs to abstain from further risky behaviors during that interval.
  —The patient needs to protect partners during that interval.
- Discuss the possibility of false-negative tests, which are most likely to occur during the window period.
- Explain that a positive test shows HIV infection, not AIDS.
- Explain that the test does not establish immunity, regardless of the results.

- Assess support systems; provide telephone numbers and resources as needed.
- Discuss patient's personally anticipated responses to test results (positive and negative).
- Outline assistance that will be offered if the test is positive.

POSTTEST COUNSELING
- If the test is negative, reinforce pretest counseling and prevention education. Remind patient that test needs to be repeated at intervals for 6 months after the most recent exposure risk.
- If the test is positive, understand that the patient may be in shock and not hear what is said.
  —Provide resources for medical and emotional support, and help the patient get immediate assistance.
  —Evaluate suicide risk and follow up as needed.
  —Determine need to test others who have had risky contact with the patient.
  —Discuss retesting to verify results. This tactic provides hope for the patient, but more important it keeps the patient in the system. While waiting for the second test result, the patient has time to think about and adjust to the possibility of being HIV infected.
  —Encourage optimism:
    - Remind patient that treatments are available.
    - Review health habits that can improve the immune system.
    - Arrange for patients to speak to HIV-infected people who are willing to share and assist the newly diagnosed patients during the transition period.
- Reinforce that an HIV-positive test means the patient is infected, but a positive test does not necessarily mean that the patient has AIDS.

Modified from Bradley-Springer, L.A., & Fendrick, R. (1994). *HIV instant instructor cards.* El Paso, Tex: Skidmore-Roth.

when trying to identify HIV in people who have a negative ELISA (antibody) test.

Important characteristics include the following:
- In all clinical stages of illness, HIV viral detection techniques identify measurable viral RNA copies in the plasma of most HIV-infected individuals.
- Viral load can provide significant information used to predict the course of disease progression, initiate ART, measure the degree of antiretroviral effect achieved, and note the failure of a drug regimen.
- Plasma HIV RNA levels fall dramatically after effective ART.
- Detection of HIV RNA levels in plasma does not indicate whether any virus is present in lymphoid or other tissues.

Viral load and CD_4^+ cell counts are distinct markers that provide different information. Viral load can predict disease progression and long-term clinical outcome; CD_4^+ cell measurements can indicate the damage sustained by the immune system (the loss of CD_4^+, or T cells) and the short-term risk for developing OIs. Each is an independent predictor of clinical outcome, and when used in combination they can give a more complete indication of clinical status, treatment response, and prognosis. A metaphor used by John Coffin describes the asymptomatic, infected patient as a train rushing along a track, heading for a bridge that has been destroyed. The time the crash will occur is determined by two variables: (1) where the train is at this instant (CD_4^+), and (2) how fast it is going (viral load) (Coffin, 1996).

A baseline determination of viral burden is recommended, with subsequent measurements every 3 to 4 months, in conjunction with CD_4^+ cell monitoring and clinical evaluations such as a history and physical examination. Guidelines will continue to be revised as the implications of viral measurement evolve and its interpretation and use become better understood. In the future, OI prophylaxis may be based on viral load as well as CD_4^+ cell counts.

RESISTANCE TESTING

Drug resistance to HAART can make effective treatment of HIV challenging. In North America and Europe, approximately, 6% to 16% of HIV has at least one resistant mutation (Yerly et al., 2007). HIV mutates easily, and this makes it hard to treat and contain. After multiple genetic mutations, the replication of HIV is "sloppy," which makes it more resistant to medication treatment and has prevented the development of an effective vaccine. ART resistance is based in the patients' inability to adhere to ART protocols. Assay tests are available that can detect HIV genetic mutations that result in ART resistance. Results of these tests are available in less than a month. A list of ART-resistant mutations has been developed by the International AIDS Society–USA. Phenotyping is available to help estimate how well the specific virus will respond to treatment in people who have been on ART for a long time. To perform phenotyping, the patient must have a high viral load (Panel on Antiretroviral Guidelines for Adults and Adolescents, 2008).

During the acute stage of HIV, resistance testing can be important so that appropriate ART can be used to prevent extensive replication of HIV. Some health care providers identify baseline genetic mutations before starting ART. A patient-specific ART regimen can be created to avoid medications that would not work. When patients are resistant to some medications used in ART, they may have cross-resistance issues with other ART medications. Resistant HIV strains are found in people who have undergone ART as well as in other people who are newly infected and often treatment naïve. Resistance to some ART drugs and the ability to transmit resistance to newly infected people are important issues for public health officials who are battling to control and prevent HIV.

OTHER LABORATORY PARAMETERS

Hematological abnormalities are common in HIV infections and may be caused by the HIV itself, by OIs, or by drug or radiation therapy. A decreased WBC count is often seen, usually in conjunction with lymphopenia (decreased lymphocytes). Thrombocytopenia (decreased platelet count) may be caused by antiplatelet antibodies. Anemia is related to the chronic disease process and to HIV invasion of the bone marrow; it is a common adverse effect of antiretroviral agents.

Alterations in liver function tests are not uncommon. Abnormalities may be caused by viral hepatitis, alcohol abuse, OIs, neoplasms, or medications. Early identification of hepatitis B and hepatitis C viral infections is important because these infections may follow a more serious course in the patient with HIV disease. Patients who are HIV positive are often also positive for hepatitis B, since both infections are bloodborne and sexually transmitted. In addition, about one fourth of HIV-infected people in the United States are coinfected with hepatitis C, one of the most important causes of chronic liver disease.

Syphilis testing is important because syphilis is more complicated and aggressive in the HIV-infected individual. It is also more difficult to treat with standard therapies and more likely to advance quickly to neurosyphilis. If a person is positive for syphilis, begin assessment and treatment immediately.

THERAPEUTIC MANAGEMENT

Therapeutic management of the HIV-infected patient focuses on monitoring HIV disease progression and immune function, preventing the development of opportunistic diseases, initiating and monitoring ART, detecting and treating opportunistic diseases, managing symptoms, and preventing complications of treatment.

HIV-positive individuals need to be linked to various points of intervention, depending on their individual needs. Individuals often deny the infection, neglect their mental and physical health, and continue behaviors that put themselves and others at risk. Interventions need to be sustained and reinforced; the emotional impact of such devastating news ("you are HIV positive") can overshadow any initial information or education provided. Stress safer behaviors and the need for medical and emotional support, such as assistance in family planning, treatment for substance abuse, treatment for STIs, treatment for tuberculosis, and immunizations.

A transdisciplinary care approach is most appropriate for patients with HIV disease because of their complex medical and psychosocial needs. The HIV-infected individual should be the primary member of this team, working along with a physician who specializes in HIV/AIDS, a social worker, a case manager, a dietitian, and a nurse. Other team members may include a dentist, a primary care provider (medical doctor, doctor of osteopathy, nurse practitioner, or physician assistant), a mental health worker, a substance abuse counselor, a nontraditional therapist (such as a massage therapist or acupuncturist), and the individual's family and significant other.

PHARMACOLOGIC MANAGEMENT

Opportunistic Diseases Associated with HIV

Probably the most difficult aspect of the medical management of HIV is dealing with the many opportunistic diseases that develop as the immune system degenerates. Although it is usually impossible to totally eradicate opportunistic diseases, the use of antiretrovirals and prophylactic interventions can control their emergence or progression. However, these regimens must continue throughout the patient's life, or the disease will return. Advances in the diagnosis and treatment of opportunistic diseases have contributed significantly to increased life expectancy and decreased morbidity. Table 16-5 lists common opportunistic diseases associated with HIV disease. Table 16-6 lists common prophylactic regimens in the HIV-infected individual.

Antiretroviral Therapy

Combination active retroviral therapy (ART) is an important component in the management of HIV infection (Table 16-7). In 1987 zidovudine was the only medica-

tion available to treat patients with HIV disease, but now the U.S. Food and Drug Administration (FDA) has approved 20 antiretroviral medications (Table 16-8). Six different classes of ART are used to prevent the viral replication process. There are integrase inhibitors, fusion inhibitors, CCR5 antagonists, NRTIs and NtRTIs (nucleoside and nucleotide reverse transcriptase inhibi-

Table 16-5 Common Opportunistic Diseases Associated with HIV/AIDS

ORGANISM OR DISEASE	CLINICAL MANIFESTATIONS	DIAGNOSTIC TESTS	TREATMENT
RESPIRATORY SYSTEM			
Pneumocystis jiroveci (formerly *carinii*) pneumonia (PCP)	Fever, night sweats, nonproductive cough, progressive SOB	Chest radiograph, induced sputum for culture, bronchoalveolar lavage	Trimethoprim-sulfamethoxazole, dapsone + pyrimethamine + leucovorin, clindamycin, atovaquone, pentamidine, steroids, trimetrexate, folinic acid
Cryptococcus species	Pneumonia, fever, cough, malaise	Sputum culture, serum antigen assay	Fluconazole, itraconazole, amphotericin B
Histoplasmosis	Pneumonia, fever, cough	Sputum culture, serum antigen assay	Amphotericin B, itraconazole, fluconazole
Mycobacterium tuberculosis	Productive cough, fever, night sweats, fatigue, weight loss	Chest radiograph, sputum for AFB stain and culture, skin test	Isoniazid, ethambutol, rifabutin, pyrazinamide, streptomycin, azithromycin, clarithromycin
Coccidioidomycosis	Fever, weight loss, cough	Sputum culture, serology	Amphotericin B, fluconazole, itraconazole
Herpes simplex virus (HSV) I	Vesicular eruptions on tracheobronchial mucosa	Viral culture or PCR	Acyclovir, famciclovir, valacyclovir
Toxoplasma gondii	Fever, SOB, nonproductive cough	Antibody test	See Neurological System section
Rhodococcus equi	Chest pain, productive cough, SOB, fever, hemoptysis	Culture from sputum or bronchoalveolar lavage	Vancomycin + imipenem + ciprofloxacin with or without rifampin, erythromycin
Aspergillosis	Fever, cough, SOB, chest pain, hemoptysis, occasional CNS symptoms	Stain of respiratory secretions of biopsy	Amphotericin B, itraconazole
INTEGUMENTARY SYSTEM			
HSV-I	Vesicular eruptions on mouth	Viral culture or PCR	Acyclovir, foscarnet, famciclovir, valacyclovir
HSV-II	Vesicular eruptions around perianal area	Viral culture or PCR	Acyclovir, foscarnet, valacyclovir, famciclovir
Varicella-zoster virus (VZV)	Shingles: erythematous macules, rash, pain, pruritus	Viral culture	Acyclovir, foscarnet, valacyclovir
Kaposi's sarcoma	Firm, flat, raised, or nodular, hyperpigmented, multicentric lesions	Biopsy of lesions	HAART, radiation, chemotherapy, alpha-interferon, palliative care, bleomycin, daunorubicin
Bacillary angiomatosis	Erythematous papules and nodules	Biopsy of lesions	Erythromicin, doxycycline, clarithromycin, azithromycin
EYE			
Cytomegalovirus (CMV) retinitis	Lesions on the retina, blurred vision, loss of vision	Ophthalmoscopic examination	Valganciclovir, foscarnet, cidofovir

AFB, Acid-fast bacilli; *CNS,* central nervous system; *CSF,* cerebrospinal fluid; *CT,* computed tomography; *GI,* gastrointestinal; *HAART,* highly active antiretroviral therapy; *IV,* intravenous; *LDH,* lactate dehydrogenase; *LOC,* level of consciousness; *MRI,* magnetic resonance imaging; *PCR,* polymerase chain reaction; *SOB,* shortness of breath.

Table 16-5	Common Opportunistic Diseases Associated with HIV/AIDS—cont'd			

ORGANISM OR DISEASE	CLINICAL MANIFESTATIONS	DIAGNOSTIC TESTS	TREATMENT
EYE—cont'd			
HSV-I	Blurred vision, corneal lesions, acute retinal necrosis	Ophthalmoscopic examination, culture	Acyclovir, foscarnet, famciclovir, valacyclovir
VZV	Ocular lesions, acute retinal necrosis	Ophthalmoscopic examination, culture	Acyclovir, foscarnet, valacyclovir, famciclovir
Toxoplasma gondii	Visual field defects	Antibody test	See Neurological System section
GASTROINTESTINAL SYSTEM			
Cryptosporidium muris	Watery diarrhea, abdominal pain, weight loss, nausea, fever	Stool examination	Antidiarrheals, paromomycin, azithromycin
CMV	Stomatitis, esophagitis, gastritis, colitis, bloody diarrhea, pain, weight loss	Endoscopic visualization, culture, biopsy; rule out other causes	Valganciclovir, foscarnet, cidofovir
HSV-I	Vesicular eruptions on tongue, buccal, pharyngeal, or perioral esophageal mucosa	Viral culture or PCR	Acyclovir, foscarnet, famciclovir, valacyclovir
Candida albicans	Whitish yellow patches in mouth, esophagus, GI tract	Microscopic examination of scraping from lesion	Nystatin, clotrimazole, ketoconazole, fluconazole, itraconazole, amphotericin B
Mycobacterium avium complex (MAC)	Watery diarrhea, weight loss, fever, fatigue, night sweats, anemia, ↑LDH, ↓alkaline phosphatase	Small bowel biopsy with AFB stain and culture; Blood cultures	Azithromycin or clarithromycin + rifabutin, ofloxacin, rifampin, clofamizine, rifabutin amikacin, ciprofloxa-
Isospora belli	Diarrhea, weight loss, nausea, abdominal pain	Stool examination	Trimethoprim-sulfamethoxazole, pyrimethamine + folic acid
Salmonella species	Gastroenteritis, fever, diarrhea	Blood and stool culture	Ampicillin, amoxicillin, ciprofloxacin, trimethoprim-sulfamethoxazole
Kaposi's sarcoma	Diarrhea, hyperpigmented lesions of mouth and GI tract, GI bleeding	GI series, biopsy	Radiation, chemotherapy, HAART
Non-Hodgkin's lymphoma	Abdominal pain, fever, night sweats, weight loss	Lymph node biopsy	Chemotherapy, HAART
NEUROLOGIC SYSTEM			
Toxoplasma gondii	Cognitive dysfunction, motor impairment, fever, headache, seizures, ↓LOC, hemiparesis	MRI, CT scan, toxoplasma serology	Pyrimethamine + leucovorin + sulfadiazine, clindamycin, azithromcycin, clarithromycin
Jamestown Canyon virus	Progressive multifocal leukoencephalopathy, mental and motor declines	MRI, CT scan, brain biopsy, autopsy	No proven therapy, but HAART may help, IV alpha-interferon or cytosine arabinoside
Cryptococcal meningitis	Cognitive impairment, motor dysfunction, fever, seizures, stiff neck, nausea and vomiting	CT scan, serum antigen test, CSF analysis	Amphotericin B + 5-flucytosine, fluconazole, itraconazole
CNS lymphomas	Cognitive dysfunction, motor impairment, aphasia, seizures, personality changes, headache	MRI, CT scan	Radiation, chemotherapy
HIV-associated cognitive motor complex (dementia)	Triad of cognitive, motor, and behavioral dysfunction (progressive)	Neurologic examination, CT or MRI, CSF analysis	Use of HAART, or stimulants

| Table 16-6 | Opportunistic Illness Prophylaxis Guidelines |

| PROBLEM | INDICATION | PREVENTIVE REGIMENS | | |
		FIRST CHOICE	ALTERNATIVE CHOICES	COMMENTS
STRONGLY RECOMMENDED AS STANDARD OF CARE				
Pneumocystis jiroveci (formerly *carinii*) pneumonia (PCP)	CD_4^+ cell count <200/mm^3 or CD_4^+ % <14%, presence of oral thrush or other AIDS-defining illness	Trimethoprim-sulfamethoxazole (TMP-SMX), 1 DS tablet/day; consider desensitization protocol for patients with non–life-threatening allergy	Dapsone, aerosolized pentamidine, atovaquone	May stop if CD_4^+ cell count >200/mm^3 for 3 months; check patients receiving dapsone for G6PD deficiency
Mycobacterium tuberculosis	Skin test (PPD) ≥5 mm or prior positive skin test	Isoniazid + pyridoxine for 9 months	Rifampin 600 mg qid for 6 months	Rule out active or extrapulmonary disease, which requires multidrug therapy; remember that a negative PPD in the presence of HIV does not exclude a diagnosis of tuberculosis
Toxoplasma gondii	CD_4^+ cell count <100/mm^3, and positive IgG antibody; check for antibodies soon after diagnosis	TMP-SMX, 1 DS tablet qid	Dapsone + pyrimethamine	If using dapsone, check for G6PD deficiency; may stop if CD_4^+ cell count >200/mm^3 for at least 3 months
Mycobacterium avium complex	CD_4^+ cell count <50/mm^3	Azithromycin 1,200 mg once each week; or clarithromycin 500 mg po bid	Rifabutin 300 mg po every day or; azithromycin 1,200 mg once weekly	
Varicella zoster virus (VZV)	Significant exposure to chickenpox or shingles for patients who have no history of either illness	Varicella zoster immune globulin IM ≤96 hours after exposure	VZV vaccine not well studied, though undergoing trials	
GENERALLY RECOMMENDED				
Streptococcus pneumoniae	CD_4^+ cell count ≥200/mm^3	Pneumovax every 5-6 years		
Hepatitis B virus	All susceptible patients	Hepatitis B vaccine series	Combination hepatitis A and B vaccine (Twinrix)	Provide as soon as possible during course of infection; antibody response is optimal with CD_4^+ cell count >200/mm^3
Influenza	All patients before influenza season	Inactivated trivalent influenza vaccine, dosed each year	Oseltamivir 75 mg po qid; rimantidine 100 mg po bid, or amantadine 100 mg po bid (active against influenza A only)	
Hepatitis A virus (HAV)	All susceptible patients at risk for HAV infection: illicit drug users, men who have sex with men, hemophiliacs, chronic liver disease	Hepatitis A vaccine (2 doses)		Combination vaccine available for hepatitis A and hepatitis B (Twinrix)

G6PD, Glucose-6-phosphate dehydrogenase; *IgG*, immunoglobulin G; *PPD*, purified protein derivative.

tors), NNRTIs (nonnucleoside reverse transcriptase inhibitors), and protease inhibitors. Each class of medication interrupts HIV at different stages of the infectious process. When health care providers prescribe three drugs from at least two different classes, this is called HAART (highly active antiretroviral therapy).

Scientists have found that the most effective medication regimen is the use of **cocktails** (at least two, but generally three or more compounds given together). Using medication combinations makes it much more difficult for the virus to develop resistance to the drugs. Such intervention may also slow the progression from asymptomatic or mildly symptomatic HIV infection to a more advanced disease. Recent developments include therapies that can dramatically reduce the quantity of circulating virus in the blood; in many cases, blood cir-

Table 16-7   Pros and Cons of Highly Active Antiretroviral Therapy (HAART)

PROS	CONS
• Minimize chance of emergence of resistant virus • May play a role in the reduction of HIV transmission • Slows disease progression • Improves quality of life	• Drugs can be toxic • Frequent side effects • Complexity of drug and dosing regimens • Impact of nonadherence on treatment failure • Expensive

Table 16-8   Medications for HIV Disease (Antiretrovirals)

Generic (Brand)	Side Effects	Comments
NUCLEOSIDE REVERSE TRANSCRIPTASE INHIBITORS (NRTIs, NUCLEOSIDE ANALOGS, "NUKES")		
Zidovudine (ZDV, Retrovir) 300 mg po q12h	Anemia, fever, malaise, headache, rash, nausea, insomnia, myalgia, confusion, agitation, seizures, bone marrow suppression, anemia, granulocytopenia, thrombocytopenia, hepatomegaly	Side effects, such as headache and nausea, typically resolve within 1 month. Bone marrow suppression side effects occur after long-term use (6 months to 2 years). Treat anemia with blood transfusions or erythropoietin (Procrit); consider treating granulocytopenia or neutropenia with colony-stimulating factor, such as filgrastim (Neupogen).
Didanosine (ddl, Videx) >60 kg: 400 mg/day <60 kg: 250 mg/day po, or if used with tenofovir (Viread)	Pancreatitis, painful peripheral neuropathy (dose related and reversible), nausea, abdominal pain, diarrhea, rash, hyperglycemia, hyperuricemia, hepatic failure, headache, insomnia, seizures, thrombocytopenia	Take on an empty stomach 2 hours apart from other drugs, such as dapsone, itraconazole, or ketoconazole. Need alkaline environment for absorption. Avoid use with H_2 blockers, alcohol, and proton pump inhibitors (PPIs). Do not cut, crush, or chew.
Stavudine (Zerit, d4T) >60 kg: 40 mg po q12h <60 kg: 30 mg po q12h	Painful peripheral neuropathy, elevations in AST/ALT anemia, headache, rash, abdominal pain, diarrhea, nausea, vomiting, myalgia	Crosses the blood-brain barrier. Use in combination therapy Decrease dosage in patients with impaired renal function. Monitor for lactic acidosis.
Lamivudine (3TC, Epivir) 300 mg/day or 150 mg po q12h	Neutropenia, rash, insomnia, fever, headache, fatigue, diarrhea, vasculitis, photophobia, paresthesias	Generally well tolerated, with most patients reporting no side effects. Pancreatitis has been reported in 15% of children taking lamivudine. Never use alone, since HIV develops resistance rapidly. Typically used with zidovudine, stavudine, abacavir, or didanosine.
Abacavir (Ziagen, ABC) 300 mg po q12h or 600 mg/day po	Nausea, vomiting, headache, fatigue, rash	About 3% of people develop a hypersensitivity, which results in flulike symptoms. Life-threatening development of Stevens-Johnson syndrome may occur; stop drug immediately and do not rechallenge, since death may occur. Avoid alcohol (increases abacavir levels in blood). No dietary restrictions. Check for HLA-B5701 type before initiating therapy.

Continued

Table 16-8 Medications for HIV Disease (Antiretrovirals)—cont'd

Generic (Brand)	Side Effects	Comments
NUCLEOSIDE REVERSE TRANSCRIPTASE INHIBITORS (NRTIs, NUCLEOSIDE ANALOGS, "NUKES")—cont'd		
Emtricitabine (FTC, Emtriva) 200 mg/day po	Headache, diarrhea, nausea, rash, lactic acidosis, "fatty liver"	No food restrictions; also active against hepatitis B virus infection. Do not combine with lamivudine.
Tenofovir (TDF, Viread) 300 mg/day po	Mild side effects, some nausea, vomiting, loss of appetite, potential for renal failure, bone mineral density loss	Do not combine with lamivudine and abacavir. Take tenofovir 2 hours before or 1 hour after didanosine. No food restrictions.
COMBINATION MEDICATIONS		
Zidovudine plus lamivudine plus abacavir (Trizivir, TZV) 1 tablet po q12h	See zidovudine, lamivudine, and abacavir	Combination of 300 mg zidovudine, 150 mg lamivudine, and 300 mg abacavir. No food restrictions. Monitor for rash.
Tenofovir plus emtricitabine (Truvada, TRV) 1 tablet/day	See emtricitabine and tenofovir	No food restrictions.
Abacavir plus lamivudine (Epzicom, EP2) 1 tablet/day	See abacavir and lamivudine	No food restrictions. Blood levels may be increased by trimethoprim-sulfamethoxazole (Bactrim, Septra); do not take with zalcitabine or stavudine.
Zidovudine plus lamivudine (Combivir, CBV) 1 tablet q12h	See zidovudine and lamivudine	Do not take with zalcitabine or stavudine. Combination of 300 mg zidovudine and 150 mg lamivudine; significantly reduces the number of pills a patient has to take.
Tenofovir plus emtricitabine plus efavirenz (Atripla) 1 tablet po q24h	See tenofovir, emtricitabine, and efavirenz	Take on an empty stomach, preferably at bedtime.
NUCLEOTIDE REVERSE TRANSCRIPTASE INHIBITORS (NtRTIs)		
Tenofovir (Viread, TDF) 300 mg/day po	Renal insufficiency and failure; lactic acidosis	
NONNUCLEOSIDE REVERSE TRANSCRIPTASE INHIBITORS (NNRTIs)		
Nevirapine (Viramune, MP) 200 mg/day po for 14 days, then 200 mg po q12h	Rash, thrombocytopenia, fever, headaches, nausea	Use in combination therapy. Report any new rash immediately; rash may progress to Stevens-Johnson syndrome, which may result in death.
Delavirdine (Rescriptor, DLV) 400 mg po q8h	Rash, elevated liver function tests	Use in combination therapy.
Efavirenz (Sustiva, EFV) 600 mg once daily (initially at bedtime)	Initial dizziness, insomnia, transient rash, vivid dreams, nightmares, difficulty concentrating	This drug may cause hyperlipidemia; monitor cholesterol and triglycerides regularly. Take on an empty stomach. Contradicted in pregnancy.
Etravirine (Intelence, ETV) 200 mg po q12h	Skin rash, lipid abnormalities, elevated liver enzymes	Give after meals; multiple drug-drug interactions.
PROTEASE INHIBITORS		
Ritonavir (Norvir, RTV) 600 mg po q12h or used as boosting agent with other protease inhibitors	Nausea, vomiting, diarrhea, circumoral paresthesias (numbness and tingling), peripheral paresthesias, taste perversions, asthenia (weakness), increased liver enzymes, elevated cholesterol and triglyceride levels	Because of side effects, institute dose escalation. Start with 300 mg po q12h and increase by 100 mg every 3-4 days until at full dose of 600 mg po q12h. Take with food to decrease gastrointestinal side effects. Ritonavir has many drug interactions: benzodiazepines, opiates, long-acting nonsedating antihistamines (terfenadine [Seldane], astemizole [Hismanal], loratadine [Claritin]), antidysrhythmics, calcium channel blockers, rifabutin, clarithromycin levels increased by 80%. Medication must be refrigerated.

Table 16-8 Medications for HIV Disease (Antiretrovirals)—cont'd

Generic (Brand)	Side Effects	Comments
PROTEASE INHIBITORS—cont'd		
Indinavir (Crixivan, DV) 800 mg po q8h, or 1,200 mg po q12h	Headache, nausea (for the first few weeks), kidney stones, (signs include kidney pain, fever, abdominal tenderness, and painful urination), asymptomatic elevation of bilirubin and liver enzymes	Take on an empty stomach (1 hour before or 2 hours after meal); recommend six to eight glasses of water per day; take 1 hour before or after didanosine; ketoconazole increases indinavir levels by 60%; should not be used with rifampin. Taken in combination with nucleoside analogs or NNRTIs.
Nelfinavir (Viracept, NFV) 1,250 mg po q12h	Diarrhea most common side effect	Can be taken without regard to food. Use in combination with nucleoside analogs or NNRTIs. Manage diarrhea with antidiarrheals (atropine-diphenoxylate [Lomotil] or loperamide [Imodium]) and increased fiber in diet.
Lopinavir plus ritonavir (Kaletra, LPVr) 2 pills q12h	Diarrhea, nausea, headaches, lipid abnormalities	Combination drug of 400 mg lopinavir and 100 mg ritonavir. Can be taken without regard to food. Dose of lopinavir should be increased to three tablets twice a day if taken with efavirenz or nevirapine.
Atazanavir (Reyataz, ATZ) 300 to 400 mg/day (2 capsules) po	High levels of bilirubin, nausea, headache, rash, stomach pain, vomiting, diarrhea, tingling in hands or feet, depression, changes in heart rhythm	Take with food. If taken with didanosine, take 2 hours before or after atazanavir. Efavirenz and tenofovir lower levels of atazanavir (take with ritonavir to compensate). Do NOT take PPIs (e.g., omeprazole [Prilosec], esomeprazole [Nexium]). Take H_2 blockers such as famotidine (Pepcid) and ranitidine (Zantac) 12 hours apart from atazanavir.
Saquinavir (Invirase, SQV) hard gel capsule 1,000 mg (5 capsules) plus 100 mg ritonavir q12h	Minimal nausea, diarrhea, vomiting, headache, fatigue	Take up to 2 hours after a full meal. Take with high-fat food. Refrigerate in hot climates. Give with 100 mg ritonavir.
Fosamprenavir (Lexiva, FPV) 1,400 mg (two 700-mg tablets) bid; may be combined with ritonavir: 1,400 mg fosamprenavir plus 200 mg ritonavir once daily, or 700 mg fosamprenavir plus 100 mg ritonavir bid	Nausea, diarrhea, vomiting, rash, numbness around mouth, abdominal pain	No food restrictions. Less than 1% of people get serious skin reactions, including Stevens-Johnson syndrome. No other side effects seem to be serious. The diarrhea in most cases can be controlled with over-the-counter medications. Fosamprenavir can increase triglycerides (a blood fat). However, it might cause less of an increase in cholesterol than other protease inhibitors. Fosamprenavir is a sulfa drug; do not administer to patients who are allergic to sulfa drugs.
Darunavir (Prezista, DRV) 600 mg po with 100 mg ritonavir q12h	Diarrhea, lipid abnormalities, nausea, vomiting	Give with food. Use with caution in patients with sulfa allergy. Monitor lipid profile regularly.
Tipranavir (Aptivus, TPV) 500 mg po with 200 mg ritonavir q12h	Intracranial hemorrhage (rare), lipid abnormalities, diarrhea	Use with caution in patients with hepatitis; monitor lipid profile.

Continued

Table 16-8   Medications for HIV Disease (Antiretrovirals)—cont'd

Generic (Brand)	Side Effects	Comments
FUSION INHIBITORS		
Enfuvirtide (T-20, Fuzeon) 90 mg (1 mL) injected subQ bid in the upper arm, thigh, or abdomen (for patients weighing >94 pounds [42.6 kg])	Skin reactions where drug is injected, ranging from redness and itching to hard lumps; headache, pain and numbness in feet or legs, dizziness, loss of sleep	Almost everybody who uses enfuvirtide gets a skin reaction, ranging from mild (slight redness) to itching, swelling, pain, hardened skin, or hard lumps. Each reaction might last up to a week. With two injections each day, reactions might occur at several spots at the same time. Long term adherence is poor because of side effects (skin).
INTEGRASE INHIBITOR		
Raltegravir (Isentress, RAL) 400 mg po q12h	Uncommon, but renal dysfunction, anemia, hepatitis described	Very well tolerated. Some drug-drug interactions.

culating levels become undetectable. Protease inhibitors directly reduce the ability of HIV to replicate, or make copies of itself inside cells. As increasing numbers of therapeutic agents and clinical trial results become available, decisions about ART have become increasingly complex. For now, these combination therapies offer optimism for successful disease management and improvements in the quality and duration of life.

It is important to administer anti-HIV medications around the clock. For example, a medication ordered three times per day should be given as close to every 8 hours as possible, not three times while the patient is awake. When medications are not given regularly, the drug levels in the blood fall low enough to allow HIV to develop resistance. This is a critical teaching point to communicate to patients.

Considerations for antiretroviral therapy include the following:
- Previous antiretroviral experience may affect the efficacy of a proposed therapy, since the HIV may have become resistant to those medications taken by the patient in the past (e.g., zidovudine, lamivudine).
- Certain combinations of antiretrovirals may reverse the resistance to a single drug. Recycling drugs previously taken can sometimes lead to improved viral suppression. Incorrect dosing (timing) or usage (missed doses) can cause drug resistance.
- Drug incompatibilities, similar side effect profiles, and toxicities must be considered when choosing a regimen.
- Consider the individual's commitment and ability to adhere to complex drug regimens. Inadequate adherence can lead to drug resistance and, ultimately, to drug failure. Stress this point to the patient. Adherence is paramount to survival and success of treatment.

Opinions differ as to when to initiate ART. The increasing number of antiretroviral agents and rapid evolution of new information have introduced extraordinary complexity into the treatment of HIV-infected people. A provider with expertise in HIV should supervise the care. Treatment should be offered to all patients with acute HIV syndrome (seroconversion illness), those within 6 months of HIV seroconversion, and all patients with symptoms credited to HIV infection. In general, treatment should be offered to individuals with fewer than 350 CD_4^+ cells/mm^3 or plasma HIV viral loads exceeding 30,000 copies/mL (bDNA method) or 55,000 copies/mL (PCR method).

Health care providers are beginning to start ART on patients with higher CD_4^+ counts than before. This strategy results in fewer prescribed medications, that are taken less often, and fewer side effects. The U.S. Public Health Service has provided guidelines for health care providers to help with decision making regarding ART. Also, the National Institutes of Health's treatment strategies have helped decrease morbidity and mortality rates for HIV-infected patients (Panel on Antiretroviral Guidelines for Adults and Adolescents, 2008).

Current HIV treatment is aimed at preventing the immune system damage that results from HIV replication. If HIV replication can be halted, then viral mutation can be prevented, and drug resistance issues can be decreased. ART is aimed at limiting viral loads to undetectable levels. With early ART, the patient's CD_4^+ counts will remain normal for a longer time. It is better to start ART when CD_4^+ counts are higher because they will drop less and recover more quickly (Paredes et al., 2000). The recommendation to treat an asymptomatic patient should be based on the patient's willingness and readiness to begin therapy; the degree of existing immunodeficiency as determined by the CD_4^+ cell count; the risk of progression as determined by the CD_4^+ cell count and viral load; the potential benefits and risks of initiating therapy; and the likelihood, after counseling and education, of adherence to the prescribed treatment regimen. Once the decision has been made to begin ART, the goal should be maximal and durable suppression of viral load, restoration or preservation of immunologic function, improvement in quality of life, and reduction of HIV-related morbidity and mortality.

Clinical trials being conducted by the ACTG and the National Institutes of Health in conjunction with universities, pharmaceutical companies, and other agencies may be important considerations for people with HIV disease. Patients may be able to participate in clinical trials or may benefit from the results of such research studies. Benefits include access to new and potentially effective treatments for HIV disease before they are released to the public, and the chance to have physician visits and laboratory work paid for by the research study.

Alternative and Complementary Therapies

People with HIV disease often use nontraditional or complementary therapies, such as massage, acupuncture or acupressure, and biofeedback. Some patients use nutritional supplements or herbal remedies with the hope of alleviating the side effects of the disease and the medications. Many patients prefer these therapies because of the limitations or side effects of approved drugs, mistrust of the health care system, easier access, lack of adequate insurance coverage, or the high cost of anti-HIV medications. These alternatives are best used in conjunction with approved therapeutic intervention.

Encourage patients to use complementary therapies as long as they do not cause undue harm and are not part of quackery medicine, which tends to drain financial resources. Warn patients about unproven drugs and the potential for fraud and quackery in a manner that does not discount their efforts at self-care. Patients may need guidance to avoid expensive and particularly dangerous forms of alternative treatments. However, remember that alternative forms of therapy may be beneficial and should always be thoroughly ex-plored. An open relationship and good communication with the patient build trust, creating a positive atmosphere for addressing difficult issues. They also reinforce the philosophy that the patient is an important member of the health care team.

Vaccine Development

Unfortunately, a vaccine for HIV is not yet available. This is because the virus easily mutates, many different viral strains exist, and poor adherence to ART has led to drug resistance issues. However, with greater understanding of the immune response to HIV and more effective ways to administer antigens, an aggressive push to create a vaccine is currently under way. Since the mid-1980s, many trials of possible vaccines have been performed with thousands of healthy people (WHO, 2006). Almost $700 million each year has been spent on this type of research (International AIDS Vaccine Initiative, 2005). Researchers have taken many approaches: live attenuated vaccinations, live recombinant vaccines, and subunit vaccines. The results have left the researchers surprised and disappointed. One initially promising study involving a vaccine that was supposed to increase cellular immune function (with an adenovirus used in place of HIV) showed that the vaccine offered no protection against HIV and in fact increased viral infection rates (Sekaly, 2008) (see Heath Promotion Box).

NURSING INTERVENTIONS

Establish a comfort level in interacting with people with HIV disease. Treat patients in a nonjudgmental, empathic, and caring manner regardless of their sexual practices or history of drug use. Your attitudes, values,

---

♦ Health Promotion

Healthy People 2010

OBJECTIVE 13-05: THE NUMBER OF HIV/AIDS CASES THAT ARE NEWLY DIAGNOSED IN ADULTS AND ADOLESCENTS WILL DECREASE.

When obtaining health histories from any client, ask questions regarding safety of sex practices and sexual activities.

- All patients should be assessed for bloodborne pathogen and sexually transmitted disease exposures.
- All patients should be encouraged to know their HIV status.
- All patients should know their partner's HIV status.
- Patients should be educated about sex practices that are "safer."
- Injection drug users should be referred to support groups and rehabilitation programs.
- Patients should be provided with culturally appropriate and age-specific educational resources that promote HIV prevention.
- Seek assistance from community-based groups when disseminating educational resources.
- HIV-infected people should be educated about ways to prevent transmitting the infection by:
  - Avoiding sharing any item that could be contaminated with the patient's blood (razors, toothbrushes, etc.)

- Not donating any body fluid or tissues
- Notifying all health care providers about HIV status
- Cleaning any body fluid that has spilled on an inanimate object with freshly mixed bleach and water solution (10 parts water to 1 part bleach)

OBJECTIVE 21.11: THE PERIOD OF TIME BETWEEN HIV INFECTION AND DEVELOPING AIDS, AND BETWEEN THE DIAGNOSIS OF AIDS AND DEATH, WILL INCREASE.

- Asymptomatic HIV-infected people should continue to receive regular evaluation by health care providers.
- Education must focus on the importance of adhering to antiretroviral therapy.
- HIV-infected people should work to improve the function of their immune system by eating nutrient-dense foods with the appropriate amount of calories and vitamins. Diet should be high in protein and low in fat content. They should reduce stress levels in all areas of life and get adequate amounts of exercise and rest.
- HIV-infected people should practice safer sexual practices to protect themselves and their partners.
- HIV-infected women should not get pregnant.

and beliefs should not interfere with the care of a patient with HIV disease. Patients are aware when their caregiver is not comfortable dealing with HIV disease. Knowledge of HIV transmission and competence in standard precautions and body substance isolation will minimize the fear of caring for HIV-infected patients. Box 16-4, Table 16-9, and Box 16-5 list appropriate nursing assessments, activities, and interventions for HIV infection and disease.

Nursing diagnoses and interventions for the patient with HIV disease include but are not limited to the following:

Nursing Diagnoses	Nursing Interventions
Risk for caregiver role strain, related to advancing disease in care receiver and inadequate caregiver coping patterns	Assess needs and capabilities of patient and caregiver.
	Assess factors that contribute to caregiver strain.
	Develop supportive and trusting relationship with caregiver.
	Enlist the help of family members, significant others, and friends to assist caregiver.

Nursing Diagnoses	Nursing Interventions
	Encourage interaction in support groups for caregivers.
	Teach stress reduction techniques to caregiver.
	Encourage caregiver to attend to own personal and health care needs.
Diarrhea, related to: • gastrointestinal infections • malabsorption • medication side effects	Document quantity, quality, and frequency of stools.
	Monitor intake and output, vital signs, and daily weight.
	Assess for skin impairment.
	Administer antidiarrheals on a routine schedule.
	Encourage increased electrolyte-rich fluid intake (fruit juices, Gatorade, Pedialyte).
	Encourage high-protein, high-calorie, and low-residue diet.

Box 16-4 Nursing Assessment of the Patient with HIV Infection

SUBJECTIVE DATA

Important Health Information

Past health history: Route of infection, risk factors, history of hepatitis or other sexually transmitted infections, frequent viral infections, parasitic infections, tuberculosis, alcohol and drug use, foreign travel

Medications: Use of immunosuppressive drugs

Functional Health Patterns

Health perception–health management: Chronic fatigue, malaise, weakness

Nutritional-metabolic: Unexplained weight loss; low-grade fevers, night sweats; anorexia, nausea, vomiting; oral lesions, bleeding, ulcerations; abdominal cramping; lesions of lips, mouth, tongue, throat; sensitivity to acidic, salty, or spicy foods; problems with teeth or bleeding gums, difficulty swallowing; skin rashes or color changes, lesions (painful or nonpainful), blisters; nonhealing wounds, pruritus

Elimination: Persistent diarrhea, constipation, painful urination

Activity-exercise: Muscle weakness, difficulty with ambulation; cough, shortness of breath

Cognitive-perceptual: Headaches, stiff neck, chest pain, rectal pain, retrosternal pain; blurred vision, photophobia, loss of vision, diplopia; confusion, forgetfulness, attention deficit, changes in mental status, memory loss; hearing impairment, personality changes, paresthesias; hypersensitivity in feet

Sexuality-reproductive: Lesions on genitalia (internal or external), pruritus, or burning in vagina or on penis; painful sexual intercourse; changes in menstruation; vaginal or penile discharge

OBJECTIVE DATA

General: Vital signs, weight, general status, diaphoresis

Eyes: Exudate, retinal lesions or hemorrhage, papilledema, pupillary response, extraocular muscle movements

Oral: A variety of mouth lesions, including blisters (herpes simplex virus–1 lesions), white-gray patches (*Candida* organisms), painless white lesions on lateral aspects of tongue (oral hairy leukoplakia), discolorations (Kaposi's sarcoma), gingivitis, tooth decay or loosening

Neck: Enlarged lymph nodes, nuchal rigidity, enlarged thyroid

Throat: Redness or white patchy lesions

Integumentary: Impaired skin integrity and skin turgor; general appearance; lesions, eruptions, discolorations; enlarged lymph nodes, bruises, cyanosis, dryness, delayed wound healing, alopecia

Respiratory: Crackles or rhonchi, dyspnea, cough (productive or nonproductive, color and amount of sputum), wheezing, tachypnea, intercostal retractions, use of accessory muscles

Lymphatic: Generalized lymphadenopathy

Abdominal: Tenderness, masses, enlarged liver or spleen, hyperactive bowel sounds

Genitourinary-rectal: Lesions or discharge, abdominal pain denoting pelvic inflammatory disease, difficult or painful urination

Neuromuscular: Aphasia, ataxia, lack of coordination, sensory loss, tremors, slurred speech, memory loss, apathy, agitation, social withdrawal or isolation, pain, inappropriate behavior, changes in level of consciousness, depression, seizures, paralysis, coma

Table 16-9 Nursing Activities in HIV Disease

LEVELS OF CARE AND GOALS	ASSESSMENT	INTERVENTIONS
HEALTH PROMOTION AND MAINTENANCE Prevention of HIV infection Early detection of HIV infection	Risk factors: What behavioral, social, physical, emotional, pathologic, and immune factors place patient at risk? Does patient need to be tested?	Educate patient, including knowledge, attitudes, and behaviors, with an emphasis on risk reduction to: • General population (cover general information) • Individual patient (specific to assessed need) Empower patient to take control of prevention measures. Provide HIV-antibody testing with pretest and posttest counseling.
ACUTE INTERVENTION Promotion of health and limitation of disability Successful management of problems caused by HIV infection	Physical health: Is patient experiencing problems? Mental health status: How is the patient coping? Resources: Does the patient have family and social support? Is patient accessing community services? Is money and insurance a problem? Does patient have access to spiritual support?	Provide case management. Educate regarding HIV, the spectrum of infection, options for care, signs and symptoms to watch for. Educate regarding immune enhancement and harm reduction. Establish long-term, trusting relationship with patient, family, and significant others. Refer to needed resources. Provide emotional and spiritual support. Provide care during acute exacerbations: recognition of life-threatening developments, life support, rapid intervention with treatments and medications, patient and family emotional support during crisis, comfort and hygiene needs. Develop resources for legal needs: discrimination prevention, wills and powers of attorney, child care wishes. Empower patient to identify needs, direct care, seek services.
CHRONIC AND HOME MANAGEMENT Maximizing quality of life Resolution of life and death issues	Physical health: Are new symptoms developing? Is patient experiencing drug side effects or interactions? Mental health status: How is patient coping? What adjustments have been made? Finances: Can patient maintain health care and basic standards of living? Family, social, and community supports: Are these supports available? Is patient using supports in an effective manner? Spirituality issues: Does patient desire support from an established religious organization? Are spirituality issues private and personal? What assistance does patient need?	Continue case management. Educate regarding treatment options. Empower patient to continue to direct care and to make desires known to family members and significant others. Continue physical care for chronic disease process: treatments, medications, comfort and hygiene needs. Refer to resources that will assist in meeting identified needs. Promote health maintenance measures. Assist with end-of-life issues: resuscitation orders, funeral plans, estate planning, child care continuation.

Box 16-5	Nursing Interventions for the Patient with HIV Infection or HIV Disease

PREVENT INFECTION

- Wash hands frequently and use skin lubricants for patient and caregiver to prevent skin breakdown.
- Use a gentle liquid soap (such as Castile); avoid bar soaps, which may irritate skin.
- Provide for daily showering or basin bath; avoid tub bath if rashes are present; avoid extremely hot temperatures.
- Use a separate washcloth for lesions.
- Use soft toothbrushes; nonabrasive toothpaste; and mouth rinses with sodium bicarbonate, saline, or lemon and hydrogen peroxide before meals and at bedtime.
- Use measures to prevent skin impairment, such as turning sheets, air mattresses.
- Elevate and support areas of edema.
- Observe biopsy sites and intravenous insertion sites daily for signs of infection.
- Change dressings at least every other day; avoid plastic occlusive dressings.
- Avoid sources of microbes, such as plants or ingestion of uncooked fresh fruits and vegetables.
- Carry out measures to prevent spread of infection: use gloves for contact with bodily secretions, double plastic bags to dispose of bodily secretions, use bleach and water (1:10) for cleaning contaminated areas.

MODIFY ALTERATIONS IN BODY TEMPERATURE

- Administer prescribed antibiotics, intravenous fluids, or antipyretics.
- Encourage fluid intake of more than 2500 mL/day.
- Maintain daily intake and output records.
- Weigh daily.
- Provide tepid sponge baths and linen changes as necessary.
- Instruct patient in deep-breathing and coughing exercises to prevent atelectasis and additional fever.

PROMOTE GOOD NUTRITION

- Provide instruction for high-calorie, high-protein, high-potassium, low-residue diet.

- Encourage high-calorie, high-potassium snacks.
- Suggest foods that are easy to swallow (gelatin, yogurt, puddings) when dysphagia is present.
- Advise patient to avoid foods that are spicy or acidic, rare meats, and raw fruits and vegetables.
- Provide oral care before patient eats.
- Encourage patient to get out of bed and sit up for meals if possible.
- Avoid odors by aerating room.
- Make appropriate dietary consultations.

PROMOTE SELF-CARE

- Assess realistic functional ability.
- Plan, supervise, and assist with activities of daily living as necessary.
- Encourage patient to be as active and independent as possible.
- Assist patient with range-of-motion exercise to prevent contractures.
- Provide equipment such as assistive eating devices, walkers, and commodes to promote patient independence.
- Pace activities and schedule rest periods to prevent fatigue.

PROVIDE COUNSELING

- Assess and support patient coping mechanisms.
- Explore with patient and significant others normalcy of grief.
- Assist patient and significant others in acknowledging and planning for anticipated losses.
- Provide information as desired and necessary, depending on patient's ability to understand.
- Suggest appropriate religious support.
- Facilitate participation in support groups or individual counseling as appropriate.

Health care needs can be unpredictable and assessment difficult because of the clinical diversity of HIV infection. HIV disease may require alternating periods of long-term and acute care. The patient may fear isolation from the community or family and friends because of the social stigma associated with HIV disease.

The disease primarily affects young people who are at the most productive time in their lives, a time when they are expected to take control. For this reason, they often want an active role in the decision-making and planning stages of their care. Patients may experience bouts of serious, debilitating illness, then recover enough to function effectively for an unpredictable amount of time. People with HIV disease often prefer to stay at home as long as possible, and some prefer to die at home. But long-term care in an inpatient setting (e.g., long-term care facility) is not compatible with the social needs of the young patient. Prolonged care is

expensive, and many patients with HIV disease do not have health insurance; alternative care is an important consideration. Church and community-based organization volunteers, such as AIDS project workers, provide support and care services for patients and families. Friends, family, and significant others are also important resources to be considered when planning care for the patient with HIV disease.

ADHERENCE

As Dr. Margaret Chesney has noted, with regard to HIV disease, "There is no point in medical history where we have ever expected any patient to adhere to a regimen this complex, as an ambulatory patient, for an indefinite period of time." Adherence (following a prescribed regimen of therapy or treatment for disease) to a prescribed regimen is paramount to survival and the success of treatment. The nurse is in a unique position to help patients adapt and maintain vigilance in their treatment. Help patients understand that ART is a lifelong, complex undertaking. The ability to incorporate anti-HIV treatment into a lifestyle is affected by multiple factors, including treatment knowledge or misinformation, underlying psychiatric or psychological pathologic conditions, physical status, family and caregiver support, health care views, socioeconomic status, culture, fear of side effects, denial, and skills (memory, impaired function) necessary to carry out a medical regimen.

Patients with higher level of motivation to take their medications as ordered can have much better outcomes compared with patients who are less compliant. Drug resistance to ART can occur over a weekend of missing doses. Typical adherence to ART is poor even when patients only have to take one or two pills each day. One study performed by the Veterans Administration indicated that only 76% of that population was up to date with their drug refills (Braithwaite et al., 2007).

Strategies to increase adherence include assessing your level of comfort with HIV, learning to listen, having knowledge and skills, giving permission to grieve and feel sad, acknowledging frustration and helplessness, providing a safe environment, and seeking expert assistance as needed. All of these can help patients incorporate this difficult treatment into their lifestyles (Table 16-10).

PALLIATIVE CARE

The WHO defines palliative care as helping patients and families deal with possibly fatal illnesses and quality-of-life issues. Palliative care's focus is on preventing and relieving suffering by quickly identifying and treating pain. Palliative care also focuses on all physical, spiritual, psychological, and social issues that affect the patient or the family (WHO, 2008a).

Palliative care is not seen as hastening the dying process or postponing death. Nurses realize that death is a natural process of life, but others may believe that a patient's death signifies the failure of medicine. The goal of palliative care is to address physical, psychological, social, spiritual, and existential needs of patients with progressive, life-threatening illnesses, with the overall goal of improving the quality of life. Most hospice programs use a palliative care approach, understanding that impending death means a shift from curing to caring. Remember that the goal is to relieve suffering through pain and symptom management at *any* point in the patient's disease process. Not surprisingly, care for dying people in the United States often does not meet the needs or expectations of the patient or family.

Palliative care for the patient with HIV disease is different from the care provided to a patient with a cancer diagnosis. Patients are treated for the chronic debilitating conditions associated with HIV disease, but also for superimposed acute exacerbations of OIs and related symptoms. Intravenous therapy, blood transfusions, and antibiotic usage may be considered palliative in the end stage of HIV disease because these interventions keep the patient comfortable and help maintain quality of life. In AIDS care, short-term aggressive, curative therapy is often important in treating acute infections such as pneumonia, while the overall goal remains palliation.

The complex needs of patients with HIV disease require a multidisciplinary team of physicians, nurses, social workers, dietitians, physical therapists, and clergy. The nurse is the "voice and advocate" for the patient who may or may not be able to communicate his or her treatment desires. Because of this unique role, it is important to be comfortable discussing treatment issues and options with patients, as well as respecting their decisions. Families and significant others of patients with end-stage HIV disease can experience what is called **disenfranchised grief,** which occurs when a loss is not openly acknowledged, publicly mourned, or socially supported (Sherman, 2001). Symptoms such as pain, fatigue, anorexia, fever, shortness of breath, diarrhea, and insomnia are common. Become familiar with the causes and interventions necessary to alleviate these symptoms. Remember that symptoms such as pain are a subjective experience and must be treated appropriately until the patient indicates the treatment has worked. Although this phase of life is difficult for both patient and nurse, many nurses express significant satisfaction with these interactions, relationships, and their outcomes.

As the HIV pandemic has changed over time with health care providers using ART and aggressive approaches to treatment, fewer HIV-infected people are requiring hospice or palliative care. However, some

Table 16-10	Factors Related to Nonadherent Behavior
FACTOR	**EXAMPLES**
Psychosocial factors	Locus of control
	Ineffective communication
	Mental health problems
	Trust
	Internal conflict, social stress, stigma
	Paternalistic behavior of the health care provider
Medications and treatments	Complex regimens
	Inconvenient dosing schedules
	Skepticism about treatment effectiveness
Cultural issues	Lack of understanding of cultural influences
	Differing worldview
Substance use	Continuing substance use
	Lack of social support
	Tenuous living arrangements
	Negative view of addiction

Modified from Crespo-Fierro, M. (1997). Compliance/adherence and care management in HIV disease. *Journal of the Association of Nurses in AIDS Care,* 8(4), 43-54.

patients are not diagnosed with HIV until they are in later stages of the disease process. These patients may choose palliative or hospice care instead of treatment.

PSYCHOSOCIAL ISSUES

People who have been diagnosed with HIV deal with a more complex set of psychosocial issues than people diagnosed with another long-term or fatal disease. Often, they are uncertain, fearful, depressed, and isolated. HIV can be treated, but it is incurable and contagious. Many people feel isolated and abandoned by friends and family because of the stigma associated with HIV. Most patients are diagnosed at an early age and do not have adequate resources to pay for the treatment. When ART is initiated when CD_4^+ counts are over 350 cells/mm^3, the cost of care over an HIV-infected person's life is approximately $620,000. When ART is initiated when CD_4^+ are under 200 cells/mm^3, the cost of care over the patient's lifetime is $567,000 (Schackman et al., 2006). The patient may be struggling with homosexuality and issues related to family acceptance. The patient may be trying to raise a family with limited resources and inadequate emotional support. Some patients are dealing with drug abuse.

Nurses and health care providers must be empathic during contact with these patients. Listening is an important skill to help convey compassion. Use therapeutic communication skills to further develop rapport with this patient. Help the patient plan and decide about health care options. The patient has the right to be supported even when the decision seems imprudent.

Assisting with Coping

Individuals who have been exposed to HIV infection, but who are without any symptoms or complications, live with uncertainty, anxiety, denial, and hopefulness (Box 16-6). The nurse's role in this stage of the disease process is to provide continued education about HIV disease and prevention and to assist in realistic goal setting. Make every effort to include the patient and the support system in planning care. Early in the care process, assess past coping styles and support sys-

| Box 16-6 | Psychological Crisis Intervals in the Course of HIV Disease |

- Diagnosis of HIV infection
- Viral load testing
- Increases in viral load
- Initiation of antiretroviral therapy
- Signs of treatment failure
- Adding prophylaxis therapies (e.g., *Pneumocystis jiroveci* [formerly *carinii*] pneumonia)
- Occurrence of opportunistic illnesses
- Change in antiretroviral treatment regimen
- Illness or death in support networks
- New treatment advances

tems, and continually reevaluate these issues. Encourage healthy patterns of coping, such as talk therapy, relaxation, and meditation. Relationships with family, friends, and significant others should be maintained, and in fact may become stronger during the HIV crisis. However, prior family conflicts amongst family members may get worse due to the stress of the illness. Families with poor communication skills are at particular risk for this outcome.

As HIV disease progresses through the clinical complications of infections and cancers, patients experience multiple losses, including the loss of energy; a self-care deficit requiring assistance with ADLs; and the loss of independence, employment, finances, and hope. The reality of death emerges. Nursing interventions should focus on a philosophy of facing life a day at a time and living each day to its fullest. This may be a time for strengthening personal and spiritual relationships and resolving any conflicts.

Anxiety and depression can become chronic, ultimately interfering with daily functioning, relationships, communication, and even the ability to make even simple decisions. Although anxiety and depression are normal with a significant health care threat, refer patients to mental health professionals for possible pharmacologic or verbal counseling when these feelings affect daily functioning for more than 3 months. Assess patients with HIV disease and depression regularly for suicidal ideation, since this phenomenon occasionally occurs in terminally ill patients. Early recognition of depression and anxiety is critical because most cases respond to medications, psychotherapy, or a combination.

Severe anxiety can cause individuals to believe they have no control over the events in their lives. Helping the patient develop a schedule of activities may decrease anxiety and feelings of powerlessness. Explore opportunities for spiritual support and comfort. Community support groups for patients and significant others may contribute to healthy coping. Arrange to spend time with the patient and the support system, in hopes this will decrease anxiety and promote better coping.

Empathic listening and helping patients find meaning in life are critical nursing interventions. Assisting families and significant others in providing support to the terminally ill patient despite their own anger and grief is a unique nursing challenge. Such care, although emotionally draining, can provide great satisfaction.

Minimizing Social Isolation

The psychosocial aspects of HIV infection are devastating. Although it is treatable, no cure exists which promotes denial, fear, depression, and anger (much as a cancer diagnosis does). The social stigma of homosexuality or injection drug use, and the fact HIV is primarily an STI, cannot be underestimated. The first stressful issue a newly diagnosed person must face is disclosure of HIV status. A tremendous fear of family, significant others, and friends reacting with anger, rejection, or abandonment is a real concern. On occasion, families and friends of the newly diagnosed individual have misinformation and unfounded fears. This can result in abandonment, though this is uncommon. Should this occur, assist the patient in identifying other sources of support or refer him or her to a mental health provider familiar with HIV infection. In larger cities, support groups for both patients and significant others can help. HIV-infected individuals who have been exposed through contaminated blood or women with HIV contracted from homosexual or heterosexual spouses may feel anger and hostility. These patients are usually supported by their families and friends, but can be isolated by other people who do not understand that HIV is not unique to MSM.

Assisting with Grieving

Many patients diagnosed with HIV infection benefit simply from listening and exploring in detail the feelings, unfounded fears, and treatment options. On the other hand, many of them need the more structured support found in therapeutic relationships or formal support groups. Significant others and family members also may need assistance to provide support to their loved one. Formal counseling can help a patient address issues such as continued employment, health insurance concerns, preparations for disability, and feelings related to death. Referral to medical or clinical social workers and appropriate community agencies is part of the nurse's responsibility in addressing psychosocial needs. For some patients, referral to clergy is another option for counseling.

CONFIDENTIALITY

Respect for the patient's right to confidentiality is particularly important for the patient with HIV disease. The diagnosis needs to be carefully protected and shared only with caregivers who need to know for the purpose of assessment and treatment.

Do health care providers have a right to know a patient's HIV status? The answer to that depends on the circumstances. If the question is whether a phlebotomist needs to know so he or she can wear two pairs of latex gloves, then the answer is no. But if it concerns whether an oncoming shift nurse needs to know so he or she can develop an appropriate care plan, then the answer is yes. Ancillary personnel such as laboratory or radiograph technicians, dietary personnel, and housekeeping staff generally do not need to know a patient's diagnosis. The use of standard precautions by all staff members for all patients all the time simplifies this issue. Knowing a patient's HIV status merely provides a false sense of security; for every patient who is known to be HIV positive, there are an additional four to seven whose seroconversion status is unknown (perhaps even to the patient).

The patient should be in control of who is told of the diagnosis. Have the utmost respect for the patient's right to confidentiality, meaning *never* discuss the patient or the diagnosis at mealtime, during breaks, in the elevator with co-workers, or with friends or family.

DUTY TO TREAT

A nurse's professional obligation to treat patients in need transcends concerns about the patients' diseases or conditions. As infectious disease health care providers note, it is not the known HIV-infected patient who is of concern; the patient whose HIV or infectious status is not known presents the greatest risk. If a nurse's primary concern is personal safety, the nurse needs to reexamine his or her commitment to the profession. The patient with HIV disease can provide valuable lessons in issues related to infectious disease control, the stereotyping of patients, and an understanding of the dedication of health care providers.

ETHICAL AND LEGAL PRINCIPLES

- The Rehabilitation Act of 1973 and the Americans with Disabilities Act (ADA) prohibit discrimination against the handicapped and the disabled. People with HIV infection or AIDS are included under these acts.
- Refusal to treat or care for people who are HIV infected or have AIDS, when that refusal is not based on a medical judgment, is as unethical as discrimination based on race, gender, or other characteristics.
- Health care professionals may not pick and choose their patients, if they are true to their oaths to provide care to all those in need.

ACUTE INTERVENTION

Early intervention after detection of an HIV infection can promote health and limit or delay disability. Because the course of HIV is extremely variable, assessment is of primary importance. Nursing interventions are tailored to any patient needs noted during assessment. The nursing assessment of HIV disease should focus on the early detection of constitutional symptoms, opportunistic diseases, and psychosocial problems (Box 16-7).

HIV disease progression may be delayed by promoting a healthy immune system. Useful interventions for the HIV-infected patient include (1) nutritional changes that maintain lean body mass, increase weight, and ensure appropriate levels of vitamins and micronutrients; (2) elimination of smoking and drug use; (3) elimination or moderation of alcohol intake; (4) regular exercise; (5) stress reduction; (6) avoidance of exposure to new infectious agents; (7) mental health counseling; (8) involvement in support groups; and (9) safer sexual practices.

Teach the patient to recognize clinical manifestations that may indicate progression of the disease; this

| Box 16-7 | Conducting a Risk Assessment |

Risk assessment specific to HIV and sexually transmitted infections (STIs), as well as bloodborne diseases, is crucial in health care delivery today. Perform regular risk assessments on all patients and when evaluating any new patient. Determine sexual and drug use risks along with other risks during routine history taking.

KEY QUESTIONS TO ASK

- Any "yes" responses require further assessment and evaluation
  - "Have you ever had a blood transfusion? Have you ever received any other kind of blood product? Before 1985?"
  - "Do you now or have you ever shared injection equipment?"
  - "Are you now or have you ever been sexually active?"

KEY POINTS TO CONSIDER

- Begin by assuring confidentiality and telling the patient why asking these questions is important:
  - "I am going to ask some personal questions. I ask all of my patients these questions so I can provide better care. All of your responses will be kept confidential. Is it OK to proceed?"
- Ask direct questions about specific behaviors:
  - "When was the last time you . . .?"
  - "How often do you . . .?"
  - "Have you ever exchanged sex for money or drugs?"
- Exploratory questions may help (especially with adolescents and young adults):
  - "Do your friends use condoms?"
  - "What happens at parties?"
  - "How easy is it to get drugs?"
- Honest responses may be more forthcoming if the behaviors are normalized:
  - "Some of my patients who use drugs inject them. Do you inject drugs or other substances?"
  - "Sometimes people have anal intercourse. Have you ever had anal intercourse?"

DRUG USE ASSESSMENT

- It is important to be nonjudgmental and nonmoralistic:
  - Injection drug use is illegal in the United States and many patients are afraid to be honest unless trust is established.
- Start with less threatening questions:
  - "What over-the-counter or prescription medications are you taking?"
  - "How often do you use alcohol? Tobacco?"
  - "Have you ever used drugs from a nonmedical source?"
  - "Have you ever injected any kind of drug?"
- Do not assume anything.
  - Drug use occurs in all socioeconomic strata. Do not forget that people inject substances such as insulin, steroids,

and vitamins. Any sharing, even one time, can result in HIV exposure.
- Look for other clues in the history and physical examination, including antisocial behavior, recurrent criminal arrests, and needle tracks.
- If there is a positive history of drug injection use, get more information:
  - "Do [did] you share needles or other equipment?"
  - "Is [was] the equipment you use(d) clean? How did you know it was clean?"
  - "What drugs did you inject?"

SEXUAL RISK ASSESSMENT

- Direct and nonjudgmental questions work best:
  - "Do you have sex with men, women, or both?"
  - "Do you have oral sex? Vaginal sex? Anal sex?"
  - "What do you know about the sexual activities of your partners?"
  - "What do you do to protect yourself during sex?"
  - "Do you use condoms? How often?"
  - "Have you ever had sex with someone you didn't know or just met?"
- Ask for an explanation of sexual practices:
  - "When you say you had sex, what exactly do you mean?"
  - "I don't know what you mean; could you explain . . .?"
- Do not assume anything.
  - Marriage does not always mean an individual is monogamous or heterosexual.
  - People who identify as homosexual may also have heterosexual sex.
- Use specific terms:
  - Use "men who have sex with men" or "women who have sex with women" instead of gay.
  - Some men do not consider themselves "gay" if they practice anal insertive intercourse, but their receptive partners are considered to be gay (can be culturally related).

CLINICAL RISK ASSESSMENT

- Assess the patient for constitutional signs, history of chronic infection and HIV, and associated problems:
  - Headaches
  - Diarrhea
  - Fatigue
  - Shingles
  - History of STI, hepatitis, or tuberculosis
  - Fever, chills, night sweats
  - Skin lesions
  - Weight loss
  - Oral thrush
  - Generalized lymphadenopathy

Modified from Mountain Plains AIDS Education and Training Center. (2009). *HIV risk assessment, a quick reference guide.* Denver: Author.

will ensure that prompt medical care is initiated. Early manifestations that need to be reported include unexplained weight loss, night sweats, diarrhea, persistent fever, swollen lymph nodes, OHL, oral candidiasis (thrush), and persistent vaginal yeast infections. Additionally, the patient should report unusual headaches, changes in vision, nausea and vomiting, and numbness or tingling in the extremities. Give the patient as much information as needed to make health care decisions. These decisions will dictate the appropriate medical and nursing interventions.

Nursing interventions become more complicated as the patient's immune system deteriorates and new problems arise to compound existing difficulties. The nursing focus should be on quality-of-life issues and symptom management, rather than on issues regarding a cure.

When opportunistic diseases develop, provide symptomatic nursing interventions, education, and emotional support. For example, an acute case of PCP requires intensive nursing interventions, including monitoring the respiratory status, administering medications and oxygen, positioning the patient to facilitate breathing, managing anxiety, promoting nutritional support, and helping the patient conserve energy to decrease oxygen demand. Because advanced HIV disease can lead to death, emotional support for the patient, caregiver, or significant other is particularly important (see Nursing Care Plan 16-1, p. 768).

Diarrhea is often a long-term problem for HIV-infected people. Damage to the intestinal villi, malabsorption, infections of the gastrointestinal tract, and the side effects of medications all contribute to a large number of patients developing diarrhea. Nursing interventions include recommending dietary interventions (Table 16-11), encouraging adequate fluid intake to prevent dehydration, instructing the patient about skin care, and managing excoriation around the perianal area. In some cases, administer antidiarrheals to help control diarrhea and prevent further complications. Recommend the use of incontinence products to prevent soiling of the clothes and bed linens. In addition, assess for factors that may trigger the diarrhea, such as anxiety, medications, or lactose intolerance.

Wasting and Lipodystrophy Syndromes

AIDS wasting has been a common clinical manifestation of HIV disease since early in the epidemic. Wasting is due to disturbances in metabolism, which interfere with the effective use of nutrients, resulting in the loss of lean (muscle) body mass, often without reduction of body fat. This loss of lean body mass is a primary cause of functional decline in wasting, resulting in increased risk of OIs, reduced quality of life, and reduced survival.

The causes of wasting are most likely multifactorial. Food intake may be inadequate because of mechanical difficulties (e.g., thrush or esophageal ulcers), loss of

appetite (e.g., side effect of medications or neurologic disease), or psychological factors such as depression and anxiety. The patient may also have decreased absorption in the intestine due to infections and a damaged mucosal barrier, which may lead to diarrhea. Some patients stop eating to decrease the number of bowel movements per day.

Wasting disturbs self-concept and self-image and can be one of the most difficult consequences of HIV infection to accept. Useful interventions for these disturbances include creating an atmosphere of acceptance and reassurance, encouraging a focus on past accomplishments and personal strengths, and facilitating the use of positive affirmations.

Decreased levels of testosterone have been reported in HIV-infected men. Testosterone has two distinct biologic properties: virilizing activity (androgenic effect) and protein building (anabolic effect). Because testosterone is an anabolic hormone, a deficiency may cause a loss of body cell mass, contributing to HIV wasting. The role of gonadotropic hormones in women with wasting has not been studied sufficiently. Women who are wasted tend to lose a lot of body fat, but body cell mass is not significantly decreased. Conversely, men tend to lose a significant amount of lean body mass (e.g., skinny arms and legs), with preservation of fat, particularly in the truncal area.

With the advances in HIV treatment and OI prophylaxis, serious malnutrition is less evident. However, nutrition does not return to normal after anti-HIV treatment begins. A syndrome of increased truncal obesity (visceral, abdominal), subcutaneous fat loss on the extremities and face (also called lipoatrophy), and metabolic abnormalities such as hyperlipidemia and insulin resistance has been reported in both men and women.

The management of wasting and lipodystrophy is difficult and generally requires multiple nursing interventions. Assess for and document the presence of diminished appetite and weight. Encourage nutritional supplementation (see Table 16-9) and increased protein intake, provide enteral supplements (through nasogastric or gastric tubes if necessary), and assist with total parenteral nutrition when needed. Administering medications to stimulate appetite, such as dronabinol (Marinol), can help. Unfortunately, these medications tend to increase body fat and not lean muscle mass. Testosterone (anabolic steroid) can be administered by mouth, intramuscularly, or transdermally to increase lean body mass and weight. The effect of testosterone can be enhanced by a low-weight resistance-training program (e.g., weightlifting), which maintains muscle tone and improves appetite.

Nutrition counseling is vital to ensure that individuals with HIV disease maintain a well-balanced diet, including supplements if necessary. The dietitian can assist in counseling, provide the patient with high-protein and high-calorie diets, and suggest meal plans

Table 16-11	Nutritional Management: HIV Infection	
CONDITION	**DIETARY RECOMMENDATION**	**INTERVENTION**
Diarrhea	Lactose-free, low-fat, low-fiber, and high-potassium foods	Avoid dairy products, red meat, margarine, butter, eggs, dried beans, peas, raw fruits and vegetables. Cooked or canned fruits and vegetables provide needed vitamins. Eat potassium-rich foods such as bananas and apricot nectar. Discontinue foods, nutritional supplements, and medications that may make diarrhea worse (Ensure, antacids, stool softeners). Avoid gas-producing foods. Serve warm, not hot, foods. Plan small, frequent meals. Drink plenty of fluids between meals.
Constipation	High-fiber foods	Eat fruits and vegetables (beans, peas), cereal, and whole wheat breads. Gradually increase fiber. Drink plenty of fluids. Exercise.
Nausea and vomiting	Low-fat foods	Avoid dairy products and red meat. Plan small, frequent meals. Prepare nonodorous foods. Eat dry, salty foods. Serve food cold or at room temperature. Drink liquids between meals. Avoid gas-producing, greasy, spicy foods. Eat slowly in a relaxed atmosphere. Rest after meals with head elevated. Take antiemetics 30 minutes before meals.
Candidiasis	Soft or pureed foods	Serve moist foods. Drink plenty of fluids. Avoid acidic and spicy foods. Use straw and tilt head back and forth when drinking. To decrease discomfort, eat soft foods, such as puddings and yogurt.
Fever	High-calorie, high-protein foods	Use nutritional supplements. Increase fluid intake.
Altered taste	Diet as tolerated	Try herbs and spices. Marinate meat, poultry, and fish. Serve food cold or at room temperature. Drink plenty of fluids. Add salt or sugar. Introduce alternative protein sources.
Anemia	High-iron foods	Eat organ meats and raisins. Drink orange juice when taking iron supplements to facilitate absorption.
Fatigue	High-calorie foods	Cook in large quantities and freeze in meal-size packets. Use microwave and convenience foods. Use easy-to-fix snack foods. Use social support system to assist with meal planning and preparation. Access in-home homemaker services and Meals-on-Wheels programs.

that fit the patient's lifestyle. Smaller, more frequent meals can be less overwhelming than larger meals. Of course, teaching about food safety is of paramount concern because enteric infections (e.g., cryptosporidiosis, microsporidiosis, and amebas) in HIV disease are often not treatable or are relapsing. In some cases, enteral or parenteral feeding becomes necessary.

Management of elevated triglycerides and lipids (cholesterol) is becoming common in HIV disease. As in other patient populations, these elevations can lead to cardiovascular disease and, in some cases, diabetes. Lipid-lowering agents such as the statins may be effective in treating this complication. However, because the liver metabolizes many of the antilipid agents, it is important to choose a statin that is safer than those that must pass through the liver to be activated; safer

anticholesterol drugs include pravastatin (Pravachol), fluvastatin (Lescol), and possibly atorvastatin (Lipitor). A program of diet, exercise, and medications can safely lower lipids and reduce the chances of a cardiovascular event.

Insulin resistance or diabetes sometimes respond to oral hypoglycemic agents (e.g., metformin or rosiglitazone [Avandia]). In some cases, the anti-HIV therapy needs to be changed to a protease-sparing combination. Managing diet, stopping smoking, losing weight, and exercising can help control the elevated blood glucose that can occur with the use of anti-HIV medications. Studies are being conducted to determine the appropriate interventions for HIV-infected individuals who are experiencing fat redistribution body changes.

Unfortunately, as with any overwhelming viral infection, HIV infection increases the patient's metabolic needs. This hypermetabolism and consequent higher energy expenditure frequently exceed the number of calories taken in by the patient. Malnutrition, weight loss, and generalized wasting are common problems in patients with HIV disease (Nursing Care Plan). As many as 70% to 90% of patients with HIV disease experience wasting. When a patient's weight is reduced to 60% of his or her ideal body weight, death can occur, regardless of the underlying condition. Malnutrition may influence morbidity and mortality in several ways. Malnutrition contributes to wasting, and wasting hastens the negative immune consequences of HIV infection. HIV wasting contributes to slower recovery from infection, impaired wound healing, increased risk of secondary infection, and decreased cardiac and respiratory function. Thus wasting can lead to an earlier death. The weight loss associated with HIV disease is often severe and debilitating, producing a vicious cycle of anorexia, malnutrition, loss of tissue mass, muscle wasting, profound fatigue, and increased susceptibility to infections and drug interactions. Although typically seen in later stages of HIV disease, malnutrition and wasting can occur in the early stages of HIV infection.

Neurologic Complications
HIV-Associated Cognitive Motor Complex
HIV-associated cognitive motor complex (previously known as AIDS dementia) is the term preferred by the WHO and the American Academy of Neurology to describe a common central nervous system complication of HIV disease. It occurs in 20% to 33% of all adults and as many as 50% of children with end-stage disease (AIDS). This condition is a complex combination of signs and symptoms, including dementia; impaired motor function; and, at times, characteristic behavioral changes that resemble those accompanying a stroke or head trauma. The disease generally does not cause alterations in the level of consciousness or psychiatric disturbances. It is usually described as a triad of cognitive, motor, and behavioral dysfunction that slowly progresses over a period of weeks to months. The cognitive changes primarily involve a mental slowing and inattention. Patients typically lose their train of thought and complain of slowed thinking. They may miss appointments and find themselves making lists of tasks and chores that need completing. The symptoms of motor dysfunction ordinarily develop after those of cognitive impairment. They include poor balance and coordination (e.g., falling and tripping, dropping things); slower hand activities (e.g., writing, eating); and, ultimately, leg weakness that can limit ambulation. The diagnosis of this type of dementia can be made by conducting a simple physical examination, neuro-

logic testing, magnetic resonance imaging and computed tomography examinations, and cerebrospinal fluid analysis.

Nursing interventions for neurocognitive dysfunction include the administration of anti-HIV and psychotropic medications (cautiously). Supervision of the patient, which includes a home safety assessment, is imperative. Ensure that orientation cues such as clocks and calendars are present, hallways and living areas are brightly lit, walkways are clear of electrical cords or throw rugs, and potentially dangerous objects (e.g., knives, poisons) are safely stored.

Caring for patients with dementia is a collaborative effort between the health care provider and family. It is advisable to seek advice from a social worker, the home health care department, and a psychologist in developing a plan to care for an impaired individual.

AIDS-dementia complex (ADC), caused by HIV infection in the brain, is a common neurologic disorder associated with HIV. Dementia symptoms are sometimes reversible if a treatable cause can be diagnosed. Treatable causes include dehydration, depression, and medication toxicity or side effects. Clinical manifestations of ADC include cognitive, behavioral, and motor abnormalities. Symptoms of ADC include decreased ability to concentrate, apathy, depression, social withdrawal, personality changes, confusion, hallucinations, altered levels of consciousness, and slowed response rates. ADC can lead to coma. Nursing interventions are focused on patient safety and caregiver support.

Peripheral Neuropathy
Neuropathies are diseases that affect the peripheral nervous system. They can affect sensory, motor, or autonomic nerves. The causes of neuropathies can be related to HIV disease itself or, more frequently, the side effects of many anti-HIV medications (e.g., stavudine [d4T, Zerit], zalcitabine [ddC, Hivid], and didanosine [ddI, Videx]). Symptoms include numbness, localized tingling, hypesthesia (diminished sensitivity to stimulation) or anesthesia, loss of vibration and position sense (proprioception), and decreased or increased sensitivity to pain. In most cases, patients complain of numbness in the fingers, the hands, and the feet and pain on walking. Patients may also experience autonomic neuropathy. Symptoms such as mild positional hypotension, cardiovascular collapse, and chronic diarrhea suggest autonomic neuropathy.

As new HIV medications with less neurotoxic side effects become available, fewer people are experiencing peripheral neuropathy. Older ART medications caused painful peripheral neuropathy, and people who have taken these medications in the past may develop this problem later.

⭐ **Nursing Care Plan 16-1   The Patient Who Is HIV Positive**

Ms. James is a 20-year-old who comes to the emergency department, accompanied by her mother, with complaints of severe vomiting and recent weight loss of 10 pounds. Ms. James went to the 24-hour clinic and learned that she is approximately 8 weeks pregnant and, because of risk factors for HIV exposure, gave informed consent for HIV antibody testing. The clinic determined that she is HIV positive by ELISA and Western blot testing. Ms. James is tearful and reluctant to answer questions about her recent HIV diagnosis and positive pregnancy test. She states she could not be HIV positive because she has had sexual intercourse only with her boyfriend of 5 years. Additionally, Ms. James is concerned about telling her mother about her HIV status and the pregnancy because she lives with her mother, who is also taking care of her sick elderly grandmother. Ms. James does not have a job and depends on family members to help her meet financial obligations and needs. Ms. James feels the added burden to her mother would "be too much" and is considering leaving home to live in a shelter.

NURSING DIAGNOSIS *Risk for caregiver role strain, related to advancing disease in care receiver, inadequate caregiver coping pattern*

Patient Goals and Expected Outcomes	Nursing Interventions	Evaluation
Caregiver will use available community and personal resources Caregiver will be able to complete necessary caregiving tasks Caregiver will receive effective support	Assess needs and capabilities of patient and caregiver. Assess factors that contribute to caregiver strain (unrealistic expectations, poor insight, inability to use resources, unsatisfactory relationship with care receiver, insufficient financial and psychosocial resources). Develop supportive and trusting relationship with caregiver. Enlist help of other family members or friends to assist. Teach caregiver to perform care activities in a safe, efficient, and energy-conserving manner. Teach stress-reduction techniques. Encourage caregiver to attend to own personal and health needs.	The caregiver provides safe, supportive care to the HIV-infected patient. The caregiver acknowledges the need for personal support and accesses resources in family and community. The caregiver shares frustrations about difficulty of caring for a significant other. The caregiver receives assistance from family members and/or professional caregivers.

NURSING DIAGNOSIS *Imbalanced nutrition: less than body requirements, related to chronic infections and/or malabsorption, nausea, vomiting, diarrhea, fatigue, or side effects of medications as evidenced by 10% or greater loss of ideal body mass*

Patient Goals and Expected Outcomes	Nursing Interventions	Evaluation
Patient's weight will remain stable Patient's nutritional intake will exceed metabolic needs Patient will regain lost weight	Assist with diagnosis of underlying opportunistic infections. Assess patient's knowledge of optimal nutritional intake. Increase protein, calorie, and fat intake. Offer nutritional supplements (Carnation Instant Breakfast, Boost, Sustacal, etc.). Schedule procedures that are painful, stressful, or nauseating so they do not interfere with mealtimes. Provide the patient with several small meals throughout the day as opposed to three large meals. Provide referrals to dietitians, social workers, and case managers. Weigh patient daily.	Patient's weight remains stable or increases. Patient reports increased energy level. Patient is able to complete activities of daily living. Patient experiences increase in lean muscle mass.

Critical Thinking Questions

1. Ms. James is tearful and asks the nurse if there is any treatment to prevent her baby from becoming HIV positive. What should be included in the nurse's information to Ms. James?
2. Ms. James asks the nurse if she can legally require her boyfriend to be tested for HIV. What is the most appropriate response?
3. Ms. James asks the nurse when she will develop AIDS now that she is HIV positive. What is the correct answer?

Management of Opportunistic Infections

With the advent of effective ART and better understanding of OI prophylaxis, the frequency of OIs has decreased dramatically. OIs still occur in severely immunocompromised patients, so become familiar with the recognition, treatment, and prophylaxis of these diseases. OIs are typically seen in individuals who are nonadherent to their antiretroviral regimen, nonadherent to OI prophylactic regimens, or at the end stage of HIV disease, and in individuals who do not consistently access the health care system. (See Tables 16-5 and 16-6 for common OIs, treatment, and prevention.)

Health Promotion

Because patients with HIV disease are living longer, more productive lives, attention to the promotion of health and healthy behaviors is important (see Health Promotion box). Encourage patients to eat well-balanced meals, stop or at least reduce the number of cigarettes smoked, get adequate sleep and rest periods if possible, use stress-reduction modalities (e.g., biofeedback, referral for counseling), obtain dental care regularly, and keep scheduled appointments with all health care providers. Attention to comorbid conditions, such as hypertension and diabetes, helps minimize additional health problems. Encourage patients to get all immunizations and keep them up to date; female patients should regularly receive gynecologic care. If hospitalizations are necessary, encourage the patient and the significant other(s) to participate in treatment decision making, and arrange for home care follow-up if indicated.

Although some pets can pose risks for transmission of OIs, they are, overall, therapeutic for the patient and healing. Only minor modifications need to be made for pet-owning HIV-infected people (e.g., birdcage and cat litter box cleaning). If possible, arrange pet visits to the hospital or care facility if a long separation is anticipated; do not dismiss the idea of benefit because this practice is not acceptable at your health care facility. Speak with managers and supervisors to obtain permission, or help develop policies and procedures that allow the visitation of pets.

PREVENTION OF HIV INFECTION

HIV disease is **preventable.** However, prevention takes the cooperation and efforts of public health care providers, medical providers, nurses in all specialties, families, communities, churches, and schools (Box 16-8). Education on prevention is the only truly effective "vaccine" available to curb the HIV pandemic. Many patients admitted to acute care facilities have unrecognized HIV disease or are at risk for HIV infection. Assess each patient's risk and counsel those at risk about HIV testing, the behaviors that put them at risk, and how to reduce or eliminate those risks. Today, every nurse is an HIV nurse, meaning that all nurses are responsible for teach-

Health Promotion

The Patient Infected with HIV

- Remind patients that a positive diagnosis is not an immediate "death sentence." Patients are living increasingly longer after diagnosis because of medications, more specialized care, and decreased morbidity and mortality related to opportunistic diseases.
- Stress the importance of health-promoting behaviors to reduce the risk of comorbidity.
- Encourage patients to maintain good nutritional status by eating regular, well-balanced meals that are high in protein and calories. Increased protein is necessary for cell and tissue repair, especially in patients who may be hypermetabolic.
- Encourage patients to limit their intake of alcoholic beverages and avoid the use of illicit or recreational drugs.
- Encourage patients to maintain an adequate sleep schedule.
- Encourage patients to use stress-reduction practices, such as biofeedback, massage, or progressive relaxation. They should also engage in relaxing or pleasurable activities.
- Advise patients to use safer sexual practices to avoid reinfection and exposure to other sexually transmitted infections.
- Encourage patients to establish an exercise regimen that includes aerobic activity as well as low-resistance weightlifting if possible.
- Most important, support patients in setting short- and long-term goals and assist them in achieving those goals.

ing patients methods to reduce the risk of transmission. Nurses must be able to discuss behaviors related to sexual activity and substance use in a nonjudgmental way (e.g., condom application, using clean "works"). Establish rapport with patients before asking sensitive, explicit questions related to behaviors typically not discussed.

Harm-reduction education is a fundamental element of HIV prevention methods. Harm reduction does not completely eliminate the risk of HIV transmission, but it minimizes the social harms and costs associated with certain behaviors. For example, asking patients to quit smoking two packs of cigarettes per day all at once almost always results in failure. With a harm-reduction approach, suggest that the patient reduce the number of cigarettes smoked from 40 to 30 a day. Although the ultimate goal is for the patient to stop smoking altogether, the patient has at least reduced the risk of long-term effects by limiting the number of cigarettes smoked. The same is true for HIV prevention. Encouraging patients to use protective barriers 50% of the time (although not ideal) still results in a reduced risk of HIV transmission.

HIV TESTING AND COUNSELING

An important part of preventing HIV transmission is HIV screening tests and follow-up education and counseling (see Box 16-3). However, do not coerce patients into having an HIV screening test. The process of helping patients make the decision about whether to undergo testing and how to be tested is called **test**

Box 16-8 Prevention Options

SEXUAL

No Risk
- Abstinence from sexual contact in which there is exchange of semen, vaginal secretions, or blood.
- Partners who are in a mutually monogamous (the state of having one mate) relationship in which neither partner is at risk of infection through injecting drug use, and in which neither partner was previously exposed to HIV.

Reduced Risk
- Limiting the number of partners, even though a potential risk exists if there was sexual contact with only one infected partner.
- Protective measures through consistent and correct use of latex condoms with a spermicide in every act of sexual intercourse in which there would be exchange of semen, vaginal secretions, or blood. The correct use of condoms is as follows:
  - —Put on the condom as soon as erection occurs and before any sexual contact (anal, vaginal, oral).
  - —Leave space at the tip of the condom.
  - —Use only water-based lubricants.
  - —Hold the condom firmly to keep it from slipping off; withdraw from partner immediately after ejaculation.

INJECTING DRUG USE

No Risk
- Stop the use of injectable drugs. Provide drug treatment opportunities.

- If drugs are going to be injected, use sterile needles and equipment.

Reduced Risk
- If needles and equipment are going to be shared, follow instructions on cleaning.
- Fill the syringe with sodium hypochlorite 5.25% (Clorox) bleach two times; empty two times. Fill the syringe with clean water two times; empty two times.

PERINATAL

No Risk
- Avoidance of pregnancy is the only certain way to prevent transmission of HIV to a fetus or infant.
- Counsel a woman of childbearing age of unknown HIV status about behaviors that would put her and her partner or spouse at risk for HIV infection. If risk factors are determined in either case, counsel both individuals about testing for HIV.

Reduced Risk
- Adherence to barrier birth control measures, including use of condoms, to avoid pregnancy.
- Use of antiretroviral therapy given during pregnancy and to infant for first 6 weeks of life.

decision counseling. Nurses and health care providers should counsel their patients before and after HIV testing. HIV tests require informed consent per state law before drawing blood. The informed consent is always accompanied by an explanation about the testing and implications of results. Also explain the limitations of the test.

HIV testing that is performed early in the disease is important for increasing survival rates of HIV-infected patients and preventing the transmission to others through high-risk behaviors. The U.S. Public Health Service published guidelines in 1987 regarding testing for people who were at high risk for becoming infected with HIV. Guidelines from the CDC in 2006 mandated that all patients in health care agencies be informed about HIV screening and then screened for HIV. However, these patients are allowed to refuse the test. Offer HIV antibody testing to all patients, regardless of patient-specific risk factors. Also, test results should be made available rapidly to the patient so education could be given to the patient, if needed. The CDC's recommendations state that informed consent is not needed. However, patients may opt out of testing if they wish. In rare emergency situations where health care providers need to know a patient's HIV status to make a decision regarding health care and the patient is unable

to speak, the patient may be tested without his or her consent.

More people with HIV can be identified with the current push for routine HIV screening. The FDA approved the use of ELISA for routine use during blood bank screenings. ELISA can identify antibodies for HIV-1 and HIV-2. Researchers who recently performed a study in Cameroon found that ELISA was highly sensitive even with wide variations in the genetic makeup of the HIV (Lee et al., 2007). The FDA has approved four rapid tests for HIV. Multispot and Oraquick can detect HIV-1 and HIV-2. Uni-Gold Recombigen and Reveal can only identify HIV-1 (Greenwald et al., 2006). These four tests are not yet available without a physician's order.

HIV antibody testing may take place in a physician's office or at designated HIV counseling and testing sites. Many patients feel more comfortable being tested by someone who knows their medical and social history, but others prefer to be tested in a location where they are unknown. Be aware of the various options for HIV antibody testing in your state or community in order to advise patients appropriately.

HIV antibody testing can be done one of two ways: confidentially or anonymously. In **confidential testing,** patients provide identifying information, including a name; an address; and often demographic information such as age, sex, race, and occupation. Using this information, care providers can locate and provide information to an individual who does not return for the test results or counseling. All records are strictly confidential, and testing in physicians' offices, clinics, and hospitals is conducted in a confidential manner. Health care providers who share or use this information inappropriately can be sued for negligence and invasion of privacy, and they may be disciplined by licensing boards for unauthorized disclosure or breach of confidentiality. Inform patients that the results of their HIV antibody test will be linked to the patient's medical record.

In **anonymous testing,** individuals are not asked to provide identifying information. Records are kept through assigned numbers, and the patient must retain this number to receive test results. It is not possible to locate and provide information to an individual who does not return for test results and counseling. In either form of testing, the nurse can perform pretest and posttest counseling.

RISK ASSESSMENT AND RISK REDUCTION

Testing for HIV is an important part of the public health response to HIV disease. Risk assessment should be patient centered, a joint process between the nurse and patient. The patient should take "ownership" of the risk for HIV infection. Assess patients for indications of risky behaviors, such as STIs. However, a patient will not get tested unless he or she perceives a need for testing and feels safe doing so. Help the patient assess the risks by asking some basic questions:

- Have you ever had a transfusion or used clotting factors? Was it before 1985?
- Have you ever shared needles, syringes, or other injecting equipment with anyone?
- Have you ever had a sexual experience in which your penis, vagina, rectum, or mouth came into contact with another person's penis, vagina, rectum, or mouth?

A positive response to any of the above questions requires further exploration with the patient. Be prepared to refer the patient to centers that provide testing and counseling services. All testing should include pretest and posttest counseling (see Boxes 16-3 and 16-7).

HIV infection in women has been frequently overlooked for several reasons. In the United States, the disease initially occurred mostly in men, and treatment models were developed accordingly. Providers did not assess the risks for women, and women did not seek testing and counseling because of denial or ignorance; thus interventions have not been implemented effectively. Heterosexual transmission of HIV in women surpassed injecting drug use as a vector for HIV transmission in the second decade of this pandemic and globally continues to be the highest risk factor in women (Dole, 2001). The 1993 CDC case definition includes at least one female-specific disease:

cervical carcinoma. Women now need to be assessed for different manifestations, such as vaginal candidiasis, a common presenting condition for HIV-positive women.

BARRIERS TO PREVENTION

HIV prevention has numerous barriers, not the least of which is a denial of risk, an attitude that "it won't happen to me." Because the virus initially infected the MSM population in the United States, many other subpopulations have ignored their risks. Fear, misunderstanding, and the potential for social isolation and social stigma are significant barriers. Some individuals are so fearful that they no longer give blood or eat at a restaurant if they think a homosexual food handler works there. Such reactions reinforce the need for consistent, accurate information about the virus, the risks of transmission, and HIV disease itself.

Cultural and community attitudes, values, and norms can affect the success of prevention efforts. A community may be opposed to HIV/AIDS education in the local school district because of the fear that values will be compromised. Those values may include views on sexuality, abstinence, the use of condoms, the use of drugs, and the provision of instructions on cleaning needles and syringes. Community organizations, churches, educators, and leaders can determine the community's expectations or norms. Cooperative efforts are essential for successful prevention of HIV transmission. The issues related to the HIV epidemic—sex, drug use, death, and homosexuality—are not easy issues for most cultures or communities.

Fear of alienation and discrimination are significant additional barriers to prevention. In some cases, individuals are reluctant to even pick up a pamphlet about HIV because they fear someone will believe they are gay or using illicit drugs. Some people will not go to a physician or to a testing and counseling site for HIV testing for fear of being seen. This fear is very real, particularly in rural parts of the country. Fear of discrimination includes fear of losing family, friends, prestige, job, housing, and insurance. Fortunately, many states have statutes to protect individuals with HIV disease from discrimination. Protection is also afforded by the ADA.

REDUCING RISKS RELATED TO SEXUAL TRANSMISSION

When patients have acute HIV and high viral loads, they are 10 times more likely to transmit HIV during sexual intercourse than during the chronic stage of HIV. Infection risk is also increased when sex is forceful or mucosal membranes are disrupted (often associated with STIs). Most HIV infections are transmitted during the primary stage of the infection. This is when most people are unaware of their infection because they are asymptomatic. Men are less likely to be infected with HIV during heterosexual intercourse than women. Women have more mucosal surface that can be exposed to infected body fluids when compared to men (National Institute of Allergy and Infectious Diseases, 2006). Male circumcision can also minimize a male's risk of becoming infected with HIV via heterosexual intercourse, according to the WHO (2009a).

Safer sexual activities reduce the risk of exposure to HIV through semen and cervicovaginal secretions. Abstaining from all sexual activity is the most effective way to accomplish this goal. Limiting sexual behavior to activities in which the mouth, penis, vagina, or rectum do not come into contact with the partner's mouth, penis, vagina, or rectum is also safe, since there is no contact with blood, semen, or cervicovaginal secretions. These activities may include massage, masturbation, mutual masturbation, telephone or cyber sex, and many other activities. Insertive sex is considered safe only in a mutually monogamous relationship with a partner who is not infected with, or at risk of becoming infected with, HIV. The problem with mutual monogamy is that both partners need to follow all of the rules all of the time. Unfortunately, cases of HIV infection occur in individuals who are not aware that their partner has not remained monogamous. Serial monogamy (maintaining a monogamous relationship, often including unprotected intercourse, with one partner for a short time, followed by another relationship, and then another) still presents an increased risk of HIV exposure (Box 16-9).

ART can be provided to people who have been exposed to HIV through unwanted sexual intercourse (rape) or via injecting drugs. The U.S. Department of Health and Human Services has developed some recommendations regarding these types of nonoccupational exposures. When a person has been exposed to body fluids from an HIV-infected person during high-risk activity less than 72 hours before seeking treatment, the exposed person should receive a 28-day supply of HAART. This is recommended even if the HIV-infected source of the exposure has a viral load that is undetected. However, if the activity is deemed to be low-risk exposure to body fluids, or if the exposed person seeks health care after the 72-hour window, ART is not recommended. Examine cases on an individual basis to determine the need for PEP, counseling, treatment, and education about preventing future exposures (CDC, 2005a).

The use of barriers reduces the risk of contact with HIV during sexual activity. Barriers should be used when engaging in sexual activity with a partner whose HIV status is not definitely known or with a partner who is known to be infected with HIV. The most commonly used barrier is the male condom. Although not 100% effective, when used correctly and consistently, male condoms are very effective in the prevention of HIV transmission. Other barriers include female condoms and latex dental dams. Female condoms consist of a vinyl sheath with two spring-form rings. The smaller ring is inserted into the vagina and holds the condom in place internally. The larger ring surrounds the opening to the condom. It keeps the condom in place externally while also protecting the external genitalia. The use of the female condom is complicated and cumbersome, and practice may be necessary to use this method effectively. Female condoms can also be used for anal sex, in both men and women. Dental dams or microwave-safe plastic wrap can be used to cover the external genitalia or anus during oral sexual activity ("rimming"). Although the risk of HIV transmission is significantly reduced with the use of latex

---

Box 16-9	**Risk of HIV Transmission Associated with Sexual Practices**

HIGH RISK (IN DESCENDING ORDER OF RISK)
- Receptive anal intercourse with ejaculation (no condom)
- Receptive vaginal intercourse with ejaculation (no condom)
- Insertive anal intercourse (no condom)
- Insertive vaginal intercourse (no condom)
- Receptive anal intercourse with withdrawal before ejaculation
- Insertive anal intercourse with withdrawal before ejaculation
- Receptive vaginal intercourse (with spermicidal foam, no condom)
- Insertive vaginal intercourse (with spermicidal foam, no condom)
- Receptive anal or vaginal intercourse (with a condom)*
- Insertive anal or vaginal intercourse (with a condom)*

SOME RISK (IN DESCENDING ORDER OF RISK)
- Oral sex with men with ejaculation
- Oral sex with women

- Oral sex with men with preejaculate fluid (precum)
- Oral sex with men, no ejaculation or precum
- Oral sex with men (with a condom)

NO RISK
- Masturbating with another person without touching one another
- Hugging, massage, dry kissing, frottage (rubbing against each other)
- Masturbating alone
- Abstinence

UNRESOLVED ISSUES
- The role of preejaculate in transmission
- The protection offered by covering female genitalia with a dental dam during oral sex
- The risk of transmission with wet kissing (French kissing) (though unlikely)

Modified from Schram, N.R. (1990). Redefining safer sex, *Focus* 5(7):3. In D.E. Grimes & R.M. Grimes (1994). *AIDS and HIV infection*. St. Louis: Mosby.
*Risk lower if no ejaculation and/or spermicidal foam used.

barriers, other STIs, such as human papillomavirus, warts, and HSV, can still be transmitted.

REDUCING RISKS RELATED TO DRUG ABUSE

The use of illicit or recreational drugs can cause immunosuppression, malnutrition, and emotional difficulties. Although using illicit drugs can increase one's risk for acquiring an HIV infection, drug use itself is not to blame. The major risks of HIV transmission are related to sharing injecting equipment and having unsafe sexual experiences while under the influence of mood-altering chemicals. Essentially, one can reduce the risk of HIV infection by not using drugs. If drugs are injected, equipment should not be shared with others. Sexual activity should not be engaged in while under the influence of any drug, including alcohol, that impairs decision making.

Abstaining from drugs is not always a viable option for a user who has no access to drug treatment services or chooses not to quit. The risk of HIV for these individuals can be eliminated if they can find alternatives to injecting, such as smoking, snorting, or ingesting drugs. Risk can also be eliminated if the user does not share injecting equipment, including needles, syringes, cookers, cotton, and rinse water. The safest tactic is for the user to have ready access to sterile equipment. Many states have laws that prohibit over-the-counter sale of needles and syringes, such as diabetic supplies. Some communities have needle exchange programs that supply sterile equipment to users to help reduce the risk of HIV transmission. The fear that needle exchange programs will result in increased illicit substance use has led to a lack of community support. However, studies have shown that in communities where exchange programs have been established, drug use does not increase and rates of HIV infection are controlled (Wodak & Cooney, 2006).

Cleaning the equipment before use decreases the risk for those who must share equipment, particularly in "shooting galleries." To clean the equipment, rinse used needles and syringes twice with tap water (using fresh tap water each time). Then fill syringes with full-strength household bleach, shake for 30 seconds, and squirt clean; repeat the bleaching process. Then rinse the equipment twice with tap water. This process takes time and may be difficult for a person experiencing drug withdrawal and in need of drugs.

REDUCING RISKS RELATED TO OCCUPATIONAL EXPOSURE

As previously discussed, the risk of acquiring HIV through occupational exposure is low. The CDC and Occupational Safety and Health Administration have instituted policies to protect employees from exposure to blood and other potentially infectious fluids (CDC, 2005b). The use of standard precautions and body substance isolation has been shown to reduce the risk of bloodborne pathogens, the risk of transmission of other diseases between the patient and the health care worker, and the risk of transmission between patients. Hand hygiene in the form of handwashing still remains the single most effective means of preventing the spread of infection.

Epidemiologic and laboratory studies suggest that several factors might affect the risk of HIV transmission after an occupational exposure. In a retrospective study conducted by the CDC of health care workers who had percutaneous exposure to HIV, the risk of HIV infection was found to be increased with exposure to a larger quantity of blood from the source patient as indicated by (1) a device visibly contaminated with the patient's blood, (2) a procedure that involved a needle being placed directly in a vein or artery, or (3) a deep injury. The risk is also increased for exposure to blood from a patient with terminal illness, possibly reflecting the higher viral load of the patient late in the course of HIV disease (CDC, 2001). Information about primary HIV infection (seroconversion) indicates that a systemic infection does not occur immediately. This leaves a brief window of opportunity during which initiation of antiretroviral PEP might prevent or inhibit systemic infection by limiting the proliferation of the virus in the initial target cells or lymph nodes.

For best prophylactic effect, PEP must be initiated within 36 hours—but preferably **within 1 to 4 hours**—of the exposure. Depending on the type of exposure and many other variables, either a two- or three-drug regimen is chosen (CDC, 2005a, b). In addition to possible exposure to an antiretroviral-resistant strain of HIV, other factors that might contribute to failures include a high titer or large volume of inoculum exposure, delayed initiation or short duration of PEP, and factors related to the exposed health care personnel (e.g., immune status).

Completion of a 4-week course of therapy after an occupational exposure is fundamental. The medications used have many side effects, and health care workers may stop PEP prematurely because of these. It is important to consult with experts in occupational exposure if side effects (headache, nausea, vomiting, diarrhea) become unbearable. The use of PEP regimens has been associated with new-onset diabetes mellitus, hyperglycemia, hypertriglyceridemia, pancreatitis, elevated lipids (cholesterol, low-density lipoproteins), and kidney stones. Despite these serious side effects, the exposed health care worker must continue therapy for 4 weeks, or until it is determined that the source patient is not HIV infected.

Hospitals or agencies should have policies that specifically address occupational HIV exposure, since chemoprophylaxis needs to occur immediately—even before testing the source patient's and health care worker's blood for HIV or other bloodborne pathogens. Serial testing of the health care worker for HIV occurs at baseline, 6 weeks, 3 months, and 6 months after the exposure.

Maintaining confidentiality for both the exposed health care worker and the source patient is of utmost importance. Many states and health care organizations have separate, distinct consent forms that are required before HIV antibody testing can be performed. Only in rare circumstances, such as the inability to give consent, can HIV antibody testing be completed without the patient's informed consent. Many ethical and legal issues surround HIV antibody testing, so be informed of the applicable laws in the state in which you practice. In many states, charges of assault and battery can be brought against health care workers who perform HIV testing against a patient's will. Appropriate counseling and referrals should be made for the health care worker and patient when HIV testing is indicated.

OTHER METHODS TO REDUCE RISK

Instruct HIV-infected people not to give blood, donate organs, or donate semen for artificial insemination. They should not share razors, toothbrushes, or other household items that may contain blood or other body fluids. They should also avoid infecting sexual and needle-sharing partners, consider using birth control measures, and eliminate breastfeeding to avoid spreading the virus to infants.

OUTLOOK FOR THE FUTURE

As we enter the third decade of the HIV pandemic, much has been learned about transmission of the virus and ways to prevent infection. With no cure in sight, prevention of infection through education, prevention of mother-to-child transmission, and in some cases PEP or preexposure prophylaxis can limit the effect this disease has on the human population.

The dynamics of the pandemic have changed dramatically as well. In the United States, HIV has the characteristics of any other chronic illness, in that it (1) has no cure, (2) continues throughout the patient's life, (3) causes increasing physical disability and dysfunction if not treated, and (4) ultimately results in significant morbidity and mortality. Chronic diseases are characterized by acute exacerbations of cyclic problems that compound each other. Despite a significant decrease in the number of OIs, new complications have emerged. Health care providers today must address body composition changes, cardiac disease, neuropathies, and the long-term effects of the very medications that have kept HIV at bay.

Since the discovery of HIV, significant advances have occurred in knowledge about the viral cycle, resulting immune response, and disease progression of HIV. New medication treatments are very effective and can help the host manage the disease by limiting replication of the virus. This can allow the immune system to continue to function. Survival rates of patients who have been diagnosed with late-stage HIV (and have access to HAART and are being cared for by health care providers with expertise in dealing with HIV) has increased dramatically. Patients who previously would have become disabled, quit jobs, and tended to end-of-life decisions are now reevaluating goals, returning to work, and rediscovering relative health. Now, couples who are serodiscordant have the option of having children with the use of sperm "washing" and in vitro fertilization.

In no other disease has there been such a rapid understanding and attempts at developing therapies as with HIV infection The HIV research arena has provided insight into other diseases and scientific fields, including virology, immunology, and oncology. At this point, though, scientists' ability to develop new therapies depends on the individual being nearly 100% adherent to regimens that are sometimes quite toxic. Adherence is poor even when therapy consists of only one pill per day. Even though treatment options for HIV have advanced, there is still a wide variation in disease progression. As research continues, it will be interesting to determine how psychological and social stressors alter immune system responses.

HIV has become a disease whose face is represented by women and people of color. Underdeveloped countries in Africa and Southeast Asia have been hardest hit; in fact, many villages have been destroyed because of HIV. The global threat of HIV is enormous, with nurses playing a key role in the care and treatment of HIV-infected individuals. For the best possible outcomes, always seek guidance from HIV specialists when treating an individual with HIV disease because the care is very complex, and multiple needs arise.

The field of HIV and AIDS nursing changes frequently, and nurses must constantly refresh their base of knowledge. Resources include local AIDS service organizations and state and regional AIDS education and training centers. As new therapies emerge, the nurse is in a unique position to educate patients and the public regarding what is undoubtedly the most challenging infectious disease discovered in the twentieth century.

Get Ready for the NCLEX® Examination!

Key Points

- HIV, a retrovirus, is the agent that causes HIV disease and AIDS.
- Education on prevention is the only "vaccine" for preventing HIV disease and AIDS.
- Women and people of color constitute the fastest-growing segment of the population with HIV disease.
- AIDS is the end stage of HIV infection.
- When HIV enters the body, its primary target is the immune system.
- HIV is transmitted by three major routes: (1) anal and vaginal intercourse, (2) injecting drugs with contaminated needles or works, and (3) from infected mother to child.
- Blood, semen, vaginal secretions, and breast milk are the body fluids that most readily transmit HIV.
- Assess each patient's risks for HIV infection and counsel those at risk about testing, behaviors that put them at risk, and how to eliminate or reduce those risks.
- A positive HIV antibody test does not mean the patient has AIDS.
- A multidisciplinary care approach in which the patient is a primary member of the team is the most appropriate method of caring for patients with HIV disease because of their complex needs.
- As HIV infection progresses, the immune system loses its ability to fight infectious agents and cancer cells.
- Encourage patients at risk for HIV infection to know their HIV status.
- Whether or not signs and symptoms are present, a person infected with HIV virus can transmit the virus.
- Barriers to HIV prevention include denial, fear, misinformation, and cultural and community norms.
- CD_4^+ counts are important markers of disease progression and the status of the immune system.
- The stigma of HIV disease, because of its association with drug use, homosexuality, and sexual transmission, is a major concern.
- The 1993 expanded case definition of AIDS includes all HIV-infected people who have CD_4^+ T-lymphocyte counts of less than 200 cells/mm³; includes all people who have one or more of three clinical conditions (pulmonary tuberculosis, recurrent pneumonia, or invasive cervical cancer); and retains the 23 clinical conditions listed in the 1987 AIDS case definition.
- Measuring viral load in the blood assesses effectiveness of therapy and possibly adherence.
- Adherence to medications is essential.

Additional Learning Resources

 Go to your free Companion CD for an audio glossary, animations, video clips, and more

evolve   Be sure to visit the companion Evolve site at http://evolve. elsevier.com/Christensen/adult/ for additional online resources.

Review Questions for the NCLEX® Examination

1. The virus responsible for causing the majority of HIV disease and AIDS is:
    1. human immunodeficiency virus type 1.
    2. human immunodeficiency virus type 2.
    3. African immunodeficiency virus type 1.
    4. *Pneumocystis jiroveci* (formerly *carinii*) deficiency virus.

2. Vertical transmission of HIV occurs from:
    1. male to female.
    2. female to male.
    3. father to child.
    4. mother to child.

3. The nurse is assessing a patient who has requested HIV testing. What would be considered to be the most risky behavior?
    1. Dry kissing a casual date
    2. Sharing a soda with an infected person
    3. Swimming with an infected person
    4. Having more than three sex partners in a year

4. What would be the most likely route of transmission of HIV?
    1. From infected female to noninfected male
    2. From infected male to noninfected female
    3. From infected father to child
    4. From infected mother to child

5. An 8-year-old is diagnosed with hemophilia. His mother is upset about the risk of her son acquiring HIV from blood products. What would be the nurse's best response?
    1. "All blood and blood products are screened for bloodborne diseases, so it is impossible for J. to be infected."
    2. "Many blood products are treated with heat or chemicals to inactivate the HIV virus."
    3. "We can talk about this if the patient requires transfusions or blood products."
    4. "All blood donors are asked about HIV status and risk factors before giving blood."

6. The storage area in which HIV reproduces in the human body is:
    1. lymph glands.
    2. muscle tissues.
    3. bone marrow.
    4. B cells.

7. A 34-year-old patient comes to the clinic requesting HIV testing. He is a gay man with two significant others in his lifetime. His lover was recently diagnosed with HIV. The patient asks the nurse how long it will take before the infection will show up in him. The best response would be:

   1. "Antibodies usually are detected in the blood within 4 to 12 weeks of exposure."
   2. "It takes at least a year to know if you will be infected with HIV."
   3. "You'll have to ask your doctor the next time you go in for an appointment."
   4. "We don't know how long it will take to seroconvert to being HIV positive."

8. The patient is concerned that he may be infected with HIV. Which symptom would alert the nurse to further assess the patient?

   1. Night sweats
   2. Rash on the legs only
   3. Constipation
   4. Pruritus

9. The HIV factory of the human body is:

   1. infected CD_4^+ cells.
   2. infected macrophages.
   3. infected sweat glands.
   4. infected parotid glands.

10. The patient is diagnosed with symptomatic HIV disease. The nurse would assess her regarding which of the following?

    1. T-cell count greater than $800/mm^3$
    2. WBC greater than 20,000/mL
    3. Thrush
    4. Weight gain

11. The diagnosis of AIDS is assigned based on which test?

    1. ELISA test
    2. CD_4^+ counts
    3. B-cell count
    4. Western blot test

12. The patient is diagnosed with HIV disease. She visits the physician today for her prescriptions. The nurse would expect the physician to order:

    1. tenofovir and emtricitabine (Truvada).
    2. efavirenz (Sustiva).
    3. lopinavir and ritonavir (Kaletra).
    4. combination of these drugs.

13. The nurse should instruct the patient with HIV to follow which diet?

    1. High calorie, high fiber, low protein
    2. Low calorie, low fiber, high protein
    3. High calorie, high protein, low residue
    4. Low calorie, high fiber, high protein

14. The progression of HIV disease is predictable in all patients. True or False?

15. HIV disease is diagnosed when the CD_4^+ cell count is 200 cells/mm^3 or fewer. True or False?

16. HIV disease in men who have sex with men is decreasing. True or False?

17. Ninety-nine percent seroconversion of exposed individuals occurs within 6 months of the exposure. True or False?

18. An HIV-infected person may appear to be healthy. True or False?

19. It is not possible to become infected with HIV after one unprotected sexual encounter. True or False?

20. Most of the children infected with the HIV virus were infected during pregnancy. True or False?

21. The most common opportunistic infection and malignant neoplasm in the patient with advanced HIV disease (AIDS) are:

    1. streptococcal pneumonitis, myeloma.
    2. *Pneumocystis jiroveci* (formerly *carinii*) pneumonia, Kaposi's sarcoma.
    3. *Streptococcus pneumoniae*, malignant melanoma.
    4. *Mycoplasma*, pneumonitis, Kaposi's sarcoma.

22. For most people who are HIV positive, marker antibodies are usually present 10 to 12 weeks after exposure. The development of these antibodies is called:

    1. immunocompetence.
    2. seroconversion.
    3. immunodeficient.
    4. viral load.

23. The expanded definition for AIDS is that the person will:

    1. have the HIV virus present.
    2. have a dysfunction of the immune system and be HIV positive.
    3. be HIV positive and have an opportunistic disease.
    4. be HIV positive with CD_4^+ lymphocyte count less than $200/mm^3$.

24. "Why should I use condoms? They don't work," retorts a young gay patient being treated for his third sexually transmitted infection. The nurse's most appropriate response would be:

    1. "Condoms may not provide 100% protection, but when used correctly and consistently with every act of sexual intercourse, they reduce your risk of getting infected with HIV or other sexually transmitted infections."
    2. "You are correct: condoms don't always work. So your best protection is to limit your number of partners."
    3. "Condoms do not provide 100% protection, so you should always discuss with your sexual partners their HIV status or ask if they have any STIs."
    4. "Condoms do not provide 100% protection, but when used with a spermicide, you can be assured of complete protection against HIV and other STIs."

25. The patient has been advised to be tested for HIV because of multiple sexual partners and intravenous illicit drug use. The nurse should make certain that the patient understands the test by informing him that:

   1. the blood is tested with the highly sensitive test called the Western blot, then with ELISA.
   2. the blood is tested with ELISA; if positive, it is tested again with ELISA and then the Western blot.
   3. a series of HIV tests are performed to determine whether the patient has AIDS.
   4. if the HIV tests are seronegative, the patient can be assured that he is not infected.

26. When the human immunodeficiency retrovirus enters the body, it attacks primarily which cells, resulting in an immunocompromised status?

   1. T-cell lymphocytes
   2. B-cell lymphocytes
   3. Neutrophils
   4. Monocytes

27. A 21-year-old patient has been treated for chlamydia and has a history of recurrent vaginal herpes. What would be the most appropriate action by the nurse?

   1. Counsel the patient about her sexual and drug use history, risk reduction measures, and HIV testing.
   2. Refer the patient to a family planning clinic.
   3. Counsel the patient about testing for HIV and what the test results mean.
   4. Counsel the patient about abstinence and a monogamous relationship.

28. If a person is infected with HIV and has not seroconverted to the HIV-specific antibody and will not test HIV antibody positive, this is referred to as:

   1. a "window-period."
   2. negative CD_4^+ count.
   3. positive CD_4^+ count.
   4. viral load.

29. In people who are HIV positive, the highest viral load is seen:

   1. at seroconversion time with CD_4^+ count less than $500/mm^3$.
   2. in symptomatic phase of HIV spectrum.
   3. at seroconversion time and in advanced HIV disease (AIDS).
   4. None of the above

30. The purpose of doing a viral load study once every 3 to 4 months in the HIV-positive person is to determine:

   1. the CD_4^+ count.
   2. the progression of the disease.
   3. effectiveness of the medication regimen.
   4. the results of the Western blot test.

31. The physician asks the nurse to talk with a patient about how HIV is transmitted. Which route of transmission should be discussed with the patient?

   1. Receiving blood, donating blood
   2. Food, water, air
   3. Sexual intercourse, sharing needles, mother-to-child transmission
   4. Dirty toilets, swimming pools, mosquitoes

32. The patient asks the nurse, "How does HIV cause AIDS?" The nurse's response should be:

   1. "HIV attacks the immune system, a system that protects the body from foreign invaders, making it unable to protect the body from organisms that cause diseases."
   2. "HIV breaks down the circulatory system, making the body unable to assimilate oxygen and nutrients."
   3. "HIV attacks the respiratory system, making the lungs more susceptible to organisms causing pneumonia."
   4. "HIV attacks the digestive system, decreasing the absorption of essential nutrients and resulting in weight loss and fatigue."

33. The pathophysiology of advanced HIV disease results from: (Select all that apply.)

   1. T-helper lymphocytes decreasing.
   2. T-suppressor lymphocytes dominating.
   3. profound immunosuppression.
   4. B lymphocytes unable to help with infection and antibody formation.
   5. T-helper lymphocytes increasing.

34. People at high risk for contracting HIV virus include: (Select all that apply.)

   1. a monogamous partner.
   2. homosexuals.
   3. drug users.
   4. heterosexual partners of homosexuals or bisexuals.
   5. prostitutes.

Objectives

1. Discuss the incidence of cancer as one of the leading causes of death in the United States.
2. Compare the three most common sites for cancer in men and women.
3. Discuss development, prevention, and detection of cancer.
4. List seven risk factors for the development of cancer.
5. Discuss the American Cancer Society's recommendations for preventive behaviors and screening tests for men and women.
6. State seven warning signs of cancer.
7. Explain common reasons for delay in seeking medical care when a diagnosis of cancer is suspected.
8. Define the terminology used to describe cellular changes, characteristics of malignant cells, and types of malignancies.
9. Describe the pathophysiology of cancer, including the characteristics of malignant cells and the nature of metastasis.
10. Describe the process of metastasis.
11. Define the systems of tumor classification: grading and staging.
12. List common diagnostic tests used to identify cancer.
13. Explain why biopsy is essential in confirming a diagnosis of cancer.
14. Describe nursing interventions for the individual undergoing surgery, radiation therapy, chemotherapy, bone marrow transplantation, or peripheral stem cell transplantation.
15. Describe the major categories of chemotherapeutic agents.
16. Explain the etiology, pathophysiology, clinical manifestations, diagnostic tests, medical management, nursing interventions, and prognosis for tumor lysis syndrome.
17. Discuss six general pain relief guidelines for the patient with advanced cancer.

Key Terms

alopecia (ăl-ō-PĒ-shē-ă, p. 796)
autologous (aw-TŎL-ŏ-gŭs, p. 800)
benign (bĕ-NĪN, p. 785)
biopsy (BĪ-ŏp-sē, p. 786)
cachexia (kă-KĔK-sē-ă, p. 801)
carcinogen (kăr-SĬN-ō-jĕn, p. 780)
carcinogenesis (kăr-sĭn-ō-JĔN-ĕ-sĭs, p. 780)
carcinoma (kăr-sĭ-NŌ-mă, p. 785)
differentiated (dĭf-ĕr-ĔN-shē-ā-tĕd, p. 786)
immunosurveillance (ĭm-ū-nō-sĕr-VĀ-lĕns, p. 785)
leukopenia (lū-kō-PĒ-nē-ă, p. 791)

malignant (mă-LĬG-nănt, p. 785)
metastasis (mĕ-TĂS-tă-sĭs, p. 785)
neoplasm (NĒ-ō-plăzm, p. 785)
oncology (ŏn-KŎL-ŏ-jē, p. 778)
palliative (PĂL-ē-ă-tĭv, p. 789)
Papanicolaou's test (smear) (pă-pĕ-NĬ-kō-lūz tĕst, smēr, p. 786)
sarcoma (săr-KŌ-mă, p. 786)
stomatitis (stō-mă-TĪ-tĭs, p. 796)
thrombocytopenia (thrŏm-bō-sīt-ō-PĒ-nē-ă, p. 796)
tumor lysis syndrome (TŪ-mŏr LĪ-sĭs SĬN-drōm, p. 799)

ONCOLOGY

Oncology is the sum of knowledge about tumors; it is the branch of medicine concerning the study of tumors. Oncology nursing is the care of people with cancer.

Until the appearance of acquired immunodeficiency syndrome (AIDS), probably no other medical diagnosis produced as much fear as a diagnosis of cancer. Cancer is feared far more than heart disease. The word *cancer* is viewed as synonymous with death, pain, and disfigurement. However, attitudes toward cancer have not kept pace with advances in the treatment and control of cancer. Education of health care professionals and the public is essential to promote more positive and realistic attitudes about cancer and cancer treatment (Lewis et al., 2007). The American Cancer Society (ACS) indicates that in the United States men have a 1 in 2 lifetime risk of developing cancer; for women, the risk is 1 in 3. The leading cancer sites for the male are prostate, lung, colon, and rectum. The leading cancer sites for the female are breast, lung, colon, and rectum (ACS, 2008a). Of every five deaths in the United States, one is from cancer, making it the second leading cause of death (heart disease is the most common).

Cancer is not one disease, but a group of more than 200 diseases characterized by the uncontrolled and unregulated growth and spread of abnormal cells.

Life Span Considerations
Older Adults

Cancer

- More cases of cancer occur among older adults than people of any other age-group.
- The incidence of cancer increases with aging, possibly as a result of decreased effectiveness of the immune system and changes in deoxyribonucleic acid.
- The types of cancers seen in older adults are prostate, lung, breast, and colorectal cancer. Cancers of the skin, urinary bladder, vagina, and vulva are seen primarily in older adults. Chronic lymphocytic leukemia and multiple myeloma are seen more frequently in older adults than in younger people.
- Many early signs and symptoms of cancer may be misdiagnosed as normal changes of aging. Stress the importance of routine medical screening and self-examination.
- Because of fear or experience, older adults may adopt a fatalistic frame of mind after hearing the diagnosis of cancer. Use of the terms *tumor* or *growth* may be more acceptable.
- The type of treatment for cancer should be based on the older person's wishes and overall state of health. Older individuals, their family members, and significant others should be presented with all options so that they can make informed decisions regarding treatment.

 Cultural Considerations
Cancer

- Blacks have a higher incidence of cancer than whites.
- The death rate from the four most common cancers (lung, colorectal, breast, prostate) is higher among minorities (except Asian Americans) than among whites.
- Asian Americans have the lowest death rate from cancer of any ethnic group.
- Black men have almost twice the rate of prostate cancer as white men and are more than twice as likely to die from the disease.
- Hispanic women have the highest rate of invasive cervical cancer of any group other than Vietnamese, and twice the incidence rate of non-Hispanic white women.
- Although black women are less likely than white women to develop breast cancer, they are more likely to die from the disease if they develop it.
- Native Americans have a lower incidence of cancer than any other group in the United States but have the poorest survival rate when they do get cancer.

Source: American Cancer Society. (2008). *Cancer facts and figures*. Atlanta: American Cancer Society.

Early detection and prompt treatment can cure some cancers and slow the progression of others. If not detected and controlled, cancer can result in death. Overall, it affects people of all ages, but most cases (76%) are diagnosed in those over the age of 55 (see Life Span Considerations box). Cancer incidence is higher in blacks than in whites and other minority groups (see Cultural Considerations box). An estimated 30% of Americans now living will experience cancer at some point in their lives. In 2006, 564,830 Americans died from cancer, which is more than 1500 persons per day (ACS, *Cancer facts and figures*, 2009).

The death rate from all cancers combined has decreased by 2.6% per year among men and by 1.8% per year among women since 2002. Cancer death rates have been decreasing since 1991 in men and since 1992 in women. Compared to the peak rates in 1990 for men and 1991 for women, the cancer death rate for all sites combined in 2004 was 18.4% lower in men and 10.5% lower in women (ACS, 2009). The 5-year survival rate is now 65%.

Lung cancer is the leading cause of cancer-related death in both men and women. Other cancers, such as breast and prostate, occur more often than lung cancer, but they have better cure and survival rates because of early detection and treatment (Figures 17-1 and 17-2).

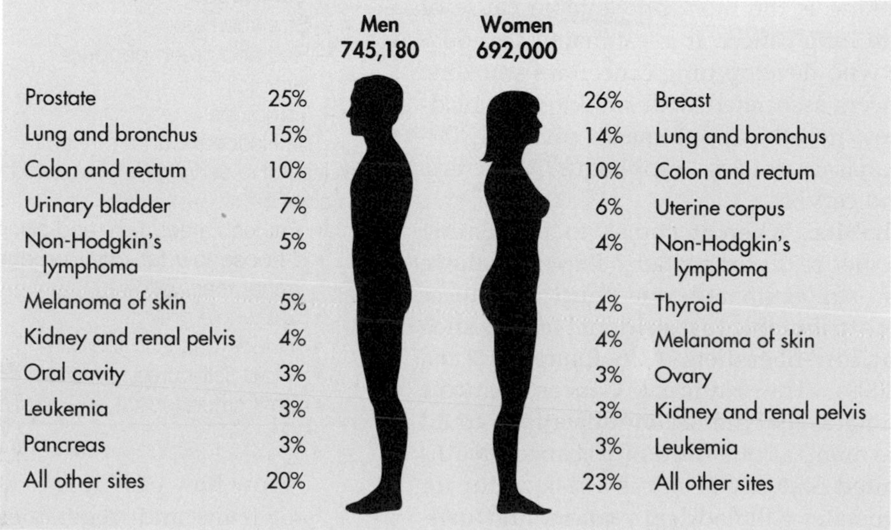

	Men 745,180		Women 692,000	
Prostate	25%		26%	Breast
Lung and bronchus	15%		14%	Lung and bronchus
Colon and rectum	10%		10%	Colon and rectum
Urinary bladder	7%		6%	Uterine corpus
Non-Hodgkin's lymphoma	5%		4%	Non-Hodgkin's lymphoma
Melanoma of skin	5%		4%	Thyroid
Kidney and renal pelvis	4%		4%	Melanoma of skin
Oral cavity	3%		3%	Ovary
Leukemia	3%		3%	Kidney and renal pelvis
Pancreas	3%		3%	Leukemia
All other sites	20%		23%	All other sites

FIGURE 17-1 Estimated cancer cases in the United States (2008 estimates). Excludes basal and squamous cell skin cancers and in situ carcinomas except urinary bladder.

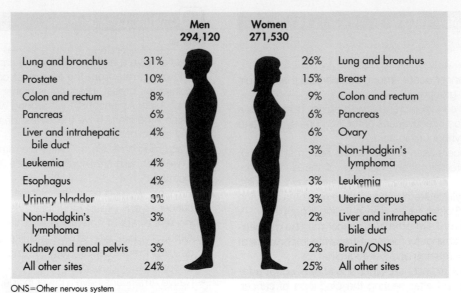

	Men 294,120			Women 271,530	
Lung and bronchus	31%		26%		Lung and bronchus
Prostate	10%		15%		Breast
Colon and rectum	8%		9%		Colon and rectum
Pancreas	6%		6%		Pancreas
Liver and intrahepatic bile duct	4%		6%		Ovary
Leukemia	4%		3%		Non-Hodgkin's lymphoma
Esophagus	4%		3%		Leukemia
Urinary bladder	3%		3%		Uterine corpus
Non-Hodgkin's lymphoma	3%		2%		Liver and intrahepatic bile duct
Kidney and renal pelvis	3%		2%		Brain/ONS
All other sites	24%		25%		All other sites

ONS = Other nervous system

FIGURE 17-2 Estimated cancer deaths in the United States (2008 estimates). Excludes basal and squamous cell skin cancers in situ carcinomas except urinary bladder.

DEVELOPMENT, PREVENTION, AND DETECTION OF CANCER

Carcinogenesis is the process by which normal cells are transformed into cancer cells. Although numerous theories have been proposed to explain it, no single cause has been accepted. The exact cause of most human cancers is still unknown, but most types are likely to have multiple causes. It is not known how many tumors have a chemical, environmental, genetic, immunologic, or viral origin. Cancers may arise spontaneously from causes that are thus far unexplained.

Primary prevention of cancer consists of changes in lifestyle habits to eliminate or reduce exposure to **carcinogens**, substances known to increase the risk for developing cancer. Risk factors include the following:

- **Smoking:** According to the American Cancer Society, smoking is the most preventable cause of death from lung cancer. It is estimated that 90% of people who develop lung cancer are smokers. Other cancers associated with smoking are bladder, kidney, mouth, lip, stomach, pharynx, larynx, paranasal sinuses, esophagus, pancreas, uterus, and cervix.
- **Dietary habits:** When it comes to preventing cancer, is diet really important? Experts believe that it is. An estimated one third of cancer deaths are attributable to nutritional factors such as high-fat, low-fiber diets (ACS, *Cancer facts and figures,* 2009). The National Cancer Institute (NCI) estimates that dietary modifications could prevent as many as one third of all cancer deaths in the United States. Obesity is a risk factor for breast, prostate, gallbladder, ovarian, and uterine cancer (National Cancer Institute, 2004). Diet also plays a role in the development of colon, rectal, and breast cancer. The NCI has launched a program called "5 a Day for Better Health" to

Health Promotion

Foods to Reduce Cancer Risk

- Vegetables from the cabbage family, such as:
  —Broccoli
  —Cauliflower
  —Brussels sprouts
  —All types of cabbage and kale
- Vegetables and fruits high in beta-carotene, such as:
  —Carrots
  —Peaches
  —Apricots
  —Squash
  —Broccoli
- Rich sources of vitamin C, such as:
  —Grapefruit
  —Oranges
  —Cantaloupe
  —Strawberries
  —Red and green peppers
  —Broccoli
  —Tomatoes

The National Cancer Institute has recommended including at least five servings of fruits and vegetables in the daily diet. In addition:

- Eat lean meat, fish, and skinned poultry.
- Choose low-fat dairy products, including white cheese rather than yellow.
- Eat whole grains.
- Include beans in the diet.
- Avoid salt-cured, smoked, or nitrite-cured foods.
- Limit saturated fat and added sugars.

show how easy it is to add at least five servings of fruits and vegetables to the daily diet as a way of reducing the risks of cancer (see Health Promotion box). Fruit and vegetable consumption may protect against cancers of the mouth and pharynx, esophagus, lung, stomach, and colon and rectum. However, consumption has seen little improvement since the mid-1990s. Less than one in four adults was eating the recommended servings in 2005 (ACS, 2009). At present only 20% of the U.S. population consumes five daily servings of fruits and vegetables.

- **Ultraviolet (UV) radiation:** Excessive exposure to the sun's UV rays is a factor in the development of basal and squamous cell skin cancers and melanoma. Sunlamps and tanning booth beds also emit UV rays and have the same risks as sunlight. (In addition, the effects of radiation commonly used for medical diagnosis and treatment are known to be carcinogenic. Exposure should be limited and monitored.)
- **Environmental and chemical carcinogens:** Some of these include fumes from rubber and chlorine and dust from cotton, coal, nickel, chromate, asbestos, and vinyl chloride. There is a greater incidence of bladder cancer among people who live in urban areas and among those who work with dyes, rubber, or leather.
- **Smokeless tobacco:** Use of smokeless tobacco increases the risk of cancer of the mouth, larynx, pharynx, and esophagus. Long-term snuff users have as much as a 50-fold greater risk of cheek and gum cancers.
- **Frequent heavy consumption of alcohol:** Alcohol may result in oral cancer and cancer of the larynx, throat, esophagus, and liver.

HEREDITARY CANCERS

About 90% of cancers are not inherited. Hereditary cancers arise from germline mutations. They are diagnosed usually 15 to 20 years earlier than cancers that are not inherited. Often, several relatives have the same or related cancers. They are more likely to be bilateral, and the same person may have multiple cancers. These multiple cancers are often seen in unusual organ combinations, such as breast and sarcoma, breast and thyroid, leukemia and brain tumors. Hereditary cancers are characterized by precursor lesions, such as polyps in colorectal cancer and dysplastic nevi in melanoma (Lewis et al., 2007).

GENETIC SUSCEPTIBILITY

For many years scientists have searched for genetic patterns in the most common cancer sites. Only 10% of cancers have an etiology of a strong genetic link (Tannock et al., 2005). The following patterns have emerged:

- The incidence of postmenopausal breast cancer is three times higher and the incidence of premenopausal breast cancer is five times higher in women with a family history of this disease. If a female has genes *BRCA1* or *BRCA2*, she has a 40% to 80% risk of having breast cancer during her lifetime. Of all women who develop breast cancer, 95% do not carry these genes (Tannock et al.,

2005). Breast cancer is rare in Asian women and common in white women.
- The incidence of lung cancer is greater in smokers with a family history of this disease than in smokers without a family history of the disease.
- The incidence of leukemia is greater in an identical twin of a person with the disease.
- Neuroblastoma occurs with increased frequency among siblings.
- Colon cancer is more likely to occur in women who have a history of breast cancer.

CANCER RISK ASSESSMENT AND GENETIC COUNSELING

When an individual or family is suspected of having a mutation in a cancer-causing gene, a cancer risk assessment is performed. This is the first step toward identifying hereditary cancer predisposition. The assessment begins with a comprehensive family history, included information on first-, second-, and third-degree relatives. Next obtain medical records to confirm the cancer diagnoses identified in the family history. The records usually requested include pathology reports, autopsy reports, death certificates, and discharge summaries from hospitalizations. Confirmation of cancer diagnoses through medical record analysis provides the patient with the most accurate risk analysis possible.

Genetic counseling is an essential component of the genetic evaluation. It is comprehensive and includes obtaining informed consent and proving education, health promotion, and support to individuals and families facing the uncertainty of hereditary cancer and cancer syndromes.

CANCER PREVENTION AND EARLY DETECTION

Prevention and early detection of cancer includes recognition of cancer's warning signals (Box 17-1). The American Cancer Society advises specific preventive behaviors and screening tests for men and women (Table 17-1). The nurse plays a prominent role in prevention and detection of cancer. Early detection and prompt treatment are directly responsible for increased survival rates in patients with cancer (see Health Promotion box). It is reported that 65% of patients who are diagnosed with cancer today will be alive 5 years after diagnosis.

| Box **17-1** | Cancer's Seven Warning Signals |

If you have a warning signal, see your physician.
1. **C**hanges in bowel or bladder habits
2. **A** sore that does not heal
3. **U**nusual bleeding or discharge
4. **T**hickening or lump in breast or elsewhere
5. **I**ndigestion or difficulty swallowing
6. **O**bvious change in warts or moles
7. **N**agging cough or hoarseness

Table 17-1	Cancer Prevention and Early Detection in Women and Men

The American Cancer Society recommends that all people get a cancer-related checkup every 3 years between the ages of 20 and 40, and every year thereafter. This checkup, depending on a person's age, might include examinations for cancer of the skin, thyroid, mouth, and lymph nodes. Screening for colorectal cancer begins at age 50. For women, examination for cancer of the ovaries begins at age 20, and screening for breast cancer begins at age 40. For males, examination for testicular cancer begins at puberty, and screening for prostate cancer begins at age 50.

PREVENTIVE BEHAVIORS	SCREENING TESTS

MEN AND WOMEN

Colorectal Cancer

- Follow screening guidelines to remove adenomatous polyps before they become cancer.
- Get at least 30 minutes of physical activity on most days.
- Achieve and maintain a healthy weight.
- Eat plenty of fruits, vegetables, and whole-grain foods, and limit intake of high-fat foods.
- Quit smoking.

Beginning at age 50, a person should follow one of the four screening options below;
- Yearly fecal occult blood test (FOBT)
- Stool DNA tests (SDNA)
- Flexible sigmoidoscopy every 5 years
- Yearly FOBT plus flexible sigmoidoscopy every 5 years

Of the options above, the American Cancer Society prefers yearly FOBT combined with flexible sigmoidoscopy every 5 years, or one of the following examination schedules:
- Double-contrast barium enema every 5 years
- Colonoscopy every 10 years
- CT colonography (also known as virtual colonoscopy) every 5 years

Talk to physician about beginning screening earlier and/or more often if a patient has any of the following risk factors:
- Strong family history of colorectal cancer or polyps (cancer of polyps in a first-degree relative younger than 60 or in two first-degree relatives of any age). NOTE: A first-degree relative is a parent, sibling, or child.
- Known family history of colorectal cancer syndromes.
- Personal history of colorectal cancer or adenomatous polyps.
- Personal history of chronic inflammatory bowel disease.

Skin Cancer

- Stay out of the sun, especially between 10 AM and 4 PM.
- Wear a broad-brimmed hat, a shirt, and sunglasses when out in the sun.
- Use sunscreen with an SPF of 15 or higher; reapply it often.
- In addition to seeking shade, the American Cancer Society recommends the "Slip! Stop! Slap! Wrap!" method of prevention: *Slip* on a shirt, *Slop* on 15 SPF (or higher) sunscreen, *Slap* on a hat, and *Wrap* on sunglasses before any exposure to the sun.
- Do not use tanning beds or sunlamps.
- Protect young children from excessive sun exposure.
- Check your skin regularly for abnormal or changing areas, especially moles, and have them examined by a physician.

- Skin examination
  - Older than age 20: Every 3 years
  - Older than age 40: Every year
- Self-examination (monthly)
  - Become familiar with any moles, freckles, or other abnormalities on the skin; use a mirror or have a family member or close friend look at areas one cannot see (ears, scalp, lower back).
  - Check for changes once a month; show any suspicious or changing areas to the physician.

Lung Cancer

- Quit smoking.
- Encourage those you live with or work with to quit.
- If you smoke, let your physician know if you develop any of the following symptoms (some may have causes other than cancer):
  - A cough that does not go away
  - Chest pain, often aggravated by deep breathing
  - Hoarseness
  - Weight loss and loss of appetite
  - Bloody or rust-colored sputum
  - Shortness of breath
  - Fever without a known reason
  - Recurring infections such as bronchitis and pneumonia
  - New onset of wheezing

No screening tests have been found to be effective; cancer is usually found on x-ray examination, but there are often no symptoms.
- Talk to the physician about possible screening if one has any of the risk factors listed below:
  - Smoke tobacco
  - Work around asbestos
  - Exposed to radon
  - Exposed to uranium
  - Exposed to arsenic
  - Exposed to vinyl chloride
  - Smoke marijuana
  - Regularly exposed to secondhand smoke

Table 17-1   Cancer Prevention and Early Detection in Women and Men—cont'd

PREVENTIVE BEHAVIORS	SCREENING TESTS

WOMEN
Cervical Cancer
• Abstain from sex or practice safer sex using barrier protection each time you have intercourse.
• Quit smoking.
• Eat a diet rich in fruits and vegetables.
• Watch for and report signs and symptoms (although all of these can have other causes):
  —Abnormal uterine bleeding or spotting
  —Abnormal vaginal discharge
  —Pain during intercourse
	• Have a yearly pelvic examination with Papanicolaou's (Pap) test beginning at age 18 or when sexually active, whichever is earlier.
	• A vaccine is approved for females aged 9 to 19 years to reduce cervical-related neoplasia and cervical cancer resulting from HPV types 16 to 18. Three vaccines are given over 6 months.
	• Beginning at age 30, after three or more consecutive satisfactory normal yearly examinations, the conventional or liquid-based Pap test may be screened every 2 or 3 years at the physician's discretion.
	• Alternatively, every 3 years the following should be performed: conventional or liquid-based cytology and cervical cancer screening with human papillomavirus DNA testing (American Cancer Society, 2007).

Breast Cancer • Follow recommended guidelines for early detection of breast cancer. • Talk with your physician about the risks and benefits of hormone replacement therapy for your risk of cancer and other diseases (like heart disease and osteoporosis). • Get at least 30 minutes of physical activity on most days. • Achieve and maintain a healthy weight. • Eat plenty of fruits, vegetables, and whole-grain foods, and limit intake of high-fat foods. • Decrease your alcohol intake.	**Ages 20 to 39** • Breast self-examination each month • Clinical breast examination by health care professional every 3 years **Ages 50 and over** • Mammogram every 2 years (U.S. Preventive Services Task Force, 2009) • Clinical breast examination by a health care professional, near the time of the mammogram • Breast self-examination every month • If woman is at increased risk (e.g., genetic tendency or family history), consult health care provider about benefits and limitations of baseline mammogram before age 50 and additional examinations such as breast ultrasound and MRI (ACS, 2007).
Endometrial Cancer • Watch for and report any abnormal uterine spotting or bleeding. • Use oral contraceptives for many years. • Talk with your physician about the risks and benefits of hormone replacement therapy for your risk of cancer and other diseases (like heart disease and osteoporosis). • If taking hormone replacement therapy with your uterus still intact, take estrogen with progesterone.	**Average risk:** • Talk with the physician especially at the time of menopause, about the risks and symptoms of endometrial cancer. • Report any vaginal bleeding or spotting to your physician.

Ovarian Cancer
• Use oral contraceptives for several years.
• Watch for and report signs and symptoms (although all of these can have other causes):
  —Abdominal swelling
  —Vaginal bleeding
  —Back or leg pain
  —Chronic stomach pain
• Talk with your physician about the risks and benefits of hormone replacement therapy and your risks of cancer and other diseases, like heart disease and osteoporosis.
	There are no effective and proven tests for early detection of ovarian cancer.
	• As part of one's health maintenance, undergo a periodic and thorough pelvic examination as directed by the physician.

Continued

Table 17-1	Cancer Prevention and Early Detection in Women and Men—cont'd
PREVENTIVE BEHAVIORS	**SCREENING TESTS**
WOMEN—cont'd	
Ovarian Cancer—cont'd	
• Talk with your physician about having your ovaries removed, if you are at high risk. (This surgery causes sudden menopause.)	
MEN	
Prostate Cancer	
• Eat a diet low in fat and high in vegetables, fruits, and grains. • Get at least 30 minutes of physical activity on most days. • Achieve and maintain a healthy weight.	Men should consider a yearly prostate-specific antigen (PSA) blood test and digital rectal examination starting at age 50 or at age 45 if at high risk (black men, or those with a father or brother diagnosed with prostate cancer at a young age).
Testicular Cancer	
• Eat a balanced diet which includes fresh fruits and vegetables. • Participate in a regular exercise program. • Learn and practice testicular self-examination.	Teach the male at puberty to perform a monthly testicular self-examination. Monthly self-examination should continue throughout the life span. Males at high risk are those with a history of an undescended testis or a previous testicular tumor.

Health Promotion

Prevention and Detection of Cancer

- Reduce or avoid exposure to known or suspected carcinogens and cancer-promoting agents, including cigarette smoke and sun exposure.
- Eat a balanced diet that includes vegetables (green, deep yellow, and orange), cruciferous vegetables (cabbage, broccoli, cauliflower and Brussels sprouts), fresh fruits, allium vegetables (onion and garlic), nuts, legumes, soy products, whole grains, and adequate amounts of fiber. Reduce the amount of fat and preservatives, including smoked and salt-cured meats. Limit the consumption of processed and red meats.
- Exercise regularly. The American Cancer Society recommends that adults engage in at least 30 minutes of moderate to vigorous physical activity, above usual activities, on five or more days per week.
- Obtain adequate, consistent periods of rest (at least 6 to 8 hours per night).
- Have a health examination on a regular basis that includes a health history, a physical examination, and specific diagnostic tests for common cancers in accordance with the guidelines published by the American Cancer Society (www.cancer.org) (see Table 17-1).
- Eliminate, reduce, or change the perceptions of stressors and enhance the ability to effectively cope with stressors.
- Enjoy consistent periods of relaxation and leisure.
- Know the seven warning signs of cancer (see Box 17-1). (These actually indicate fairly advanced disease.)
- Learn and practice self-examination (e.g., skin examination, breast self-examination, testicular self-examination).
- Seek immediate medical care if you notice a change in what is normal for you and if cancer is suspected. Early detection of cancer has a positive effect on prognosis.

Beginning in high school, all women should be taught to perform breast self-examination (BSE) each month, 2 or 3 days after the menstrual period ends. After menopause, a woman should choose a specific day to help her remember, such as the first day of each month. A woman needs to become familiar with the appearance and feel of her breasts. This will help her identify any change from one month to the next. Any abnormality—such as discharge from the nipples; puckering, dimpling, peau d'orange (skin appearance of an orange peel, or scaling of the skin; and the palpation of a lump or thickness)—is significant. (See Chapter 12 for instructions on BSE.) Teach BSE to all patients (men and women), emphasizing that any identifiable problem should be brought to the attention of a physician. Any delay is a waste of valuable time if cancer is present.

Teach males, beginning at puberty, to check the scrotum for enlargement, thickening, or the presence of a lump in the testicles. This should be done monthly, after a warm bath or shower. Emphasize that a physician must be contacted to determine the significance of any changes from the normal, smooth consistency of the testes (see Chapter 12). Some symptoms of testicular cancer include a lump in or enlargement of either testicle, a heavy feeling in the scrotum, dull aching in either the groin or the lower abdomen, fluid collection in the scrotum, and tenderness or enlargement of the breasts (this results from hormones produced by cancer cells) (National Cancer Institute, 2007).

Advise men over age 50 to have a prostate-specific antigen (PSA) test and rectal examination once a year. Symptoms of blood in the urine, difficulty starting to urinate, a weak flow of urine, or other urination problems should be reported to the physician.

A common reason for delay in diagnosing cancer is that early malignant changes do not produce pain. Cancer may be insidious at the onset, and it may be far advanced before the individual has any symptoms.

PATHOPHYSIOLOGY OF CANCER

CELL MECHANISMS AND GROWTH

The basic unit of structure and function in all living things is the **cell.** The adult human body contains approximately 60,000 billion cells. Although there are many different types of cells, all of them have certain common characteristics. For example, all cells need nourishment to maintain life, and all cells use almost identical nutrients. All cells use oxygen, which combines with fat, protein, or carbohydrates to release the energy needed for cells to function. The mechanisms for changing nutrients into energy are generally the same in all cells, and all cells deliver their end product of chemical reactions into the nearby fluids.

Most cells are able to reproduce. When cells are destroyed, the remaining cells of the same type reproduce until the correct number has been replenished. This orderly replacement of cells is governed by a control mechanism that stops when the loss or damage has been corrected. Dynamic, active, and orderly, the healthy cell is a small powerhouse, laboratory, factory, and duplicating machine, perfectly copying itself over and over. Our immune system helps us from developing cancer by destroying the abnormal cells. Occasionally our immune system fails to recognize these abnormal cells and cancer develops.

Cancer cells are not subject to the usual restrictions placed on cell proliferation by the host. When malignant cells change, they become unlike parent cells; they are not differentiated, or recognizable as being the same in size or shape as normal cells. Cancer cells can divide and multiply, but not in a normal manner. Instead of limiting their growth to meet specific needs of the body, they continue to reproduce in a disorderly and unrestricted manner. The cellular features of cancer cells are a local increase in the number of cells, loss of normal cellular arrangement, variation in cell shape and size, increased nuclear size, increased miotic activity, and abnormal mitosis and chromosomes.

Proliferation is not always indicative of cancer, however. Abnormal cellular growth is classified as nonneoplastic growth and neoplastic growth. The four common nonneoplastic growth patterns are hypertrophy, hyperplasia, metaplasia, and dysplasia. Though not neoplastic conditions, these may precede the development of cancer. **Anaplasia** means "without form" and is an irreversible change in which the structures of adult cells regress to more primitive levels.

Neoplasm is the term for uncontrolled or abnormal growth of cells. Neoplasms may be benign (not recurrent or progressive; nonmalignant) or malignant (growing worse and resisting treatment, as in cancerous growths [Table 17-2]). The growths are also called **tumors,** which means swelling or enlargement. They may be localized or invasive. Benign tumors may become serious because their increased size damages surrounding tissues, as in a benign brain tumor. Malignant neoplasms may progress and destroy surrounding tissues. They may also metastasize from the primary site of origin to distant sites.

Metastasis is the process by which tumor cells spread from the primary site to a secondary site. Once cancer cells have moved to another area of the body, secondary tumors may grow in that area. Metastasis can occur by (1) direct spread of tumor cells by diffusion to other body cavities or (2) circulation by way of blood and lymphatic channels.

In addition to the identified carcinogenic factors that may cause malignant cellular changes, certain viruses have been suspected. There is also evidence to suggest that certain genetic factors result in a predisposition to the development of cancer.

The body's immune system is responsible for recognizing and destroying malignant cells. The immune system may be weakened by cancer-producing substances, tumor cells, and the aging process. Some T cells are responsible for immunosurveillance (the immune system's recognition and destruction of newly developed abnormal cells). When a cell becomes malignant, it carries a tumor-specific antigen on its membranes that is recognized by the body as nonself and destroyed. If T-cell function is suppressed by age, drugs (e.g., corticosteroids), poor nutrition, alcohol, serious infections, or certain disease processes (e.g., neoplastic invasion of bone and lymph tissue), the risk of cancer increases. To suppress T-cell rejection of a transplanted organ, steroids and other drugs are given. The resultant loss of immunosurveillance increases the risk of certain cancers.

DESCRIPTION, GRADING, AND STAGING OF TUMORS

Cancers are described according to the original site of the primary tumor. Carcinoma is the term used for malignant tumors composed of epithelial cells, which

| Table 17-2 | General Characteristics of Neoplasms |

BENIGN TUMORS	MALIGNANT TUMORS
Slow, steady growth	Rate of growth varies—usually rapid
Remains localized	Metastasizes
Usually contained within a capsule	Rarely contained within a capsule
Smooth, well defined; movable when palpated	Irregular; more immobile when palpated
Resembles parent tissue	Little resemblance to parent tissue
Crowds normal tissue	Invades normal tissue
Rarely recurs after removal	May recur after removal
Rarely fatal	Fatal without treatment

Box 17-2 TNM Cancer Staging Classification System

T SUBCLASSES: PRIMARY TUMOR

T_x	Tumor cannot be adequately assessed
T_0	No evidence of primary tumor
T_{is}	Carcinoma in situ
T_1-T_4	Progressive increase in tumor size and involvement

N SUBCLASSES: REGIONAL LYMPH NODES

N_x	Regional lymph nodes cannot be assessed
N_0	No regional lymph node metastasis
N_1-N_4	Increasing involvement of regional lymph nodes

M SUBCLASSES: DISTANT METASTASIS

M_x	Not assessed
M_0	No (known) distant metastasis
M_1-M_4	Distant metastasis present, specify site(s)

HISTOPATHOLOGY

G_1	Well-differentiated grade; cells differ slightly from normal cells (mild dysplasia)
G_2	Moderately well-differentiated grade; cells are more abnormal (moderate dysplasia)
G_3	Poorly differentiated grade; cells are very abnormal (severe dysplasia)
G_4	Undifferentiated; cells are immature and primitive (anaplasia); cells difficult to determine

From American Joint Committee for Cancer. (1992). *AJCC manual for staging of cancer.* (4th ed.). Philadelphia: Lippincott.

---

tend to metastasize. Carcinomas originate from embryonal ectoderm (skin and glands) and endoderm (mucous membrane linings of the respiratory tract, gastrointestinal [GI] tract, and genitourinary tract). Sarcoma refers to malignant tumors of connective tissues; they originate from embryonal mesoderm, such as muscle, bone, or fat, usually manifesting as a painless swelling. Sarcoma may affect bone, bladder, kidneys, liver, lungs, parotids, and spleen. **Lymphomas** and **leukemias** originate from the hematopoietic system.

A tumor may be named for its location, its cellular makeup, or the person by whom it was identified.

Grading of Tumors

Tumors are classified grade 1 to grade 4 by the degree of malignancy. Grade 1 is the most differentiated (most like the parent tissue) tumor and the least malignant. Grade 4 is the least differentiated (unlike parent tissue) tumor and the most malignant (Box 17-2).

Extent of Disease Classification

Classifying the extent and spread of disease is termed **staging.** This classification system is based on a description of the extent of the disease rather than on cell appearance. Although staging for different types of cancer has similarities, there are many differences, based on a thorough knowledge of the natural history of each specific type of cancer.

Clinical Staging

The clinical staging classification system determines the extent of the disease process of cancer by stages:

Stage 0:	Cancer in situ
Stage I:	Tumor limited to the tissue of origin; localized tumor growth
Stage II:	Limited local spread
Stage III:	Extensive local and regional spread
Stage IV:	Metastasis

TNM Classification System

The **TNM classification system** represents the standardization of the clinical staging of cancer. This classification system is used to determine the extent of the disease process of cancer according to three parameters: tumor size (T), degree of regional spread to the lymph nodes (N), and metastasis (M) (see Box 17-2). This system is used to direct treatment, predict prognosis, and contribute to cancer research by ensuring reliable comparison of different patients.

Bethesda System

Exfoliative (pertaining to the shedding of something) cytology (e.g., Papanicolaou's test [smear] [Pap]) is a means of studying cells that the body has shed during the normal sequence of growth and replacement of body tissues. If cancer is present, cancer cells are also shed. The method is most commonly used to detect cancers of the cervix, but it may be used for tissue specimens from any organ.

The results of the Pap test, as given by the **Bethesda system** (the preferred system), are as follows:

Negative: Normal (formerly class I)

Probably negative: May indicate infection, atypical squamous cells, or reactive changes (formerly class II)

Suspicious, but not conclusive for malignancy: Low-grade squamous intraepithelial lesion (formerly class III)

More suspicious, strongly suggestive of malignancy: High-grade squamous intraepithelial lesion (formerly class IV)

Conclusive for malignancy: Invasive squamous cell carcinoma (formerly class V)

DIAGNOSIS OF CANCER

BIOPSY

People who show signs of cancer should undergo diagnostic testing to confirm or rule out the diagnosis. The only definitive way to determine the presence of malignant cells is to perform a tissue biopsy (the removal of a small piece of living tissue from an organ or other part of the body for microscopic examination; used to confirm or establish a diagnosis, establish prognosis, or follow the course of a disease).

In general, the purpose of a biopsy is to obtain a sample of tissue for pathologic examination. The three

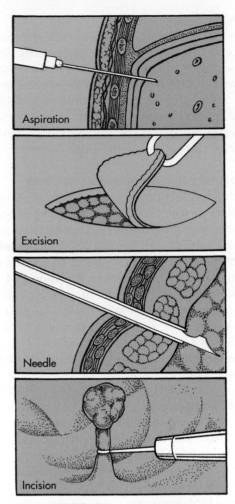

FIGURE 17-3 Types of biopsy.

types of biopsy are incisional, excisional, and needle aspiration (Figure 17-3). **Incisional** biopsy is the removal of a portion of tissue for examination, such as the bite biopsy performed during endoscopy. **Excisional** biopsy is the removal of the complete lesion, with little or no margin of surrounding normal tissue removed, as in polypectomy. Another example of excisional biopsy is the dissection of peripheral lymph nodes, such as those of the axilla for staging of breast cancer or those of the peritoneal region for staging of various abdominal cancers. **Needle aspiration** biopsy is the aspiration of fluid or tissue by means of a needle (breast biopsy is performed with an aspiration needle). Transcutaneous aspiration biopsy has eliminated most of the exploratory laparotomies for diagnosing metastatic cancer of the liver or for primary inoperable pancreatic cancer. Organs accessible to thin-needle biopsy under guidance of palpation include breasts, skin, thyroid gland, prostate, palpable lymph nodes, and salivary glands.

ENDOSCOPY

Cells or tissue can also be obtained using an **endoscope** to directly visualize an internal structure through a body cavity or a small incision. Endoscopes are rigid or flexible tubes containing a magnifying lens and a light. Endoscopes vary in diameter and length according to the structure being examined. The bronchoscope is used to visualize the tracheobronchial tree; upper GI endoscopy allows direct visualization of the upper GI tract (esophagus, stomach, duodenum); the colonoscope is used to visualize the entire colon; and the sigmoidoscope is used to examine the sigmoid colon, the rectum, and the anus.

DIAGNOSTIC IMAGING

Other diagnostic studies determine the depth of the specific lesion and identify other structures that may have been invaded. These include radiographs and scanning procedures. Commonly ordered radiographic studies are the chest radiograph, mammography, bone scan, GI series, barium enema, and intravenous pyelogram.

Bone scanning involves several steps. Before the scan, a radioactive material is injected into a vein in the arm. The patient is encouraged to drink water over the next 1 to 3 hours to aid renal clearance of any radioisotope not picked up by the bone. Areas of concentrated uptake may represent a tumor or an abnormality. These areas of concentration can be detected days or weeks before an ordinary radiograph could reveal a lesion. Bone scanning is indicated to detect metastatic tumors. All malignancies capable of metastasis may reach the bone, especially malignancies of breasts, kidneys, lungs, prostate, thyroid gland, and urinary bladder.

Tomography is the special technique of making multiple radiographic films at different depths of a specific area, organ, or structure. The details of each thin section can be clearly visualized.

Computed Tomography

Computed tomography (CT) scan uses radiographs and a computed scanning system to record images of specific structures at different angles. The entire body can be scanned to detect any abnormal lesion. CT scan is especially helpful in detecting small lesions that were missed by radiographs or tomography.

Radioisotope Studies

Radioisotope studies require the injection or ingestion of a radioactive substance. A scanning device is used to identify the distribution of the substance in different areas of the body. Concentration of the radioisotope in a specific organ, such as the thyroid gland or the brain, identifies a tumor in that location (may be primary or metastatic).

Ultrasound Testing

Ultrasound is a noninvasive procedure using high-frequency sound waves to examine internal structures. As a transducer is moved over the area being studied, an ultrasound beam is directed through the tissues and reflects back to the transducer. The sound waves are converted into electrical impulses, which produce an image on a display screen. Ultrasound can show the size, consistency, and shape of the structure being studied. It is most helpful in distinguishing between cystic and solid tumors. Ultrasound is not used to examine bones or air-filled organs. The procedure is painless. People having ultrasonography feel the transducer moving over their skin and may need to hold their breath for brief periods and remain still during the procedure.

Magnetic Resonance Imaging

Magnetic resonance imaging (MRI) is a painless diagnostic procedure that does not involve any exposure to radiation. The person reclines on a narrow surface that moves into a cylindrical tunnel containing magnetic coils; radiofrequency energy waves produce signals that are processed by a computer and displayed as images on a video monitor. The images can be recorded on film or magnetic tape for permanent storage. This test is currently used in the diagnosis of intracranial and spinal lesions and of cardiovascular and soft tissue abnormalities. The procedure also provides information about changes within the cells of soft tissues, arteries, veins, the brain, and the spinal column.

During the test the person having MRI must not have any metallic materials on the body, including jewelry. MRI cannot be done on patients with metallic implants, such as a pacemaker, orthopedic nail, or aneurysm clip.

During the test the patient can talk to those performing the test by means of a microphone placed inside the scanner tunnel. The patient will hear the sound waves thumping on the magnetic field and must lie still while the test is being done; it may take more than an hour to obtain the images needed.

Position Emission Tomography

Positron emission tomography (PET) is useful in many aspects of oncology. A radioactive chemical is given to the patient just before PET scanning. A PET scan can demonstrate glucose metabolism, oxygenation, blood flow, and tissue perfusion for any designated area. Alterations in the normal metabolic process in pathologic conditions are diagnosed during a PET scan (Pagana & Pagana, 2007).

PET is useful to visualize fast-growing tumors and to specify their anatomical location. PET also helps note tumor response to therapeutic intervention, identify a recurrence of a tumor after surgical intervention, and assist in differentiating a tumor from other abnormal conditions such as an infection (Pagana & Pagana, 2008). PET is extremely useful in visualizing regional and metastatic extension of a specific tumor. Oncologic staging is more accurate with PET than CT scan. PET is also used to determine the specific site to perform a biopsy of a suspected tumor (Pagana & Pagana, 2008).

LABORATORY AND DIAGNOSTIC EXAMINATIONS

Measurement of Alkaline Phosphatase Blood Levels

Alkaline phosphatase is elevated if there is metastasis to the bone or liver.

Serum Calcitonin Level

Calcitonin is a hormone secreted by the thyroid gland in response to a rising serum calcium level. The level is increased in the blood of people who have cancer of the thyroid. It may be elevated with breast cancer and oat cell cancer of the lung. Calcitonin stimulation testing may be used in addition to the baseline level testing to confirm a diagnosis. Instruct the patient to not eat or drink during the night before the test.

Carcinoembryonic Antigen Serum Level

Normally, production of carcinoembryonic antigen (CEA) stops before birth, but it may begin again if a neoplasm develops. This test cannot be used as a general indicator of cancer because CEA can be elevated for other reasons, such as smoking cigarettes. CEA is found in increased amounts in the blood of people with colorectal cancer. The test may assist in the evaluation of cancer treatment, in which a rising CEA level may indicate tumor recurrence or metastatic disease. This test is used less frequently today because research has found it less accurate than was previously thought.

Blood Markers

Many different blood studies (markers) are currently being evaluated to determine their usefulness in cancer screening and diagnosis. Three examples are the PSA for prostate cancer, CA-125 for ovarian cancer, and CA-19-9 for pancreatic or hepatobiliary cancer.

PSA is a biologic marker, specific for cellular activity in the prostate gland. PSA, the gold standard tumor marker for prostate cancer, is increasingly important in the diagnostic assessment and follow-up of patients with the disease. PSA also plays an important role in staging prostate cancer and in monitoring for recurrence. The American Cancer Society began recommending its use for screening asymptomatic men in November 1992.

Although PSA levels are usually elevated when cancer is present, PSA alone does not diagnose prostate cancer. Other common conditions, such as benign enlargement of the prostate, can also elevate PSA. The finding of elevated PSA requires further evaluation to assess the cause of the high levels. This may involve transrectal ultrasonography (TRUS) of the prostate gland.

The PSA assay requires a physician's interpretation. No specific level of PSA signals the presence or absence of prostate cancer. The PSA test is produced by different manufacturers, and the different products yield different results. Men with benign prostatic enlargement have different normal levels than men with normal prostate glands.

In 1987, to determine what role PSA might play in screening asymptomatic men, the American Cancer Society undertook its National Prostate Cancer Detection Project, a long-term study of 2425 men at 10 clinical centers across the United States. This study looked at the impact of PSA and two other screening methods—digital rectal examination (DRE) and TRUS—alone and in combination in the early detection of prostate cancer.

The American Cancer Society currently recommends that asymptomatic men older than the age of 40 be screened for prostate cancer via DRE; men older than age 50 should undergo annual PSA and DRE. Men who are at high risk for prostate cancer (black men or men with a first-degree relative, such as a father or brother, diagnosed with prostate cancer at a young age) should begin annual PSA testing at age 45 (ACS, 2009). If the result of either is suspicious, further evaluation is necessary.

A PSA is done by collecting a sample of the patient's blood before prostate palpation. The normal range for a man over the age of 40 is 0 to 4 ng/L. Even a small increase in a PSA test level needs to be carefully evaluated. Although the PSA is used to screen for prostate cancer, it is used most widely to determine the effectiveness of cancer treatment and to assess the recurrence of prostate cancer. A rising PSA after surgery for cancer of the prostate suggests recurrence.

CA-125 is a cancer antigen detected in the blood and peritoneal ascites. The normal range is 35 units/mL. CA-125 may be elevated in gynecologic cancers (including ovarian cancer) and cancer of the pancreas. A monoclonal antibody has been developed that reacts with this antigen, giving physicians a method to measure the amount of CA-125 in blood samples. This test is used mainly to signal a recurrence of ovarian cancer. It is not a way to detect primary ovarian cancer, since other conditions—such as endometriosis, hepatitis, pelvic inflammatory diseases, or pregnancy—may increase CA-125 levels in the blood.

A tumor marker, **CA-19-9** antigen, is used in the diagnosis, monitoring of a patient's response to therapeutic intervention, and surveillance of the patient with pancreatic or hepatobiliary cancer. CA-19-9 is elevated in 70% of patients with pancreatic cancer and 65% of patients with hepatobiliary cancer. CA-19-9 is not an effective screening tool for pancreatic or biliary tumors in the general population because of its lack of sensitivity and specificity (Pagana & Pagana, 2008).

Stool Examination for Occult Blood

The cause of blood in the stool must be identified to rule out the possibility of cancer. The **guaiac test** is commonly used to detect occult (hidden) blood in the stools. Other commonly used tests for occult blood in the stool are **Hematest, Occultest,** and **Hemoccult test.** Early detection self-tests are available for home use. If blood is found, the person should seek immediate medical attention. For accurate test results, it is essential that the person not ingest red meat, turnips, melons, aspirin, or vitamin C for 4 days before the test.. The test must be performed on three consecutive bowel movements. Urge people to follow through with diagnostic tests recommended by their physician as a result of preliminary examinations and laboratory tests.

CANCER THERAPIES

SURGERY

By the time it is decided that surgery is needed to remove a cancerous lesion, cancer cells may already have spread to other areas. The goal of surgery is to remove all malignant cells; this may include removal of the tumor, surrounding tissue, and regional lymph nodes. Surgery in conjunction with chemotherapy and/or radiation therapy may increase the destruction of cancer cells. The effects of cancer drugs and radiation treatments administered before, during, and after surgery are being investigated. A surgical cure may result from a well-isolated lesion removed in the very early stages, as in cancer of the skin, testicle, breast, or cervix. Surgery may be performed for many reasons: preventive, diagnostic, curative, and palliative (therapy designed to relieve uncomfortable symptoms, but that does not produce a cure).

Polyps in the colon may be removed during a colonoscopy before malignant changes occur. Occasionally, prophylactic mastectomy is done to prevent breast cancer in those identified to be at increased risk because of their family history or other factors. If the cancerous lesion has already metastasized, surgery may provide palliation by relieving some of the associated problems, such as obstruction, ulceration, hemorrhage, and pain. The pituitary, adrenal glands, ovaries, or testes may be surgically removed to help control the growth and spread of malignancies caused by hormonal stimulation.

A radical surgical approach to operable tumors is no longer routinely used because of more sensitive and accurate diagnosing methods, a greater variety of surgical procedures, more sophisticated staging techniques, and more available advanced treatment options. The more conservative surgical management of breast cancer (i.e., lumpectomy instead of total mastectomy) is an excellent example of this trend.

Reconstructive surgery may be needed to improve body functions and appearance after some types of surgery, such as modified radical mastectomy. Breast reconstruction is an option for women whose disease and treatment enable the surgeon to implant a prosthesis or to transplant tissue from other areas of the body to recreate a more natural-looking breast. When this is anticipated, preoperative counseling by the surgeon and the nurse helps the patient consider the long-range outcome instead of the immediate surgical procedure.

The use of laser beams as an alternative for some oncology surgical procedures is increasing. The laser beam vaporizes tissue with little bleeding and low risk of infection. Currently the major uses of laser surgery are in ophthalmology, gynecology, urology, neurosurgery, and otolaryngology. The chief discomfort while undergoing laser surgery is that the person must lie very still while the laser is in use.

Communication

Nurse-Patient Therapeutic Dialogue Prior to Modified Radical Mastectomy

Nurse: Good afternoon, Mrs. Snyder My name is Jill, and I will be your nurse this evening. How are you feeling? (introduction and general lead)

Patient: I'm feeling all right now. It's tomorrow I'm dreading.

Nurse: You're dreading tomorrow? (restatement)

Patient: Yes. My doctor told me he has to remove my entire breast. I dread the thought that I'll look so different.

Nurse: You're anxious about the fact that you may look different. (reflection)

Patient: I'll be embarrassed to undress in front of my husband. He may think I'm no longer attractive.

Nurse: Have you had a chance to discuss your feelings with your husband? (clarification)

Patient: No, he's out of town but will be back tonight. I guess I could talk to him then. Maybe he will accept it better than I think.

Nurse: We'll talk more after you've had a chance to talk to him about your feelings. Is there anything else on your mind that you'd like to talk about now? (showing acceptance and general lead)

Nursing Interventions

If you are not present when the physician explains recommendations for care, ask the physician what he or she has told the patient and the family. This is essential to be able to reinforce the information given. Patients and families are usually frightened and may not remember all that the physician has explained to them.

Patients should have confidence and trust in those responsible for their care. Positive feelings and attitudes promote relaxation and help reduce anxiety and fear (see Communication box). Encourage the patient to ask the physician any questions concerning potential risks of a given treatment. A patient needs to feel comfortable with the decision to follow through with the physician's recommendations.

The following are nursing guidelines to ensure that patients get the information they need:

- Be present when patient and physician are discussing treatment decisions.
- If necessary, clarify explanations of treatments, including benefits and side effects, and help the patient formulate questions and voice concerns. Address patient or family concerns and questions concerning alternative treatments.
- Afterward, talk to the patient and the family about the information the physician presented; assess their understanding of the treatment, as well as their goals and needs.
- Report any apparent misunderstandings, unrealistic expectations, or other problems to the physician.
- Communicate with the patient to verify that his or her questions were answered.
- Accept and support the patient's choice, regardless of personal opinion.

Preparing the patient for a surgical procedure must include an explanation of what to expect postoperatively. Preoperative teaching is discussed in Chapter 2.

Whatever the surgical procedure, the patient's nutritional status, both before and after surgery, has been found to be a significant factor in the amount of surgery that can be tolerated, the rate of recovery, the patient's role performance, and the adequacy of wound healing.

When surgery may result in a changed body image, as in mastectomy, laryngectomy, or the formation of an ostomy, the patient may benefit from talking with another person who has undergone the same type of surgery. The American Cancer Society sponsors support groups and prepares volunteers to visit patients who need these types of surgical procedures. Reach to Recovery; the Lost Chord Club; I Can Cope; Look Good, Feel Good; and a local chapter of the United Ostomy Associations of America are some of the special groups available in some local communities.

RADIATION THERAPY

Radiation therapy can be used to cure or control cancer that has spread to local lymph nodes or to treat tumors that cannot be removed. Radiation may be used preoperatively to reduce the size of a tumor. Postoperative radiation may be indicated to destroy malignant cells not removed by surgery. Radiation may also be used to slow the growth of malignant tumors.

Radiation may be delivered externally or internally. External therapy may be directed toward superficial lesions or toward deeper structures within the body. Because malignant cells lack the capacity for repair, more cancer cells than normal cells are damaged by radiation, and normal cells are able to recover better. However, normal cells do have a maximum dose of radiation that they can tolerate before irreversible damage occurs. Treatment plans are designed to minimize the radiation dose to normal structures. Meticulous planning and recording of the dose are essential.

External Radiation Therapy

When external radiation is planned, the specific area on the body is marked to indicate the port at which external radiation will be directed. These markings must not be washed off. If the area becomes wet while bathing, the skin should be patted with an absorbent towel. Help the patient understand the need to protect this area. Also instruct the patient to avoid using any ointments, lotions, or powder on this area. The physician may approve specific lotions or creams for drying skin. Tell the patient to protect the radiated area from direct sunlight and to avoid applications of heat or cold because these would increase erythema, drying, and pruritus of the skin, which is common over an irradiated area.

Encourage a diet high in protein and calories and a fluid intake of 2 or 3 L/day. Reassure the person undergoing radiation therapy that lethargy and fatigue are common during treatment, and that frequent rest periods are helpful.

Some 60% of all people with cancer are treated with radiation therapy at some point. For many of these, radiation therapy is the only therapy needed to destroy the cancer.

Internal Radiation Therapy

Radioactive implant (brachytherapy) is the insertion of **sealed radioactive materials** temporarily or permanently into hollow cavities, within body tissues, or on the body's surface. The radioactive source delivers a specific radiation dose continuously over hours or days. A highly concentrated radiation dose is delivered in or near a tumor. This technique is generally combined with a course of external radiation therapy to increase the dosage to a specific site. Certain organs, such as the uterus and vagina, are natural receptacles for the placement of an applicator that can be loaded with radioactive material. Radioactive needles, wires, seeds, beads, or catheters may be inserted directly into tumor tissue.

Unsealed internal radiation is administered intravenously or orally, so that it is distributed throughout the patient's body. Take special precautions to prevent exposure to radiation from direct contact with the patient or any body tissue or fluid (Box 17-3). In general, assemble materials and plan ahead to provide several nursing interventions at the same time on entering the patient's room. Stand as far away as possible from the site where an internal radiation device is in the patient's body. Limit the time needed for close contact near the irradiated site. If direct, prolonged care is needed, wear a lead apron.

Children younger than 18 years of age and pregnant women should not be allowed to visit implant patients. Advise approved visitors to limit visits to 10 minutes and to stand as far away from the patient as possible.

When cancer of the cervix is treated with the use of an applicator containing a radioactive material, the applicator is placed in the vagina. The following special nursing measures are indicated:

1. Place "Radiation in Use" sign on the patient's door.
2. Prevent dislodgment. Keep the patient on strict bed rest. Instruct the patient not to turn from side to side or onto the abdomen. Do not raise the head of the bed more than 45 degrees.
3. Do not give a complete bed bath while the applicator is in place, and do not bathe the patient below the waist. Do not change bed linen unless necessary.
4. Encourage the patient to do active range-of-motion (ROM) exercises with both arms and mild foot and leg exercises to minimize the hazards of immobility. Patient wears antiembolism stockings (thromboembolic disease hose) or pneumatic compression boots.
5. Monitor vital signs every 4 hours, observing for elevations in temperature, pulse, and respirations. Report to the physician a temperature higher than 100° F (37.7° C).
6. Observe for and report any rash or skin eruption, excessive vaginal bleeding, or vaginal discharge.
7. Keep accurate intake and output record. Encourage a fluid intake of at least 3 L/day. An indwelling catheter is in place to reduce the size of the bladder and decrease the effects of radiation on the bladder. Check to be sure it is draining well.
8. Serve diet as ordered—usually a low-residue diet to minimize peristalsis and bowel movement, which might lead to dislodgment of the applicator.
9. Check position of applicator every 4 hours.
10. Keep long-handled forceps and a special lead container in the patient's room for use by the radiologist, should the implant become dislodged. Never touch a dislodged applicator or any other materials that have fallen out of the patient. These may contain the radioactive sources. Any bed linens, dressings, or pads that have been changed for the patient must be checked with a radiation survey meter before they are removed from the patient's room.
11. After the applicator is removed, the indwelling catheter is usually removed, and a douche and enema are generally prescribed.
12. Precautions are no longer needed after removal of the applicator. Encourage ambulation and gradual resumption of activities.
13. Sexual intercourse is usually delayed for 7 to 10 days.
14. Instruct the patient to notify the physician of nausea, vomiting, diarrhea, frequent or painful urination, or a temperature more than 100° F (37.7° C).

CHEMOTHERAPY

Chemotherapy drugs are used to reduce the size or slow the growth of metastatic cancer. Most chemotherapeutic agents work by interfering with the cells' **replication** process (ability to multiply or reproduce). These drugs damage the cell and cause cellular death. Both malignant and normal cells are affected by chemotherapy. Cells that multiply rapidly, such as cells of the **hematopoietic system,** the **hair follicles,** and the **GI system,** are affected the most. The majority of the side effects from chemotherapeutic agents result from the destruction of normal cells in these systems (Table 17-3).

Hematopoietic System
Leukopenia

Leukopenia (reduction in the number of circulating white blood cells [WBCs] due to depression of the bone marrow) is a common problem for patients receiving chemotherapy. It can lead to life-threatening

Box 17-3	**Instructions for Nursing Interventions for Patients Treated with (Unsealed Internal Radiation) ^{131}I for Thyroid Cancer**

Spend as little time as possible for ordinary nursing care. The patient must be as self-sufficient as possible. The patient is radioactive and exposes the nurse to radiation while caring for the patient. The radioactive ^{131}I leaves the patient through urine and perspiration. Therefore the patient contaminates everything he or she touches and can spread contamination to the nurse in this way.

PRECAUTIONS TO REDUCE EXPOSURE TO THE NURSE

a. Limit the time spent in the room. Work quickly and enter only as necessary.
b. When in the room, maintain as much distance from the patient as possible. A few feet of distance makes a lot of difference in the amount of exposure to the nurse.
c. Wear shoe covers and disposable, fluid-proof gloves, and avoid contact with all surfaces in the room.
d. When leaving the room:
   1. Wash hands with gloves on.
   2. Remove one shoe cover at the door, step that foot out, and drop that shoe cover into the trash.
   3. Remove the other shoe cover and step that foot out and drop that shoe cover into the trash.
   4. Remove gloves and drop them into the trash.
   5. Do not remove shoe covers or gloves from the room. All trash must stay in the room.
e. Always wear the dosimeter while in the room and log the exposure you receive at each visit. The dosimeter, log, and instructions are kept outside the door.
   1. No visitors are allowed.
   2. The patient is confined to the room.
   3. Nothing is to leave the room unless checked for contamination and released by the radiation safety officer (RSO)/designee. All trash and laundry are to remain in the special containers.
   4. Pregnant, nursing, or nuclear medicine personnel will not enter the area.
   5. Shoe covers and fluid-proof disposable gloves (nonsterile type) are to be worn when entering the room. Gowns will be available.
   6. The dosimeter is to be worn in the room, and exposure is to be logged when leaving the room.
   7. All clothes and bed linens used by the patient should be placed in the laundry bag provided and should be left in the patient's room to be checked by the RSO/designee.
   8. No housekeeping is allowed until the room is officially released.
   9. Food is delivered only by nursing. It is delivered to the door and picked up by the patient. Mail, flowers, and other items are delivered in the same way.
   10. Whenever possible, only disposable items may be used in the care of these patients. These items

should be placed in the designated waste container. Contact the RSO/designee for proper disposal of the contents of the designated waste container.

11. Except in emergencies, urine collection or blood draws are not allowed after the patient has been dosed with ^{131}I. The urine and blood are radioactive.
12. The patient is to flush the toilet three times after each use, and males should sit down to void.
13. If the nurse helps to collect the excreta, disposable gloves should be worn. Afterward, hands should be washed with the gloves on and again after the gloves are removed. The gloves should be placed in the designated waste container for disposal by the RSO/designee.
14. Utmost precautions must be taken to see that no urine or vomitus is spilled on the floor or the bed. If any part of the patient's room is suspected to be contaminated, notify the RSO/designee in the Nuclear Medicine Department.
15. If a nurse, attendant, or anyone else knows or suspects that his or her skin or clothing, including shoes, is contaminated, notify the RSO/designee immediately. The potentially contaminated person should remain in an area adjacent to the patient's room and should not walk about the hospital. If the hands become contaminated, wash them immediately with soap and water.
16. If a therapy patient should need emergency surgery or should die, notify the RSO or the Nuclear Medicine Department immediately.
17. Vomiting within 24 hours after oral administration, urinary incontinence, or excessive sweating within the first 48 hours may result in contamination of linen and floor. In any such situation, or if radioactive urine or feces is spilled during collection, call the RSO/designee. Meanwhile, handle all contaminated material with disposable gloves and avoid spreading contamination.
18. All vomitus must be kept in the patient's room for disposal by the RSO/designee only if the patient has vomited over the bed or the surrounding area. Otherwise, it will be flushed down the toilet with at least three volumes of water or more after it. Feces need not be routinely saved unless ordered on the chart. The same toilet should be used by the patient at all times, and it should be well flushed (at least three times).
19. The patient may not be discharged without prior approval of the RSO/designee. The room may not be remade, used, or entered by unauthorized people until released by the RSO. Nothing may leave the room unless it is checked for contamination and released by the RSO.

Courtesy Great Plains Regional Medical Center Nuclear Medicine Department, North Platte, Nebraska.

Table 17-3   Medications for Chemotherapy

Drug and Class	Mode of Action	Disease for Which Commonly Used	Common Side Effects
ALKYLATING AGENTS			
Cyclophosphamide (Cytoxan)	Interferes with DNA replication, cell-cycle nonspecific	Leukemia, breast, lymphoma, lung, ovarian, myeloma	Myelosuppression, alopecia, hemorrhagic cystitis, nausea, vomiting, cardiotoxicity
Cisplatin (Platinol)	Interferes with DNA replication, cell-cycle nonspecific	Testicular, ovarian, lung, cervical, head and neck	Nephrotoxicity, neurotoxicity, nausea, vomiting, ototoxicity
Carboplatin (Paraplatin)	Interferes with DNA replication, cell-cycle nonspecific	Ovarian, leukemia, lung	Myelosuppression, nausea, vomiting, nephrotoxicity, neurotoxicity
Chlorambucil (Leukeran)	Interferes with DNA replication, cell-cycle nonspecific	Lymphoma, chronic lymphocytic leukemia	Myelosuppression, sterility, stomatitis, pulmonary infiltrates
ANTITUMOR ANTIBIOTICS			
Bleomycin (Blenoxane)	Inhibits DNA and RNA synthesis, cell-cycle nonspecific	Testicular, cervical, Hodgkin's lymphoma	Anaphylaxis, nausea, vomiting, rash, pulmonary fibrosis, alopecia, stomatitis
Doxorubicin (Adriamycin)	Inhibits DNA and RNA synthesis, cell-cycle nonspecific	Breast, endometrial, leukemia, Hodgkin's melanoma, lymphoma	Myelosuppression, cardiotoxicity, extravasation, nausea, vomiting, alopecia, stomatitis, red urine (24-48 hours)
Mitoxantrone (Novantrone)	Inhibits DNA and RNA synthesis, cell-cycle nonspecific	Hodgkin's lymphoma, leukemia, breast cancer	Myelosuppression, cardiotoxicity, nausea, vomiting, blue urine (immediate to 24 hours)
ANTIMETABOLITES			
Cytarabine (Ara-C, Cytosar)	Damages cell in S phase, cell-cycle specific	Leukemia, lymphoma	Myelosuppression, neurotoxicity, rash, nausea, vomiting, stomatitis, alopecia, anaphylaxis
Fludarabine (Fludara)	Damages cell in S phase, cell-cycle specific	Leukemia (chronic lymphocytic leukemia, hairy cell), low-grade lymphoma	Myelosuppression, CNS toxicity, visual disturbance, nausea and vomiting, renal damage (tumor lysis syndrome)
Fluorouracil (5-FU)	Damages cell in S phase, cell-cycle specific	Breast, colorectal, liver, endometrial, esophageal, pancreatic, bladder	Myelosuppression, nausea, vomiting, stomatitis, alopecia, diarrhea
Gemcitabine (Gemzar)	Damages cell in S phase, cell-cycle specific	Pancreatic, lung	Myelosuppression, fatigue
Methotrexate (MXT, amethopterin)	Damages cell in S phase, cell-cycle specific	Breast, lymphoma, leukemia, bladder, head and neck, esophageal	Myelosuppression, diarrhea, oral and GI ulcerations, pulmonary infiltrates, nausea and vomiting
HORMONAL AGENTS			
Corticosteroids (dexamethasone [Decadron], hydrocortisone [Solu-Cortef], methylprednisolone [Solu-Medrol, Medrol], prednisone)	Alter hormonal environment that promotes cancer growth	Used in many chemotherapy disease protocols	Fluid and electrolyte disturbances, neuromuscular imbalances, changes in appetite and energy, requires glucose and insulin adjustment
Megestrol (Megace)	Alters hormonal environment that promotes cancer growth	Breast, prostate	Menstrual changes, hot flashes, nausea, vomiting, headache, weight gain, edema

CNS, Central nervous system; *DNA,* deoxyribonucleic acid; *GI,* gastrointestinal; *RNA,* ribonucleic acid.

Continued

Table 17-3   Medications for Chemotherapy—cont'd

Drug and Class	Mode of Action	Disease for Which Commonly Used	Common Side Effects
HORMONAL AGENTS—cont'd			
Leuprolide (Lupron)	Alters hormonal environment that promotes cancer growth	Prostate	Impotence, testicular atrophy, hot flashes, gynecomastia, peripheral edema
Tamoxifen (Nolvadex)	Competes with estrogen for binding sites in breast and other tissues	Breast	Vaginal bleeding, hot flashes, rash, hypercalcemia, peripheral edema
VINCA ALKALOIDS			
Etoposide (VP-16)	Inhibits cell division, cell-cycle specific	Lung, testicular, leukemia, lymphoma, small cell carcinoma of the lung	Myelosuppression, nausea, vomiting, diarrhea, fever, hypotension, phlebitis, alopecia
Vinblastine (Velban)	Inhibits cell division, cell-cycle specific	Testicular, Hodgkin's, lung, lymphoma, bladder, renal	Myelosuppression, extravasation, nausea, vomiting, alopecia, loss of deep tendon reflex
Vincristine (Oncovin)	Inhibits cell division, cell-cycle specific	Leukemia (acute lymphocytic leukemia, chronic myelogenous leukemia)	Extravasation, alopecia, stomatitis, constipation, peripheral neuropathy, optic atrophy
Vinorelbine (Navelbine)	Inhibits cell division, cell-cycle specific	Breast, lung, Hodgkin's, head and neck	Myelosuppression, alopecia, injection site reaction (phlebitis), nausea, anorexia, constipation, peripheral neuropathy
MISCELLANEOUS ANTINEOPLASTIC AGENTS			
Asparaginase (Elspar)	Cell-cycle specific (G phase)	Acute lymphocytic leukemia	Nausea, vomiting, chills, headache, CNS depression, abdominal pain, anaphylaxis
Paclitaxel (Taxol)	Mitotic inhibitor	Breast, lung, ovarian	Myelosuppression, dyspnea, hypotension, alopecia, cardiotoxicity, peripheral neuropathy, anaphylaxis
Docetaxel (Taxotere)	Miotic inhibitor	Breast, lung, ovarian	Myelosuppression, fluid retention, mucositis, phlebitis, vomiting, diarrhea, anaphylaxis
Topotecan (Hycamtin)	Interrupts DNA synthesis	Lung, breast, esophagus, tumor, lymphoma	Myelosuppression, nausea, vomiting, diarrhea, fever, fatigue, alopecia, elevated liver enzymes
Irinotecan (CPT-11, Camptosar)	Interrupts DNA synthesis	Colorectal, pancreatic	Severe diarrhea, myelosuppression, nausea and vomiting

infections. Normal value for WBCs is 5000 to 10,000/mm³. A total WBC less than 4000/mm³ is leukopenia. Lack of neutrophils, the type of WBC most often suppressed in the differential WBC count, is called **neutropenia.** Normal value for neutrophils is 60% to 70%, or 3000 to 7000/mm³. The neutrophil count is less than 1000/mm³ in neutropenia and less than 500/mm³ in severe neutropenia. A patient with severe neutropenia should be placed on neutropenic precautions. Without enough neutrophils, the body's

first line of defense collapses, opening the way for pneumonia, septicemia, or other potentially overwhelming infections.

Protect the patient against pathogens, monitor the patient for signs of infection, and respond aggressively if an infection occurs. Monitor the patient's vital signs every 4 hours and notify the physician if temperature starts to rise. A temperature of 100.4° F (38° C) or more is considered a sign of impending infection (see Safety Alert box).

⚠ Safety Alert!

Neutropenic Precautions

- Monitor for fever and neutrophil count to identify signs of and potential for infection.
- Evaluate for presence of chills. Take vital signs every 4 hours because fever may be the only indication of infection and septic shock.
- Report temperature elevations of more than 100.4° F (38° C) to the health care provider immediately so that antibiotic therapy can be initiated promptly to avoid the rapidly lethal effects of infection.
- Institute good hand hygiene technique with antiseptic solution for all people in contact with patient; place patient in private room; limit or screen visitors and hospital staff members with colds or potentially communicable illness to prevent transmission of harmful pathogens to patient.
- Teach patient necessary personal hygiene techniques (e.g., hand hygiene, oral care, skin hygiene, pulmonary hygiene, and potential infection risks).
- Avoid invasive procedures (e.g., venipuncture, urinary catheter) as much as possible.
- Administer hematopoietic growth factors (e.g., granulocyte colony-stimulating factors [G-CSFs] such as filgrastim [Neupogen] or pegfilgrastim [Neulasta]) to increase patient's WBC count and reduce infection risk during periods of neutropenia. Maintain neutropenic diet (avoid fresh fruits and vegetables because of presence of microscopic pathogens in uncooked produce). Discourage fresh flowers or live plants in the room. Mites, gnats, and other microscopic organisms could be a potential source of infection for the patient.

Take the following systematic approach to assessing the patient for infection.

Assessing the mouth. Stomatitis (inflammation of the oral mucosa) is one of the most common complications of chemotherapy and can lead to severe swallowing problems and systemic infections. Use a penlight and tongue blade to look for lesions, ulcers, or white plaque.

Teach the patient the importance of performing regular, but gentle, mouth care. Have the patient use a soft toothbrush and rinse the mouth with normal saline or sodium bicarbonate solution every 2 to 4 hours. A sponge-tipped applicator (Toothette) may help prevent bleeding gums, a common adverse effect of chemotherapy and radiation.

To reduce the risk of an oral *Candida* infection, the physician may order prophylactic antifungal medications such as an oral nystatin (Mycostatin) suspension, clotrimazole (Lotrimin) lozenges, or fluconazole (Diflucan). A soft or liquid diet may also be ordered

Assessing the skin. A rash or eruption may indicate that the patient has an infection or is predisposed to one. Bacteria may flourish in skinfolds, such as in the groin and axillae, so clean these areas twice a day with soap and water. Water-soluble moisturizers may be used to keep the patient's skin from drying. To prevent cuts, advise the patient to shave with an electric razor.

Vascular access sites are common gateways to infection. Monitor central and peripheral intravenous (IV) catheters carefully. Check for edema, drainage, erythema, or pain around catheter entry sites. Organisms can also grow along catheter tracts and infect the blood, resulting in septicemia. Signs and symptoms of a catheter tract infection include tenderness around the catheter site and referred pain in the shoulder.

Administer oral drugs whenever possible. Try to avoid subcutaneous or intramuscular injections because they can cause abscesses in patients with neutropenia. Excessive bleeding is also a risk for these patients because of the potential for associated decreases in platelets and other formed elements in the blood.

Puncturing the skin is sometimes unavoidable, as when the patient needs a bone marrow biopsy. After a biopsy, carefully assess the site, swab it with an antibacterial solution (such as povidone-iodine [Betadine]), and apply an occlusive dressing until the skin heals.

Assessing for pulmonary function. Many neutropenic patients with lung infections do not have common signs and symptoms, such as sputum production or infiltrates demonstrable on chest radiographs. Therefore be alert for other indications of an impending infection, including changes in lung sounds, respiratory rate and rhythm, and breathing effort. The patient may also complain of pain during inspiration or expiration.

To help prevent a lung infection, encourage the patient to perform deep-breathing and coughing exercises and to be as active as possible. Use of an incentive spirometer can help by maximizing ventilatory capacity.

Assessing urinary and bowel function. Changes in urinary function can also warn of infection in a neutropenic patient. Assess for decreased urinary output, changes in the urine's odor or color, hematuria, or glycosuria. The patient may also complain of urinary frequency, urgency, or pain.

To reduce the risk of urinary tract infection, avoid bladder catheterization. If catheterization is absolutely indicated, follow strict aseptic technique when inserting the catheter and perform catheter care according to the agency's guidelines.

Also routinely assess the patient's bowel function. Assess stool samples for color, consistency, and the presence of blood, and ask the patient to report any changes in bowel habits.

Does the patient need to strain when defecating? If so, the physician may prescribe a stool softener such as docusate (Colace). Straining can cause ulcerations or fissures in the rectum, creating ports of entry for bacteria. Avoid enemas, rectal medications, and rectal thermometers, which can break the mucosal lining. Be aware that neutropenia predisposes a patient to rectal abscesses. If the patient complains of perirectal pain, notify the physician immediately.

Medical management. A breakthrough in treating patients with neutropenia is commercially made colony-stimulating factors (CSFs), the only therapy that can actually prevent or manage neutropenia. The two types of CSFs are G-CSF (filgrastim, pegfilgrastim) and granulocyte-macrophage colony-stimulating factors (GM-CSF) (sargramostim [Leukine, Prokine]). These CSFs are given subcutaneously or intravenously. Although CSFs are extremely expensive, they are used prophylactically for patients at increased risk for neutropenia, such as those with a history of developing severe or prolonged neutropenia after chemotherapy.

Anemia

Anemia is a reduction in the number of circulating red blood cells (RBCs), hemoglobin, or volume of packed RBCs (hematocrit) due to depression of the bone marrow. Normal values are as follows:

	Male	Female
Erythrocytes (RBCs)	4.7 to 6.1 million/mm^3	4.2 to 5.4 million/mm^3
Hemoglobin	14 to 18 g/dL	12 to 16 g/dL
Hematocrit	42% to 52%	37% to 47%

Hemoglobin levels of 10 to 14 g/dL indicate mild anemia, 6 to 10 g/dL indicate moderate anemia, and less than 6 g/dL indicate severe anemia. Fatigue is a major problem for persons with anemia because of the decreased oxygenation to tissues from the decreased hemoglobin. For the hospitalized patient, plan to balance activities and rest to prevent increased oxygen expenditure and hypoxemia. Persons at home need to plan activities of daily living to allow rest periods.

Recombinant human erythropoietin, or epoetin alfa (EPO; Epogen, Procrit), was initially approved by the U.S. Food and Drug Administration (FDA) in 1987 for management of chronic anemia associated with end-stage renal disease. In 1993 the FDA approval was expanded to include management of chemotherapy-related anemia. EPO is given subcutaneously or intravenously.

Transfusion of packed RBCs is indicated if there is evidence of cardiac decompensation or if low hemoglobin levels are combined with low platelet counts. The transfusion improves oxygen-carrying capacity, which provides for more efficient use of blood components and less risk of volume overload.

Thrombocytopenia

Thrombocytopenia is a reduction in the number of circulating platelets due to the depression of the bone marrow. Normal platelet values are 150,000 to 400,000/mm^3. When the platelet count is less than 20,000/mm^3, spontaneous bleeding can occur. Platelet transfusions may be necessary.

Patient teaching measures to prevent injury and hemorrhage due to decreased platelets include (1) use soft toothbrush or swab for mouth care; (2) keep mouth clean and free of debris; (3) avoid intrusions into rectum (such as rectal medications or enemas); (4) use electric shaver; (5) apply direct pressure for 5 to 10 minutes if any bleeding occurs; (6) avoid contact sports, elective surgery, and tooth extraction; (7) avoid picking or blowing nose forcefully; (8) avoid trauma, falls, bumps, and cuts; (9) avoid use of aspirin or aspirin preparations; and (10) use adequate lubrication and gentleness during sexual intercourse.

Integumentary System

Alopecia

Alopecia is loss of hair due to the destruction of hair follicles. It may occur by two mechanisms. If the hair roots are atrophied, alopecia occurs readily. The hair falls out either spontaneously or during hair combing, often in large clumps. If the hair shaft is constricted because of atrophy or necrosis, the hair will break off very near the scalp. The root remains in the scalp, and a patchy, thinning pattern of hair loss occurs. Hair loss may also occur on other parts of the body. Loss of leg, arm, pubic, axillary, and facial hair is less common than loss of eyebrows and eyelashes.

The pattern and extent of hair loss cannot be accurately predicted for a given patient. When treatment is given with a drug known to cause alopecia, tell the patient that severe hair loss can begin within a few days or weeks of treatment and that partial or complete baldness can quickly ensue. Drug-induced alopecia is never permanent. The patient may experience a change in hair color or texture when the hair grows back. Occasionally, hair growth may return while chemotherapy treatment continues. Because hair loss is temporary, and the drugs are necessary to control or cure the cancer, most patients tolerate the hair loss with minimal distress. However, many patients have difficulty adjusting to the change in body image due to hair loss.

To meet the patient's needs, provide an education program, written materials, and educational sessions with a hair stylist. Inform the patient about health care measures for scalp protection, such as using gentle shampoos; avoiding hair dryers, curling irons, permanents, and hair coloring; protecting the scalp in winter and summer (cold or heat loss); and wearing protective covering when outdoors. The patient with long or thick hair may wish to trim or cut hair short to delay hair loss as long as possible. Provide sincere concern and emotional support for the patient.

Gastrointestinal System

Stomatitis

Stomatitis is a mouth inflammation due to destruction of normal cells of the oral cavity. It may range from erythema of the oral mucosa to mild or severe ulceration. Methotrexate, 5-fluorouracil (5-FU), doxorubicin, dactinomycin, and bleomycin are the chemotherapeutic drugs that most frequently cause stomatitis. Patients may also develop a superimposed fungal infection of the mouth and esophagus, and oral nystatin or fluconazole is usually prescribed. Good mouth care is important.

Viscous lidocaine (Xylocaine) is used when stomatitis becomes intolerable. Light topical application can decrease pain so the patient may eat and drink. Usually a soft or liquid diet is encouraged to help maintain nutritional status.

Nausea, Vomiting, and Diarrhea

Nausea, vomiting, and diarrhea are disorders of the GI tract caused by the excessive breakdown of normal GI cells. Nausea and vomiting are among the most uncomfortable and distressing side effects of chemotherapy. The onset and duration vary greatly among patients and with the drug given. For the ambulatory patient, nausea may interfere with the ability to continue daily work. Persistent vomiting may result in fluid and electrolyte imbalance, general weakness, and weight loss. Decline of nutritional status renders the patient more susceptible to infection and perhaps less able to tolerate therapy. Such physiologic symptoms can accompany or precipitate psychological responses such as depression and withdrawal. Every effort must be made to minimize chemotherapy-induced nausea and vomiting.

Antiemetics vary in success. Tetrahydrocannabinol (THC) (a chemical found in marijuana) taken in pill form produces an antiemetic effect in some patients who have not benefited from the commonly prescribed prochlorperazine (Compazine). Metoclopramide (Reglan), ondansetron (Zofran), and granisetron (Kytril) are often helpful for people receiving chemotherapy, and lorazepam (Ativan) may produce a relaxed state during which an individual is less sensitive to nausea-inducing stimuli (Table 17-4). The patient may receive antiemetics orally,

Table 17-4	Medications for Symptom Control of Cancer Treatment		
Generic (Brand)	**Action**	**Side Effects**	**Nursing Implications**
Ondansetron (Zofran)	Antiemetic	Headache, diarrhea, constipation, abdominal pain, transient increase in aspartate aminotransferase (AST) or alanine aminotransferase (ALT)	Dilute intravenous dose with D_5W or NaCl and give total dose (approximately 32 mg) 30 minutes before chemotherapy. Give 8 mg po before chemotherapy and three times a day for 2 days.
Granisetron (Kytril)	Antiemetic	Headache, constipation, somnolence, diarrhea, mild changes in blood pressure	Administer dose over 5-minute period, beginning 30 minutes before chemotherapy. Give once a day in a 5-minute infusion, or give 2 mg po 1 hour before chemotherapy and 1 mg bid for 2 days.
Metoclopramide (Reglan)	Antiemetic	Drowsiness, extrapyramidal reactions, restlessness, dysrhythmias, anxiety	Administer IV dose 30 minutes before administration of chemotherapeutic agent. Administer oral doses 30 minutes before meals and at bedtime.
Prochlorperazine (Compazine)	Antiemetic	Extrapyramidal symptoms, orthostatic hypotension, ocular changes (blurred vision), dry mouth, constipation, urine retention, photosensitivity	Use cautiously with other CNS depressants (e.g., alcohol) and medications that decrease blood pressure, as well as patients with liver disease. Decrease dose in older adults. Do not exceed recommended dose. Protect from light.
Diphenoxylate with atropine (Lomotil)	Antidiarrheal	Sedation, dizziness, dry mouth, urinary retention, rash	Watch for physical dependence. It should work within 48 hours. Give naloxone as antidote for respiratory depression.
Morphine (Roxanol, MS Contin)	Opioid analgesic	Decreased respiratory rate, euphoria, seizures, physical dependence, hypotension, bradycardia, miosis, drowsiness, dizziness, urinary retention, constipation, rash	Use cautiously with other CNS depressants (e.g., alcohol). Monitor respirations, heart rate, and mental status closely. Have naloxone available as antidote. Do not give sustained-release tablets for acute pain.
Hydromorphone (Dilaudid)	Opioid analgesic	Decreased respiratory rate, euphoria, seizures, physical dependence, hypotension, bradycardia, miosis, drowsiness, dizziness, urinary retention, constipation, rash	Use cautiously with other CNS depressants (e.g., alcohol). Monitor respirations, heart rate, and mental status closely. Have naloxone available as antidote. Do not give sustained-release tablets for acute pain. Have Dilaudid-HP (10 mg/mL) available for chronic pain.

GI, Gastrointestinal; *NaCl,* sodium chloride.

Continued

Table 17-4   Medications for Symptom Control of Cancer Treatment—cont'd

Generic (Brand)	Action	Side Effects	Nursing Implications
Naproxen (Naprosyn, Anaprox)	Nonsteroidal antiinflammatory agent	Agranulocytosis, headache, dizziness, drowsiness, peripheral edema, visual disturbances, GI upset (occult blood loss and peptic ulcers), prolonged bleeding time, tinnitus	Concurrent use of alcohol, acetylsalicylic acid, and steroids increases chance of GI bleeding. It may interact with warfarin sodium (Coumadin). Avoid use in patient allergic to acetylsalicylic acid. Give with food. Advise patient that it may take 4 weeks to show benefit.
Diphenhydramine (Benadryl)	Antihistamine; may also be used for antiemetic and sedation purposes	Drowsiness, dry mouth	Anticholinergic effect; used as an antiemetic.
Metoclopramide (Reglan)	Antiemetic	Restlessness, dry mouth, delayed gastric emptying, gastroesophageal reflux	Assess patient for nausea, vomiting, abdominal distention, and bowel sounds before and after administration
Amitriptyline (Elavil)	Tricyclic antidepressant	Tremors, orthostatic hypotension, urinary retention	Use in combination with narcotics in neuropathies and postherpetic neuralgia (especially with burning pain). Therapeutic effect takes 2 to 3 weeks.
Dexamethasone (Decadron)	Antiinflammatory and immune modifier	Hyperglycemia, mood swings, depression	Effective as antiemetic in chemotherapy: immunosuppression, palliation of selected neoplasms.
Lorazepam (Ativan)	Antianxiety agent, antiemetic	Drowsiness, headache, diarrhea, respiratory depression	Smoking decreases effectiveness. Decreases nausea, especially when given before and during chemotherapy.

intramuscularly, rectally, or intravenously, as well as via pumps in patient-controlled analgesia.

The development and use of the 5-HT$_3$ antagonists (ondansetron, granisetron) has resulted in effective antiemetic therapy. Prevention of nausea and vomiting increases patient comfort while decreasing or eliminating anxiety and fear. These antiemetics are given before chemotherapy and afterward, as directed by the physician. The drugs have mild side effects and can be used safely in the outpatient setting. Metoclopramide, a dopamine antagonist, has proven effective in controlling mild to moderate nausea and vomiting. Metoclopramide blocks dopamine receptors in the chemoreceptor trigger zone of the central nervous system, stimulates motility of the upper GI tract, and accelerates gastric emptying (see Table 17-4).

Changes in bowel habits commonly occur but usually do not require intervention. If diarrhea becomes marked or persistent, an antidiarrheal medication such as diphenoxylate with atropine (Lomotil) may be prescribed.

Nursing Interventions

Combinations of chemotherapy agents, as well as chemotherapy combined with other treatments, have increased the number of cures, remissions, and palliative outcomes. Many of the problems experienced by people undergoing chemotherapy are the same as those that may result from radiation therapy (depending on the target site and amount of radiation). Help the patient realize that some of the problems are the result of therapy and not a sign that the cancer is getting worse.

Nursing diagnoses and interventions for the patient undergoing chemotherapy include but are not limited to the following:

Nursing Diagnoses	Nursing Interventions
Impaired tissue integrity: oral mucous membrane, related to: • stomatitis (inflammation of the mouth) • xerostomia (decreased salivation)	Assist with frequent, careful oral hygiene and hydration; use very soft toothbrush. Provide meticulous mouth care. Administer prescribed antifungal medication such as fluconazole. Give soothing oral lozenges, ice chips, and frequent sips of ice water; avoid hot beverages; use lip balm for dryness.

Nursing Diagnoses	Nursing Interventions
Imbalanced nutrition: less than body requirements, related to: <ul><li>anorexia (from changes in taste and smell)</li><li>nausea and vomiting</li><li>dysphagia (difficulty swallowing)</li><li>aspiration</li><li>diarrhea</li><li>malabsorption</li><li>cachexia (general ill health and malnutrition, marked by weakness and emaciation, usually associated with a serious disease such as cancer)</li></ul>	Provide adequate, easily digestible, soft, bland diet; avoid spicy foods. Keep room free of odors and clutter. Administer prescribed antiemetic medications. Give small, frequent, highly nutritional meals to meet the extra demands created by energy used by malignant cells; allow extra time to eat.
Risk for infection, related to: <ul><li>weakened immune system</li><li>leukopenia</li></ul>	Protect against infections, especially from other people. Advise patient to avoid crowds. Observe and promptly report to physician any signs of inflammation at injection sites or insertion sites of any peripheral or central IV lines; report any temperature greater than 100° F (37.7° C). Use sterile technique whenever possible. Initiate reverse isolation as indicated. Monitor temperature, leukocyte count. Discourage fresh-cut flowers. Avoid indwelling catheters and performing rectal procedures or examinations. Administer antibiotics as prescribed.

Tumor Lysis Syndrome

Tumor lysis syndrome (TLS) is an oncologic emergency with rapid lysis of malignant cells.

Etiology and Pathophysiology

TLS may occur spontaneously in patients with inordinately high tumor burdens. However, it is usually a result of chemotherapy or, less commonly, radiation therapy. It may occur anywhere from 24 hours to 7 days after antineoplastic therapy is initiated. Patients most at risk are those who have large tumor cell burdens (e.g., high-grade lymphomas) or markedly elevated WBC level (acute leukemias). TLS is also seen in chronic lymphocytic leukemia and metastatic breast cancer.

The syndrome develops when chemotherapy or irradiation causes the destruction (or lysis) of a large number of rapidly dividing malignant cells. As malignant cells are lysed, intracellular contents are rapidly released into the bloodstream. This results in high levels of potassium (hyperkalemia), phosphate (hyperphosphatemia), and uric acid (hyperuricemia). These conditions, plus secondary hypocalcemia, all put the patient at risk for renal failure and alterations in cardiac function.

Clinical Manifestations

Early signs include nausea, vomiting, anorexia, and diarrhea; these may be accompanied by muscle weakness and cramping. Later signs may progress to tetany, paresthesias, seizures, anuria, and cardiac arrest.

Diagnostic Tests

TLS is diagnosed by observation of the signs and symptoms and by confirmation of abnormal laboratory values. Early symptoms of TLS may not be readily apparent, and clinical manifestations appear rapidly; the syndrome is most frequently detected by abnormalities in blood chemistry. Serum potassium, phosphate, calcium, and uric acid are diagnostic. Other important values include serum creatinine, blood urea nitrogen, and urine pH.

Medical Management

The best way to treat TLS is to prevent it by recognizing the patient population who is at risk and initiating prophylactic measures before beginning antineoplastic therapy. This includes pretreatment **hydration** to maintain a urinary output of 150 mL/hr. Hydration should begin 24 to 48 hours before treatment and continue for at least 72 hours after treatment. **Diuretics** may be used to promote the excretion of phosphate and uric acid, to prevent volume overload, and to promote the excretion of potassium in the urine. **Allopurinol** prevents uric acid formation. It is begun a few days before treatment and should be continued for 3 to 5 days after treatment is completed. **Sodium bicarbonate** is used to maintain an alkaline urine (pH over 7) to prevent uric acid crystallization. Cation-exchange resins, such as kayexalate, are used to bind with potassium so it can be excreted through the bowel. **Calcium gluconate** is given intravenously to correct hypocalcemia. Cardiac monitoring is required. Phosphate-binding gels, such as aluminum hydroxide, are given to form an insoluble complex that is excreted by the bowel. When these measures are not successful, renal dialysis may be necessary.

Nursing Interventions

Nursing interventions include identifying patients at risk for TLS and initiating hydration 24 to 48 hours before chemotherapy. Administer allopurinol before and during chemotherapy to maintain alkaline urine. Assess medications for those that contain phosphate or spare potassium and discuss discontinuation with physician. Monitor potassium, phosphorus, calcium, and uric acid levels. Also assess patient for signs and symptoms of TLS, including the following:

- **Hyperkalemia:** electrocardiographic changes, muscle weakness, twitching, paresthesia, paralysis, muscle cramps, nausea, vomiting, lethargy, and syncope
- **Hyperphosphatemia:** azotemia, oliguria, hypertension, and renal failure
- **Hypocalcemia:** electrocardiographic changes (heart block, dysrhythmias, and cardiac arrest), tetany, confusion, and hallucinations
- **Hyperuricemia:** renal failure, nausea, vomiting, flank pain, gout, and pruritus

If hyperuricemia is detected, administer diuretics, sodium bicarbonate, cation-exchange resins, and phosphate-binding gels as appropriate. Monitor intake and output and notify physician if urinary output is less than 100 mL/hr. Monitor urine pH and maintain at greater than 7 with sodium bicarbonate. Prepare the patient and family for dialysis if other measures are not effective.

Prognosis

Successful treatment of TLS depends on preventing renal failure. TLS typically resolves within 7 days, once appropriate treatment is initiated.

Chemotherapy has proven effective in treatment of many cancer patients. Many cancer patients can be cured with chemotherapy, whereas others experience cancer-free intervals or control of cancer pain. Learn about each drug being administered to anticipate the expected side effects and plan the nursing interventions needed.

Follow safety guidelines in preparing and administering chemotherapeutic agents because they may be absorbed into the skin or inhaled. The major types of chemotherapeutic agents used to treat cancer are given in Table 17-3.

BIOTHERAPY

The observation of interactions between the immune system and malignant cells led to the development of therapies that could manipulate this natural process. Traditionally, this field has been known as immunotherapy. It has led to the modern era of biotherapy. Since the 1980s, biotherapy, or biologic therapy, has emerged as an important fourth modality for treating cancer. **Biotherapy** may be defined as treatment with agents derived from biologic sources or affecting biologic responses.

Biologic response modifiers (BRMs) work through three major mechanisms. The first mechanism increases, restores, or modifies the host defenses against the tumor (CSFs, filgrastim, erythropoietin, GM-CSFs). The second mechanism uses agents that are directly toxic to tumors (interleukins, bacille Calmette-Guérin vaccine [BCG]). The third mechanism modifies the tumor biology (interferons alpha, beta, and gamma).

Most of these therapies are intramuscular or subcutaneous injections and need to be given over an extended time. Compliance and motivation are important considerations when monitoring these patients. Side effects common to BMRs include fatigue, flulike symptoms, leukopenia, nausea, and vomiting.

Health care professionals must understand these therapies to help give the cancer patient the best chance available. These therapies and research are leading to the development of gene therapy today; this will lead to improved cancer therapy in the future.

BONE MARROW TRANSPLANTATION

Bone marrow transplantation is the process of replacing diseased or damaged bone marrow with normally functioning bone marrow. Bone marrow transplants (BMTs) are used in the treatment of a variety of diseases and offer a chance for long-term survival.

Stem cell transplants are being used in some solid tumor cancers, such as high-risk breast cancer. Bone marrow harvests are becoming less frequent because many centers have turned to peripheral stem cell transplants for hematopoietic support after high-dose chemotherapy (Lewis et al., 2007).

Most transplantation bone marrow is obtained by multiple needle aspirations from the posterior iliac crest while the patient is under general or spinal anesthesia. The anterior iliac crest and sternum may also be used. The amount of marrow extracted ranges from 600 to 2500 mL for the average adult. After processing, the marrow is given to the patient intravenously through a transfusion bag, or it can be frozen (cryopreservation). Marrow may be kept for 3 or more years. When the bone marrow is infused, it is via a central line without a filter over 1 to 4 hours.

Bone marrow may be removed from an individual for personal use (autologous, indicating something that has its origin within an individual, especially a factor present in tissues or fluids) at a later time. Alternatively, an individual may be given **allogenic** bone marrow (meaning the transplant came from someone else). Three types of allogenic BMTs are (1) **syngeneic** (donation from the patient's identical twin), (2) **related** (donation from a relative, usually a sibling), and (3) **unrelated** (donation from a nonrelative). The patient is at increased risk for developing infection during the process of transplant because the immune defenses are weakened. These patients are cared for in special bone marrow units so they can be monitored closely.

Interventions to prevent infections include protective isolation or laminar airflow rooms; prophylactic systemic antibiotics and antiviral agents (primarily acyclovir); and routine cultures of blood, urine, throat, and stool. Despite these and other interventions, the patient can become septic in hours, with multisystem failure.

Survival after bone marrow transplantation depends on the patient's age, remission, and clinical status at the time of transplantation.

PERIPHERAL STEM CELL TRANSPLANTATION

An emerging and promising alternative to BMT is peripheral stem cell transplant (PSCT). This procedure is based on the fact that peripheral or circulating stem cells are capable of repopulating the bone marrow. PSCT is a type of transplant that differs from BMT primarily in the method of collection of stem cells. Because there are fewer stem cells in the blood than in the bone marrow, mobilization of stem cells from the bone marrow into the peripheral blood can be done using chemotherapy or hematopoietic growth factors, such as GM-CSF and G-CSF.

The donor's blood is collected via pheresis, in which the person is attached to a cell separator machine that removes peripheral stem cells and then returns the blood to the person. This procedure, called **leukapheresis,** usually takes 2 to 4 hours. In autologous transplants the stem cells are purged to kill any cancer cells and then frozen and stored until used for transplantation. Although many of the same steps (harvesting, intensive chemotherapy, reinfusion) of BMT are used in PSCT, the hematologic recovery period in PSCT is shorter, and fewer, less severe complications are seen (Lewis et al., 2007).

NURSING INTERVENTIONS

Communicate genuine concern for cancer patients by reinforcing information explained to patients by their physicians regarding the expectations of their specific treatments. Patients may become discouraged by toxic side effects and other problems they experience while undergoing conventional cancer therapies. Allow extra time to listen to patients with cancer express their feelings, and encourage them to follow the guidelines of conventional medical practice that offer the most hope.

ADVANCED CANCER

PAIN MANAGEMENT

Patients with cancer may have pain at any point during the course of the disease and its treatment. In fact, of the 4 million people throughout the world who die from cancer each year, 70% experience pain as a primary symptom. Unfortunately, many people believe that pain is an early symptom of cancer and do not seek diagnosis until pain occurs. In fact, pain is almost always a late symptom and indicates tumor obstruction, pressure on the nerves, invasion of bone, phantom sensation, peripheral neuropathy, and neuralgia.

It is estimated that 85% of patients with cancer pain can be managed effectively with appropriate therapy. The American Cancer Society, the American Pain Society, the World Health Organization, the Oncology Nursing Society, and many other organizations consider pain control a major issue in the management of a person with cancer.

One of the many challenges in caring for the patient with pain is the assessment. Accept the definition of pain as whatever the person experiencing the pain says it is, existing whenever the patient says it does. It is extremely important not to be judgmental concerning the patient's complaints of pain.

Cultural and religious practices in one's family play an important role in the perception of pain or suffering as a weakness. Some families tend to minimize pain. Other cultures expect the expression of pain; therefore they may have a greater overt expression of pain.

Opioids used in the management of cancer pain include morphine (the prototype), hydromorphone (Dilaudid), fentanyl, and methadone. Sustained-release morphine in an oral form, such as MS Contin, Oramorph SR, Avinza, Kadian, or Roxanol SR, is particularly effective in the management of the terminally ill person with pain. Administering opioids via transdermal method, inhalation, IV drips, intrathecally, and epidurally enhances the analgesic effect. Avoiding the peaks and valleys of pain relief with bolus injections provides more constant pain relief. The need for around-the-clock dosage is clear. Fixed dosage schedules with adequate doses for pain relief provide more constant blood levels and predictable pain relief. Some patients have breakthrough pain that requires additional doses, but the fixed dosage schedule should be maintained. Monitor and treat any opioid side effects such as constipation, vomiting, and respiratory and central nervous system depression.

In addition to opioids, valuable nonopioid analgesics used in the treatment of certain levels of cancer pain are acetaminophen; aspirin; and nonsteroidal antiinflammatory drugs, such as ibuprofen, indomethacin, and naproxen.

Patient self-control methods include distraction, massage, relaxation, biofeedback, hypnosis, and imagery. Many patients find that self-care measures enhance the effectiveness of other prescribed pain interventions. Adequate rest, sleep, diversion, and other meaningful activities also help manage the patient's pain. The patient with advanced cancer often experiences cachexia, a profound state of ill health, and malnutrition, marked by weakness and emaciation. Positioning, giving meticulous skin care, offering nutritious fluids and foods, and using other comfort measures to promote relaxation and rest will help to reduce pain and severe fatigue.

The nurse's unique role in pain management involves acting as link between the patient and the health care team, spending time with the patient, assessing the patient's response to the pain and its management, and educating the patient and the family. In addition, be able to articulate a concise pain assessment as well as anticipate and address patient, family, and health care provider misconceptions about pain management. For example, many patients and their families have opioid phobia, the irrational and undocumented fear that even the appropriate use of opioids causes addiction. This fear of addiction among both health care providers and the public seems to be a major reason for the undertreatment of pain. Understand and be able to state why opioids are needed for terminally ill patients. Appropriate use of pain management strategies enables patients and families to accept the therapeutic value of drugs such as opioids. Ensure that patients are not subjected to severe suffering from potentially controllable pain.

General guidelines for the use of pain relief measures are (1) use a variety of pain relief measures; (2) use pain relief measures before the pain becomes severe; (3) include pain relief measures that the patient believes will be helpful; (4) determine the patient's ability or willingness to participate actively in the use of pain relief measures; (5) rely on patient behavior to indicate pain severity rather than relying on known physical stimuli; (6) encourage the patient to try a pain relief measure at least two times before abandoning it as ineffective; (7) have an open mind as to what may relieve the patient's pain, including nonpharmacologic measures; and (8) keep trying to relieve the pain; do not become discouraged and do not stop working with the patient.

Fear and anxiety increase as a result of pain. Many cancer patients believe increased pain is a sign their condition is worsening and death is imminent. Pain increases their fear, and the cycle of pain continues. The most effective pain relief is probably a combination of (1) appropriate pain relief methods, (2) the opportunity to make personal and spiritual peace if there are unresolved conflicts in relationships with others, and (3) someone to listen and offer comfort.

NUTRITIONAL THERAPY

Nutritional problems that most frequently occur in the patient with cancer are malnutrition, anorexia, altered taste sensation, nausea, vomiting, diarrhea, stomatitis, and mucositis. These problems can be caused by a combination of factors, including drug toxicity, effects of radiation therapy, tumor involvement, recent surgery, emotional distress, or difficulty with ingestion or digestion of food. If the patient is inadequately nourished, the normal cells will not be able to recover from the effects of therapy, and the immune system will be depressed because of depletion of protein stores.

Malnutrition

The patient with cancer usually experiences protein and calorie malnutrition characterized by fat and muscle depletion. Encourage the patient to eat foods that increase protein intake and facilitate repair and regeneration of cells, as well as high-calorie foods that provide energy and minimize weight loss.

Suggest to the physician the need for a nutritional supplement as soon as a 5% weight loss is noted or the patient has the potential for protein and caloric malnutrition. Monitor albumin and prealbumin levels. Once a 10-pound (4.5-kg) weight loss occurs, it is difficult to maintain the nutritional status. Instruct the patient to use nutritional supplements in place of milk when cooking or baking. Nutritional supplements can be easily be added to scrambled eggs, pudding, custard, mashed potatoes, cereal, and cream sauces. Packages of instant breakfast can be used as indicated or sprinkled on cereals, desserts, and casseroles. If the malnutrition cannot be treated with dietary intake, it may be necessary to use enteral or parenteral nutrition as an adjunct nutritional measure.

Anorexia

The anorexia experienced by a patient with cancer is a challenging problem. An intervention may be effective one day and ineffective the next. Continual assessment and intervention are necessary to successfully manage this problem. Adopt the philosophy that something can be done to prevent or minimize anorexia, evaluate each intervention, and continue to use those interventions that have been successful in the past. Megestrol (Megace) is used in cachexia anorexia to stimulate the appetite.

Altered Taste Sensation

Cancer cells are believed to release substances that resemble amino acids and stimulate the bitter taste buds. The patient may also experience an alteration in the sweet, sour, and salty taste sensations. Meat may taste bitter. At this time the physiologic basis of these varied taste alterations is unknown. Instruct the patient with an altered taste problem to avoid foods he or she dislikes. Frequently the patient may feel compelled to eat certain foods because they are "healthy." Advise the patient to experiment with spices and other seasoning agents to mask the taste alterations. Lemon juice, onion, mint, basil, and fruit juice marinades may improve the taste of certain meats and fish. Bacon bits, onion, and pieces of ham may enhance the taste of vegetables. Just adding more spice or seasoning agent is usually not an effective way to enhance the taste.

COMMUNICATION AND PSYCHOLOGICAL SUPPORT

The patient and the family may become irritable and angry with caregivers when the patient is suffering and has progressive problems. Understand that these feelings are not directed toward the caregivers personally but have emerged from the circumstances associated with the patient's disease. A display of anger toward the staff may be caused by deep-seated frustration or anxiety. Understanding and continued warm, responsive caring are the best approaches. The patient may not hear the explanations that are given when feelings are at a high level. Listening and administering kind, gentle nursing care may communicate more effectively than words. Touch may also be appropriate, letting the patient know that someone else is aware of the emotional distress being experienced.

Nurses are able to make cancer's effects less traumatic through sensitivity and creativity. Understand how much each patient needs a sense of control; some need it more than others. The health care system encourages dependency by stripping away most traces of a patient's identity. An adult is told when to get out of bed, have a drink, wash up, and even urinate. Be aware of what is happening to the patient and provide as many avenues of patient control as possible. Learn the art of talking to patients, not *at* patients.

Psychological support of the patient is an important aspect of cancer care. Because of the effectiveness of cancer treatment, many patients with cancer are cured or their disease is controlled for long periods. Thus emphasis must be placed on maintaining an optimal quality of life after the diagnosis of cancer. A positive attitude of patient, family, and caregivers toward cancer and cancer treatment has a significant positive effect on the quality of life that the patient experiences. A positive attitude may also influence the patient's prognosis.

Most people view the diagnosis of cancer as a crisis. Cancer affects the quality of life of all cancer patients in some way. Four quality-of-life factors affecting cancer patients and their families are social, psychological, physical, and spiritual (American Cancer Society, 2008a). The most common concerns voiced by the patient are (1) fear of recurrence, (2) chronic or acute pain, (3) sexual problems, (4) fatigue, (5) guilt for delaying screening or treatment, (6) behavior that may have increased the risk for cancer, (7) changes in physical appearance, (8) depression, (9) sleep problems, (10) change in role performance, and (11) being a financial burden on their loved ones (American Cancer Society, 2008a).

Coping with these fears exposes the patient to a range of emotions and behaviors: shock, anger, denial, bargaining, depression, helplessness, hopelessness, rationalization, acceptance, and intellectualization. These behavioral patterns may occur at any time during the process of cancer. However, some patterns appear to occur more frequently or at a greater intensity at certain specific stages of the disease process. The following factors may determine how the patient will cope with the diagnosis of cancer:

- **Ability to cope with stressful events in the past** (e.g., loss of job, major disappointment): Ask how the patient has coped with stressful events to gain an understanding of the patient's coping patterns, their effectiveness, and the usual coping time frame.
- **Availability of significant others:** The patient who has effective support systems tends to cope more effectively than the patient who does not.
- **Ability to express feelings and concerns:** The patient who is able to express feelings and needs

and who seeks and asks for help appears to cope more effectively than the patient who internalizes feelings and needs.
- **Age at the time of diagnosis:** Age determines the coping strategies to a great degree. For example, a young mother with cancer has different concerns than a 70-year-old woman with cancer.
- **Extent of disease:** Cure or control of the disease process is usually easier to cope with than the reality of terminal illness.
- **Disruption of body image:** Disruption of the body image (e.g., radical neck dissection, alopecia, mastectomy) may intensify the psychological effect of cancer.
- **Presence of symptoms:** Symptoms such as fatigue, nausea, diarrhea, and pain may intensify the psychological effect of cancer.
- **Experience with cancer:** If experiences with cancer have been negative, the patient will probably view the present status as negative.
- **Attitude associated with cancer:** A patient who feels in control and has a positive attitude about cancer and cancer treatment is better able to cope with the diagnosis and treatment than one who feels hopeless, helpless, and out of control.

To facilitate the development of a hopeful attitude about cancer and to support the patient and the family during the various stages of the process of cancer, continue to be available, especially during difficult times. Exhibit a caring attitude, and listen actively to fears and concerns. Maintain a relationship based on trust and confidence; be open, honest, and caring in the approach. Use touch to exhibit caring; a squeeze of the hand may at times be more effective than words.

Provide essential information regarding cancer and cancer care. Provide relief from distressing symptoms. Assist the patient in setting realistic, reachable short- and long-term goals. Assist the patient in maintaining usual lifestyle patterns. Above all, maintain hope, which is the key to effective cancer care. Hope varies, depending on the patient's status—hope that the symptoms are not serious, hope that the treatment is curative, hope for independence, hope for relief of pain, hope for a longer life, or hope for a peaceful death. Hope provides control over what is occurring and is the basis of a positive attitude toward cancer and cancer care (Lewis et al., 2007) (see Evidence-Based Practice box).

TERMINAL PROGNOSIS

Coping with the multiple problems associated with advanced cancer can lead to a sense of helplessness and hopelessness in spite of all efforts. The patient and the family may look forward to death as a relief from unrelenting suffering.

Most patients with advanced cancer know that they are dying. They recognize attempts to avoid the truth and may distrust and feel hostile toward the person who makes such attempts. Honesty and openness are

Evidence-Based Practice   The Burden of Illness for Cancer Survivors

Evidence Summary

A group of researchers wanted to learn about the burden of illness among cancer survivors. They studied more than 1800 cancer survivors, as well as individuals without cancer (control group) who were matched with cancer survivors by age, sex, and educational attainment. The study examined several measures of burden or stress, including a person's sense of utility or feeling useful, a perception of overall health, and days lost from work. The results of the study showed that cancer survivors had poorer outcomes across all measures: lower utility, higher levels of lost productivity, and more likely to report their health as fair or poor when matched with control subjects.

Application to Nursing Practice

As a nurse, learn to assess the many ways in which cancer affects the lives of patients who are survivors. Because can-

cer causes long-term effects, spend time assessing patients' symptoms, the effects of symptoms on lifestyle and self-care ability, the effects on patient relationships, the patients' ability to remain productive and successful in their jobs, their economic security, and their physical well-being. Patients' self-perceptions are also important to understand when you attempt any intervention that requires the patient to be motivated and involved.

Reference

Yabroff, K.R., et al. (2004). Burden of illness in cancer survivors: findings from a population-based national sample, *J Natl Cancer Inst* 96(17):1322.

From Potter, P.A., & Perry, A.G. (2009). *Fundamentals of nursing: concepts, process, and practice.* (7th ed.). St. Louis: Mosby.

the best approaches. Most patients surprise caregivers by expressing relief at a willingness to discuss what is foremost in their minds: their imminent death.

Spiritual activities may provide mental and emotional strength in spite of physical deterioration. The patient may ask the nurse to read the Bible or to pray with him or her, or the patient may request that a minister, priest, or rabbi visit. Spiritual strength may help the patient and the family cope with the continuing problems encountered in the cancer experience.

The hospital social worker assists the patient and family in planning for home care. Arrangements for any special supplies and equipment are made before discharge. The nurse plays a major role in teaching the patient and at least one family member or significant other how to continue any special care needed at home, such as dressing changes, irrigations, the management of a feeding tube, or the care of a central venous line for administration of parenteral nutrition or medications.

Throughout the hospital stay, take advantage of time available to promote self-care to the greatest extent possible. Assess the patient's readiness to learn and ability to actively participate in self-care. If necessary, consult advanced clinical nursing specialists to provide individualized guidelines for teaching patients. Include plans for patient education in the nursing care plan. Document evidence of the patient's comprehension of and ability to handle self-care, and plan for any assistance needed from others. Continuity of care is the goal in discharge planning. Hospice services can be arranged in most communities for those who have advanced cancer. There are freestanding hospices, hospices within a hospital or skilled nursing facility, or at-home arrangements. The primary focus of a hospice is enhancing the patient's quality of life, not prolonging it. Efforts are directed toward relief from pain and other problems. Skilled professional care and voluntary support services are provided to assist the patient and the family in living life to the fullest each day.

Get Ready for the NCLEX® Examination!

Key Points

- It is currently estimated that one of every five people in the United States will get cancer. The 5-year survival rate is 65%.
- There is strong evidence that what people eat or drink or their lifestyle habits may predispose them to the development of cancer.
- The American Cancer Society recommends specific preventive behaviors and screening tests for cancer prevention and early detection for men and women.
- It is imperative for the person to perform self-examination to detect any changes and report them to the physician immediately.
- It is important to have periodic physical examinations and to seek medical attention promptly if one of the warning signs of cancer develops.

- A common reason for a delay in diagnosing cancer is that early malignant changes are not accompanied by pain.
- Seeking medical attention when warning signs occur is also frequently delayed because people fear the possible diagnosis of cancer and hope the signs and symptoms will just go away.
- The diagnosis of cancer has a profound effect on family members, as well as on the patient. They experience shock, disbelief, denial, anger, fear, anxiety, and a sense of helplessness.
- Most of the side effects from chemotherapeutic agents result from the destruction of normal cells from the hematopoietic system, hair follicles, and the GI system.
- TLS is an oncologic emergency that occurs in cancer patients with heavy tumor burdens after they receive chemotherapy or irradiation, which causes rapid lysis of malignant cells.

- The American Cancer Society sponsors organized support groups for individuals with the same types of cancer; some of these are Reach to Recovery; the Lost Chord Club; I Can Cope; Look Good, Feel Good; and the Ostomy Club. Prepared volunteer visitors are available in most communities to visit a newly diagnosed patient.
- Spiritual strength assists the patient and the family in coping with the problems experienced as a result of cancer. Based on the patient's preference, religious counsel may be helpful.
- The American Cancer Society, the American Pain Society, the World Health Organization, and the Oncology Nursing Society consider pain control a major issue in the management of a person with cancer.
- The concept of rehabilitation should be applied in planning care for the patient with cancer to promote the highest level of functioning possible.

Additional Learning Resources

 Go to your Companion CD for an audio glossary, animations, video clips, and more.

evolve Be sure to visit the Evolve site at http://evolve.elsevier.com/Christensen/adult/ for additional online resources.

Review Questions for the NCLEX® Examination

1. The patient has mouth pain 10 days after receiving chemotherapy. On inspection, the nurse finds the inside of the mouth is erythematous, edematous, and dry. The most likely problem is:
   1. candidiasis.
   2. hypercalcemia.
   3. stomatitis.
   4. esophagitis.

2. The patient has metastatic breast cancer with involvement in her L5 vertebral body. She is paralyzed from the waist down with incontinence of stool and urine. She is undergoing radiation therapy for spinal cord compression. What is an appropriate nursing diagnosis?
   1. Risk for disturbed body image, related to alopecia
   2. Risk for deficient fluid volume, related to stool incontinence
   3. Risk for impaired skin integrity, related to prolonged immobility and incontinence
   4. All of the above

3. A 58-year-old patient with colon cancer is receiving combined radiation and chemotherapy. He has diarrhea; this is related to the:
   1. diagnosis.
   2. patient's inability to eat and drink during treatment.
   3. treatment's irritating effect on the mucosa of the GI tract.
   4. fluid and electrolyte imbalance.

4. The current recommendation for first-time baseline mammogram in asymptomatic women is:
   1. at the onset of menopause.
   2. that it is not necessary if the patient has had a previous biopsy.
   3. at ages 35 to 39.
   4. at age 50.

5. What are considered cancer-screening activities? *(Select all that apply.)*
   1. Performing a risk factor assessment and physical examination
   2. Giving a patient instructions for performing the test for fecal occult blood
   3. Instructing a patient in self-examination of the skin or oral cavity
   4. Laboratory examinations for CA-125 and CA-19-9

6. The patient has terminal lung cancer. To maintain optimal pain control, oral analgesics generally should be given:
   1. at scheduled intervals.
   2. every 2 hours.
   3. as required.
   4. in relation to the patient's activity level.

7. Cancer prevention and health promotion behaviors for patients with cancer:
   1. will not decrease the risk of developing a second malignancy.
   2. will not be affected by personal choices related to diet and smoking.
   3. are increasingly important with the growing population of cancer survivors.
   4. would include only routine physical examinations.

8. The patient has been diagnosed with stage I breast cancer. She is receiving adjuvant chemotherapy and radiation therapy following a lumpectomy. Which point about alopecia should not be made? *(Select all that apply.)*
   1. Chemotherapy-related hair loss is reversible and temporary.
   2. All chemotherapeutic agents result in alopecia.
   3. Hair that grows back may have a different texture and color.
   4. Gentle shampooing is recommended.

9. A 61-year-old patient is receiving chemotherapy. The patient becomes anemic and has petechiae and ecchymoses scattered over her upper trunk, especially her arms. What side effect is the patient experiencing?
   1. Bone marrow suppression
   2. Cardiac suppression
   3. Liver toxicity
   4. Pulmonary toxicity

10. Before the insertion of a cervical implant, the nurse tells the patient what to expect while it is in place. Which statement is accurate?

    1. "Nurses will always be available, but they will spend only a short time at your bedside."
    2. "Personal cleanliness is essential, so you will be given a complete bed bath each day."
    3. "Pain or discomfort is a common side effect of this type of radiation."
    4. "Your bed linens will be completely changed each day to minimize radioactive contamination."

11. A 24-year-old patient has been receiving chemotherapy for acute lymphoblastic leukemia. Which statement indicates that he understands discharge teaching concerning leukopenia?

    1. "I am cured and have no limitations."
    2. "My family can catch leukopenia, so I need to be careful to not get too close to any of them."
    3. "I should avoid close contact with people who might give me an infection."
    4. "I need to be careful not to cut myself when shaving because I may not be able to stop the bleeding."

12. A 42-year-old patient has palpated a small lump on her left breast during her monthly BSE. She has scheduled an appointment with her physician. Which test will be used to make a definite diagnosis of a benign or malignant tumor of her breast?

    1. Biopsy
    2. Mammography
    3. Tomography
    4. Ultrasound

13. The nurse educator is discussing the importance of the reduction of carcinogens in primary prevention of cancer. Which risk factor is considered significant in numerous types of cancer?

    1. Diet low in fat
    2. Occasional moderate use of alcohol
    3. High pollen count in the environment
    4. Smoking

14. A therapeutic approach by the nurse to assist a terminally ill cancer patient in the management of his pain is that:

    1. antiinflammatory agents are effective analgesics for severe pain.
    2. opioids should be withheld because they are addictive.
    3. pain is what the patient says it is.
    4. one can increase one's tolerance for pain.

15. Which statement by a chemotherapy patient who has a low WBC count, a low platelet count, and a hemoglobin measurement of 5.6 g/dL, would indicate the need for further teaching?

    1. "I check my mouth and teeth after each meal."
    2. "I've been very constipated and need an enema."
    3. "My husband and I have been using a vaginal lubrication before intercourse."
    4. "My lips are dry and cracking. I need some lubricant."

16. Which is a biologic modifier that is a breakthrough in treating patients with neutropenia and is used prophylactically for patients at risk for neutropenia?

    1. Lymphopenic stimulating factor (LSF)
    2. Erythropoietic stimulating factor (ESF)
    3. Neutropenic stimulating factor (NSF)
    4. Colony-stimulating factor (CSF)

17. According to the American Cancer Society, what would have the greatest influence in reducing the risk of lung cancer?

    1. Five fruits and vegetables a day
    2. Yearly chest radiograph for those 50 years and older
    3. Cessation of smoking
    4. Reduction of environmental and chemical carcinogens

18. Aggressive chemotherapy to decrease the growth of rapidly progressive malignant tumors causes destruction of a large number of rapidly dividing malignant cells and increases the risk of which complication? (The drug allopurinol and hydration help control the metabolic complication that may occur.) _____

19. The nursing diagnosis of *imbalanced nutrition: less than body requirements* is often seen in chemotherapy patients as a result of:

    1. impaired tissue integrity, related to damage to integumentary tissue.
    2. alopecia and leukopenia.
    3. stomatitis, anorexia, vomiting, and diarrhea.
    4. myelosuppression.

20. What points are important in educating the patient and the family in prevention of constipation? (Select all that apply.)

    1. Opioids may cause constipation, so laxatives must be given with opioids.
    2. Patients who are not eating continue to produce waste in the bowel and get impacted with feces.
    3. High fluid intake should be maintained.
    4. The patient should have a bowel movement at least every day.
    5. If possible, eating foods high in fiber is helpful.

21. A patient has a vaginal radiation implant in place. The nurse would:

    1. instruct her to turn from side to side for comfort.
    2. restrict fluid intake to prevent bladder distention.
    3. promote intake of a high-residue diet to prevent constipation.
    4. monitor vital signs every 4 hours and report temperature greater than 100° F.

22. In the nursing interventions of a patient receiving external radiation therapy for a malignancy, the nurse must remember to:

    1. vigorously scrub the areas of entry of "ports" marked by the radiologist.
    2. apply some form of ointment with a metallic base to the area of entry each time the patient goes for radiation treatments.

3. instruct the patient to avoid irritating the "ports" by not lying on that part of the body and not wearing constricting clothing.
4. isolate the patient so he or she will not expose others to radiation.

23. The patient has a history of oat cell carcinoma of the lung and is being treated with chemotherapy. His WBC count is 2.5/mm^3. The nurse's primary concern would be:

1. prevention of hemorrhage.
2. prevention of infection.
3. prevention of dehydration.
4. prevention of electrolyte imbalance.

24. A 63-year-old patient has a diagnosis of cancer of the prostate gland with metastasis and is experiencing cachexia. This state is best described by which characteristic?

1. Poor health, malnutrition, weakness, and emaciation
2. Increased appetite and nervousness
3. Irritability and anger
4. Depression, fear, and anxiety

Matching

25. _____ Carcinogen
26. _____ Mammography
27. _____ Pathogenesis
28. _____ Thrombocytopenia
29. _____ Leukopenia

A. Reduction of WBCs
B. Radiographic examination of the breast
C. The development of morbid conditions or of disease
D. Decrease in platelets
E. Any agent or substance that causes cancer

30. Metoclopramide (Reglan) is an antiemetic that is helpful in preventing chemotherapy-induced emesis. Choose all the correct answers that describe its action.

1. Blocks dopamine receptors in chemoreceptor trigger zone of CNS
2. Accelerates gastric emptying
3. Blocks the effects of serotonin at 5-HT$_3$ receptor sites
4. Stimulates motility of the upper GI tract

31. The destruction of cancer cells results in the release of what factors into systemic circulation? *(Select all that apply.)*

1. Linoleic acid
2. Potassium
3. Uric acid
4. Phosphorus

32. The TNM staging classification stages cancer according to:

1. absence of atypical or abnormal cells.
2. cytology suggestive of but not conclusive for malignancy.
3. tumor size, lymph node involvement, any metastasis.
4. cytology conclusive for malignancy.

33. The medication of choice for pain control in the hospice setting is usually:

1. ibuprofen.
2. morphine.
3. meperidine.
4. codeine.

34. Using the TNM staging classification system, a tumor staged as T4N3M1 would mean:

1. no evidence of primary tumor, lymph node involvement, or distant metastasis.
2. carcinoma in situ, regional lymph node involvement, and metastasis to one site.
3. large tumor, lymph node involvement, and distant metastasis.
4. medium-sized tumor, no lymph node involvement, and distant metastasis.

°C	degrees Centigrade	ECG, EKG	electrocardiogram
°F	degrees Fahrenheit	EEG	electroencephalogram
ʒ	dram	elix	elixir
@*	at	ER	emergency room
♀	female	ESR	erythrocyte sedimentation rate
♂	male		
>*	greater than	ETOH	ethyl alcohol
<*	less than	Fʒ	fluid ounce
↑	increase	FUO	fever of unknown origin
↓	decrease	Fx, fx	fracture; fractional urine test
1°	primary	g, gm, Gm	gram
2°	secondary	GI	gastrointestinal
Δ	change	gr	grain
aa	indicating equal amounts of each	gt; gtt	drop; drops
		GTT	glucose tolerance test
ABGs	arterial blood gases	h, hr	hour
ac	before meals	H&P	history and physical examination
ad lib	freely as desired		
ADL	activities of daily living	HCT, Hct	hematocrit
ama, AMA	against medical advice	Hgb	hemoglobin
AND	allow natural death	HIV	human immunodeficiency virus (AIDS)
BE	barium enema		
bid	two times a day	hs	at bedtime
BP	blood pressure	I&O	intake and output
BRP	bathroom privileges	IDDM	insulin-dependent diabetes mellitus
BUN	blood urea nitrogen		
c̄	with	IM	intramuscular
cap	capsule	IV	intravenous
CBC	complete blood count	IVP	intravenous push; intravenous pyelogram
cc*	cubic centimeter		
CDC	Centers for Disease Control and Prevention	IVU	intravenous urogram
		K	potassium
cm	centimeter	kg	kilogram
c/o	complains of	KUB	kidney, ureters, and bladder (radiograph)
CO	carbon monoxide		
CO₂	carbon dioxide	KVO	keep vein open
CPR	cardiopulmonary resuscitation	L	liter
		LOC	laxative of choice; level of consciousness
CT	computed tomography		
D₅W	5% dextrose in water	m	meter
dL	deciliter	mcg, μg*	microgram
DNR	do not resuscitate	mg	milligram
Dx, dx	diagnosis	mL	milliliter

*On The Joint Commission's Lists of Dangerous Abbreviations, Acronyms, and Symbols (see Appendix B).

mm	millimeter	qd*	every day
mm Hg	millimeters of mercury	qh	every hour
MRI	magnetic resonance imaging	qid	four times a day
Ndx	nursing diagnoses	qod*	every other day
NPO	nothing per os, nothing by mouth	ROM	range of motion
		Rx	take; treatment
O_2	oxygen	s̄	without
OD	optical density; overdose	SC, SQ, Sub-Q, subQ	subcutaneous
O.D.	right eye	ss	half
O.S.	left eye	SSE	soapsuds enema
O.U.	both eyes	stat	immediately
oz, ʒ̄	ounce	tid	three times a day
pc	after meals	TKO	to keep open
PERRLA	pupils equal, round, and reactive to light and accommodation	TLC	tender loving care
		TPN	total parenteral nutrition
		TPR	temperature, pulse, and respirations
pH	hydrogen ion concentration (acidity and alkalinity)		
		U*	unit
PO, po	orally, per os	IU*	international unit
prn	as often as necessary, when required	WBC	white blood cell, white blood count
q	every		

The Joint Commission's Lists of Dangerous Abbreviations, Acronyms, and Symbols

A "minimum list" of dangerous abbreviations, acronyms, and symbols has been approved by The Joint Commission (TJC). Beginning March 5, 2009 the items in Table 1 must be included on each accredited organization's Do Not Use list:

Table 1 Minimum Do-Not-Use List of Abbreviations

ABBREVIATION	POTENTIAL PROBLEM	PREFERRED TERM
U (for unit)	Mistaken as *zero (0)*, *four (4)*, or cc	Write *unit*
IU (for international unit)	Mistaken for IV (intravenous) or 10 (ten)	Write *international unit*
Q.D., Q.O.D., Q.I.D. (Latin abbreviations for once daily, every other day, and 4 times daily)	Mistaken for each other The period after the "Q" can be mistaken for an "I," and the "O" can be mistaken for "I"	Write *daily, every other day,* and *4 times daily*
Trailing zero (X.0 mg) (NOTE: prohibited only for medication-related notations) Lack of leading zero (.X mg)	Decimal point is missed	Never write a zero by itself after a decimal point (X mg), and always use a zero before a decimal point (0.X mg)
MS MSO$_4$ MgSO$_4$	Confused for one another Can mean morphine sulfate or magnesium sulfate	Write *morphine sulfate* or *magnesium sulfate*

© 2009 The Joint Commission. Used with permission.

Additional abbreviations, acronyms, and symbols for *possible* future inclusion in the official "Do Not Use" list are provided in Table 2.

Table 2 Additional Abbreviations to Avoid

ABBREVIATION	POTENTIAL PROBLEM	PREFERRED TERM
Greater than (>) Less than (<)	Mistaken for the letter "L" or the number "7" (seven)	Write "greater than" or "less than"
Abbreviations for drug names	Mistaken for abbreviations for similar drugs	Write out full drug names
Apothecary units	Confused with metric units Uncommon term	Use metric units
@	Mistaken for the number "2" (two)	Write "at"
cc	Mistaken for U (units)	Write "ml" or "milliliters" or "mL" (preferred)
µg	Mistaken for mg (milligrams)	Write "micrograms" or "mcg"

© 2009 The Joint Commission. Used with permission.

Recommended precautions: Two nurses must double-check the following before administration: heparin, insulin, parental chemotherapeutic agents, patient-controlled analgesia, and epidural pumps.

Health Insurance Portability and Accountability Act (HIPAA) privacy requirements: Patient information concerning name, age, diagnosis, and so forth should not be posted. Charts and medication records must be kept in confidential area.

Also, the Institute for Safe Medication Practices (ISMP) has published a list of dangerous abbreviations relating to medication use that it recommends should be explicitly prohibited. This list is available on its website, www.ismp.org (revised 2007).

Laboratory Reference Values*

Reference Intervals for Hematology

TEST	CONVENTIONAL UNITS	SI UNITS
Acid hemolysis (Ham test)	No hemolysis	No hemolysis
Alkaline phosphatase, leukocyte	Total score, 14-100	Total score, 14-100
Cell counts		
Erythrocytes		
Males	4.6-6.2 million/mm^3	4.6-6.2 × 10^{12}/L
Females	4.2-5.4 million/mm^3	4.2-5.4 × 10^{12}/L
Children (varies with age)	4.5-5.1 million/mm^3	4.5-5.1 × 10^{12}/L
Leukocytes, total	4500-11,000/mm^3	4.5-11.0 × 10^9/L
Leukocytes, differential counts*		
Myelocytes	0%	0/L
Band neutrophils	3%-5%	150-400 × 10^6/L
Segmented neutrophils	54%-62%	3000-5800 × 10^6/L
Lymphocytes	25%-33%	1500-3000 × 10^6/L
Monocytes	3%-7%	300-500 × 10^6/L
Eosinophils	1%-3%	50-250 × 10^6/L
Basophils	0%-1%	15-50 × 10^6/L
Platelets	150,000-400,000/mm^3	150-400 × 10^9/L
Reticulocytes	25,000-75,000/mm^3	25-75 × 10^9/L
	(0.5%-1.5% of erythrocytes)	
Coagulation tests		
Bleeding time (template)	2.75-8.0 min	2.75-8.0 min
Coagulation time (glass tube)	5-15 min	5-15 min
D-Dimer	<0.5 mcg/mL	<0.5 mg/L
Factor VIII and other coagulation factors	50%-150% of normal	0.5-1.5 of normal
Fibrin split products (Thrombo-Welco test)	<10 mcg/mL	<10 mg/L
Fibrinogen	200-400 mg/dL	2.0-4.0 g/L
Partial thromboplastin time, activated (aPTT)	20-25 sec	20-35 sec
Prothrombin time (PT, Pro-time, International normalized ratio [INR])	12.0-14.0 sec	12.0-14.0 sec
Coombs' test		
Direct	Negative	Negative
Indirect	Negative	Negative
Corpuscular values of erythrocytes		
Mean corpuscular hemoglobin (MCH)	26-34 pg/cell	26-34 pg/cell
Mean corpuscular volume (MCV)	80-96 μm^3	80-96 fL
Mean corpuscular hemoglobin concentration (MCHC)	32-36 g/dL	320-360 g/L
Haptoglobin	20-165 mg/dL	0.20-1.65 g/L
Hematocrit		
Males	40-54 mL/dL	0.40-0.54
Females	37-47 mL/dL	0.37-0.47
Newborns	49-54 mL/dL	0.49-0.54
Children (varies with age)	35-49 mL/dL	0.35-0.49
Hemoglobin		
Males	13.0-18.0 g/dL	8.1-11.2 mmol/L
Females	12.0-16.0 g/dL	7.4-9.9 mmol/L
Newborns	16.5-19.5 g/dL	10.2-12.1 mmol/L
Children (varies with age)	11.2-16.5 g/dL	7.0-10.2 mmol/L

*Conventional units are percentages; SI units are absolute cell counts.
SI, International System of Units.

Continued

---

*From Rakel, R.E., & Bope, E.T. (2009). *Conn's current therapy 2009*. Philadelphia: Saunders.

Reference Intervals for Hematology—cont'd

TEST	CONVENTIONAL UNITS	SI UNITS
Hemoglobin, fetal	<1.0% of total	<0.01 of total
Hemoglobin A_{1C}	3%-5% of total	0.03-0.05 of total
Hemoglobin A_2	1.5%-3.0% of total	0.015-0.03 of total
Hemoglobin, plasma	0.0-5.0 mg/dL	0.0-3.2 μmol/L
Methemoglobin	30-130 mg/dL	19-80 μmol/L
Erythrocyte sedimentation rate (ESR)		
Wintrobe		
Males	0-5 mm/hr	0-5 mm/hr
Females	0-15 mm/hr	0-15 mm/hr
Westergren		
Males	0-15 mm/hr	0-15 mm/hr
Females	0-20 mm/hr	0-20 mm/hr

Reference Intervals* for Clinical Chemistry (Blood, Serum, and Plasma)

ANALYTE	CONVENTIONAL UNITS	SI UNITS
Acetoacetate plus acetone		
Qualitative	Negative	Negative
Quantitative	0.3-2.0 mg/dL	30-200 μmol/L
Acid phosphatase, serum (thymolphthalein mono-phosphate substrate)	0.1-0.6 units/L	0.1-0.6 units/L
ACTH (see Corticotropin)		
Alanine aminotransferase (ALT, serum (SGPT)	1-45 units/L	1-45 units/L
Albumin, serum	3.3-5.2 g/dL	33-52 g/L
Aldolase, serum	0.0-7.0 units/L	0.0-7.0 units/L
Aldosterone, plasma		
Standing	5-30 ng/dL	140-830 pmol/L
Recumbent	3-10 ng/dL	80-275 pmol/L
Alkaline, phosphatase (ALP), serum		
Adult	35-150 units/L	35-150 units/L
Adolescent	100-500 units/L	100-500 units/L
Child	100-350 units/L	100-350 units/L
Ammonia nitrogen, plasma	10-50 μmol/L	10-50 μmol/L
Amylase, serum	25-125 units/L	25-125 units/L
Anion gap, serum calculated	8-16 mEq/L	8-16 mmol/L
Ascorbic acid, blood	0.4-1.5 mg/dL	23-85 μmol/L
Aspartate aminotransferase (AST), serum (SGOT)	1-36 units/L	1-36 units/L
Base excess, arterial blood, calculated	0 ± 2 mEq/L	0 ± 2 mmol/L
Bicarbonate		
Venous plasma	23-29 mEq/L	23-29 mmol/L
Arterial blood	21-27 mEq/L	21-27 mmol/L
Bile acids, serum	0.3-3.0 mg/dL	0.8-7.6 μmol/L
Bilirubin, serum		
Conjugated	0.1-0.4 mg/dL	1.7-6.8 μmol/L
Total	0.3-1.1 mg/dL	5.1-19.0 μmol/L
Calcium, serum	8.4-10.6 mg/dL	2.10-2.65 mmol/L
Calcium, ionized, serum	4.25-5.25 mg/dL	1.05-1.30 mmol/L
Carbon dioxide, total, serum or plasma	24-31 mEq/L	24-31 mmol/L
Carbon dioxide tension (P_{CO_2}), blood	35-45 mm Hg	35-45 mm Hg
β-Carotene, serum	60-260 mcg/dL	1.1-8.6 μmol/L
Ceruloplasmin, serum	23-44 mg/dL	230-440 mg/L

*Reference values may vary depending on the method and sample source used.
SI, International System of Units.

Reference Intervals for Clinical Chemistry (Blood, Serum, and Plasma)—cont'd

ANALYTE	CONVENTIONAL UNITS	SI UNITS
Chloride, serum or plasma	96-106 mEq/L	96-106 mmol/L
Cholesterol, serum or EDTA plasma		
Desirable range	<200 mg/dL	<5.20 mmol/L
Low-density lipoprotein (LDL) cholesterol	60-180 mg/dL	1.55-4.65 mmol/L
High-density lipoprotein (HDL) cholesterol	30-80 mg/dL	0.80-2.05 mmol/L
Copper	70-140 mcg/dL	11-22 μmol/L
Corticotropin (ACTH), plasma, 8 AM	10-80 pg/mL	2-18 pmol/L
Cortisol, plasma		
8:00 AM	6-23 mcg/dL	170-630 nmol/L
4:00 PM	3-15 mcg/dL	80-410 nmol/L
10:00 PM	<50% of 8:00 AM value	<50% of 8:00 AM value
Creatine, serum		
Males	0.2-0.5 mg/dL	15-40 μmol/L
Females	0.3-0.9 mg/dL	25-70 μmol/L
Creatine kinase (CK), serum		
Males	55-170 units/L	55-170 units/L
Females	30-135 units/L	30-135 units/L
Creatinine kinase MB isoenzyme, serum	<5% of total CK activity	<5% of total CK activity
	<5% of ng/mL by immunoassay	<5% of ng/mL by immunoassay
Creatinine, serum	0.6-1.2 mg/dL	50-110 μmol/L
Erythrocytes	145-540 ng/mL	330-120 nmol/L
Estradiol-17β, adult		
Males	10-65 pg/mL	35-240 pmol/L
Females		
Follicular	30-100 pg/mL	110-370 pmol/L
Ovulatory	200-400 pg/mL	730-1470 pmol/L
Luteal	50-140 pg/mL	180-510 pmol/L
Ferritin, serum	20-200 ng/mL	20-200 mcg/L
Fibrinogen, plasma	200-400 mg/dL	2.0-4.0 g/L
Folate, serum	3-18 ng/mL	6.8-4.1 nmol/L
Follicle-stimulating hormone (FSH), plasma		
Males	4-25 mU/mL	4-25 units/L
Females, premenopausal	4-30 mU/mL	4-30 units/L
Females, postmenopausal	40-250 mU/mL	40-250 units/L
Gastrin, fasting, serum	0-100 pg/mL	0-100 mg/L
Glucose, fasting, plasma or serum	70-115 mg/dL	3.9-6.4 nmol/L
γ-Glutamyltransferase (GGT), serum	5-40 units/L	5-40 units/L
Growth hormone (hGH), plasma, adult, fasting	0-6 ng/mL	0-6 mcg/L
Haptoglobin, serum	20-165 mg/dL	0.20-1.65 g/L
Immunoglobulins, serum (see table of Reference Intervals for Tests of Immunologic Function)		
Iron, serum	75-175 mcg/dL	13-31 μmol/L
Iron-binding capacity, serum		
Total	250-410 mcg/dL	45-73 μmol/L
Saturation	20%-55%	0.20-0.55
Lactate		
Venous whole blood	5.0-20.0 mg/dL	0.6-2.2 mmol/L
Arterial whole blood	5.0-15.0 mg/dL	0.6-1.7 mmol/L
Lactate dehydrogenase (LD), serum	110-220 units/L	110-220 units/L
Lipase, serum	10-140 units/L	10-140 units/L
Lutropin (LH), serum		
Males	1-9 units/L	1-9 units/L
Females		
Follicular phase	2-10 units/L	2-10 units/L
Midcycle peak	15-65 units/L	15-65 units/L
Luteal phase	1-12 units/L	1-12 units/L
Postmenopausal	12-65 units/L	12-65 units/L
Magnesium, serum	1.3-2.1 mg/dL	0.65-1.05 mmol/L
Osmolality	275-295 mOsm/kg water	275-295 mOsm/kg water

EDTA, ethylenediaminetetraacetic acid.

Continued

Reference Intervals for Clinical Chemistry (Blood, Serum, and Plasma)—cont'd

ANALYTE	CONVENTIONAL UNITS	SI UNITS
Oxygen, blood, arterial, room air		
Partial pressure (PaO$_2$)	80-100 mm Hg	80-100 mm Hg
Saturation (SaO$_2$)	95%-98%	95%-98%
pH, arterial blood	7.35-7.45	7.35-7.45
Phosphate, inorganic, serum		
Adult	3.0-4.5 mg/dL	1.0-1.5 mmol/L
Child	4.0-7.0 mg/dL	1.3-2.3 mmol/L
Potassium		
Serum	3.5-5.0 mEq/L	3.5-5.0 mmol/L
Plasma	3.5-4.5 mEq/L	3.5-4.5 mmol/L
Progesterone, serum, adult		
Males	0.0-0.4 ng/mL	0.0-1.3 mmol/L
Females		
Follicular phase	0.1-1.5 ng/mL	0.3-4.8 mmol/L
Luteal phase	2.5-28.0 ng/mL	8.0-89.0 mmol/L
Prolactin, serum		
Males	1.0-15.0 ng/mL	1.0-15.0 mcg/L
Females	1.0-20.0 ng/mL	1.0-20.0 mcg/L
Protein, serum, electrophoresis		
Total	6.0-8.0 g/dL	60-80 g/L
Albumin	3.5-5.5 g/dL	35-55 g/L
Globulins		
α_1	0.2-0.4 g/dL	2.0-4.0 g/L
α_2	0.5-0.9 g/dL	5.0-9.0 g/L
β	0.6-1.1 g/dL	6.0-11.0 g/L
γ	0.7-1.7 g/dL	7.0-17.0 g/L
Pyruvate, blood	0.3-0.9 mg/dL	0.03-0.10 mmol/L
Rheumatoid factor	0.0-30.0 IU/mL	0.0-30.0 kIU/L
Sodium, serum or plasma	135-145 mEq/L	135-145 mmol/L
Testosterone, plasma		
Males, adult	300-1200 ng/dL	10.4-41.6 nmol/L
Females, adult	20-75 ng/dL	0.7-2.6 nmol/L
Pregnant females	40-200 ng/dL	1.4-6.9 nmol/L
Thyroglobulin	3-42 ng/mL	3-42 mcg/L
Thyrotropin (hTSH), serum	0.4-4.8 μIU/mL	0.4-4.8 mIU/L
Thyrotropin-releasing hormone (TRH)	5-60 pg/mL	5-60 ng/L
Thyroxine (FT$_4$), free, serum	0.9-2.1 ng/dL	12-27 pmol/L
Thyroxine (T$_4$), serum	4.5-12.0 mcg/mL	58-154 nmol/L
Thyroxine-binding globulin (TBG)	15.0-34.0 mcg/mL	15.0-34.0 mg/L
Transferrin	250-430 mg/dL	2.5-4.3 g/L
Triglycerides, serum, after 12-hr fast	40-150 mg/dL	0.4-1.5 g/L
Triiodothyronine (T$_3$), serum	70-190 ng/dL	1.1-2.9 nmol/L
Triiodothyronine uptake, resin (T$_3$RU)	25%-38%	0.25-0.38
Troponin I	0.05-0.50 ng/mL	0.05-0.5 ng/mL
Urate		
Males	2.5-8.0 mg/dL	150-480 μmol/L
Females	2.2-7.0 mg/dL	130-420 μmol/L
Urea, serum or plasma	24-49 mg/dL	4.0-8.2 nmol/L
Urea, nitrogen, serum or plasma	11-23 mg/dL	8.0-16.4 nmol/L
Viscosity, serum	1.1-1.8 × water	1.1-1.8 × water
Vitamin A, serum	20-80 mcg/dL	0.70-2.80 mcmol/L
Vitamin B$_{12}$, serum	180-900 pg/mL	133-664 pmol/L

Reference Intervals for Therapeutic Drug Monitoring (Serum or Plasma)*

ANALYTE	THERAPEUTIC RANGE	TOXIC CONCENTRATIONS	PROPRIETARY NAME(S)
ANALGESICS			
Acetaminophen	10-40 mcg/mL	>150 mcg/mL	Tylenol
			Datril
Salicylate	100-250 mcg/mL	>300 mcg/mL	Aspirin
			Bufferin
ANTIBIOTICS			
Amikacin	20-30 mcg/mL	Peak >35 mcg/mL	Amkin
		Trough >10 mcg/mL	
Gentamicin	5-10 mcg/mL	Peak >10 mcg/mL	Garamycin
		Trough >2 mcg/mL	
Tobramycin	5-10 mcg/mL	Peak >10 mcg/mL	Nebcin
		Trough >2 mcg/mL	
Vancomycin	5-35 mcg/mL	Peak >40 mcg/mL	Vancocin
		Trough >10 mcg/mL	
ANTICONVULSANTS			
Carbamazepine	5-12 mcg/mL	>15 mcg/mL	Tegretol
Ethosuximide	40-100 mcg/mL	>250 mcg/mL	Zarontin
Phenobarbital	15-40 mcg/mL	40-100 ng/mL (varies widely)	Luminal
Phenytoin	10-20 mcg/mL	>20 mcg/mL	Dilantin
Primidone	5-12 mcg/mL	>15 mcg/mL	Mysoline
Valproic acid	50-100 mcg/mL	>100 mcg/mL	Depakene
ANTINEOPLASTICS AND IMMUNOSUPPRESSIVES			
Cyclosporine A	150-350 ng/mL	>400 ng/mL	Sandimmune
Methotrexate, high-dose, 48 hr	Variable	>1 μmol/L, 48 hr after dose	
Sirolimus (within 1 hr of 2-mg dose)	4.5-14 ng/mL	Variable	Rapamune
Sirolimus (within 1 hr of 5-mg dose)	10-28 ng/mL	Variable	Rapamune
Tacrolimus (FK-506), whole blood	3-20 mcg/L	>15 mcg/L	Prograf
BRONCHODILATORS AND RESPIRATORY STIMULANTS			
Caffeine	3-15 ng/mL	>30 mcg/mL	Elixophyllin
Theophylline (aminophylline)	10-20 mcg/mL	>30 mcg/mL	Quibron
CARDIOVASCULAR DRUGS			
Amiodarone (obtain specimen more than 8 hr after last dose)	1.0-2.0 mcg/mL	>2.0 mcg/mL	Cordarone
Digoxin (obtain specimen more than 6 hr after last dose)	0.8-2.0 mcg/mL	>2.4 ng/mL	Lanoxin
Disopyramide	2-5 mcg/mL	>7 mcg/mL	Norpace
Flecainide	0.2-1.0 mcg/mL	>1 mcg/mL	Tambocor
Lidocaine	1.5-5.0 mcg/mL	>6 mcg/mL	Xylocaine
Mexiletine	0.7-2.0 mcg/mL	>2 mcg/mL	Mexitil
Procainamide	4-10 mcg/mL	>12 mcg/mL	Pronestyl
Procainamide plus NAPA (*N*-acetyl procainamide)	8-30 mcg/mL	>30 mcg/mL	
Propranolol	50-100 ng/mL	Variable	Inderal
Quinidine	2-5 mcg/mL	>6 mcg/mL	Cardioquin
			Quinaglute
Tocainide	4-10 ng/mL	>10 ng/mL	Tonocard
PSYCHOPHARMACOLOGICAL DRUGS			
Amitriptyline	120-150 ng/mL	>500 ng/mL	Elavil
			Triavil
Bupropion	25-100 ng/mL	Not applicable	Wellbutrin
Desipramine	150-300 ng/mL	>500 ng/mL	Norpramin
Imipramine	125-250 ng/mL	>400 ng/mL	Tofranil
Lithium (obtain specimen 12 hr after last dose)	0.6-1.5 mEq/L	>1.5 mEq/L	Lithobid
Nortriptyline	50-150 ng/mL	>500 ng/mL	Aventyl
			Pamelor

*Values may vary depending on the method and sample collection device used. Always consult the reference values provided by the laboratory performing the analysis.

Reference Intervals* for Clinical Chemistry (Urine)

ANALYTE	CONVENTIONAL UNITS	SI UNITS
Acetone and acetoacetate, qualitative	Negative	Negative
Albumin		
Qualitative	Negative	Negative
Quantitative	10-100 mg/24 hr	0.15-1.5 μmol/day
Aldosterone	3-20 mcg/24 hr	8.3-55 nmol/day
δ-Aminolevulinic acid (δ-ALA)	1.3-7.0 mg/24 hr	10-53 μmol/day
Amylase	<17 units/hr	<17 units/hr
Amylase-to-creatinine clearance ratio	0.01-0.04	0.01-0.04
Bilirubin, qualitative	Negative	Negative
Calcium (regular diet)	<250 mg/24 hr	<6.3 nmol/day
Catecholamines		
Epinephine	<10 mcg/24 hr	<55 nmol/day
Norepinephine	<100 mcg/24 hr	<590 nmol/day
Total free catecholamines	4-126 mcg/24 hr	24-745 nmol/day
Total metanephrines	0.1-1.6 mg/24 hr	0.5-8.1 μmol/day
Chloride (varies with intake)	110-250 mEq/24 hr	110-250 mmol/day
Copper	0-50 mcg/24 hr	0.0-0.80 μmol/day
Cortisol, free	10-100 mcg/24 hr	27.6-276 nmol/day
Creatine		
Males	0-40 mg/24 hr	0.0-0.30 mmol/day
Females	0-80 mg/24 hr	0.0-0.60 mmol/day
Creatinine	15-25 mg/kg/24 hr	0.13-0.22 mmol/kg/day
Creatinine clearance (endogenous)		
Males	110-150 mL/min/1.73 m^2	110-150 mL/min/1.73 m^2
Females	105-132 mL/min/1.73 m^2	105-132 mL/min/1.73 m^2
Cystine or cysteine	Negative	Negative
Dehydroepiandrosterone		
Males	0.2-2.0 mg/24hr	0.7-6.9 μmol/day
Females	0.2-1.8 mg/24hr	0.7-6.2 μmol/day
Estrogens, total		
Males	4-25 mcg/24 hr	14-90 nmol/day
Females	5-100 mcg/24 hr	18-360 nmol/day
Glucose (as reducing substance)	<250 mg/24 hr	<250 mg/day
Hemoglobin and myoglobin, qualitative	Negative	Negative
Hemogentisic acid, qualitative	Negative	Negative
17-Hydroxycorticosteroids		
Males	3-9 mg/24 hr	8.3-25 μmol/day
Females	2-8 mg/24 hr	5.5-22 μmol/day
5-Hydroxyindoleacetic acid		
Qualitative	Negative	Negative
Quantitative	2-6 mg/24 hr	10-31 μmol/day
17-Ketogenic steroids		
Males	5-23 mg/24 hr	17-80 μmol/day
Females	3-15 mg/24 hr	10-52 μmol/day
17-Ketosteroids		
Males	8-22 mg/24 hr	28-76 μmol/day
Females	6-15 mg/24 hr	21-52 μmol/day
Magnesium	6-10 mEq/24 hr	3-5 mmol/day
Metanephrines	0.05-1.2 ng/mg creatinine	0.03-0.70 mmol/mmol creatinine
Osmolality	38-1400 mOsm/kg water	38-1400 mOsm/kg water
pH	4.6-8.0	4.6-8.0
Phenylpyruvic acid, qualitative	Negative	Negative
Phosphate	0.4-1.3 g/24 hr	13-42 mmol/day
Porphobilinogen		
Qualitative	Negative	Negative
Quantitative	<2 mg/24 hr	<9 μmol/day
Porphyrins		
Coproporphyrin	50-250 mcg/24 hr	77-380 nmol/day

*Values may vary depending on the method used.
SI, International System of Units.

Reference Intervals for Clinical Chemistry (Urine)—cont'd

ANALYTE	CONVENTIONAL UNITS	SI UNITS
Uroporphyrin	10-30 mcg/24 hr	12-36 nmol/day
Potassium	25-125 mEq/24 hr	25-125 mmol/day
Pregnanediol		
Males	0.0-1.9 mg/24 hr	0.0-6.0 μmol/day
Females		
Proliferative phase	0.0-2.6 mg/24 hr	0.0-8.0 μmol/day
Luteal phase	2.6-10.6 mg/24 hr	8-33 μmol/day
Postmenopausal	0.2-1.0 mg/24 hr	0.6-3.1 μmol/day
Pregnanetriol	0.0-2.5 mg/24 hr	0.0-7.4 μmol/day
Protein, total		
Qualitative	Negative	Negative
Quantitative	10-150 mg/24 hr	10-150 mg/day
Protein-to-creatinine ratio	<0.2	<0.2
Sodium (regular diet)	60-260 mEq/24 hr	60-260 mmol/day
Specific gravity		
Random specimen	1.003-1.030	1.003-1.030
24-hr collection	1.015-1.025	1.015-1.025
Urate (regular diet)	250-750 mg/24 hr	1.5-4.4 mmol/day
Urobilinogen	0.5-4.0 mg/24 hr	0.6-6.8 μmol/day
Vanillylmandelic acid (VMA)	1.0-8.0 mg/24 hr	5-40 μmol/day

Reference Intervals for Toxic Substances

ANALYTE	CONVENTIONAL UNITS	SI UNITS
Arsenic, urine	<130 mcg/24 hr	<1.7 μmol/day
Bromides, serum, inorganic	<100 mg/dL	<10 mmol/L
Toxic symptoms	140-1000 mg/dL	14-100 mmol/L
Carboxyhemoglobin, blood	Saturation, percent	
Urban environment	<5%	<0.05
Smokers	<12%	<0.12
Symptoms		
Headache	>15%	>0.15
Nausea and vomiting	>25%	>0.25
Potentially lethal	>50%	>0.50
Ethanol, blood	<0.05 mg/dL, <0.005%	<1.0 mmol/L
Intoxication	>100 mg/dL, >0.1%	>22 mmol/L
Marked intoxication	300-400 mg/dL, 0.3%-0.4%	65-87 mmol/L
Alcoholic stupor	400-500 mg/dL, 0.4%-0.5%	87-109 mmol/L
Coma	>500 mg/dL, >0.5%	>109 mmol/L
Lead, blood		
Adults	<20 mcg/dL	<1.0 μmol/L
Children	<10 mcg/dL	<0.5 μmol/L
Lead, urine	<80 mcg/24 hr	<0.4 μmol/day
Mercury, urine	<10 mcg/24 hr	<150 nmol/day

SI, International System of Units.

Reference Intervals for Tests Performed on Cerebrospinal Fluid

TEST	CONVENTIONAL UNITS	SI UNITS
Cells	<5 mm³; all mononuclear	<5 × 106/L; all mononuclear
Protein electrophoresis	Albumin predominant	Albumin predominant
Glucose	50-75 mg/dL (20 mg/dL less than in serum)	2.8-4.2 mmol/L (1.1 mmol/L less than in serum)
IgG		
Children <14 yr	<8% of total protein	<0.08 of total protein
Adults	<14% of total protein	<0.14 of total protein
IgG index	0.3-0.6	0.3-0.6
Oligoclonal banding on electrophoresis	Absent	Absent
Pressure, opening	70-180 mm H₂O	70-180 mm H₂O
Protein, total	<15-45 mg/dL	150-450 mg/L

SI, International System of Units.

Reference Intervals for Tests of Gastrointestinal Function

TEST	CONVENTIONAL UNITS
Bentiromide	6-hr urinary arylamine excretion >57% excludes pancreatic insufficiency
β-Carotene, serum	60-250 ng/dL
Fecal fat estimation	
Qualitative	No fat globules seen by high-power microscope
Quantitative	<6 g/24 hr (>95% coefficient of fat absorption)
Gastric acid output	
Basal	
Males	0.0-10.5 mmol/hr
Females	0.0-5.6 mmol/hr
Maximum (after histamine or pentagastrin)	
Males	9.0-48.0 mmol/hr
Females	6.0-31.0 mmol/hr
Ratio: basal/maximum	
Males	0.0-0.31
Females	0.0-0.29
Secretion test, pancreatic fluid	
Volume	>1.8 mL/kg/hr
Bicarbonate	>80 mEq/L
D-Xylose absorption test, urine	>20% of ingested dose excreted in 5 hr

Reference Intervals for Tests of Immunologic Function

TEST	CONVENTIONAL UNITS	SI UNITS
AUTOANTIBODIES, SERUM, ADULT		
Anti-CCP antibody	0-19 units	
Anti-dsDNA antibody	0-40 international units	0-40 international units
Antinuclear antibody	<1:40	
Rheumatoid factor (total IgG, IgA, IgM)	0-30 mg/dL	
COMPLEMENT, SERUM		
C3	85-175 mg/dL	0.85-1.75 g/L
C4	15-45 mg/dL	150-450 mg/L
Total hemolytic (CH₅₀)	150-250 units/mL	150-250 units/mL
IMMUNOGLOBULINS, SERUM, ADULT		
IgA	70-310 mg/dL	0.70-3.1 g/L
IgD	0.0-6.0 mg/dL	0.0-60 g/L
IgE	0.0-430 mg/dL	0.0-430 mg/L
IgG	640-1350 ng/dL	6.4-13.5 mcg/L
IgM	90-350 mg/dL	0.90-3.5 g/L

Anti-CCP, Anticyclic citrullinated peptide; *dsDNA,* double-stranded DNA; *Ig,* immunoglobulin; *SI,* International System of Units.

Reference Intervals for Lymphocytes Subsets, Whole Blood, Heparinized

ANTIGEN(S) EXPRESSED	CELL TYPE	PERCENTAGE (%)	ABSOLUTE CELL COUNT
CD2	E rosette T cells	73-87	860-1880
CD3	Total T cells	56-77	140-370
CD3 and CD4	Helper-inducer cells	32-54	550-1190
CD3 and CD8	Suppressor-cytotoxic cells	24-37	430-1060
CD3 and DR	Activated T cells	5-14	70-310
CD16 and CD56	Natural killer (NK) cells	8-22	130-500
CD 19	Total B cells	7-17	140-370

Helper-to-suppressor ratio: 0.8-1.8.

Reference Values for Semen Analysis

TEST	CONVENTIONAL UNITS	SI UNITS
Volume	2-5 mL	2-5 mL
Liquefaction	Complete in 15 min	Complete in 15 min
pH	7.2-8.0	7.2-8.0
Leukocytes	Occasional or absent	Occasional or absent
Spermatozoa		
Count	$60\text{-}150 \times 10^6$ mL	$60\text{-}150 \times 10^6$ mL
Motility	>80% motile	>0.80 motile
Morphology	80%-90% normal forms	>0.80-0.90 normal
Fructose	>150 mg/dL	>8.33 mmol/L

SI, International System of Units.

Chapter 1
1. 2
2. 3
3. 1
4. 4
5. 2
6. 4
7. 1
8. 3
9. 2
10. 2
11. 3
12. 4
13. 3
14. 2
15. e
16. d
17. a
18. c
19. b
20. f
21. k
22. a
23. i
24. b
25. g
26. c
27. j
28. d
29. e
30. h

Chapter 2
1. 4
2. 2
3. 3
4. 1
5. 1
6. 4
7. 3
8. 2
9. 1
10. 2
11. 3
12. 2
13. 4
14. 3

15. 3
16. 2
17. 3
18. 2
19. 2
20. 1
21. 3
22. 2
23. 3
24. 4
25. 2

Chapter 3
1. 1
2. 2
3. 3
4. 3
5. 2
6. 1
7. 1
8. 1
9. 4
10. 2
11. 1
12. 2
13. 3
14. 1
15. 2
16. 1
17. 2
18. 2
19. 2
20. 1
21. 2
22. 2
23. 1, 2
24. 1
25. 3
26. papule
27. 2
28. 3
29. 2
30. 1, 2, 4
31. 4
32. 1, 2, 4

Chapter 4
1. 2
2. 4
3. 4
4. 2
5. 3
6. 4
7. 2
8. 4
9. 3
10. 3
11. 2
12. 2
13. 1
14. 2
15. 2
16. 3
17. 3
18. 4
19. 1
20. 4
21. 3
22. 3
23. 4
24. 3, 4
25. 4

Chapter 5
1. 2
2. 3
3. 2
4. 2
5. 2
6. 2
7. 4
8. 2
9. 2
10. 1
11. 1
12. 3
13. 3
14. 4
15. 4
16. 3
17. 3
18. 1
19. 3

20. 2
21. 4
22. 3
23. 4
24. 1
25. 1
26. 4
27. 4
28. 2
29. 1
30. 1, 2, 4

Chapter 6
1. 1
2. 1
3. 2, 3, 4
4. 4
5. 2
6. 3
7. 2
8. 3
9. 3
10. 1, 2, 3
11. 4
12. 2
13. 3
14. 3
15. 2
16. 2
17. 4
18. 1
19. Reinfection, cirrhosis
20. 4
21. 1
22. 1, 3
23. 2
24. 3
25. 1, 2, 3
26. 2
27. 1, 4
28. 4
29. 1

Chapter 7
1. 3
2. 1

3. 2
4. 3
5. 4
6. 2
7. 3
8. 2
9. 4
10. 3
11. 1
12. 4
13. 3
14. 2
15. 3
16. 2
17. 2
18. 1
19. 2
20. 4
21. 3
22. 1
23. 2
24. 1
25. 1, 2, 3
26. 1, 2, 3, 5
27. 1, 2, 3, 5
28. 1, 2, 4, 5
29. 2
30. 4
31. 1
32. 2
33. 1, 4
34. 2

Chapter 8
1. 1
2. 2
3. 1
4. 3
5. 4
6. 3
7. 4
8. 1
9. 4
10. 4
11. 2
12. 2
13. 4

14. 2
15. 1
16. 3
17. 1
18. 2
19. 2
20. 2
21. 4
22. 3
23. 1
24. Troponin I
25. 3
26. 2
27. 1
28. 1, 2, 3
29. 1, 2, 4
30. 4
31. 2
32. 3
33. 4
34. 3
35. 1, 2, 4
36. 1, 3, 4
37. 4

Chapter 9
1. 2
2. 3
3. 3
4. 4
5. 4
6. 1
7. 2
8. 3
9. 3
10. 3
11. 2
12. 1
13. 2
14. 4
15. 1
16. 3
17. 4
18. 3
19. 1
20. 3
21. 4

22. 1
23. 3
24. 3
25. 1
26. 1, 3, 4
27. 1, 2, 4
28. 2, 3, 4, 5
29. 1, 2, 4
30. 2
31. 1, 2, 3, 5
32. 1, 3, 4
33. 2, 3, 4, 5
34. 1, 2, 3, 4
35. 1, 2, 4, 5
36. 1, 2, 3, 5
37. 1

Chapter 10
1. 4
2. 3
3. 1
4. 4
5. 1
6. 3
7. 4
8. 1
9. 3
10. 2
11. 2
12. 3
13. 1
14. 1
15. 1
16. 4
17. 2
18. 3
19. 2
20. 4
21. 4
22. 1
23. 1
24. 2
25. 2
26. 4
27. 1, 2, 3
28. 1, 2, 3
29. 1, 2, 4
30. 1, 3, 4
31. 1
32. 1

Chapter 11
1. 3
2. 1
3. 4
4. 3
5. 3
6. 4
7. 1
8. 4
9. 4
10. 1
11. 1
12. 4
13. 4
14. 2
15. 2
16. 4
17. 3
18. 4
19. 4
20. 3
21. 3
22. Regular or
    rapid acting
23. 1, 2, 3
24. 3
25. 1
26. 2, 3, 4
27. 2
28. 1, 2, 3
29. 2
30. 1
31. 1
32. 1, 2, 3
33. 3
34. 3
35. Glycosylated
    hemoglobin
    (HgA$_{1c}$)
36. 1, 2, 4

Chapter 12
1. 1
2. 2
3. 3
4. 4

33. 3
34. 1
35. 2

Chapter 11

5. 3
6. 4
7. 2
8. 1
9. 1, 3, 4
10. 3
11. 2
12. 1
13. 3
14. 4
15. 1
16. 3
17. 4
18. 2, 3
19. 2
20. 4
21. 1
22. 1
23. 3
24. 1
25. 2
26. 2
27. 3
28. 2
29. 4
30. 1, 2

Chapter 13
1. 3
2. 2
3. 1
4. 4
5. 3
6. 4
7. 1
8. 1
9. 2
10. 1, 2, 3
11. 2
12. 2
13. 1
14. 2
15. 3
16. 1
17. 3
18. 2
19. 3
20. 3
21. 2, 3, 4
22. 1

23. 1
24. 3
25. 3
26. 1
27. 1
28. 2
29. 4
30. Cochlear
    implant
31. 4
32. 1
33. 2
34. 1

Chapter 14
1. 4
2. 3
3. 2
4. 2
5. 1
6. 4
7. 3
8. 1
9. 3
10. 3
11. 1
12. 1
13. 1, 2, 3
14. 1
15. 2
16. 2
17. 1
18. 4
19. 1
20. 3
21. 2, 3, 4
22. C
23. E
24. D
25. B
26. A
27. 1, 2, 3, 4
28. 2, 3, 4
29. 1, 2, 3, 5
30. 3
31. 4
32. 2
33. 4
34. 3
35. 1, 2, 3

36. 2
37. 1

Chapter 15
1. 4
2. 2
3. 1
4. 2
5. 2
6. 1
7. 3
8. 3
9. 4
10. 2
11. 1
12. 1
13. 2, 3, 4
14. 3
15. 4
16. 3
17. Natural
    rubber latex
    proteins
18. 2, 3, 4
19. 1, 3, 4

Chapter 16
1. 1
2. 4
3. 4
4. 2
5. 2
6. 1
7. 1
8. 1
9. 1
10. 3
11. 2
12. 4
13. 3
14. False
15. True
16. True
17. True
18. True
19. False
20. False
21. 2
22. 2
23. 4

24. 1
25. 2
26. 1
27. 1
28. 1
29. 3
30. 2
31. 3
32. 1
33. 1, 2, 3, 4
34. 2, 3, 4, 5

Chapter 17
1. 3
2. 3
3. 3
4. 3
5. 1, 2, 3
6. 1
7. 3
8. 1, 3, 4
9. 1
10. 1
11. 3
12. 1
13. 4
14. 3
15. 2
16. 4
17. 3
18. Tumor lysis
    syndrome
19. 3
20. 1, 2, 3, 5
21. 4
22. 3
23. 2
24. 1
25. E
26. B
27. C
28. D
29. A
30. 1, 2, 4
31. 2, 3, 4
32. 3
33. 2
34. 3

Chapter 1 Introduction to Anatomy and Physiology

Herlihy, B., & Maebius, N.K. (2008). *The human body in health and illness*. Philadelphia: Saunders.

Jarvis, C. (2008). *Physical examination and health assessment*. (5th ed.). Philadelphia: Saunders.

Langford, R.W., & Thompson, J.M. (2008). *Mosby's handbook of diseases*. (4th ed.). St. Louis: Mosby.

Lewis, S.L., Heitkemper, M.M., Dirksen, S.R., et al. (2007). *Medical-surgical nursing: assessment and management of clinical problems*. (7th ed.). St. Louis: Mosby.

Memmler, R.L., et al. (2008). *Structure and function of the human body*. (9th ed.). Philadelphia: Lippincott.

Monahan, F.D., Sands, J.K., Neighbors, M., et al. (2007). *Phipps' medical-surgical nursing: health and illness perspectives*. (8th ed.). St. Louis: Mosby.

Mosby's dictionary of medicine, nursing, and health professions. (2009). (8th ed.). St. Louis: Mosby.

Patton, K.T., & Thibodeau, G.A. (2008). *Mosby's handbook of anatomy and physiology*. St. Louis: Mosby.

Petti, K. (2007). *Anatomy and physiology*. (6th ed.). St. Louis: Mosby.

Swisher, L. (2008). *Structure and function of the body*. (13th ed.). St. Louis: Mosby.

Thibodeau, G.A., & Patton, K.T. (2007). *Anatomy and physiology*. (6th ed.). St. Louis: Mosby.

Thibodeau, G.A., & Patton, K.T. (2008). *Structure and function of the body*. (13th ed.). St. Louis: Mosby.

Thibodeau, G.A., & Patton, K.T. (2009). *The human body in health and disease*. (5th ed.). St. Louis: Mosby.

Thompson, J.M., McFarland, G.K., Hirsch, J.E., et al. (2001). *Mosby's clinical nursing*. (5th ed.). St. Louis: Mosby.

Chapter 2 Care of the Surgical Patient

Ackley, B.J., & Ladwig, G.B. (2009). *Nursing diagnosis handbook*. (7th ed.). St. Louis: Mosby.

Beattie, S. (2007). Wound dehiscence. *RN*, 70(6):34-38.

Bulechek, G.M., Butcher, H.K. & Dochterman, J.M. (2008). *Nursing interventions classifications (NIC)*. (5th ed.). St. Louis: Mosby.

Blaney-Koen, L. (2007). Safe surgery a patient's guide. *Journal of Patient Surgery*, 3(1):56.

Centers for Disease Control and Prevention (CDC). (2002). *Guideline for hand hygiene in healthcare settings*. Available at www.cdc.gov/handhygiene. Accessed November, 2009.

Cofer, M. (2005). Unwelcome companion to older patients: postoperative delirium. *Nursing*, 35(1):32.

Crum, E., & Valinti, J. (2007). Can a bloodless surgery program work in a trauma setting? *Nursing*, 37(3):54-56.

D'Arcy, Y. (2006). How to care for a surgical patient with chronic pain. *Nursing*, 36(3):17.

Daniels, S.M. (2007). Improving hospital care for surgical patients. *Nursing*, 37(8):36-42.

Dunn, D. (2006). Age smart care. Preventing perioperative complications in older adults. *Nursing Made Incredibly Easy!* 4(3):30-41.

Elkin, M.K., Perry, A.G., & Potter, P.A. (2007). *Nursing interventions and clinical skills*. (4th ed.). St. Louis: Mosby.

Giger, J.M., & Davidhizar, R.E. (2007). *Transcultural nursing: assessment and intervention*. (5th ed.). St. Louis: Mosby.

Harkreader, H., Hogan, M.A., & Thobaben, M. (2007). *Fundamentals of nursing: care and clinical judgment*. (3rd ed.). St. Louis: Mosby.

Hunter, S., Thompson, P., Langemo, D., et al. (2007). Understanding wound dehiscence. *Nursing*, 37(9):28, 30.

The Joint Commission (2009a). *Universal protocol*. Available at www.jointcommission.org/PatientSafety/UniversalProtocol/up_facts.htm. Accessed November, 2009.

The Joint Commission. (2009b). *Universal protocol for preventing wrong site, wrong procedure and wrong person surgery*. Available at www.jointcommission.org/PatientSafety/NationalPatientSafetyGoals. Accessed November, 2009.

Lewis, S.L., Heitkemper, M.M., Dirksen, S.R., et al. (2007). *Medical-surgical nursing: assessment and management of clinical problems*. (7th ed.). St. Louis: Mosby.

McCaffery, M., Grimm, M.A., Pasero, C., et al. (2005). On the meaning of "drug seeking." *Pain Management Nursing*, 6(4):122-136.

McCaffery, M., & Pasero, C. (1999). *Pain: clinical manual*. (2nd ed.). St. Louis: Mosby.

Monahan, F.D., Sands, J.K., Neighbors, M., et al. (2007). *Phipps' medical-surgical nursing: health and illness perspectives*. (8th ed.). St. Louis: Mosby.

Moorhead, S., Johnson, M., Maas, M., et al. (2008). *Nursing outcomes classification (NOC)*. (4th ed.). St. Louis: Mosby.

Mosby's dictionary of medicine, nursing, and health professions. (2009). (8th ed.). St. Louis: Mosby.

Nichols, R.L. (2001). Preventing surgical site infections: a surgeon's perspective. *Emerging Infectious Diseases*, 7(2):220-224.

North American Nursing Diagnosis Association International (NANDA-I). (2009). *NANDA-I nursing diagnoses: definitions and classification 2009-2011*. Oxford, United Kingdom: Author.

Occupational Safety and Health Administration (OSHA). (n.d.). *Healthcare wide hazards: infection*. Available at www.cdc.gov/handhygiene. Accessed November, 2009.

Odom-Forren, J. (2006). Preventing surgical site infections. *Nursing 2006*, 36(16):59-64.

Pagana, K.D., & Pagana, T.J. (2008). *Mosby's diagnostic and laboratory test reference*. (9th ed.). St. Louis: Mosby.

Patient education series. (2007). *Nursing*, 37(8):43.

Pearce, J.M. (2006). Documenting preoperative education. *Nursing*, 36(8):71.

Potter, P.A., & Perry, A.G. (2007). *Basic nursing: essentials for practice*. (6th ed.). St. Louis: Mosby.

Potter, P.A., & Perry, A.G. (2009). *Fundamentals of nursing: concepts, process, and practice*. (7th ed.). St. Louis: Mosby.

Ridge, R.A. (2008). Doing it right to prevent wrong-site surgery. *Nursing*, 38(3):24,25.

Rothrock, J.C. (2007). *Alexander's care of the patient in surgery*. (13th ed.). St. Louis: Mosby.

Sarvis, C. (2006). Postoperative wound care. *Nursing*, 36(12):56-57.

Schwartz, A., Jr. (2006). Learning the essentials of epidural anesthesia. *Nursing*, 36(1):44-50.

Skidmore-Roth, L. (2010). *Mosby's 2010 nursing drug reference*. (23rd ed.). St. Louis: Mosby.

Tabor, W. (2007). Cutting edge of robtic surgery. *Nursing*, 37(2):48-50.

Chapter 3 Care of the Patient with an Integumentary Disorder

Anderson, L.M. (2005). Atopic dermatitis: More than a simple skin disorder. *Journal of the American Academy of Nurse Practitioners,* 17(7):249, 251.

Aschenbrenner, D.S. (2007). A new topical ointment for impetigo. *American Journal of Nursing,* 107(9):31.

Black, J.M., & Hawks, H.J. (2009). *Medical-surgical nursing: clinical management for positive outcomes.* (8th ed.). Philadelphia: Saunders.

Bresett, J. (2006). Would you suspect this skin eating infection? *RN,* 69(3):31-35.

Burn Care Central. (2007). *Nursing Made Incredibly Easy!* 5(4):17-20.

Centers for Disease Control and Prevention (CDC). (2009). Fire deaths and injuries: fact sheet. Available at www.cdc.gov/Home-andRecreationalSafety/Fire-Prevention/fires-factsheet.html. Accessed November, 2009.

DeBoer, S., Felty, C., Seaver, M. (2004). Burn care in EMS. *Emergency Medical Services,* 33(2):69, 72, 87.

Dulak, S.B. (2006). Stop: the assault on the skin in HIV. *RN,* 69(6):25-30.

GlaxoSmithKline (GSK). (2007). *SGK announces FDA approval of Altabax (retapamulin ointment), 1%.* Available at www.gsk.com/media/pressreleases/2007/2007_04_12GSK1014.htm. Accessed November, 2009.

Hess, C.T. (2003). Treating a fungal rash. *Nursing,* 33(9):9.

Hockenberry, M.J., & Wilson, D. (2007). *Wong's nursing care of infants and children.* (8th ed.). St. Louis, Mosby.

Holcomb, S.S. (2006). Nonmelanoma skin cancer. *RN,* 36(6):56-58.

Kent, H. (2000). PDT effective for inflammatory, viral skin lesions. *Dermatology Times,* 22(8):19.

Kleinpell, R. (2003). The role of the critical care nurse in the assessment and management of the patient with severe sepsis. *Critical Care Nursing Clinics of North America,* 15(1):27.

Lee, M., & Kalb, R.E. (2008). Systemic therapy for psoriasis. *Dermatology Nursing,* 20(8):105-108.

Lewis, S.L., Heitkemper, M.M., Dirksen, S.R., et al. (2007). *Medical-surgical nursing: assessment and management of clinical problems.* (7th ed.). St. Louis: Mosby.

Linton, A.D. (2007). *Introduction to medical surgical nursing.* (4th ed.). Philadelphia: Saunders.

McCance, K.L., & Huether, S.E. (2010). *Pathophysiology: the biologic basis for disease in adults and children.* (6th ed.). St. Louis: Mosby.

Melnyk, B.M., & Ebling, A.M. (2001). Effectiveness of oral antibiotics and topical retinal therapy in the treatment of acne in adolescents. *Pediatric Nursing,* 27(4):41.

Monahan, F.D., Sands, J.K., Neighbors, M., et al. (2007). *Phipps' medical-surgical nursing: health and illness perspectives.* (8th ed.). St. Louis: Mosby.

Mosby's dictionary of medicine, nursing, and health professions. (2009). (8th ed.). St. Louis: Mosby.

Mower-Wade, D., & Kang, T.M. (2004). Sepsis: when defense turns deadly. *Nursing 2004,* 34(7):30.

Novatnack, E. (2007). Shingles: what you should know. *RN,* 70(6):27-32.

Nowlin, A. (2006). The delicate business of burn care. *RN,* 69(1):51-58.

Quillen, T.F. (2004). Easing the heartbreak of psoriasis. *Nursing,* 34(11):18.

Quillen, T.F. (2007). Myths and facts ... about shingles. *Nursing,* 7:29-32.

Roy, D.E., & Stotts, N.A. (2002). Targeting cellulitis. *Nursing,* 32(12):32.

Sheridan R., & Tompkins, R. (2004). What's new in burns and metabolism. *Journal of the American College of Surgeons,* 198:243.

Stalbow, J. (2004). Preventing cellulitis in older people with persistent lower limb edema. *British Journal of Nursing,* 13(12):725.

Chapter 4 Care of the Patient with a Musculoskeletal Disorder

American Academy of Orthopaedic Surgeons (AAOS). (2006). *Total hip replacement.* Available at http://orthoinfo.aaos.org/fact/thr_report.cfm?thread_ID=504&topcategory=Joint%20Replacement. Accessed October, 2009.

American Association of Hip and Knee Surgeons (AAHKS). *Minimally invasive and small incision joint replacement surgery: What surgeons should consider.* Available at www.aahks.org/member/resources/MIS_Surgeons.pdf. Accessed October, 2009.

American Society for Surgery of the Hand (ASSH). *Wrist arthroscopy.* Available at www.assh.org/Public/HandConditions/Pages/Wristarthroscopy.aspx. Accessed October, 2009.

Bergstrom I, Froyochuss, D., & Landgren, B.M. (2005). Physical training and hormone replacement therapy reduce the decrease in bone mineral density in peri-menopausal women: a pilot study. *Osteoporosis International,* 16(7):823-828.

Bezaitis, A. (2008). Successful strategies for fall prevention. *AgingWell.* 1(1):28-31.

Bonner, S. (2007a). Fixate on pin site care. *Nursing Made Incredibly Easy!* 5(4):22-25.

Bonner, S. (2007b). TKO knee pain with total knee replacement. *Nursing Made Incredibly Easy!* 5(2):30-39.

Brookhart, M.A., Avorn, J., Katz, J.N., et al. (2007). Gaps in treatment among users of osteoporosis medications: the dynamics of noncompliance. *American Journal of Medicine,* 120(3):251-256.

Capo, J.T., Swan, K.G., Jr., & Tan, V. (2006). External fixation techniques for distal radius fractures. *Clinical Orthopaedics and Related Research,* 445(3):30-41.

Centers for Disease Control and Prevention. National Center for Injury Prevention and Control. Division of Unintentional Injury Prevention. (2007). *Falls among older adults: an overview.* Available at www.cdc.gov/HomeandRecreationalSafety/Falls/adultfalls.html. Accessed October, 2009.

Chou, R., Qaseem, A., Snow, V., et al. (2007). Diagnosis and treatment of low back pain pain: a joint clinical practice guideline from the American College of Physicians and the American Pain Society. *Annals of Internal Medicine,* 147(7):478-491.

Cleveland Clinic. (2007). *Osteomyelitis.* Available at http://my.clevelandclinic.org/disorders/osteomyelitis/hic_osteomyelitis.aspx. Accessed October, 2009.

Crowley, L.V. (2004). *An introduction to human disease: pathology and pathophysiology considerations.* Sunbury, Mass: Jones & Bartlett.

D'Arcy, Y. (2006a). Phantom limb pain: what it is, how to treat it. *LPN,* 2(6):15-17.

D'Arcy, Y. (2006b). Treating pain after a total joint replacement. *Nursing,* 36(5):26-28.

D'Arcy, Y. (2007). Latest pain relief a combination of new and old. *The Nurse Practitioner,* 32(1):11-12.

D'Arcy, Y. (2008). Getting a grip on neuropathic pain. *LPN,* 4(2):14-19.

Dell, D.D. (2007). Getting the point about fibromyalgia. *Nursing,* 36(2):61-64.

Dubuisson, W.C. (2009). Orthopedic measures. In A.G. Perry & P.A. Potter, *Clinical nursing skills and techniques.* (7th ed.). St. Louis: Mosby.

Editorial. (2007). The path to managing neuropathic pain. *Nursing Made Incredibly Easy!* 5(1):26-29.

Geerts, W.H., Pineo, G.F., Heit, J.A., et al. (2004). Prevention of venous thromboembolism: the Seventh ACCP Conference on Antithrombotic and Thrombolytic Therapy. *Chest,* 126(3 Suppl):338S-400S.

Goldenberg, D.I., Burckhardt, C., & Crofford, L. (2006). Management of fibromyalgia syndrome. *Journal of the American Medical Association,* 292(19):2388-2395.

Gowall, B. (2007). Joint surgery paving the way to a smooth recovery. *RN,* 70(1):37.

Habel, M. (2006). Fibromyalgia: looking good and feeling awful. *Nursing Spectrum,* 15(12):17-18.

Hairon, N. (2007). Improving falls prevention and standards of fracture care. *Nursing Times*, 103(47):23-24.

Helmann D., & Stone, J.H. (2007). Arthritis and musculoskeletal disorders. In L. Tierney, S.J. McPhee, & M.A. Papadakis (Eds.): *Current medical diagnosis and treatment.* (44th ed.). New York: McGraw-Hill.

Hendrich, A. (2007). Predicting patient falls. *American Journal of Nursing*, 107(11):50-58.

Holcomb, S. (2006). Osteoporosis. *Nursing*, 36(4):48-49.

Kelly, A.M. (2006). Managing osteoarthritis pain. *Nursing*, 36(11): 20-21.

Keskin, D., Borman, P., Ersöz, M., et al. (2008). The risk factors related to falling in elderly females. *Geriatric Nursing*, 29(1):58-63.

Kneale, J., & Davis, P. (2005). *Orthopaedic and trauma nursing.* (2nd ed.). Edinburgh, London: Churchhill Livingstone.

Leavitt, F., & Katz, R.S. (2006). Distraction as a key determinant of impaired memory in patients with fibromyalgia. *Journal of Rheumatology*, 33(1):127-132.

Lewis, S.L., Heitkemper, M.M., Dirksen, S.R., et al. (2007). *Medical-surgical nursing: assessment and management of clinical problems.* (7th ed.). St. Louis: Mosby.

Majithia, V., & Geraci, S. (2007). Rheumatoid arthritis: diagnosis and management. *American Journal of Medicine*, 129(2):936-939.

Mauck, K.F., & Clarke, B.L. (2006). Diagnosis, screening, prevention and treatment of osteoporosis. *Mayo Clinic Proceedings*, 81(15): 662-672.

Mayo Clinic staff (n.d.). *Phantom pain.* Available at www.mayoclinic.com/health/phantom-pain/DS00444. Accessed October, 2009.

McCarberg, B., & D'Arcy, Y. (2007). Target pain with topical peripheral analgesics. *The Nurse Practitioner*, 32(7):44-49.

National Institute of Arthritis and Musculoskeletal and Skin Disease (n.d.). *Arthritis.* Available at www.niams.nih.gov/Health_Info/Arthritis/default.asp. Accessed October, 2009.

National Institute on Aging. (2008). *Osteoporosis: the bone thief.* Available at www.nia.nih.gov/HealthInformation/Publications/osteoporosis.htm. Accessed October, 2009.

Olson, A. (2007). Osteoporosis detection. *The Nurse Practitioner*, 32(6):20-27.

Patkar, A., Masand, P.S., Krulewicz, S., et al. (2007). A randomized, controlled, trial of controlled release paroxetine in fibromyalgia. *The American Journal of Medicine*, 120(5):448-454.

Potter, P.A., & Perry, A.G. (2009). *Fundamentals of nursing: concepts, process, and practice.* (7th ed.). St. Louis: Mosby.

Ricks, E. (2007). Wrist arthroscopy. *AORN Journal*, 86(2):181-188.

Seabolt, J. (2007). Bone up on osteoporosis. *LPN*, 3(6):30-37.

Seabolt, J. (2008). An overview of osteomyelitis. *LPN*, 4(2):45-48.

Smeltzer, S.C., Bare, B.G., Hinkle, J.L., et al. (2007). *Brunner & Suddarth's textbook of medical-surgical nursing,* (11th ed.). Philadelphia: Lippincott, Williams and Wilkins.

Springhouse. (2007). *Surgical care made incredibly visual!* Philadelphia: Lippincott Williams & Wilkins.

Sweeney, J., & Ardisson, M. (2006). What's fat embolism? *Nursing*, 36(11):22.

Sze, P.-C., Cheung, W.H., Qin, L., et al. (2008). Biomechanical study of an anthropometrically designed hip protector for older Chinese women. *Geriatric Nursing*, 29(1):64-69.

Taylor, J. (2007). What's happened to pain management. *Nursing Times*, 103(48):18-19.

U.S. Food and Drug Administration (FDA). (2006). *FDA Talk Paper: FDA approved artificial disc: another alternative to treat low back pain.* Available at www.fda.gov/MedicalDevices/ProductsandMedicalProcedures/DeviceApprovalsandClearances/PMAApprovals/ucm110875.htm. Accessed November, 2009.

Webb, R. (2007). Bone up proton pump inhibitors and fracture risk. *Nursing*, 37(10):60-61.

Yeom, H., Fleury, J., & Keller, C. (2008). Risk factors for mobility limitation in community-dwelling older adults: a social ecological perspective. *Geriatric Nursing*, 29(2):133-140.

Chapter 5 Care of the Patient with a Gastrointestinal Disorder

Abdel-Rahman, W.M., Mecklin, J.P., Peltomäki, P. (2006). The genetics of HNPCC: application to diagnosis and screening. *Critical Reviews in Oncology/Hematology*, 58(3):208-220.

Ackley, B.J., & Ladwig, G.B. (2009). *Nursing diagnosis handbook.* (7th ed.). St. Louis: Mosby.

Agrawal, J., & Syngal, S. (2005). Colon cancer screening strategies. *Current Opinions in Gastroenterology*, 21(1):59.

Alspach, J. (2006). *Core curriculum for critical care nursing.* (6th ed.). Philadelphia: Saunders.

American Cancer Society (ACS). (2007). *Cancer facts and figures 2007.* Atlanta: Author.

American Cancer Society (ACS). (2008). *Cancer facts and figures 2008.* Atlanta: Author.

American Cancer Society (ACS). (2009). *Cancer facts and figures 2009.* Available at www.cancer.org/docroot/STT/STT_0.asp. Accessed November, 2009.

American Gastroenterological Association (AGA). Available at www.gastro.org. Accessed October, 2009.

Amerine, E. (2007). Preventing and managing acute diverticulitis. *Nursing*, 37(9):56.

Austin, N. (2007). Spores, babies and alcohol. A nurses battle with *C. diff. RN*, 70(3):39-43.

Baker, D.E. (2005). Rationale for using serotonergic agents to treat irritable bowel syndrome. *American Journal of Health-System Pharmacology*, 62(7):700-711.

Barkauskas, V., Baumann, L.C., & Darling-Fisher, C. (2006). *Health and physical assessment.* (4th ed.). St. Louis: Mosby.

Black, J.M., & Hawks, H.J. (2009). *Medical-surgical nursing: clinical management for positive outcomes.* (8th ed.). Philadelphia: Saunders.

Brush, K. (2007). Abdominal compartment syndrome. *Nursing*, 37(7):37.

Carlo, J.T., DeMarco, D., Smith, B.A., et al. (2005). The utility of capsule endoscopy and its role for diagnosing pathology in the gastrointestinal tract. *American Journal of Surgery*, 190(6):886.

Chan, H.L., Wu, J.C., Chan, F.K., et al. (2001). Is non-*Helicobacter pylori*, non-NSAID peptic ulcer a common cause of upper GI bleeding? *Gastrointestinal Endoscopy*, 53:438.

Deglin, J., & Vallerand, A. (2005). *Davis' drug guide for nurses.* (13th ed.). Philadelphia: Davis.

Dicken, B.J., Bigam, D.L., Cass, C., et al. (2005). Gastric adenocarcinoma review and considerations for future directions. *Annals of Surgery*, 241(1):27.

Ebersole, P.E., Touhy, T.A., Hess, P., et al. (2008). *Toward healthy aging: human needs and nursing response.* (7th ed.). St. Louis: Mosby.

Elkin, M.K., Perry, A.G., & Potter, P.A. (2007). *Nursing interventions and clinical skills.* (4th ed.). St. Louis: Mosby.

Freeman, L. (2007). Responding to small-bowel obstruction. *Nursing*, 37(5):56.

Fry, D. (2007). Exposing the source of peptic ulcer disease. *LPN*, 3(3):6.

Gabriel, S. (2006). Bariatric surgery basics, getting to the heart of a weighty matter. *Nursing Made Incredibly Easy!* 4(1):43.

Gallagher, S. (2004). Taking the weight off with bariatric surgery. *Nursing*, 34(3):59.

Greenwald, B. (2005). Comparison of three stool tests for colorectal cancer screening. *Medsurg Nursing*, 14:292.

Hahn, J. (2007). The bottom line on hemorrhoids. *Nursing Made Incredibly Easy!* 5(5):13.

Hara, A.K., Leighton, J.A., Heigh, R.I., et al.: (2006). Crohn disease of the small bowel: preliminary comparison among CT enterography, capsule endoscopy, small bowel follow-through, and ileoscopy. *Radiology*, 238(1):128-134.

Harris, H. (2006). *C. difficile,* attack to killer diarrhea. *Nursing Made Incredibly Easy!* 4(3):13.

Heitkemper, M., & Jarrett, M. (2005). Overlapping conditions in women with irritable bowel syndrome. *Urologic Nursing*, 25:25-30.

Hill, R. (2007). Conquering constipation. *LPN*, 3(4):48.

Hirano, I., Richter, J.E.; Practice Parameters Committee of the American College of Gastroenterology. (2007). ACG practice guidelines: esophageal reflux testing. *American Journal of Gastroenterology*, 102(3):668.

Jarvis, C. (2008). *Physical examination and health assessment*. (5th ed.). Philadelphia: Saunders.

Johanson, J.F. (2004). Options for patients with irritable bowel syndrome: contrasting traditional and novel serotonergic therapies. *Neurogastroenterology and Motility*, 16(6):701-711.

Kang, J.Y., Meville, D., Maxwell, J.D. (2004). Epidemiology and management of diverticular disease of the colon. *Drugs & Aging*, 21(4):211, 2004.

Karlowicz, D. (2004). An endoscopic approach to GERD. *RN*, 66(12):56.

Kent, V. (2007). Caring for a patient with a bowel obstruction. *LPN*, 3(5):31.

Lawrence, B. (2007). Esophageal pH monitoring goes wireless. *Nursing*, 37(10):26.

Legnani, P., & Kornblut, A. (2005). Video capsule endoscopy in inflammatory bowel disease 2005. *Current Opinions in Gastroenterology*, 21:438.

Lewis, S.L., Heitkemper, M.M., Dirksen, S.R., et al. (2007). *Medical-surgical nursing: assessment and management of clinical problems*. (7th ed.). St. Louis: Mosby.

Livingston, C.D., Jones, H.L., Jr., Askew, R.E., Jr., et al. (2001). Laparoscopic hiatal hernia repair in patients with poor esophageal motility or paraesophageal herniation, *The American Surgeon*, 67:987, 2001.

Matthew, C.G., & Lewis, C.M. (2004). Genetics of inflammatory bowel disease: progress and prospects *Human Molecular Genetics*, 13:R161, 2004.

Memmler, R.L., et al. (2008). *Structure and function of the human body*. (9th ed.). Philadelphia: Lippincott.

Monahan, F.D., Sands, J.K., Neighbors, M., et al. (2007). *Phipps' medical-surgical nursing: health and illness perspectives*. (8th ed.). St. Louis: Mosby.

Mosby's dictionary of medicine, nursing, and health professions. (2009). (8th ed.). St. Louis: Mosby.

Pagana, K.D., & Pagana, T.J. (2008). *Mosby's diagnostic and laboratory test reference*. (9th ed.). St. Louis: Mosby.

Perry, A.G., & Potter, P.A. (2009). *Clinical nursing skills and techniques*. (7th ed.). St. Louis: Mosby.

Potter, P.A., & Perry, A.G. (2007). *Basic nursing: essentials for practice*. (6th ed.). St. Louis: Mosby.

Sansbury, L.B., Millikan, R.C., Scroeder, J.C., et al. (2005). Use of nonsteroidal anti-inflammatory drugs and risk of colon cancer in a population-based, case-control study of African-Americans and whites. *American Journal of Epidemiology*, 162(6):548-558.

Seidel, H.M., Ball, J.W., Dains, J.E., et al. (2007). *Mosby's guide to physical examination*. (6th ed.). St. Louis: Mosby.

Smeltzer, S.C., Bare, B.G., Hinkle, J.L., et al. (2007). *Brunner & Suddarth's textbook of medical-surgical nursing*, (11th ed.). Philadelphia: Lippincott, Williams and Wilkins.

Thibodeau, G.A., & Patton, K.T. (2007). *Anatomy and physiology*. (6th ed.). St. Louis: Mosby.

Thibodeau, G.A., & Patton, K.T. (2008). *Structure and function of the body*. (13th ed.). St. Louis: Mosby.

Thibodeau, G.A., & Patton, K.T. (2009). *The human body in health and disease*. (5th ed.). St. Louis: Mosby.

Thompson, J.M., McFarland, G.K., Hirsch, J.E., et al. (2001). *Mosby's clinical nursing*. (5th ed.). St. Louis: Mosby.

Tucker, S.M., Cannobio, M.M., Paquette, E.V., et al. (2007). *Patient care standards: collaborative planning and nursing interventions*. (7th ed.). St. Louis: Mosby.

Vglente, S. (2007). Keep *C. difficile* infection at bay. *Nursing*, 37(10):56.

Walker, B. (2004). Assessing gastrointestinal infections. *Nursing*, 34(5):48.

Young-Fadok, T., et al. *Treatment of acute diverticulitis and clinical manifestations of colonic diverticular disease*. Available at www.uptodate.com. Accessed July 8, 2007.

Additional Resources

Crohn's and Colitis Foundation of America, 386 Park Ave. South, 17th Floor, New York, NY 10016-8804. 800-932-2423 or 212-685-3440. Information hotline: 800-343-3637. Available at www.ccfa.org. Accessed November, 2009.

United Ostomy Association, 19772 MacArthur Blvd., Suite 200, Irvine, CA 92612-2405. 800-826-0826. Available at www.uoaa.org. Accessed November, 2009.

Chapter 6 Care of the Patient with a Gallbladder, Liver, Biliary Tract, or Exocrine Pancreatic Disorder

Ackley, B.J., & Ladwig, G.B. (2009). *Nursing diagnosis handbook*. (7th ed.). St. Louis: Mosby.

American Cancer Society (ACS). (2007). *Cancer facts and figures 2007*. Atlanta: Author.

American Cancer Society (ACS). (2007). Detailed guide: pancreatic cancer. Available at www.cancer.org/docroot/CRI/CRI_2_3x.asp?dt=34. Accessed October, 2009.

Black, J.M., & Hawks, H.J. (2009). *Medical-surgical nursing: clinical management for positive outcomes*. (8th ed.). Philadelphia: Saunders.

Boyer, M.J. (2008). *Study guide to Brunner and Suddarth's textbook of medical-surgical nursing*. (11th ed.). Philadelphia: Lippincott.

Centers for Disease Control and Prevention (CDC). (2009). *Recommended immunization schedule for persons aged 1 through 6 years*. Available at www.cdc.gov/vaccines/recs/schedules/downloads/child/2009/09_0-6yrs_schedule_pr.pdf. Accessed November, 2009.

Centers for Disease Control and Prevention (CDC), & National Center for Infectious Diseases. (2008). *Viral hepatitis*. Available at www.cdc.gov/hepatitis/index.htm. Accessed October, 2009.

Durston, S. (2004). The ABCs and more of hepatitis. *Nursing Made Incredibly Easy!* 2(4):22-32.

Editorial. (2007). Function junction: testing your patient in liver function. *Nursing Made Incredibly Easy!* 5(1):17-19.

Giger, J.M., & Davidhizar, R.E. (2007). *Transcultural nursing: assessment and intervention*. (5th ed.). St. Louis: Mosby.

Holcomb, S. (2007). Stopping the destruction of acute pancreatitis. *Nursing*, 37(6):43.

Hussar, D. (2007). New drugs07, part 2. *Nursing*, 37(8):46.

Jacobson, I. (2006). Therapeutic options for chronic hepatitis B: considerations and controversies. *American Journal of Gastroenterology*, 101:51.

Jones, S. (2003). When the liver fails: new help and hope. *RN*, 66(11):33.

Lewis, S.L., Heitkemper, M.M., Dirksen, S.R., et al. (2007). *Medical-surgical nursing: assessment and management of clinical problems*. (7th ed.). St. Louis: Mosby.

Madsen, D., Sebolt, T., Cullen, L., et al. (2005). Listening to bowel sounds: an evidence-based practice project. *American Journal of Nursing*, 105(12):40.

McCarron, K. (2007). Jaundice: more than meets the eye. *Nursing Made Incredibly Easy!* 5(3):25.

McCaughan, G.W., Koorey, D.J., & Strasser, S.I. (2005). Liver transplantation for viral hepatitis, *Hospital Medicine*, 66(1):8-12.

Monahan, F.D., Sands, J.K., Neighbors, M., et al. (2007). *Phipps' medical-surgical nursing: health and illness perspectives*. (8th ed.). St. Louis: Mosby.

Mosby's dictionary of medicine, nursing, and health professions. (2009). (8th ed.). St. Louis: Mosby.

Pagana, K.D., & Pagana, T.J. (2008). *Mosby's diagnostic and laboratory test reference*. (9th ed.). St. Louis: Mosby.

Pellegrino, A. (2006). Looking at liver cancer. *Nursing*, 36(10), 52.

Perry, A.G., & Potter, P.A. (2009). *Clinical nursing skills and techniques*. (7th ed.). St. Louis: Mosby.

Phillips, R.A. (2006). Acute pancreatitis: inflammation gone wild. *Nursing Made Incredibly Easy!* 4(5):18-28.

Potter, P.A., & Perry, A.G. (2007). *Basic nursing: essentials for practice*. (6th ed.). St. Louis: Mosby.

Potter, P.A., & Perry, A.G. (2009). *Fundamentals of nursing: concepts, process, and practice*. (7th ed.). St. Louis: Mosby.

Riehl, M. (2007). Help your patient cope with pancreatic cancer. *Nursing*, 37(4):54.

Seidel, H.M., Ball, J.W., Dains, J.E., et al. (2007). *Mosby's guide to physical examination*. (6th ed.). St. Louis: Mosby.

Shaheen, N., Hansen, R.A., Morgan, D.R., et al. (2006). The burden of gastrointestinal and liver diseases. *American Journal of Gastroenterology*, 101(9):2128-2138.

Thibodeau, G.A. & Patton, K.T. (2007). *Anatomy and physiology*. (6th ed.). St. Louis: Mosby.

Thibodeau, G.A. & Patton, K.T. (2008). *Structure and function of the body*. (13th ed.). St. Louis: Mosby.

Thibodeau, G.A., & Patton, K.T. (2009). *The human body in health and disease*. (5th ed.). St. Louis: Mosby.

Thompson, J.M., McFarland, G.K., Hirsch, J.E., et al. (2001). *Mosby's clinical nursing*. (5th ed.). St. Louis: Mosby.

Tucker, S.M., Cannobio, M.M., Paquette, E.V., et al. (2007). *Patient care standards: collaborative planning and nursing interventions*. (7th ed.). St. Louis: Mosby.

Venes, D. (2009.) *Taber's cyclopedic medical dictionary*. (21st ed.). Philadelphia: Davis.

Verna, E.C., & Brown, R.S., Jr., (n.d.). *Liver transplantation for hepatitis C virus infection*. Available at www.uptodate.com/patients/content/topic.do?topicKey=~aJJa1SKQK2jouT&selectedTitle=3~150&source=search_result. Accessed November, 2009.

Chapter 7 Care of the Patient with a Blood or Lymphatic Disorder

Ackley, B.J., & Ladwig, G.B. (2009). *Nursing diagnosis handbook*. (7th ed.). St. Louis: Mosby.

Aster, J. (2005). Diseases of white blood cells, lymph nodes, spleen and thymus. In V. Kumar, A. Abbas, N. Fausto, et al., (Eds.): *Robbins and Cotran pathologic basis of disease*, Philadelphia: Elsevier.

Baehner, R. (n.d.) *Overview of neutropenia*. Available at www.uptodate.com. Version 13.2. Accessed June 20, 2006.

Barkauskas, V., Baumann, L.C., & Darling-Fisher, C. (2006). *Health and physical assessment*. (4th ed.). St. Louis: Mosby.

Beattie, S. (2007a). Bedside emergency-hemorrhage. *RN*, 70(8):32-36.

Beattie, S. (2007b). Hands-on-help, bone marrow aspiration and biopsy. *RN*, 70(2):41.

Black, J.M., & Hawks, H.J. (2009). *Medical-surgical nursing: clinical management for positive outcomes*. (8th ed.). Philadelphia: Saunders.

Borton, D. (1996). WBC count and differential. *Nursing*, 26:11.

Burruss, N., & Holz, S. (2005). Managing the risks of thrombocytopenia. *Nursing*, 35:32hn5.

Canellos, G. (2004). Lymphoma: present and future challenges. *Seminars in Hematology*, 41(suppl 17):26.

Damsky, D. (2006). Caring for a patient with lymphedema. *Nursing 2006*, 36(6):49.

Deglin, J., & Vallerand, A. (2009). *Davis's drug guide for nurses*. (17th ed.). Philadelphia: Davis.

Deitch, E. (2006). Intensive care management of the trauma patient. *Critical Care Medicine*, 34(9):2294.

Geiter, H. (2003). Disseminated intravascular coagulopathy. *Dimensions of Critical Care Nursing*, 22(3):108.

Giger, J.M., & Davidhizar, R.E. (2008). *Transcultural nursing: assessment and intervention*. (5th ed.). St. Louis: Mosby.

Hebbel, R. (2005). Pathobiology of sickle cell disease. In R. Hoffman, B. Furie, E. Benz, et al. (Eds.), *Hematology: basic principles and practice*. (4th ed.). Philadelphia: Saunders.

Holcomb, S.S. (2006). Putting the squeeze on lymphedema. *Nursing Made Incredibly Easy!* 4(2):26-34.

Kim, M.J., McFarland, G.K., & McLane, A.M. (1989). *Pocket guide to nursing diagnoses*. (3rd ed.). St. Louis: Mosby.

Lewis, S.L., Heitkemper, M.M., Dirksen, S.R., et al. (2007). *Medical-surgical nursing: assessment and management of clinical problems*. (7th ed.). St. Louis: Mosby.

Lipschitz, D. (2003). Medical and functional consequences of anemia in the elderly. *Journal of the American Geriatrics Society*, 51(suppl 3):510.

March, J.C. (2005). Management of acquired aplastic anemia. *Blood Reviews*, 19:143.

Mauch, P. (2006). *Staging and selection of treatment modality in patients with Hodgkin's disease*. Available at www.uptodate.com. Accessed June 20, 2006.

McCarron, K. (2004). Deciphering diagnostics. Clues in the blood: know your CBCs. *Nursing Made Incredibly Easy!* 5(3):13-17.

MedlinePlus. (2009). *Sickle cell anemia*. Available at www.nlm.nih.gov/medlineplus/sicklecellanemia.html. Accessed October, 2009.

Monahan, F.D., Sands, J.K., Neighbors, M., et al. (2007). *Phipps' medical-surgical nursing: health and illness perspectives*. (8th ed.). St. Louis: Mosby.

Montoya, V.L, Wink, D., Sole, M.L. (2004). Anemia, what lies beneath. *Nursing Made Incredibly Easy!* 2(1):37-45.

Mosby's dictionary of medicine, nursing, and health professions. (2009). (8th ed.). St. Louis: Mosby.

Munson, B. (2005). Myths and facts . . . about polycythemia vera. *Nursing*, 35(5):28.

North American Nursing Diagnosis Association International (NANDA-I). (2009). *NANDA-I nursing diagnoses: definitions and classification 2009-2011*. Oxford, United Kingdom: Author.

Pagana, K.D., & Pagana, T.J. (2008a). *Diagnostic testing and nursing implications: a case study approach*. (6th ed.). St. Louis: Mosby.

Pagana, K.D., & Pagana, T.J. (2008b). *Mosby's diagnostic and laboratory test reference*. (9th ed.). St. Louis: Mosby.

Perry, A.G., & Potter, P.A. (2009). *Clinical nursing skills and techniques*. (7th ed.). St. Louis: Mosby.

Platt, A. (2007). How much do you know about sickle-cell disease? *LPN*, 3(4):32.

Portielje, J.E., Westendorp, R.G., Kluin-Nelemans, H.C., et al. (2001). Morbidity and mortality in adults with immune thrombocytopenic purpura. *Blood*, 97:2549.

Potter, P.A., & Perry, A.G. (2007). *Basic nursing: essentials for practice*. (6th ed.). St. Louis: Mosby.

Redaelli, A. (2005). A systematic literature review of the clinical and epidemiological burden of acute lymphoblastic leukemia (ALL). *European Journal of Cancer Care*, 14:53.

Robinson, P. (2005). Is surgery safe for a patient with hemophilia? *Nursing*, 35:32.

Seidel, H.M., Ball, J.W., Dains, J.E., et al. (2007). *Mosby's guide to physical examination*. (6th ed.). St. Louis: Mosby.

Seiter, K. (2002). Treatment of acute myelogenous leukemia in the elderly patients. *Clinical Geriatrics*, 10:41.

Skidmore-Roth, L. (2010). *Mosby's 2010 nursing drug reference*. (23rd ed.). St. Louis: Mosby.

Stone, R., O'Donnell, M.R., & Sekeres, M.A. (2004). Acute myeloid leukemia. *American Society of Hematology*, 1:98.

Thibodeau, G.A., & Patton, K.T. (2007). *Anatomy and physiology*. (6th ed.). St. Louis: Mosby.

Thibodeau, G.A., & Patton, K.T. (2008). *Structure and function of the body*. (13th ed.). St. Louis: Mosby.

Thompson, J.M., McFarland, G.K., Hirsch, J.E., et al. (2001). *Mosby's clinical nursing*. (5th ed.). St. Louis: Mosby.

Weiss, G., & Goodnough, L.T. (2005). Anemia of chronic disease. *New England Journal of Medicine*, 352(10):1011-1023.

Chapter 8 Care of the Patient with a Cardiovascular or a Peripheral Vascular Disorder

Agruss, J.C., & Garrett, K. (2006). The stealth factor in cardiovascular disease risk. *Nursing Made Incredibly Easy!* 4(2):51-55.

American College of Obstetrics and Gynecologists (ACOG) Women's Health Care Physicians. (2004). Coronary artery disease. *Obstetrics and Gynecology*, 104(4 Suppl):415.

American Heart Association. (2005). *2005 heart and stroke facts statistics*. Dallas: Author.

Antman, E.M., Anbe, D.T., Armstrong, P.W., et al. (2004). ACC/AHA guidelines for the management of patients with ST-elevation myocardial infarction: a report of the American College of Cardiology/American Heart Association Task Force on Practice Guidelines (Committee to Revise the 1999 Guidelines for the Management of Patients with Acute Myocardial Infarction). *Circulation*, 110(9):e82-292.

Bartley, M. (2006). Keeping thromboembolism at bay. *Nursing*, 36(10), 36.

Belch, J.J., Topol, E.J., Agnelli, G., et al. (2003). Critical issues in peripheral arterial disease detection and management: a call to action. *Archives of International Medicine*, 163(8):884-892.

Bentz, B. (2006). Gaining control over A-fib. *RN*, (12):35.

Black, J.M., & Hawks, H.J. (2009). *Medical-surgical nursing: clinical management for positive outcomes*. (8th ed.). Philadelphia: Saunders.

Bozkurt, A.K., Koksal, C., & Ercan, M. (2004). The altered hemorheologic parameter in thromboangitis obliterans: a new insight, *Clinical and Applied Thrombosis/Hemostasis*, 10:45.

Calianno, C., & Holton, S.J. (2007). Fighting the triple threat of lower extremity ulcers. *Nursing*, 37(3):57-63.

Cheek, D. (2006). New respect for the humble endothelium. *Nursing*, 36(3):44.

Cheek, D. (2008). Women's heart disease: what's new? *Nursing*, 38(1):36.

Chojnowski, D. (2004). Putting together the pieces of cardiomyopathy. *Nursing Made Incredibly Easy!* 2(3):18-28.

Chojnowski, D. (2006). Managing systolic heart failure. *Nursing*, 36(7):36.

Chojnowski, D. (2007). Protecting patients from harm: taking aim at heart failure. *Nursing*, 37(11):50-55.

Cooper, L.T. (2004). Long-term survival and amputation risk in thromboangitis obliterans (Buerger's disease). *Journal of the American College of Cardiologists*, 44:2410.

Cotter, J., Bixby, M., & Morse, B. (2006). Helping patients who need a permanent pacemaker. *Nursing*, 36(8):50-54.

Craig, K. (2006). Heart attack. *Nursing*, 36(5):43.

Croce, H. (2007). Aortic problems. *RN*, 70(3):26.

Cuddy, P. (2006). Lipid lowerers. *RN*, 69(8):27.

Fink, A. (2006). Endocarditis after valve replacement surgery. *American Journal of Nursing*, 106(2):40.

Gahan, L. (2005). Using compression therapy for venous insufficiency. *Nursing*, 35(12):24.

Giger, J.M., & Davidhizar, R.E. (2008). *Transcultural nursing: assessment and intervention*. (5th ed.). St. Louis: Mosby.

Hayes, D. (2007). New guidelines for preventing infective endocarditis. *Nursing*, 37(8):22.

Hirsch, A.T., & Duprez, D. (2003). The potential role of angiotension-converting enzyme inhibition in peripheral arterial disease. *Vascular Medicine*, 8:273-278.

Hobbs, R.E. (2003). Using BNP to diagnose, manage, and treat heart failure. *Cleveland Clinics Journal of Medicine*, 70(4):333.

Holcomb, S. (2006). Carditis hearts afire. *Nursing Made Incredibly Easy!* 4(4):14-24.

Hussar, D. (2008). New drugs. *Nursing*, 38(2):49.

Irwin, G. (2007). How to protect a patient with aortic aneurysm. *Nursing*, 37(2):36.

Iyer, P.W., & Camp, N.H. (2007). *Nursing documentation: a nursing process approach*. (5th ed.). St. Louis: Mosby.

Kasper, D.L., Braunwald, E., Hauser, S., et al. (2004). *Harrison's principles of internal medicine*. (16th ed.). New York: McGraw-Hill.

Lackey, S. (2006). Suppressing the scourge of AMI. *Nursing*, 36(5):36.

Langford, R., & Thompson, J. (2008). *Mosby's handbook of diseases*. (4rd ed.). St. Louis: Mosby.

Lewis, S.L., Heitkemper, M.M., Dirksen, S.R., et al. (2007). *Medical-surgical nursing: assessment and management of clinical problems*. (7th ed.). St. Louis: Mosby.

McCarron, K. (2006). Puzzled about atherosclerosis? *Nursing Made Incredibly Easy!* 4(6):11-14.

McFarland, G., & McFarland, E. (2005). *Nursing diagnosis and intervention: planning for patient care*. (5th ed.). St. Louis: Mosby.

Miller, J. (2007). Keeping your patient hemodynamically stable. *Nursing*, 37(5):36.

Moriarty, M. (2004). Heart disease. *RN*, 67(1):33.

Mosby's dictionary of medicine, nursing, and health professions. (2009). (8th ed.). St. Louis: Mosby.

Moz, T. (2007). Cardiovascular disease: the heart of the matter. *LPN*, 3(2):35.

National Heart, Lung and Blood Institute. Available at www.nhlbi.nih.gov. Accessed November, 2009.

Nienaber, C., & Eagle, K. (2003). Aortic dissection: new frontiers in diagnosis and management. Part II: therapeutic management and follow-up. *Circulation*, 108(5):772.

Pagana, K.D., & Pagana, T.J. (2008). *Mosby's diagnostic and laboratory test reference*. (9th ed.). St. Louis: Mosby.

Palatnik, A. (2005). And the beat goes on. *Nursing Made Incredibly Easy!* 3(1):30-41.

Ponce, C., et al. (2005). Anticoagulation self-monitoring. *American Journal of Nursing*, 105(10):62.

Pope, B. (2004). What's at the heart of your patient's chest pain? *Nursing Made Incredibly Easy!* 8:18.

Riggs, J. (2004). New therapies for heart failure. *RN*, 67(3):29.

Riggs, J. (2006). Too pooped to pump: managing chronic heart failure. *Nursing Made Incredibly Easy!* 4(1):28-39, 41, 42.

Roca, J. (2007). Responding to atrial fibrillation. *Nursing*, 37(4):37.

Roman, L., & Metules, T.J. (2007). Door-to-balloon time: the race is on. *RN*, 70(2):35-38.

Shatzer, M., & Saul, L. (2004). What does BNP tell you? *Nursing Made Incredibly Easy!* 2(3):7.

Sherrod, M.M., Albarez, Y., Brookshire, A., et al. (2007). A woman's worst enemy. *American Nurse Today*, 2(2):26.

Sunderlin, M. (2006). Keeping pace with cardiac devices. *RN*, 69(7):40.

Thibodeau, G.A. & Patton, K.T. (2008). *Structure and function of the human body*. (13th ed.). St. Louis: Mosby.

Thibodeau, G.A., & Patton, K.T. (2009). *The human body in health and disease*. (5th ed.). St. Louis: Mosby.

Thomas, C.L. (2009). *Taber's cyclopedic medical dictionary*. (21st ed.). Philadelphia: Davis.

Thompson, J.M., McFarland, G.K., Hirsch, J.E., et al. (2001). *Mosby's clinical nursing*. (5th ed.). St. Louis: Mosby.

Tran, H., & Anand, S.S. (2004). Oral antiplatelet therapy in cerebrovascular disease, coronary artery disease, and peripheral artery disease. *Journal of the American Medical Association*, 292:1867-1874.

Treat-Jackson, D., & Walsh, M.E. (2003). Treating patients with peripheral arterial disease and claudication. *Journal of Vascular Nursing*, 21:5-14, 2003.

Trujillo-Santos, J., Perea-Milla, E., Jimenez-Puente, A., et al. (2005). Bedrest or ambulation in the initial treatment of patients with acute deep vein thrombosis or pulmonary embolism: findings from RIETE registry. *Chest*, 127:1631-1636.

Tucker, S.M., Cannobio, M.M., Paquette, E.V., et al. (2007). *Patient care standards: collaborative planning and nursing interventions*. (7th ed.). St. Louis: Mosby.

Turka, J. (2006). Is this on the level? *Nursing Made Incredibly Easy!* 4(4):7, 9.

Turner, L. (2006). Keeping warfarin therapy in balance. *Nursing*, 36(11):43.

U.S. Department of Health and Human Services, National Institutes of Health, & National Heart, Lung, and Blood Institute. (2003). *The seventh report of the Joint National Committee on Prevention, Detection, Evaluation, and Treatment of High Blood Pressure*, Bethesda, Md.: Author.

Willigendael, E.M., Teijink, J.A., Bartelink, M.L., et al. (2004). Influence of smoking on increase and prevalence of peripheral arterial disease. *Journal of Vascular Surgey*, 40:1158.

Willis, K. (2001). Gaining perspective on peripheral vascular disease. *Nursing*, 31:2.

Wipke-Tevis, D.D., & Sae-Sia, W. (2004). Caring for vascular leg ulcers: a best approach practice update. *Home Healthcare Nurse*, 22(4):237.

Wright, J. (2006). Cardiovascular meds. *RN*, 69(5):33.

Xu, Y., & Whitmer, K. (2006). C-reactive protein and cardiovascular disease in people with diabetes. *American Journal of Nursing*, 106(8):66.

Chapter 9 Care of the Patient with a Respiratory Disorder

American Cancer Society (ACS). (2009). *Cancer facts and figures.* Available at www.cancer.org/downloads/STT/500809web.pdf. Accessed November, 2009.

American Lung Association. (2007). *Chronic obstructive pulmonary disease.* Available at www.lungusa.org/lung-disease/copd. Accessed November, 2009.

Astle, S. (2007). Taking your patient off of a ventilator. *RN,* 70(5):34.

Balas, M. (2009). Prone positioning of patients with acute respiratory distress syndrome: applying research to practice. *Critical Care Nurse,* 20(1), 24-36.

Barkauskas, V., Baumann, L.C., & Darling-Fisher, C. (2006). *Health and physical assessment.* (4th ed.). St. Louis: Mosby.

Bauldoff, G.S., & Diaz, P.T. (2006). Improving outcomes for COPD patients. *Nurse Practitioner,* 31(8):26-28.

Beattie, S. (2007). Bedside emergency. *RN,* 70(7):34.

Black, J.M., & Hawks, H.J. (2009). *Medical-surgical nursing: clinical management for positive outcomes.* (8th ed.). Philadelphia: Saunders.

Carr, E. (2005). Nursing care of the patient with head and neck cancer. In J. Itano, & K. Taoka, (Eds.):, *Core curriculum for oncology nursing.* (4th ed.). St. Louis: Elsevier.

Centers for Disease Control and Prevention (CDC). (2006). *Reported TB in U.S.* U.S. Department of Health and Human Services, Atlanta: Author.

Coughlin, A. (2007a). Coping with COPD. *Nursing Made Incredibly Easy!* 5(6):40.

Coughlin, A. (2007b). Helping patients cope with COPD. *LPN,* 3(3):46.

Coughlin, A., & Parchinsky, C. (2006). Go with the flow of chest tube therapy. *Nursing,* 36(3):36.

Crawford, A., & Harris, H. (2008). *COPD: help your patients breathe easier.* Available at http://rn.modernmedicine.com/rnweb/article/articleDetail.jsp?id=482654. Accessed November, 2009.

Deglin, J., & Vallerand, A. (2009). *Davis's drug guide for nurses.* (17th ed.). Philadelphia: Davis.

Dest, V. (2000). Oncology today: lung cancer. *RN,* 63(5):32.

Dest, V. (2006). Lung cancer, the battle continues. *RN,* 69(11):30.

Dugan, M. (2007). A tale of sleep apnea. *Nursing Made Incredibly Easy!* 5(3):28-37.

Edmondson, D. (2008). Smoke out lung cancer. *LPN,* 4(1):39, 2008.

ExcellentHealth.com. (n.d.). *Anthrax drugs.* Available at www.excellenthealth.com/news011102a.htm. Accessed November, 2009.

Giger, J.M., & Davidhizar, R.E. (2008). *Transcultural nursing: assessment and intervention.* (5th ed.). St. Louis: Mosby.

Global initiative for chronic obstructive lung disease. (n.d.). Available at http://goldcopd.com. Accessed November, 2009.

Goldrick, B. (2004). 21st-century emerging and reemerging infections. *American Journal of Nursing,* 104(1):67.

Goldrick, B. (2005). Emerging infections—update TB in the United States. *American Journal of Nursing,* 105(7):85.

Holcomb, S.S. (2006). The stuffy head blues. *Nursing Made Incredibly Easy!* 4(2):64.

Ignatavicius, D.D., & Workman, M.L. (2006). *Medical-surgical nursing: patient-centered collaborative care.* (6th ed.). Philadelphia: Saunders.

Jacobs, M. (2005). Ease the stress of managing ARDS. *Made Incredibly Easy!* 3(1):6.

Jacobs, M., & Meyer, T. (2006). The push is on in pulmonary hypertension. *Made Incredibly Easy!* 4(3):42-52.

Jeffries, M. (2007). Helping your patient combat lung cancer. *Nursing,* 37(12):36.

Kamangar, N., Nikhanj, N.S., & Sharma, S. (2006). *Chronic obstructive pulmonary disease.* Available at www.emedicine.com/med/topic373/htm. Accessed November, 2009.

Kamienski, M. (2007). When sore throat gets serious. *American Journal of Nursing,* 107(10):35.

Kattan, M., et al. (2005). Asthma outcomes: you get what you pay for. *Journal of Allergy and Clinical Immunology,* 116(5):1058-1063.

Katz, J., & Hirsch, A. (2003). When global health is local health (SARS). *American Journal of Nursing,* 103(12):75.

Koschel, M. (2004). Pulmonary embolism. *American Journal of Nursing,* 104(6):46.

Kucik, C.J., et al. (2005). Management of epistaxis. *American Family Physician,* 71:305.

Langford, R., & Thompson, J. (2008). *Mosby's handbook of diseases.* (4th ed.). St. Louis: Mosby.

Lewis, S.L., Heitkemper, M.M., Dirksen, S.R., et al. (2007). *Medical-surgical nursing: assessment and management of clinical problems.* (7th ed.). St. Louis: Mosby.

Manno, M. (2005). Managing mechanical ventilation. *Nursing,* 35(12):36, 2005.

McCarron, K. (2006). Puzzled about the state of airlessness? (Atelectasis). *Nursing Made Incredibly Easy!* 4(10):60.

McFarland, G., & McFarland, E. (2007). *Nursing diagnosis and intervention: planning for patient care.* (5th ed.). St. Louis: Mosby.

Miracle, V., & Winston, M. (2000). Take the wind out of asthma. *Nursing,* 30(8):34.

Monahan, F.D., Sands, J.K., Neighbors, M., et al. (2007). *Phipps' medical-surgical nursing: health and illness perspectives.* (8th ed.). St. Louis: Mosby.

Mosby's dictionary of medicine, nursing, and health professions. (2009). (8th ed.). St. Louis: Mosby.

Otto, S. (2005). *Oncology nursing.* (5th ed.). St. Louis: Mosby.

Pagana, K.D., & Pagana, T.J. (2008). *Mosby's diagnostic and laboratory test reference.* (9th ed.). St. Louis: Mosby.

Parini, S. (2003). Severe acute respiratory syndrome. *Nursing,* 33(9):96.

Potter, P.A., & Perry, A.G. (2007). *Basic nursing: essentials for practice.* (6th ed.). St. Louis: Mosby.

Potter, P.A., & Perry, A.G. (2009). *Fundamentals of nursing: concepts, process, and practice.* (7th ed.). St. Louis: Mosby.

Price, S., & Wilson, L. (2007). *Pathophysiology: clinical concepts of disease processes.* (7th ed.). St. Louis: Mosby.

Pruitt, B. (2006). Weaning patients from mechanical ventilation. *Nursing,* 36(9):36.

Pruitt, B. (2007a). Clearing the air with chest tubes. *LPN,* 3(5):50.

Pruitt, B. (2007b). Fending off influenza. *Nursing,* 37(10):44.

Pruitt, B., et al. (2006). Ventilation associated pneumonia. *Nursing,* 36(2):36.

Ruppel, G. (2007). *Manual of pulmonary function testing.* (9th ed.). St. Louis: Mosby.

Rushing, J. (2007). Clinical do's and don'ts—managing a water-seal chest drainage unit. *Nursing,* 37(12):12.

Scheff, B. (2006). Avian influenza. *Nursing,* 37(5):51.

Schiech, L. (2007). Looking at laryngeal cancer. *Nursing,* 37(5):50.

Schleder, B. (2004). Keeping hospital bugs at bay: how you can protect your patients from noscomial pneumonia. *Nursing Made Incredibly Easy!* 2(2):36-42.

Seidel, H.M., Ball, J.W., Dains, J.E., et al. (2007). *Mosby's guide to physical examination.* (6th ed.). St. Louis: Mosby.

Skidmore-Roth, L. (2010). *Mosby's 2010 nursing drug reference.* (23rd ed.). St. Louis: Mosby.

Swearingen, P.L. (2007). *Manual of medical-surgical nursing.* (6th ed.). St. Louis: Mosby.

Tate, T.J., & Tasota, F. (2002). More than a snore: recognizing the danger of sleep apnea. *Nursing,* 32(8):46.

Thibodeau, G.A., & Patton, K.T. (2008). *Structure and function of the body.* (13th ed.). St. Louis: Mosby.

Thibodeau, G.A., & Patton, K.T. (2009). *The human body in health and disease.* (5th ed.). St. Louis: Mosby.

Thompson, B.T., et al. (2006). *Clinical manifestations of and diagnostic strategies for acute pulmonary embolism.* Available at www.uptodate.com.

Thompson, J.M., McFarland, G.K., Hirsch, J.E., et al. (2001). *Mosby's clinical nursing.* (5th ed.). St. Louis: Mosby.

Todd, B. (2006). The Quantiferon-TB Gold Test. *American Journal of Nursing,* 106(6):33.

Valentine, K.A., et al. (2006). *Treatment of acute pulmonary embolism.* Available at www.uptodate.com.

Wisniewski, A. (2004). When air is rare—helping patients with chronic bronchitis or emphysema breathe easier. *Nursing Made Incredibly Easy!* 2(1):20-27, 35.

Woodruff, D. (2006). Take these 6 easy steps to ABG analysis. *Nursing Made Incredibly Easy!* 4(1):4-7.

Chapter 10 Care of the Patient with a Urinary Disorder

Abrams, A.C. (2006). *Clinical drug therapy.* (8th ed.). Philadelphia: Lippincott.

Ackley, B.J., & Ladwig, G.B. (2009). *Nursing diagnosis handbook.* (7th ed.). St. Louis: Mosby.

Adam, L., Kassouf, W., & Dinney, C. (2005). Clinical applications for targeted therapy in bladder cancer. *Urologic Clinics of North America*, 32(2):239-246.

American Institute of Cancer Research (AICR). (2007). *Concerns over the increasing incidence of kidney cancer.* Available at www.elements-4health.com/concerns-over-the-increasing-incidence-of-kidney-cancer.html. Accessed November, 2009.

Aparicio, A., et al. (2005). The current and future application of adjuvant systemic chemotherapy in patients with bladder cancer following cystectomy. *Urologic Clinics of North America*, 32(2):217-230.

Barton-Burke, M., & Gustason, C. (2007). Sexuality in women with cancer. *Nursing Clinics of North America*, 42(4):531-554.

Berry, A. (2006). Helping children with nocturnal enuresis. *American Journal of Nursing*, 106(8):56-64.

Beuscart-Azephir, A., Pelayo, S., Anceaux, F., et al. (2005). Impact of CPOE on doctor-nurse cooperation for the medication ordering and administration process. *International Journal of Medical Informatics*, 74(7-8):629-641.

Black, J.M., & Hawks, H.J. (2009). *Medical-surgical nursing: clinical management for positive outcomes.* (8th ed.). Philadelphia: Saunders.

Breiterman-White, R. (2005). Functional ability of patients on dialysis: the crital role of anemia. *Nephrology Nursing Journal*, 32(1):79-82.

Bruner, D., & Calvano, T. (2007). The sexual impact of cancer and cancer treatments in men. *Nursing Clinics of North America*, 42(4):555-580.

Burrows-Hudson, S. (2005). Chronic kidney disease: an overview. *American Journal of Nursing*, 105(2):40-50.

Campbell, B. (2006). Bladder cancer. *Nursing*, 36(4):54-64.

Campoy, S., & Elwell, R. (2005). Pharmacology & CKD. *American Journal of Nursing*, 105(9):60-72.

Chang, S., & Cookson, M. (2005). Radical systectomy for bladder cancer: the case for early intervention. *Urologic Clinics of North America*, 32(2):147-155.

Coca, S., Krumholz, H., Garg, A., et al. (2006). Underrepresentation of renal disease in randomized controlled trials of cardiovascular disease. *Journal of the American Medical Association*, 296(11):1377-1384.

Collins, K. (2009). *Concerns over kidney cancer grow.* Available at www.aicr.org/site/News2?page=NewsArticle&id=14447&news_iv_ctrl=0&abbr=pr_hf_. Accessed November, 2009.

Costantini, L., Beanlands, H., McCay, E., et al. (2008). The self-management experience of people with mild to moderate chronic kidney disease. *Nephrology Nursing Journal*, 35(2):147-156.

Curtin, R., Johnson, H., & Shatell, D. (2004). The peritoneal dialysis experience: insights from long-term patients. *Nephrology Nursing Journal*, 31(6):615-625.

De Geest, S., Schäfer-Keller, P., Denhaerynck, K., et al. (2006). Supporting medication adherence in renal transplantation (SMART): a pilot RCT to improve adherence to immunosuppressive regimens. *Clinical Transplantation*, 20:359-368.

Editorial. (2007). Fast facts about loop diuretics. *Nursing*, 37(10):56hn7-56hn8.

Eeles, R., Kote-Jarai, Z., Giles, G.G., et al. (2008). Multiple newly identified loci associated with prostate cancer susceptibility. *Nature Genetics*, 40:316-321.

Ficorelli, C., & Weeks, B. (2006). Facing up to prostate cancer. *Nursing*, 36(5):66-67.

Frey, K., Ed. (2008). *Surgical technology for the surgical technologist.* (3rd ed.). Clifton Park, NY: Delmar Cengage.

Gesek, F., & Desmond, J. (2008). Improved patient outcomes in chronic kidney disease: optimizing vitamin D therapy. *Nephrology Nursing Journal*, 35(2S):5A-23S.

Gilchrist, K. (2007). BPH. *LPN*, 3(1):32-39.

Goldstein, S.L, Graham, N., Warady, B.A., et al. (2008). Measuring health-related quality of life in children with ESRD: performance of the generic and ESRD-specific instrument of the pediatric quality of life inventory. *American Journal of Kidney Diseases*, 51(2):285-297.

Greenlings-Coppin, C., Porzolt, F., Autenrieth, M., et al. (2006). Targeted therapy for advanced renal cell carcinoma (Protocol). *Cochrane Data Base of Systematic Reviews*, Issue 2, Art. No. CD006017.DOI:101002/14651858.CD006017.

Hautmann, R., & Stein, J. (2005). Neobladder with prostatic capsule and seminal-sparing cystectomy for bladder cancer: a step in the wrong direction. *Urologic Clinics of North America*, 32(2):177-185.

Hedayati, T., & Keegan, M. (2009). *Prostatitis.* Available at http://emedicine.medscape.com/article/785418-overview. Accessed November, 2009.

Herr, H. (2005). Surgical factors in the treatment of superficial and invasive bladder cancer. *Urologic Clinics of North America*, 32(2):157-164.

Hinds, A. (2004). Obstructive uropathy: considerations for the nephrology nurse. *Nephrology Nursing Journal*, 31(2):166.

Hlebovy, D. (2006). Hemodailysis special interest group networking session: fluid management: moving and removing fluid during hemodialysis. *Nephrology Nursing Journal*, 33(4):441-446.

Israel, G., & Bosniak, M. (2003). Renal imaging for diagnosis and staging of renal cell carcinoma. *Urologic Clinics of North America*, 30(3):499-514.

Jamison, R., Hartigan, P., Kaufman, J.S., et al. (2008). Effect of homocysteine lowering on mortality and vascular disease in advanced chronic kidney disease and end-stage renal disease. *Journal of the American Medical Association*, 298(10):1163-1170.

Janos, V., & Higgins, L. (2007). Interstitial cystitis. *ADVANCE for Nurse Practitioners*, 15(3):55-57.

Jemal, A., Siegal, R., Ward, E., et al. (2006). *Cancer statistics.* Available at http://caonline.amcancersoc.org/cgi/content/abstract/56/2/106. Accessed November, 2009.

Johns Hopkins Children's Center. (2006). *Kidney stones occurring more often in children.* Available at www.hopkinschildrens.org/Kidney-Stones-Occuring-More-Often-in-Children.aspx. Accessed November, 2009.

Karch, A. (2008). *2009 Lippincott's nursing drug guide.* Philadelphia: Lippincott.

Kessler, T., Burkhard, F., & Studer, U. (2005). Clinical indications and outcomes with nurse-sparing cycstectomy in patients with bladder cancer. *Urologic Clinics of North America*, 32(2):165-175.

Khera, M., & Lipshultz, L. (2007). The role of testosterone replacement therapy following radical prostatectomy. *Urologic Clinics of North America*, 34(4):549-553.

Kidney Disease Outcomes Quality Initiative (KDOQI). (2007). Clinical practice guidelines and clinical practice recommendations for diabetes and chronic kidney disease. *American Journal of Kidney Diseases*, 49(suppl2):2.

Koivula, B., & Minielly, B. (2006). The Canadian introduction to the Greenlight laser. *Canadian Operating Room Nursing Journal*, 24(1):30-34.

Kontak, J., & Campbell, S. (2003). Prognostic factors in renal cell carcinoma. *Urologic Clinics of North America*, 30(3):467-480.

Krebs, L. (2007). Sexual assessment: research and clinical. *Nursing Clinics of North America*, 42(4):515-529.

Legg, V. (2005). Complications of chronic kidney disease. *American Journal of Nursing*, 105(6):40-50.

Leibovich, B., Pantuck, A., Bui, M., et al. (2003). Current staging of renal cell carcinoma. *Urologic Clinics of North America*, 30(3):481-498.

Lewis, S.L., Heitkemper, M.M., Dirksen, S.R., et al. (2007). *Medical-surgical nursing: assessment and management of clinical problems.* (7th ed.). St. Louis: Mosby.

Lilley, L., Harrington, S., & Snyder, J. (2007). *Pharmacology and the nursing process.* (5th ed.). St. Louis: Mosby, Inc.

Lu, D.F., McCarthy, A.M., Lanning, L.D., et al. (2007). A descriptive study of individuals with membranoproliferative glomerulonephritis. *Nephrology Nursing Journal,* 34(3):295-303.

Mahoney, C. (2007). Should patients eat during dialysis? *Nursing,* 37(10):57-58.

Matsuoka, S., Tominaga, Y., Uno, N., et al. (2006). Surgical significance of undescended parathyroid gland in renal hyperparathyroidism. *Surgery,* 139(6):815-820.

MayoClinic.com.(2009). *Urinary incontinence.* Available at http://mayoclinic.com/health/urinary-incontinence/DS00404. Accessed November, 2009.

McCarley, P., & Salai, P. (2005). Cardiovascular disease in chronic kidney disease. *American Journal of Nursing,* 105(4):40-53.

Medtronic, Inc. (n.d.). *About overactive bladder.* Available at www.medtronic.com/your-health/overactive-bladder/index.htm. Accessed November, 2009.

Middelton, L., & Essick, M. (2003). Inherited urologic malignant disorders: nursing implications. *Urologic Nursing,* 23(1):15-29.

Miller, D., Macdonald, D., Kolnacki, K., et al. (2004). Challenges for nephrology nurses in the management of children with chronic kidney disease. *Nephrology Nursing Journal,* 31(3):287.

Monoharan, M., & Soloway, M. (2005). Optimal management of the T1G3 bladder cancer. *Urologic Clinics of North America,* 32(2):133-145.

Moore, P., Farney, A., Sundberg, A., et al. (2006). Experience with dual kidney transplants from donors at the extremes of age. *Surgery,* 140(4):597-606.

Morgentaler, A. (2007). Testosterone replacement therapy and prostate cancer. *Urologic Clinics of North America,* 34(4):555-563.

Moyad, M. (2003). Calcium oxalate kidney stones: another reason to encourage moderate calcium intakes and other dietary changes. *Urologic Nursing,* 23(4):310.

Mulders, P., Bleumer, I., & Oosterwijk, E. (2003). Tumor antigens and markers in renal call carcinoma. *Urologic Clinics of North America,* 39(3):455-465.

Muruve, N., Steinbecker, K., & Willard, T.B. (2008). *Transurethral needle ablation of the prostate.* Available at www.emedicine.com/MED/topic3069.htm. Accessed November, 2009.

National Cancer Institute (NCI). (2008). *Bladder cancer.* Available at www.cancer.gov/cancertopics/pdq/treatment/bladder/Patient. Accessed November, 2009.

National Kidney Foundation (NKF). (2004). *Sexuality and chronic kidney disease.* Available at www.kidney.org/atoz/content/sexuality.cfm. Accessed November, 2009.

Nicholson, L., & Smith, D. (2007). Dysfunctional elimination syndrome. *ADVANCE for Nurse Practitioners,* 15(3):27-32.

Nieder, A., & Taneja, S. (2003). The role of partial nephrectomy for renal cell carcinoma. *Urologic Clinics of North America,* 30(3):529-542.

O'Donnell, M. (2005). Practical applications of intravesical chemotherapy and immunotherapy in high-risk patients with superficial bladder cancer. *Urologic Clinics of North America,* 32(2):121-131.

Pagana, K.D., & Pagana, T.J. (2008). *Mosby's diagnostic and laboratory test reference.* (9th ed.). St. Louis: Mosby.

Page, S., Rosenberg, M., & Hazzard, M. (2005). Interstitial cystitis: current diagnosis and management strategies, *ADVANCE for Nurse Practitioners,* 13(12):18.

Palmer, M.H., & Newman, D.K. (2006). Bladder control: educational needs of older adults, *Journal of Gerontologic Nursing,* 32(1):28.

Pasche, B. (2006). A new strategy in the war on renal cell cancer. *Journal of the American Medical Association,* 295(21):2537-2538.

Pavkov, M., Bennett, P.H., Knowler, W.C., et al. (2006). Effect of youth-onset type 2 diabetes mellitus on incidence of end-stage renal disease and mortality in young and middle-aged Pima Indians. *Journal of the American Medical Association,* 296(4):421-426.

Pelusi, J. (2006). Sexuality and body image. *American Journal of Nursing,* 106(3suppl):32-38.

Phillips, M. (2007). *Berry & Kohn's operating room technique.* (11th ed.). St. Louis, Mosby.

Pilkey, R., Morton, A., Boffa, M., et al. (2007). Subclinical vitamin K deficiency in hemodialysis patients. *American Journal of Kidney Disease,* 49(3):432-439.

Polt, C. (2006). Taking the pressure off for women with stress incontinence. *Nursing 2006,* 36(2):49-51.

Potter, P.A., & Perry, A.G. (2009). *Fundamentals of nursing: concepts, process, and practice.* (7th ed.). St. Louis: Mosby.

Purcell, W., Manias, E., Williams, A., et al. (2004). Accurate dry weight assessment: reducing the incidence of hypertension and cardiac disease in patients on hemodialysis. *Nephrology Nursing Journal,* 31(6):631-638.

Rossi, S., Ed. (2004). *Australian medicine handbook.* Adelaide: Australian Medicines Handbook.

Rubenstein, J., & McVary, K.T. (2008). *Transurethral microwave thermotherapy of the prostate (TUMT).* Available at http://emedicine.medscape.com/article/449623-followup. Accessed November, 2009.

Saccomano, S., & DeLuca, D. (2008). Managing acute renal failure. *Men in Nursing,* 3(2):32-42.

Schiffl, H., Lang, S.M., & Fischer, R. (2002). Daily hemodialysis and the outcome of acute renal failure. *New England Journal of Medicine,* 346(5):305.

Shiller, J., & Gonzalez, R. (2007). Green light laser: BPH treatment shows promise. *RN,* 70(11):28-32.

Smith, J. (2008). *Robotic versus open radical prostatectomy: "What is the real story?"* Available at http://www1.gotomeeting.com/en_US/island/webinare/registration0Post.temp1Z_sid=12178969%3A. Accessed May 3, 2008.

Stafford, H.S., Saltzstein, S.L., Shimasaki, S., et al. (2008). Oncology: adrenal/renal/upper tract/bladder. *Journal of Urology,* 179(5):1704-1708.

Stewart, M. (2006). Narrative literature review: sexual dysfunction in the patient on hemodialysis. *Nephrology Nursing Journal,* 33(6):631-641.

Stratta, R., Sundberg, A., Rohr, M., et al. (2006). Optimal use of older donors and recipients in kidney transplantation. *Surgery,* 139(3):324-333.

Thomas-Hawkins, C., & Zazworsky, D. (2005). Self-management of chronic kidney disease. *American Journal of Nursing,* 105(10):40-49.

U.S. Department of Agriculture (USDA). (2009). *MyPyramid.* Available at www.mypyramid.gov. Accessed November, 2009.

Uzzo, R., Cairns, P., Al-Saleem,T., et al. (2003). The basic biology and immunobiology of renal cell carcinoma: considerations for the clinician. *Urologic Clinics of North America,* 39(3):423-436.

Vasavada, S., & Rackley, R. (2006). How effective is pharmacotherapy for overactive bladder? *Patient Care,* January 1, 2006. Available at www.modernmedicine.com/modernmedicine/Urology/How-effective-is-pharmacotherapy-for-overactive-bl/ArticleStandard/Article/detail/283042. Article now available only to registered Modern Medicine members.

Vaughn, D., & Malkowicz, S. (2005). Neoadjuvant chemotherapy in patients with invasive bladder cancer. *Urologic Clinics of North America,* 32(2):231-237.

Vogel, S., & Rossert, J. (2005). A clinical review of antibody-mediated pure red cell aplasia. *Nephrology Nursing Journal,* 32(1):17-27.

Wijeysundera, D., Karkouti, K., Dupuis, J.Y., et al. (2007). Derivation and validation of simplified predictive index for renal replacement therapy after cardiac surgery. *Journal of the American Medical Association,* 297(16):1801-1809.

Wilmoth, M. (2007). Sexuality: a critical component of quality of life in chronic disease. *Nursing Clinics of North America,* 42(4):507-514.

Wilson, R.T., Silverman, D.T., Fraumeni, J.F., Jr., et al. (2008). *New malignancies following cancer of the urinary tract.* Available at http://seer.cancer.gov/publications/mpmono/Ch11_Bladder.pdf. Accessed November, 2009.

Wood, L., & Manchen, B. (2007). Sorafenib: a promising new targeted therapy for renal cell carcinoma. *Clinical Journal of Oncology Nursing*, 11(5):649-656.

Chapter 11 Care of the Patient with an Endocrine Disorder

American Diabetes Association. (2006). Standards of medical care for patients with diabetes mellitus. *Diabetes Care*, 29(suppl 1):54-542.

American Diabetes Association. (2007a). *Insulin pumps*. Available at www.diabetes.org/living-with-diabetes/treatment-and-care/medication/insulin/insulin-pumps.html. Accessed November, 2009.

American Diabetes Association. (2007b). Standards of medical care in diabetes. *Diabetes Care*, 30(suppl 1):540-541.

Anthony, M. (2006). When the blood glucose level takes a dive. *Nursing Made Incredibly Easy!* 4(6):15-17.

Appel, S. (2005). Sizing up metabolic syndrome. *Nursing*, 35(12):20.

Aschenbrenner, D. (2005). New drug for diabetes approved. *American Journal of Nursing*, 105(7):25.

Barkauskas, V., Baumann, L.C., & Darling-Fisher, C. (2006). *Health and physical assessment*. (4th ed.). St. Louis: Mosby.

Bass, A., Will, T., Todd, M., et al. (2007). The latest tools for patients with diabetes. *RN*, 70(6):39-43.

Bauer, J. (2006). Drug update: manufacturer breathes new life into delivery of insulin. *RN*, 69(31):64.

Black, J.M., & Hawks, H.J. (2009). *Medical surgical nursing: clinical management for positive outcomes*. (8th ed.). Philadelphia: Saunders.

Bode, B., Weinstein, R., Bell, D., et al. (2002). Comparison of insulin aspart with buffered regular insulin and insulin lispro in continuous subcutaneous infusion: a randomized study in type 1 diabetes. *Diabetes Care*, 25(3):439-444.

Brozenec, S. (1998). *Coping with multisystem complications*. St. Louis: Mosby.

D'Arcy, Y. (2007). Getting a grip on neuropathic pain. *LPN*, 4(2):14.

Davidson, M., Mehta, A.E., Siraj, E.S. (2006). Inhaled human insulin: an inspiration for patients with diabetes mellitus? *Cleveland Clinic Journal of Medicine*, 73(6):569-578.

Funnel, M., & Barlage, D. (2002). Managing diabetes with "agent oral." *Nursing*, 34(3):36.

Gattullo, B. (2007). Diabetic retinopathy. *Nursing*, 37(7):51.

Griffing, G.T., Odeke, S., Nagelberg, S.B. (2009). *Addison's disease*. Available at http://emedicine.medscape.com/article/116467-diagnosis. Accessed November, 2009.

Hieronymus, L., & O'Connell, B. (2004). Diabetes basics: managing hyperglycemia. *Diabetes Self-Management*, 21(6):44, 46-48.

Holcomb, S.S. (2005). Detecting thyroid disease. *Nursing*, 35(10):4-8.

Holcomb, S.S. (2007). A delicate balance: keeping thyroid hormones in check. *LPN*, 3(2):46.

Hussar, D. (2007). New drugs-insulin glulisine and insulin determir. *Nursing*, 37(2):52.

Hypoglycemia Support Foundation. Available at www.hypoglycemia.org. Accessed November, 2009.

Jacques, S. (2004). Diabetes under control: diabetes and depression. *American Journal of Nursing*, 104(9):56.

Jones, H., Edwards, L., Vallis, T.M., et al. (2003). Changes in diabetes self-care behaviors make a difference in glycemic control: the Diabetes Stages of Change (DiSC) study, *Diabetes Care* 26(3):732-737.

Levine, A., & Brennan, A.P. (2007). Rethinking sliding-scale insulin: one hospital's efforts in the ICU and elsewhere. *American Journal of Nursing*, 107(10):74-79.

Lewis, S.L., Heitkemper, M.M., Dirksen, S.R., et al. (2007). *Medical-surgical nursing: assessment and management of clinical problems*. (7th ed.). St. Louis: Mosby.

LoBiondo-Wood, G., & Haber, J. (2009). *Nursing research: methods and critical appraisal for evidence-based practice*. (7th ed.). St. Louis:Mosby.

Maddox, T., & Parker, D.M. (2006). Going up? Rapid ACTH screening. *Nursing Made Incredibly Easy!* 4(3):62-53.

McCance, K.L., & Huether, S.E. (2010). *Pathophysiology: the biologic basis for disease in children and adults*. (6th ed.). St Louis: Mosby.

Medical Letter, Inc. (2006). Drugs for hypothyroidism and hyperthyroidism. *Treatment Guidelines from Medical Letter*, 44(4):17, 2006.

Monahan, F.D., Sands, J.K., Neighbors, M., et al. (2007). *Phipps' medical-surgical nursing: health and illness perspectives*. (8th ed.). St. Louis: Mosby.

Mosby's dictionary of medicine, nursing, and health professions. (2009). (8th ed.). St. Louis: Mosby.

National Diabetes Education Program. Available at www.ndep.nih.gov. Accessed November, 2009.

Pagana, K.D., & Pagana, T.J. (2008). *Mosby's diagnostic and laboratory test reference*. (9th ed.). St. Louis: Mosby.

Perry, A.G., & Potter, P.A. (2009). *Clinical nursing skills and techniques*. (7th ed.). St. Louis: Mosby.

Potter, P.A., & Perry, A.G. (2007). *Basic nursing: essentials for practice*. (6th ed.). St. Louis: Mosby.

Ridge, R. (2007). Boosting insulin safety. *Nursing*, 37(2):14.

Scemons, D. (2007). Are you up-to-date on diabetes medications? *Nursing*, 37(7):45.

Skidmore-Roth, L. (2010). *Mosby's 2010 nursing drug reference*. St. Louis: Mosby.

Thibodeau, G.A., & Patton, K.T. (2008). *Structure and function of the body*. (13th ed.). St. Louis: Mosby.

Thibodeau, G.A., & Patton, K.T. (2009). *The human body in health and disease*. (5th ed.). St. Louis: Mosby.

Thompson, J.M., McFarland, G.K., Hirsch, J.E., et al. (2001). *Mosby's clinical nursing*. (5th ed.) .St. Louis: Mosby.

Tierney L., McPhee, S.J., Papadakis, M.A. (2007). *Current medical diagnosis and treatment*. (44th ed.). New York: McGraw-Hill.

U.S. Food and Drug Administration (US FDA). (2009). Byetta (exenatide)—renal failure. Available at www.fda.gov/Safety/MedWatch/SafetyInformation/SafetyAlertsforHumanMedicalProducts/ucm188703.htm. Accessed November, 2009.

Watts, S.A., Anselmo, J. (2006). Nutrition for diabetes—all of day's work. *Nursing*, 36(6):45-48.

White, R. (2007). Insulin pump therapy (continuous subcutaneous insulin infusion). *Primary Care*, 34(4):845.

Whiteman, K. (2006). ACTH stimulation: testing the adrenals. *Nursing*, 36(7):24.

Wilson, S.F., & Gidden, J.F. (2009). *Health assessment for nursing practice*. (4th ed.). St Louis: Mosby.

Wright, M., & Appel, S.J. (2007). Inhaled insulin: breathing new life into diabetes therapy. *Nursing*, 37(1):46.

Chapter 12 Care of the Patient with a Reproductive Disorder

Ackley, B.J., & Ladwig, G.B. (2009). *Nursing diagnosis handbook*. (7th ed.). St. Louis: Mosby.

Akert, J. (2003). Hormone replacement therapy, *RN*, 66(12):40.

American Cancer Society (ACS). (2007a). *Cancer facts and figures, 2007*. Available at www.cancer.org/downloads/STT/CAFF-2007PWsecured.pdf. Accessed November, 2009.

American Cancer Society (ACS). (2007b). Guidelines for breast screening with MRI as an adjunct to mammography. *CA: A Cancer Journal for Clinicians*, 57:75-89.

American Cancer Society (ACS). (2007c). *Ovarian cancer has early symptoms*. Available at www.cancer.org/docroot/NWS/content/NWS_1_1x_Ovarian_Cancer_Symptoms_The_Silence_Is_Broken.asp. Accessed November, 2009.

American Cancer Society (ACS). (2008a). *Cancer facts and figures, 2008*. Available at www.cancer.org/docroot/stt/content/stt_1x_cancer_facts_and_figures_2008.asp. Accessed November, 2009.

American Cancer Society (ACS). (2008b). *Cancer statistics*. Atlanta: Author.

American Cancer Society (ACS). (2009a). *American Cancer Society guidelines for the early detection of cancer*. Available at www.cancer.org/docroot/PED/content/PED_2_3X_ACS_Cancer_Detection_Guidelines_36.asp?sitearea=PED. Accessed November, 2009.

American Cancer Society (ACS). (2009b). *American Cancer Society responds to changes to USPSTF mammography guidelines.* Available at www.cancer.org/docroot/MED/content/MED_2_1x_American_Cancer_Society_Responds_to_Changes_to_USPSTF_Mammography_Guidelines.asp?sitearea=MED. Accessed November, 2009.

American Cancer Society (ACS). (2009c). *Cancer facts and figures.* Available at www.cancer.org/downloads/STT/500809web.pdf. Accessed November, 2009.

American Cancer Society (ACS). (2009d). *How is breast cancer staged?* Available at www.cancer.org/docroot/CRI/content/CRI_2_4_3X_How_is_breast_cancer_staged_5.asp?rnav=cri. Accessed November, 2009.

American Congress of Obstetricians and Gynecologists (ACOG). (2004). *Menopausal bleeding.* Available at www.acog.org/publications/patient_education/bp162.cfm. Accessed November, 2009.

American Congress of Obstetricians and Gynecologists (ACOG). (2009). *Response of the American Congress of Obstetricians and Gynecologists to new breast cancer screening recommendations from the U.S. Preventive Services Task Force.* Available at www.acog.org/from_home/Misc/uspstfResponse.cfm. Accessed November, 2009.

American Society for Reproductive Medicine Practice Committee (ASRM). (2006). *Report on varicocele and infertility.* Available at www.asrm.org/Media/Practice/Report_on_varicocele.pdf. Accessed November, 2009.

Aschenbrenner, D. (2004). Hormone replacement therapy (HRT): what should you tell patients about it now? *American Journal of Nursing,* 104(6):51.

Balzer-Riley, J. (2008). *Communication in nursing.* (6th ed.). St. Louis: Mosby.

Barkauskas, V., Baumann, L.C., & Darling-Fisher, C. (2006). *Health and physical assessment.* (4th ed.). St. Louis: Mosby.

Barton, D., & Loprinzi, C.L. (2004). Making sense of the evidence regarding nonhormonal treatments for hot flashes. *Clinical Journal of Oncology Nursing,* 8:39.

Black, J.M., & Hawks, H.J. (2009). *Medical-surgical nursing: clinical management for positive outcomes.* (8th ed.). Philadelphia: Saunders.

Carroll, C. (2006). Sorting out breast biopsy options. *Nursing,* 36(3):70.

Centers for Disease Control and Prevention (CDC). (2006). *New estimates of U.S. HIV prevalence, 2006.* Available at www.cdc.gov/hiv/topics/surveillance/resources/factsheets/prevalence.htm. Accessed November, 2009.

Centers for Disease Control and Prevention (CDC), Division of STD Prevention. (2007a). *Sexually transmitted diseases surveillance, 2007: chlamydia.* Available at www.cdc.gov/std/stats07/chlamydia.htm. Accessed November, 2009.

Centers for Disease Control and Prevention (CDC), Division of STD Prevention. (2007b). *Sexually transmitted diseases surveillance, 2007: gonorrhea.* Available at www.cdc.gov/std/stats07/gonorrhea.htm. Accessed November, 2009.

Centers for Disease Control and Prevention (CDC), Division of STD Prevention. (2007c). *Sexually transmitted diseases surveillance, 2007: syphilis.* Available at www.cdc.gov/std/stats07/syphilis.htm. Accessed November, 2009.

Centers for Disease Control and Prevention (CDC), Division of STD Prevention. (2007d). *Sexually transmitted diseases surveillance, 2007: trichomoniasis.* Available at www.cdc.gov/STD/Trichomonas/STDFact-Trichomoniasis.htm. Accessed November, 2009.

Centers for Disease Control and Prevention. (CDC). (2008). HIV prevalence estimates—United States, 2006. *MMWR Mortality and Morbidity Weekly Report,* 57(39):1073-1076.

Centers for Disease Control and Prevention (CDC). (n.d.). *Sexually transmitted diseases: genital herpes—CDC fact sheet.* Available at www.cdc.gov/std/herpes/STDFact-herpes.htm. Accessed November, 2009.

Chlebowski, R., Hendrix, S.L., Langer, R.D., et al. (2003). Influence of estrogen plus progestin on breast cancer and mammography in healthy postmenopausal women: the Women's Health Initiative Randomized Trial. *Journal of the American Medical Association,* 289:3243-3253.

Cleveland Clinic. (2009). *Image guided biopsy.* Available at http://my.clevelandclinic.org/services/biopsy/hic_Minimally_Invasive_Breast_Biopsy.aspx. Accessed November, 2009.

Cullen, P., & Cameron, C. (2006). Progress towards an effective syphilis vaccine: the past, present, and future. *Expert Review of Vaccines,* 5(1):65.

Deglin, J., & Vallerand, A. (2008). *Davis's drug guide for nurses.* (16th ed.). Philadelphia: Davis.

Elkin, M.K., Perry, A.G., & Potter, P.A. (2007). *Nursing interventions and clinical skills.* (4th ed.). St. Louis: Mosby.

Editorial. (2005). Who should use hormone therapy? *Nursing Made Incredibly Easy!* 3(1):64.

Facts at a glance. (n.d.). *Regional/global HIV/AIDS statistics.* Available at www.statehealthfacts.org. Accessed November, 2009.

Ficorelli, C. (2007). Untangling the complexities of male infertility. *Nursing,* 37(1):24.

Gardner, J. (2006). What you need to know about genital herpes. *Nursing,* 36(10):26.

Giger, J.M., & Davidhizar, R.E. (2007). *Transcultural nursing: assessment and intervention.* (5th ed.). St. Louis: Mosby.

Greifzu, S. (2004). Breast cancer. *RN,* 67(2):35.

Hockenberry, M.J., & Wilson, D. (2007). *Wong's nursing care of infants and children.* (8th ed.). St. Louis, Mosby.

Holcomb, S. (2008). Assessing the cause of postmenopausal bleeding. *LPN,* 4(2):50.

Hollingsworth, A.B., Singletary, S.E., Morrow, M. et al. (2004). Current comprehensive assessment and management of women at increased risk for breast cancer. *American Journal of Surgery,* 187(3):349-362.

Katz, A. (2005). Sexuality and hysterectomy: finding the right words: responding to patients'concerns about the potential effects of surgery. *American Journal of Nursing,* 105(12):65-68.

Kudachadkar, R., O'Regan, R.M. (2005). Aromatase inhibitors as adjuvant therapy for post menopausal patients with early stage breast cancer. *CA: A Cancer Journal for Clinicians,* 55(3):145-163.

Lehman, M. (2007). It whispers, so listen—ovarian cancer. *RN,* (10):28.

Lewis, J.H., Rosen, R., & Goldstein, I. (2005). Erectile dysfunction. *Nursing,* 35:64.

Lewis, S.L., Heitkemper, M.M., Dirksen, S.R., et al. (2007). *Medical-surgical nursing: assessment and management of clinical problems.* (7th ed.). St. Louis: Mosby.

Mahoney, S.F., & Armstrong, A. (2005). Accurate diagnosis of postmenopausal bleeding. *Nursing,* 30(8):61-63.

Martin, V. (2006). Shining a light on ovarian cancer, the hidden tumor. *Nursing Made Incredibly Easy!* 4(6):28-37.

McCaffery, M., & Pasero, C. (1999). *Pain: clinical manual.* (2nd ed.). St. Louis: Mosby.

McDaniel, C. (2007). Uterine fibroid embolization: the less invasive alternative. *Nursing,* 37(7):26-27.

Memmler, R.L., et al. (2008). *Structure and function of the human body.* (9th ed.). Philadelphia: Lippincott.

Mirshahidi, H. (2004). Managing early breast cancer. *Postgraduate Medicine,* 116:23.

National Cancer Institute (NCI). (2006a). *Clinical announcement: intraperitoneal chemotherapy for ovarian cancer.* Available at http://ctep.cancer.gov/highlights/docs/clin_annc_010506.pdf. Accessed November, 2009.

National Cancer Institute (NCI). (2006b). *NCI issues clinical announcement for preferred method of treatment for advanced ovarian cancer.* Available at www.cancer.gov/newscenter/IPchemotherapyQandA. Accessed November, 2009.

National Cancer Institute (NCI). (2009a). *A closer look: does mammography sometimes detect too much breast cancer?* Available at www.cancer.gov/ncicancerbulletin/102009/page6. Accessed November, 2009.

National Cancer Institute (NCI). (2009b). *Factsheet: testicular cancer: questions and answers.* Available at www.cancer.gov/cancertopics/factsheet/Sites-Types/testicular. Accessed November, 2009.

National Institutes of Health (NIH). (n.d.). *Women's Health Initiative hormone therapy study: menopausal hormone therapy information.*

Available at www.nih.gov/PHTindex.htm. Accessed November, 2009.

O'Rourke, E. (2007). Syphilis, still a public health danger. *RN*, 70(7):26.

Pagana, K.D., & Pagana, T.J. (2008). *Mosby's diagnostic and laboratory test reference*. (9th ed.). St. Louis: Mosby.

Park, A. (2007). Breast-cancer basics: diagnosis and treatment keep changing: here's what you need to know now. *Time*, 170(16):46.

Potter, P.A., & Perry, A.G. (2009). *Fundamentals of nursing: concepts, process, and practice*. (7th ed.). St. Louis: Mosby.

Santoro, N., & Chervenak, J.L. (2004). The menopause transition. *Endocrinology and Metabolism Clinics of North America*, 33:627.

Saslow, D., Castle, P.E., Cox, J.T., et al. (2007). American Cancer Society guideline for human papillomavirus (HPV) vaccine use to prevent cervical cancer and its precursors. *CA: A Cancer Journal for Clinicians*, 57(1):7-28.

Seidel, H.M., Ball, J.W., Dains, J.E., et al. (2007). *Mosby's guide to physical examination*. (6th ed.). St. Louis: Mosby.

Skidmore-Roth, L. (2010). *Mosby's 2010 nursing drug reference*. (23rd ed.). St. Louis: Mosby.

Snow, M. (2007). HPV vaccine: new treatment for an old disease. *Nursing*, 37(3):67.

Thibodeau, G.A. & Patton, K.T. (2007). *Anatomy and physiology*. (6th ed.). St. Louis: Mosby.

Thibodeau, G.A. & Patton, K.T. (2008). *Structure and function of the body*. (13th ed.). St. Louis: Mosby.

Thompson, J.M., McFarland, G.K., Hirsch, J.E., et al. (2001). *Mosby's clinical nursing*. (5th ed.).St. Louis: Mosby.

Timby, B.K., & Lewis, L.W. (2008). *Fundamental skills and concepts in patient care*. (9th ed.). Philadelphia: Lippincott.

Ulbricht, C.E., & Basch, E.M. (2005). Natural standard herb and supplement reference: evidence based clinical reviews. St. Louis: Mosby.

U.S. Food and Drug Administration (FDA). (2009a). *Cervarix. Product information: package insert*. Available at www.fda.gov/downloads/BiologicsBloodVaccines/Vaccines/ApprovedProducts/UCM186981.pdf. Accessed November, 2009.

U.S. Food and Drug Administration (FDA). (2009b). *FDA approved first DNA test for two types of human papillomavirus: agency also approved second DNA test for wider range of HPV types*. Available at www.fda.gov/NewsEvents/Newsroom/PressAnnouncements/ucm149544.htm. Accessed November, 2009.

U.S. Food and Drug Administration (FDA). (2004). *Timeline of breast implant activities*. Available at www.fda.gov/MedicalDevices/ProductsandMedicalProcedures/ImplantsandProsthetics/BreastImplants/ucm064242.htm. Accessed November, 2009.

U.S. Preventive Services Task Force (USPSTF). (2009). *Screening for breast cancer*. Available at www.ahrq.gov/clinic/USpstf/uspsbrca.htm. Accessed November, 2009.

Villa, I.I., Costa, R.L., Petta, C.A., et al. (2005). Prophylactic quadrivalent human papillomavirus (types 6, 11, 16, and 18) L1 virus-like particle vaccine in young women: a randomized double-blind placebo-controlled multicentre phase II efficacy trial. *Lancet Oncology*, 6(5):271-278.

Weaver, C. (2007). Compassionate care for the mastectomy patient. *Nursing Made Incredibly Easy!* 5(6):36.

Yeh, I.T. (2007). Post menopausal hormone replacement therapy: endometrial and breast effects. *Advances in Anatomic Pathology*, 14(1):17.

Additional Resource

American Cancer Society. Available at www.cancer.org. Accessed November, 2009.

Chapter 13 Care of the Patient with a Visual or Auditory Disorder

Albert, D., Miller, J.W., Azar, D.T, et al. (2008). *Albert and Jakobiec's principles and practice of ophthalmology*. (3rd ed.). Philadelphia: Saunders.

American Foundation for the Blind. (2009). *Facts and figures on Americans with vision loss*. Numbers of legally blind Americans. Available at www.afb.org/Section.asp?SectionID=15&DocumentID=4398#legal. Accessed December, 2009.

American Society of Ophthalmic Registered Nurses (ASORN). (2004). *Core curriculum for ophthalmic nursing*. (3rd ed.). Dubuque, Iowa: Kendall/Hunt.

Ball, K. (2007). *The perioperative challenge*. (5th ed.). St. Louis: Mosby.

Black, J.M., & Hawks, H.J. (2009). *Medical-surgical nursing: clinical management for positive outcomes*. (8th ed.). Philadelphia: Saunders.

Brandt, J.T., et al. (2008). Community resources for the ophthalmic practice. In D. Albert, J.W. Miller, D.T. Azar, et al. (Eds.), *Albert and Jakobiec's principles and practice of ophthalmology*. (3rd ed., vol. 5). Philadelphia: Saunders.

Burke, M., & Walsh, M. (2009). *Gerontologic nursing*. (5th ed.). St Louis: Mosby.

Corell, C. (2007). New outlook for age-related macular degeneration. *Nursing*, 37(3):27.

Gallagher, R.P., & Lee, T.K. (2006). Adverse effects of ultraviolet radiation: a brief review. *Progress in Biophysics and Molecular Biology*, 92(1):119-31.

Giger, J.M., & Davidhizar, R.E. (2007). *Transcultural nursing: assessment and intervention*. (5th ed.). St. Louis: Mosby.

Hard of Hearing Advocates. Available at www.hohadvocates.org. Accessed November, 2009.

Jaffe, M., & Skidmore-Roth, L. (2005). *Home health nursing*. (5th ed.). St. Louis: Mosby.

Johns Hopkins University. (2004). New strategies for preventing vision loss. *John Hopkins Medical Letter*, 15:4.

Lewis, S.L., Heitkemper, M.M., Dirksen, S.R., et al. (2007). *Medical-surgical nursing: assessment and management of clinical problems*. (7th ed.). St. Louis: Mosby.

Leyland M., & Zinicola, E. (2003). Multifocal versus monofocal intraocular lenses after cataract extraction. *Cochrane Data Base of Systematic Reviews*, Issue 3, Art No. CD003169.

Mayo Clinic staff. *Cataracts*. Available at www.mayoclinic.com/health/cataracts/DS00050. Accessed November, 2009.

McGwin, G., Jr., Gewant, H.D., Modjarrad, K., et al. (2006). Effect of cataract surgery on falls and mobility in independently living older adults. *Journal of the American Geriatric Society*, 54(7):1089-1094.

Monahan, F.D., Sands, J.K., Neighbors, M., et al. (2007). *Phipps' medical-surgical nursing: health and illness perspectives*. (8th ed.). St. Louis: Mosby.

Monk, H. (2005). Bring common eye emergencies into focus. *Nursing*, 35(12):46.

Monk, H. (2006). Presbyopia and cataract. *LPN*, 2(6):27.

Monk, H. (2007). Glaucoma and macular degeneration. *LPN*, 3(10):47.

Mosby's dictionary of medicine, nursing, and health professions. (2009). (8th ed.). St. Louis: Mosby.

Munson, B. (2006). Now, listen up! Understanding hearing loss and deafness. *Nursing Made Incredibly Easy!* 4(2):38.

National Eye Institute (NEI). National Institutes of Health (NIH). (2008). *Age-Related Eye Disease Study: results*. Available at www.nei.nih.gov/amd. Accessed November, 2009.

National Institute on Deafness and other Communication Disorders. (n.d.). *Cochlear implants*. Available at www.nidcd.nih.gov/health/hearing/coch.asp. Accessed November, 2009.

National Institutes of Health (NIH), & National Eye Institute. (2006). *Cataract: what you should know*. NIH Publication No. 03-201. Bethesda, MD: Author.

Novak, J.C., & Broom, B.L. (2008). *Ingalls and Salerno's maternal and child health nursing*. (11th ed.). St Louis: Mosby.

Potter, P.A., & Perry, A.G. (2009). *Fundamentals of nursing: concepts, process, and practice*. (7th ed.). St. Louis: Mosby.

Pullen, R. (2006). Spin control, caring for a patient with inner ear disease. *Nursing*, 36(5):48.

Rosenthal, B. (2009). *Age-related macular degeneration (AMD): an overview*. Available at www.healthandage.com/?q=archive/2233. Accessed November, 2009.

Rothrock, J. (2007). *Alexander's care of the patient in surgery*. (13th ed.). St. Louis: Mosby.

Seidel, H.M., Ball, J.W., Dains, J.E., et al. (2007). *Mosby's guide to physical examination*. (6th ed.). St. Louis: Mosby.

Skidmore-Roth, L. (2010). *Mosby's 2010 nursing drug reference*. (23rd ed.). St. Louis: Mosby.

Thibodeau, G.A., & Patton, K.T. (2007). *Anatomy and physiology*. (6th ed.). St. Louis: Mosby.

Thibodeau, G.A., & Patton, K.T. (2008). *Structure and function of the body*. (13th ed.). St. Louis: Mosby.

Thompson, J.M., McFarland, G.K., Hirsch, J.E., et al. (2001). *Mosby's clinical nursing*. (5th ed.). St. Louis: Mosby.

Zhou, B. Wang, B. (2006). Pegaptanib for the treatment of age-related macular degeneration. *Experimental Eye Research*, 83(3):615-619.

Additional Resources

"The Aging Eye," a special report, is available from Harvard Health Publications, P.O. Box 421073, Palm Coast, FL 32142-1073. E-mail: harvardpro@palmcoastd.com.

American Academy of Ophthalmology, P.O. Box 7424, San Francisco, CA 94120-7424. Available at www.aao.org. Accessed November, 2009.

American Academy of Otolaryngology, Head and Neck Surgery, *Meniere's disease*. Available at www.entnet.org/HealthInformation/menieresDisease.cfm. Accessed November, 2009.

American Foundation for the Blind, 15 West 16th St., New York, NY 10011. A list of free brochures.

American Optometric Association Communications Division, 243 North Lindbergh Blvd., St. Louis, MO 63141. Free brochures on eye care for the elderly.

Captioned Films for the Deaf, 800-237-6213.

The EAR Foundation. Available at www.earfoundation.org. Accessed November, 2009.

Glaucoma Research Foundation. Available at www.glaucoma.org. Accessed November, 2009.

Macular Degeneration Partnership. Available at www.amd.org. Accessed November, 2009.

MD support. Available at www.mdsupport.org/support.html. Accessed November, 2009.

National Eye Institute, 2020 Vision Place, Bethesda, MD 20892. 301-496-5248. Available at www.nei.nih.gov. Accessed November, 2009.

National Eye Institute, Office of Scientific Reporting, Bldg. 31, Rm. 6A32, Bethesda, MD 20205. A list of free brochures on eye disorders.

National Institute on Deafness and Other Communication Disorders Balance Disorders. Available at www.nidcd.nih.gov/health/balance/balance_disorders.htm. Accessed November, 2009.

National Institute to Prevent Blindness, 79 Madison Ave., New York, NY 10016. Free pamphlets on specific diseases affecting the eye.

Vision Foundation, 2 Mt. Auburn St., Watertown, MA 02172. Free vision inventory list.

Vestibular Disorders Association (VEDA). Available at www.vestibular.org. Accessed November, 2009.

Chapter 14 Care of the Patient with a Neurologic Disorder

Alexander, D. (2007). Controlling pain, facing the pain of trigeminal neuralgia. *Nursing*, 37(11):18.

Alverzo, J. (2007). Improving stroke outcomes. *American Journal of Nursing*, 107(110):72B.

Alzheimer's Disease Education and Referral Center, 800-438-4380. Available at www.alzheimers.org. Accessed November, 2009.

American Parkinson Disease Association. Available at www.apdaparkinson.org. Accessed November, 2009.

American Stroke Association. Available at www.strokeassociation.org/presenter.jhtml?identifier=1200037. Accessed November, 2009.

Avalos-Bock, S. (2005). West Nile virus and the U.S. blood supply. *American Journal of Nursing*, 105(2):34.

Awakenings. Available at www.parkinsonsdisease.com.

Baldwin, K. (2006). It's a knock-out punch. *Nursing Made Incredibly Easy!* 42(2):11.

Barker, E. (2006). A new weapon to combat stroke. *RN*, 69(3):26.

Beattie, S. (2007). Bedside emergency, unconscious patients. *RN*, 70(9):32.

Bender, K. (2003). West Nile virus: a growing challenge. *American Journal of Nursing*, 103(6):32.

Black, J.M., & Hawks, H.J. (2009). *Medical-surgical nursing: clinical management for positive outcomes*. (8th ed.). Philadelphia: Saunders.

Brandes, J.L. (2005). Practical use of topiramax for migraine prevention. *Headache*, 45 (suppl 1):566.

Centers for Disease Control and Prevention (CDC). (2008). *Division of vector-borne infectious diseases: West Nile virus*. Available at www.cdc.gov/ncidod/dvbid/westnile/index.htm. Accessed November, 2009.

Czaplinski, A., Yen, A.A., & Appel, S.H. (2006). Amyotrophic lateral sclerosis: early predictors of prolonged survival. *Journal of Neurology*, 253(11):1428-1436.

Deuschl, G., Schade-Brittinger, C., Krack, P., et al. (2006). A randomized trial of deep-brain stimulation for Parkinson's disease. *The New England Journal of Medicine*, 355:896-908.

Editorial. (2004). Drug for migraine: eletriptan hydobromide (Replax). *Nursing*, 34(2):58.

Epilepsy Foundation. (n.d.). *Epilepsy and seizure statistics*. Available at www.epilepsyfoundation.org/about/statistics.cfm. Accessed November, 2009.

Fagley, M. (2007). Taking charge of seizure activity. *Nursing*, 37(9):42.

Fisher, D. (2004). Help your patient manage myasthenia gravis. *Nursing Made Incredibly Easy!* 2(1):28-35.

Giger, J.M., & Davidhizar, R.E. (2007). *Transcultural nursing: assessment and intervention*. (5th ed.). St. Louis: Mosby.

Goetz, C. (2007). *Textbook of clinical neurology*. (3rd ed.). Philadelphia: Saunders.

Goldrick, B. (2003). Keeping West Nile virus at bay. *Nursing*, 33(8):44.

Goldstein, L.B., Adams, R., Alberts, M.J., et al. (2006). Primary prevention of ischemic stroke: a guideline from the American Heart Association/American Stroke Association Stroke Council, *Stroke*, 37(6):1583-1633.

Gusa, D., Miers, A., & Wijdicks, E. (2007). More than meets the eye. *RN*, 70(12):43-47.

Hayes, D. (2006). Viral meningitis in adults. *Nursing*, 36(2):64.

Hess, D., & Highes, M. (2005). Multiple sclerosis: when to suspect—keys to diagnosis. *Consultant*, 45(8):844-852.

Jarvis, C. (2008). *Physical examination and health assessment*. (5th ed.). Philadelphia: Saunders.

Kim, S.U. (2004). Human neural stem cells genetically modified for brain repair in neurological disorders. *Neuropathology*, 24:159.

King, K., & Olson, D.M. (2007). What you should know about neurogenic shock. *American Nurse Today*, 2(2):36, 2007.

Lawes, R. (2007). Uncovering the layers of meningitis and encephalitis. *Nursing Made Incredibly Easy!* 5(4):26-35.

Lewis, S.L., Heitkemper, M.M., Dirksen, S.R., et al. (2007). *Medical-surgical nursing: assessment and management of clinical problems*. (7th ed.). St. Louis: Mosby.

Loder, E., & Biondi, D. (2005). General principles of migraine management: the changing role of prevention. *Headache*, 45(suppl 1):533.

Lower, J. (2007). Fearlessly facing neurologic evaluation. *LPN*, 3(2):11.

Mathews, C. (2007). Getting ahead of acute meningitis and encephalitis. *Nursing*, 37(11):36-39.

Mauk, K. (2006). Heeding TIAs: stroke's early warning system. *Nursing*, 36(5):20.

McCarron, K. (2006). The shakedown on Parkinson's disease. *Nursing Made Incredibly Easy!* 4(6), 2006.

Michael J. Fox Foundation for Parkinson's Research. Available at www.michaeljfox.org. Accessed November, 2009.

Mosby's dictionary of medicine, nursing, and health professions. (2009). (8th ed.). St. Louis: Mosby.

Nadalo, L.A., & Walters, M.C. (2009). *Carotid artery, stenosis.* Available at http://emedicine.medscape.com/article/417524-media. Accessed November, 2009.

National Guideline Clearinghouse. (n.d.). *Practice guidelines for the management of bacterial meningitis.* Available at www.guidelines.gov/summary/summary.aspx?doc_id=5946. Accessed November, 2009.

National Institute of Neurological Disorders and Stroke. (n.d.a). *Know stroke. Know the signs. Act in time.* Available at www.ninds.nih.gov/disorders/stroke/knowstroke.htm. Accessed November, 2009.

National Institute of Neurological Disorders and Stroke. (n.d.b). *Parkinson's disease: hope through research.* Available at www.ninds.nih.gov/disorders/parkinsons_disease/detail parkinsons_disease.htm.

National Institute of Neurological Disorders and Stroke. (n.d.c) Available at www.ninds.nih.gov. Accessed November, 2009. Accessed November, 2009.

National Institute on Aging. (2007). *Progress report on Alzheimer's disease.* Available at www.nia.nih.gov/Alzheimers/Publications/ADProgress2007. Accessed November, 2009.

Nowlin, A. (2006). The dysphagia dilemma: how you can help. *RN*, 69(6):44-48.

Overstreet, M. (2004). When mosquitoes attack—an update on West Nile virus. *Nursing Made Incredibly Easy!* 2(3):42-45.

Pagana, K.D., & Pagana, T.J. (2008). *Mosby's diagnostic and laboratory test reference.* (9th ed.). St. Louis: Mosby.

Palmieri, R. (2006). Cerebral artery stenosis paves the way for a stroke. *Nursing*, 36(6):36-41.

Palmieri, R. (2007a). Piecing together the puzzle of Guillain-Barré syndrome. *Nursing Made Incredibly Easy!* 5(6):52-55.

Palmieri, R. (2007b). Responding to primary brain tumor. *Nursing*, 37(1):36.

Palmieri, R. (2007c). Unraveling the mystery of amyotrophic lateral sclerosis. *LPN*, 3(3):29.

Patient education series. (2007). Alzheimer's disease. *Nursing*, 37(6):50.

Phillips, R. (2007). Treating carotid artery stenosis to prevent stroke. *Nursing Made Incredibly Easy!* 5(1):41.

Rice, R. (2008). *Home health nursing practice.* (5th ed.). St. Louis: Mosby.

Rietberg, M.B., Brooks, D., Uitdehaaga, B.M., et al. (2005). Exercise therapy for multiple sclerosis. *Cochrane Data Base of Systematic Reviews*, Issue 1, Art. No. CD003980.

Schutte, D.L. (2006). Alzheimer disease and genetics. *American Journal of Nursing*, 106(12):40-48.

Serdans, B. (2005). A nurse with dystonia chooses DBS. *American Journal of Nursing*, 105(9):54.

Seshadri, S., Beiser, A., Selhub, J., et al. (2002). Plasma homocysteine as a risk factor for dementia and Alzheimer's disease. *New England Journal of Medicine*, 346:476.

Smith, M., & Buckwalter, K. (2005). Behaviors associated with dementia. *American Journal of Nursing*, 105(7):40-53.

Spinal Cord Information Network. (2009). *Spinal cord injury: facts and figures at a glance.* University of Alabama at Birmingham. Available at www.spinalcord.uab.edu/show.asp?durki=119513. Accessed November, 2009.

Parkinson's Disease Foundation. Available at www.pdf.org. Accessed November, 2009.

Thomure, A. (2006). Helping your patient manage Parkinson's disease. *Nursing*, 36(8):20.

Tian, G.F., Amzi, H., Takano, T., et al. (2005). An astrocytic basis of epilepsy. *Nature Medicine*, 11:973.

U.S. Food and Drug Administration (FDA). (2003). *Memantine approved for Alzheimer's disease.* FDA Patient Safety News: Show #22. Available at www.accessdata.fda.gov/psn/printer.cfm?id=182. Accessed November, 2009.

Weir, C.J., Muir, S.W., Walters, M.R., et al. (2003). Serum urate as an independent predictor of poor outcome and future vascular events after acute stroke. *Stroke*, 34(8):1951.

Wijdicks, E.F. (2006). Clinical scales for comatose patients: The Glasgow Coma Scale in historical context and the new FOUR score. *Reviews in Neurological Diseases*, 3(3), 109.

Wijdicks, E.F., & Bamlet, W.R., et al. (2005). Validation of a new coma scale: the FOUR Score. *Annals of Neurology*, 58(4), 585.

Wolf, C.A., Wijdicks, E.F., Bamlet, W.R., et al. (2007). Further validation of the FOUR score coma scale by intensive care nurses. *Mayo Clinic Proceedings*, 82(4):435-438.

Chapter 15 Care of the Patient with an Immune Disorder

American Autoimmune Related Diseases Association. Available at www.aarda.org. Accessed November, 2009

Darkauskas, V., Baumann, L.C., & Darling-Fisher, C. (2006). *Health and physical assessment.* (4th ed.). St. Louis: Mosby.

Black, J.M., & Hawks, H.J. (2009). *Medical-surgical nursing: clinical management for positive outcomes.* (8th ed.). Philadelphia: Saunders.

Colletti, M., et al. (2002). Immunologic system. In J.M. Thompson, G.K. McFarland, J.E. Hirsch, et al., (Eds.): *Mosby's clinical nursing.* (5th ed.). St. Louis: Mosby.

Durston, S. (2006). Caring for the immune compromised patient. *LPN*, 2(4):31.

Durston, S. (2007). Uncompromising immunocompromised patient care. *Nursing Made Incredibly Easy!* 5(4):52-61.

Global Initiative for Asthma (GINA). *Guidelines. 2004 Update: workshop report, global strategy for asthma management and prevention.* Available at www.ginasthma.org/GuidelineItem.asp:intId-987. Accessed November, 2009.

Gulanick, M., & Myers, J.L. (2006). *Nursing care plans: nursing diagnoses and interventions.* (6th ed.). St. Louis: Mosby.

Hayden, M. (2004). In defense of the body: how the immune system protects us from harm. *Nursing Made Incredibly Easy!* 2(3):30-41.

Hoffman, R., Benz, E.J., Jr., Shattil, S., et al. (2004). *Hematology: basic principles and practice.* (4th ed.). Philadelphia: Churchill Livingstone.

Immune Deficiency Foundation (IDF). (2007). *IDF guide for nurses: on immune globulin therapy for primary immunodeficiency diseases.* Available at www.primaryimmune-org/pubs/book_nurse/nurses_guide_pdf. Accessed November, 2009.

Lewis, S.L., Heitkemper, M.M., Dirksen, S.R., et al. (2007). *Medical-surgical nursing: assessment and management of clinical problems.* (7th ed.). St. Louis: Mosby.

Lupus Foundation of America. Available at www.lupus.org. Accessed November, 2009.

Male, D., Brostoff, J., Roth, D., et al. (2006). *Immunology.* (7th ed.). St. Louis: Mosby.

Monahan, F.D., Sands, J.K., Neighbors, M., et al. (2007). *Phipps' medical-surgical nursing: health and illness perspectives.* (8th ed.). St. Louis: Mosby.

Mosby's dictionary of medicine, nursing, and health professions. (2009). (8th ed.). St. Louis: Mosby.

National Institute of Allergy and Infectious Diseases. (2009). *The immune system.* Available at http://www3.niaid.nih.gov/topics/immuneSystem. Accessed November, 2009.

Pagana, K.D., & Pagana, T.J. (2008). *Mosby's diagnostic and laboratory test reference.* (9th ed.). St. Louis: Mosby.

Potter, P.A., & Perry, A.G. (2007). *Basic nursing: essentials for practice.* (6th ed.). St. Louis: Mosby.

Pullen, R. (2007a). Managing cutaneous vaxculitis in a patient with lupus erythematosus. *Dermatology Nursing*, 19(2):21.

Pullen, R. (2007b). Understanding systemic lupus erythematosus. *LPN*, 3(6):41.

Rooney, J. (2005). Systemic lupus erythematosus. Unmasking a great imitator. *Nursing*, 35(11):54.

Rote, N.S. (2010). Alternations in immunity and inflammation. In K.L. McCance, & S.E. Huether, *Pathophysiology: the biologic basis for disease in adults and children.* (6th ed.). St. Louis: Mosby.

Scherf, R., & White-Reid, K. (2008). Giving intravenous immunoglobulin. *RN*, 71(1):29-34.

Seidel, H.M., Ball, J.W., Dains, J.E., et al. (2007). *Mosby's guide to physical examination.* (6th ed.). St. Louis: Mosby.

Shearer, W., & Fleisher, T. (2007). The immune system. In N.F. Adkinson, W. Busse, B. Bochner, et al. (Eds.), *Middleton's allergy: principles and practice.* (7th ed.). Philadelphia: Mosby.

Thompson, J.M., McFarland, G.K., Hirsch, J.E., et al. (2002). *Mosby's clinical nursing.* (5th ed.). St. Louis: Mosby.

Venes, D. (2009.) *Taber's cyclopedic medical dictionary.* (21st ed.). Philadelphia: Davis.

Wysocki, L. (2007). Anaphylaxis doesn't have to be a shock. *Nursing Made Incredibly Easy!* 5(6):9-13.

Chapter 16 Care of the Patient with HIV/AIDS

AIDS Education Global Information System, (2002). *CDC fact sheet: human Immunodeficiency virus type 2.* Available at: www.aegis.com/default.asp?req=http://www.aegis.com/pubs/cdc_fact_sheets/2002/HIV-2.html. Accessed November, 2009.

Andrews G, Skinner D, & Zuma K. (2006) Epidemiology of health and vulnerability among children orphaned and made vulnerable by HIV/AIDS in sub-Saharan Africa. *AIDS Care* 2006;18:269-276.

Barré-Sinoussi, F., Chermann, J.C., Rey, F., et al. (1983). Isolation of a T-lymphotropic retrovirus from a patient at risk for acquired immune deficiency syndrome (AIDS), *Science,* 220(4599):868-871.

Black, J.M., & Hawks, H.J. (2009). *Medical-surgical nursing: clinical management for positive outcomes.* (8th ed.). Philadelphia: Saunders.

Braithwaite, R.S., Kozal, M.J., Chang, C.C., et al. (2007). Adherence, virological and immunological outcomes for HIV-infected veterans starting combination antiretroviral therapies. *AIDS,* 21:1579-1589.

Buonaguro, L., Tornesello, M.L., & Buonaguro, F.M., (2007). Human immunodeficiency virus type 1 subtype distribution in the worldwide epidemic: pathogenetic and therapeutic implications, *Journal of Virology,* 81(19):10209-10219.

Centers for Disease Control (CDC). (1981). MMWR: recommendations and reports. *MMWR: Morbidity and Mortality Weekly Report,* 30 (RR-21):1-3.

Centers for Disease Control and Prevention (CDC). (1998). *Human immunodeficiency virus type 2.* Available at www.cdc.gov/hiv/resources/factsheets/hiv2.htm. Accessed November, 2009.

Centers for Disease Control and Prevention (CDC). (2001). Updated U.S. Public Health Service guidelines for the management of occupational exposures to HBV, HCV, and HIV and recommendations forpostexposure prophylaxis. *MMWR: Morbidity and Mortality Weekly Report,* 50(RR-11):1.

Centers for Disease Control and Prevention (CDC). (2005a). Antiretroviral postexposure prophylaxis after sexual, injection-drug use, or other nonoccupational exposure to HIV in the United States. *MMWR: Morbidity and Mortality Weekly Report,* 54(RR-02):1-20.

Centers for Disease Control and Prevention (CDC). (2005b). Updated U.S. Public Health Service guidelines for the management of occupational exposures to HIV and recommendations for postexposure prophylaxis. *MMWR: Morbidity and Mortality Weekly Report,* 54(RR-09):1-17.

Centers for Disease Control and Prevention (CDC). (2006). Revised recommendations for HIV testing of adults, adolescents, and pregnant women in health-care settings. *MMWR: Morbidity and Mortality Weekly Report,* 22:55(RR-14):1-17.

Centers for Disease Control and Prevention (CDC). (2007a). *HIV/AIDS Surveillance Report, 2005.* Atlanta: US Department of Health and Human Services.

Centers for Disease Control and Prevention (CDC). (2007b). *HIV/AIDS among women.* Available at www.cdc.gov/hiv/topics/women/resources/factsheets/women.htm. Accessed November, 2009.

Centers for Disease Control and Prevention (CDC). (2007c). *HIV/AIDS among youth.* Available at www.cdc.gov/hiv/resources/factsheets/youth.htm. Accessed November, 2009.

Centers for Disease Control and Prevention (CDC). (2007d). *Sexually transmitted siseases surveillance, 2006.* Atlanta: U.S. Department of Health and Human Services.

Centers for Disease Control and Prevention (CDC). (2007e). *Surveillance of occupationally acquired HIV/AIDS in healthcare personnel, as of December, 2006.* Available at www.cdc.gov/ncidod/dhqp/bp_hcp_w_hiv.html. Accessed November, 2009.

Centers for Disease Control and Prevention (CDC). (2008). *HIV/AIDS surveillance report, 2006.* Available at www.cdc.gov/hiv/topics/surveillance/resources/reports/. Accessed November, 2009.

Centers for Disease Control and Prevention (CDC). (2009a). *HIV/AIDS among gay and bisexual men.* 2007. Available at www.cdc.gov/nchhstp/newsroom/docs/FastFacts-MSM-FINAL-508COMP.pdf. Accessed November, 2009.

Centers for Disease Control and Prevention (CDC). (2009b). *HIV/AIDS surveillance report,* Available at www.cdc.gov/hiv/topics/surveillance/resources/reports/index.htm#surveillance. Accessed November, 2009.

Cheng, D.M., Nunes, D., Libman, H., et al. (2007). Impact of hepatitis C on HIV progression in adults with alcohol problems. *Alcoholism, Clinical and Experimental Research,* 31(5):829-836.

Donnegan, E. (2003). *Transmission of HIV by blood, blood products, tissue transplantation and artificial insemination.* Available at http://hivinsite.ucsf.edu/InSite?page=kb-00&doc=kb-07-02-09. Accessed November, 2009.

Fletcher, M.A., & Klimas, N.G. (2007). Cytotoxic lymphocytes. In G. Fink, (Ed.), *Encyclopedia of stress.* (2nd ed.) Oxford: Academic Press.

Gallo, R.C., Salahuddin, S.Z,. Popovic, M., et al. (1984). Frequent detection and isolation of cytopathic retroviruses (HTLV-III) from patients with AIDS and at risk for AIDS. *Science,* 224 (4648):500-503.

Garry, R.F., Witte, M.H., Gottlieb, A.A., et al. (1988). Documentation of an AIDS virus infection in the United States in 1968, *Journal of the American Medical Association,* 260(14): 2085-2087.

Greenwald, J.L., Burstein, G.R., Pincus, J., et al. (2006). A rapid review of rapid HIV antibody tests. *Current Infectious Disease Report,* 8(2):125-131.

Hall, H.R., Song, R., Rhodes, P., et al. (2008). Estimation of HIV incidence in the United States, *Journal of the American Medical Association,* 300(5):520-529.

Henry J. Kaiser Family Foundation (2007). *The global HIV/AIDS epidemic. HIV/AIDS policy fact sheet, November 2007.* Available at www.kff.org/hivaids/upload/3030-103.pdf. Accessed November, 2009.

International AIDS Vaccine Initiative. (2005). *Tracking funding for preventive HIV vaccine research & development: estimates of annual investments and expenditures, 2000-2005.* International AIDS Vaccine Initiative. Available at www.iavi.org/lists/iavipublications/attachments/bf4f74f0-95b1-446c-9da9-78ca1bb40ecf/hvmrtwg_tracking_funding_for_preventive_hiv_vaccine_research_and_development_2006_eng.pdf. Accessed November, 2009].

Ironson, G., & Hayward, H. (2008) Do positive psychosocial factors predict disease progression in HIV? A review of the evidence. *Psychosomatic Medicine,* 70(5):546-554.

Joint United Nations Programme on HIV/AIDS (UNAIDS) & World Health Organization (WHO). (n. d.). *AIDS epidemic update report update.* Available at www.unaids.org/en/KnowledgeCentre/HIVData/EpiUpdate/EpiUpdArchive. Accessed November, 2009.

Kalichman, S.C. (2008). Co-occurrence of treatment nonadherence and continued HIV transmission risk behaviors: implications for positive prevention interventions. *Psychosomatic Medicine,* 70(5): 593-597.

Klimas, N., Koneru, A.O., & Fletcher, M.A. (2008). Overview of HIV. *Psychosomatic Medicine,* 70(5):523-530.

Lee, S., Wood, O., Tang, S., et al. (2007). Detection of emerging HIV variants in blood donors from urban areas of Cameroon. *AIDS Research and Human Retroviruses,* 23(10):1262-1267.

Lekkerkerker A.N., van Kooyk Y., & Geijtenbeek T.B. (2006). Viral piracy: HIV-1 targets dendritic cells for transmission. *Current HIV Research,* 4(2):169-176.

Leserman, J. (2008). Role of depression, stress, and trauma in HIV disease progression. *Psychosomatic Medicine,* 70(5):539-545.

National Institute of Allergy and Infectious Diseases. National Institutes of Health (NIH). (2009). *HIV infection in women.* Available at http://www3.niaid.nih.gov/topics/HIVAIDS/Understanding/Population+Specific+Information/womenHiv.htm. Accessed November, 2009.

Panel on Antiretroviral Guidelines for Adult and Adolescents (2008). *Guidelines for the use of antiretroviral agents in HIV-1-infected adults and adolescents.* Available at www.aidsinfo.nih.gov/ContentFiles/AdultandAdolescentGL.pdf. Accessed November, 2009.

Paredes, R., Mocroft, A., Kirk, O., et al. (2000). Predictors of virological success and ensuing failure in HIV-positive patients starting highly active antiretroviral therapy in Europe: results from the EuroSIDA study. *Archives of Internal Medicine,* 24(160):1123-1132.

Perinatal HIV Guidelines Working Group (2008). *Public Health Service Task Force recommendations for use of antiretroviral drugs in pregnant HIV-infected women for maternal health and interventions to reduce perinatal HIV transmission in the United States.* Available at aidsinfo.nih.gov/ContentFiles/PerinatalGL.pdf. Accessed November, 2009.

Potter, S.J., Lacabaratz, C., Lambotte, O., et al. (2007) Preserved central memory and activated effector memory CD4+ T-cell subsets in human immunodeficiency virus controllers: an ANRS EP36 study. *Journal of Virology,* 81(24):13904-13915.

Rowland-Jones, S., & Whittle, H.C. (2007). Out of Africa: what can we learn from HIV-2 about protective immunity to HIV-1? *Nature Immunology,* 8(4):329-331.

Schackman, B.R., Gebo, K.A., Walensky, R.P., et al. (2006). The lifetime cost of current human immunodeficiency virus care in the United States. *Medical Care,* 44(11):990-997.

Sekaly, R.P. (2008). The failed HIV Merck vaccine study: a step back or a launching point for future vaccine development? *Journal of Experimental Medicine,* 205(1):7-12.

Sepkowitz, K.A., & Eisenberg, L. (2005). *Occupational deaths among healthcare workers.* Available at www.cdc.gov/ncidod/EID/vol11no07/04-1038.htm. Accessed November, 2009.

Sherman, D. (2001). Palliative care. In C.A. Kirton, D. Talotta, & K. Zwolski (Eds.), *Handbook of HIV/AIDS nursing.* St. Louis: Mosby.

Smith, J., & Daniel, R. (2006). Following the path of the virus: the exploitation of host DNA repair mechanisms by retroviruses. *ACS Chemical Biology,* 1(4):217-226.

Temoshok, L.R., Wald, R.L., Synowski, S., et al. (2008). Coping as a multisystem construct associated with pathways mediating HIV-relevant immune function and disease progression. *Psychosomatic Medicine,* 70(5):555-561.

Wodak, A., & Cooney, A., (2006). Do needle syringe programs reduce HIV infection among injecting drug users: a comprehensive review of the international evidence. *Substance Use and Misuse,* 41(6-7):777-813.

World Health Organization (WHO). (2006). *State of the art of new vaccines: research and development.* 2006. Available at www.who.int/vaccines-documents/DocsPDF06/814.pdf. Accessed November, 2009.

World Health Organization (WHO). (2007). *Male circumcision for HIV prevention.* Available at www.who.int/hiv/topics/malecircumcision/en/index.html. Accessed November, 2009.

World Health Organization (WHO). (2008). *WHO definition of palliative care.* Available at www.who.int/cancer/palliative/definition/en. Accessed November, 2009.

World Health Organization (WHO). (2009). *Initiative for Vaccine Research (IVR): zoonotic infections.* Available at www.who.int/vaccine_research/diseases/zoonotic/en/index.html. Accessed: June 15, 2009.

Yerly, S., von Wyl, V., Ledergerber, B., et al. (2007). Transmission of HIV-1 drug resistance in Switzerland: a 10-year molecular epidemiology survey. *AIDS,* 21(18):2223-2229.

Chapter 17 Care of the Patient with Cancer

Ackley, B.J., & Ladwig, G.B. (2009). *Nursing diagnosis handbook.* (7th ed.). St. Louis: Mosby.

Alfaro-Lefevre, R. (2007). *Critical thinking in nursing: a practical approach.* (4th ed.). St. Louis: Mosby.

American Cancer Society (ACS). (2003). *Tamoxifen and raloxifene to reduce breast cancer risk: questions and answers.* Available at www.cancer.org/docroot/CRI/content/CRI_2_6Xtamoxifen_ and_Raloxifene_Question_and_Answers_5.asp. Accessed May, 2008.

American Cancer Society (ACS). (2008a). *Cancer statistics.* Atlanta: Author.

American Cancer Society (ACS). (2008b). *Understanding chemotherapy.* www.cancer.gov/cancertopics/chemo-side-effects/understandingchemo. Accessed November, 2009.

American Cancer Society (ACS). (2009). *Cancer facts and figures.* Available at www.cancer.org/downloads/STT/500809web.pdf. Accessed November, 2009.

American Cancer Society (ACS). (n.d.). *Kidney cancer.* Available at www.cancer.gov/cancertopics/types/kidney. Accessed November, 2009.

American Cancer Society. (n.d.). *Testicular cancer.* Available at www.cancer.gov/cancertopics/types/testicular. Accessed November, 2009.

Balzer-Riley, J. (2008). *Communication in nursing.* (6th ed.). St. Louis: Mosby.

Barkauskas, V., Baumann, L.C., & Darling-Fisher, C. (2006). *Health and physical assessment.* (4th ed.). St. Louis: Mosby.

Black, J.M., & Hawks, H.J. (2009). *Medical-surgical nursing: clinical management for positive outcomes.* (8th ed.). Philadelphia: Saunders.

Calle, E.E., Rodriguez, C., Walker-Thurmond, K., et al. (2003). Overweight, obesity, and mortality from cancer in a prospectively studied cohort of US adults. *New England Journal of Medicine,* 348(17):1625-1638.

Cantril, C. (2004). Emergency tumor lysis syndrome. *American Journal of Nursing,* 104(4):49.

Carroll, C. (2006). Sorting out breast biopsy options. *Nursing,* 36(3):70.

Correa, P. (2003). *Helicobacter pylori* infection and gastric cancer. *Cancer Epidemiology, Biomarkers, and Prevention,* 12(3):238S.

Coyne, B. (2004). Chemo's toll on memory. *RN,* 67(4):40.

Curtis, C. (2006). Improving the care of cancer survivors. *American Journal of Nursing,* 106(3):48.

D'Arcy, Y. (2005). Conquering pain: have you tried these new techniques? *Nursing,* 35(3):36-41.

Dell, D.D. (2005). Battling breast cancer. *Nursing Made Incredibly Easy!* 3(5):4-20.

Dest, V. (2006a). Cancer therapies. *RN,* 69(6):31.

Dest, V. (2006b). Lung cancer, the battle continues. *RN,* 69(11):30.

Edmondson, D. (2008). Smoke out lung cancer. *LPN,* 4(1):39.

Freedman, G.M., & Anderson, P.R. (2003). Routine mammography is associated with earlier stage disease and greater eligiblity for breast conservation in breast carcinoma patients age 40 years and older. *Cancer,* 98(5):918.

Giger, J.M., & Davidhizar, R.E. (2007). *Transcultural nursing: assessment and intervention.* (5th ed.). St. Louis: Mosby.

Gordon, M. (2009). *Manual of nursing diagnosis.* (11th ed.). St. Louis: Mosby.

Held-Warmkessel, J. (2005). Managing three critical cancer complications. *Nursing,* 35(1):58.

Higdon, M.L., & Higdon, J.A. (2006). *Treatment of oncologic emergencies.* Available at www.aafp.org/afp/20061201/1873.html. Accessed November, 2009.

Jeffries, M. (2007). Helping your patient combat lung cancer, *Nursing,* 37(2):36-41.

Kehoe, C. (2007). Getting to know oncologic emergencies. *Nursing Made Incredibly Easy!* 5(5):49-56.

Lehman, M. (2007). *It whispers, ovarian cancer.* Available at www.rnweb.com, 28, 2007.

Lewis, S.L., Heitkemper, M.M., Dirksen, S.R., et al. (2007). *Medical-surgical nursing: assessment and management of clinical problems.* (7th ed.). St. Louis: Mosby.

Lilley, L., Harrington, S., & Snyder, J. (2007). *Pharmacology and the nursing process.* (5th ed.). St. Louis: Mosby, Inc.

Mayo Clinic staff. (2009). *Chemotherapy.* Available at www.mayoclinic.com/health/chemotherapy/MY00536. Accessed November, 2009.

McCaffery, M., & Pasero, C. (2007). *Pain: clinical manual*. (4th ed.). St. Louis: Mosby.

Mee, C.L. (2007). Hospice care. *Nursing*, 37(11):43.

Monahan, F.D., Sands, J.K., Neighbors, M., et al. (2007). *Phipps' medical-surgical nursing: health and illness perspectives*. (8th ed.). St. Louis: Mosby.

Mosby's dictionary of medicine, nursing, and health professions. (2009). (8th ed.). St. Louis: Mosby.

National Cancer Institute (NCI). (n.d.a). *Cancer health disparities*. Available at www.cancer.gov/cancertopics/types/disparities. Accessed November, 2009.

National Cancer Institute (NCI). (n.d.b). *Renal cell cancer treatment (PDQ): health professional version*. Available at www.cancer.gov/cancertopics/pdq/treatment/renalcell/healthprofessional. Accessed November, 2009.

National Cancer Institute (NCI). (n.d.c). *Targeted cancer therapies*. Available at www.cancer.gov/cancertopics/factsheet/Therapy/targeted. Accessed November, 2009.

National Comprehensive Cancer Network. (2006). *Breast cancer treatment guidelines for patients: Version VIII*. Available at www.nccn.org/patients/patient_gls_english/_breast/contents/asp. April 2008.

National Guidelines Clearinghouse. (n.d.). *Management of breast cancer in women: a national clinical guideline*. www.guideline.gov/summary/summary.aspx?doc_id=8510. Accessed November, 2009.

Netherbee, S. (2006). New weapons to snuff out kidney cancer. *Nursing*, 36(12):59.

Ngo-Metzger, Q., McCarthy, E.P., Burns, R.B., et al. (2003). Older Asian American and Pacific Islanders dying of cancer use hospice less frequently than older white patients. *American Journal of Medicine*, 115(1):47.

Otto, S. (2005). *Oncology nursing*. (5th ed.). St. Louis: Mosby.

Pagana, K.D., & Pagana, T.J. (2008). *Mosby's diagnostic and laboratory test reference*. (9th ed.). St. Louis: Mosby.

Shinn, S. (2004). Cervical cancer. *Nursing*, 34(5):36.

Skidmore-Roth, L. (2010). *Mosby's 2010 nursing drug reference*. (23rd ed.). St. Louis: Mosby.

Smeltzer, S.C., Bare, B.G., Hinkle, J.L., et al. (2007). *Brunner & Suddarth's textbook of medical-surgical nursing*, (11th ed.). Philadelphia: Lippincott Williams and Wilkins.

Tannock, I.F., Hill, R., Bristow, R., et al. (2005). *The basic science of oncology*. (4th ed.). New York: McGraw-Hill.

Taylor, D.S., & Penny, A.S. *Oncologic emergencies*. Available at www.emedicine.com/ped/topic2590.htm. Accessed November, 2009.

Thompson, J.M., McFarland, G.K., Hirsch, J.E., et al. (2001). *Mosby's clinical nursing*. (5th ed.). St. Louis: Mosby.

Tucker, S.M., Cannobio, M.M., Paquette, E.V., et al. (2007). *Patient care standards: collaborative planning and nursing interventions*. (7th ed.). St. Louis: Mosby.

U.S. Department of Health and Human Services. (n.d.). *Tracking Healthy People 2010*. Washington, DC: U.S. Government Printing Office.

U.S. Food and Drug Administration (US FDA). (2006). *FDA approves new treatment for gastrointestinal and kidney cancer*. Available at www.fda.gov/NewsEvents/Newsroom/PressAnnouncements/2006/ucm108583.htm. Accessed November, 2009.

Weaver, C. (2007). Compassionate care for the patient with a mastectomy. *Nursing Made Incredibly Easy!* 5(6):26.

Workman, L. (2002). Breast cancer—new strategies to beat an old enemy. *Nursing*, 32(10):58.

Illustration Credits

Chapter 1

1-1, 1-2, 1-3, 1-4, 1-5, 1-6, 1-9, 1-13, from Thibodeau, G.A., & Patton, K.T. (2008). *Structure and function of the body.* (13th ed.). St. Louis: Mosby. 1-7, from Herlihy, B., & Maebius, N.K. (2007). *The human body in health and illness.* (3rd ed.). Philadelphia: Saunders. 1-8, 1-10, 1-11, from Thibodeau, G.A., & Patton, K.T. (2007). *Anatomy and physiology.* (6th ed.). St. Louis: Mosby.

Chapter 2

2-1, 2-6, 2-9, 2-12, 2-17, 2-18, from Harkreader, H., & Hogan, M.A. (2007). *Fundamentals of nursing: caring and clinical judgment.* (3rd ed.). Philadelphia: Saunders. 2-2, from Cole, G. (1996). *Fundamental nursing: concepts and skills.* (2nd ed.). St. Louis: Mosby. 2-3, 2-4, 2-7, 2-16, from Elkin, M.K., et al. (2007). *Nursing interventions and clinical skills.* (4th ed.). St. Louis: Mosby. 2-5, from Potter, P.A., & Perry, A.G. (2006). *Basic nursing: essentials for practice.* (6th ed.). St. Louis: Mosby. 2-8, from Meeker, M.H., & Rothrock, J.C. (1999). *Alexander's care of the patient in surgery.* (11th ed.). St. Louis: Mosby. 2-10, 2-14, courtesy of Great Plains Regional Medical Center, North Platte, Nebraska. 2-11, from Lewis, S.L., et al. (2007). *Medical-surgical nursing: assessment and management of clinical problems.* (7th ed.). St. Louis: Mosby. 2-13, from Potter, P.A., & Perry, A.G. (2009). *Fundamentals of nursing.* (7th ed.). St. Louis: Mosby. Skill 2-1, step 14, from Sorrentino, S.A. (2008). *Mosby's textbook for nursing assistants.* (7th ed.). St. Louis: Mosby. Skill 2-2, step 9a, step 10c; Skill 2-3, step 10; Skill 2-4, step 17, step 20, from Potter, P.A., & Perry, A.G. (2009). *Fundamentals of nursing.* (7th ed.). St. Louis: Mosby. Skill 2-3, step 8, from Elkin, M.K., et al. (2007). *Nursing interventions and clinical skills.* (4th ed.). St. Louis: Mosby.

Chapter 3

3-1, from Thibodeau, G.A., & Patton, K.T. (2005). *The human body in health and disease.* (4th ed.). St. Louis: Mosby. 3-2, 3-7, 3-8, 3-13, 3-18, from Habif, T.P. (2004). *Clinical dermatology.* (4th ed.). St. Louis: Mosby. 3-3, 3-4, 3-5, 3-6, 3-10, 3-17, courtesy of the Department of Dermatology, School of Medicine, University of Utah. 3-9 from Weston, W.L., et al. (2007). *Color textbook of pediatric dermatology.* (4th ed.). St. Louis: Mosby. 3-11, from Habif, T.P., et al. (2005). *Skin disease: diagnosis and treatment.* (2nd ed.). St. Louis: Mosby. 3-12, from Baran, R., et al. (1991). *Color atlas of the hair, scalp, and nails.* St. Louis: Mosby. 3-14, courtesy of Department of Derma-

tology, University of North Carolina at Chapel Hill. 3-15, from Zitelli, B.J., & Davis, H.W. (2007). *Atlas of pediatric physical diagnosis.* (5th ed.). St. Louis: Mosby. 3-16, from Belcher, A.E. (1992). *Cancer nursing.* St. Louis: Mosby. 3-19, from Hockenberry, M.J., & Wilson, D. (2007). *Wong's nursing care of infants and children.* (8th ed.). St. Louis: Mosby. 3-20, 3-21, courtesy of Intermountain Burn Center, University of Utah. 3-22, from Thibodeau, G.A., & Patton, K.T. (2007). *Anatomy and physiology.* (6th ed.). St. Louis: Mosby. 3-23, 3-24, 3-25, courtesy of Burn Center, Cleveland Metropolitan General Hospital, Cleveland, Ohio.

Chapter 4

4-1, 4-4, from Thibodeau, G.A., & Patton, K.T. (2008). *Structure and function of the body.* (13th ed.). St. Louis: Mosby. 4-2, 4-3, 4-5, 4-6, 4-22, 4-24, 4-39, 4-41, from Thibodeau, G.A., & Patton, K.T. (2005). *The human body in health and disease.* (4th ed.). St. Louis: Mosby. 4-7, 4-8, from Kamal, A., & Brocklehurst, J.C. (1991). *Color atlas of geriatric medicine.* (2nd ed.). St. Louis: Mosby. 4-9, 4-17, 4-25, from Lewis, S.L., et al. (2007). *Medical-surgical nursing: assessment and management of clinical problems.* (7th ed.). St. Louis: Mosby. 4-10, 4-23, 4-34, from Ignatavicius, D.D., & Workman, M.L. (2009). *Medical-surgical nursing across the healthcare continuum.* (6th ed.). Philadelphia: Saunders. 4-11, 4-16, 4-20, 4-31, B; Skill 4-1, step 8a, from Monahan, F.D., et al. (2007). *Phipps' medical-surgical nursing: health and illness perspectives.* (8th ed.). St. Louis: Mosby. 4-12, 4-15, 4-32, courtesy of Zimmer, Inc., Warsaw, Indiana. 4-13, courtesy of Orthologic Corporation, Phoenix, Arizona. 4-18, 4-31, A, modified from Mourad, L. (1991). *Orthopedic disorders.* St. Louis: Mosby. 4-26, 4-29, courtesy of Dr. Henry Bohlman, Cleveland, Ohio. 4-27, 4-40, from Beare, P.G., & Myers, J.L. (1998). *Adult health nursing.* (3rd ed.). St. Louis: Mosby. 4-28, A, from Stryker Howmedica Osteonics, Inc., Mahway, New Jersey. 4-28, 4-38, from Thompson, J.M., et al. (2002). *Mosby's clinical nursing.* (5th ed.). St. Louis: Mosby. 4-30, from Elkin, M.K., et al. (2008). *Nursing interventions and clinical skills.* (4th ed.). St. Louis: Mosby. 4-33, from Harkness, G.A., & Dincher, J.R. (1999). *Medical-surgical nursing: total patient care.* (10th ed.). St. Louis: Mosby. 4-34, 4-36, from Potter, P.A., & Perry, A.G. (2006). *Basic nursing: essentials for practice.* (6th ed.). St. Louis: Mosby. 4-35, from Elkin, M.K., et al. (2004). *Nursing interventions and clinical skills.* (3rd ed.). St. Louis: Mosby.

4-37, courtesy of Roll-a-Bout Corporation, Frederica, Delaware.

Chapter 5
5-1, 5-2, 5-4, from Thibodeau, G.A., & Patton, K.T. (2007). *Anatomy and physiology.* (6th ed.). St. Louis: Mosby. **5-3,** from Thibodeau, G.A., & Patton, K.T. (2008). *Structure and function of the body.* (13th ed.). St. Louis: Mosby. **5-5, 5-20,** from Monahan, F.D., et al. (2007). *Phipps' medical-surgical nursing: health and illness perspectives.* (8th ed.). St. Louis: Mosby. **5-6,** from Lewis, S.L., et al. (2007). *Medical-surgical nursing: assessment and management of clinical problems.* (7th ed.). St. Louis: Mosby. **5-8, 5-12, 5-13, 5-14, 5-16,** from Beare, P.G., & Myers, J.L. (1998). *Adult health nursing.* (3rd ed.). St. Louis: Mosby.

Chapter 6
6-1, courtesy of Olympus America, Inc., Melville, New York. **6-2, 6-4, 6-7, 6-9,** from Lewis, S.L., et al. (2007). *Medical-surgical nursing: assessment and management of clinical problems.* (7th ed.). St. Louis: Mosby. **6-3, 6-8,** from Beare, P.G., & Myers, J.L. (1998). *Adult health nursing.* (3rd ed.). St. Louis: Mosby. **6-5,** from Kamal, A., & Brockelhurst, J.C. (1991). *Color atlas of geriatric medicine.* (3rd ed.). St. Louis: Mosby. **6-6,** from Monahan, F.D., et al. (2007). *Phipps' medical-surgical nursing: health and illness perspectives.* (8th ed.). St. Louis: Mosby.

Chapter 7
7-1, 7-4, from Thibodeau, G.A., & Patton, K.T. (2007). *Anatomy and physiology.* (6th ed.). St. Louis: Mosby. **7-2, 7-3,** from Thibodeau, G.A., & Patton, K.T. (2007). *The human body in health and disease.* (3rd ed.). St. Louis: Mosby. **7-5,** from Belcher, A.E. (1992). *Mosby's clinical nursing series: blood disorders.* St. Louis: Mosby.

Chapter 8
8-1 from Thibodeau, G.A., & Patton, K.T. (2004). *Structure and function of the human body.* (12th ed.). St. Louis: Mosby. **8-2, 8-3,** from Thibodeau, G.A., & Patton, K.T. (2007). *Anatomy and physiology.* (6th ed.). St. Louis: Mosby. **8-4, 8-5, 8-6, 8-17,** from Canobbio, M. (1990). *Mosby's clinical nursing series: cardiovascular disorders.* St. Louis: Mosby. **8-9, A,** courtesy of Medtronic, Inc., Minneapolis, Minnesota. **8-9, B, 8-10, 8-11, 8-12, B, 8-16, 8-19, 8-20, A, B, 8-21, 8-23,** from Lewis, S.L., et al. (2007). *Medical-surgical nursing: assessment and management of clinical problems.* (7th ed.). St. Louis: Mosby. **8-12, A,** from Urden, L.D., et al. (2006). *Thelan's critical care nursing: diagnosis and management.* (5th ed.). St. Louis: Mosby. **8-13, 8-25,** from Monahan, F.D., et al. (2007). *Phipps' medical-surgical nursing: health and illness perspectives.* (8th ed.). St. Louis: Mosby. **8-14,** from Beare, P.G., & Myers, J.L. (1998). *Adult health nursing.* (3rd ed.). St. Louis: Mosby. **8-15,** from *Heart disease and stroke,* 2:99, 1993. Copyright American Heart Association. **8-23, 8-24,** from Kamal, A., & Brockelhurst, J.C.

Color atlas of geriatric medicine. (3rd ed.). St. Louis: Mosby–Year Book, Europe.

Chapter 9
9-1, 9-2, 9-3, 9-4, 9-6, from Thibodeau, G.A., & Patton, K.T. (2008). *Structure and function of the body.* (13th ed.). St. Louis: Mosby. **9-5,** from Thibodeau, G.A., & Patton, K.T. (2005). *The human body in health and disease.* (4th ed.). St. Louis: Mosby. **9-7, A,** courtesy of Olympus America, Inc., Melville, New York. **9-7, B,** from Meduri, G.U., et al. Protected bronchoalveolar lavage. *American Review of Respiratory Disease,* 143.855, 1991, official journal of the American Thoracic Society, copyright American Lung Association. **9-8,** from Lewis, S.L., et al. (2007). *Medical-surgical nursing: assessment and management of clinical problems.* (7th ed.). St. Louis: Mosby. **9-9, 9-12,** from Potter, P.A., & Perry, A.G. (2009). *Fundamentals of nursing.* (7th ed.). St. Louis: Mosby. **9-13,** from Wilson, S., & Thompson, J. (1991). *Mosby's clinical nursing series: respiratory disorders.* St. Louis: Mosby. **9-14,** from Lewis, S.L., et al. (1996). *Medical-surgical nursing: assessment and management of clinical problems.* (4th ed.). St. Louis: Mosby. **9-15,** from McCance, K.L., & Huether, S.E. (2006). *Pathophysiology: the biologic basis for disease in adults and children.* (5th ed.). St. Louis: Mosby.

Chapter 10
10-1, 10-2, 10-3, 10-5, from Thibodeau, G.A., & Patton, K.T. (2007). *Anatomy and physiology.* (6th ed.). St. Louis: Mosby. **10-6,** from Lewis, S.L., et al. (2007). *Medical-surgical nursing: assessment and management of clinical problems.* (7th ed.). St. Louis: Mosby. **10-7, 10-9,** from Beare, P.G., & Myers, J.L. (1998). *Adult health nursing.* (3rd ed.). St. Louis: Mosby. **10-10, 10-11,** from Tucker, S., et al. (1996). *Patient care standards: collaborative practice planning guides.* (6th ed.). St. Louis: Mosby. **10-12,** from Belcher, A.E. (1992). *Cancer nursing.* St. Louis: Mosby. **10-14,** from Thibodeau, G.A., & Patton, K.T. (2008). *Structure and function of the body.* (13th ed.). St. Louis: Mosby.

Chapter 11
11-1, 11-2, 11-4, from Thibodeau, G.A., & Patton, K.T. (2008). *Structure and function of the body.* (13th ed.). St. Louis: Mosby. **11-5,** from Thibodeau, G.A., & Patton, K.T. (2007). *Anatomy and physiology.* (6th ed.). St. Louis: Mosby. **11-6,** courtesy of the Group for Research in Pathology Education. **11-7, 11-8,** from Seidel, H.M., et al. (2003). *Mosby's guide to physical examination.* (5th ed.). St. Louis: Mosby. **11-9,** from Schneeburg, N.G. (1979). *Essentials of clinical endocrinology.* St. Louis: Mosby. **11-10,** courtesy of L.V. Bergman & Associates, Inc., Cold Springs, New York. **11-14, 11-15, A, B, 11-17, 11-18,** from Lewis, S.L., et al. (2007). *Medical-surgical nursing: assessment and management of clinical problems.* (7th ed.). St. Louis: Mosby. **11-16,** from Potter, P.A., & Perry, A.G. (2003). *Basic nursing: essentials for practice.* (5th ed.). St. Louis: Mosby.

Glossary

Pronunciation of Terms*

The markings ¯ and ˘ above the vowels (a, e, i, o, and u) indicate the proper sounds of the vowels.

When ¯ is above a vowel, its sound is long, that is, exactly like its name. For example:

ā as in āpe
ē as in ēven
ī as in īce
ō as in ōpen
ū as in ūnit

The ˘ marking indicates a short vowel sound, as in the following examples:

ă as in ăpple
ĕ as in ĕvery
ĭ as in ĭnterest
ŏ as in pŏt
ŭ as in ŭnder

A

ablation Amputation or excision of any part of the body; removal of a growth or harmful substance.

achalasia Abnormal condition characterized by the inability of a muscle, particularly the cardiac sphincter of the stomach, to relax.

achlorhydria Abnormal condition characterized by the absence of hydrochloric acid in the gastric secretions.

acquired immunodeficiency syndrome (AIDS) Acquired condition that impairs the body's ability to fight infection; the end stage of the continuum of HIV infection, in which the infected person has a CD_4^+ (lymphocyte) count of 200 cells/mm^3 or fewer.

active transport The movement of materials across the membrane of a cell by means of chemical activity, which allows the cell to admit larger molecules than would otherwise be able to enter.

acute coryza Acute rhinitis, also known as the common cold; an inflammatory condition of the mucous membranes of the nose and accessory sinuses.

adaptive immunity Protection that provides a specific reaction to each invading antigen and has the unique ability to remember the antigen that caused the attack.

adherence Following a prescribed regimen of therapy or treatment for disease.

adventitious Abnormal sounds superimposed on breath sounds.

agnosia Total or partial loss of the ability to recognize familiar objects or people through sensory stimuli; results from organic brain damage.

air embolism An abnormal circulatory condition in which air travels through the bloodstream and becomes lodged in a blood vessel.

allergen A substance that can produce a hypersensitive reaction in the body but that is not necessarily inherently harmful.

alopecia Loss of hair resulting from destruction of hair follicles.

amenorrhea Absence of menstrual flow.

anaphylactic shock Severe, life-threatening hypersensitivity reaction to a previously encountered antigen.

anasarca Severe, generalized edema.

anastomosis Surgical joining of two ducts or blood vessels to allow flow from one to the other.

anatomy The study, classification, and description of structures and organs of the body.

anemia Blood disorder characterized by red blood cell, hemoglobin, and hematocrit levels below normal range.

anesthesia Absence of sensation (*an-*, meaning "without," and -*esthesia*, meaning "awareness or feeling").

aneurysm A localized dilation of the wall of a blood vessel, usually caused by atherosclerosis, hypertension, and less commonly by a congenital weakness in a vessel wall.

angina pectoris Paroxysmal thoracic pain and choking feeling caused by decreased oxygen (anoxia) of the myocardium.

ankylosis Fixation of a joint, often in an abnormal position, usually resulting from destruction of articular cartilage and subchondral bone.

antigen A substance recognized by the body as foreign that can trigger an immune response.

anuria Urinary output of less than 100 to 250 mL in 24 hours.

aphasia Abnormal neurologic condition in which language function is defective or absent because of an injury to certain areas of the cerebral cortex.

aplasia In hematology, a failure of the normal process of cell generation and development.

apraxia Impairment of the ability to perform purposeful acts; inability to use objects properly.

arteriosclerosis Common arterial disorder characterized by thickening, loss of elasticity, and calcification of arterial walls, resulting in a decreased blood supply.

arthrocentesis Puncture of a joint with a needle to withdraw fluid; performed to obtain synovial fluid for diagnostic purposes.

arthrodesis Surgical fusion of a joint.

arthroplasty Surgical repair or refashioning of one of both sides, parts, or specific tissues within a joint.

ascites An accumulation of fluid and albumin in the peritoneal cavity.

---

*From Chabner, D. (2004). *The language of medicine.* (7th ed.). Philadelphia: Saunders.

asterixis Hand-flapping tremor usually induced by extending the arm and dorsiflexing the wrist; frequently seen in hepatic coma.

asthenia General feeling of tiredness and listlessness.

astigmatism Defect in the curvature of the eyeball surface.

ataxia Abnormal condition characterized by impaired ability to coordinate movement.

atelectasis Collapse of lung tissues, preventing the respiratory exchange of carbon dioxide and oxygen.

atherosclerosis A common arterial disorder characterized by yellowish plaques of cholesterol, lipids, and cellular debris in the inner layer of the walls of large and medium-sized arteries.

attenuation The process of weakening the degree of virulence of a disease organism.

audiometry Testing of hearing acuity.

aura Sensation, as of light or warmth, that may precede the onset of a migraine or an epileptic seizure. An epileptic aura may be psychic, or it may be sensory with olfactory, visual, auditory, or taste hallucinations.

autograft Surgical transplantation of any tissue from one part of the body to another location in the same individual.

autoimmune/autoimmunity Immune response (autoantibodies or cellular immune response) to one's own tissues.

autologous Something that has its origin within an individual, especially a factor present in tissues or fluids.

azotemia Retention of excessive amounts of nitrogenous compounds in the blood.

B

bacteriuria Presence of bacteria in the urine.

benign Not recurrent or progressive; opposite of malignant.

biopsy The removal of a small piece of living tissue from an organ or another part of the body for microscopic examination to confirm or establish a diagnosis, estimate a prognosis, or follow the course of a disease.

bipolar hip replacement (hemiarthroplasty) Prosthetic implant used to replace the femoral head and neck in hip fractures when the vascular supply to the femoral head is or may become compromised.

blanching test A test of the rate of capillary refill; blanching means to cause to become pale by applying digital pressure.

bradycardia Slow rhythm characterized by a pulse rate of fewer than 60 beats per minute.

bradykinesia An abnormal condition characterized by slowness of voluntary movements and speech.

bronchoscopy Visual examination of the larynx, trachea, and bronchi using a standard rigid, tubular metal bronchoscope or a narrower, flexible fiberoptic bronchoscope.

B-type natriuretic peptide (BNP) A neurohormone secreted by the heart in response to ventricular expansion.

C

cachexia General ill health and malnutrition marked by weakness and emaciation; usually associated with a serious disease such as cancer.

callus Bony deposits formed between and around the broken ends of a fractured bone during healing.

candidiasis Mild fungal infection that appears in men and women; usually caused by *Candida albicans* and *C. tropicalis.*

carcinoembryonic antigen (CEA) Oncofetal glycoprotein antigen found in colonic adenocarcinoma and other cancers; also found in nonmalignant conditions.

carcinogen Substance known to increase the risk for the development of cancer.

carcinogenesis Various factors that are possible origins of cancer.

carcinoma The term used for a malignant tumor composed of epithelial cells; it displays a tendency to metastasize.

carcinoma in situ Preinvasive, asymptomatic carcinoma that can be diagnosed only by microscopic examination of cervical cells.

cardiac arrest Sudden cessation of functional circulation.

cardioversion Restoration of the heart's normal sinus rhythm by delivery of a synchronized electric shock through two metal paddles placed on the patient's chest.

catabolism Breakdown or destructive phase of metabolism. Catabolism occurs when complex body substances are broken down to simpler ones; opposite of anabolism.

cataract Opacity or clouding of the lens.

CD$_4^+$ lymphocyte A type of white blood cell; a protein on the surface of cells that normally helps the body's immune system combat disease.

cell The fundamental unit of all living tissue.

cellular immunity Acquired immunity characterized by the dominant role of small T lymphocytes; also called *cell-mediated immunity.*

Centers for Disease Control and Prevention (CDC) Federal agency that provides facilities and services for investigation, identification, prevention, and control of disease; headquartered in Atlanta, Georgia.

chancre Painless erosion of a papule that ulcerates superficially with a scooped-out appearance.

Chlamydia trachomatis A gram-negative intracellular bacterium that causes several common sexually transmitted diseases.

Chvostek's sign Abnormal spasm of the facial muscles elicited by light taps on the facial nerve in patients who are hypocalcemic; seen in tetany.

circumcision Surgical procedure in which a part of the foreskin is removed, leaving the glans penis uncovered.

climacteric Phase of the aging process marking the transition from the reproductive phase to a nonreproductive stage of life.

Colles' fracture A fracture of the distal portion of the radius within 1 inch of the joint of the wrist.

colporrhaphy Surgical correction of cystocele and rectocele by shortening the muscles that support the bladder and repair the rectocele.

colposcopy Examination of the cervix and vagina using a colposcope.

compartment syndrome Pathologic condition caused by progressive development of arterial compression and reduced blood supply to an extremity. Increased pressure from external devices (casts, bulky dressings) causes decreased blood flow, resulting in ischemic tissue necrosis; most often occurs in the extremities.

conjunctivitis Inflammation of the conjunctiva.

conscious sedation Administration of central nervous system depressant drugs and/or analgesia to relieve anxiety and/or provide amnesia during surgical, diagnostic, or interventional procedures.

contracture Abnormal, usually permanent condition of a joint characterized by flexion and fixation and caused by atrophy and shortening of muscle fibers.

coronary artery disease (CAD) Variety of conditions that obstruct blood flow in the coronary arteries.

cor pulmonale Abnormal cardiac condition characterized by hypertrophy of the right ventricle of the heart as a result of hypertension of the pulmonary circulation.

coryza Acute inflammation of the mucous membranes of the nose and accessory sinuses, usually accompanied by edema of the mucosa and nasal discharge.

costovertebral angle Pertaining to a rib and a vertebra; one of two angles that outline a space over the kidneys.

crackle(s) Short, discrete, interrupted crackling or bubbling adventitious breath sounds heard on auscultation of the chest, most commonly upon inspiration. They are produced by passage of air through the bronchi that contain secretions of exudate or are constricted by spasms or thickening; usually heard during inspiration; formerly called rales.

crepitus Sound that resembles the crackling noise heard when rubbing hair between the fingers or throwing salt on an open fire. It is associated with gas gangrene, the rubbing of bone fragments, or the crackles of a consolidated area of the lung in pneumonia.

cryosurgery Procedure to "freeze" the border of a retinal hole with a frozen-tipped probe.

cryotherapy A procedure in which a topical anesthetic is used so that a cryoprobe can be placed directly on the surface of the eye.

cryptorchidism Failure of testes to descend into the scrotum.

culdoscopy Diagnostic procedure that provides visualization of the uterus and adnexa (uterine appendages that include the ovaries and fallopian tubes).

curettage Scraping of material from the wall of a cavity or other surface; performed to remove tumors or other abnormal tissue for microscopic study.

Curling's ulcer Duodenal ulcer that develops 8 to 14 days after severe burns on the surface of the body; the first sign is usually vomiting of bright red blood.

cyanosis Slightly bluish, gray, slatelike, or dark purple discoloration of the skin resulting from the presence of abnormally reduced amounts of oxygenated hemoglobin in the blood.

cytology/cytologic evaluation Study of cells and their formation, origin, structure, biochemical activities, and pathology.

cytoplasm "Living matter"; a substance that exists only in cells, composed largely of a gel-like substance that contains water, minerals, enzymes, and other specialized materials.

D

debridement Removal of damaged cellular tissue from a wound or burn to prevent infection and promote healing.

deep brain stimulation (DBS) Involves placing an electrode in either the thalamus, globus pallidus, or subthalamic nucleus and connecting it to a generator placed in the upper chest (like a pacemaker).

defibrillation The termination of ventricular fibrillation by delivering a direct electrical countershock to the precordium.

dehiscence Partial or complete separation of a surgical incision or rupture of a wound closure.

dendrite Branching process that extends from the cell body of a neuron and receives impulses.

diabetes mellitus (See type 1 diabetes mellitus; type 2 diabetes mellitus.)

diabetic retinopathy Disorder of retinal blood vessels characterized by capillary microaneurysms, hemorrhage, exudates, and formation of new vessels and connective tissue.

dialysis Medical procedure for the removal of certain elements from the blood or lymph by virtue of the difference in their rates of diffusion through an external semipermeable membrane or, in the case of peritoneal dialysis, through the peritoneum.

differentiated Describes a tumor that is most like the parent tissue.

diffusion A process in which solid particles in a fluid move from an area of higher concentration to an area of lower concentration.

diplopia Double vision.

disseminated intravascular coagulation (DIC) Acquired hemorrhage syndrome of clotting, cascade overstimulation, and anticlotting processes.

diuresis Secretion and passage of large amounts of urine.

dorsal Toward the back.

drainage Free flow or withdrawal of fluids from a wound or cavity by some sort of system (such as a urinary catheter or T-tube).

dysarthria Difficult, poorly articulated speech resulting from interference in the control over the muscles of speech.

dysmenorrhea Painful menstruation.

dysphagia Difficulty swallowing.

dyspnea Shortness of breath or difficulty in breathing; may be caused by disturbances in the lungs, certain heart conditions, and hemoglobin deficiency.

dysrhythmia Any disturbance or abnormality in a normal rhythmic pattern, specifically irregularity in the normal rhythm of the heart; also called *arrhythmia*.

dysuria Painful or difficult urination.

E

embolism An abnormal circulatory condition in which an embolus (e.g., a foreign substance, blood clot, fat, air, or amniotic fluid) travels through the bloodstream and becomes lodged in a blood vessel.

embolus A foreign object, quantity of air or gas, bit of tissue or tumor, or a piece of thrombus that circulates in the bloodstream until it becomes lodged in a vessel.

empyema Accumulation of pus in a body cavity, especially the pleural space, as a result of infection.

endarterectomy Surgical removal of the intimal lining of an artery.

endocrinologist Physician who specializes in endocrinology.

endometriosis Condition in which endometrial tissue appears outside the uterus.

enucleation Surgical removal of the eyeball.

enzyme-linked immunosorbent assay (ELISA) Antibody test that uses a rapid enzyme immunochemical assay method to detect HIV antibodies.

epididymitis Infection of the cordlike excretory duct of the testicles.

epistaxis Hemorrhage from the nose; nosebleed.

erythrocytosis Abnormal increase in the number of circulating red blood cells.

erythropoiesis The process of red blood cell production.

eschar Black, leathery crust; a slough that the body forms over burned tissue.

esophageal varices A complex of longitudinal, tortuous veins at the lower end of the esophagus.

evisceration Protrusion of an internal organ through a disrupted wound or surgical incision.

exacerbation An increase in the seriousness of a disease or disorder; marked by greater intensity in the signs or symptoms of the patient being treated.

excoriation Injury to the surface layer of skin caused by scratching or abrasion.

exophthalmos An abnormal condition characterized by a marked protrusion of the eyeballs.

extravasation The escape of fluids into surrounding tissue.

extrinsic Caused by external factors.

extubate To remove an endotracheal tube from an airway.

exudate Fluid, cells, or other substances that have been slowly exuded or discharged from body cells or blood vessels through small pores or breaks in cell membrane.

F

fibromyalgia A musculoskeletal chronic pain syndrome of unknown etiology that causes pain in muscles, bones, or joints.

filtration The transfer of water and dissolved substances from an area of higher pressure to an area of lower pressure.

fistula Abnormal opening between two organs.

flaccid Weak, soft, and flabby; lacking normal muscle tone.

flail chest Two or more ribs fractured in two or more places resulting in instability in part of the chest wall with associated hemothorax, pneumothorax, and pulmonary contusion.

flatulence Excessive formation of gases in the stomach or intestine.

G

Glasgow coma scale A quick, practical, standardized system for assessing the degree of conscious impairment in the critically ill; also used for predicting the duration and ultimate outcome of coma, primarily in patients with head injuries.

glaucoma An abnormal condition of elevated pressure within an eye because of obstruction of the outflow of aqueous humor.

global cognitive dysfunction Generalized impairment of intellect, awareness, and judgment.

glycosuria Abnormal presence of sugar, especially glucose in the urine.

H

heart failure (HF) Syndrome characterized by circulatory congestion due to the heart's inability to act as an effective pump; it should be viewed as a neurohormonal problem in which pathology progresses as a result of chronic release in the body of substances such as catecholamines (epinephrine and norepinephrine).

hemarthrosis Bleeding into a joint space, a hallmark of severe disease usually occurring in the knees, ankles, and elbow.

hematemesis Vomiting blood.

hematuria Blood in the urine.

hemianopia Defective vision or blindness in half of the visual field.

hemiplegia Paralysis of one side of the body.

hemophilia A Hereditary coagulation disorder; caused by a lack of antihemophilic factor VIII, which is needed to convert prothrombin to thrombin through thromboplastin component.

hemoptysis Expectorating blood from the respiratory tract.

hepatic encephalopathy A type of brain damage caused by a liver disease and consequent ammonia intoxication.

hepatitis Inflammation of the liver resulting from several causes, including several types of viral agents or exposure to toxic substances.

heterograft (xenograft) Tissue from another species, used as a temporary graft.

heterozygous Having two different genes.

hirsutism Excessive body hair in a masculine distribution.

HIV disease Symptomatic human immunodeficiency virus (HIV) infection that is not severe enough for a diagnosis of acquired immunodeficiency syndrome (AIDS); symptoms of HIV disease are persistent unexplained fever, night sweats, diarrhea, weight loss, and fatigue.

HIV infection The state in which HIV enters the body under favorable conditions and multiplies, producing injurious effects.

homeostasis A relative constancy in the internal environment of the body, naturally maintained by adaptive responses that promote healthy survival.

homograft (allograft) The transfer of tissue between two genetically dissimilar individuals of the same species, such as a skin transplant between two humans who are not identical twins.

homozygous Having two identical genes, inherited from each parent, for a given hereditary characteristic.

human immunodeficiency virus (HIV) An obligate virus; a retrovirus that causes AIDS.

humoral immunity One of the two forms of immunity that respond to antigens such as bacteria and foreign tissue. It is mediated by B cells.

hydronephrosis The dilation of the renal pelvis and calyces.

hypercapnia Greater than normal amounts of carbon dioxide in the blood.

hyperglycemia A greater than normal amount of glucose in the blood.

hyperopia Farsightedness; inability to see objects at close range.

hyperreflexia Neurologic condition characterized by increased reflex reactions.

hypersensitivity An abnormal condition characterized by an excessive reaction to a particular stimulus.

hypocalcemia A deficiency of calcium in serum.

hypoglycemia A lower than normal amount of glucose in the blood; usually caused by administration of too much insulin, excessive secretion of insulin by the islet cells of the pancreas, or dietary deficiency.

hypokalemia A condition in which an inadequate amount of potassium, the major intracellular cation, is found in the circulatory bloodstream.

hypoventilation An abnormal condition of the respiratory system that occurs when the volume of air is not adequate for the metabolic needs of the body.

hypoxemia An abnormal deficiency of oxygen in the arterial blood.

hypoxia An inadequate, reduced tension of cellular oxygen.

I

idiopathic Cause unknown.

idiopathic hyperplasia Increase, without any known cause, in the number of cells.

ileal conduit Ureters are implanted into a loop of the ileum that is isolated and brought to the surface of the abdominal wall.

immunity The quality of being unsusceptible to or unaffected by a particular disease condition.

immunization A process by which resistance to an infectious disease is induced or increased.

immunocompetence/immunocompetent The ability of an immune system to mobilize and deploy its antibodies and other responses to stimulation by an antigen.

immunodeficiency An abnormal condition of the immune system in which cellular or humoral immunity is inadequate and resistance to infection is increased.

immunogen Any agent or substance capable of provoking an immune response or producing immunity.

immunology Study of the immune system; the reaction of tissues of the immune system of the body of antigenic stimulation.

immunosuppression/immunosuppressive Administration of agents that significantly interfere with the ability of the immune system to respond to antigenic stimulation by inhibiting cellular and humoral immunity.

immunosurveillance The immune system's recognition and destruction of newly developed abnormal cells.

immunotherapy A special treatment of allergic responses; involves the administration of increasingly larger doses of the offending allergens to gradually develop immunity.

incentive spirometry A procedure in which a device (spirometer) is used at the bedside at regular intervals to encourage a patient to breathe deeply.

incision Surgical cut produced by a sharp instrument to create an opening into an organ or space in the body.

infarct Localized area of necrosis in tissue, a vessel, or an organ resulting from tissue anoxia; caused by an interruption in the blood supply to an area.

informed consent Permission obtained from the patient to perform a specific test or procedure.

innate immunity The body's first line of defense; provides physical and chemical barriers to invading pathogens and protects the body against the external environment.

intermittent claudication A weakness of the legs accompanied by cramplike pains in the calves; caused by poor arterial circulation of the blood to the leg muscles.

intraoperative Pertaining to a period of time during a surgical procedure.

intrinsic Caused by internal factors.

introitus An entrance to a cavity (e.g., the vaginal introitus).

intussusception Infolding of one segment of the intestine into the lumen of another segment; occurs in children.

ischemia Decreased blood supply to a body organ or part; often marked by pain and organ dysfunction.

J

jaundice Yellowish discoloration of the skin, mucous membranes, and sclera of the eyes caused by greater than normal amounts of bilirubin in the blood.

K

Kaposi's sarcoma (KS) Rare cancer of the skin or mucous membranes; characterized by blue, red, or purple raised lesions and seen mainly in middle-aged Mediterranean men and those with HIV disease.

keloids Overgrowths of collagenous scar tissue at the site of a skin wound.

keratitis An inflammation of the cornea.

keratoplasty Excision of the corneal tissue, followed by surgical implantation of a cornea from another human donor.

ketoacidosis Acidosis accompanied by an accumulation of ketone in the blood resulting from faulty carbohydrate metabolism.

ketone bodies Normal metabolic products, β-hydroxybutyric and aminoacetic acid, from which acetone may spontaneously arise.

kyphosis An abnormal condition of the vertebral column; characterized by increased convexity in the curvature of the thoracic spine.

L

labyrinthitis Inflammation of the labyrinthine canals of the inner ear.

laparoscopy The examination of the abdominal cavity with a laparoscope through a small incision beneath the umbilicus.

leukemia Malignant disorder of the hematopoietic system in which an excess of leukocytes accumulates in the bone marrow and lymph nodes.

leukopenia An abnormal decrease in the number of white blood cells to fewer than 5000 cells/mm^3 due to depression of the bone marrow.

leukoplakia A white patch in the mouth or on the tongue.

lipodystrophy Abnormality in the metabolism or deposition of fats. Insulin lipodystrophy is the loss of local fat deposits in diabetic patients as a complication of repeated insulin injections.

lordosis An increase in the curve at the lumbar space region that throws the shoulder back, making the appearance "lordly or kingly."

lumen Space within an artery, vein, intestine, or tube such as a needle or catheter.

lymphangitis Inflammation of one or more lymphatic vessels or channels; usually results from an acute streptococcal or staphylococcal infection in an extremity.

lymphedema Primary or secondary disorder characterized by the accumulation of lymph in soft tissue and edema.

lymphokine One of the chemical factors produced and released by T lymphocytes that attract macrophages to the site of infection or inflammation and prepare them for attack.

M

macules Small, flat, discolored blemishes; flush with the skin surface.

malignant Growing worse, resisting treatment; said of cancerous growths. Also tending or threatening to produce death; harmful.

mammography Radiography of the soft tissue of the breast to allow identification of various benign and neoplastic processes.

mastoiditis Infection of one of the mastoid bones.

melena Abnormal, black, tarry stool containing digested blood.

membrane Thin sheet of tissue that serves many functions in the body; it covers surfaces, lines and lubricates hollow organs, and protects and anchors organs and bones.

menorrhagia Excessive menstrual flow.

metastasis The process by which tumor cells are spread to distant parts of the body.

metrorrhagia Excessive spotting between cycles.

micturition Urination.

miotic Causing constriction of the pupil of the eye.

mitosis Type of cell division of somatic (i.e., nonreproductive) cells in which each daughter cell contains the same number of chromosomes as the parent cell.

multiple myeloma A malignant neoplastic immunodeficiency disease of the bone marrow; the tumor is composed of plasma cells.

mydriatic Causing pupillary dilation.

myeloproliferative Excessive bone marrow production.

myocardial infarction An occlusion of a major coronary artery or one of its branches; it is caused by atherosclerosis or an embolus resulting in necrosis of a portion of cardiac muscle.

myopia Condition of nearsightedness; inability to see objects at a distance.

myringotomy A surgical incision of the tympanic membrane to relieve pressure and release purulent exudate from the middle ear.

N

neoplasm Uncontrolled or abnormal growth of cells.

nephrotoxin Substances with specific destructive properties for the kidneys, such as certain antibiotics, heavy metals, solvents, and chemicals.

neuropathy Any abnormal condition characterized by inflammation and degeneration of the peripheral nerves.

nevi Pigmented, congenital skin blemishes that are usually benign but may become cancerous.

nocturia Excessive urination at night.

nucleus Largest organelle within the cell; it is responsible for cell reproduction and control of the other organelles.

nystagmus Involuntary, rhythmic movement of the eyes. Oscillations may be horizontal, vertical, rotary, or mixed.

O

occlusion An obstruction or closing off in a canal, vessel, or passage of the body.

occult blood Blood that is hidden or obscured from view.

oliguria A diminished capacity to form and pass urine (less than 500 mL in 24 hours); result is that the end products of metabolism cannot be excreted efficiently.

oncology The sum of knowledge regarding tumors; the branch of medicine that deals with the study of tumors.

open reduction with internal fixation (ORIF) A surgical procedure allowing fracture alignment under direct visualization while using various internal fixation devices applied to the bone.

opportunistic Disease characteristic caused by a normally nonpathogenic organism in a host whose resistance has been decreased by a disorder such as AIDS.

organ A group of several different kinds of tissue arranged so that they can work together to perform a special function.

orthopnea An abnormal condition in which a person must sit or stand to breathe deeply or comfortably.

osmosis Passage of water across a selectively permeable membrane; the water moves from a less concentrated solution to a more concentrated solution.

P

palliative Designed to relieve pain and distress and to control the signs and symptoms of disease; not designed to produce a cure.

pancytopenia Deficient condition of all three major blood elements (red cells, white cells, and platelets); results from the bone marrow being reduced or absent.

panhysterosalpingo-oophorectomy Removal of the uterus, fallopian tubes, and ovaries; also called total abdominal hysterectomy with bilateral salpingo-oophorectomy.

Papanicolaou test (Pap smear) A simple smear method of examining stained exfoliative cells; used most commonly to detect cancers of the cervix.

papules Palpable, circumscribed, red solid elevations in the skin; smaller than 0.5 cm.

paracentesis A procedure in which fluid is withdrawn from the abdominal cavity.

paralytic (adynamic) ileus Most common type of intestinal obstruction; a decrease in or absence of intestinal peristalsis and bowel sounds that may occur after abdominal surgery.

parenchyma Tissue of an organ as distinguished from supporting or connective tissue.

paresis A lesser degree of movement deficit from partial or incomplete paralysis.

paresthesia Any subjective sensation, such as a prickling "pins and needles" feeling or numbness.

passive transport The movement of small molecules across the membrane of a cell by diffusion; no cellular energy is required.

pathognomonic Sign or symptom specific to a disease condition.

pediculosis Lice infestation.

perioperative Entire surgical inpatient period occurring immediately before, during, and immediately after surgery.

peripheral Pertaining to the outside, surface, or surrounding area of an organ, other structure or fluid of vision.

pernicious Capable of causing great injury or destruction; deadly, fatal.

phagocytic Refers to the ingestion and digestion of bacteria.

phagocytosis The process that permits a cell to surround or engulf any foreign material and digest it.

phimosis A condition in which the prepuce is too small to allow retraction of the foreskin over the glans penis.

physiology Explanation of the processes and functions of the various structures of the body and how they interrelate.

pinocytosis The process by which extracellular fluid is ingested by the cells.

plasmapheresis Removal of plasma that contains components causing or thought to cause disease. Also called *plasma exchange* because when the plasma is removed, it is replaced by substitution fluids such as saline or albumin.

pleural effusion An abnormal accumulation of fluid in the thoracic cavity between the visceral and parietal pleurae.

pleural friction rub Low-pitched, grating, or creaking lung sounds that occur when inflamed pleural surfaces rub together during respiration.

***Pneumocystis jiroveci* (formerly *carinii*) pneumonia (PCP)** An unusual pulmonary disease caused by a parasite that is primarily associated with people who have suppressed immune systems, especially in people with AIDS.

pneumothorax A collection of air or gas in the pleural space, causing the lung to collapse.

polycythemia Abnormal increase in the number of red blood cells in the blood.

polydipsia Excessive thirst.

polyphagia Eating to the point of gluttony.

polyuria Excretion of an abnormally large quantity of urine.

postictal period A rest period of variable length after a tonic-clonic seizure.

postoperative Pertaining to a period of time after surgery.

preoperative Pertaining to a period of time before surgery.

procidentia Protrusion of the entire uterus through the introitus.

proliferation Reproduction or multiplication of similar forms.

proprioception Sensation pertaining to stimuli originating from within the body regarding spatial position and muscular activity stimuli or to the sensory receptors that those stimuli activate. This sensation gives one the ability to know the position of the body without looking at it and the ability to "know objectively the sense of touch."

prostatodynia Pain in the prostate gland.

prosthesis Artificial replacement for a missing body part.

pruritus The symptoms of itching; an uncomfortable sensation leading to the urge to scratch; scratching often leads to secondary infection. Some causes of pruritus are allergy, infection, elevated serum urea, jaundice, and skin irritation.

pulmonary edema Accumulation of extravascular fluid in lung tissues and alveoli; caused most commonly by left-sided heart failure.

pustulant vesicles Small, circumscribed pus-containing elevations of the skin.

pyuria Pus in the urine.

R

radial keratotomy Microscopic incisions on the surface of the cornea outside the optical area. These eight spokelike incisions flatten the cornea to a more normal curvature, thus reducing or eliminating myopia.

Reed-Sternberg cells Atypical histocytes; large, abnormal, multinucleated cells in the lymphatic system, found in Hodgkin's lymphoma.

remission A decrease in the severity of a disease or any of its symptoms.

residual urine Urine remaining in the urinary tract after voiding.

retention The inability to void even in the presence of an urge to void.

retinal detachment Separation of the retina from the choroid in the posterior of the eye.

retrovirus Lentivirus that contains reverse transcriptase, which is essential for reverse transcription (the production of a deoxyribonucleic acid [DNA] molecule from a ribonucleic acid [RNA] model).

rule of nines Division of the body into multiples of nine; used to determine the total body surface area (BSA) involved in burn trauma.

S

sarcoma Malignant tumor of connective tissues such as muscle or bone; usually presents as a painless swelling.

scoliosis Curvature of the spine usually consisting of two curves: the original abnormal curve and a compensatory curve in the opposite direction.

sentinel lymph node mapping Diagnostic tool used before therapeutic surgery, which identifies the first lymph node most likely to drain cancerous cells; used in axillary lymph node biopsy, specifically in breast cancer staging.

sequestrum A fragment of necrotic bone that is partially or entirely detached from the surrounding or adjacent healthy bone.

seroconversion The development of detectable levels of antibodies; a change in serologic tests (e.g., ELISA and Western blot) from negative to positive as antibodies develop in reaction to an infection.

seronegative Negative result on serologic examination. The state of lacking HIV antibodies; confirmed by blood tests.

sibilant wheeze Musical, high-pitched, squeaking, or whistlelike sound caused by the rapid movement of air through narrowed bronchioles.

singultus Hiccup.

Sjögren syndrome Dry eye syndrome; an immunologic disorder characterized by low fluid production by lacrimal (tear), salivary, and other glands, resulting in abnormal dryness of mouth, eyes, and other mucous membranes.

Snellen's test Eye chart test for visual acuity; letters, numbers, or symbols are arranged on the chart in decreasing size from top to bottom.

sonorous wheeze Low-pitched, loud, coarse, snoring sound.

spastic Involuntary, sudden movements or muscular contractions with increased reflexes.

spider telangiectases Dilated superficial arterioles.

stapedectomy The removal of the stapes of the middle ear and insertion of a graft and prosthesis.

steatorrhea Excessive fat in the feces.

stertorous Pertaining to a respiratory effort that is strenuous and struggling, which provokes a snoring sound.

stoma Combining form meaning a mouth or opening.

stomatitis Inflammation of the mouth due to destruction of normal cells of the oral cavity that may result from infection by bacteria, viruses, or fungi from exposure to certain chemicals or drugs, vitamin deficiency, or systemic inflammatory disease.

strabismus Condition in which the eyes are unable to focus in the same direction; commonly called *cross-eyed*.

stroke An abnormal condition of the blood vessels of the brain characterized by hemorrhage into the brain; formation of an embolus or thrombus resulting in ischemia of the brain tissues normally perfused by the damaged vessels. The sequelae depend on the location and extent of ischemia.

subluxation Partial dislocation.

suppuration To produce purulent material.

surgery Branch of medicine concerned with diseases and trauma requiring operative procedures.

surgical asepsis A group of techniques that destroy all microorganisms and their spores (sterile technique).

system An organization of varying numbers and kinds of organs arranged so that they can work together to perform complex functions for the body.

T

tachycardia An abnormal condition in which the myocardium contracts regularly but at a rate greater than 100 beats per minute.

tachypnea An abnormally rapid rate of breathing.

tenesmus Persistent, ineffectual spasms of the rectum or bladder, accompanied by the desire to empty the bowel or bladder.

thoracentesis The surgical perforation of the chest wall and pleural space with a needle for the aspiration of fluid for diagnostic or therapeutic purposes.

thrombocytopenia An abnormal hematologic condition in which the number of platelets is reduced to fewer than 100,000/mm^3.

thrombus Of or pertaining to a clot.

tinnitus A subjective noise sensation in one or both ears; ringing or tinkling sound in the ear.

tissue An organization of many similar cells that act together to perform a common function.

tophi Calculi containing sodium urate deposits that develop in periarticular fibrous tissue; typically found in patients with gout.

trichomoniasis A sexually transmitted disease caused by the protozoan *Trichomonas vaginalis*.

Trousseau's sign A test for latent tetany in which carpal spasms are induced by inflating a sphygmomanometer cuff on the upper arm to a pressure exceeding systolic blood pressure for 3 minutes; used in hypocalcemia and hypomagnesemia.

tumor lysis syndrome Oncologic emergency that occurs with rapid lysis of malignant cells; most frequently associated with chemotherapy treatment. It is most commonly a result of treatment-related malignant cell death in patients with large tumor cell burdens.

turgor The normal resiliency of the skin caused by the outward pressure of the cells and interstitial fluid; may be assessed as increased or decreased skin turgor.

tympanoplasty One of several operative procedures on the eardrum or ossicles of the middle ear designed to restore or improve hearing in patients with conductive hearing loss.

type 1 diabetes mellitus Condition in which impaired glucose tolerance results because of destruction of beta cells in the pancreatic islets; results in deficient insulin production, but the patient retains normal sensitivity to insulin action; also called insulin-dependent diabetes mellitus.

type 2 diabetes mellitus Condition in which impaired glucose tolerance results from an abnormal resistance to insulin action; also called non–insulin-dependent diabetes mellitus.

U

unilateral neglect Condition in which an individual is perceptually unaware of and inattentive to one side of the body.

urolithiasis Formation of urinary calculi.

urticaria Itching skin eruption characterized by welts of varying sizes with well-defined inflamed margins and pale centers (also called *hives*).

V

ventral Facing forward; the front of the body.

verruca Benign, viral, warty skin lesion with a rough, papillomatous (nipplelike) growth.

vertical transmission Transmission of HIV from a mother to a fetus; can occur during pregnancy, during delivery, or through postpartum breastfeeding.

vertigo The sensation that the outer world is revolving about oneself or that one is moving in space.

vesicle Circumscribed elevation of skin filled with serous fluid.

viral load Amount of measurable HIV virions.

virulent Having the power to produce disease; of or pertaining to a very pathogenic or rapidly progressive condition.

Volkmann's contracture A permanent contracture with clawhand, flexion of wrist and finger, and atrophy of the forearm; can occur as a result of compartment syndrome.

volvulus Twisting of the bowel on itself, causing intestinal obstruction.

W

Western blot A laboratory blood test to detect the presence of antibodies to a specific antigen; used in diagnosing HIV.

wheals Irregularly shaped, elevated areas, white in the center with a pale red periphery, with superficial localized edema; vary in size (hives, mosquito bite).

Index

A

Abacavir, 753-756t
Abacavir/lamivudine, 753-756t
Abaracept, 119-122t
ABCDE mnemonic
    for preoperative patient, 20b
    for skin lesions, 67-68
ABCDs of melanoma, 93f
ABCs of immediate recovery, 45t
Abdomen, regions of, 3, 3f
Abdominal aorta, atherosclerotic
    lesions in, 355f
Abdominal aortic aneurysm repair,
    360f
Abdominal cavity, 2, 3f, 3t
Abdominal distention, postopera-
    tive, 52
Abdominal hysterectomy, 569-570
Abdominal surgery, areas for surgi-
    cal skin preparation, 27f
Abduction, 113
    after total hip replacement, 135,
    136f
Abduction splint, 140
Ablation, 18, 18t
Abnormal spinal curvatures, 170,
    170f
Abnormal uterine bleeding, 548-550
ABO blood types, 266-267, 267f
Abrasion, corneal, 628
Abscess
    brain, 706
    in diverticulosis and diverticuli-
    tis, 214
    hepatic, 247-248
    pancreatic, 253
Absence seizure, 677-678t
Acanthamoebic keratitis, 615
Acarbose, 520, 520t
Acceleration-deceleration injury, 708
Accessory glands
    of female reproductive system,
    537, 537f
    of male reproductive system,
    534-535
Accessory organs, 12-14t
    of digestive system, 175-176, 179,
    179f
Accommodation, vision and, 604
Acebutolol, 318-319t
Acetaminophen
    for fibromyalgia syndrome, 132t
    hepatotoxicity of, 240
    for neuropathic pain, 668
Acetazolamide, 444, 625-627, 625-626t
Acetic acid, 637-638t
Acetylcholine, 652
Acetylcysteine, 401-403t
Acetylsalicylic acid; See Aspirin
Achalasia, 189-190, 190b
Achlorhydria, 180, 275-276
Acid-base disturbances, 383t
Acid-fast bacillus isolation, 400
Acidosis in end-stage renal disease,
    471
Acid-perfusion test, 181
Acne, 62f, 83-84, 83f
    in premenstrual syndrome,
    550-551

Acoustic nerve, 604f, 605f, 656f, 657f
Acquired aplastic anemia, 273
Acquired immunity, 720-721, 720t,
    721f
Acquired immunodeficiency syn-
    drome; See Human immunode-
    ficiency virus infection
Acral lentiginous melanoma, 92-93
Acromegaly, 489-491, 489f
Active transport, 8-9, 8t
Activities of daily living
    epilepsy and, 678, 678b
    paralyzed patient and, 673f, 674,
    674f
    vision loss and, 610
Activity
    after total knee replacement, 134
    motor function disturbances and,
    673
    multiple sclerosis and, 682
    Parkinson's disease and, 685
Acute abdominal inflammations,
    212-216, 213b, 214f, 215f
Acute intervention in HIV infection,
    759t, 763-769, 764b
Acute otitis media, 636-639
Acute phase of burn, 98-101, 99f,
    102b
Acute respiratory distress syn-
    drome, 418-420
Acute retroviral syndrome, 745,
    745t
Acyclovir, 70-71t, 549-550t
    for Bell's palsy, 702
    for genital herpes, 588
    for herpes simplex infection, 69
    for herpes simplex virus enceph-
    alitis, 705
    for keratitis, 615
    for shingles, 72
Adalimumab, 119-122t
Adaptive immunity, 720-721, 720t,
    721f
Addisonian crisis, 507
Addison's disease, 506-508, 507t
Adduction, 113
Adductor muscles, 113t, 114f
Adenocarcinoma, 459, 572
Adenohypophysis, 485
Adenoids, 374, 375f
Adenopathy in HIV infection, 745-
    746, 745t
Adenosine, 318-319t
Adenosine triphosphate, 6
Adrenal cortex, 486, 488f
Adrenal crisis, 506-507
Adrenal glands, 435, 435f, 486-487,
    488f
Adrenal medulla, 486-487, 488f
Adrenalectomy, 506
Adrenocortical steroids, preopera-
    tive, 36-37t
Adrenocorticotropic hormone, 486f
    Cushing's syndrome and, 504
    functions of, 487f
    for multiple sclerosis, 681
Advanced cardiac life support, 319
Adventitious breath sounds, 379,
    379t

Adynamic ileus, 218-219
Age-related macular degeneration,
    606, 621-622
Agglutination, 267
Aging
    cardiovascular system and, 312
    immune system and, 722-723
    integumentary system and, 103b
    nervous system and, 655
    peripheral vascular system and,
    348
    reproductive system and, 538
    thrombophlebitis and, 362
    urinary system and, 439
Agnosia, 675
Agranulocytosis, 281-282
AIDS; See Human immunodefi-
    ciency virus infection
AIDS-dementia complex, 767
Airbag deployment injury, 163
Airway
    burn injury and, 97, 98f
    immediate postoperative phase
    and, 45t
    laryngeal cancer and, 390
Akinetic seizure, 677-678t
Alanine aminotransferase, 231
Albumin, 232
    hypoalbuminemia and, 467
    in urine, 438
Albumin/globulin ratio, 232
Albuterol, 401-403t
Alcohol
    cancer risk and, 781
    hypertension and, 352, 354
    laryngeal cancer and, 389
    pancreatitis and, 253
Aldosterone, 435
Aldosteronism, 352t
Alendronate, 129, 129t
Alimentary canal, 175-180, 176f,
    177b
Aliskiren hemifumarate, 353
Alkaline phosphatase, 232, 545
    for cancer diagnosis, 788
    in musculoskeletal disorders,
    117t
Alkaline-ash foods, 445b
Alkylating agents, 793-794t
Allergen, 722, 727b
Allergic conjunctivitis, 386-387
Allergic rhinitis, 386-387
Allergy, 724, 725b, 727b, 728-729
    skin test for, 81
Allogenic bone marrow transplan-
    tation, 800
Allograft, 100, 729
Allopurinol, 127, 280, 458, 799
Almotriptan, 666
Alopecia, 94
    chemotherapy-related, 796
Alosteron, 204
Alpha cell, 487-488
Alpha-fetoprotein, 242
Alpha-glucosidase inhibitors, 520,
    520t
Alteplase, 329t, 698
Aluminum acetate solution, 70-71t
Alveolar disease, 421

Alveolar duct, 374f, 377
Alveolus, 308, 377, 377f
Alzheimer's disease, 688-690, 689f,
    690b, 691b
Amantadine, 685, 686-687t
Ambulation after surgery, 51-52,
    51b, 51f
    in musculoskeletal trauma,
    170-171
Ambulatory electrocardiography,
    309
Ambulatory surgery, 18t, 55-56
Amenorrhea, 489, 546-547
Amino acids, erythropoiesis and,
    277b
Aminoglutethimide, 576
Aminophylline, 401-403t
Amiodarone, 318-319t
Amitriptyline
    for cancer treatment symptoms,
    797-798t
    for fibromyalgia syndrome, 132t
    for interstitial cystitis, 454
    for premenstrual syndrome, 551
Amlopidine, 329t
Ammonia in urine, 438
Amoxicillin, 195, 202, 636, 637-638t
Amphiarthrosis, 110
Amphotericin B, 184
Ampicillin, 202
Amputation stump, bandaging of,
    168f
Amrinone, 329t
Amsler's grid test, 606-607, 608-609t
Amylase, 179
Amylopsin, 179
Amyotrophic lateral sclerosis, 693
Anakinra, 119-122t
Anal fissure and fistula, 226
Analgesics
    for acute otitis media, 636
    after pelvic surgery, 570
    for burn, 97-98
    for cancer pain, 801
    for external otitis, 635
    for gallstones, 249
    for keratitis, 615
    for myocardial infarction, 329t
    for pancreatitis, 254
    for pericarditis, 344
    for peritonitis, 216
    for pleurisy, 407
    preoperative, 36-37t
    for pulmonary edema, 416
Anaphase, 7f, 8
Anaphylaxis, 727-728
Anaplasia, 785
Anasarca, 467
Anastomosis, 19t
    in Billroth procedures, 195f
    in esophagogastrectomy, 189
Anastrozole, 576
Anatomy and physiology, 1-16
    abdominal regions and, 3, 3f
    abdominopelvic quadrants and,
    3, 4f
    body cavities and, 2, 3f, 3t
    body planes and, 2, 2f
    cardiovascular, 304-307

Page numbers followed by b indicate boxes; f, figures; t, tables.

Anatomy and physiology (Continued)
  cells and, 5-9
  endocrine, 485-489
  musculoskeletal, 109-113
  neurologic, 651-657
  organs and systems in, 12, 12-14t
  reproductive, 534-538
  respiratory, 374-378
  of skin, 59-61, 59b, 60f
  structural levels of organization
    and, 3-12, 4f
  tissues and, 9-12, 10t, 11f
  urinary, 12-14t, 434-439, 435f
  effects of surgery on, 23t
Anemia, 269-281
  aplastic, 273-274, 275b
  chemotherapy-related, 796
  in cirrhosis, 237
  in hepatic abscess, 247
  in HIV infection, 749, 766t
  in Hodgkin's lymphoma, 294-295
  hypovolemic, 271-272
  iron deficiency, 275-276, 276b,
    277b
  in non-Hodgkin's lymphoma,
    297
  pernicious, 272-273
  in renal tumor, 459
  in rheumatic heart disease, 343
  sickle cell, 276-279
  in stomach cancer, 200
  in systemic lupus erythematosus,
    86
Anesthesia, 37-41
  conscious sedation, 40
  general, 37-39, 39f
  local, 40
  regional, 39-40, 39f
  urinary function and, 50
Aneurysm, 359-360
  clipping and wrapping of, 697-
    698, 697f
  hemorrhagic stroke and, 696
Angina pectoris, 321-325, 322f,
    325b, 326b, 327t
  in cardiomyopathy, 347
  in polycythemia, 279-280
Angioedema, 81-82
  in anaphylaxis, 727
Angiography, 305-306, 308
  cerebral, 664
  fluorescein, 606-607
  magnetic resonance, 662-663
  in peripheral vascular disease,
    351
  pulmonary, 380, 417
  renal, 442
Angioma, 91
Angiotensin II receptor blockers,
    353
Angiotensin-converting enzyme
    inhibitors
  for atherosclerosis, 356
  for heart failure, 336-337t
  for hypertension, 353
  for myocardial infarction, 329t
Anisocoria, 669f
Ankle sprain, 161
Ankle-brachial index, 356
Ankylosing spondylitis, 123-125
Anoscopy in hemorrhoids, 224
Antacids, 193-195t
  for acute gastritis, 191
  for gastroesophageal reflux
    disease, 187
  for pancreatitis, 254
  for peptic ulcer disease, 193
  [f]rior pituitary, 485, 486f, 487f
  [f]ior rectosigmoid resection,
    22, 222f
  [f]r tibial artery, 355f, 357f
  [p]osterior colporrhaphy, 562-
    563
  398
  [f]associated pseudomem-
  [ou]s colitis, 202-203, 203

Antibiotics
  for acne vulgaris, 83
  for acute follicular tonsillitis, 392
  for acute otitis media, 636
  for acute respiratory distress
    syndrome, 419
  for anthrax, 398
  antitumor, 793-794t
  for brain abscess, 706
  for bronchiectasis, 429
  for cellulitis, 75
  for cystitis, 453
  for ear infection, 637-638t
  effects during surgery, 38t
  for epididymitis, 584
  for external otitis, 635
  for Helicobacter pylori infection,
    195
  for hepatic abscess, 247
  for impetigo contagiosa, 76
  inhibition of normal intestinal
    bacteria and, 202
  for laryngitis, 393
  for Legionnaire's disease, 396
  for lymphangitis, 293
  for meningitis, 704
  for osteomyelitis, 131
  for pelvic inflammatory disease,
    558
  for peritonitis, 216
  for pharyngitis, 394
  for pleurisy, 407
  for pneumonia, 406
  preoperative, 36-37t
  for prostatitis, 455
  for pyelonephritis, 455-456
  for sinusitis, 395
  for syphilis, 589
  for systemic lupus erythemato-
    sus, 87
  for toxic shock syndrome, 559
  for urinary tract infection, 444-
    445, 452
Antibody, B-cell production of, 721
Anticholinergics
  for emphysema, 422
  for irritable bowel syndrome,
    204
  for pancreatitis, 254
  preoperative, 36-37t
Anticoagulants, 318-319t
  herbal remedies and, 356
  for myocardial infarction, 329t
  preoperative, 36-37t
  for pulmonary embolism, 417-
    418, 418
  safety guidelines for, 364b
Anticonvulsants
  for head injury, 709
  for increased intracranial pres-
    sure, 671
  for neuropathic pain, 668
  for seizures, 679t
  for trigeminal neuralgia, 701
Antidepressants
  for migraine prophylaxis, 666
  for neuropathic pain, 668
  for premenstrual syndrome, 551
Antidiarrheal agents
  for Crohn's disease, 211
  for intestinal infection, 203
  for ulcerative colitis, 207
Antidiuretic hormone, 437-438, 485,
    486f
  diabetes insipidus and, 492
  syndrome of inappropriate antid-
    iuretic hormone secretion
    and, 493
Antidysrhythmics, 318-319t, 329t
  effects during surgery, 38t
Antiemetics
  for acute gastritis, 191
  for chemotherapy-related vomit-
    ing, 797-798
  for vomiting in cirrhosis, 237
Antifungal agents, 70-71t, 78

Antigen, 721
Antigen-antibody allergic rhinitis,
    386-387
Antigen-antibody complexes, 731
Antihistamines
  for allergic rhinitis and conjuncti-
    vitis, 386
  for allergy symptoms, 725
  for angioedema, 81
  for skin disorders, 70-71t
  for transfusion reaction, 729
  for urticaria, 81
Antihypertensives, 354b
  effects during surgery, 38t
Antiinflammatory agents
  for cancer pain, 801
  for Crohn's disease, 210
  for neuropathic pain, 668
  for osteoarthritis, 126
  for rheumatoid arthritis, 119-122t
  for systemic lupus erythemato-
    sus, 87
  for ulcerative colitis, 207
Antimalarial drugs
  for rheumatoid arthritis, 119-122t
  for systemic lupus erythemato-
    sus, 87
Antimetabolites, 793-794t
Antineoplastic agents, 793-794t
  for rheumatoid arthritis, 119-122t
Antinuclear antibody
  plasmapheresis and, 731
  in rheumatoid arthritis, 119
Antiplatelet agents
  for myocardial infarction, 329t
  for transient ischemic attack, 696
Antipyrine and benzocaine,
    637-638t
Antiretroviral therapy
  drug resistance to, 749
  in HIV infection, 750-757, 753t,
    753-756t
  perinatal transmission of HIV
    and, 741
Antisecretory agents, 195
Antispasmodics, 193-195t
  for gallstones, 249
  for intestinal infection, 203
Antitumor antibiotics, 793-794t
Antiviral agents
  for Bell's palsy, 702
  for genital herpes, 588
  for herpes simplex infection, 69
  for herpes simplex virus enceph-
    alitis, 705
  for keratitis, 615
  for shingles, 72
Antrectomy, 195
Anuria in end-stage renal disease,
    471
Aorta, 178f, 307, 304f, 305f, 306f,
    307f
  coronary artery bypass graft and,
    323f
Aortic aneurysm, 359, 360f
Aortic semilunar valve, 305, 305f,
    342t
Aortogram, 308
Aortoiliac aneurysm, 360f
Aphasias, 659
  in stroke, 696-697
Aplastic anemia, 273-274, 275b
Apnea, 387-388, 388f
Appendicitis, 212-216, 213b
Appendicular skeleton, 110, 110b,
    111f
Applanation tonometry, 624-625,
    625f
Apraxia in Alzheimer's disease, 689
Aqueous humor, 602-603, 603
Arachnoid membrane, 654
Arcus senilis, 607
Areola, 10t, 11, 537-538, 538f, 582
Armour Thyroid, 490t
Aromatase inhibitors, 576
Arrector pili muscle, 60f, 61

Arrhythmias, 314-319, 315f,
    318-319t
  in acromegaly, 491
  after myocardial infarction, 329
  in hyperparathyroidism, 502
Arterial aneurysm, 359-360, 359f,
    360f
Arterial assessment, 349-350, 349b
Arterial blood gases, 311
  in acute respiratory distress syn-
    drome, 419
  in asthma, 427
  in atelectasis, 411
  in chronic bronchitis, 424
  in emphysema, 422
  in neurologic disorders, 661
  normal values for, 150
  in pulmonary embolism, 417
  in respiratory disorders, 382-383,
    383b, 383t
Arterial blood pressure, 351
Arterial disorders, 355-362, 355f
Arterial embolism, 357-359
Arterial oxygen tension, 382, 383b
Arterial oxygenation saturation,
    382, 383b
Arteries, 306
Arteriography, cerebral, 664
Arteriosclerosis, 355
Arthritis, 117-128, 118t
  gouty, 127-128
  in systemic lupus erythematosus,
    86
Arthrocentesis, 116
Arthrodesis, 133
Arthroplasty, 133
  hip, 135-136, 135f, 136f
  knee, 133-135, 133f, 134b
Arthroscopy, 116
Articulation, 110, 110f
Artificial disk replacement, 165
Artificial tears replacement, 616
Aschoff's nodule, 343
Ascites
  in cirrhosis, 236
  in ovarian cancer, 568
  in peritonitis, 215
Ascorbic acid
  erythropoiesis and, 277b
Asepsis, iron absorption and, 276
Asparaginase, 793-794t
Aspart insulin, 515-516t
Aspartate aminotransferase, 231
Aspergillosis, 750-751t
Aspiration procedure, 116
Aspirin (acetylsalicylic acid)
  for angina pectoris, 322
  for headache, 666
  for myocardial infarction, 329t
  for rheumatoid arthritis, 119-122t
  for systemic lupus erythemato-
    sus, 87
  for transient ischemic attack,
    696
Assisted reproductive technologies,
    556
Asterixis in cirrhosis, 240
Asthenia, 451, 471
Asthma, 420f, 426-428
  contact dermatitis and, 79
Astigmatism, 608-609t, 611, 611t
Astringents, 70-71t
Ataxia in multiple sclerosis, 681
Ataxic breathing, 669
Atazanavir, 753-756t
Atelectasis, 49, 409, 410-411
Atenolol, 329t
Atherosclerosis, 320, 321f
  migraine and, 665
  thrombotic stroke and, 695
Atonic bladder, 450
Atopic dermatitis, 82
Atracurium besylate, 671
Atrial fibrillation, 315-316, 694-695
Atrial pacing, 315f
Atrioventricular block, 316

Atrioventricular node, 306f
Atrioventricular valve, 305
Atrophic vaginitis, 557-558
Atrophy, 62f, 62t
Atropine, 36-37t, 254
Attenuated vaccine, 723
Audio books, 610
Audiometric testing, 632
Auditory association area of brain, 653f
Auditory disorders, *see* Sensory system disorders
Aura in seizure, 676
Auranofin, 119-122t
Auricle, 604, 604f
Autograft, 100, 729
Autoimmune disorders, 724, 730-731
    Addison's disease in, 506-508
    immune thrombocytopenic purpura in, 286
    pernicious anemia in, 272-273
    systemic lupus erythematosus in, 85-87, 85f
Autologous bone marrow transplantation, 800
Autologous transfusion, 729
Automaticity, 305, 677-678t
Autonomic dysreflexia, 710-712, 712b, 712f
Autonomic nervous system, 655
Axial skeleton, 110, 110b, 111f
Axillary lymph nodes, 268f, 572f
    breast cancer and, 574
Axon, 651f, 652
Azatadine, 401-403t
Azathioprine
    for Crohn's disease, 210
    for liver transplantation, 246
    for myasthenia gravis, 692
    for rheumatoid arthritis, 119-122t
    for systemic lupus erythematosus, 87
    for thrombocytopenia, 287
Azithromycin
    for cervicitis, 558
    for *Chlamydia trachomatis*, 592
Azotemia, 471
    in acute pyelonephritis, 455

B

B cell, 265-266, 721, 721f
    autoimmune disorders and, 730
    humoral immunity and, 721
    involvement in HIV infection, 743t
B cell lymphoma, 297-298
Bacillary angiomatosis, 750-751t
Bacillus anthracis, 398
Baclofen
    for motor problems, 672
    for neurologic disorders, 686-687t
Bacteriuria, 451
Balkan frame, 157
Balloon tamponade for epistaxis, 385
Balsalazide
    for Crohn's disease, 210
    for ulcerative colitis, 207
Bandemia, 265
Barium enema, 182
Barium swallow, 181, 188
Barrel chest, 421, 421f
Barrett's esophagus, 187
Barrier methods of contraception, 593-595t
Bartholin's gland, 537, 537f
Basal cell carcinoma, 91, 91f
Basal ganglia, 652
Basiliximab, 246
Basophil, 263f, 263-264t, 265, 743t
Battle's sign, 709, 709f
Bell's palsy, 701-702
Benazepril, 336-337t
Benign prostatic hypertrophy, 462-464, 463b, 463f, 545

Benign tumor, 90-93, 166-167, 785, 785t
Benzodiazepines, 36-37t
Benzoyl peroxide, 70-71t, 83
Benztropine, 685, 686-687t
Bernstein test, 181
Beta cell, 487-488
Beta-adrenergic blockers, 318-319t
    for glaucoma, 625-627
    for heart failure, 336-337t
    for hypertension, 353
    for migraine prophylaxis, 666
    for myocardial infarction, 329t
Betamethasone, 70-71t, 85
Betaxolol hydrochloride, 625-626t
Bethanechol chloride, 443t
Bethesda system, 543t, 786
Bicalutamide, 465
Bicarbonate ion, 383, 383b
Biguanide, 520-521, 520t
Bilateral orchiectomy, 465
Bile duct, primary biliary cirrhosis and, 190, 236
Bi-level positive airway pressure, 388
Bilirubin, 440t
Billroth procedures, 195, 195f
Bimanual pelvic examination, 541-542, 568
Biofeedback techniques, 226, 362
Biologic identity, 539
Biologic response modifiers, 800
Biopsy, 543-544
    bone marrow, 269
    breast, 543, 574
    in cancer diagnosis, 786-787, 787f
    cervical, 543-544
    endometrial, 544, 567
    liver, 233-234
    lung, 382
    renal, 468
    skin, 90, 93
    synovial fluid, 119
    testicular, 545
Biotherapy for cancer, 800
Bismuth subsalicylate, 193-195t
Bisphosphonates, 129t, 577
Biventricular pacemaker, 319, 335
Bladder, 435f, 438-439, 438f
    cancer of, 461-462
    cystitis and, 453, 453b
    interstitial cystitis and, 453-454
    neurogenic, 450-451
Bladder training, 447-448
Blanching test, 170
Bleeding, abnormal uterine, 548-550
Bleeding time, 263-264t
Bleomycin, 793-794t
Blepharitis, 613-614, 613t
Blind spot, 603
Blindness, 607-610, 610b, 610f
    diabetes mellitus-related, 526, 526f
    in multiple sclerosis, 681
Blister, 62f, 62t, 94
Blood, 10t, 11, 262-267, 263f, 266f
    blood types and, 266-267
    formation in red bone marrow, 110
    hemostasis and, 266
    red blood cells and, 263-265, 263f
    Rh factor and, 267
    thrombocytes and, 266
    white blood cells and, 265-266
Blood alkaline phosphatase, 788
Blood clotting, 266f
Blood creatinine, 440
Blood culture, 310, 405-406
Blood disorders, 262-302
    agranulocytosis in, 281-282
    anemia in, 269-281; *See also* Anemia
    coagulation disorders in, 284-286
    diagnostic blood studies in, 263-264t, 269
    disseminated intravascular coagulation in, 289-291, 290b

Blood disorders (*Continued*)
    drug therapy for, 283t
    hemophilia in, 287-289, 289b
    leukemia in, 282-284, 283t, 285b
    multiple myeloma in, 291-292
    nursing process for, 298-299
    older adult and, 298b
    polycythemia in, 279-281
    thrombocytopenia in, 286-287, 286b
    von Willebrand's disease in, 289
Blood gas analysis, 150
Blood glucose, diabetes mellitus and, 511, 514
Blood markers for cancer diagnosis, 788-789
Blood poisoning, 75
Blood pressure
    hypertension and, 351-354
    renin and, 437
Blood products, transmission of HIV via, 740
Blood transfusion, 729
    in agranulocytosis, 281
    Jehovah's Witness opposition to, 270b
Blood types, 266, 267f
Blood urea nitrogen, 440, 472
Blood vessels, 306-307, 365-366
Blown pupil, 669
Bobath approach, 699
Body section roentgenography, 115
Bone
    effects of bed rest on mineral content in, 117
    fracture of, 137-148
    mineral storage in, 110
    structure of, 110
Bone density measurement, 502
Bone marrow aspiration, 269
Bone marrow transplantation
    for aplastic anemia, 274
    for breast cancer, 577
    for cancer, 800-801
    for leukemia, 283
Bone scan, 116, 787
Bone tumor, 166-167
Bosniak Classification of Renal Cysts, 460-461
Bouchard's nodes, 125
Bowel preparation, 182-183, 183b
Bowel sounds, postoperative, 52
Bowel training, in fecal incontinence, 226
Bowman's capsule, 436, 436f, 437f
Brachytherapy, 465, 576
Bradford frame, 157
Bradycardia, 315
Bradydysrhythmias, 320
Bradykinesia, 683, 684-685
Brain, 652-654
    abscess of, 706
    Alzheimer's disease and, 688-690, 689f, 690b
    anatomy of, 652, 653, 654, 653f, 654b
    encephalitis and, 705-706
    hepatic encephalopathy and, 240
    in regulation of food intake, 180
    in regulation of respiration, 378
    tumor of, 352t, 707-708
Brain attack; *See* Stroke
Brain scan, 662
Brainstem, 654, 670
Breast, 537-538, 538f
    biopsy of, 543, 574
    fibrocystic breast condition and, 570-571
Breast cancer, 571-583; *See also* Female reproductive disorders
    genetics in, 781
    nursing care plan for mastectomy in, 577-578b
    patient teaching in, 579-581, 580b

Breast cancer (*Continued*)
    preventing muscle contractures after mastectomy, 579-580, 580f, 581b
    prevention and early detection of, 782-784t
    prognosis in, 583, 583t
    staging of, 574, 575b
Breast conservation surgery, 574-575
Breast reconstruction surgery, 581-582, 789
Breast self-examination, 573b, 573f, 784
Breath sounds, 379, 379t
Breathing, 374, 377-378
    immediate postoperative phase and, 45t
Breathing techniques
    for chronic bronchitis, 426
    for pneumonia, 407
    for pulmonary edema, 416
Bricker's procedure, 478-479
Bromocriptine, 490t, 556
Bronchiectasis, 428-429
Bronchiole, 374f, 377
Bronchitis
    acute, 395-396
    chronic, 424-426
Bronchodilators
    for bronchiectasis, 429
    for chronic bronchitis, 426
    for emphysema, 422
Bronchoscopy, 381, 381f
Bronchus, 374f, 376f, 377
Brudzinski's sign, 704
Bruising, postauricular, 709f
Brush biopsy, 441
B-type natriuretic peptide, 311, 335
Buck's traction, 156, 157f
Buerger's disease, 360-361
Bulbar conjunctiva, 607
Bulla, 62f, 62t
Bumetanide
    for heart failure, 336-337t
    for increased intracranial pressure, 671
Bundle of His, 305, 306f
Burn, 94-103, 94b, 102b, 104b
    classification of severity, 97b
    corneal, 628
    topical medications for, 101t
Burn shock, 95
Burow's solution, 70-71t
Bursae, 12
Buspirone, 551
Busulfan, 280
Butenafine, 78
Butoconazole, 549-550t

C

CA 19-9 tumor antigen, 256, 789
CA-125 tumor antigen, 545, 568, 789
Cabergoline, 489
Cachexia, 48, 221, 801
Caffeine, 452
Calamine lotion, 70-71t
Calcitonin, 486
Calcitonin-salmon, 129t
Calcitriol, 504
Calcium values in musculoskeletal disorders, 117t
Calcium channel blockers, 318-319t
    for hypertension, 353
    for migraine prophylaxis, 666
    for myocardial infarction, 329t
Calcium pump, 8t, 9
Calcium salts, 490t
Calculus, urinary, 457-459, 458f
Caldwell-Luc operation, 394-395
Callus, 144
Canal of Schlemm, 602
Cancer, 778-807
    biotherapy for, 800
    bladder, 461-462
    bone marrow transplantation for, 800-801

Cancer (Continued)
  breast, 571-583; See also Female
    reproductive disorders
    genetics in, 781
    prognosis in, 583, 583t
    cell mechanisms and growth
      of, 785
  cervical, 543, 565-567, 782-784t
  chemotherapy in, 791-800, 793-
    794t; See also Chemotherapy
  colorectal, 220-224, 221b, 222f,
    782-784t
  communication support in,
    802-803
  cultural considerations in, 779b
  description, grading, staging of,
    786, 786b
  development, prevention, detec-
    tion of, 780-785, 782-784t,
    781b
  diagnosis of, 786-789
  disseminated intravascular coag-
    ulation and, 290
  endometrial, 567, 782-784t
  esophageal, 188-189, 188b
  Hodgkin's lymphoma, 293-297,
    294b, 295f, 296b, 730
  laryngeal, 389-390
  liver, 241-243
  lung, 413-415, 414b, 782-784t
  multiple myeloma, 291-292
  non-Hodgkin's lymphoma, 297-
    298, 750-751t
  oral cavity, 184-186
  ovarian, 545, 567-569, 782-784t, 789
  pancreatic, 255-257, 257f
  penile, 586
  prostate, 464-466, 464b, 782-784t,
    788
  skin, 91, 91f, 92-93, 93f
  stomach, 200-201
  terminal prognosis in, 803-804
  testicular, 585-586, 586b, 586f,
    782-784t
  thyroid, 501-502, 792b
Candidiasis, 591
  associated with HIV infection,
    750-751t, 766t
  chemotherapy-related, 795
  in external otitis, 635
  oral, 184
  peristomal area integrity and, 209
  vaginal, 557, 591
Capillary, 306
Capillary refill time, 349b
Capsaicin cream, 119-122t
Capsule endoscopy, 181, 181f, 210
Captopril, 329t, 336-337t
Carbamazepine, 668, 679t, 701
Carbamide peroxide, 637-638t
Carbidopa-levodopa, 686-687t
Carbon dioxide, mechanics of
  breathing and, 377-378
Carbon monoxide poisoning, 97
Carbonic anhydrase inhibitor di-
  uretics, 444
Carbonic anhydrase inhibitors,
  625-627
Carboplatin, 793-794t
Carbuncle, 77, 602f, 603f
Carcinoembryonic antigen, 200, 221,
  788
Carcinogenesis, 780
Carcinoma, 785-786
Carcinoma in situ, 565
Cardiac arrest, 319-320
Cardiac catheterization, 308, 335
Cardiac cirrhosis, 236
Cardiac cycle, 306, 306f, 307f
Cardiac disease; See Heart disease
Cardiac dysrhythmias, 314-319, 318-
  319t; See also Cardiovascular
  disorders
  in acromegaly, 491
  after myocardial infarction, 329
  in hyperparathyroidism, 502

Cardiac enzymes, 311
Cardiac monitor, 309-310
Cardiac muscle, 10t, 11, 11f
Cardiac rehabilitation, 331-332
Cardiac tamponade, 344
Cardiac transplantation, 347-348,
  347b
Cardiogenic shock, 329, 330t
Cardioglycosides, 318-319t, 336-337t
Cardiomyopathy, 346-348, 347b
Cardiomyotomy, 190
Cardiopulmonary resuscitation, 319
Cardiospasm, 189
Cardiovascular disorders, 303-372
  angina pectoris in, 321-325, 322f,
    325b, 326b, 327t
  cardiac arrest in, 319-320
  cardiac dysrhythmias in, 314-319
    atrial fibrillation in, 315-316
    atrioventricular block in, 316
    drug therapy for, 318-319t
    patient teaching in, 317-319
    premature ventricular con-
      tractions in, 316
    sinus bradycardia in, 315, 315f
    sinus tachycardia in, 314
    supraventricular tachycardia
      in, 315
    ventricular fibrillation in, 317
    ventricular tachycardia in,
      316-317
  cardiomyopathy in, 346-348, 347b
  coronary artery disease in, 320-
    321, 321f, 327t; See also Cor-
    onary artery disease
  endocarditis in, 345-346
  laboratory tests in, 310-311
  myocardial infarction in, 326-332,
    326f; See also Myocardial
    infarction
  myocarditis in, 346
  normal aging patterns and, 312
  nursing process for, 367-369
  older adult and, 312b
  pericarditis in, 343-345
  peripheral vascular disorders in,
    348-367; See also Peripheral
    vascular disorders
  pulmonary edema in, 340, 340b,
    341t
  rheumatic heart disease in,
    342-343
  risk factors for, 312-314, 313b
  valvular heart disease in, 340-
    342, 342t
Cardiovascular syphilis, 589
Cardiovascular system, 12-14t,
  304-307
  adrenal disorders and, 507t
  blood vessels and, 306-307
  effects of surgery on, 23t
  heart and, 304-306, 304f
  pulmonary circulation and, 308
  systemic lupus erythematosus
    and, 86
Cardioversion, 310
Carditis, 343
Caries, 183-184
Carotid artery disease, 694-695
Carotid duplex study, 664
Carotid endarterectomy, 696
Carpal tunnel syndrome, 163-164,
  163f
Carpopedal spasm after thyroidectomy, 497-498
Cast for fracture, 153-159, 153f, 155f
  mobilization and, 155
  neurovascular problems and, 155
  patient teaching in, 154
  removal of, 156
  skin care and, 155
  toileting and, 155
  turning patient and, 155

Casts in urine, 440t
Catabolism, 52
Cataracts, 617-618, 617f, 618f, 619b
Catheter ablation for atrial fibrilla-
  tion, 316
Caudal, term, 1, 2f
CD4+ cell
  diagnostic criteria for acquired
    immunodeficiency syn-
    drome and, 736t, 744
  early symptomatic HIV disease
    and, 745-746
  monitoring in HIV infection,
    747
Cecum, 176f, 178, 178f
Cefaclor, 637-638t
Cefazolin, 36-37t
Cefdinir, 590
Cefotaxime, 36-37t
Cefoxitin, 558
Ceftriaxone, 36-37t, 590
Celecoxib, 119-122t
Celiac artery, atherosclerotic lesions
  in, 355f
Cell, 4-9, 4f
Cell membrane, 8-9, 8t, 9f, 9t, 10f
Cell-mediated immunity, 722-723,
  722b, 723
Cellular immunity, 722-723, 722b,
  723
Cellulitis, 74-75
Central hearing loss, 634
Central nervous system, 651,
  652-654
  infection and inflammation of,
    702-703
  brain abscess in, 706
  encephalitis in, 705-706
  Guillain-Barré syndrome in,
    703-704
  meningitis in, 704-705
  West Nile virus in, 705-706
  spinal cord in, 654, 655f
Centriole, 5f, 6, 6t
Cephalosporins
  inhibition of normal intestinal
    bacteria and, 202
  for pneumonia, 406
Cerebellum, 653f, 654
Cerebral arteriography, 664
Cerebral cortex, 652
  Alzheimer's disease and, 688
Cerebral edema
  in encephalitis, 705
  in head trauma, 709
Cerebrospinal fluid
  increased intracranial pressure
    and, 669
  lumbar puncture and, 661-662,
    662f
  normal characteristics of, 661t
  ventricles of brain and, 654
Cerebrum, 652, 653f, 654b
Cerumen, 61, 604
Ceruminous gland, 61, 604
Cervical cap, 593-595t
Cervical intraepithelial neoplasia
  classification, 543t
Cervical spine, whiplash injury of,
  160-161
Cervicitis, 558, 591-592
Cervix, 536-537, 536f
  biopsy of, 543-544
  cancer of, 565-567
    early detection and prevention
      of, 782-784t
    human papillomavirus and, 543
    conization of, 542, 544
Chalazion, 613-614, 613t
Chambers of eye, 603
Chancre, 589
Chemical messenger, 7
Chemonucleolysis, 165
Chemotherapy, 791-800, 793-794t
  alopecia and, 796
  anemia and, 796

Chemotherapy (Continued)
  in bladder cancer, 461
  in bone tumor, 167
  in breast cancer, 576
  in colorectal cancer, 221-222
  in esophageal cancer, 188
  in Hodgkin's lymphoma, 295
  immunosuppression and, 730
  in laryngeal cancer, 390
  in leukemia, 283
  leukopenia and, 791-796
  in lung cancer, 414
  medications for symptom control
    in, 797-798t
  mouth assessment in, 795
  in multiple myeloma, 292
  nausea, vomiting, and diarrhea
    and, 797-798
  neutropenia and, 795-796, 795b
  in non-Hodgkin's lymphoma,
    297-298, 298
  nursing interventions in, 798
  in oral cavity cancer, 185
  in ovarian cancer, 568
  in pancreatic cancer, 257
  pulmonary function and, 795
  skin assessment in, 795
  in stomach cancer, 201
  stomatitis and, 796
  thrombocytopenia and, 796
  tumor lysis syndrome and, 799,
    799-800
  urinary and bowel function and,
    795
Chest, computed tomography of,
  380
Chest physiotherapy, 411, 422
Chest tube
  guidelines for, 410b
  in lung cancer, 414
  in pleural effusion or empyema,
    408, 409f
  in pneumothorax, 412
Cheyne-Stokes respirations, 669
Chlamydia trachomatis, 558, 591-592
  in conjunctivitis, 614
  in prostatitis, 583
Chlorambucil, 87, 793-794t
Chlorhexidine gluconate, 70-71t
Chloride in cerebrospinal fluid, 661t
Chlorothiazide, 336-337t, 443
Choked disk, 670
Cholangiography, 232-233
Cholecystectomy, 250
  laparoscopic, 251
Cholecystitis, 248-253
Choledocholithiasis, 250
Cholelithiasis, 248-253
Cholesteatoma, 636
Cholesterol
  elevation in HIV disease, 766
  hyperlipidemia and, 313-314,
    313b
  hypertension and, 352
Cholesterol-lowering drugs, 314
Cholestyramine, 255-256t
Choline magnesium trisalicylate,
  119-122t
Choline salicylate, 119-122t
Cholinesterase, 113
Chorea in Huntington's disease, 694
Choroid, 602-603, 603f
Chronic bronchitis, 420f, 424-426
Chronic constipation, 225b
Chronic glomerulonephritis,
  469-470
Chronic lymphocytic leukemia, 282
Chronic myelogenous leukemia, 282
Chronic obstructive pulmonary
  disease, 420-429, 420f
Chronic otitis media, 636
Chronic pelvic pain, 453
Chronic renal failure, 471-472,
  473-474b
  in hyperparathyroidism, 502
  nursing care plan for, 473-474b

Chvostek's sign, 497-498, 503
Cigarette smoking; *See* Smoking
Cilia, 5f, 6t
    tracheal, 375-377
Ciliary body, 602-603, 603f
Cilostazol, 356
Cimetidine, 193-195t
    for acute gastritis, 191
    for gastroesophageal reflux
        disease, 187
    for hypoparathyroidism, 504
    for pancreatitis, 254
Ciprofloxacin
    for Crohn's disease, 211
    for gonorrhea, 590
    for prostatitis, 455, 583
Circulation, 307-308
    immediate postoperative phase
        and, 45t
Circulation check, 139b
Circulatory system, 12-14t
Circumcision, 535, 584
Circumferential aneurysm, 359
Cirrhosis, 236-241
    home care considerations in,
        241b
    nursing care plan for, 242b
Cisplatin, 793-794t
    for esophageal cancer, 188
    for laryngeal cancer, 390
    for ovarian cancer, 568
Clarithromycin
    for Crohn's disease, 211
    for *Helicobacter pylori*, 195
Claudication, 355
Clean-catch specimen, 439-440
Climacteric
    male, 553-554
    menopause as, 551
Clindamycin, 202
Clinical staging, 786
Clipping of aneurysm, 697-698,
    697f
Clomiphene citrate, 556
Clonazepam
    for fibromyalgia syndrome, 132t
    for seizures, 679t
Clonidine, 353, 553
Clopidogrel, 696
Closed fracture, 142f, 143f, 145
Closed head injury, 708-709
Clostridium difficile colitis, 202
Clostridium perfringens, 150
Clotrimazole, 452, 549-550t
Clotting defects, 287-291
    hemophilia A in, 287-289, 289b
    von Willebrand's disease in, 289
Clotting time, 263-264f
Clubbing, 421-422, 428
Cluster headache, 666
CMS mnemonic, 139
Coagulation disorders, 284-286
Coagulation studies, 310
Coal tar products, 70-71t, 82, 85
Coarctation of aorta, 352t
Coarse crackles, 379f
Coccidioidomycosis, 750-751t
Cochlea, 604f, 605, 605f
Cochlear implant, 634, 645, 645f
Cocktail, antiretroviral, 753-756
Cogwheel rigidity, 684
Colchicine, 127
Cold sore, 68, 69f
Colistin, 637-638t
Colitis, antibiotic-associated pseu-
    domembranous, 202
Collecting tubule, 436, 436f, 437f
Colles' fracture, 144
Colloid goiter, 500-501, 501f
Colon, 178-179
Colon resection, 207
Colonoscopy, 182-183, 183b, 207,
    210, 214, 219, 221
Colony-stimulating factors, 795-796
Color perception, 607t
Color vision, 608-609t

Colorectal cancer, 220-224, 221b,
    222f, 782-784t
Colostomy, 214-215, 214f, 215f
Colposcopy, 542
Coma, diabetic, 511, 523, 525t
Combination chemotherapy
    in Hodgkin's lymphoma, 295
    in leukemia, 283
Combination medications for HIV
    disease, 753-756t
Comedone, 83, 83f
Comminuted fracture, 143f, 144
Common bile duct, 176f, 179f
    gallstones in, 248f
    intravenous cholangiography
        and, 232
    operative cholangiography and,
        232-233
    T-tube in, 250, 250f
Common cold, 391-392
Communication
    in angina pectoris, 325b
    with blind person, 610b
    in cancer, 790b, 802-803
    in chronic obstructive pulmonary
        disease, 424b
    in diabetes mellitus, 527b
    in dialysis, 476b
    in gastrointestinal disorders,
        197b
    in headache, 665b
    hearing loss and, 633b
    in Hodgkin's lymphoma, 296b
    in postoperative eye surgery,
        620b
    stroke and, 699-700
Compartment syndrome, 148-149,
    149f
Compensatory mechanisms, 383t
Complement system, 722
Complementary and alternative
    therapies
    for cardiovascular and peripheral
        vascular disorders, 356b
    for endocrine disorders, 521b
    for HIV infection, 757
    for integumentary disorders,
        105b
    for irritable bowel syndrome,
        205b
    for musculoskeletal disorders,
        126b
    for reproductive disorders, 597b
    for urinary disorders, 452b
Complete blood count, 263-264t,
    269
    in asthma, 427
    in cardiovascular disorders, 310
    in cellulitis, 75
    in chronic bronchitis, 424
    in peritonitis, 216
Complete fracture, 143f, 144
Compression techniques for venous
    stasis ulcer, 366
Computed tomography, 115-116
    in appendicitis, 212
    in atelectasis, 411
    for cancer diagnosis, 787
    in colorectal cancer, 221
    in diverticulosis and diverticuli-
        tis, 214
    in esophageal cancer, 188
    in hematologic and lymphatic dis-
        orders, 269
    in hepatobiliary disorders, 235
    in Hodgkin's lymphoma, 294-295
    in hydronephrosis, 457
    in intestinal obstruction, 219
    in laryngeal cancer, 389
    in lung cancer, 413-414
    in non-Hodgkin's lymphoma,
        297
    in peritonitis, 216
    in pulmonary embolism, 417
    in pyelonephritis, 455
    in respiratory disorders, 380

Computed tomography (*Continued*)
    in stomach cancer, 200
    in stroke, 697
    in urinary disorders, 442
Conchae, 374, 375f
Condom, 593-595t, 772-773
Conductive hearing loss, 633
Confidential testing, 770-771
Congenital cataracts, 617
Congenital hearing loss, 633
Congenital hypothyroidism, 498,
    499f
Conization, 542, 544, 566
Conjugated equine estrogen,
    549-550t
Conjunctiva, 602, 603f
    inflammation of, 614-615
    normal findings of, 607t
Conjunctivitis, 386-387, 614-615
Connective tissue, 10t, 11
Connective tissue membrane, 12
Conscious sedation, 40
Consciousness, immediate postop-
    erative phase and, 45t
Contact dermatitis, 79, 729
    type IV allergic, 728
Contact lenses, 609, 613b
Continent ileal urinary reservoir,
    479, 479f
Continuous closed bladder irriga-
    tion, postprostatectomy, 464
Continuous passive motion
    machine, 134, 134f
Contraception, 592-593, 593-595t,
    593f
    after onset of menopause, 553
Contracture
    after mastectomy, 579-580, 580f,
        581b
    burn-related, 98
    in osteomyelitis, 131
    Volkmann's, 148-149
Contralateral hemianopia, 696
Controlled coughing technique, 30-
    31b, 30b, 30f
Contusion, 160
Convergence, vision and, 604
Coombs' test, 297
Coping-stress tolerance pattern in
    neurologic disorders, 675
Cor pulmonale, 421
Cordotomy, 668
Cornea, 602, 603f, 607t
    inflammation of, 615
    transplantation of, 629-630
    trauma to, 627-629
Corneal ring segments, 612
Coronary arteries, 305f
Coronary artery bypass graft, 322-
    323, 323f
Coronary artery disease, 320-321,
    321f, 327f
    angina pectoris in, 321
    coronary artery bypass graft for,
        322-323, 323f
    hypothyroidism and, 499
    patient teaching in, 324
    percutaneous transluminal coro-
        nary angioplasty for, 323,
        324f
    stent placement for, 323, 324f
Coronary atherosclerotic heart
    disease, 320-321
Corpus albicans, 538, 539f
Corpus cavernosa, 535
Corpus spongiosum, 535
Corticosteroids
    for acute respiratory distress syn-
        drome, 419
    for angioedema, 81
    for Bell's palsy, 702
    for cancer treatment, 793-794t
    for chronic bronchitis, 426
    for Crohn's disease, 211
    effects during surgery, 38t
    for emphysema, 422

Corticosteroids (*Continued*)
    for external otitis, 635
    for gouty arthritis, 127
    for Guillain-Barré syndrome, 703
    for increased intracranial pres-
        sure, 671
    for liver transplantation, 246
    for meningitis, 704
    for multiple sclerosis, 681
    for myasthenia gravis, 692
    for nephrotic syndrome, 468
    for pelvic inflammatory disease,
        558
    preoperative, 36-37t
    for respiratory disorders,
        401-403t
    for rheumatoid arthritis, 119-122t
    for shingles, 72
    for systemic lupus erythemato-
        sus, 87
    for thrombocytopenia, 286
    topical, 70-71t
    for ulcerative colitis, 207
Coryza, 391-392
Cosmetic surgery, 18t
Costovertebral angle pain, 455
Coude catheter, 445-446, 446f
Cough, surgeries contraindicating
    coughing, 33b
Coughing techniques, 30-31b, 30b,
    30f
    for lung cancer, 415
    for pneumonia, 407
Cowper's gland, 534-535, 534f
Cox-2 inhibitor, 119-122t
C-peptide test, 512
Crackles, 379, 379t
    in atelectasis, 411
    in bronchiectasis, 428
    in pulmonary edema, 415
Cranial, term, 1
Cranial cavity, 3f, 3t
Cranial nerves, 655, 656f, 657t,
    659-660
Craniectomy, 707-708
Craniocerebral trauma, 708-710,
    709f
Craniotomy, 707-708
C-reactive protein, 311
    in pericarditis, 343
    in rheumatoid arthritis, 119
Creatine kinase, 311
Creatine phosphokinase, 397
Creatinine, 434
Creatinine clearance, 440, 469-470
Crepitus, fracture-related, 144
Cretinism, 498, 499f
Crohn's disease, 206t, 209-212
Crotamiton, 70-71t, 90
Crust, 62f, 62t
    in impetigo contagiosa, 75-76,
        76f
Crutch walking, 111f, 158-159, 158b,
    159f
Crutchfield tongs, 712, 713f
Cryoprecipitate
    for disseminated intravascular
        coagulation, 290
    for von Willebrand's disease, 289
Cryopreserved embryo transfer,
    556
Cryotherapy
    in diabetic retinopathy, 620
    in retinal detachment, 623
Cryptococcal infection, 750-751t
Cryptorchidism, 585
Cryptosporidial infection, 750-751t
Crystalline lens, 603
Culdoscopy, 542
Cultural considerations
    in cancer, 779b
    in cardiovascular disease, 312,
        321b
    in diabetes mellitus, 528b
    in female reproductive cancer,
        565b

Cultural considerations (Continued)
   in gastrointestinal disorders, 227b
   in hepatobiliary disorders, 258b
   in HIV infection, 738b
   in nonadherence to HIV drug regimen, 761
   in osteoporosis, 128b
   in sensory disorders, 618b
   in skin care, 68b
   in skin disorders, 68b
   in stroke, 694b
   of surgical patient, 20-21, 22b
   in tuberculosis, 399b
   in urinary disorders, 439b
Curling's ulcer, burn-related, 98
Cushing's response, 669
Cushing's syndrome, 352t, 504-506, 505f, 507t
Cutaneous anthrax, 398
Cutaneous ureterostomy, 477t
Cyanocobalamin, 272-273, 283t
Cyclobenzaprine, 132t
Cyclopentolate hydrochloride, 625-626t
Cyclophosphamide, 793-794t
   for breast cancer, 576
   for myasthenia gravis, 692
   for rheumatoid arthritis, 119-122t
   for systemic lupus erythematosus, 87
Cyclosporine
   for Crohn's disease, 210
   for interstitial cystitis, 454
   in liver transplantation, 246
   for myasthenia gravis, 692
Cyst, 62f, 62t
   chalazion, 613-614, 613t
   in fibrocystic breast condition, 570
   ovarian, 564
   renal, 460-462
Cystectomy, 477t, 478
Cystitis, 453, 453b
   interstitial, 453-454
   menopause-related, 552
   vaginal fistula and, 561
Cystocele, 562-563, 563f
Cystolithiasis, 457
Cystometrogram, 442
Cystoscopy, 441, 545
   in bladder cancer, 461
   in hydronephrosis, 457
   in renal tumor, 459
   in urinary tract trauma, 467
   in urolithiasis, 458
Cystostomy catheter, 445-446
Cytarabine, 793-794t
Cytologic studies
   in bladder tumor, 461
   in respiratory disorders, 382
Cytomegalovirus infection
   associated with HIV infection, 750-751t
   in encephalitis, 705
Cytoplasm, 5f, 6
Cytoprotective agents, 195
Cytotoxic T cell, 743t

D
Daclizumab, 246
Dakin's solution, 101t
Dalteparin, 417
Danazol, 549-550t, 560-561, 571
Dantrolene, 672
Dark skin assessment, 67
Darunavir, 753-756t
Daughter cell, 7, 7f
Davol drain, 250
D-dimer test, 290, 417
   in peripheral vascular disease, 351
   in thrombophlebitis, 363
Deafness, 633-635, 633b, 640
Debridement
   of burn wound, 99
   of venous stasis ulcer, 366

Decompression in intestinal obstruction, 219-220
Decongestants, 386-387
Decorticate response, 670f
Deep brain stimulation, 685
Deep breathing exercises
   after mastectomy, 580
   in pneumonia, 407
Deep femoral artery, atherosclerotic lesions in, 355f
Deep vein thrombosis, 50, 362, 363f
DEET insect repellent, 705
Defibrillation, 317
Degenerative joint disease, 125-127, 125b, 125f, 126f
Dehiscence, 48, 48f, 200-201
Dehydration
   in burn, 95
   in diabetes insipidus, 492
   in meningitis, 704
   in toxic shock syndrome, 559
Delavirdine, 753-756t
Delayed healing of fracture, 152
Delayed hypersensitivity, 723, 729-730
Delayed union, 152
Delegation considerations in perioperative nursing, 19b
Demeclocycline, 494
Dementia, 589, 750-751t
Demyelination in multiple sclerosis, 680, 681f
Dendrite, 651f, 652
Dental plaque and caries, 183-184
Deoxyribonucleic acid, 7, 7f
de Pezzer catheter, 445-446, 446f
Depolarization, 308, 309f
Dermatitis, 79, 80-81
   atopic, 82
   contact, 79
Dermatophytoses, 78, 78f
Dermis, 60f, 61
Descending colon, 176f, 178, 178f
Descending colostomy, 222f
Desmopressin, 283t
   for diabetes insipidus, 493
   for von Willebrand's disease, 289
Detemir, 515-516t
Deviated nasal septum, 385-386
Dexamethasone, 625-626t
   for cancer, 793-794t
   for chemotherapy symptoms, 797-798t
   for immune disorders, 726t
   for increased intracranial pressure, 671
Diabetes insipidus, 492-493
Diabetes mellitus, 509-528, 510t
   acute complications in, 523-526
   cardiovascular disease risk and, 314
   chronic complications in, 526-528, 526f
   clinical manifestations of, 511
   coma in, 525t
   cultural considerations in, 528b
   diabetic ketoacidosis in, 525b
   diabetic retinopathy and, 618-620
   diagnosis of, 511-512, 512b, 512f
   diet and, 513-514
   emergency care for hypoglycemic reaction in, 524b
   exercise and, 514
   foot care in, 522b, 527b
   home care considerations in, 528b
   insulin therapy for, 514-520, 514f
   insulin-enhancing drugs for, 521, 521t
   malignant external otitis and, 635
   medications for, 514, 520-521, 520t
   nursing care plan for, 523-524b
   older adult and, 523b
   pathophysiology of, 510-511
   patient teaching in, 521-528
   peripheral vascular diseases and, 349

Diabetes mellitus (Continued)
   renal failure and, 470
   risk for stroke, 694-695
   self-care behaviors in, 513b
   sexual dysfunction and, 541
   stress of acute illness, surgery and, 514
   type 1, 509-510
   type 2, 510
Diabetic coma, 511
Diabetic ketoacidosis, 511, 525b, 525t
Diabetic neuropathy, 526, 526f, 667
Diabetic retinopathy, 526, 526f, 618-620
Diagnostic blood studies, 263-264t
Diagnostic surgery, 18t
Diagnostic tests
   for blood disorders, 269
   for cancer, 787-788
   cardiovascular, 308, 310
      for cardiac arrhythmias, 317
      for heart failure, 334-335
      for myocardial infarction, 328
      for valvular heart disease, 341
   for diabetes mellitus, 512b
   for ear disorders, 631-632
      audiometric testing in, 632
      otoscopy in, 631
      tuning fork tests in, 631-632, 632f
      vestibular testing in, 632
      whispered voice test in, 631
   for female reproductive disorders, 544-545
   gastrointestinal, 180-183
      barium enema in, 182
      barium swallow and Gastrograffin studies in, 181
      capsule endoscopy in, 181, 181f
      colonoscopy in, 182-183, 183b
      esophageal function studies in, 181
      esophagogastroduodenoscopy in, 180-181, 180f
      obstruction series in, 183
      sigmoidoscopy in, 182
      tube gastric analysis in, 180
      upper gastrointestinal study in, 180
   hepatobiliary, 231-236
      abdominal computed tomography in, 235
      endoscopic retrograde cholangiopancreatography in, 235-236, 235f
      gallbladder scanning in, 233
      hepatitis virus studies in, 234
      intravenous cholangiography in, 232
      liver enzyme tests in, 231-232
      needle liver biopsy in, 233-234
      operative cholangiography in, 232-233
      oral cholecystography in, 232
      pancreatic ultrasonography in, 235
      radioisotope liver scanning in, 234
      serum ammonia test in, 234
      serum amylase test in, 234
      serum bilirubin test in, 231
      serum lipase test in, 235
      serum protein test in, 232
      T-tube cholangiography in, 233
      ultrasonography in, 233
      urine amylase test in, 234-235
   for human immunodeficiency virus, 747-749
      CD4+ cell monitoring in, 747
      drug resistance testing and, 749
      HIV antibody testing for, 747, 747b

Diagnostic tests (Continued)
      laboratory parameters and, 749
      pretest and posttest counseling and, 748b
      viral load monitoring in, 747-748
   for hyperthyroidism, 496b
   for male reproductive disorders, 545, 546b
   for musculoskeletal disorders, 113-117
   neurologic, 662-665
      angiogram in, 664
      brain scan in, 662
      carotid duplex study in, 664
      computed tomography in, 662
      echoencephalogram in, 665
      electroencephalogram in, 663, 663f
      electromyogram, 664-665
      magnetic resonance angiography in, 662-663
      magnetic resonance imaging in, 662
      myelogram in, 664
      positron emission tomography in, 663
   for oral cavity disorders, 185
   for peripheral vascular disease, 350-351
   preoperative, 24
   respiratory, 379-429
      arterial blood gases in, 382-383, 383b, 383t
      bronchoscopy in, 381, 381f
      chest radiography in, 379-380
      computed tomography in, 380
      cytologic studies in, 382
      laryngoscopy in, 381
      lung biopsy in, 382
      mediastinoscopy in, 380-381
      pulmonary function tests in, 380
      pulse oximetry in, 383-384, 384f
      sputum specimen in, 381, 381b, 382b
      thoracentesis in, 382, 382f
   for stroke, 697
   for urinary disorders
      computed tomography in, 442
      endoscopic procedures in, 441
      intravenous pyelography or urography in, 441
      kidney-ureter-bladder radiography in, 441
      magnetic resonance imaging in, 442
      renal angiography in, 442
      renal biopsy in, 442
      renal scan in, 442
      renal venogram in, 442
      retrograde pyelography in, 441
      transrectal ultrasound in, 442
      ultrasonography in, 442
      urodynamic studies in, 442-443
      voiding cystourethrography in, 441
   for visual disorders, 606-607, 608-609t
Dialysis, 474-477
Diaphragmatic hernia, 217-218
Diarrhea
   after gastric surgery, 196
   chemotherapy-related, 797-798
   in HIV infection, 745, 745t, 765, 766t
   infectious, 201
Diarthrosis, 110, 110f
Diastole, 306, 307f
Diastolic blood pressure, hypertension and, 351
Diatrizoate, 181

Diazepam
    for motor problems, 672
    for myocardial infarction, 329t
    preoperative, 36-37t
    for seizures, 679t
Didanosine, 753-756t
Didanosine/tenofovir, 753-756t
Diencephalon, 653
Diet history, 20
Differential white blood cell count, 265
Differentiated, term, 786
Diffusion, 3t, 9, 9f
    epidermis and, 60
Digestive system, 12-14t, 175-180, 176f, 177b
Digital examination, 221, 224
Digital mammography, 544
Digital subtraction angiography, 350
Digitalis, 336-337t
Digoxin, 318-319t, 329t
Dihydrotachysterol, 504
Dilated cardiomyopathy, 346
Dilation and curettage, 544
Diltiazem, 318-319t, 329t
Dimenhydrinate, 193-195t, 637-638t
Diphenhydramine, 70-71t, 726t
    for anaphylaxis, 727
    for angioedema, 81
    for cancer treatment symptoms, 797-798t
    for contact dermatitis, 79
Diphenoxylate with atropine, 193-195t, 797-798t
Diplopia, 681, 692
Dipyridamole, 696
Direct bilirubin, 231
Direct fluorescent antibody test for Chlamydia trachomatis, 592
Direct laryngoscopy, 381, 389
Discharge instructions
    in bipolar hip replacement, 140f
    in pelvic inflammatory disease, 559
    in total hip replacement, 136
    in total knee replacement, 134
Discharge of surgical patient, 55-56, 56b, 56f
Discoid lupus, 85
Disease-modifying antirheumatic drugs, 119-122t, 123
Diskectomy, 165
Dislocation, 162-163
Disopyramide, 318-319t
Displaced fracture, 143f
Dissecting aneurysm, 359f
Disseminated intravascular coagulation, 289-291, 290b
Distal convoluted tubule, 436, 436f, 437f, 437t
Disturbed sensory and perceptual function, 675-676
Diuretics
    for acute renal failure, 471
    for cirrhosis, 237-238
    effects during surgery, 38t
    to enhance urinary output, 443-444
    for glaucoma, 627
    for heart failure, 336-337t
    for hypertension, 353
    for increased intracranial pressure, 671
    for myocardial infarction, 329t
    for syndrome of inappropriate antidiuretic hormone secretion, 494
    for tumor lysis syndrome, 799
Divalproex, 679t
Diverticulitis, 176f, 213-215, 214f, 215f
Diverticulosis, 176f, 213-215, 214f, 215f
Division of cell, 7-8, 7f
Dobutamine, 318-319t
    for heart failure, 336-337t
    for myocardial infarction, 329t

Docetaxel, 793-794t
Donazepril, 686-687t
Dopamine, 652
    for anaphylaxis, 727
    for cardiovascular disorders, 318-319t
    for heart failure, 336-337t
    Huntington's disease and, 694
    for myocardial infarction, 329t
    Parkinson's disease and, 683-684
Dopamine agonists for acromegaly, 489
Doppler ultrasound, 350
Dorsal body cavity, 2, 3f, 3t
Dorsiflexion, 113
Double vision, 681, 692
Double-barrel transverse colostomy, 214-215, 214f
Doubling time of tumor, 572
Doxorubicin, 576, 793-794t
Doxycycline
    for anthrax, 398
    for cervicitis, 558
    for Chlamydia trachomatis, 592
    for interstitial cystitis, 454
    for pelvic inflammatory disease, 558
    for prostatitis, 455
Drain, postoperative care of, 223
Drainage
    of hepatic abscess, 247
    postoperative, 45
Dressing
    for burn, 100
    for enucleation, 629
    for keratitis, 615
Droperidol, 36-37t
Drug holiday, 685
Drug resistance testing in HIV infection, 749
Drusen, 621
Dry eye disorders, 615-616
Dry tap, 274
Ductus deferens, 534, 534f
Duloxetine hydrochloride, 132t
Dumping syndrome, 196
Duodenal ulcer, 192-200
Duodenum, 176f, 177f, 178, 179f, 180-181
Duplex scanning, 351
Dura mater, 654
    lumbar puncture and, 662f
Dutasteride, 462
Dwarfism, 492, 499f
Dysarthria, 659
    in amyotrophic lateral sclerosis, 693
    in stroke, 697
Dysgraphia, 689
Dysmenorrhea, 546, 547-548, 590-591
Dyspareunia
    in endometriosis, 560
    in uterine prolapse, 562
Dyspepsia, 244, 270
Dysphasia, 189
Dysplasia cytologic classification of Pap test, 543t
Dyspnea
    in emphysema, 421, 422-423
    respiratory assessment and, 378
Dysrhythmias, 314-319
    atrial fibrillation in, 315-316
    atrioventricular block in, 316
    drug therapy for, 318-319t
    patient teaching in, 317-319
    premature ventricular contractions in, 316
    sinus bradycardia in, 315, 315f
    sinus tachycardia in, 314
    supraventricular tachycardia in, 315
    ventricular fibrillation in, 317
    ventricular tachycardia in, 316-317
Dysuria, 441

E

Ear, 604-605, 604f, 605f
    external, 604
    inner, 605, 605f
    middle, 604-605
Ear disorders, 631; See also Sensory system disorders, auditory
    cultural considerations in, 618b
    diagnostic examinations in, 631-632
    ear infection in, 639b
    foreign body obstruction in, 639-640
    nursing process for, 645-646
Ear surgery
    cochlear implant in, 645, 645f
    coughing contraindication in, 33
    in Ménière's disease, 642t
    myringotomy in, 645
    patient teaching in, 644b
    stapedectomy in, 644
    tympanoplasty in, 644-645
Earwax, 604
Echinacea, 22t, 452
Echocardiography, 310
Echoencephalography, 665
Ectropion, 616-617
Eczema, 82
Edema
    in cardiovascular disorders, 368
    cast-related, 155
    pitting, 333, 334f, 334t
    pulmonary, 340, 340b, 341t, 415-416, 419
    venous assessment in, 350
Efavirenz, 753-756t
Ejaculation, 534-535
Ejection fraction, 310
Elective surgery, 18t
Electrical burn, 97
Electrical conduction system of heart, 305-306
Electrocardiography, 309f, 310
Electrode, electrocardiographic, 308
ElectroDiathermy, 623
Electroencephalography, 663, 663f
Electrolytes, postoperative management of, 52-53
Electromyography, 117, 664-665
    in carpal tunnel syndrome, 163-164
Eletriptan, 666
Embolectomy, 358
Embolic stroke, 695, 695f
Embolization of uterine artery, 564
Embolus, 32-33
    arterial, 357-359
    in endocarditis, 345
    myocardial infarction and, 326
    pulmonary, 50, 380, 416-418
Emergence phase of general anesthesia, 38
Emergency care
    for autonomic dysreflexia or hyperreflexia, 712b
    for diabetic ketoacidosis, 525b
    for hypoglycemic reaction, 524b
Emergency surgery, consent for, 25
Emergent phase of burn, 97-98, 98b, 98f
Emollients, 70-71t
Emphysema, 420f, 421-423, 421f, 422b, 425b
Empyema, 388f, 408-410, 409f, 410b
    in pneumonia, 406
Emtricitabine, 753-756t
Enalapril
    for heart failure, 336-337t
    for myocardial infarction, 329t
Encephalitis, 683, 705
Endarterectomy, 358
Endocarditis, 345-346
Endocardium, 304
Endocrine disorders, 484-532
    adrenal, 504-509

Endocrine disorders (Continued)
    complementary and alternative therapies for, 521b
    diabetes mellitus in, 509-528, 510t
    medications for, 490t
    nursing process for, 528-529
    parathyroid, 495-504
    pituitary, 489-495
    thyroid, 495-504
Endocrine glands, 485, 485f
Endocrine system, 12-14t, 485-489
    effects of surgery on, 23t
Endolymph, 605, 605f, 642t
Endometrial biopsy, 544, 567
Endometrial cancer, 567, 782-784t
Endometriosis, 560-561, 560f
Endometritis, 558
Endoplasmic reticulum, 5f, 6, 6t
Endoscopic retrograde cholangio-pancreatography, 235-236, 235f
Endoscopic sphincterotomy, 250f
Endoscopic spinal microsurgery, 116-117
    in herniated nucleus pulposus, 165
    in rheumatoid arthritis, 124
Endoscopic ultrasonography in esophageal cancer, 188
Endoscopy
    in cancer diagnosis, 787
    capsule, 181, 181f
    in gastrointestinal disorders, 180-181, 180f
    lower gastrointestinal, 182
    in musculoskeletal disorders, 116-117
    of pelvic organs, 542b
    in stomach cancer, 200
    in urinary disorders, 441
Endotracheal intubation, 97, 98f, 671
End-stage renal disease, 471-472, 473-474b
Enema, 25
Enfuvirtide, 753-756t
Enoxaparin
    preoperative, 36-37t
    for pulmonary embolism, 417
Enteroscopy, 180
Entropion, 616-617
Enucleation, 629
Enzyme-linked immunosorbent assay, for human immunodeficiency virus, 768
Enzymes in complement system, 722
Eosinophil, 263-264t, 263f, 265
Ephedra, 22t
Epidermis, 60
Epididymis, 534, 534f, 584
Epidural anesthesia, 40
Epidural hematoma, 708-709
Epigastric region, 3, 3f
Epiglottis, 374, 375f, 376f
Epilepsy, 676-680
Epimysium, 111
Epinephrine, 486-487
    for anaphylaxis, 724, 727
    for angioedema, 81
    for immune disorders, 726t
    for respiratory disorders, 401-403t
    for transfusion reaction, 729
    for urticaria, 81
Epistaxis, 384-385
Epithelial membrane, 12
Epithelial tissue, 10t, 11
Epithelioma of lip, 185
Epoetin alfa, 576, 796
Erectile dysfunction, 554-555, 555f
Erosion, 62f, 62t
Erysipelas, 75
Erythrocyte, 263-265, 263f
    anemia and, 269-281
    polycythemia and, 279-281
    in urine, 438, 440t

Erythrocyte indexes, 269
Erythrocyte sedimentation rate, 263-264t
Erythrocytosis, 279-281
Erythromycin, 396, 406, 592
Erythropoiesis, 265
  food sources needed for, 277b
Erythropoietin, 265
Eschar, 99
Escharotomy, 99, 99f
Escherichia coli O157:H7, 201-202
  in cystitis, 453
  in epididymitis, 584
  in prostatitis, 583
  in urinary tract infection, 451
  in vaginitis, 557
Esmolol, 318-319t
Esomeprazole, 187
Esophageal function studies, 101
Esophageal hernia, 217-218
Esophageal varices
  in cirrhosis, 238-239
  in polycythemia, 279-280
Esophagoenterostomy, 189
Esophagogastrectomy, 189
Esophagogastroduodenoscopy, 192
Esophagogastrostomy, 189
Esophagoscopy, 189
Esophagus, 176f, 177, 177f, 180-181, 186-190, 375f
  upper gastrointestinal series and, 180
Esotropia, 611t
Essential hypertension, 352, 352b
Estradiol transdermal system, 549-550t
Estrogen, 488, 574
Estrogen receptor modulator, 129t
Etanercept, 119-122t, 124
Ethacrynic acid, 671
Ethambutol, 401t
Ethmoid sinus, 374
Ethosuximide, 679t
Etidronate, 129
Etoposide, 793-794t
Etravirine, 753-756t
Eustachian tube, 374, 604-605
Evidence-based practice
  in burden of illness for cancer survivors, 804
  in changes in diabetes self-care behaviors, 513b
  in exercise training in chronic obstructive pulmonary disease, 422b
  in treatment of chronic constipation in older adult, 225b
  in urinary incontinence, 449b
Evisceration, 48, 48f, 200-201
Excisional biopsy, 786-787, 787f
Exemestane, 576
Exenatide, 521, 521t
Exercise
  after mastectomy, 579-580, 580f, 581b
  in cardiac rehabilitation, 331, 332b
  diabetes mellitus and, 514
  for hypertension reduction, 353
  multiple sclerosis and, 682
  to reduce myocardial oxygen needs, 326
Exercise-stress electrocardiography, 310
Exfoliative dermatitis, 80-81
Exocrine glands, 485
Exophthalmos, 495, 495f, 606-607
Expressive aphasia, 654, 696-697
Extensors, 113t
External auditory canal, 604
External beam radiation, 576
External condom catheter, 446
External fixation devices, 152-153, 152f
External hernia, 216-217

External otitis, 635-640
External radiation therapy, 790-791
Extracapsular hip fracture, 137-138, 137f
Extracapsular surgery, 617
Extracorporeal shock wave lithotripsy, 249-250, 458
Extrapyramidal system, 652
Eye, 602-603, 602f, 603f, 607t
  Bell's palsy and, 702
  care in paralyzed patient, 672
  FOUR Score Coma Scale and, 660t
  Graves' disease and, 495, 495f
  increased intracranial pressure and, 669, 669f
  safety measures for, 629b
Eye disorders, 606; *See also* Sensory system disorders, visual
Eye surgery, 629-631
  in cataracts, 617, 618f
  coughing contraindication in, 33
  enucleation in, 629
  for glaucoma, 625-627
  in injured punctal sac, 616
  keratoplasty in, 629-630
  patient teaching after, 620b
  photocoagulation in, 630
  postoperative communication in, 620b
  refractive, 612
  in retinal detachment, 622-623, 622f
  vitrectomy in, 630-631
Eyedrops, 616
Eyelid, 603f, 607t, 613-614, 613t, 616-617

F
Face
  acromegaly and, 489, 489f
  Bell's palsy and, 701-702
  Cushing's syndrome and, 504-505, 505f
Facial muscles, 114f
Facial nerve, 604f, 656f, 657f
  Bell's palsy and, 701-702
Factor IX for hemophilia, 288
Factor VIII
  for hemophilia, 288
  for von Willebrand's disease, 289
Fallopian tube, 536, 536f
Famciclovir, 588, 702
Famotidine, 193-195t
  for gastroesophageal reflux disease, 187
  preoperative, 36-37t
Farsightedness, 611, 611t
Fasciae, 111
Fasciculations, 660
Fasciotomy, 148, 149f
Fasting blood glucose, 512
Fat embolism, 150
Fat intake
  after myocardial infarction, 332
  hypertension and, 353
Fat tissue, 10t, 11
Fecal incontinence, 226-227
Felbamate, 679t
Felon, 77
Female condom, 593-595t
  risk of HIV transmission and, 772-773
Female reproductive disorders, 533-600
  abnormal uterine bleeding in, 548-550
  acute mastitis in, 571
  amenorrhea in, 547
  atrophic vaginitis in, 557-558
  breast cancer in, 571-583
    body image acceptance after mastectomy, 580
    bone marrow and stem cell transplantation for, 577
    breast reconstruction and, 581-582

Female reproductive disorders (Continued)
    chemotherapy in, 576
    clinical manifestations of, 572, 573f
    diagnostic tests for, 572-574
    etiology and pathophysiology of, 571-572, 571b, 572f
    genetics in, 781
    home care considerations in, 583b
    hormonal therapy for, 576-577
    monoclonal antibody therapy for, 577
    nursing care plan for mastectomy in, 577-578b
    ovarian ablation in, 577
    patient teaching in, 579-581, 580b
    preventing muscle contractures after mastectomy, 579-580, 580f, 581b
    prevention and early detection of, 782-784b
    prognosis in, 583, 583t
    radiation therapy in, 575-576
    reconstructive surgery in, 789
    staging of, 574, 575b
    surgical intervention in, 574-575
  cervical cancer in, 565-567
  cervicitis in, 558
  chronic mastitis in, 571
  complementary and alternative therapies for, 597b
  cystocele and rectocele in, 562-563, 563f
  displaced uterus in, 562
  dysmenorrhea in, 547-548
  endometrial cancer in, 567
  endometriosis in, 560-561, 560f
  fibrocystic breast condition in, 570-571
  hysterectomy for, 569-570
  Kegel exercises and, 553
  laboratory and diagnostic examinations in, 541-545, 542b, 543t, 546b
  medications for, 549-550t
  menopause and, 551-553
  ovarian cancer in, 567-569
  ovarian cyst in, 564
  pelvic inflammatory disease in, 558-559
  premenstrual syndrome in, 550-551
  toxic shock syndrome in, 559-560
  uterine leiomyomas in, 563-564, 563f
  uterine prolapse in, 562, 562f
  vaginal fistula in, 561-562, 561f
  vaginitis in, 557
Female reproductive system, 12-14t, 535-538, 536f
  cirrhosis and, 238f
Female sex glands, 488
Female urethra, 439
Femoral hernia, 216
Femoral-popliteal bypass graft, 357f
Femur, 111f
  hip fracture and, 137-142, 138f
Fentanyl
  for cancer pain, 801
  preoperative, 36-37t
Ferrous sulfate, 283t
Fetal hemoglobin, 277
Feverfew, 22t
Fexofenadine, 726t
Fiberoptic endoscopy, 180, 180f, 192
Fibrillation, 315-316, 317
Fibrinolytics, 356
Fibrocystic breast condition, 570-571
Fibroid tumors, uterine, 563-564, 563f
Fibromyalgia syndrome, 131, 132t

Fibromyositis, 131-132
Fibrosis, 131-132
Fibrous connective tissue, 10t, 11
Filgrastim, 283t
Filtration, 9, 9t
Finasteride, 443t
Fine crackles, 379t
Fine scaling, 62f
Fine-needle aspiration biopsy of breast, 543, 574
First-degree burn, 95t, 96f
Fissure, 62f, 62t, 226
Fistula
  anal, 226
  arteriovenous, 475f
  in Crohn's disease, 210
  in diverticulosis and diverticulitis, 214
  in esophageal cancer, 188
  vaginal, 561-562, 561f
Flaccid, term, 660, 672
Flaccid bladder, 450
Flagella, 6t
Flat plate of abdomen, 183, 216, 219
Flavoxate, 443t
Flexion, 113
Flexors, 113t
Floor of mouth cancer, 185
Flow-oriented inspiratory spirometer, 28-30
Fluconazole, 70-71t, 184
Fludarabine, 793-794t
Fludrocortisone, 490t, 507
Fluid balance, 52-53, 507t
Fluid deficit, postoperative, 50
Fluid deprivation test, 493
Fluid excess, postoperative, 50
Fluid overload
  in burn, 95
  in syndrome of inappropriate antidiuretic hormone secretion, 493
Fluid retention in heart failure, 334
Fluid therapy
  in burn, 97, 98b
  in hypovolemic anemia, 271-272
  for shock, 149
Flunisolide, 726t
Fluocinolone, 70-71t
Fluorescein angiography, 606-607
Fluoroquinolone, 445
Fluoroscopy, 308
5-Fluorouracil, 793-794t
  for breast cancer, 576
  for esophageal cancer, 188
  for laryngeal cancer, 390
Fluoxetine
  for menopause, 553
  for premenstrual syndrome, 551
Flutamide, 465
Fluticasone, 401-403t
Foley catheter, 445-446, 446f
Folic acid
  for blood and lymphatic disorders, 283t
  erythropoiesis and, 277b
  for pernicious anemia, 272-273
  sulfasalazine and, 207
Follicle-stimulating hormone, 486f
  functions of, 487f
  menstrual cycle and, 538
Folliculitis, 77
Food diary, 207
Foot
  acromegaly and, 489
  diabetes mellitus and, 522b, 527b
  muscles of, 113t
  osteoarthritis and, 125f
  postoperative venous stasis and, 50
Footboard for paralyzed patient, 673
Foreign body
  in ear, 639-640
  in eye, 628

Foreskin, 535
  phimosis and paraphimosis and, 584
Fosamprenavir, 753-756t
Fosinopril, 336-337t
Fosphenytoin
  for increased intracranial pressure, 671
  for seizures, 679t
Foster bed, 157
Foster frame, 712
FOUR Score Coma Scale, 658-659, 660t
Fourchette, 537f
Four-point gait in crutch walking, 111f
Fourth ventricle of brain, 653f
Fovea centralis, 603, 603f
Fracture, 137-148
  capillary refill test in, 153-154, 154f
  cast brace for, 153, 154f
  cast for, 153-159, 153f, 155f
  clinical manifestations of, 144
  complications of, 148-152
  etiology and pathophysiology of, 142-144, 142f, 143f
  hip, 137-142, 138f
  medical management of, 145
  open reduction with internal fixation in, 142b
  orthopedic devices for, 157-159
  pelvic, 147-148
  prevention of, 160b
  rapid orthopedic and peripheral vascular assessment in, 144-145
  skeletal pin external fixation in, 152-153, 152f
  traction for, 156, 156-157, 156f, 157b, 157f
  vertebral, 145-147, 146f
Free thyroxine, 496
Frontal lobe, 654
Frontal sinus, 374, 375f
Frovatriptan, 666
Full-thickness burn, 95t, 96f
Functional health patterns in HIV infection, 758
Functional hearing loss, 633
Functional neck dissection, 185
Fundoplication, 187
Fundus, uterine, 536, 536-537, 536f
Fungal infection
  cutaneous, 78-79, 78f
  in external otitis, 635
Furosemide, 443-444
  for cirrhosis, 237-238
  for heart failure, 336-337t
  for hyperparathyroidism, 503
  for increased intracranial pressure, 671
  for myocardial infarction, 329
  for syndrome of inappropriate antidiuretic hormone secretion, 494
Furuncle, 77, 77f
Fusiform aneurysm, 359, 359f, 697f
Fusion inhibitors, 753-756t

G

Gabapentin
  for neuropathic pain, 668
  for seizures, 679t
  for trigeminal neuralgia, 701
Gallbladder, 176f, 179f, 190
  cholecystitis and cholelithiasis and, 248-253
  intravenous cholangiography and, 232
  operative cholangiography and, 232-233
  oral cholecystography of, 232
  T-tube cholangiography and, 233
  ultrasonography of, 233
Gallbladder scan, 233

Gallbladder series, 232
Gallstones, 248-253
Gamete intrafallopian transfer, 556
Gamma delta T cell, 680
Gamma globulin
  cerebrospinal fluid, 661t
  for hepatitis A, 245
Gamma glutamyl transferase, 232
Gardasil, 566
Gardnerella vaginitis, 557
Garlic, 356
Gas exchange, 378, 380
Gas gangrene, 150-151
Gastric analysis, 269, 272
Gastric lavage, 239
Gastric outlet obstruction, 192
Gastric surgery, 195-196, 195f, 196f
Gastric tumor, 200-201
Gastric ulcer, 191-192
Gastrin, 192
Gastritis, 190-191
Gastrocnemius, 114f
Gastroduodenostomy, 195, 195f
Gastroesophageal reflux disease, 186-188
  asthma and, 426
Gastrogaffin study, 181
Gastrointestinal anthrax, 398
Gastrointestinal disorders, 175-230
  achalasia in, 189-190, 190b
  acute gastritis in, 190-191
  anal fissure and fistula in, 226
  appendicitis in, 212-216, 213b
  associated with HIV infection, 750-751t
  barium enema studies in, 182
  barium swallow and Gastrogaffin studies in, 181
  capsule endoscopy in, 181, 181f
  chronic constipation in, 225b
  colonoscopy in, 182-183, 183b
  colorectal cancer in, 220-224, 221b, 222f
  Crohn's disease in, 209-212
  cultural considerations in, 227b
  dental plaque and caries in, 183-184
  diverticulosis and diverticulitis in, 176f, 213-215, 214f, 215f
  endoscopic studies in, 180-181, 180f
  esophageal carcinoma in, 188-189, 188b
  esophageal function studies in, 181
  examination of stool for occult blood in, 182
  external hernias in, 216-217
  fecal incontinence in, 226-227
  gastroesophageal reflux disease in, 186-188
  gastrointestinal bleeding in, 197b, 198b
  hemorrhoids in, 224-226, 224f
  hiatal hernia in, 217-218, 217f, 218f
  intestinal infections in, 201-203
  intestinal obstruction in, 218-220, 219f
  irritable bowel syndrome in, 203-205, 205b
  nursing process for, 227-228
  obstruction series in, 183
  older adult and, 218b
  oral candidiasis in, 184
  oral cavity carcinoma in, 184-186
  peptic ulcer disease in, 190-201
  peritonitis in, 215-216
  sigmoidoscopy in, 182
  stomach cancer in, 200-201
  stool culture in, 183
  tube gastric analysis in, 180
  ulcerative colitis in, 205-209, 206t, 207b, 208f, 209b
  upper gastrointestinal series in, 180

Gastrointestinal system, 175-180, 176f, 177b
  chemotherapy-related complications of, 796-798
  cirrhosis and, 238f
  effects of surgery on, 23t
  postoperative status of, 52
  preoperative preparation of, 25
  systemic lupus erythematosus and, 86
Gastrojejunostomy, 195-196, 195f
Gastroscopy, 180-181, 180f
Gastrostomy, 189
Gefitinib, 414
Gemcitabine, 255-256t, 257, 793-794t
Gender identity, 539
Gender role, 540
General anesthesia, 37-39, 39f
Generalized tonic-clonic seizure, 677-678t
Genetic counseling
  in cancer, 781
  in Huntington's disease, 694
Genetics
  in cancer, 781
  in Huntington's disease, 693
  immunity and, 722
  in risk for breast cancer, 571
Genioglossal advancement and hyoid myotomy, 388
Genital herpes, 69, 587-588, 588f
Gentamicin
  for burn, 101t
  for eye infection, 625-626t
Gigantism, 491
Ginger
  effects during surgery, 38t
  preoperative considerations for, 22t
Gingival bleeding
  in coagulation disorders, 285
  in von Willebrand's disease, 289
Ginkgo biloba, 356
  effects during surgery, 38t
  preoperative considerations for, 22t
Ginseng
  effects during surgery, 38t
  preoperative considerations for, 22t
Glargine insulin, 515-516t
Glasgow Coma Scale, 658, 659t
Glatiramer acetate, 681
Glaucoma, 623-627, 624f, 625f, 627f
Gleason Grading System, 465
Glial cell, 11-12, 651
Glimepiride, 520, 520t
Glipizide, 520, 520t
Glomerulonephritis
  acute, 468-469
  chronic, 469-470
  in hyperparathyroidism, 502
Glomerulus, 436, 436f, 437f, 437t
Glossopharyngeal nerve, 656f, 657t
Glucagon, 487-488
  for hypoglycemic reaction in diabetes mellitus, 521
Glucocorticoids, 486
Glucosamine, 126
Glucose
  cerebrospinal fluid, 661t
  diabetes mellitus and, 510-511
  in urine, 438, 440t
Glucose intolerance, 471
Glucose loading test, 491
Glulisine, 515-516t
Glyburide, 520, 520t
Glycemic index, 513
Glycogen, diabetes mellitus and, 510-511
Glycopyrrolate, 36-37t
Glycosuria, 511
Glycosylated hemoglobin, 512
Goiter, 500-501, 501f
Gold salts, 119-122t

Goldmann perimetry test, 606-607
Golgi apparatus, 5f, 6, 6t, 651f
GoLYTELY bowel preparation, 182-183, 183b
Gonadotropic hormones, 486f
Goniometer, 110
Gonococcal infection, 394, 614
Gonorrhea, 589-590
Goserelin, 465
Gout, 127-128
Graafian follicle, 538
Graft rejection, 729-730
Gram stain
  in cellulitis, 75
  in pelvic inflammatory disease, 558
Granisetron, 576
  for chemotherapy-related vomiting, 797-798t, 797-798
Granulocyte, 265
Granulocyte-colony stimulating factor, 283t, 795-796
Granulocyte-macrophage colony-stimulating factors, 795-796
Granuloma in Crohn's disease, 210
Graves' disease, 495-498, 495f, 496b
Gravidity, 596
Greenstick fracture, 143f, 144
Griseofulvin, 70-71t, 78
Growth hormone, 486f
  acromegaly and, 489
  dwarfism and, 492
  gigantism and, 491
Growth hormone suppression test, 491
Guaiac test, 789
Guarana, 22t
Gyrus, 652

H

Habit training, 447-448
Haemophilus influenzae
  in acute otitis media, 636
  in cellulitis, 74-75
  in conjunctivitis, 614
  in meningitis, 704
  in pneumonia, 404-405, 405
Hair, 60f, 61
  alopecia and, 94
  chemotherapy-related complications of, 796
  Cushing's syndrome and, 505, 505f
  folliculitis and, 77
  hypertrichosis and, 94
  hypothyroidism and, 499
  hypotrichosis and, 94
Halo brace, 146, 146f
Halo traction, 712
Haloperidol
  for Alzheimer's disease, 689
  drug-induced parkinsonism and, 683
Harris flush, 52
Hartmann's procedure, 214-215, 214f
Head and neck
  principal muscles of, 112t
  trauma to, 352t, 708-710, 709f
Head-tilt/chin-lift technique, 388-389
Health promotion
  in allergies, 725b
  in communication for people with impaired hearing, 633b
  in contact lens care, 613b
  in foods to reduce cancer risk, 780b
  in foot care in diabetes mellitus, 522b
  for healthy skin, 84b
  in hip fracture, 137b
  in HIV infection, 759t, 769, 769b
  in iron administration, 277b
  in Kegel exercises, 553b
  in menstruation education, 546b

Health promotion (Continued)
in myocardial infarction, 332b
in nephritis, 469b
in neurologic disorders, 675b
in pneumonia, 404b
in prevention and detection of cancer, 784b
in prevention of esophageal cancer, 188b
in renal failure, 472b
in screening for colorectal cancer, 221b
in sexual health, 540b
Healthy People 2010, HIV infection and, 757b
Hearing aid care, 634b
Hearing loss, 633-635, 633b
in acute otitis media, 636
behavioral clues indicating, 601b
in brain tumor, 707
cochlear implant for, 645, 645f
cultural considerations in, 618b
hearing aid care and, 634b
in otosclerosis, 640
Heart, 304-306, 304f; See also Cardiovascular disorders and Cardiovascular system
diagnostic imaging of, 308
cardiac catheterization and angiography in, 308
cardiac monitors and, 309-310
echocardiography in, 310
electrocardiography in, 309f, 310
thallium scanning in, 310
electrical conduction system of, 305-306
myocardial infarction and, 326-332, 326f. See also Myocardial infarction.
Heart disease
cardiomyopathy in, 346-348, 347b
coronary artery disease in, 320-321, 321f, 327t
dysrhythmias in, 314-319
atrial fibrillation in, 315-316
atrioventricular block in, 316
drug therapy for, 318-319t
patient teaching in, 317-319
premature ventricular contractions in, 316
sinus bradycardia in, 315, 315f
sinus tachycardia in, 314
supraventricular tachycardia in, 315
ventricular fibrillation in, 317
ventricular tachycardia in, 316-317
endocarditis in, 345-346
hypertension and, 351-354
drug therapy for, 353, 354b
essential, 352, 352b
etiology and pathophysiology of, 351-352
malignant, 353
nonpharmacologic therapy for, 353-354
secondary, 352-353, 352t
myocarditis in, 346
pericarditis in, 343-345
rheumatic, 342-343
valvular, 340-342, 342t
Heart failure, 332-348
in acromegaly, 491
after myocardial infarction, 329
classification and staging of, 333b
diagnostic tests for, 334-335
left ventricular failure in, 333
medical management of, 335, 336-337t
nursing care plan for, 338-339b
nursing guidelines for, 339
patient teaching in, 339
pitting edema in, 333, 334f, 334t
in polycythemia, 279-280

Heart failure (Continued)
pulmonary edema and, 340
right ventricular failure in, 333-334
signs and symptoms of, 334b
Heart sounds, 306
Heart transplantation, 347-348, 347b
Heartburn, 186-187
Heberden's nodes, 125, 126f
Helical computed tomography chest scan, 380
Helicobacter pylori in peptic ulcer disease, 191
antibiotics for, 195
Hemangioma, 62f
Hemarthrosis in hemophilia, 287
Hematemesis, 192
Hematest, 789
Hematocrit, 263-264t, 265
Hematologic disorders; See Blood disorders
Hematologic system, 10t, 11, 262-269, 266f
blood formation in, 110
blood types and, 266-267
chemotherapy effects on, 791-796
hemostasis and, 266
red blood cells and, 263-265, 263f
Rh factor and, 267
systemic lupus erythematosus and, 86
thrombocytes and, 266
white blood cells and, 265-266
Hematopoiesis, 110
Hematopoietic stem cell transplantation
for aplastic anemia, 274
for sickle cell anemia, 278
Hemianopia, 661
Hemiarthroplasty, 138f, 139
Hemiparesis, 696
Hemiplegia, 673, 696
Hemoccult test, 789
Hemodialysis
in end-stage renal disease, 474-475, 475f
in systemic lupus erythematosus, 87
Hemoglobin, 263-264t, 265
Hemolyzation, 267
Hemophilia A, 287-289, 289b
Hemorrhagic stroke, 695-696, 695f
Hemorrhoidectomy, 224-225
Hemorrhoids, 224-226, 224f
Hemostasis, 266
Henle's loop, 436, 436f, 437f, 437t
Heparin
for disseminated intravascular coagulation, 290
for myocardial infarction, 329t
preoperative, 36-37t
for pulmonary embolism, 417
Hepatic abscess, 247-248
Hepatic disorders; See Hepatobiliary disorders
Hepatic encephalopathy, 240
Hepatitis, 243-247
clinical manifestations of, 244, 244f
liver transplantation in, 245-246
medical management of, 244-246
modes of transmission, 244b
nursing interventions for, 246-247
prevention of, 243b
viral studies in, 234
Hepatitis A virus, 243, 244
prophylaxis guidelines for, 752t
Hepatitis B vaccine, 245
Hepatitis B virus, 243, 244, 245
associated with HIV infection, 749
liver cancer and, 241
prophylaxis guidelines for, 752t
Hepatitis C virus, 243, 244, 245
associated with HIV infection, 749
liver cancer and, 241
Hepatitis viruses, 243, 244

Hepatobiliary disorders, 231-261
cholecystitis and cholelithiasis in, 248-253
laparoscopic cholecystectomy for, 251
lithotripsy for, 249-250
cirrhosis in, 236-241
complementary and alternative therapies for, 249b
cultural considerations in, 258b
drug therapy for, 255-256t
hepatitis in, 243-247
laboratory and diagnostic examinations in, 231-236
abdominal computed tomography in, 235
endoscopic retrograde cholangiopancreatography in, 235-236, 235f
gallbladder scanning in, 233
hepatitis virus studies in, 234
intravenous cholangiography in, 232
liver enzyme tests in, 231-232
needle liver biopsy in, 233-234
operative cholangiography in, 232-233
oral cholecystography in, 232
pancreatic ultrasonography in, 235
radioisotope liver scanning in, 234
serum ammonia test in, 234
serum amylase test in, 234
serum bilirubin test in, 231
serum lipase test in, 235
serum protein test in, 232
T-tube cholangiography in, 233
ultrasonography in, 233
urine amylase test in, 234-235
liver abscess in, 247-248
liver cancer in, 241-243
nursing process for, 257-258
older adult and, 253b
pancreatic cancer in, 255-257, 257f
pancreatitis in, 253-255
Hepatomegaly
in hepatic abscess, 247
in Hodgkin's lymphoma, 294
in polycythemia, 279-280
Herald patch, 74, 74f
Herbal therapies
for cardiovascular and peripheral vascular disorders, 356b
effects during surgery, 38t
for endocrine disorders, 521
for hepatobiliary disorders, 249b
for HIV infection, 757
for integumentary disorders, 86
for irritable bowel syndrome, 205b
for menopause, 552-553
for respiratory disorders, 391b
review before surgery, 21, 22t
Hernia, 216-227
external, 216-217
hiatal, 217-218, 217f, 218f
Herpes simplex virus, 68-72, 69f
associated with HIV infection, 750-751t
Bell's palsy and, 701-702
in encephalitis, 705
in genital herpes, 587-588
in keratitis, 615
Herpes zoster, 72-74, 72f, 73b
Heterograft, 100
Hiatal hernia, 217-218, 217f, 218f
HIDA scanning, 233
High-ceiling diuretics, 443-444
High-density lipoproteins 311, 313, 313b
Highly active antiretroviral therapy, 737-738
drug resistance to, 749
pros and cons of, 753t

Hip
arthroplasty of, 135-136, 135f, 136f
fracture of, 137-142, 138f
Hirsutism, 94, 505
Histamine2 receptor antagonists
for gastroesophageal reflux disease, 187
for pancreatitis, 254
for peptic ulcer disease, 193
preoperative, 36-37t
Histoplasmosis, 750-751t
Hodgkin's lymphoma, 293-297, 294b, 295f, 296b, 730
Hoffman external fixation device, 152f
Holter monitor, 309
Homans' sign, 50, 362
Home care considerations
in burn, 102b, 104b
in chronic oxygen therapy, 424b
in cirrhosis, 241b
in diabetes mellitus, 528b
guidelines for baths and soaks, 104b
in hemophilia, 289b
in HIV infection, 759t
in lung cancer, 414b
in myocardial infarction, 332b
in peptic ulcer disease, 199b
in urinary diversion, 480b
Home unit, 309
Homeostasis, 5
Homocysteine, 311
Alzheimer's disease and, 688-689
Homograft, 100
Homonymous hemianopia, 696
Homozygous, term, 276-277
Hordeolum, 613-614, 613t
Hormonal agents in chemotherapy, 793-794t
Hormonal deprivation therapy in prostate cancer, 465
Hormonal therapy in breast cancer, 576-577
Hormone replacement therapy
postmenopausal, 552
risk for endometrial cancer and, 567
Hormones, 485
anterior pituitary, 485, 486f, 487f
electrical conduction system of heart and, 305
influence on kidney, 437-438
Host defense system, 719
Huff coughing, 28-29b, 30b
Humalog, 515-516t
Human chorionic gonadotropin, 545
Human immunodeficiency virus antibody testing, 747, 747b
Human immunodeficiency virus infection, 734-778
acute intervention in, 763-769
acute retroviral syndrome and, 745, 745t
assisting with grieving in, 763
confidentiality and, 763
cultural considerations in, 738b
dementia in, 706-707
diagnostic criteria for, 736t
diagnostic tests for, 747-749
CD4+ cell monitoring in, 747
drug resistance testing and, 749
HIV antibody testing for, 747, 747b
laboratory parameters and, 749
pretest and posttest counseling and, 748b
viral load monitoring in, 747-748
duty to treat and, 763
early infection in, 745, 745f
early symptomatic disease in, 745-746, 746b, 746f

Human immunodeficiency virus infection (Continued)
  ethical and legal principles and, 763
  etiology of, 587
  future of, 774
  health promotion in, 769
  Healthy People 2010 and, 757b
  historical background of, 734-738
  HIV-associated cognitive motor complex in, 767
  nursing care plan for, 768b
  nursing interventions in, 757-769, 759t, 760b
  nutrition management in, 766t
  older adult and, 737b
  pathophysiology of, 742-744
  peripheral neuropathy in, 767
  prevention of, 769-774, 769b, 770b
  significance of problem, 737
  spectrum of, 744-746
  terminal phase of, 746
  terms related to, 745t
  therapeutic management of, 749-757
  transmission of, 738-742, 739f
  trends and affected populations, 737-738
  tuberculosis and, 399
  viral load and disease progression in, 742-744, 744f
  wasting and lipodystrophy syndromes in, 765-767
  white blood cell involvement in, 743t
Human papillomavirus, 543, 565
Human papillomavirus vaccine, 566
Humoral immunity, 721-723
Huntington's disease, 693-694
Hydrocele, 585
Hydrochlorothiazide
  for cirrhosis, 237-238
  for heart failure, 336-337t
Hydrocortisone
  for Addison's disease, 507
  for cancer treatment, 793-794t
  for ear infection, 637-638t
  for external otitis, 635
  for psoriasis, 85
  for respiratory disorders, 401-403t
Hydromorphone, 797-798t
  for cancer pain, 801
  for sickle cell crisis, 278
Hydronephrosis, 457
Hydroxychloroquine
  for rheumatoid arthritis, 119-122t
  for systemic lupus erythematosus, 87
Hydroxyurea
  for polycythemia, 280
  for sickle cell anemia, 278
Hydroxyzine, 70-71t
Hypercalcemia
  in hyperparathyroidism, 502
  in multiple myeloma, 291
  in renal tumor, 459
Hypercapnia
  in chronic bronchitis, 424
  in obstructive sleep apnea, 387
Hyperextension, 113
Hyperglycemia
  in diabetes mellitus, 510-511
  diabetic coma and, 525t
  diabetic ketoacidosis and, 525b
  insulin therapy and, 516
Hyperglycemic hyperosmolar nonketotic coma, 525t
Hyperkalemia
  in Addison's disease, 506-507
  in tumor lysis syndrome, 800
Hyperlipidemia
  cardiovascular disease and, 317-319
  in nephrotic syndrome, 467
  peripheral vascular diseases and, 349

Hyperopia, 608-609t, 611, 611t
Hyperparathyroidism, 502-503
Hyperphosphatemia in tumor lysis syndrome, 800
Hyperreflexia
  emergency care for, 712b
  in spinal cord injury, 710-712
Hypersensitivity disorders, 724-730, 725b, 726b
Hypersensitivity reaction, 723-724, 724,
  in anaphylaxis, 727
  safety issues in, 726b
Hypertension, 351-354
  cardiovascular disease risk and, 314
  drug therapy for, 353, 354b
  essential, 352, 352b
  malignant, 353
  nonpharmacologic therapy for, 353-354
  peripheral vascular diseases and, 349
  and risk for stroke, 694-695
  secondary, 352-353, 352t
Hyperthermia, postoperative, 46, 46t
Hyperthyroidism, 495-498, 495f, 496b
Hypertrichosis, 94
Hypertrophic arthritis, 125-127, 125b, 125f, 126f
Hypertrophic cardiomyopathy, 346
Hypertrophic scar, 62f
Hypoalbuminemia in nephrotic syndrome, 467
Hypocalcemia, 503
Hypochloremic alkalosis, 443
Hypogastric region, 3, 3f
Hypoglossal nerve, 656f, 657t
Hypoglycemia, insulin therapy and, 517-518, 522, 524b, 525t
Hypokalemia in Cushing's syndrome, 504-505
Hyponatremia, in syndrome of inappropriate antidiuretic hormone secretion, 493
Hypoparathyroidism, 503-504
Hypophysis, 485
Hypopituitary dwarfism, 492
Hypopnea, 387
Hypotension
  in anaphylaxis, 727
  in intestinal obstruction, 219
  in pancreatitis, 253
  plasmapheresis-related, 731
  in toxic shock syndrome, 559
Hypothalamus, 485f, 653, 653f
Hypothermia, postoperative, 45-46, 46t
Hypothyroidism, 498-500, 499f
  levothyroxine-related, 496
  medications for, 497t
Hypotrichosis, 94
Hypoventilation, atelectasis and, 410
Hypovolemic anemia, 271-272
Hypovolemic shock, 271
Hypoxia, 380b
Hysterectomy, 569-570
  in cervical cancer, 566
  as contraception, 593-595t
  in endometrial cancer, 567
  vaginal, 569
Hysterosalpingogram, 544

I
Ibandronate, 129t
Ibritumomab, 297
Ibuprofen
  for rheumatoid arthritis, 119-122t
  for systemic lupus erythematosus, 87
Idiopathic aplastic anemia, 273
Idiopathic hyperplasia, 489

Ileal conduit (ileal loop), 478-479, 479f
Ileoanal anastomosis, 207
Ileostomy, 207, 208f
Ileum, 176f, 178, 178f
Ilizarov apparatus, 152f
Imaging studies, diagnostic
  of breast, 574
  in breast cancer screening, 573
  for cancer diagnosis, 787, 787-788
  in cardiovascular disorders, 311-312
  in hematologic and lymphatic disorders, 269
  in hepatobiliary disorders, 233, 235
  in musculoskeletal disorders, 113-116
  in neurologic disorders, 662
  of pancreas, 235
  in respiratory disorders, 380
  of skull, 662
  in spinal cord injury, 712
  in stomach cancer, 200
  in stroke, 697
  in urinary disorders, 442
Immediate postoperative phase, 44-46, 45f, 45t
Immune disorders, 719-733
  adaptive immunity and, 720-721, 720t, 721f
  anaphylaxis in, 727-728, 727b
  autoimmune disorders in, 730-731
  delayed hypersensitivity in, 729-730
  effects of aging on immune system and, 722-723
  hypersensitivity disorders in, 724-730, 725b, 726b
  immune response and, 723-724, 723b
  immunodeficiency disorders in, 730
  latex allergy in, 728-729
  medications for, 726t
  nature of immunity and, 719-722, 720f
  nephritis in, 468-470, 469b
  nephrotic syndrome in, 467-468
  transfusion reactions in, 729
Immune response, 722b, 723-724, 723b
Immune system, 719
  effects of surgery on, 23t
  human immunodeficiency virus and, 742-744
  malignant cells and, 785
  organs and tissues of, 721f
Immunity, nature of, 719-722, 720f
Immunization, 723
  for hepatitis, 245
Immunocompetence, 719, 721-722
Immunodeficiency disorders, 723, 724, 730
Immunogen, 722
Immunoglobulin E, 724
Immunoglobulin M test for West Nile virus, 705
Immunosuppressives
  for cardiac transplantation, 348
  for Crohn's disease, 210
  for graft rejection, 729
  for liver transplantation, 246
  for rheumatoid arthritis, 119-122t
  for thrombocytopenia, 287
Immunosurveillance, malignant cells and, 785
Immunotherapy, 723
Impacted fracture, 137f, 143f, 144
Impetigo contagiosa, 75-76, 76f
Implantable cardioverter-defibrillator, 335
Impotence
  after spinal cord injury, 712
  obstructive sleep apnea and, 387

In vitro fertilization, 556
Incentive spirometry, patient teaching in, 28, 28-29b, 28b, 29f
Incision
  postoperative care of, 48
  preoperative teaching about, 35
Incisional biopsy, 786-787, 787f
Incisional hernia, 216
Incomplete fracture, 143f
Incontinence
  bowel, 226-227
  urinary, 448-450, 449b
Incus, 604f, 605
Indinavir, 753-756t
Indirect bilirubin, 231
Indirect laryngoscopy, 185, 381
Indomethacin, 119-122t
Induction phase of general anesthesia, 38
Infarct, 32-33
Infective endocarditis, 345-346
Infertility, 555-556
  endometriosis and, 561
Infiltrative anesthesia, 40
Inflammatory bowel disease, 205-212
Inflammatory cutaneous disorders, 79-87
Inflammatory eyelid disorders, 613-615, 613t
Inflammatory heart disorders, 342-348
Inflammatory musculoskeletal disorders, 117-171
Inflammatory urinary disorders, 451-456
Infliximab
  for Crohn's disease, 211
  for rheumatoid arthritis, 119-122t
Influenza, prophylaxis guidelines for, 752t
Informed consent, 24-25
Inguinal hernia, 216
Inhalational anthrax, 398
Injection drug abuse, transmission of HIV via, 738-740
Innate immunity, 720, 720t
Inner ear, 604f, 605, 605f
Inotropic agents, 318-319t
  for heart failure, 336-337t
  for myocardial infarction, 329t
Inpatient surgery, 18t, 19
Insensible fluid loss in end-stage renal disease, 472
Inspiratory capacity, 380
Instep claudication, 360
Insufficiency in valvular heart disease, 340
Insulin
  diabetes mellitus and, 509
  effects during surgery, 38t
  islets of Langerhans and, 487-488
Insulin pen, 517, 517f
Insulin pump, 518-520, 519f
Insulin resistance, 510
Insulin therapy, 514-520, 514f
Insulin-enhancing drugs, 521, 521t
Intacs, 612
Integra Dermal Regeneration Template, 99
Integrase inhibitor, 753-756t
Integumentary disorders, 59-108
  alopecia in, 94
  appendages of skin and, 61
  associated with HIV infection, 750-751b
  bacterial, 74-77
  burns in, 94-103
  chief complaint in, 67-68
  complementary and alternative therapies for, 105b
  cultural considerations in, 68b
  effects of aging on skin, 103b
  functions of skin and, 59-60, 59b
  fungal, 78-79, 78f
  healthy skin promotion and, 84b

Integumentary disorders (Continued)
    hypertrichosis in, 94
    hypotrichosis in, 94
    inflammatory, 79-87
    inspection and palpation in, 61-67
    medications for, 70-71t
    nursing process for, 103-105
    parasitic, 87-90
    paronychia in, 94
    primary skin lesions in, 62t
    psychosocial assessment in, 68
    structure of skin and, 60-61, 60f
    tumors in, 90-93
    viral, 68-74
Integumentary system, 12-14t
Interatrial node, 306f
Interbrain, 653
Interferon beta-1a, 681
Interferon beta-1b, 681
Intermediate acting insulin, 515-516t
Intermittent claudication, 349, 355
Intermittent irrigation, postprostatectomy, 464
Internal monitoring in increased intracranial pressure, 671
Internal radiation therapy, 791, 792b
    in breast cancer, 576
International normalized ratio, 263-264t
Interstitial cystitis, 453-454
Intertrochanter hip fracture, 137-138, 137f
Intervertebral disk herniation, 164-166, 164f
Intestinal disorders, 201-227
    anal fissure and fistula in, 226
    appendicitis in, 212-213, 213b
    colorectal cancer in, 220-224, 221b, 222f
    Crohn's disease in, 209-212
    diverticulosis and diverticulitis in, 176f, 213-215, 214f, 215f
    external hernias in, 216-227
    hemorrhoids in, 224-226, 224f
    hiatal hernia in, 217-218, 217f, 218f
    infections in, 201-203
    intestinal obstruction in, 218-220, 219f
    irritable bowel syndrome in, 203-205, 205b
    ulcerative colitis in, 205-209, 206t, 207b, 208f, 209b
Intestinal infection, 201-203
Intestinal obstruction, 218-220, 219f
Intracapsular hip fracture, 137-138, 138f
Intracranial pressure elevation, 668-672, 669f, 670f
Intracranial surgery, coughing contraindication in, 33
Intradermal skin testing, 79
Intramedullary rod, 138f, 139
Intraocular lens, 617
Intraocular pressure, glaucoma and, 623
Intraoperative phase of surgery, 43-44, 43f
    circulating nurse and scrub nurse roles in, 44, 44b, 44f
    holding area and, 43-44
Intrauterine device, 593-595t
Intravenous cholangiography, 232
Intravenous immunoglobulin
    for myasthenia gravis, 692
    for thrombocytopenia, 286-287
Intravenous pyelography, 441
Intravenous regional anesthesia, 40
Intravenous saline for hypovolemic anemia, 271-272
Intravenous urography, 441
Intrinsic factor, 177-178
    pernicious anemia and, 272

Involuntary nervous system, 651
Iodine dye in myelogram, 664
Iopamidol, 664
Ipsilateral pupil, 669, 669f
Irinotecan, 793-794t
Iris, 602-603, 603f, 607t
Iron, 276, 277b
Iron deficiency anemia, 275-276, 276b, 277b
Iron dextran, 283t
Irreducible hernia, 216
Irritability, electrical conduction system of heart and, 305
Irritable bowel syndrome, 203-205, 205b
Ischemia, 321, 326
Ischemic stroke, 695
Islets of Langerhans, 487-488
Isograft, 729
Isoniazid, 400, 401-403t
Isosorbide, 329t
Isospora belli, 750-751t
Isotretinoin, 70-71t, 83
Itraconazole, 70-71t

J
Jackknife position, 41f
Jacksonian-focal seizure, 677-678t
Jackson-Pratt drain, 250
Jamestown Canyon virus, 750-751t
Jaundice, serum bilirubin test for, 231
Jehovah's Witness, 270b
Jejunum, 178
Jock itch, 78
Joint, 110, 110f
    dislocation of, 162-163
    sprain of, 160
Joint pain in rheumatic heart disease, 343
Juxtaglomerular apparatus, 436, 437f

K
Kaolin-pectin, 193-195t
Kaposi's sarcoma, 185, 298, 734, 750-751t
Kava, 22t
Kegel exercises, 447, 450, 553, 553b
Keloid, 62f, 62t, 90-91, 91f
Kelp, 521
Keratin, 60-61, 61
Keratitis, 615
Keratoconjunctivitis sicca, 615-616
Keratolytic agents, 85
Keratoplasty, 629-630
Keratorefractive surgery, 612
Kernig's sign, 704
Ketoacidosis, diabetic, 511
Ketoconazole, 193-195t
Ketone bodies, 438, 440t, 510-511
Ketonuria, 512
Ketorolac, 36-37t
Kidney, 434-438, 435f; See also renal entries
    acute glomerulonephritis and, 468-469
    chronic glomerulonephritis and, 469-470
    diuretics to enhance urinary output and, 443-444
    effects of aging on, 439
    gross anatomical structure of, 435, 435f
    hormonal influence on, 437-438
    hydronephrosis and, 457
    hypertension and, 351
    major functions of, 438b
    medication considerations for renal function and, 443-445
    microscopic structure of, 435-438, 436f
    nephritis and, 468-470
    nephrotic syndrome and, 467-468
    pyelonephritis and, 455-456
    renal failure and, 470-472, 472b

Kidney (Continued)
    systemic lupus erythematosus and, 86
    transplantation of, 478, 478f
Kidney stones, 457-459, 458f
Kidney-ureter-bladder radiography, 441
Klebsiella
    in acute otitis media, 636
    in pneumonia, 405
    in prostatitis, 583
Knee arthroplasty, 133-135, 133f, 134b
Kock pouch, 207, 207-208, 208f, 479, 479f
Küntscher nail, 138f, 139
Kyphoplasty, 130
Kyphosis, 170, 170f

L
Labia majora, 536f, 537, 537f
Labia minora, 536f, 537, 537f
Laboratory tests
    in auditory disorders, 631-632, 632f
    in blood disorders, 269
    in cancer diagnosis, 788-789
    in cardiovascular disorders, 310-311, 335
    in female reproductive disorders, 541-545
    in gastrointestinal disorders, 180-183
    in hepatobiliary disorders, 231-236
    in musculoskeletal disorders, 117, 117t
    in neurologic disorders, 661-665
    preoperative, 24
    in respiratory disorders, 379-429
    in urinary disorders, 439-443
    in visual disorders, 606-607, 608-609t
Labyrinth, 605
Labyrinthitis, 639
Lacrimal apparatus, 602, 602f
Lactate dehydrogenase, 232
Lactiferous duct, 537-538, 538f
Lactulose, 255-256t
Laminectomy, 165
Laminography, 115
Lamivudine, 753-756t
Lamotrigine
    for seizures, 679t
    for trigeminal neuralgia, 701
Language, neurologic assessment and, 659
Lansoprazole, 187, 193-195t
Lantus, 515-516t
Laparoscopic cholecystectomy, 250-251, 251
Laparoscopy
    in endometriosis, 560
    in female reproductive disorders, 542
Large intestine, 178-179, 178f
Laryngeal edema in anaphylaxis, 727
Laryngitis, 393
Laryngopharynx, 374, 375f
Laryngoscopy, 381, 393
Larynx, 176f, 374, 376f
    cancer of, 389-390
Laser in-situ keratomileusis, 612
Laser photocoagulation, 622
Laser surgery
    in cancer, 789
    in macular degeneration, 621
Laser trabeculoplasty, 625-627
Later postoperative phase, 46-52, 46t, 47f
Latex agglutination test, 119
Latex allergy, 26-27, 28b, 728-729
Latissimus dorsi musculocutaneous flap, 582, 582f
Lavage, 25

Leflunomide, 119-122t
Left atrium, 304, 304f, 305f, 307f
Left bronchus, 374f, 376f, 377
Left ventricular failure, 333-334, 334,
Left-sided stroke, 696-697, 697f
Leg exercises, 32, 32f
Legionnaire's disease, 396-397
Leiomyoma, uterine, 563-564, 563f
Lens, 603f
    cataracts and, 617-618, 617f, 618f, 619b
Lente insulin, 515-516t
Lentigo melanoma, 92-93
Lentivirus, 742
Letrozole, 576
Leukapheresis, 801
Leukemia, 282-284, 283t, 285b, 785-786
Leukocyte, 263f, 265-266
    agranulocytosis and, 281-282
    leukemia and, 282-284, 283t, 285b
    in urine, 438
Leukopenia, 281, 791-796
Leukoplakia, 185
Leukorrhea, 587-588
Leukotriene modifiers
    for asthma, 427
    for respiratory disorders, 401-403t
Leukotriene receptor antagonists, 401-403t, 725-726
    for allergic rhinitis and conjunctivitis, 386
    for asthma, 427
Leuprolide, 465, 793-794t
    for endometriosis, 560-561
LeVeen continuous peritoneal jugular stent, 238, 238f
Level of consciousness, 658, 658t, 659t
Levetiracetam, 679t
Levodopa, 685, 686-687t
Levofloxacin, 590, 592
Levonorgestrel, 593-595t
Levothyroxine, 490t
Lice infestation, 87-89, 89f
Lichenification, 62f, 62t
Lidocaine
    for cardiac dysrhythmias, 318-319t
    for myocardial infarction, 329t
    for pain in genital herpes, 588
    for stomatitis, 796
Lindane, 70-71t, 89
Liothyronine, 490t
Liotrix, 490t
Lipase, 179
Lipodystrophy syndromes, 765-767
Lisinopril, 336-337t
Lispro insulin, 515-516t, 516
Lithiasis, 457
Lithium carbonate, 494
Lithotripsy, 249-250
Liver, 176f, 179, 179f. See also Hepatobiliary disorders.
    abscess of, 247-248
    cancer of, 241-243
    cirrhosis of, 236-241
    hepatitis and, 243-247
Liver enzyme tests, 231-232
Liver transplantation, 245-246
Lobectomy
    in liver cancer, 242-243
    in lung cancer, 414
Local anesthesia, 40
Local seizure, 677-678t
Lodoxamide, 387
Long-acting insulin, 515-516t
Loop diuretics, 443-444
    for increased intracranial pressure, 671
Loperamide, 193-195t, 207
Lopinavir/ritonavir, 753-756t
Loratidine, 726t

Lorazepam
for Alzheimer's disease, 689
for cancer treatment symptoms, 797-798t
for chemotherapy-related vomiting, 797-798
preoperative, 36-37t
Lordosis, 170, 170f
Lou Gehrig's disease (amyotrophic lateral sclerosis), 693
Low-density lipoproteins
hyperlipidemia and, 313, 313b
serum lipid tests and, 311
Lower airway disorders; See Respiratory disorders, lower airway
Lower extremities
amputation of, 167-169, 168f
peripheral arterial disease of, 355-357, 355f
principal muscles of, 112t
venous stasis ulcer and, 366-367, 366f
Lower gastrointestinal endoscopy, 182
Lower gastrointestinal series, 182
Low-molecular-weight heparins, 364
Lumbar puncture, 661-662, 662f
Lumen, 320
Lumpectomy, 574-575
Lung, 374f, 376f, 382, 395-420; See also Respiratory disorders, lower airway
Lung biopsy, 382
Lung volume tests, 380
Luteinizing hormone, 486f, 487f, 538
Lymph, 267-268
Lymph nodes, 268, 268f, 721f
in breast, 572f
involvement in breast cancer and, 583t
Lymph vessels, 267-268
Lymphangitis, 292-293
Lymphatic disorders, 292-298
drug therapy for, 283t
laboratory and diagnostic tests in, 269
nursing process for, 298-299
older adult and, 298b
Lymphatic system, 12-14t, 267-269, 268f
Lymphedema, 293
Lymphocyte, 263f, 265-266, 720-721
white blood cell count and, 263-264t
Lymphokine, 721
Lymphoma, 785-786
associated with HIV infection, 750-751b
Hodgkin's, 293-297, 294b, 295f, 296b
non-Hodgkin's, 297-298
Lypressin, 493
Lysis, 19t
Lysosome, 5f, 6, 6t
Lysozyme, 176-177, 602

M

Macrophage, 720-721
involvement in HIV infection, 743t
Macula, 603
Macula densa cell, 436-437
Macula lutea, 603f
Macular degeneration, 621
Macule, 62f, 62t, 75-76
Mafenide, 101t
Magnesium, 311, 354
Magnetic resonance angiography, 662-663
Magnetic resonance imaging, 115
in breast cancer screening, 573
for cancer diagnosis, 788
in esophageal cancer, 188
in female reproductive disorders, 544-545

Magnetic resonance imaging (Continued)
in hematologic and lymphatic disorders, 269
in Hodgkin's lymphoma, 294-295
in laryngeal cancer, 389
in lung cancer, 413-414
in neurologic disorders, 662
in stroke, 697
in urinary disorders, 442
Maintenance phase of general anesthesia, 38
Major surgery, 18t
Male climacteric, 553-554
Male condom, 593-595t
Male infertility testing, 555
Male reproductive disorders, 533-600
complementary and alternative therapies for, 597b
epididymitis in, 584
erectile dysfunction in, 554-555, 555f
hydrocele in, 585
laboratory and diagnostic examinations in, 545, 546b
male climacteric and, 553-554
penile cancer in, 586
phimosis and paraphimosis in, 584-585
prostatitis in, 583-584
testicular cancer in, 585-586, 586b, 586f
varicocele in, 585
Male reproductive system, 12-14t, 534-535, 534f, 535f
Male sex glands, 488
Malecot catheter, 445-446, 446f
Malignant hypertension, 353
Malignant hyperthermia, 46, 46t
Malignant melanoma, 92-93, 93f
Malignant tumor, 785
Malleus, 604f, 605
Mammography, 544, 571, 573
Mannitol, 444, 625-626t
for glaucoma, 627
Mantoux test, 400
Marijuana, 797-798
Mast cell, 743t
Mastectomy
arm exercises after, 581b
breast prosthesis and, 580-581
lymphedema related to, 579
nursing care plan for, 577-578b
sexual dysfunction after, 541
therapeutic dialogue before, 790b
Mastitis, 571
Mastoiditis, 636
Maxillary sinus, 374, 375f
McBurney's point, 212
Mean corpuscular hemoglobin, 269
Measles, 62f
Meclizine hydrochloride, 637-638t
Meclofenamate, 119-122t
Median nerve, carpal tunnel syndrome and, 163-164, 163f
Mediastinoscopy, 380-381
Mediastinum, 2, 3f, 3t, 304
Medical nutrition therapy for diabetes mellitus, 513
Medium crackles, 379t
Medroxyprogesterone acetate, 549-550t, 593-595t,
Medulla oblongata, 653f, 654
Megaloblastic anemia profile, 269
Megestrol, 793-794t
Meglitinides, 520, 520t
Meissner's corpuscle, 60f
Melanin, 60-61
Melanocyte, 60-61
Melanocyte-stimulating hormone, 486f
Melatonin, 488-489
Melena, 192
Meloxicam, 119-122t
Melphalan, 280

Memantine, 686-687t, 689
Membrane, 8-9, 8t, 9f, 9t, 12
Menarche, 538, 546
Ménière's disease, 641-644, 642t, 643b
Meninges, 654
Meningitis, 704-705
West Nile virus in, 705
Meningococcal vaccine, 704-705
Menopause, 538, 551-553
risk for breast cancer, 571
Menorrhagia, 546, 548-550
in hypothyroidism, 499
Menstrual cycle, 538, 539f
Menstruation, disturbances of, 546-556
health teaching for, 546b
Mental status, 658-659, 658t, 659t, 660t
Meperidine, 249, 255-256t
Mephenytoin, 679t
MERCI Retriever, 698, 698f
Mesalamine, 193-195t
for Crohn's disease, 210
for ulcerative colitis, 207
Mesentery, 178f
Mesocaval shunt, 239-240
Metabolic acidosis, 383t
Metabolic alkalosis, 383t
Metaphase, 7f, 8
Metastasis, 785
Metformin, 520-521, 520t
Methadone, 801
Methenamine mandelate, 445
Methimazole, 496
Methotrexate, 793-794t
for breast cancer, 576
for Crohn's disease, 210
for psoriasis, 85
for rheumatoid arthritis, 119-122t
Methoxsalen, 70-71t, 85
Methyldopa, drug-induced parkinsonism and, 683
Methylprednisolone
for cancer treatment, 793-794t
preoperative, 36-37t
for respiratory disorders, 401-403t
Metoclopramide
for chemotherapy-related vomiting, 797-798t, 797-798
preoperative, 36-37t
Metoprolol, 318-319t
for heart failure, 336-337t
for myocardial infarction, 329t
Metronidazole, 549-550t
for Crohn's disease, 211
for Helicobacter pylori, 195
for trichomoniasis, 591
for urethritis, 452
Metrorrhagia, 546, 548-550
Mexiletine, 318-319t
Miconazole, 78, 549-550t
Midazolam
for increased intracranial pressure, 671
preoperative, 36-37t
Midbrain, 653f, 654
Middle ear, 604-605, 604f
Miglitol, 520, 520t
Migraine headache, 665
Miller-Abbott tube, 219-220
Mineralocorticoids, 486
Minerals, storage in bone, 110
effects of bed rest of content in bone, 117
Minor surgery, 18t
Miotics, 625-627
Misoprostol, 193-195t
Mite infestation, 89-90, 89f
Mitochondrion, 5f, 6, 6t, 651f
Mitosis, 7, 7f
Mitotane, 490t, 505
Mitoxantrone, 681, 793-794t
Mitral valve, 305, 305f
Mixed hearing loss, 633

Mixed insulins, 515-516t
Mobile surgery unit, 19
Mobility
after burn, 102
cast and, 155
Modified radical mastectomy, 575, 577-578b, 790b
Moexipril, 336-337t
Moniliasis, 184, 591
Monoclonal antibody therapy
for breast cancer, 577
for Crohn's disease, 211
Monocyte, 263f, 265
involvement in HIV infection, 743t, 744
white blood cell count and, 263-264t
Montelukast, 401-403t, 725-726
Monticello-Spinelli Circular Fixator, 152f
Morning-after pill, 593-595t
Morphine
for acute respiratory distress syndrome, 419
after pelvic surgery, 570
for cancer pain, 797-798t, 801
for heart failure, 336-337t
for myocardial infarction, 329t
preoperative, 36-37t
for sickle cell crisis, 278
Motor function, assessment, 660
Motor function disturbances, 672-675
Motor unit, 113
Mouth, 176, 183-186
Mucin, 177-178
Mucolytics, 429
Mucous membranes, 12
Mucus, 12
MUGA scanning, 335
Multiorgan system disease in polycythemia, 279
Multiple myeloma, 291-292
Multiple sclerosis, 680-683, 681f
Mupirocin, 76
Murmur, 306
in rheumatic heart disease, 343
Muscle, 10t, 11, 11f
contraction of, 113
of eye, 602
functions of, 110-113, 113b, 113t, 114f
principal muscles of body, 112t, 114f
Muscle contracture
after mastectomy, 579-580, 580f, 581b
burn-related, 98
in osteomyelitis, 131
Volkmann's, 148-149
Muscle relaxants, 672
Muscle tone, 113
Muscular system, 12-14t
Musculocutaneous flap procedure in breast reconstruction, 582
Musculoskeletal disorders, 109-174
bone tumors in, 166-167
electrographic procedures in, 117
endoscopic examination in, 116-117
fibromyalgia syndrome in, 131, 132t
fracture in, 137-148; See also Fracture
cast for, 153-159, 153f, 155f
compartment syndrome and, 148-149, 149f
delayed healing of, 152
fat embolism and, 150
gas gangrene and, 150-151
orthopedic devices for, 157-159
prevention of, 160b
shock and, 149-150
skeletal pin external fixation in, 152-153, 152f
thromboembolus and, 151, 151b

Musculoskeletal disorders (Continued)
traction for, 156, 156-157, 156f, 157b, 157f
hip arthroplasty in, 135-136, 135f, 136f
inflammatory, 117-171
ankylosing spondylitis in, 123-125
arthritis in, 117-128, 118t
gout in, 127-128
osteoarthritis in, 125-127, 125b, 125f, 126f
rheumatoid arthritis in, 118-123, 118t, 119-122t, 119f
knee arthroplasty in, 133-135, 133f, 134b
laboratory tests in, 117, 117t
nursing process for, 169-171, 170f
osteomyelitis in, 131
osteoporosis in, 128-133, 129f, 129t
radiographic studies in, 113-116
traumatic injuries in, 160-169
Musculoskeletal system
adrenal disorders and, 507t
articulations and, 110, 110f
divisions of skeleton and, 110, 110b, 111f
effects of bed rest on mineral content in bone, 117
effects of surgery on, 23t
functions of muscle and, 110-113, 112t, 113b, 113t, 114f
functions of skeletal system and, 109-110
structure of bone and, 110
systemic lupus erythematosus and, 86
Mushroom catheter, 445-446, 446f
Myasthenia gravis, 690-693, 693b
Mycobacterium avium complex
associated with HIV infection, 750-751t
prophylaxis guidelines for, 752t
Mycobacterium tuberculosis, 398, 752t
Mycophenolate mofetil
for liver transplantation, 246
for thrombocytopenia, 287
Mycoplasmal pneumonia, 405
Myelin, 652
Myelography, 115, 664
Myocardial infarction, 326-332, 326f
in anaphylaxis, 727
cardiac rehabilitation in, 331-332
cardiogenic shock and, 329, 330t
clinical manifestations of, 327, 327t
diagnostic tests for, 328
health promotion and, 332b
home care considerations in, 332b
medical management of, 328-329, 329t
patient teaching in, 330-332
serum cardiac markers in, 311
signs and symptoms of, 327t
Myocarditis, 346
Myocardium, 304
Myoclonic seizure, 677-678t
Myofascial pain syndrome, 131-132
Myoglobin, 117t
Myoma, 563-564, 563f
Myomectomy, 564
Myopia, 608-609t, 611, 611t
Myringotomy, 636, 645
Myxedema, 498, 499f
Myxedema ileus, 499

N

Nabumetone, 119-122t
Nadolol, 329t
Nails, paronychia and, 94
Nalidixic acid, 444-445
Naproxen
for cancer treatment symptoms, 797-798t
for rheumatoid arthritis, 119-122t

Naratriptan, 666
Nasal continuous positive airway pressure, 388, 388f
Nasal polyp, 385-386
Nasogastric tube
after gastric surgery, 196, 197t
for burn victim, 97
in gallstones, 249
in intestinal obstruction, 219-220
in pancreatitis, 254
in peritonitis, 216
Nasojejunal tube, 219-220
Nasopharynx, 374, 375f
Nasoseptoplasty, 385-386
Natalizumab, 211
Nateglinide, 520, 520t
Natural immunity, 720, 720t
Natural killer cell, 721
involvement in HIV infection, 743t
Nausea, chemotherapy-related, 576, 797-798
Near blindness, 607-610, 610b, 610t
Necrosis
in intestinal obstruction, 219
in myocardial infarction, 326
Necrotizing pneumonia, 404
Needle-aspiration biopsy, 786-787, 787f
Needle liver biopsy, 233-234
Needlestick injury, HIV and, 741
Negative feedback, 485
Neisseria gonorrhoeae
in epididymitis, 584
in gonococcal pharyngitis, 394
in gonorrhea, 589
in pelvic inflammatory disease, 558
in prostatitis, 583
Neisseria meningitidis meningitis, 704
Nelfinavir, 753-756t
Neomycin, 255-256t
for burn, 101t
for ear infection, 637-638t
Neoplasm, 785; See also Tumor
Neostigmine, 692
Nephrectomy, 477, 477t
Nephritis, 468-470
Nephrolithiasis, 457
Nephrolithotomy, 458, 458f
Nephron, 435-437, 436f
Nephroscopy, 441
Nephrostomy, 477-478, 477t
Nephrotic syndrome, 467-468
Nerve block, 39
for neuropathic pain, 667
Nervous system; See Neurologic system
Nervous tissue, 10t, 11-12
Nesiritide, 336-337t
Neufeld nail and screws, 138f, 139
Neuralgia, trigeminal, 700-701, 701b, 701f
Neurectomy, 668
Neurilemma, 651f, 652
Neurogenic bladder, 450-451
Neuroglial cell, 651
Neurohypophysis, 485
Neurologic disorders, 650-718
AIDS dementia in, 706-707
Alzheimer's disease in, 688-690, 689f, 690b
amyotrophic lateral sclerosis in, 693
associated with HIV infection, 750-751t, 767
Bell's palsy in, 701-702
brain abscess in, 706
brain tumor in, 707-708
central nervous system infection and inflammation in, 702-703
disturbed sensory and perceptual function in, 675-676
encephalitis in, 705-706

Neurologic disorders (Continued)
epilepsy or seizures in, 676, 678b, 679t
Guillain-Barré syndrome in, 703-704
head injury in, 708-710, 709f
headache in, 665-667, 665b
health promotion in, 675b
Huntington's disease in, 693-694
increased intracranial pressure in, 668-672, 669f, 670f
laboratory and diagnostic tests in, 661-665
medications for, 686-687t
meningitis in, 704-705
multiple sclerosis in, 680-683, 681f
muscle tone and motor function disturbances in, 672-675
myasthenia gravis in, 690-693, 693b
neurologic assessment in, 657-661
neuropathic pain in, 667-668
nursing process for, 713-714
older adult and, 656b
Parkinson's disease in, 683-688, 683f, 684f
prevention of, 656-657, 657b
spinal cord trauma in, 710-713
stroke in, 695-696
trigeminal neuralgia in, 667, 700-701, 701b, 701f
Neurologic examination, 657-661
cranial nerve assessment in, 659-660
history in, 657-658
language and speech in, 659
mental status in, 658-659, 658t, 659t, 660t
motor function in, 660
sensory and perceptual status in, 661
in stroke, 699
Neurologic system, 12-14t, 651-657
adrenal disorders and, 507t
autonomic nervous system and, 655
brain and, 652-654, 653f, 654b
cells of, 651-652, 651f
in control of respiration, 378
cranial nerves and, 655, 656f, 657t
effects of aging on, 655
effects of surgery on, 23t
HIV infection and, 746, 758
spinal cord and, 654, 655f
spinal nerves and, 655
structural divisions of, 651
systemic lupus erythematosus and, 86
Neuromuscular junction, 652
Neuron, 11-12, 651-652, 651f, 652
Neuropathic pain, 667-668
Neuropathy, diabetic, 522, 526, 526f, 667
Neurotransmitters, 113, 652
Neurovascular assessment, 139b, 170
Neurovascular problems, cast-related, 155
Neutropenia, 791-794, 795b
Neutrophil, 263f, 265
involvement in HIV infection, 743t
white blood cell count and, 263-264t
Nevirapine, 753-756t
Nevus, 91
Nifedipine, 329t
Nilutamide, 465
Nissen fundoplication, 218, 218f
Nitrates
for angina pectoris, 326
for heart failure, 336-337t
for myocardial infarction, 329t

Nitrofurantoin, 445
Nitrofurazone, 101t
Nitroglycerin
for angina pectoris, 321
for heart failure, 336-337t
for myocardial infarction, 329t
for ruptured esophageal varix, 239
Nitroprusside, 416
Nizatidine, 187, 193-195t
Node of Ranvier, 651f, 652
Nodular melanoma, 92-93
Nodule, 62f, 62t
Aschoff's, 343
in thyroid cancer, 501
Non-Hodgkin's lymphoma, 297-298, 750-751t
Nonnucleoside reverse transcriptase inhibitors, 753-756t
Non–small cell lung cancer, 413
Nonsteroidal antiinflammatory drugs
for cancer pain, 801
for cancer treatment symptoms, 797-798t
effects during surgery, 38t
for fibromyalgia syndrome, 132t
hepatotoxicity of, 240
for neuropathic pain, 668
for osteoarthritis, 126
preoperative, 36-37t
for rheumatoid arthritis, 119-122t
for systemic lupus erythematosus, 87
Nonunion, 152
Norepinephrine, 486-487, 652
Norfloxacin, 445
Norplant, 593-595t
Nortriptyline, 454
Nose, 374, 375f
allergic rhinitis and, 386-387
deviated septum and nasal polyps and, 385-386
epistaxis and, 384-385
Nose surgery, coughing contraindication in, 33
Nosebleed, 384-385
Nosocomial urinary tract infection, 452
Novolin R, 515-516t
NovoLog, 515-516t
NPH insulin, 515-516t
Nuclear scanning, 115
Nucleic acid amplification for Chlamydia trachomatis, 592
Nucleoside reverse transcriptase inhibitors, 753-756t
Nucleotide reverse transcriptase inhibitors, 753-756t
Nucleus, 5f, 6, 6t
Numerical system for Pap test interpretation, 543t
Nursing care plan
for Alzheimer's disease, 691b
for cataracts, 619b
for cirrhosis, 242b
for diabetes mellitus, 523-524b
for emphysema, 425b
for end-stage renal disease, 473-474b
for gastrointestinal bleeding, 198b
for heart failure, 338-339b
for herpes zoster, 73b
for hip fracture, 141b
for HIV infection, 768b
for leukemia, 285b
for Ménière's disease, 643b
for modified radical mastectomy, 577-578b
for surgical patient, 54-55b
Nursing diagnoses
postoperative, 54b
preoperative, 53b
Nursing process
for blood or lymphatic disorders, 298-299

Nursing process (Continued)
for cardiovascular disorders, 367-369
for endocrine disorders, 528-529
for gastrointestinal disorder, 227-228
for integumentary disorders, 103-105
for musculoskeletal disorders, 169-171, 170f
for reproductive disorders, 596-597
for respiratory disorders, 429-430
for sensory disorders, 645-646
for surgical patient, 53, 53b, 54b
for urinary disorders, 480-481
Nutrition
burn victim and, 100
cancer and, 802
chronic obstructive pulmonary disease and, 423
diabetes mellitus and, 513
factor in perioperative nursing, 20
HIV infection and, 760, 765, 766t
macular degeneration and, 621
multiple sclerosis and, 682
paralyzed patient and, 673-674
Parkinson's disease and, 685-688
polycythemia and, 290
renal disease and, 445, 445b
stroke and, 699
ulcerative colitis and, 207
Nystagmus
in Ménière's disease, 641
in multiple sclerosis, 681
Nystatin, 193-195t, 549-550t
for candidiasis, 591
for thrush, 184
for urethritis, 452

O
Obesity
cancer and, 780-781
cardiovascular disease risk and, 314
diabetes mellitus and, 509
hypertension and, 352
multiple sclerosis and, 682
obstructive sleep apnea and, 387
peripheral vascular diseases and, 349
risk for breast cancer, 571
Obligate virus, 738
Oblique fracture, 143f, 144
Oblique muscle layer of stomach, 177f
Obstruction
ear, 639-640
esophageal cancer-related, 188
gastric outlet, 192
intestinal, 218-220, 219f
upper airway, 388-389
urinary, 456-457
Obstruction series, 183
Obstructive sleep apnea, 387-388, 388f
Occipital lobe, 654
Occlusion
myocardial infarction and, 326
of pancreatic duct, 253
Occultest, 789
Occupational exposure transmission of HIV, 740-741, 773-774
Octreotide, 489, 490t
Oculomotor nerve, 656f, 657t
Ofloxacin
for Chlamydia trachomatis, 592
for gonorrhea, 590
for prostatitis, 455, 583
Older adult
blood or lymphatic disorders and, 298b
cancer and, 779b
cardiac disease and, 312b
chronic constipation and, 225b
diabetes mellitus and, 523b

Older adult (Continued)
gastrointestinal disorders and, 218b
hepatobiliary disorders and, 253b
hip fracture and, 137-142, 138f
HIV infection and, 737b
immune disorders and, integumentary system of, 103b
musculoskeletal disorders and, 137b
neurologic disorders and, 656b
obstructive sleep apnea and, 387
reproductive disorders and, 539b
respiratory disorders and, 405b
sensory disorders and, 607b
surgery and, 20b
urinary disorders and, 439b
Olfactory nerve, 656f, 657t
Oliguria
in acute renal failure, 470
in nephrotic syndrome, 467
Olsalazine, 193-195t
for Crohn's disease, 210
for ulcerative colitis, 207
Omeprazole, 187, 193-195t
Oncology, 778-779
Ondansetron
for chemotherapy-related vomiting, 576, 797-798t, 797-798
preoperative, 36-37t
One and one-half leg-hip spica cast, 153, 153f
One-day surgery, 19
Open fracture, 142f, 143f
Open reduction with internal fixation, 142b, 145
Operating room, 43, 43f
Operative cholangiography, 232-233
Ophthalmoscopy, 608-609t
Opioid analgesics
for cancer pain, 801
preoperative, 36-37t
Opportunistic infections
in HIV infection, 735-736, 749-750, 750-751t, 752t, 769
prophylaxis guidelines for, 752t
Optic disk, 603, 603f
cupping in glaucoma, 624, 624f
normal findings of, 607t
Optic nerve, 603f, 656f, 657t
Oral airways, 39f
Oral candidiasis, 184
in HIV infection, 746, 746f
Oral cavity carcinoma, 184-186
Oral cholecystography, 232
Oral contraceptives, 549-550t
essential hypertension and, 352
Oral glucose challenge test, 489
Oral glucose tolerance test, 512
Oral hairy leukoplakia, 746
Oral hypoglycemics, 520-521, 520t
Orchiectomy, 465
Organ of Corti, 605, 605f
Organ systems, 12, 12-14t
Oropharyngeal cancer, 184-186
Oropharynx, 374, 375f
Orthopedic devices, 157-159, 158b, 159f
Orthopnea, 378-379
in cardiovascular disorders, 368
in heart failure, 334
in valvular heart disease, 341
Osmosis, 9, 9t, 10f
Osmotic diuretics, 444, 671
Osteoarthritis, 125-127, 125b, 125f, 126f
arthroplasty in, 133
rheumatoid arthritis versus, 118t
Osteochondroma, 166
Osteogenic sarcoma, 166
Osteogenic tumor, 166
Osteomyelitis, 131
Osteoporosis, 128-133, 129f, 129t
in Cushing's syndrome, 504-505
postmenopausal, 552

Otitis media, 386
Otosclerosis, 640-641
Otoscopy, 631
Outpatient surgery, 19
Ova and parasites, 183
Ovarian ablation, 577
Ovarian cancer, 567-569, 782-784t
CA-125 tumor antigen in, 545, 789
Ovarian cyst, 564
Ovary, 485f, 488, 536, 536f
Oxcarbazepine, 679t, 701
Oxybutynin chloride, 443t
Oxygen saturation, 382, 383b
Oxygen therapy
in anaphylaxis, 727
in asthma, 427
in bronchiectasis, 429
in emphysema, 422
home care considerations in, 424b
in hypovolemic anemia, 271-272
in increased intracranial pressure, 671
in pulmonary edema, 416
Oxymetazoline, 401-403t
Oxytocin, 485, 486f

P
P wave, 308, 309f
Pacemaker
sinoatrial node as, 305, 306f
for sinus bradycardia, 315, 315f
Paclitaxel, 793-794t
for esophageal cancer, 188
for ovarian cancer, 568
Palliative surgery, 18, 18t
Palliative therapy
in esophageal cancer, 188
in HIV infection, 761-762
in Huntington's disease, 694
in liver cancer, 242-243
in prostate cancer, 465
Palmar-Schatz stent, 324f
Palpation
of breast, 573f
in skin disorders, 61-67
Palpebral conjunctiva, 607
Palpitations, in cardiovascular disorders, 368
Pamidronate
for breast cancer, 577
for osteoporosis, 129
Pancreas, 176f, 179, 179f, 485f, 487-488
cancer of, 255-257, 257f
diabetes mellitus and, 509-528, 510t; See also Diabetes mellitus
endoscopic retrograde cholangiopancreatography and, 235-236, 235f
pancreatitis and, 253-255
serum amylase test and, 234
serum lipase test and, 235
ultrasonography of, 235
urine amylase test and, 234-235
Pancreatic duct, 179f
Pancrelipase, 255-256t
Pancytopenic aplastic anemia, 273
Panhysterosalpingo-oophorectomy, 569
Pantoprazole, 187
Papanicolaou test, 542-543, 543t
Bethesda system and, 786
cervical cancer and, 565
Papilla
renal, 435, 435f
of tongue, 176
of Vater, 179
Papillary muscle, 305, 305f
Papillary thyroid cancer, 501-502
Papilledema, 670
Papule, 62f, 62t
Para-aminosalicylate sodium, 401-403t

Paracentesis, 237-238, 238
Paralysis, 660, 672-675
Paralytic ileus, 52, 218-219, 223
Paranasal sinuses, 374, 375f
Paraphimosis, 584-585
Paraplegia, 710, 711t
Parasitic infection, 87-90
Parasympathetic nervous system, 655
Parathyroid, 485f, 486, 487f
Parathyroid disorders, 502-503
Parathyroid hormone, 129t, 486
Paraurethral glands, 537, 537f
Parenchyma, 236
Paresis, 660
in stroke, 696
Paresthesia
in diabetic neuropathy, 526
in peripheral arterial disease of lower extremities, 355
in premenstrual syndrome, 550-551
Parietal lobe, 654
Parietal membrane, 12
Parietal pleura, 378
Parity, 596
risk for breast cancer and, 571
Parkinsonian syndrome, 503
Parkinson's disease, 683-688, 683f, 684f
Paronychia, 94
Paroxysmal nocturnal dyspnea, 334
Partial cystectomy, 461
Partial laryngectomy, 389
Partial pressure of arterial oxygen, 382, 383b
Partial pressure of carbon dioxide, 382-383, 383b
Partial seizure, 677-678t
Partial thromboplastin time, 263-264t
Partial-thickness burn, 95t, 96f
Passive transport, 9, 9f, 9t
PATCHES mnemonic, 349
Pathologic fracture
effects of bed rest of content in bone and, 117
in hyperparathyroidism, 502
in multiple myeloma, 291
Patient positioning
after total knee replacement, 134
of burn victim, 99-100
for lumbar puncture, 661, 662f
of paralyzed patient, 673
for surgery, 40-41, 41f
Patient teaching
after eye surgery, 620b
in amputation, 168-169, 168f
in angina pectoris, 326b
in breast cancer, 579-581, 580b
in breast self-examination, 573b
in cardiac dysrhythmias, 317-319
in cast care, 154
in controlled coughing technique, 30-31b, 30b, 30f
in coronary artery disease, 324
in diabetes mellitus, 521-528
in dietary needs in osteoporosis, 130b
before discharge of burn victim, 102
in ear infection, 639b
in ear surgery, 644b
in glaucoma, 627b
in heart failure, 339
in hypertension, 354
in ileostomy care, 209
in incentive spirometry, 28b
in liver transplantation, 246-247
in myasthenia gravis, 693b
in myocardial infarction, 330-332
in open reduction with internal fixation, 142b
in pacemaker, 320
in postoperative breathing techniques, 31-32

Patient teaching (Continued)
  postprostatectomy, 464b
  in preoperative care, 21b
  in quadriceps setting exercises, 140b
  in retinal detachment, 623b
  in seizures, 678b
  in skin graft, 100b
  in sleep hygiene, 133b
  in stroke, 700
  in testicular self-examination, 586b
  in urinary catheterization, 446-448
  in use of thromboembolic deterrent stockings and sequential compression devices, 33-34b, 33b, 34f
  in valvular heart disease, 342
  in vertigo, 640b
Patient-controlled analgesia, 278
Peak expiratory flow in asthma, 427-428
Pediculosis, 87-89, 89f
Pelvic cavity, 2, 3f, 3t
Pelvic examination, 567, 568
Pelvic fracture, 147-148
Pelvic inflammatory disease, 558-559
Pelvic ultrasonography, 545
Penicillamine, 119-122t
Penicillin
  for anthrax, 398
  for pneumonia, 406
  for syphilis, 589
Penile prosthesis, 555, 555f
Penis, 534f, 535
  cancer of, 586
  candidiasis and, 591
  genital herpes and, 587-588, 588f
  phimosis and paraphimosis and, 584-585
Penrose drain, 250
Pentosan polysulfate sodium, 454
Pentoxifylline, 356
Peptic ulcer disease, 190-201
  older adult and, 218
Percutaneous cordotomy, 668
Percutaneous drainage of hepatic abscess, 247
Percutaneous endoscopic gastrostomy, 185
Percutaneous renal biopsy, 442
Percutaneous transluminal angioplasty, 696
Percutaneous transluminal coronary angioplasty, 323, 324f, 328
Perforation
  in diverticulosis and diverticulitis, 214
  in duodenal ulcer, 192
  in esophageal cancer, 188
Pergolide, 685
Pericardial friction rub, 343-344
Pericardiocentesis, 344
Pericarditis, 343-345
Pericardium, 304
Perilymph, 605, 605f
Perindopril, 336-337t
Perineum, 537
Perioperative nursing, 18-23
  education and experience of patient and, 23
  intraoperative phase of surgery and, 43-44, 43f
    circulating nurse and scrub nurse roles in, 44, 44b, 44f
    holding area and, 43-44
  medications and, 21-23, 22t
  nutritional status and, 20
  patient age and, 19
  physical condition of patient and, 19, 20b
  postoperative phase of surgery and, 44-53; See also Postoperative phase of surgery

Perioperative nursing (Continued)
  preoperative phase of surgery and, 23-43, 23t; See also Preoperative phase of surgery
  psychosocial needs and, 20, 21b, 21f
  socioeconomic and cultural needs and, 20-21, 22b
Peripheral arterial disease, 355-357, 355f, 356b, 357f
Peripheral facial paralysis, 701-702
Peripheral nervous system, 651, 655
Peripheral neuropathy in HIV infection, 767
Peripheral smear, 269
Peripheral stem cell transplantation, 801
Peripheral vascular disorders, 348-367
  arterial aneurysm in, 359-360, 359f, 360f
  arterial embolism in, 357-359
  arteriosclerosis and atherosclerosis in, 355
  Buerger's disease in, 360-361
  diagnostic tests for, 350-351
  normal aging patterns and, 348
  peripheral arterial disease in, 355-357, 355f, 356b, 357f
  Raynaud's disease in, 361-362
  risk factors for, 348-349
  thrombophlebitis in, 362-365, 363f, 363t
  varicose veins in, 363t, 365-366
  venous stasis ulcer in, 366-367, 366f, 367f
Peristomal area integrity, 209
Peritoneal dialysis, 475-477, 476f, 477b
Peritonitis, 215-216
Pernicious anemia, 272-273
  after total gastrectomy, 196
  in Crohn's disease, 210
Pessary, 449
Petechiae, 279-280, 286
pH
  blood, 378
  cerebrospinal fluid, 661t
  urine, 440t
Phacoemulsification, 617, 618f
Phagocyte, 720-721
  involvement in HIV infection, 744
Phagocytosis, 8, 8t, 265
Phalen's maneuver, 163
Phantom limb pain, 168, 667
Pharyngitis, 394
Pharyngoplasty, 388
Phenazopyridine, 443t
Phenobarbital, 679t
Phenothiazine, drug-induced parkinsonism and, 683
Phenytoin, 679t
Pheochromocytoma, 352t, 508-509
Phimosis, 535, 584-585
Phlebotomy in polycythemia, 280
Phosphorus values in musculoskeletal disorders, 117t
Photochemotherapy for psoriasis, 85
Photocoagulation, 630
Photophobia, 386, 623
Photorefractive keratectomy, 612
Photoselective vaporization of prostate, 462-463
Pia mater, 654
Pilocarpine, 625-626t, 625-627
Pineal gland, 485f, 488-489
Pinkeye, 614-615
Pinocytosis, 8, 8t
Pioglitazone, 520, 520t
Pitting edema
  in heart failure, 333-334, 334f, 334t
  in peripheral vascular disease, 350
Pituitary gland, 485, 485f, 486f, 487f, 653f

Pituitary gland disorders, 489-495
  acromegaly in, 489-491, 489f
  diabetes insipidus in, 492-493
  dwarfism in, 492
  gigantism in, 491
  syndrome of inappropriate antidiuretic hormone secretion in, 493-495
Pituitary tumor
  in acromegaly, 489
  in Cushing's syndrome, 505
Pityriasis rosea, 74, 74f
Placenta, 488
Planography, 115
Plantar flexion, 113
Plaque, 62f, 62t
  dental, 183-184
  in psoriasis, 84
Plasma, 263
Plasma cell disorder, 291-292
Plasma membrane, 5, 5f, 6t
Plasmapheresis
  for autoimmune disorders, 731
  for myasthenia gravis, 692
Platelet, 263f, 266, 266f
  thrombocytopenia and, 286-287
Platelet count, 263-264t
Plethysmography, 350
Pleural cavity, 2, 3f, 3t
Pleural effusion, 333, 378, 388f, 408-410, 409f, 410f
Pleural friction rub, 379, 379t
Pleur-Evac, 409f
Pleurisy, 407-408
Pneumatic retinopexy, 623
Pneumococcal infection
  in conjunctivitis, 614
  in keratitis, 615
  in meningitis, 704
  in pneumonia, 404
Pneumococcal vaccine, 406, 704-705
Pneumocystis jiroveci pneumonia, 734, 750-751t, 752t
Pneumonectomy, 414
Pneumonia, 403-407, 404b
  Haemophilus influenzae, 404-405, 405
  necrotizing, 404
  older adult and, 405b
  pneumococcal, 404
  Pneumocystis jiroveci, 734, 750-751t, 752t
Pneumothorax, 411-413, 412f
Polycystic kidney disease, 460
Polycythemia, 279-281, 310
Polydipsia, 492, 511
Polymenorrhea, 552
Polymorphonuclear leukocyte, 265
Polymyxin B, 635
Polymyxin B, neomycin, bacitracin, and hydrocortisone, 637-638t
Polyneuritis, 703-704
Polyphagia in diabetes mellitus, 511
Polysomnography, 387
Polyuria, 492, 511
Polyvinyl alcohol, 625-626t
Pons, 653f, 654
Portal hypertension, 236, 238-239
Portocaval shunt, 239-240
Position and movement, 606
Positioning
  after total knee replacement, 134
  of burn victim, 99-100
  for lumbar puncture, 661, 662f
  of paralyzed patient, 673
  for surgery, 40-41, 41f
Positive expiratory pressure therapy, 28-29b
Positron emission tomography
  for cancer diagnosis, 788
  in cardiovascular disorders, 310
  in Hodgkin's lymphoma, 295
  in laryngeal cancer, 389
  in lung cancer, 413-414
  in neurologic disorders, 663
Postanesthesia care unit, 44-46, 45f

Posterior pituitary, 485
Postexposure prophylaxis
  for anthrax, 398
  for human immunodeficiency virus, 745
Postherpetic neuralgia, 667
Postictal period, 676
Postinfectious polyneuritis, 703-704
Postmenopause palpable ovary syndrome, 568
Postoperative ambulation, 51-52, 51b, 51f
Postoperative assessment form, 47f
Postoperative care
  in amputation, 168-169, 168f
  in brain tumor, 708
  in cardiac transplantation, 348
  in cataract surgery, 618
  in colorectal cancer, 223-224
  in corneal transplant, 630
  in esophageal surgery, 190
  in gallbladder surgery, 251
  in hernia repair, 217
  in hysterectomy, 569-570
  in intestinal obstruction, 220
  in laparoscopic cholecystectomy, 251
  in liver transplantation, 246
  in thyroidectomy, 497
  in total knee replacement, 134
  in ulcerative colitis, 208, 209b
Postoperative pain, 49-50, 49b
Postoperative phase of surgery, 44-53
  ambulation and, 51-52, 51b, 51f
  fluids and electrolytes in, 52-53
  gastrointestinal status in, 52
  immediate assessments in, 46-48, 46t, 47f, 48b
  immediate postoperative care in, 44-46, 45f, 45t
  incision care in, 48, 48f
  pain management in, 49-50, 49b, 50f
  urinary function in, 50
  venous stasis and, 50-51
  ventilation and, 48-49
Postoperative shock, 46-48, 48b
Postprandial blood glucose, 512
Potassium
  Cushing's syndrome and, 504-505
  hypertension and, 354
  postoperative management of, 52
  serum electrolyte tests and, 311
  supplementation for heart failure, 336-337t
Potassium iodide, 401-403t, 490t
Potassium-sparing diuretics, 444
Pott's fracture, 144
Povidone-iodine, 70-71t
PQRST mnemonic, 67
Pramipexole, 685
Pramlintide, 521, 521t
Preanesthesia care unit, 43
Prednisone
  for cancer treatment, 793-794t
  for multiple sclerosis, 681
  for nephrotic syndrome, 468
  for respiratory disorders, 401-403t
  for rheumatoid arthritis, 119-122t
Pregebalin, 132t
Pregnancy test, 545
Pregnancy-induced hypertension, 352t
Prehypertension, 351
Premature ventricular contractions, 316
Premenstrual dysphoric disorder, 550
Premenstrual syndrome, 550-551
Prenatal infection
  in syphilis, 589
  in trichomoniasis, 590

Preoperative assessment form, 42f
Preoperative care
   in brain tumor, 708
   in cataract surgery, 618
   in colorectal cancer, 222-223
   in corneal transplant, 630
   in esophageal surgery, 190
   in gallbladder surgery, 251
   in hysterectomy, 569
   in thyroidectomy, 497
   in ulcerative colitis, 208
Preoperative checklist, 41, 42f
Preoperative medications, 35-37, 36-37t, 38t
Preoperative phase of surgery, 23-43, 23t
   applying sequential compression devices in, 34, 34f
   applying thromboembolic deterrent stockings in, 33-34, 34f
   cardiovascular considerations in, 32-33
   conscious sedation and, 40
   eliminating wrong site and procedure surgery in, 43
   explaining of surgical wound in, 35
   fear of pain and, 35
   gastrointestinal preparation and, 25
   general anesthesia and, 37-39, 39f
   genitourinary considerations in, 35, 35f
   informed consent and, 24-25
   laboratory tests and diagnostic imaging in, 24
   latex allergy considerations in, 26-27, 28b
   local anesthesia and, 40
   positioning patient for surgery in, 40-41, 41f
   preoperative checklist for, 41, 42f
   preoperative medication and, 35-37, 36-37t, 38t
   preoperative teaching and, 24
   preparing for postoperative patient in, 43
   regional anesthesia and, 39-40
   respiratory preparation and, 28-29b, 28-32, 28b, 29f, 30f
   skin preparation and, 25-26, 26b, 27f
   transport to operating room in, 43
   vital signs measurement in, 33-35
Preoperative teaching, 24
   in controlled coughing technique, 30-31b, 30b, 30f
   in incentive spirometry, 28, 28-29b, 28b, 29f
   in postoperative breathing techniques, 31-32
   in postoperative leg exercises, 32, 32f
   in postoperative turning exercises, 32, 32f
Prepuce, 535
Presbycusis, 606
Presbyopia, 608-609t
Primary aldosteronism, 352t
Primary open-angle glaucoma, 623, 624f
Primary polycythemia, 279
Primary survey in burn, 97
Primidone, 679t
Probenecid, 127
Procainamide, 318-319t
Prochlorperazine
   for acute gastritis, 191
   for chemotherapy-related vomiting, 576, 797-798t, 797-798
Procidentia, 562, 562f
Proctocolectomy, 207
Progesterone, 488
   breast cancer and, 574

Progestin-only contraceptive pill, 593-595t
Prolactin, 485, 486f, 487f
Prolapse
   in hemorrhoids, 224
   uterine, 562, 562f
Promethazine, 191
Pronation, 113
Propafenone, 318-319t
Propantheline, 254, 255-256t
Prophase, 7f, 8
Propranolol, 318-319t, 329t
Proprioception, 661
Proprioceptor, 606
Propylthiouracil, 496
Prostadynia, 454
Prostate, 438f, 534-535, 534f, 535
   benign prostatic hypertrophy and, 462-464, 463b, 463f
   diagnostic studies of, 545
   prostatitis and, 454-455, 583-584
Prostate cancer, 464-466, 464b
   blood marker for, 788
   prevention and early detection of, 782-784t
Prostatectomy, 463, 463b, 463f
Prostate-specific antigen, 440, 465, 545, 788
Prostatic smear, 545
Prostatitis, 454-455, 583-584
Prosthesis
   breast, 580-581
   penile, 555, 555f
   preoperative management of, 41
Protease, 179
Protease inhibitors, 753-756t
Proteinuria, 440t
   in glomerulonephritis, 469
   in nephrotic syndrome, 467
Proteus spp.
   in acute otitis media, 636
   in prostatitis, 583
   in urinary tract infection, 451
Prothrombin time, 263-264t
Proton pump inhibitors
   for gastroesophageal reflux disease, 187
   for peptic ulcer disease, 193
Protozoal infection in trichomoniasis, 590-591
Proximal convoluted tubule, 436, 436f, 437f, 437t
Pruritus, 61
Pseudocyst, pancreatic, 253
Pseudomonal infection
   in acute otitis media, 636
   in external otitis, 635
   in keratitis, 615
   in prostatitis, 454, 583
   of urinary tract, 451
Psoriasis, 84-85, 84f
Psychogenic hearing loss, 633
Psychomotor seizure, 677-678t
Psychosocial factors
   in cardiovascular disease risk, 314
   in nonadherence to HIV drug regimen, 761
Psychosocial needs, of patient, 20, 21b, 21f
Ptosis in myasthenia gravis, 692
Ptyalin, 176-177
Pubococcygeal exercises, 447
Pulmonary angiography, 380
Pulmonary arteriography, 380
Pulmonary artery, 304, 304f, 377-378
Pulmonary circulation, 308
Pulmonary disorders, 395-420; *See also* Respiratory disorders
   chemotherapy-related, 795
Pulmonary edema, 340, 340b, 341t, 415-416
Pulmonary embolism, 416-418
   postoperative, 50
   pulmonary angiography in, 380

Pulmonary function tests, 380
Pulmonary semilunar valve, 305
Pulmonary spirometry tests, 380
Pulmonary trunk, 305f
Pulmonary veins, 304, 304f, 305f
Pulse oximetry
   in atelectasis, 411
   in chronic bronchitis, 424
   in respiratory disorders, 383-384, 384f
Pupil, 602-603, 603f
   constriction of, 604
   increased intracranial pressure and, 669, 669f
   normal findings of, 607t
Purkinje fibers, 305, 306f
Purpura
   in cirrhosis, 237
   thrombocytopenic, 286
Purulent otitis media, 636
Pustulant vesicle, 75-76, 76f
Pustule, 62f, 62t
   in tinea capitis, 78, 78f
PUVA therapy for psoriasis, 85
Pyelolithotomy, 458, 458f
Pyelonephritis, 455-456, 502
Pyloroplasty, 196
Pyrazinamide, 401-403t
Pyrethrin, 70-71t, 89
Pyridostigmine, 686-687t, 692
Pyrosis, 186-187
Pyuria, 451, 453

Q

Quad cane, 159f
Quadrants, abdominopelvic, 3, 4f
Quadriceps setting exercises, 140b
QuantiFERON-TB Gold test, 400
Quinapril, 336-337t
Quinolone, 444-445

R

Rabeprazole, 187
Raccoon eyes, 709, 709f
Race
   hypertension and, 352
   risk for breast cancer and, 571
Radial keratotomy, 612
Radiation therapy, 790-791, 792b
   in bladder cancer, 461
   in bone tumor, 167
   in colorectal cancer, 221
   in esophageal cancer, 188
   in Hodgkin's lymphoma, 295
   immunosuppression and, 730
   in lung cancer, 414
   in multiple myeloma, 292
   in non-Hodgkin's lymphoma, 297-298
   in oral cavity cancer, 186
   in prostate cancer, 465
   tumor lysis syndrome and, 799
Radical neck dissection, 185, 389-390
Radical perineal prostatectomy, 463, 463f
Radical prostatectomy, 465
Radicular pain, 164
Radioactive iodine uptake test, 496
Radiography
   cardiovascular, 308
   in deviated septum and nasal polyps, 385
   in intestinal obstruction, 219
   in musculoskeletal disorders, 113-116
   in oral cavity disorders, 185
   in sinusitis, 394
   of skull, 662
   in spinal cord injury, 712
Radioisotope liver scanning, 234
Radioisotope studies for cancer diagnosis, 787
Rales, 379, 379t
Raloxifene, 129t, 577
Raltegravir, 753-756t

Ranitidine, 193-195t
   for acute gastritis, 191
   for gastroesophageal reflux disease, 187
   preoperative, 36-37t
Rapid orthopedic and peripheral vascular assessment, 144-145
Rapid plasma reagin test, 589
Rapid-acting insulin, 515-516t
Rasagiline, 685
Raynaud's disease, 361-362
Rebound tenderness, 212, 215
Receptive aphasia, 654, 659
Recombinant human erythropoietin, 796
Reconstruction surgery, 18t, 789
   in breast cancer, 581-582
Rectal examination
   in benign prostatic hypertrophy, 462
   in endometrial cancer, 567
   in prostate cancer, 464-465
Rectocele, 562-563, 563f
Rectovaginal fistula, 561, 561f
Rectum, 176f, 178-179, 178f, 179
Red blood cell, 263-265, 263f
   anemia and, 269-281; *See also* Anemia
   polycythemia and, 279-281
   in urine, 440t
Red blood cell count, 263-264t
Reed-Sternberg cell, 294
Reflexes, 660t
   spinal cord and, 654, 655f
   testing of, 660
Refraction, 604, 608-609t
Refractive surgery, 612
Refractory errors, 610-613, 611t
Regional anesthesia, 39-40, 39f
Regular Humulin R, 515-516t
Relaxation techniques
   for hypertension, 354
   for Raynaud's disease, 362
Relaxed pelvic muscles, 562-563, 562f
Renal adenocarcinoma, 459
Renal angiography, 442
Renal biopsy, 442
Renal calculus, 457-459, 458f
Renal capsule, 435, 435f
Renal corpuscle, 436, 436f, 437f
Renal cortex, 435, 435f
Renal cyst, 460-462
Renal disorders, 434-483; *See also* Kidney disorders and Urinary disorders
Renal failure, 470-472
   acute, 470-471
   chronic, 471-472, 473-474b
   health promotion in, 472b
   hemodialysis in, 474-475, 475b, 475f
   peritoneal dialysis in, 475-477, 476f, 477b
   psychosocial aspects of, 476b
Renal medulla, 435, 435f
Renal pelvis, 435, 435f
Renal scan, 442
Renal system, 12-14t, 434-439, 435f
   effects of aging on, 439
   effects of surgery on, 23t
   kidney in, 434-438, 435f, 436f, 437f, 437t, 438b
   postoperative management of, 50
   systemic lupus erythematosus and, 86
   ureters in, 438
   urethra in, 439
   urinary bladder in, 438-439, 438f
   urine abnormalities and, 438
   urine composition and characteristics and, 438
Renal transplantation, 478, 478f
Renal tubule, 436, 436f, 437f
Renal tumor, 459-460
Renal vein, 435f

Renal venogram, 442
Renin, 437
Repaglinide, 520, 520t
Replication of cell, 791
Repolarization, 308, 309f
Reproductive cycle, 546-556
Reproductive disorders, 533-600;
    See also Female reproductive
    disorders and Male reproduc-
    tive disorders
Reproductive system, 12-14t
    anatomy and physiology of,
        534-538
    effects of aging on, 538
    female, 535-538, 536f, 537f,
        538f, 539f
    male, 534-535, 534f, 535f
    cirrhosis and, 238f
Rescue process, 274
Rescue therapy in asthma, 427
Reserpine, drug-induced parkin-
    sonism and, 683
Residual urine, 448
Respiration, neurologic control of,
    378
Respiratory acidosis, 383t
Respiratory alkalosis, 383t
Respiratory disorders, 373-433
    associated with HIV infection,
        750-751t
    complementary and alternative
        therapies for, 391b
    infections in, 391-395
        acute follicular tonsillitis in,
            392-393
        acute rhinitis in, 391-392
        laryngitis in, 393
        pharyngitis in, 394
        sinusitis in, 394-395
    laboratory and diagnostic exami-
        nations in, 379-429
        arterial blood gases in, 382-
            383, 383b, 383t
        bronchoscopy in, 381, 381f
        chest radiography in, 379-380
        computed tomography in, 380
        cytologic studies in, 382
        laryngoscopy in, 381
        lung biopsy in, 382
        mediastinoscopy in, 380-381
        pulmonary function tests in,
            380
        pulse oximetry in, 383-384,
            384f
        sputum specimen in, 381,
            381b, 382b
        thoracentesis in, 382, 382f
    lower airway, 395-420
        acute bronchitis in, 395-396
        acute respiratory distress syn-
            drome in, 418-420
        anthrax in, 398
        asthma in, 426-428
        atelectasis in, 410-411
        bronchiectasis in, 428-429
        chronic bronchitis in, 424-426
        emphysema in, 421-423, 421f,
            422b, 425b
        Legionnaire's disease in,
            396-397
        lung cancer in, 413-415, 414b
        pleural effusion or empyema
            in, 388f, 408-410, 409f,
            410b
        pleurisy in, 407-408
        pneumonia in, 403-407, 404b
        pneumothorax in, 411-413,
            412f
        pulmonary edema in, 415-416
        pulmonary embolism in,
            416-418
        severe acute respiratory syn-
            drome in, 397
        tuberculosis in, 398-403, 399b
        medications for, 401-403t
    nursing process for, 429-430

Respiratory disorders (Continued)
    older adult and, 405b
    upper airway, 384-390
        allergic rhinitis and conjuncti-
            vitis in, 386-387
        deviated septum and nasal
            polyps in, 385-386
        epistaxis in, 384-385
        laryngeal cancer in, 389-390
        obstructive sleep apnea in,
            387-388, 388f
        upper airway obstruction in,
            388-389
Respiratory distress
    in angioedema, 81
    in pleural effusion or empyema,
        408
    in pneumothorax, 412
Respiratory system, 12-14t
    assessment of, 378-379, 379t, 380b
    effects of surgery on, 23t
    lower respiratory tract and, 377,
        377f
    mechanics of breathing and,
        377-378
    nervous control of respiration
        and, 378
    nursing assessment in HIV infec-
        tion and, 758
    upper respiratory tract and,
        374-377
        larynx and, 374, 376f
        nose and, 374, 375f
        pharynx and, 374
        trachea and, 374-377, 376f
Restrictive cardiomyopathy, 346
Retapamulin, 76
Rete testis, 534
Reticulocyte count, 263-264t
Retina, 603, 603f
    diabetic retinopathy and, 526,
        526f, 618-620
    normal findings of, 607t
    retinal detachment and, 622-623,
        622f
Retrograde cystography, 441
Retrograde pyelography, 441
Retrograde urethrography, 441
Retropubic prostatectomy, 463, 463f
Retrovirus, human immunodefi-
    ciency virus as, 742
Rh factor, 267
Rheumatic heart disease, 342-343
Rheumatoid arthritis, 118-123, 118t,
    119f
    arthroplasty in, 133
    medications for, 119-122t
Rheumatoid factor, 117t, 119
Rheumatoid spondylitis, 123-124
Rhinitis
    acute, 391-392
    allergic, 386-387
Rhodococcus equi, 750-751t
Rhonchus, 379, 379t
    in acute bronchitis, 395
Rhythm method of contraception,
    593-595t
Ribosome, 5f, 6, 6t
Rifampin, 400, 401-403t
Rifapentine, 400, 401-403t
Right ventricular failure, 333-334
Rigidity in Parkinson's disease, 684,
    684f
Riluzole, 693
Ring sign, 709f
Ringworm, 78, 78f
Risedronate, 129t, 130
Ritonavir, 753-756t
Rituximab, 119-122t, 287
Rizatriptan, 666
Robinson catheter, 445-446, 446f
Roll-A-Bout walker, 159, 159f
Ropinirole, 685
Rosiglitazone, 520, 520t
Rotigotine, 685
RotoRest bed, 157

Rotter's nodes, 572f
Rubber-band ligation of hemor-
    rhoids, 224, 224f
Rubin's insufflation test, 545,
    555-556
Rule of nines, 95-96, 96f
Russell's traction, 156, 157f

S
Saccular aneurysm, 359, 359f
Sacral nerve modulation and stimu-
    lation, 450-451
Safety
    Alzheimer's disease and, 690
    anticoagulant therapy and, 364b
    aplastic anemia and, 275b
    appendicitis and, 213b
    blindness and, 610, 610f
    crutches and, 158b
    cystitis and, 453b
    diabetic ketoacidosis and, 525b
    emergency care for hypoglyce-
        mic reaction, 524b
    hypersensitivity reaction and,
        726b
    neutropenic precautions and, 795b
    paralysis and, 673
    prevention and
        of burns, 94b
        of hepatitis, 243b
        of musculoskeletal trauma,
            160b
        of neurologic injuries, 657b
    sexually transmitted infections
        and, 587b
    in sprains and strains, 161b
    in thromboembolus, 151b
Sagittal plane, 2, 2f
Saint John's wort, 22t
Salicylates
    for myocardial infarction, 329t
    for rheumatoid arthritis, 119-122t
Salicylic acid, 70-71t
Saliva, 176-177
Salivary gland, 176-177
Salmeterol, 401-403t
Salmonella, 750-751t
Salpingitis, 558
Salsalate, 119-122t
Same-day admit surgery, 18t, 19
Saphenous aortocoronary artery
    bypass, 323f
Saphenous vein
    for coronary artery bypass graft,
        323f
    ligation and stripping of, 365
Saquinavir, 753-756t
Sarcoma, 785-786
    Kaposi's, 185, 298, 734, 750-751t
    osteogenic, 166
Sarcoptes scabiei, 89-90, 89f
Scabies, 62f, 89-90, 89f
Scale, 62f, 62t
Scanography, 115
Scar, 62f, 62t
Scarlet red, 101t
Schiller's iodine test, 544
Schilling test, 269, 272
Schiøtz tonometry, 624-625, 625f
Schirmer's tear test, 606-607,
    608-609t
Schwann cell, 651f, 652
Schwartz' sign, 641
Sclera, 602, 603f, 607t
Scleral buckling, 622f, 623
Sclerotherapy, 224, 365
Scoliosis, 170, 170f
Scotomata, 681
Scott inflatable prosthesis, 555f
Scrotum, 488, 534, 534f
Scrub nurse, 44b, 44f
Sebaceous cyst, 62f
Sebaceous gland, 60f, 61
    acne vulgaris and, 83
Sebum, 61
Second-degree burn, 95t, 96f

Secondary hypertension, 352-353,
    352t
Segmental neutrophil, 265
Seizure, 676-680
    activities of daily living and, 678,
        678b
    in brain abscess, 706
    in brain tumor, 707
    care during, 679-680
    clinical manifestations of, 676,
        677-678t
    in increased intracranial pres-
        sure, 670
    medications for, 678, 679t
Selective serotonin reuptake ago-
    nists, 666
Selective serotonin reuptake
    inhibitors
    for menopause, 553
    for migraine prophylaxis, 666
    for premenstrual syndrome, 551
Selectively permeable, term, 5
Selegiline, 685, 686-687t
Self-Cath Closed System, 450
Self-catheterization, 447
Self-monitoring of blood glucose,
    511-512, 512, 512f
Semen analysis, 545
Semicircular canal, 604f, 605, 605f
Semilunar valve, 305
Seminal vesicle, 534-535, 534f
Senescent arthritis, 125-127, 125b,
    125f, 126f
Sengstaken-Blakemore tube, 239,
    239f
Senile vaginitis, 557-558
Sensorineural hearing loss, 633
Sensory examination, 661
Sensory system
    ear in, 604-605, 604f
    eye in, 602-603
    normal aging of, 606
    position and movement in, 606
    taste and smell in, 606
    touch in, 606
Sensory system disorders, 601-649
    auditory, 631
        acute otitis media in, 636-639
        behavioral clues indicating
            hearing loss and, 631b
        cochlear implant for, 645, 645f
        deafness in, 633-635, 633b, 634b
        external otitis in, 635-640
        laboratory and diagnostic ex-
            aminations for, 631-632,
            632f
        labyrinthitis in, 639
        medications for, 637-638t
        Ménière's disease in, 641-644,
            642t, 643b
        myringotomy for, 645
        obstructions of ear in, 639-640
        otosclerosis in, 640-641
        patient teaching in ear infec-
            tion and, 639b
        patient teaching in ear surgery
            and, 644b
        stapedectomy for, 644
        tympanoplasty for, 644-645
        vertigo in, 640b
    cultural considerations in, 618b
    nursing process for, 645-646
    visual, 606
        age-related macular degenera-
            tion in, 621-622
        allergic conjunctivitis in,
            386-387
        anatomy of eye and, 602-603,
            602f, 603f
        associated with HIV infection,
            750-751t
        astigmatism, strabismus,
            myopia, and hyperopia
            in, 611, 611t
        blindness and near blindness
            in, 607-610, 610b, 610f

Sensory system disorders (Continued)
cataracts in, 617-618, 617f, 618f, 619b
communication in postoperative eye surgery and, 620b
conjunctivitis in, 614-615
corneal inflammation in, 615
corneal injuries in, 627-629
corneal transplant for, 629-630
cultural considerations in, 618b
diabetic retinopathy in, 618-620
dry eye disorders in, 615-616
ectropion and entropion in, 616-617
enucleation for, 629
glaucoma in, 623-627, 624f, 625f, 627b
hordeolum, chalazion, and blepharitis in, 613-614, 613t
laboratory and diagnostic examinations for, 606-607, 608-609t
medications for, 625-626t
nursing process for, 645-646
patient teaching after eye surgery, 620b
photocoagulation for, 630
refractory errors in, 610-613, 611t
retinal detachment in, 622-623, 622f, 623b
vitrectomy for, 630-631
Sentinel lymph node mapping, 574
Sequential compression devices, 34, 34f
Seroconversion, human immunodeficiency virus and, 740, 745
Seronegative test for human immunodeficiency virus, 747
Serotonin, 652
Serous membrane, 12
Sertraline, 551
Serum ammonia test, 234
Serum amylase test, 234
Serum bilirubin test, 231
Serum CA-125 tumor antigen, 545
Serum calcitonin, 788
Serum cardiac markers, 311
Serum creatinine, 440
Serum electrolyte tests, 311
Serum insulin, 512
Serum lipase test, 235
Serum lipids, 311
Serum protein test, 232
Serum thyroxine, 496
Serum triiodothyronine, 496
Severe acute respiratory syndrome, 397
Sex hormones, 486
Sexual health, 540b
Sexual history, 540-541, 540b, 541b
Sexual identity, 539-540
Sexual transmission of human immunodeficiency virus, 739-740, 771-773
Sexuality, 538-539, 541, 541b
Sexually transmitted infections, 586-592, 587b
candidiasis in, 591
cervical cancer and, 565
chlamydial infection in, 591-592
genital herpes in, 587-588, 588f
gonorrhea in, 589-590
prevention of, 592b
risk for penile cancer and, 586
syphilis in, 588-589
trichomoniasis in, 590-591
Shaving, preoperative, 25
Shingles, 72-74, 72f, 73b
Shock
anaphylactic, 727
cardiogenic, 329, 330t
fracture-related, 149-150
hypovolemic, 271
postoperative, 46-48, 48b

Short-acting insulin, 515-516t
Short-leg walking cast, 154f
Short-stay surgical center, 19
Shoulder spica cast, 153, 153f
Sibilant wheezes, 379, 379t
Sickle cell anemia, 276-279
Sickle cell crisis, 278
Sigmoid colostomy, 222f
Sigmoidoscopy, 182
Sildenafil citrate, 554-555
Silver nitrate, 101t
Silver sulfadiazine, 101t
Simple mastectomy, 575
Simple vaginitis, 557
Singultus, 52
Sinoatrial node, 305, 306f
Sinus bradycardia, 315, 315f
Sinus tachycardia, 314
Sinusitis, 394-395
Sitting position for surgery, 41f
Sjögren syndrome, 615-616
Skeletal fixation devices, 152-153, 152f
Skeletal muscle, 10t, 11, 11f
functional groups of, 113, 113t, 114f
structure of, 111
Skeletal pin external fixation, 152-153, 152f
Skeletal system, 12-14t
divisions of, 110, 110b, 111f
functions of, 109-110
multiple myeloma and, 291
Skeletal traction, 156, 156f
in spinal cord injury, 712
Skene's gland, 537, 537f
Skin
Addison's disease and, 506-507
appendages of, 61
chemotherapy-related complications of, 795
coagulation disorders and, 285
diabetes mellitus and, 511
effects of aging on, 103b
functions of, 59-60, 59b
healthy skin promotion and, 84b
hypothyroidism and, 499
hypovolemic anemia and, 271
immune response and, 723
of older adult, 103b
peripheral vascular disease and, 350, 351b
polycythemia and, 280
preoperative preparation of, 25, 27f
structure of, 60-61, 60f
thrombocytopenia and, 286
Skin biopsy, 90, 93
Skin cancer
basal cell carcinoma in, 91, 91f
malignant melanoma in, 92-93, 93f
prevention and early detection of, 92b, 782-784t
squamous cell carcinoma in, 91-92, 91f
Skin care
cast and, 155
in diabetes mellitus, 522
in multiple sclerosis, 682
paralyzed patient and, 673
Skin disorders, 59-108
alopecia in, 94
associated with HIV infection, 750-751t
bacterial, 74-77
burns in, 94-103
complementary and alternative therapies for, 105b
cultural considerations in, 68b
fungal, 78-79, 78f
inflammatory, 79-87
medications for, 70-71t
nursing process for, 103-105
parasitic, 87-90
psychosocial assessment in, 68
tumors in, 90-93
viral, 68-74

Skin graft, 100, 100b
Skin lesion, 62t
in genital herpes, 588, 588f
Skin replacement therapy, 99
Skin traction, 156, 157f
Skull radiography, 662
Sleep apnea, 387-388, 388f
Sleep hygiene, 133b
Sliding hernia, 217f
Sliding nails, 139
Slit-lamp examination, 606-607
Small cell lung cancer, 413
Small intestine, 178
Small intestine disorders, 201-227
anal fissure and fistula in, 226
appendicitis in, 212-213, 213b
capsule endoscopy in, 181, 181f
colorectal cancer in, 220-224, 221b, 222f
Crohn's disease in, 209-212
diverticulosis and diverticulitis in, 176f, 213-215, 214f, 215f
external hernias in, 216-227
hemorrhoids in, 224-226, 224f
hiatal hernia in, 217-218, 217f, 218f
infections in, 201-203
intestinal obstruction in, 218-220, 219f
irritable bowel syndrome in, 203-205, 205b
ulcerative colitis in, 205-209, 206t, 207b, 208f, 209b
Smell, 606
Smoke inhalation damage, 95
Smoking
Buerger's disease and, 360
cancer and, 780
cardiovascular disease and, 312-313
cataracts and, 617
emphysema and, 421, 423
hypertension and, 352, 354
peptic ulcer disease and, 195
peripheral vascular diseases and, 349
Smooth muscle, 10t, 11, 11f
Snellen's test, 608-609t
Snoring in obstructive sleep apnea, 387
Socioeconomic needs of surgical patient, 20-21
Sodium
hypertension and, 354
postoperative management of, 52
restriction of
after myocardial infarction, 332
in cirrhosis, 237-238, 240
in lymphedema, 293
serum electrolyte tests and, 311
Sodium bicarbonate, 799
Sodium hypochlorite, 101t
Sodium oxybate, 132t
Sodium-potassium pump, 8-9
Somatostatin analogs, 489, 490t
Sonorous wheezes, 379t
Sotalol, 318-319t
Specific gravity
cerebrospinal fluid, 661t
urine, 440, 440t
Speech
after stroke, 699-700
Glasgow Coma Scale and, 659t
neurologic assessment and, 659
Sperm, 534-535, 535, 536f
Spermatic cord, 534
Spermatogenesis, 535
Sphenoid sinus, 374, 375f
Spica cast, 153, 153f
Spinal accessory nerve, 656f, 657t
Spinal anesthesia, 39f, 40
Spinal cavity, 2, 3f, 3t
Spinal column
curvature abnormalities of, 170, 170f
spinal anesthesia and, 39f, 40

Spinal cord, 653f, 654, 655f
coverings of, 654
trauma to
clinical manifestations of, 710-712, 712f
emergency care for autonomic dysreflexia in, 712b
etiology and pathophysiology of, 710, 710f, 711f
medical management of, 712, 713f
patient teaching in, 712-713
Spinal fusion, 165
Spinal nerves, 655
Spinal surgery, coughing contraindication in, 33
Spine
fracture of, 145-147, 146f
herniated nucleus pulposus and, 164-166, 164f
myelogram of, 115
osteoporosis and, 128-133, 129f, 129t
Spiral computed tomography chest scan, 380
Spiral fracture, 143f, 144
Spirometry tests, 380
Spironolactone, 255-256t, 444
Spleen, 176f, 268, 268f, 721f
Splenectomy, 274
Splint, 158
Sprain, 160
ankle, 161
strain versus, 161b
Sputum specimen, 381, 381b, 382b
Squamous cell carcinoma, 91-92, 91f
Staging, 786, 786b
of breast cancer, 574, 575b
of heart failure, 333b
of Hodgkin's lymphoma, 294b, 295f
Stapedectomy, 644
Stapes, 604f, 605
Staphylococcal infection
in acute mastitis, 571
in brain abscess, 706
in cellulitis, 74-75
in conjunctivitis, 614
in epididymitis, 584
in external otitis, 635
in folliculitis, 77
in impetigo contagiosa, 75-76
in keratitis, 615
in meningitis, 704
in pelvic inflammatory disease, 558
in pneumonia, 404
in toxic shock syndrome, 559
Stasis ulcer, 62f, 350
Status asthmaticus, 427
Status epilepticus, 676
Stavudine, 753-756t
Steapsin, 179
Steinmann pin, 156f
Stem cell transplantation
for aplastic anemia, 274
for breast cancer, 577
for sickle cell anemia, 278
Stenosis in valvular heart disease, 340
Stent
in coronary artery disease, 323, 324f
LeVeen, 238, 238f
in urinary obstruction, 456
Steroid hormones, 486
Steroid therapy; See Corticosteroids
Stoma care, 209
Stomach, 176f, 177-178, 177f, 190-201
acute gastritis and, 190-191
cancer of, 200-201
gastroscopy and, 180-181, 180f
peptic ulcer disease and, 190-201
tube gastric analysis and, 180
upper gastrointestinal series and, 180

Stomatitis, 795-796, 796
Stool culture, 183, 202
Stool examination for occult blood, 182, 789
Stool softeners after myocardial infarction, 329t
Strabismus, 611, 611t
Strain, 161, 161b
Stratum corneum, 60, 60f
Stratum germinativum, 60, 60f
Strep throat, 394
Streptococcal infection
    in acute follicular tonsillitis, 392
    acute glomerulonephritis following, 468
    in acute mastitis, 571
    in acute otitis media, 606
    in brain abscess, 706
    in cellulitis, 74-75
    in conjunctivitis, 614
    in epididymitis, 584
    in keratitis, 615
    in meningitis, 704
    in pelvic inflammatory disease, 558
    in pharyngitis, 394
    in pneumonia, 404
    prophylaxis guidelines for, 752t
    in prostatitis, 583
Streptococcus pneumoniae, 404
Streptococcus pyogenes, 635
Streptokinase, 329t
Stress
    cardiovascular disease risk and, 314
    diabetes mellitus and, 514
    hypertension and, 352, 354
    irritable bowel syndrome and, 204
    peripheral vascular diseases and, 349
    premenstrual syndrome and, 551
    ulcerative colitis and, 207
Striae, 505
Stridor
    after thyroidectomy, 497-498
    in hypoparathyroidism, 503
Stroke, 695-700
    assessment of, 696-697, 697f
    communication problems in, 699-700
    cultural considerations in, 694b
    diagnostic tests for, 697
    embolic, 695
    etiology and pathophysiology of, 694-695, 695f
    hemorrhagic, 695-696
    ischemic, 695
    medical management of, 697-699, 697f, 698f
    nursing interventions in, 699-700
    patient teaching in, 700
    thrombotic, 695
    transient ischemic attack and, 696
Stryker frame, 157, 712
Stump care, 168f
Stye, 613-614, 613f
Subcutaneous fatty tissue, 60f, 61
Subcutaneous insulin injection, 516-517, 519b, 519f
Subdural hematoma, 708-709
Sublingual gland, 176f
Subluxation, 162
Substantia nigra, Parkinson's disease and, 683-684, 683f
Sucralfate, 193-195t
Sudoriferous glands, 61
Sulcus, 652
Sulfacetamide sodium, 625-626t
Sulfasalazine, 193-195t
    for Crohn's disease, 210
    for rheumatoid arthritis, 119-122t
    for ulcerative colitis, 207
Sulfinpyrazone, 127
Sulfonamides, 336-337t
Sulfonylureas, 520, 520t

Sumatriptan, 666
Sundowning, 689
Superficial burn, 95t, 96f
Superficial fascia, 61
Superior vena cava syndrome, 413
Supination, 113
Supine position for surgery, 41f
Suppuration, 77
Suprapubic catheter, 445-446
Suprapubic prostatectomy, 463, 463f
Supratentorial shift, 669
Supraventricular tachycardia, 315
Surgery, 17
    for cancer, 789-790
    classification of procedures, 18t
    common fears associated with, 21b
    common settings for, 19b
    coughing contraindications in, 33b
    effects on body systems, 23t
    positioning for, 40-41, 41f
    possible airways used during, 39f
    skeletal fixation devices and, 152-153, 152f
    skin preparation for, 26b, 27f
    surgical terminology and, 19t
    wrong site and wrong procedure, 43
Surgical asepsis, 44
Surgical patient, 17-58
    ambulatory surgery discharge and, 55-56
    discharge of, 55-56, 56b, 56f
    intraoperative phase of surgery and, 43-44, 43f
        circulating nurse and scrub nurse roles in, 44, 44b, 44f
    holding area and, 43-44
    nursing care plan for, 54-55b
    nursing process for, 53, 53b, 54b
    perioperative nursing and, 18-23
    postoperative phase of surgery and, 44-53
    preoperative phase of surgery and, 23-43, 23t
Surgical skin preparation, 26b, 27f
Surgical wound
    postoperative care of, 48
    preoperative teaching about, 35
Sutilains ointment, 101t
Sweat gland, 60-61, 60f, 61
Swimmer's ear, 635
Sympathectomy, 362
Sympathetic nervous system, 655
Synaptic cleft, 113
Synarthrosis, 110
Syncope, in cardiovascular disorders, 368
Syndrome of inappropriate antidiuretic hormone secretion, 493-495
Synergistic bone marrow transplantation, 800
Synovial fluid, 12
Synovial fluid aspiration, 119, 140f
Synovial membrane, 12
Syphilis, 588-589, 749
System review in immediate postoperative phase, 45t
Systemic circulation, 307-308
Systemic lupus erythematosus, 85-87, 85f
Systems of body, 12, 12-14t
    effects of surgery on, 23t
Systole, 304, 306f
Systolic blood pressure, 351

T

T cell, 265-266, 721
    autoimmune disorders and, 730
    cell-mediated immunity and, 722
    humoral immunity and, 721
    immunosurveillance and, 785
    thymus gland and, 488

T wave, 308, 309f
Tachycardia
    sinus, 314
    supraventricular, 315
    ventricular, 316-317
Tachydysrhythmias, 320
Tacrine, 686-687t
Tacrolimus, 246
Tactile receptor, 606
Tadalafil, 554-555
Tamoxifen, 793-794t
    for breast cancer, 576
    risk for endometrial cancer and, 567
Taste, 606
Teeth, 176
Tegaserod, 204
Telangiectasis, 62f, 62t, 91
Telemetry, 309
Telophase, 7f, 8
Temazepam, 336-337t
Temporal lobe, 653f, 654
Tendon, 111
Tendon sheath, 111
Tenesmus, 202
Tenofovir, 753-756t
Tenofovir/emtricitabine, 753-756t
Tenofovir/emtricitabine/efevirenz, 753-756t
Tension headache, 665-666, 666
Tension pneumothorax, 412f
Terazosin hydrochloride, 443t, 462
Terbinafine, 70-71t
Terconazole, 549-550t
Teriparatide, 129t, 130
Terminal bronchiole, 377
Terminal prognosis in cancer, 803-804
Test decision counseling, 769-770
Testes, 485f, 488, 534, 534f
    hydrocele and, 585
Testicular biopsy, 545
Testicular cancer, 585-586, 586b, 586f, 782-784t
Testicular self-examination, 585-586, 586b, 586f
Testosterone, 488, 534
Testosterone cypionate, 549-550t
Tetany, 486
    after removal of parathyroid glands, 503
    after thyroidectomy, 497-498
Tetracycline, 70-71t
    for acne vulgaris, 83
    for Chlamydia trachomatis, 592
    for Helicobacter pylori, 195
    for pneumonia, 406
Tetrahydrocannabinol, 797-798
Tetraplegia, 710, 711t
Texas condom catheter, 446
Thalamus, 653, 653f
Thallium scanning, 310
T-helper cell, 721
Theophylline, 401-403t
Thiazide diuretics, 443
Thiazolidinediones, 520, 520t
Third-degree burn, 95t, 96f
Thonzonium, 637-638t
Thoracentesis, 378, 382, 382f, 408
Thoracic cavity, 2, 3f, 3t
Thoracic surgery, 27f
Thoracotomy
    in pleural effusion or empyema, 408
    in pneumothorax, 412
Thrombin, 266f
Thromboangiitis obliterans, 360-361
Thrombocyte, 266, 266f
Thrombocytopenia, 286-287, 286b
    chemotherapy-related, 796
    in HIV infection, 749
Thrombocytopenic purpura, 286
Thromboembolic deterrent stockings, 33-34, 34f
Thromboembolus, fracture-related, 151, 151b

Thrombolytic agents
    for acute ischemic stroke, 698
    for atherosclerosis, 356
    for myocardial infarction, 329t
Thrombophlebitis, 362-365, 363f, 363t
    pelvic surgery and, 570
    in polycythemia, 279-280
Thrombotic stroke, 695, 695f
Thrombus, 32-33, 50
Thrush, 184, 591
Thymectomy, 692
Thymosin, 488
Thymus, 268-269, 268f, 485f, 488, 721f
Thyroid, 485-486, 485f, 487f
Thyroid cartilage, 374, 375f, 376f
Thyroid crisis, 498
Thyroid disorders, 495-504
    cancer in, 792b
    hyperthyroidism in, 495-498, 495f, 496b
    hypothyroidism in, 498-500, 499f
    medications for, 497t
    simple goiter in, 500-501, 501f
    thyroid cancer in, 501-502
Thyroid hormones, 485-486
Thyroid scan, 496
Thyroid storm, 498
Thyroidectomy, 496-497
Thyroid-stimulating hormone, 486f
    for evaluation of thyroid disease, 496
    functions of, 487f
Thyroxine, 485-486
Tiagabine, 679t
Tibial pin traction with Steinmann pin, 156f
Tic douloureux, 700-701, 701b, 701f
Ticlopidine
    for myocardial infarction, 329t
    for transient ischemic attack, 696
Tiludronate, 129
Timolol maleate, 625-626t
Tinea capitis, 78, 78f
Tinea corporis, 78, 78f
Tinea cruris, 78
Tinea pedis, 78
Tinel's sign, 163
Tinnitus, 606
Tioconazole ointment, 549-550t
Tipranavir, 753-756t
Tissue, 4f, 5, 9-12, 10t, 11f
Tissue plasminogen activator
    for acute ischemic stroke, 698
    for myocardial infarction, 329t
Tissue typing, 5
Tizanidine, 132t
TNM staging system, 786, 786b
    in breast cancer, 574, 575b
Tocainide, 318-319t
Tolcapone, 685
Tolmetin sodium, 119-122t
Tolnaftate, 70-71t, 78
Tongue, 176f, 375f, 376f
    cancer of, 185
Tonometry, 608-609t
Tonsil, 268, 268f, 374
Tonsillectomy and adenoidectomy, 392
Tonsillitis, 392-393
Tooth decay, 183-184
Tophi, 127
Topical amphotericin B, 549-550t
Topiramate
    for migraine prophylaxis, 666
    for seizures, 679t
    for trigeminal neuralgia, 701
Topotecan, 793-794t
Toremifene, 576
Total body surface area, 94
Total cholesterol, 313b
Total joint replacement
    hip, 135-136, 135f, 136f
    knee, 133-135, 133f, 134b

Total lung capacity, 380
Touch, 606
Toxic megacolon, 206
Toxic shock syndrome, 559-560
Toxoplasma gondii
  associated with HIV infection, 750-751t
  prophylaxis guidelines for, 752t
Trabeculectomy, 625-627
Tracheostomy, 388
Traction, 146, 146f, 156-157
Traction-inflammatory headache, 665
TRAM flap, 582, 582f
Tramadol, 132t
Trandolapril, 336-337t
Transcutaneous aspiration biopsy, 786-787, 787f
Transcutaneous electrical nerve stimulation, 49-50, 50f
Transdermal oxybutynin, 450
Transfusion reactions, 729
Transgender, 540
Transient ischemic attack, 696
Transplantation, 18t
  corneal, 629-630
  heart, 347-348, 347b
  kidney, 478, 478f
  liver, 245-246
  pancreatic, 521
  rejection of, 729-730
Transport to operating room, 43
Transrectal ultrasound, 442
Transurethral prostatectomy, 463, 463f
Transverse loop colostomy, 214-215, 215f
Transverse rectus abdominis musculocutaneous flap, 582, 582f
Trastuzumab, 577
Treadmill test, 350
Tremor in Parkinson's disease, 684, 684f
Trendelenburg's test, 365
Treponema pallidum, 588-589
Triamcinolone, 70-71t
Triamterene, 444
Trichomonas vaginalis, 557, 590, 590-591
Tricuspid valve, 305, 305f
Tricyclic antidepressants
  for migraine prophylaxis, 666
  for premenstrual syndrome, 551
Triethanolamine polypeptide oleate, 637-638t
Trigeminal nerve, 656f, 657t
Trigeminal neuralgia, 667, 700-701, 701b, 701f
Trigger points of trigeminal nerve, 701
Trihexyphenidyl, 685, 686-687t
Triiodothyronine, 485-486
Trimethadione, 679t
Trimethobenzamide, 191
Trimethoprim-sulfamethoxazole
  for ear infection, 637-638t
  for prostatitis, 455, 583
  for urethritis, 452
Triptans, 666
Trochlear nerve, 656f, 657t
Tropic hormones, 485
Troponin I, 311, 327
Trousseau's sign, 497-498
Trunk muscles, 112t
Trypsin, 179
T-suppressor cell, 721
T-tube
  care of, 251-252
  for gallstones, 250, 250f
T-tube cholangiography, 233
Tubal insufflation, 545
Tubal ligation, 593f
Tube gastric analysis, 180
Tubercle, 399
Tuberculin skin test, 400
Tuberculosis, 398-403, 399b

prophylaxis guidelines for, 752t
Tumor, 62f, 62t, 785, 785t
  adrenal, 504
  bladder, 461-462
  bone, 166-167
  brain, 352t, 707-708
  breast, 571-583
    body image acceptance after mastectomy, 580
    bone marrow and stem cell transplantation for, 577
    breast reconstruction and, 581-582
    chemotherapy in, 576
    clinical manifestations of, 572, 573f
    diagnostic tests for, 572-574
    etiology and pathophysiology of, 571-572, 571b, 572f
    home care considerations in, 583b
    hormonal therapy for, 576-577
    monoclonal antibody therapy for, 577
    nursing care plan for mastectomy in, 577-578b
    ovarian ablation in, 577
    patient teaching in, 579-581, 580b
    preventing muscle contractures after mastectomy, 579-580, 580f, 581b
    prognosis in, 583, 583t
    radiation therapy in, 575-576
    staging of, 574, 575b
    surgical intervention in, 574-575
  cutaneous, 90-93
    angiomas in, 91
    basal cell carcinoma in, 91, 91f
    keloids in, 90-91, 91f
    malignant melanoma in, 92-93, 93f
    nevi in, 91
    prevention of, 92b
    squamous cell carcinoma in, 91-92, 91f
    warts in, 91
  gastric, 200-201
  grading of, 786, 786b
  laryngeal, 389-390
  pheochromocytoma, 508
  pituitary
    in acromegaly, 489
    in Cushing's syndrome, 505
  renal, 459-460
  salivary gland, 184-185
  testicular, 585-586
Tumor, node, metastasis staging system, 785, 786, 786b
  in breast cancer, 574, 575b
Tumor lysis syndrome, 799-800
Tuning fork tests, 631-632, 632f
Turbinates, 374, 375f
Turning exercises, 32, 32f
Tympanic membrane, 604, 604f
Tympanoplasty, 644-645
Tympanostomy tube, 636
Type 1 diabetes mellitus, 509-510, 510t
Type 2 diabetes mellitus, 510, 510t

U

Ulcer, 62f, 62t
  in peptic ulcer disease, 190-201
    drug therapy for, 193-195t, 193-195
    duodenal ulcers in, 192-200
    gastric ulcers in, 191-192
    home care considerations in, 199b
    physiologic stress ulcers in, 192
    surgical interventions for, 195-196, 195f, 196f, 197t
    venous stasis, 366-367, 366f, 367f
Ulcerative colitis, 205-209, 206t, 207b,

208f, 209b
Ultralente, 515-516t
Ultrasonography
  in appendicitis, 212
  of breast, 574
  for cancer diagnosis, 787-788
  in diverticulosis and diverticulitis, 214
  in female reproductive disorders, 544
  in fibrocystic breast condition, 571
  in hepatobiliary disorders, 233
  in hydronephrosis, 457
  pancreatic, 235
  in pelvic inflammatory disease, 558
  in peritonitis, 216
  in pyelonephritis, 455
  in urinary disorders, 442
  in urolithiasis, 458
Ultraviolet radiation, cancer and, 781
Umbilical region, 3, 3f
Unicompartmental knee arthroplasty, 133-134
Unilateral neglect, 661, 699
Universal donor blood, 266-267, 267f
Universal recipient blood, 266-267, 267f
Unna's paste boot, 366, 367f
Unrelated bone marrow transplantation, 800
Unstable angina, 321
Upper airway obstruction, 388-389
Upper extremities muscles, 112t
Upper gastrointestinal endoscopy, 180-181, 180f
Upper gastrointestinal series, 180
Ureter, 435f, 438
Ureterolithiasis, 457
Ureterolithotomy, 458, 458f
Ureterosigmoidostomy, 477t
Urethra, 435f, 439
  male, 534-535, 535
Urethral catheter, 445
Urethral stricture, 466-467
Urethritis, 452-453
  Chlamydia trachomatis in, 591-592
  in gonorrhea, 589-590
Urethrovaginal fistula, 561, 561f
Urethrovesical reflux, 453
Urgent surgery, 18t
Uric acid, 117t
Urinalysis, 439-440, 440t
  in hydronephrosis, 457
  in neurologic disorders, 661
  in urinary tract trauma, 467
  in urolithiasis, 458
Urinary bladder, 435f, 438-439, 438f
  bladder training and, 447-448
  cancer of, 461-462
  cystitis and, 453, 453b
  interstitial cystitis and, 453-454
  neurogenic, 450-451
Urinary catheterization, 445-448
Urinary disorders, 434-483
  acute glomerulonephritis in, 468-469
  benign prostatic hypertrophy in, 462-464, 463b, 463f
  bladder tumor in, 461-462
  chronic glomerulonephritis in, 469-470
  complementary and alternative therapies for, 452b
  cultural considerations in, 439b
  cystitis in, 453, 453b
  end-stage renal disease in, 471-472, 473-474b
  hydronephrosis in, 457
  interstitial cystitis in, 453-454
  laboratory and diagnostic examinations in, 439-443
    blood urea nitrogen in, 440

Urinary disorders (Continued)
    computed tomography in, 442
    creatinine clearance in, 440
    endoscopic procedures in, 441
    intravenous pyelography or urography in, 441
    kidney-ureter-bladder radiography in, 441
    magnetic resonance imaging in, 442
    prostate-specific antigen test in, 440
    renal angiography in, 442
    renal biopsy in, 442
    renal scan in, 442
    renal venogram in, 442
    retrograde pyelography in, 441
    serum creatinine in, 440
    specific gravity in, 440
    transrectal ultrasound in, 442
    ultrasonography in, 442
    urinalysis in, 439-440, 440t
    urine osmolality in, 441
    urodynamic studies in, 442-443
    voiding cystourethrography in, 441
  medication considerations in, 443-445, 443t
  nephritis, 468-470
  nephrotic syndrome in, 467-468
  neurogenic bladder in, 450-451
  nursing process for, 480-481
  nutritional considerations in, 445, 445b
  older adult and, 439b
  prostate cancer in, 464-466, 464b
  prostatitis in, 454-455
  pyelonephritis in, 455-456
  renal cyst in, 460-462
  renal failure in, 470-472, 472b
  renal tumor in, 459-460
  surgical procedures in, 477-479, 477t
    kidney transplantation in, 478, 478f
    nephrectomy in, 477
    nephrostomy in, 477-478
    urinary diversion in, 478-479, 479f, 480b
  urethral strictures in, 466-467
  urethritis in, 452-453
  urinary catheterization in, 445-448
    bladder training and, 447-448
    nursing interventions and patient teaching in, 446-448
    self-catheterization and, 447
    types of catheters for, 445-446, 446f
  urinary incontinence in, 448-450, 449b
  urinary obstruction in, 456-457
  urinary retention in, 448
  urinary tract infection in, 444-445, 451-452
  urinary tract trauma in, 467
  urine abnormalities in, 438
  urolithiasis in, 457-459, 458f
Urinary diversion, 478-479, 479f, 480b
Urinary incontinence, 448-450, 449b
Urinary meatus, 439, 537, 537f
Urinary obstruction, 456-457
Urinary retention, 448
Urinary system, 12-14t, 434-439, 435f
  chemotherapy-related complications of, 795
  effects of aging on, 439
  effects of surgery on, 23t
  kidney in, 434-438, 435f, 436f, 437f, 437t, 438b
  medications affecting, 443t
  postoperative management of, 50

Urinary system (Continued)
    ureters in, 438
    urethra in, 439
    urinary bladder in, 438-439, 438f
    urine abnormalities and, 438
    urine composition and characteristics and, 438
Urine
    abnormalities of, 438
    composition and characteristics of, 438
    formation of, 437, 437t
    residual, 448
    urinalysis and, 440t
Urine amylase test, 234-235
Urine specific gravity, 440, 440t
Urodynamic studies, 442-443
Urokinase, 356
Urolithiasis, 457-459, 458f
Urosepsis, 452
Urticaria, 81, 727
Uterus, 550-557, 556f
    displaced, 562
    endometrial cancer and, 567
    leiomyoma of, 563-564, 563f
    prolapse of, 562, 562f
Uvuloplasty, 388

V

Vaccine
    attenuated, 723
    hepatitis, 245
    herpes zoster, 72
    human immunodeficiency virus, 757
    human papillomavirus, 566
    pneumococcal, 406
Vagina, 536f, 537
Vaginal fistula, 561-562, 561f
Vaginal hysterectomy, 569
Vaginal orifice, 537f
Vaginitis, 557
Vagotomy, 196, 196f
Vagus nerve, 656f, 657t
Valacyclovir, 588, 702
Valerian root, 22t
Valproic acid, 679t, 701
Valve replacement surgery, 341
Valvular heart disease, 340-342, 342t
Vamipril, 336-337t
Vanillylmandelic acid, 508
Vardenafil, 554-555
Varicella zoster virus, prophylaxis guidelines for, 752t
Varicocele, 585
Varicose veins, 363t, 365-366
Vas deferens, 534, 534f
Vasectomy, 534, 593-595t, 593f
Vasodilators for acute respiratory distress syndrome, 419
Vasopressin, 255-256t, 490t

Vasopressors
    for anaphylaxis, 727
    for myocardial infarction, 329t
Vasospasm after aneurysm clipping, 698
Vena cava, 304
Veneral Disease Research Laboratory test, 589
Venlafaxine, 553
Venography, 351
Venous disorders, 362-367
Venous insufficiency, 350
Venous stasis, 50-51, 570
Venous stasis ulcer, 366-367, 366f, 367f
Ventilation, postoperative management of, 48-49
Ventilation-perfusion scan, 380
Ventral body cavity, 2, 3f, 3t
Ventricle of brain, 654
Ventricular fibrillation, 317
Ventricular tachycardia, 316-317
Venule, 304
Verapamil, 318-319t, 329t
Verruca, 91
Vertebral fracture, 145-147, 146f
Verteporfin, 621
Vertigo, 640b
Very-low-density lipoproteins, 313, 313b
Vesicle, 62f, 62t
Vesicocervical fistula, 561f
Vesicostomy catheter, 445-446
Vesicovaginal fistula, 561, 561f
Vestibular gland, 537, 537f
Vestibular testing, 632
Vestibule
    auditory, 604f, 605, 605f
    vaginal, 537, 537f
Vestibulocochlear nerve, 656f, 657t
Villus, 178
Vinblastine, 793-794t
Vinca alkaloids, 793-794t
Vincristine, 793-794t
Vinorelbine, 793-794t
Viral infection
    in acute otitis media, 636
    in acute rhinitis, 391-392
    in Bell's palsy, 701-702
    cutaneous, 68-74
    in encephalitis, 705-706
    in external otitis, 635
    in genital herpes, 69, 587-588, 588f
    Guillain-Barré syndrome after, 703
    in hepatitis, 243-247
    human immunodeficiency virus, 734-778
    in meningitis, 704
    in pharyngitis, 394

Viral infection (Continued)
    in pneumonia, 405
    in severe acute respiratory syndrome, 397
    in sinusitis, 394
    West Nile virus in, 705-706
Viral load in human immunodeficiency virus infection, acute retroviral syndrome and, 739, 742-744, 744f, 745, 747-748
Visceral membrane, 12
Visceral muscle, 10t, 11, 11f
Visceral pleura, 378
Vision, physiology of, 604
Visual acuity, 607t
    in retinal detachment, 622
Visual disorders; See Sensory system disorders, visual
Vital capacity, 380
Vitamin A
    eye and, 603
    lung cancer prevention and, 413
Vitamin B$_6$ supplementation in premenstrual syndrome, 551
Vitamin B$_{12}$
    erythropoiesis and, 277b
    pernicious anemia and, 272
Vitamin C
    erythropoiesis and, 277b
    iron absorption and, 276
    for macular degeneration, 621
    supplementation in vaginal fistula, 561
Vitamin D
    for psoriasis, 85
    synthesis in skin, 60
    values in musculoskeletal disorders, 117t
Vitamin E
    for fibrocystic breast condition, 571
    for hot flashes, 553
    lung cancer prevention and, 413
    for macular degeneration, 621
Vitiligo, 62f
Vitrectomy, 630-631
Vitreous humor, 603
Voiding cystourethrography, 441, 466
Voiding pattern alterations, 448-451
Volkmann's contracture, 148-149
Volume-oriented spirometer, 30, 30f
Voluntary muscle, 10t, 11, 11f, 111-113
Volvulus, 218, 219f
von Hippel-Lindau disease, 459
von Willebrand's disease, 289
Vorozole, 576
Vulva, 537, 537f

W

Walker, 159, 159f
Warfarin, 318-319t
    for myocardial infarction, 329t
    preoperative, 36-37t
    for pulmonary embolism, 417
Wart, 91
Wasting in HIV infection, 765-767
Water deprivation test, 493
Water intoxication, 494
Water-seal drainage, 410b
Weight reduction
    for diverticulosis and diverticulitis, 214
    for hypertension, 353
West Nile virus, 705-706
Western blot, 747
Wheal, 62f, 62t, 81
Wheezes, 379, 379t
Whiplash, 160-161
Whipple procedure, 256, 257f
Whispered voice test, 631
Whistle-tip catheter, 445-446
White blood cell, 263f, 265-266
White blood cell count, 263-264t
White matter of spinal cord, 655f
Windpipe, 374-375
Wood's light examination, 78
Wound care
    after total knee replacement, 134
    in burn, 99
Wound dehiscence, 48, 48f
Wound evisceration, 48, 48f
Wound healing, 200-201
Wrist, carpal tunnel syndrome and, 163-164, 163f
Wrong site and wrong procedure surgery, 43

X

Xenograft, 100
Xerofoam, 101t
Xiphoid process, 111f

Z

Zafirlukast, 401-403t, 725-726
Zidovudine, 753-756t
Zidovudine/lamivudine, 753-756t
Zidovudine/lamivudine/abacavir, 753-756t
Zileuton, 401-403t, 725-726
Zinc, 621
Zolmitriptan, 666
Zonisamide, 679t
Zoonotic transmission of HIV, 735
Zygote, 536
Zygote intrafallopian transfer, 556